# DIAGNOSTIC CYTOPATHOLOGY

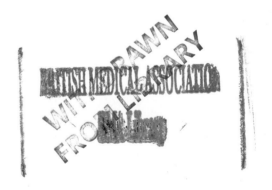

Commissioning Editor: Michael Houston
Development Editor: Joanne Scott
Project Manager: Kerrie-Anne McKinlay
Design: Charles Gray
Editorial Assistant: Rachael Harrison
Illustration Manager: Merlyn Harvey
Illustrators: Richard Tibbitts/Paul Richardson/Martin Woodwerd
Marketing Managers (UK/USA): Ria Timmerman/Brenna Christensen

## THIRD EDITION

# DIAGNOSTIC CYTOPATHOLOGY

EDITED BY

**WINIFRED GRAY,** (RETIRED), MB BS FRCPATH
Consultant Cytopathologist/Histopathologist
John Radcliffe Hospital
Oxford
UK

**GABRIJELA KOCJAN,** MB BS SPEC CLIN CYT FRCPATH
Senior Lecturer
Head of Diagnostic Cytopathology
University College Hospital
London
UK

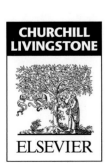

CHURCHILL
LIVINGSTONE

ELSEVIER

# CHURCHILL LIVINGSTONE
ELSEVIER

an imprint of Elsevier Limited.

First edition 1995
Second edition 2003
Third edition 2010
  Reprinted 2010 (twice)

**ISBN: 978-0-7020-3154-0**

**British Library Cataloguing in Publication Data**
Diagnostic cytopathology – 3rd ed.
     1. Cytodiagnosis.
     I. Gray, W. (Winifred) II. Kocjan, Gabrijela.
     616′ .07582-dc22

A catalogue record for this book is available from the British Library

**Library of Congress Cataloging in Publication Data**
A catalog record for this book is available from the Library of Congress

**Notice**
Medical knowledge is constantly changing. Standard safety precautions must be followed, but as new research and clinical experience broaden our knowledge, changes in treatment and drug therapy may become necessary or appropriate. Readers are advised to check the most current product information provided by the manufacturer of each drug to be administered to verify the recommended dose, the method and duration of administration, and contraindications. It is the responsibility of the practitioner, relying on experience and knowledge of the patient, to determine dosages and the best treatment for each individual patient. Neither the Publisher nor the author assume any liability for any injury and/or damage to persons or property arising from this publication.

The Publisher

Printed in China
Last dgit is the print number: 9 8 7 6 5 4 3

# Contents

# Preface

Cytopathology has seen major developments, opportunities and challenges in the first decade of 21st century. At the time of writing for the second edition of *Diagnostic Cytopathology*, the human genome had only recently been elucidated, genomics and proteomics were budding sciences, molecular markers were just coming into widespread use and vaccines for cervical cancer were still under investigation.

Today, the clinical value, diagnostic accuracy and cost effectiveness of a wide variety of applications of cytology are accepted by physicians and surgeons; in many cases a cytological diagnosis can serve as the basis for patient management without reliance on surgical procedures. Using molecular markers, so-called 'Personalised/Therapeutic Pathology' based on material obtained by fine needle aspiration, mutations diagnostic of a range of tumours, such as colorectal, lung or breast cancer, can be identified. Cervical screening still plays an important part in prevention of cervical cancer, especially with the use of liquid based cytology, but must now integrate with papillomavirus sub-typing and with the emerging programme of vaccination.

The expectation of high standards of performance amongst clinicians and the public has grown with each new development. We are under an obligation therefore to maintain our expertise, to attract and train new recruits and to educate our colleagues in the advantages and limitations of our speciality. This edition stresses not just the diagnostic cytological features of the various conditions we encounter, but also the diagnostic pitfalls and the grey areas between so as to enable the reader to give more evidence-based reports.

In recognition of their rapid expansion, there are new chapters on recent technological developments and on the cytodiagnosis of childhood tumours. A special section on the importance of multidisciplinary team meetings that include the cytopathologist as a core member of the team has also been included at the end of each chapter. As active members of this team, we can define our role in the management pathway and thus bring the patient and the microscope together as never before.

The third edition of *Diagnostic Cytopathology* hopes to contribute to all of these aspects of our working life. As editors, we have had the pleasure of seeking experts from around the world to update or rewrite each of the chapters, with particular attention to the latest developments in their own field. In some areas, the complexity of the subject has necessitated putting together a team from different laboratories, a matter of slight trepidation, which fortunately was not ever justified. We hope that readers will not just find the diagnostic answers they seek but will catch some of the dedication to cytopathology that has gone into the authorship of these chapters We would also like to think that the book will tempt would-be pathologists to embark on a training in cytology – we believe that getting to know cells will be a necessary and enjoyable skill for many years to come.

As editors again, we would like to thank all of the chapter authors for the huge amount of work that has gone into the contributions they have made. We are also well aware that none of us could have managed without the assistance of staff within our laboratories, from secretaries, technical colleagues, photographers and fellow pathologists. We are very grateful to our long-suffering families, too, for being so understanding and supportive throughout. And finally, we would never have managed without the editorial staff at Elsevier, who have been encouraging, patient and pressing, according to need, so as to ensure timely completion of the work of this third edition.

*Winifred Gray*
*Gabrijela Kocjan*
*2010*

# List of Contributors

**Måns Åkerman (retired)** MD, PhD, FIAC
Associate Professor of Pathology; Senior Cytopathologist
Department of Pathology and Cytopathology
University Hospital
Lund, Sweden

**Asmund Berner** MD, PhD, MIAC
Senior Consultant, Division of Pathology
Oslo University Hospital – Central Hospital – The
Norwegian Radium Hospital
Professor, Faculty Division Central Hospital
University of Oslo
The Medical Faculty
Oslo, Norway

**Alfred H. Böcking** MD, FIAC
Professor of Pathology
Director, Institute of Cytopathology
University of Düsseldorf
Düsseldorf, Germany

**Anna M. Bofin** MD, PhD
Associate Professor of Pathology
Norwegian University of Science and Technology
Department of Laboratory Medicine
Children's and Women's Health
Trondheim, Norway

**Anna Maria Buccoliero** MD, PhD
Pathologist
University of Florence
Department of Human Pathology and Oncology
Viale Giovan Battista Morgagni
Florence, Italy

**Ian D. Buley** MA, BM, BCh, FRCPath
Consultant Pathologist and Honorary University Fellow to
the Peninsula Medical School
Torbay Hospital
Torquay, UK

**Ashish Chandra** FRCPath, DipRCPath (Cyto)
Clinical Lead
Guy's and St. Thomas' NHS Foundation Trust
Cellular Pathology
St Thomas' Hospital
London, UK

**Eidi Christensen** MD
Consultant Dermatologist and Research Fellow
St Olav's Hospital
Department of Dermatology
Norwegian University of Science and Technology (NTNU)
Trondheim, Norway

**Beatrix Cochand-Priollet** MD, PhD
Associate Professor of Pathology
Department of Pathology and Cytopathology
Lariboisière Hospital
Paris, France

**Karin J. Denton** MB, ChB, FRCPath
Consultant Cytopathologist
Cellular Pathology Department
North Bristol NHS Trust
Bristol, UK

**John Denton** MSc
Pathology Research Fellow
Department of Clinical and Laboratory Medicine
University of Manchester
Manchester, UK

**Minaxi S. Desai** MBBS, FRCPath
Consultant Cytopathologist and Clinical Head
Manchester Cytology Centre
Director
Manchester Cytology Training Centre
Central Manchester and Manchester Children's University
Hospitals NHS Trust
Manchester, UK

**Henryk A. Domanski** MD, PhD
Associate Professor of Pathology and Consultant Pathologist
University Hospital
Department of Pathology and Cytology
Lund, Sweden

**Monique Fabre** MD
Associate Professor of Pathology
University Paris-Sud 11
Head of Liver Pathology Unit
Paul Brousse Hospital
Villejuif, France

**Mary Falzon** FRCPath
Consultant Histopathologist/Cytopathologist
Divisional Clinical Director
University College Hospital
London, UK

**Anthony J. Freemont** MD, FRCP, FRCPath
Professor of Osteoarticular Pathology
School of Biomedicine
University of Manchester
Manchester, UK

**Malcolm Galloway** BSc, MBBS, FRCPath, FAcad Med
Consultant Neuropathologist and Honorary
Senior Lecturer
Department of Cellular Pathology
Royal Free Hampstead NHS Trust and University College
London Medical School
London, UK

**Thomas E. Giles** MB, ChB, FRCPath
Consultant Cytopathologist
Department of Cytology
Royal Liverpool University Hospital
Liverpool, UK

**Winifred Gray (retired)** MB, BS, FRCPath
Consultant Cytopathologist/Histopathologist
John Radcliffe Hospital
Oxford, UK

**Amanda Herbert** MB, BS, FRCPath
Consultant Histopathologist and Cytopathologist
Guy's and St Thomas' NHS Foundation Trust
London, UK

**Ika Kardum-Skelin** MD, PhD
Associate Professor and Consultant Cytologist
Specialist in Medical/Clinical Cytology
Head of Laboratory of Cytology and Hematology
Department of Medicine
Merkur University Hospital
Zagreb, Croatia

**Jerzy Klijanienko** MD
Head of Cytopathology
Department of Tumour Biology
Curie Institute
Paris, France

**Tadao Kobayashi** MD, PhD
Head of Laboratory Medicine
Saisekai Shiga Hospital
Department of Pathology
Professor (affiliate), Cancer Education Center
Osaka University Graduate School of Medicine
Shiga, Japan

**Gabrijela Kocjan** MB, BS, Spec Clin Cyt, FRCPath
Senior Lecturer
Head of Diagnostic Cytopathology
University College Hospital
London, UK

**Irmeli Lautenschlager** MD, PhD
Senior Scientist
Helsinki University Central Hospital and
University of Helsinki
Department of Microbiology (Virology)
Helsinki, Finland

**Victor Lee** MBBS, FRCPA
Assistant Professor and Consultant
National University Health System and National University
of Singapore
Department of Pathology
Singapore, Republic of Singapore

**Tanya Levine** MA, MBBS, RCDipPath (Cyto), FRCPath
Director
London Regional Cytology Training Center
Consultant Cellular Pathologist
North West London Hospitals NHS Trust
London, UK

**Vesna Mahovlić** MD, MSc
Consultant Cytologist
Specialist in Medical/Clinical Cytology
Head of Department of Gynecologic Cytology
Zagreb University Hospital Center
University Department of Obstetrics and Gynecology
Zagreb, Croatia

**Sanjiv Manek** BSc, MBBS, FRCPath, DipRCPath (Cyto)
Consultant Gynaecological Pathologist
John Radcliffe Hospital
Department of Cellular Pathology
Oxford, UK

**Julie McCarthy** MBBS, LRCP, FRCPath, PhD, DipRCPath (Cyto)
Consultant Cytopathologist
Department of Histo/Cytopathology
Cork University Hospital
Wilton, Cork, Ireland

**Robert F. Miller** MB, BSc (Hons), FRCP, CBiol FIBiol
Reader in Clinical Infection
University College London
Research Department of Infection and Population Health
London, UK

**Siok-Bian Ng** MBBS, FRCPA
Assistant Professor and Consultant
Department of Pathology
National University Health System and National University
of Singapore
Singapore, Republic of Singapore

**Yoshiaki Norimatsu** PhD, CMIAC
Professor
Ehime Prefectural University of Health Sciences
Department of Medical Technology
Faculty of Health Sciences
Ehime, Japan

**M. Helena Oliveira** MD
Pathologist, Head of Department
Laboratory of Anatomic Pathology
HPP – Centro Hospitalar de Cascais
Cascais, Portugal

**Svante R. Orell** AM, ML (Sweden), FRCPA, FIAC
Consultant Pathologist
Clinpath Laboratories
Kent Town, Australia

**Lucio Palombini** MD
Professor of Anatomic Pathology and Cytopathology
University of Naples Federico II
Department of Biomorfological and Functional Sciences
Faculty of Medicine and Surgery
Napoli, Italy

**Martha Bishop Pitman** MD
Associate Professor of Pathology, Harvard Medical School
Assistant Director of Cytopathology, Director of the Fine
Needle Aspiration Biopsy Service
Massachusetts General Hospital
Boston, MA, USA

**Stephen S. Raab** MD
Vice Chair and Professor of Pathology
Director of Anatomic Pathology and Cytopathology
Department of Pathology
University of Colorado Denver
Aurora, CO, USA

**Ibrahim Ramzy** MD, FRCPC
Professor of Clinical Pathology and Obstetrics/Gynecology
University of California
Irvine, CA, USA
Adjunct Professor of Pathology
Baylor College of Medicine
Houston, TX, USA

**Derek E. Roskell** MA, BM, BCh, FRCPath
Consultant Pathologist
Oxford Radcliffe Hospitals NHS Trust;
Honorary Senior Lecturer
Oxford University
Oxford, UK

**Manuel Salto-Tellez** MD (LMS), FRCPath
Associate Professor and Senior Consultant
Director, Diagnostic Molecular Oncology Centre
Department of Pathology
National University Health System and National University
of Singapore
Singapore, Republic of Singapore

**Torill Sauer** MD, PhD
Professor of Pathology
Department of Pathology
Oslo University Hospital
Ulleval, Oslo, Norway

**Fernando Schmitt** MD, PhD, FIAC
Professor of Pathology
Medical Faculty of Porto University and Institute of
Molecular Pathology and Immunology
University of Porto
Porto, Portugal

**Ketan A. Shah** FRCPath
Consultant Pathologist
Department of Cellular Pathology
John Radcliffe Hospital
Oxford, UK

**Vinod B. Shidham** MD, MRCPath, FIAC
Professor
Medical College of Wisconsin
Department of Pathology
Milwaukee, MI, USA

**Jan F. Silverman** MD
Chair and Director of Anatomic Pathology
Drexel University College of Medicine
Allegheny General Hospital Pittsburch
PA, USA

**Lambert Skoog** MD, PhD
Professor of Clinical Cytology
Department of Pathology and Cytology
Karolinska University Hospital
Solna, Sweden

**Philip Sloan** BDS(Hons), FDS RCS(Eng), PhD, FRCPath
Consultant Histopathologist and Lead Clinician
Royal Victoria Infirmary
Department of Cellular Pathology
Newcastle-upon-Tyne, UK

**John H. F. Smith** BSc, MBBS, FRCPath, MIAC
Consultant Histopathologist and Cytopathologist
Director, East Pennine Cytology Training Centre
Department of Histopathology and Cytology
Royal Hallamshire Hospital
Sheffield, UK

**Peter A. Smith** BSc, MBBS, FRCPath
Consultant Cytopathologist and Clinical Director of
Pathology
Department of Pathology
Royal Liverpool University Hospital
Liverpool, UK

**Voichita M. Suciu** MD
Pathologist
Institute Gustave Roussy
Department of Medical Biology and Pathology
Villejuif, France

**Edneia Miyki Tani** MD, PhD
Associate Professor of Pathology and Head of Division of
Clinical Cytology
Karolinska University Hospital Solna
Department of Pathology and Cytology
Stockholm, Sweden

**Maria Thom** BSc, MBBS, FRCPath, MD
Senior Lecturer and Honorary Consultant in
Neuropathology
National Hospital for Neurology and Neurosurgery
UCL, Institute of Neurology
London, UK

**Paul J. Turek** MD, FACS, FRSM
Director, The Turek Clinic
Retired Endowed Chair Professor
Departments of Urology, Obstetrics, Gynecology and
Reproductive Sciences
University of California
San Francisco, CA, USA

**Philippe Vielh** MD, PhD
Pathologist, Director of Cytopathology
Department of Medical Biology and Pathology
Institute Gustave Roussy
Villejuif, France

**Eva von Willebrand** MD, PhD
Senior Scientist
Transplantation Laboratory
University of Helsinki
Helsinki, Finland

**Christine Waddell** MSc, MB, ChB, DObs, RCOG
Consultant Cytopathologist
Department of Cellular Pathology
Birmingham Women's NHS Foundation Trust
Birmingham, UK

**Martin Young** BSc, MBBS, MRCOG, FRCPath
Clinical Head of Service Histopathology
Department of Cellular Pathology
Royal Free Hampstead NHS Trust
London, UK

**Pio Zeppa** MD, PhD
Associate Professor of Pathology and Cytopathology
University of Naples Federico II
Department of Biomorfological and Functional Sciences
Faculty of Medicine and Surgery
Napoli, Italy

**Pohar Marinšek Živa** MD, PhD
Associate Professor of Pathology
Department of Cytopathology
Institute of Oncology
Ljubljana, Slovenia

# Dedication

As the editors of this third edition we would like to dedicate our book to those who introduced us to the science and art of cytopathology.

In particular we wish to thank Dr Arthur Spriggs, Dr Željka Znidarčić and Dr Naseem Husain for teaching us in the beginning how to recognise cells by their faces and for inspiring us to spend a lifetime exploring this most satisfying of disciplines.

# Section 1

## Introduction

# Cytopathology: the history, the present and the future direction

Ibrahim Ramzy and Amanda Herbert

## Chapter contents

A simplified version of historical research is that of tracing an idea or observation in a certain field to its earliest proponent or discoverer, and then citing in chronological order the names of subsequent investigators, as if their work was the direct continuation of a single line of thought. Such an approach is apt to give a false linear concept of scientific evolution by ignoring the fact that ideas and observations may often have more than one source and may extend beyond the boundaries of any particular field into related or even unrelated fields. Cytology is a good example of this.

Cytology started as a then revolutionary idea of looking at imprints of cut tumour surfaces at postmortem. It has evolved through many new methods of procuring, fixing and staining cells, but its main attribute lies in its ability to allow prompt, accurate assessment of cell changes on material taken with minimally invasive procedures and processing. As the possibilities for diagnosis and research expand, its immediacy provides a method of preliminary diagnosis, validation of sample adequacy and collection of appropriate material for tests such as flow cytometry, immunocytochemistry, molecular biology and microbiological culture, many of which require fresh unfixed cellular material. Thus, in modern clinical diagnosis, it returns to its roots, when imprints of intraoperative liver biopsies, crush preparations of brain tumours or direct smears of endoscopic ultrasound-guided fine needle aspirates (FNA) are assessed on-site by cytopathologists as members of a multidisciplinary team. As such, this is a cyclical rather than linear evolution of a technique whose roots are firmly bedded in cytomorphology.

The introductory chapter of the first edition of *Diagnostic Cytopathology* was written by Bernard Naylor and covered the development of the discipline from its beginnings in the nineteenth century to its full acceptance by pathologists and clinicians by the end of the twentieth century, using the same format as an article in *Acta Cytologica*.[1] Following his lead, we will discuss the evolution of cytopathology over four sometimes overlapping eras; the early history (1860–1940); the development and expansion of exfoliative cytology in the USA

and elsewhere (1940–1960); the consolidation of cytopathology as a discipline and the parallel developments of population screening and FNA cytology (1955–1985); the maturation of cytopathology as a discipline and its integration with new technology (1985 to the present day). Future directions are difficult to predict, but the integration of its basic principles with other disciplines and technologies, as well as the impact of changing economies will define the role cytopathology can play in the future.

## The early historical era

Microscopic observations of normal and abnormal human cells, either exfoliated or in imprints or scrapes, were steadily and independently recorded throughout the nineteenth century.[2–5] By the first decade of the twentieth century, exfoliated cancer cells had been described in all of the types of specimens in which we look for them today.[6] One fine example, published in 1861,[7] 22 years before the birth of Papanicolaou, featured an exquisite drawing of cancer cells in pharyngeal secretion obtained postmortem from a man who died with a growth in this throat (Fig. 1.1). To any of us looking at this illustration

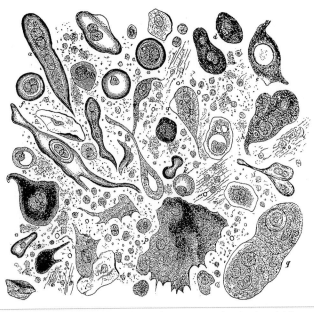

**Fig. 1.1** Pharyngeal secretion obtained postmortem showing keratinising squamous cell carcinoma. This drawing appeared in the medical literature 22 years before the birth of Papanicolaou.

*The authors wish to acknowledge the invaluable input from Professor Bernard Naylor, who coauthored the chapter in the previous edition. Dr Naylor's contribution remains visible throughout the chapter.*

today, almost 150 years later, it is obvious that the patient died from keratinising squamous cell carcinoma.

For the most part, however, these early reports were regarded as scientific curiosities, of little or no practical value. A widely prevailing attitude underlay this situation, well-expressed by Gloyne in 1919 speaking of cancer cells in pleural fluids: 'Most pathologists are now agreed that it is practically impossible to identify these cells in film preparations'[8] and by Bland-Sutton in 1922: 'in the appearance of a cell from cancer there is nothing characteristic of the disease, nothing that would lead a pathologist to identify it as a malignant cell'.[9] However, at much the same time Professor LS Dudgeon proved these statements to be incorrect and began to use cytology at St Thomas' Hospital for the diagnosis of a wide variety of neoplastic and inflammatory diseases from imprints of surgical specimens.[10] According to a later article by John Bamforth of the same hospital, in which some of the original plates are reproduced, Dudgeon considered 'that the stained films were much nicer to examine than paraffin sections'.[11] Many modern-day cytopathologists would agree and Dudgeon's beautiful illustrations demonstrate the importance of good fixation and cell preparation. He died at the outbreak of the Second World War and his prediction that 20 years or more would elapse before the cytological method would be generally accepted was sadly only too true, at least in the UK. At much the same time in the USA, FNA cytology was being developed and the first series on aspiration of neoplasms was published from Memorial Hospital for Cancer and Allied Diseases in New York City.[12–14] Yet this experience was not taken forward at the time and one wonders if the method of cell preparation, which involved heating, alcohol fixation, dehydration and clearing to mimic histological sections could have rendered the cytomorphology less than satisfactory. Nevertheless, two important principles had been established: that needle aspiration could safely be carried out in living patients and that 'diagnosis by aspiration is as reliable as the combined intelligence of the clinician and pathologist'[14]– an early example of a multidisciplinary team. Another half century had to pass before aspiration cytology became firmly established in the USA, perhaps as a testament to the importance of cell preparation.

## Development and expansion of exfoliative cytology

A second era of cytopathology began in 1941 with the publication of an article on the diagnostic value of vaginal smears in carcinoma of the uterus by George N. Papanicolaou, an anatomist, and Herbert F. Traut, a gynaecologist.[15] This article was followed in 1943 by their monograph *Diagnosis of Uterine Cancer by the Vaginal Smear*,[16] with its superbly executed watercolour drawings of exfoliated cells and tissues. Gynaecologists, especially in the USA, were quick to grasp the significance of these two publications, which were succeeded over the next two decades by many more publications by Papanicolaou and his colleagues dealing with the cytological diagnosis of cancer in a variety of other organs. Although cancer cells in vaginal smears had been recognised and briefly described and illustrated in publications of the nineteenth century,[4,5] Papanicolaou's contribution to this field was two-fold: he recognised the importance of wet fixation of cytological specimens and he systematically began to accumulate examples of cancer cells in vaginal smears,

culminating in his paper *New Cancer Diagnosis*.[17] Papanicoloau's original research was on the oestrous cycle of mammals, using cellular samples from the vaginas of guinea pigs. Later, he extended this work to humans and, inevitably, received vaginal smears from women with cervical cancer and discovered by chance that he was able to recognise cancer cells in these smears. At virtually the same time, Aurel A. Babes (1885–1961), a distinguished academic pathologist in Romania, published a major article[18] on the same subject, preceded by presentations at the Bucharest Gynaecology Society,[19,20] in which he accurately described the appearance of cells of squamous cell carcinoma in scrapings of the uterine cervix. However, these presentations made virtually no impact on the cytological scene. Babes' technique of preparing, staining and examining vaginal smears was substantially different from Papanicolaou's and would never have lent itself to mass screening for cervical cancer without modification.

The publications of Papanicolaou and Traut in 1941 and 1943 heralded the second era of cytopathology and the advent of screening for cervical cancer. The breakthrough was that 'malignant cells' could be observed in scrapings from a cervix that was entirely normal to the naked eye, taken from a healthy asymptomatic woman. The idea of pre-cancerous cell change was conceived. Concurrently with the development of cervical screening, the cytological method of cancer diagnosis began to be more widely applied to the respiratory, alimentary and urinary tracts as well as to the serous cavities and the central nervous system. In 1954, Papanicolaou published his magnum opus, the comprehensive *Atlas of Exfoliative Cytology* (Fig. 1.2).[21] This emphasis on the development of cytology by Papanicolaou and his colleagues should not detract from many carefully executed earlier or contemporary studies of the cytology of other organs, reviewed in the publications of Grunze and Spriggs.[3,4] But unquestionably, the impetus of the development of cytopathology as we know it today resulted from the painstaking research of Papanicolaou in the USA. The journey of Papanicolaou, justly referred to as the father of cytopathology, from his birthplace in Kymi on the Aegean island of Evia to his position in the Department of Anatomy at Cornell University is documented by many cytopathologists, including Naylor and Koss.[1,22]

## Consolidation of cytopathology as a discipline

From the earliest days of cytology, there was scepticism among pathologists about the validity of the diagnosis of cancer by cytology alone. It almost smacked of fraud that cancer, whose unique attribute was its ability to invade tissue and metastasise, could be diagnosed by examining cells that had dropped off from an epithelial surface. Nevertheless, during the decades that followed the pioneering work of Papanicolaou, the widespread development both of population-based cervical screening and the cytological diagnosis of tumours resulted in the development of cytopathology as an established discipline.

The era of consolidation[1] was heralded by two publications: the first issue of *Acta Cytologica* in 1957, the oldest journal devoted exclusively to cytopathology; and in 1961, by the publication of *Diagnostic Cytology and its Histopathologic Bases* by Leopold G. Koss in association with Grace R. Durfee.[23] This book (Fig. 1.3), now in its fifth edition (2005), brought together under

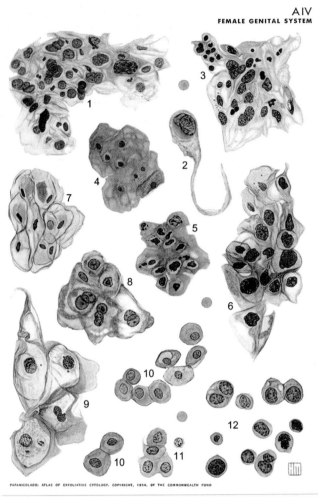

AIV
FEMALE GENITAL SYSTEM

PAPANICOLAOU: ATLAS OF EXFOLIATIVE CYTOLOGY. COPYRIGHT, 1954, BY THE COMMONWEALTH FUND

**Fig. 1.2** Reprinted by permission of the publisher from *Atlas of Exfoliative Cytology* by George N. Papanicolaou, Figure AIV, Cambridge, Mass: Harvard University Press, Copyright © 1954, 1956, 1960 by the Commonwealth Fund. Copyright © renewed 1982 by Mari Diane Murayama.

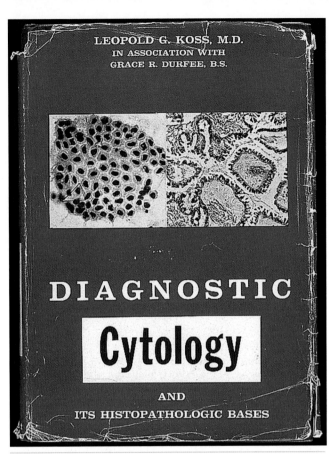

**Fig. 1.3** An important landmark in cytopathology: the first edition of *Diagnostic Cytology and its Histopathologic Bases*, published in 1961. (With kind permission from Koss Leopold G. *Diagnostic Cytology and its Histopathologic Bases*, Lippincott, Williams & Wilkins, 1961.)

one cover not only a body of theoretical and practical knowledge of cytopathology but also the correlation between cytology and histopathology, the essential basis for all pathologists who have an interest in cytopathology. As might be expected, the last 60 years have seen an explosion in the literature of cytopathology, with thousands of articles and scores of books written on the subject. In the English language alone, there are now four journals devoted exclusively to cytopathology: *Acta Cytologica, Diagnostic Cytopathology, Cytopathology* and *Cancer Cytopathology*, begun in 1957, 1985, 1990 and 1997, respectively. Societies promoting cytology were founded locally, nationally and internationally. The forerunner of these was the Inter-Society Cytology Council, founded in 1951 and later known as the American Society of Cytopathology. Many other societies developed over the next few decades, for example the International Academy of Gynecologic Cytology (1957), later known as International Academy of Cytology, the British Society for Clinical Cytology (1961), the Australian Society of Cytopathology (1969), and the European Federation of Cytology Societies (1969). These societies now have major roles in maintaining high standards in cytopathology by their educational activities, their contribution to the certification of pathologists and technologists in cytopathology, their

influence in research and their contribution to legislation that affects the practice of cytopathology.

## Population-based cervical cancer screening

Population-based cervical screening is now practiced to a greater or lesser extent in almost all countries of the developed world. Invasive cervical cancer is a rare disease in countries where screening is widely available but remains the commonest cause of death from cancer in women in countries without such programmes. Although the Imperial Cancer Research Fund Coordinating Committee on Cervical Screening made the statement in 1984 that 'with the exception of stopping smoking, cervical cytology screening offers the only major proved public health measure for significantly reducing the burden of disease',[24] its introduction was highly controversial and has remained so at every stage of its development. The 1950s in the USA saw enormous enthusiasm for the treatment of 'carcinoma *in situ*', often by hysterectomy, while the meaning of that term was hotly contested. McKelvey considered that to 'call atypical lesions malignant and treat them as cancers is to fog our own critical recesses and to harm the patient ...'[25]

The first apparently successful population-based programmes were reported in British Columbia[26] and Tennessee[27] but the reports of their success were criticised for not being controlled trials: the risk might have been lower in the screened compared with the unscreened populations and the risk of carcinoma *in situ* was not known.[28] Carcinoma *in situ* could only be diagnosed when the presence of invasion had been excluded after complete excision, meaning that its outcome became increasingly difficult to determine. By close follow-up of women with cervical abnormalities, Peterson deduced that 'we are able to recognise lesions which carry a measurable risk (30–40%) of sooner or later becoming malignant'.[29] Despite these caveats, gynaecologists faced with the clinical management of relatively young women with cervical cancer were the first to pioneer screening programmes in the UK and recognised the importance of training highly skilled non-medical scientists in screening the slides. The first population-based programme in the UK was led by Macgregor and Baird in the early 1960s.[30] Pilot centres with training schools were set up in Newcastle, Edinburgh, Birmingham and London. However, there was considerable scepticism about the necessity for mass screening,[31] which may be part of the reason why the national programme in the UK that was introduced in 1967 was so poorly funded.[32] Data from the Nordic countries demonstrated conclusively that organised programmes could substantially reduce the incidence and mortality of cervical cancer.[33] By 1986, there was sufficient evidence from an international multicentre analysis to show that 5-yearly and 3-yearly screening reduced the risk of invasive cancer by 84% and 93%, respectively, while little additional benefit was achieved by annual screening.[34] Although population screening was vindicated, its early history demonstrates the hazards of introducing health measures without clinical trials, and the difficulties in measuring outcomes of interventions based on the treatment of risk.

## FNA cytology

FNA was first introduced in Sweden by Franzen, a haematologist-oncologist by training, who used the same Romanovsky staining method as for bone marrow aspirates.[35] The technique was further developed by Soderstrom[36], Fox[37] and also by Lopes Cardoso, Von Haam, Črepinko and Hauptmann.[38–40] The rapid development of this technique relied on cytopathologists taking their own aspirates in clinics closely associated with pathology departments, thus facilitating correlation of cytology and histology. In the UK, FNA was pioneered by, among others, a surgeon, John Webb,[41] who was given enthusiastic support by some of the renowned cytopathologists of the time.[42] The technique also became popular in the USA[43] after a long interval since its early use in the 1930s.

Not only was this popularity an outcome of the spread of cytopathological expertise, but it was also fostered by the development of diagnostic angiography, ultrasound and computed tomography. These techniques have enabled the performance of FNA on virtually any deeply seated organ. This has been further enhanced by the introduction of flexible endoscopy and hybrid techniques such as ultrasound-guided endoscopic FNA. Although FNA is increasingly carried out for deep-seated lesions by radiologists and gastroenterologists, palpable masses may readily be aspirated free-hand, even without negative pressure.[44] In many centres, FNA is performed by cytopathologists who have developed a reputation for high accuracy and low inadequate rates when the procedures

are carried out in their dedicated clinics.[45] The advantages of immediate assessment of sample adequacy, the availability of cytotechnologists and biomedical scientists with skill in preparing the slides, and the presence of the patients themselves to provide proper clinical information make this the ideal setting for FNA cytology.

The development of aspiration cytology has proved to be one of the biggest advances in anatomical pathology and brought us, we believe, to the end of the era of consolidation. That ending was summarised by Dr George L. Wied, Editor of *Acta Cytologica*, in a personal communication with Dr Bernard Naylor, when he said 'The cytologic crusades are over'; sadly, as with all crusades, they never quite end.

## Responsibilities of cytology as a discipline

Until the effectiveness of cervical screening had been established in the mid-1980s, the main criticisms faced by cytopathologists had related to whether or not screening was necessary; whether it worked and whether it was ethical to treat lesions before they became invasive. There was a sudden change of emphasis in the mid–late 1980s when incidents in several different countries drew the attention of the media, public and lawyers to the consequences of cytological abnormalities being missed. In the UK, a damning editorial in the *Lancet* about the inefficiencies of the so-called national screening programme was the first indication that it was simply not working;[46] and was not controlling an increased risk of disease in young women.[47] At much the same time, a national enquiry in New Zealand followed publication of the outcome of a group of women with carcinoma *in situ* who had not received adequate treatment.[48] In 1987, the *Wall Street Journal* published an exposé about cancers being missed through the excessive demands made on their cytology technicians by certain for-profit commercial laboratories.[49] This article raised a huge outcry in the news media in the USA, resulting in stringent federal rules regulating the laboratory practice of gynaecological cytology and the imposition of proficiency testing. In the UK, a successful centrally organised NHS Cervical Screening Programme was launched in 1988, which resulted in a dramatic fall in incidence and mortality in all age groups screened (Fig. 1.4). Screening is thought to have prevented an epidemic of cervical cancer in recent generations at greater risk of disease.[50] The events of the 1980s should, however, serve as a warning to implement quality-assurance practices and not to demand excessive output from cytotechnologists, biomedical scientists and cytology screeners. Quality assurance practices are now documented in the second edition of the *European Guidelines for Quality Assurance in Cervical Cancer Screening*.[51]

The prospect of a federally mandated proficiency test provided the impetus for developing an acceptable and reproducible terminology for cervical cytology, which had been bedevilled by a variety of reporting systems that were not understandable from one institution to another. This confusion was engendered by the reporting system that Papanicolaou devised in the 1940s, which used 'classes' of cytological changes from normality to overt malignancy expressed as the Roman numerals I to V. Unfortunately, a certain class report from one laboratory often meant something different from that of another, thus vitiating comparison of their results. Prominent gynaecological cytopathologists in the USA, such as the late Drs James Reagan and Stanley Patten, never used

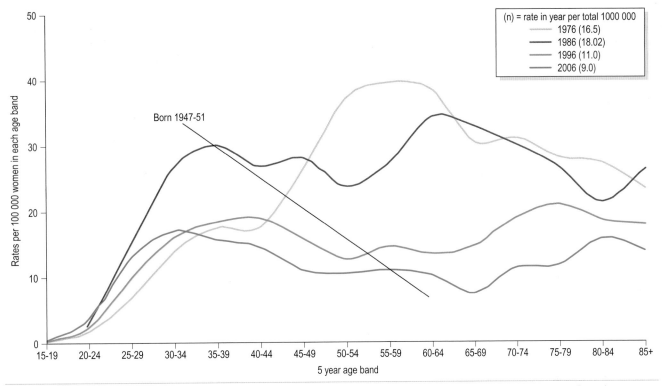

**Fig. 1.4** Incidence of invasive carcinoma of the uterine cervix before, during and after the introduction of organised screening in the United Kingdom (Source: National statistics website: www.statistics.gov.ukStatBase/Product.asp?vlnk = 7720. Crown copyright material is reproduced with the permission of the Controller Office of Public Sector Information (OPSI)).

the Papanicolaou classes, preferring to replace them with readily understandable diagnostic statements. Their pleas to others to adopt such a method of reporting were often to no avail since many clinicians believed they knew exactly what a Class III report meant, unlike cytopathologists who never had a consensus on the morphological criteria for formulating such a report.

In December 1988, a workshop was convened at the National Cancer Institute in Bethesda, Maryland to hammer out reporting terminology that would be a reflection of the development of cervical cancer and the near impossibility of discriminating with any degree of consistency between certain degrees of squamous intraepithelial neoplasia in cytological preparations. It would also take account of the qualitative difference between low-grade squamous intraepithelial lesions, most of which were already known to represent infection with the human papillomavirus (HPV), and high-grade lesions, which carried a greater risk of persistence and progression to invasive cancer. The outcome of this workshop, *the Bethesda System for Reporting Cervical/Vaginal Cytology Diagnoses*, was promulgated several months later, to be followed by a revision published in 1992. The consensus conference in 2001 resulted in a further revision, ironing out some problems.[52] Reports according to the Bethesda system (TBS) provide information as to the quality of the cellular sample, a general categorisation of the cellular findings, and a descriptive diagnosis of any abnormality. The system lends itself to computer entry and its adoption could facilitate quality assurance measures and the international exchange of data.

The Bethesda system has received general support in the USA from professional societies and has gained widespread acceptance in laboratory practice largely because of its intrinsic simplicity and the need for standardised terminology to deal

with the advent of government-mandated proficiency tests. Although many European countries have retained a three-tier system for reporting dyskaryosis (dysplasia), the recent EU guidelines have firmly recommended that all systems should at least be translatable into TBS.[53] The British Society for Clinical Cytology has recently adopted a revised terminology, which moves closer and is certainly translatable into TBS.[54]

The lessons learnt from the history of cytopathology in the twentieth century about the importance of quality control, comprehensible terminology and close cooperation between cytopathologists, non-medical cytologists and clinicians are equally relevant to gynaecological and diagnostic non-gynaecological cytology as they find their place in the rapidly expanding technological revolution of the twenty-first century.

## Cytopathology in the twenty-first century

Although it is difficult to be certain about the direction cytology will follow in the future, several factors will clearly have a major impact on the way we will, or should practice. Technological innovations in imaging, sampling, automated screening as well as the development of new tumour markers and molecular techniques are among these factors. Together with development of HPV vaccines and changes in treatment, these will alter the focus of cytopathology practice and will present opportunities as well as challenges.

One of the greatest challenges facing the present era of cytopathology is to expedite the processing of cervicovaginal specimens, while achieving maximum accuracy of interpretation. Accomplishing this goal has been a dream since the 1950s, when Mellors and colleagues studied the nucleic acid content of the squamous carcinoma cell using the fluorochrome berberine sulphate and observed measurable differences of fluorescence between benign cells and cancer cells.[5,55,56] This was followed by numerous clinical studies of cytological specimens employing the same principle, but the method eventually fell into disuse when the degree of discrimination required by observers was found to be essentially similar to that required with conventional cytology. Nevertheless, recent technical innovations in automated screening, as well as in other fields of cytopathology, have left a clear impact on the discipline, shaping the ability and application of cytopathology in the diagnosis and management of disease.

## Advances in imaging techniques

The rapidly developing technology of imaging enhances visualisation and sampling of lesions that were not easily localised by older methods. Progress in this area is expected to result in more refined and sensitive techniques that are more comfortable and carry less risk for the patient, and as such will certainly have an impact on the ability to sample areas that are now difficult or too risky to reach. Stereotactic localisation and the ability to visualise masses in three-dimensions is widely used for taking FNA and core biopsies. The implication of these improvements in imaging for cytopathology is simple: if an organ or a lesion can be reached, a demand for interpretation of material procured from it will soon be created.

## Sampling devices

Sampling devices greatly influence the diagnostic accuracy of any test and the ability to establish definitive diagnoses. The use of new brushes and similar devices is now the standard of care, not only for gynaecologists seeking to sample the endocervix or endometrium,[57,58] but also for gastroenterologists, urologists and pulmonologists. Indeed, the marriage of imaging and sampling techniques undoubtedly opens new fields. The use of flexible endoscopy and ultrasound to guide FNA by gastroenterologists and chest physicians is but one example of such development.[59] Although some of these new techniques enhance the role of cytology, others may seem to replace traditional cytology, as in the case of ultrasound-guided core needle biopsy that has all but replaced FNA cytology as the method of choice for sampling the prostate and, in some cases, the breast. However, the focus should always be on what is best for patients. Is it necessary for women, for example, to be subjected to multiple core biopsies of breast lesions that could easily be biopsied with considerably less bruising by FNA? Yes, for some lesions but certainly not for all.[60] It is in this field that George Wied's crusade continues.

## Rapid on-site evaluation

The utilisation and reliability of FNA depends on the availability of skilled, enthusiastic cytopathologists and cytotechnologists. Unlike core biopsies, FNA sample adequacy may be assessed on-site and provisional diagnoses provided. With expensive procedures such as endoscopic ultrasound guided (EUS) FNA and endobronchial ultrasound-guided (EBUS)

FNA, rapid on-site evaluation (ROSE) saves money even if an immediate diagnosis is not needed. With immediate assessment, appropriate material can be retained for microbiological culture, flow cytometry or immunocytochemistry. This is one of many areas where cytopathologists and cytotechnologists can contribute to clinical management if they are prepared to leave the apparent safety of their offices.[61]

## Automated processing and screening

Fuelled by an almost logarithmic increase in computing power, automation is playing an increasingly significant role in the practice of cytology. Several companies raced to take advantage of this tremendous computer power to enhance the speed and accuracy of processing and screening, and to relieve technicians of the burden of screening hundreds of normal smears to find the few abnormal ones. Pressures from the manufacturers were being brought to bear on the public and clinicians to demand 'State of the Art' processing and screening. Guidelines for instruments used for primary and secondary screening were developed by the International Academy of Cytology[62] and by the Intersociety Working Group (ISWG), a group that included representatives from American and other national organisations of pathologists, technologists and gynaecologists.[63,64] The group also attempted to quench the thirst of the public and physicians for balanced, truthful and unbiased information about the new liquid-based technology and computerised screening.[65]

Liquid-based technology offers *automated processing* to enhance specificity and sensitivity especially with cervicovaginal cytology.[66] Currently, two technically ingenious automated processors, the ThinPrep®[67] (Fig. 1.5) and the AutoCyte®[68] (Fig. 1.6) passed rigorous testing and are widely used throughout the world; the latter as its successor PrepStain™. The lack of cellular debris, blood and exudate makes it easier to detect cellular abnormalities and may speed up the time required for screening. Rapid cell transfer from the sampling device to the transporting fixative fluid ensures preservation of cell detail with minimal artifactual changes. Liquid-based cytology (LBC) has been introduced throughout the UK on the recommendation of the National Institute for Clinical Excellence, largely based on a Health Technology Assessment report of three pilot sites for implementation.[69] The main reason for its introduction in the UK was the dramatic fall in rates of inadequate smears seen at all the pilot sites. LBC was considered to be at least as sensitive as conventional cytology, although a subsequent meta-analysis concluded that there was no significant improvement in sensitivity for detection of high-grade CIN compared with conventional cytology.[70] Nevertheless, LBC has the major advantage of providing residual material for HPV testing as well as other molecular tests and immunocytochemistry; and it has also facilitated the development of automated screening. Cervical screening is no longer reliant on microscopic examination of a single slide and LBC has opened the door to a multitude of new approaches to improve its accuracy. Whether these new techniques save more lives has yet to be proven but they will undoubtedly shed yet more light on the pathogenesis of cervical cancer and its precursors.

Two *automated screening systems* have now been deemed satisfactory for routine screening by the US Department of Health and Human Services and the MAnual screening Versus Automated Reading In Cytology (MAVARIC) trial is in progress

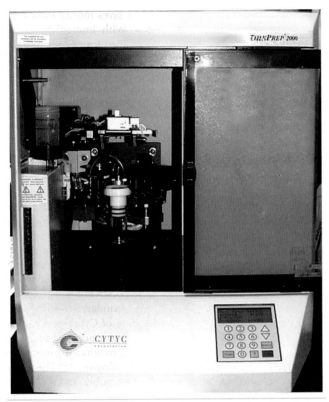

**Fig. 1.5** ThinPrep® device for liquid-based smear preparation. (With kind permission from Hologic UK Ltd.)

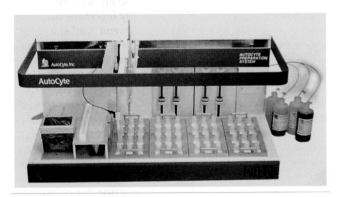

**Fig. 1.6** AutoCyte PREP® equipment.

to see whether they should be used in the NHSCSP. These devices are the latest developments in a prolonged quest for a fully automated screening system, first attempted by Tolles in 1955[71] with a machine, the Cytoanalyser. Automated screening devices met with mixed success until the increase in computing power permitted the development of several instruments.[72] The Papnet® system was designed for the analysis of conventionally prepared and stained smears, either for pre-screening or for quality assurance of slides found to be negative on prior manual screening. After training a neural network system on a series of normal smears, it recognised cells that differ from the normal reference. The abnormal cells were then displayed on a high-resolution television monitor for human assessment (Fig. 1.7). This two-stage system had great promise in that its approach did not use the traditional image analysis techniques that require image segmentation.[73] Unfortunately, for economic reasons the system has been withdrawn from the market.

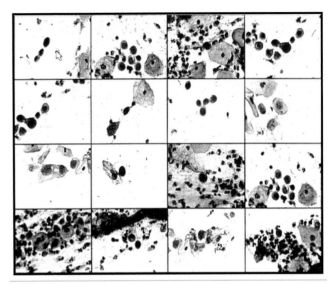

**Fig. 1.7** Panel of images displayed from the Papnet® system.

The Autopap® system was originally developed by Neopath and has been further developed as FocalPoint™. It uses multiple algorithms, which address single cells, thin cell groups and thick cell groups and evaluate multiple cellular features to assign a score between 0.0 and 1.0 to each preparation.[74] The score reflects the likelihood of having a significant abnormality and the device can localise on the slide cells or cell groups of interest. The system can be used for rescreening negative smears, thus reducing false negatives, or can be used as primary screener to eliminate the need for manual screening of a percentage of smears with the lowest score and least likely to be abnormal.

The ThinPrep Imaging System™ uses LBC slides that are stained with a modified Papanicolaou stain and scanned by the imager, which stores the coordinates of 22 cellular areas of greatest interest. It does not pretend to make a diagnosis but guides the cytotechnologist to the selected areas. Decisions are made as usual by the cytotechnologist and cytopathologist. This technology has gained FDA and CE approval for use as a primary screening method and has been shown to be more accurate than visual screening.[75] It can also be used as a powerful quality-control tool instead of rapid review or proportional rescreening of negative slides.

Both these systems accurately conform to George Wied's prediction of the direction that automated cytology would take when he wrote, 'If automation has a place in screening cytological samples, it will be in an interactive mode where the system scans the sample and shows so-called 'alarms' to a human observer for final analysis'.[5] Despite financial difficulties that led to consolidation of manufacturers and technologies, screening automation will stay in some form and economies of scale will eventually help to lower cost. Marriage of automated screening and processing will allow more standardisation of the way cells are spread and stained, thus improving the quality and reliability of screening. Cytotechnologists will continue to have an important role to play, but their job description, and consequently the training requirements, will have to change. They will need to be more computer literate and will have to spend more time examining atypical cases that the automated screener has selected for review.[76] These changes are expected to improve patient care and reduce the risk of technologists becoming victims of the deadly 'burn-out' syndrome.

## Tumour markers and molecular techniques

New tumour and proliferation markers are being developed for histological sections all the time, but many can be applied to FNAs by the use of immunocytochemistry. The specificity of many markers does not withstand the test of time, while others, such as prostate specific antigen (PSA) and CA125, continue to hold their ground. A detailed discussion of these is beyond the scope of this chapter. It is safe to predict that the armamentarium will be expanded in due time to encompass a wide variety of prognostic markers for different malignancies beyond those that we have today.

Molecular techniques undoubtedly will play a bigger role in the future in tumour diagnosis in general and in cervical cancer screening.[77] Fluorescence *in situ* hybridisation (FISH), polymerase chain reaction (PCR), gel-based analysis and diagnostic chip technology will leap forwards with the advancing knowledge of genetics of disease, derived from mapping of the human genome. The development of sensitive techniques to detect the genomes for HPV raises hope that a molecular test, capable of identifying patients with increased potential to develop cancer may offer an alternate to the Pap smear as we know it. High-risk HPV testing is already widely used for triage of cases with atypical or low-grade cytology[78] and new markers are likely to improve the specificity of markers currently available.

*Molecular probes* for non-random translocations in leukaemias, lymphomas, solid soft tissue sarcomas and for other cancer-related abnormalities are available; the growing list of genes includes p16, p53 tumour suppressor, retinoblastoma, familial polyposis, neurofibromatosis and many others. Probe detection by fluorochrome has progressed from a single colour per hybridisation to multicolour spectrally distinguishable probes for the 22 somatic chromosomes and the two sex chromosomes simultaneously. Miniaturisation of computers has also allowed the development of new generations of flow cytometers. Cell cycle analysis can now be easily performed by flow cytometry of cytology samples or by computerised image analysis.

*Microarray technologies*, based on computer chip manufacturing methods, have a great potential application, allowing high-throughput analysis of samples by the use of a large number of biological molecular markers.[79,80] These arrays can be of tissue blocks, oligonucleotides, cDNA or proteins (Fig. 1.8). Each type of array is used for a different reason and has its own limitation and potential. For example, probes made from tumour RNA can be used to test the expression levels of thousands of genes placed on a single slide to detect mutations.

To cytopathologists, these developments present a challenge and an excellent opportunity. Treatment of malignancies may require new classification by molecular techniques in addition to those of morphology. An FNA would be evaluated morphologically to assess adequacy of the sample and to identify it as being derived from a malignant neoplasm; the remainder of the specimen would then be triaged for a battery of molecular or other ancillary studies. New classifications of tumours by criteria that cannot be discerned by morphology alone may arise. It is unlikely that a single biomarker assessed by any technique, be it molecular, immunohistochemical or flow cytometric, is specific for a malignant phenotype; hence the continuous need for morphology.

## HPV vaccination

HPV vaccination is already set to revolutionise cervical cancer control throughout the world. Its integration with existing screening programmes is one of the main challenges facing cytopathology today while its benefits in terms of deaths from invasive cancer would be greater in countries without such programmes. Vaccination has the potential to prevent the majority of cases of CIN as well as invasive cancer,[81,82] but questions remain about its effectiveness at population level.[83] With current costs, uptake may be low and, although initial trials are highly encouraging, little is known about the duration of protection, its long-term risks or the relevance of HPV types not included in current vaccines. There is some concern that vaccinated women already infected with HPV may have a false sense of security and not want to be screened, although this is strongly recommended.[84] As prevalence of CIN falls in partly vaccinated populations, it may become difficult to maintain the high levels of accuracy required of primary cytological screening as sensitivity is known to be related to prevalence of abnormality in the material examined. It may become difficult to maintain the interest and enthusiasm of cytologists and primary HPV testing may be introduced at least for vaccinated women. Paradoxically, primary HPV testing might increase the need for quality control of cytology. Women and their medical advisers would need to be confident that a negative test was really negative when high-risk HPV had already been detected. The evolution of cytology into a triaging procedure may not be far off; for that to happen, however, there should be a concentrated effort by pathologists, gynaecologists, colposcopists and patients to mount an effective public relations campaign and get the attention of reluctant politicians. Economies of scale would help to lower the cost to society which, with the eventual development of polyvalent vaccines for boys as well as girls, could allow vaccination to reach its true potential in countries where it is so badly needed.[85]

## Meeting new professional challenges

## Global issues and opportunities

With the globalisation of the world economies and the potential breakdown of economic and social barriers between countries

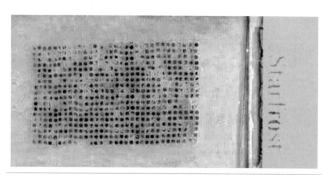

**Fig. 1.8** Tissue microarray showing an array of 576 prostatic biopsy specimens on a single glass slide (Courtesy of Dr Gustavo Ayala, Houston, Texas).

and continents, cytopathology as a discipline has to adapt to these new realities. Issues such as priorities for developing countries and the most cost-effective mechanisms of healthcare delivery, even in developed countries, cannot be ignored. It is clear that not all new technologies can be afforded by developing nations, and preventive measures such as vaccination or combating parasitic infections, would be more effective and critical. There are opportunities for cytopathology to contribute to the improvement of life for people living in such countries. As an example, FNA services can be easily integrated into the management of disease in rural settings, where biopsy or frozen section service cannot be established. Acceptance of new technologies or vaccines may be also influenced by local culture, custom or religious belief. Education may be a critical piece of the puzzle that has to be solved prior to implementing a programme, whose costs and benefits should reflect the local social, economic and medical realities.

## Matching expectations with reality

Perhaps one of the major challenges that cytopathology increasingly faces is to meet the expectations of a society that demands perfect outcomes and clinical colleagues who are becoming more dependent on cytological methods. Unfortunately, the legal profession attempts to portray cervical cytology as an exact science with well-defined criteria for what is normal and abnormal, which is an unrealistic concept. In the quest to attain perfection we have attempted to separate into clearly defined entities a condition that in reality is a continuum of change, not always easy to distinguish from normality. This unrealistic expectation carries the risk of portraying in the eyes of the public one of the most successful cancer screening tools in existence as an unreliable test. Inevitably, this leads to a temptation to report as atypical or borderline any slight deviation from the perfect prototype, thus practicing legally 'safe' cytopathology, resulting in unnecessary colposcopy, distress and expense. It is here that guidelines for practice and achievable standards are so useful, as are initiatives to harmonise these standards across different countries.[51]

## Integration of surgical pathology and cytopathology

Integration of surgical pathology and cytopathology is an inevitable outcome of acceptance of cytopathology by surgical pathologists that will gather more momentum in the future. Although some surgical pathologists are still sceptical, the success of cytology and the widening of the sphere of influence of both subspecialties have gradually eroded the barrier that separates them. More surgical pathologists will come to realise that squash techniques, touch preparations and bench aspirates, will offer them a valuable and different perspective on a resected specimen. These in-between techniques should be routine standard of care, particularly in intraoperative consultations of thyroid nodules (the best way to see nuclear changes of papillary cancer) and lymph nodes (in lymphomas) and during prostatic or cervical cancer surgery. The methods can also provide useful information about intraoperative liver core biopsies, lung biopsies (granuloma versus cancer) and brain tumours.[86] Minute fragments of valuable material, such as is

often the case with pituitary gland, pancreas and orbital needle biopsy specimens should not be sacrificed at the edge of the frozen section knife, when a touch preparation might yield the diagnosis.

## Interdisciplinary integration

Integration between pathology, in general, and other disciplines, particularly imaging, molecular technology and genetics will create more demand for optimising the information to be obtained from small samples procured by non-invasive procedures from a wider variety of organs, expanding the opportunities for FNA sampling. The ever-changing panorama of cytopathology and its scope will dictate the training of practitioners of cytopathology, both in content and methodology, to meet the demands of the future. Pathologists of the twenty-first century, particularly those who run an active FNA service, have to be capable of communicating effectively with patients and clinical colleagues, in addition to having solid training in general anatomical pathology. Taking this a step further, it would help if medical students were exposed to the world of cytopathology, including FNA procedures, early in their formative medical years. Future generations of biomedical scientists and cytotechnologists will encounter a broader practice, having to examine samples from different organs arriving on their microscopic stage. The increased accessibility to the Internet will continue to shape the future of delivery of new information, not only to physicians and technologists, but also to patients.

## Epilogue

The dawn of the third millennium opened up opportunities for cytology to grow and have an impact on patient care in many ways; some new techniques will disappear with the sunset, but others will thrive or evolve in a different format. The demand to get more information from smaller specimens will increase, clearly a golden opportunity to apply new methods to analyse cytological material. The evolution of cytopathology has been 'multicentric' in origin, which confirms the view expressed at the beginning of this chapter.

Were Dr Papanicolaou alive today, he would be amazed and gratified by the events and the advances that have taken place in cytology since he gave his paper 'New cancer diagnosis', 80 years ago: the application of cytology to diagnosis of cancer in all of the systems of the body, the development of successful screening programmes for cervical cancer, the flourishing of aspiration cytology, the application of automated screening systems, molecular technology, immunocytochemistry and other sophisticated techniques to cytology specimens, the development of education and training in cytology, the publication of journals and formation of societies devoted exclusively to cytopathology. This impressive list of achievements continues to depend on accurate sampling techniques, high-quality technical preparations, minimally invasive procedures, good medical and non-medical specialist training, quality control and direct communication between patients, clinicians and cytopathologists.

# REFERENCES

1. Naylor B. The century for cytopathology. Acta Cytol 2000;44:709–25.

2. Hajdu SI. Cytology from antiquity to Papanicolaou. Acta Cytol 1977;21:668–76.

3. Spriggs AI. History of cytodiagnosis. J Clin Pathol 1977;30:1091–102.

4. Grunze H, Spriggs AI. History of Clinical Cytology: a Selection of Documents, 2nd edn. Darmstadt: Ernst Giebler; 1983.

5. Wied GL. Clinical cytology: past, present and future. Beitr Onkol 1990;38:1–58.

6. Naylor B. The history of exfoliative cancer cytology. Univ Mich Med Bull 1960;26:289–96.

7. Beale LS. Results of the chemical and microscopic examination of solid organs and secretions: Examination of sputum from a case of cancer of the pharynx and the adjacent parts. Arch Med (London) 1861;2:44–46.

8. Gloyne SR. The clinical pathology of thoracic puncture fluids. Lancet 1919;1:935–37.

9. Bland-Sutton J. Tumours, Innocent and Malignant. 7th edn London: Cassell; 1922.

10. Dudgeon LS, Patrick CV. A new method for the rapid diagnosis of tumours. Br J Surg 1927;15:250–61.

11. Bamforth J. Pioneer work by Professor Dudgeon in cytological diagnosis. J Clin Pathol 1963;16:395–98.

12. Martin HE, Ellis HB. Biopsy by needle puncture and aspiration. Ann Surg 1930;92:169–81.

13. Coley BL, Sharp GS, Ellis EB. Diagnosis of bone tumors by aspiration. Am J Surg 1931;13:215–24.

14. Stewart FW. The diagnosis of tumors by aspiration. Am J Pathol 1933;9:801–12.

15. Papanicolaou GN, Traut HF. The diagnostic value of vaginal smears in carcinoma of the uterus. Am J Obstet Gynecol 1941;42:193–205.

16. Papanicolaou GN, Traut HF. Diagnosis of uterine cancer by the vaginal smear. New York: Commonwealth Fund; 1943.

17. Papanicolaou GN. New cancer diagnosis: In: Proceedings of the 3rd Race Betterment Conference. Battle Creek: Race Betterment Foundation, 1928: 528–534.

18. Babes A. Diagnostic du cancer du col utérin par les frottis. Presse Méd 1928;36:451–54.

19. Daniel C, Babes A. Posibilitatea diagnosticului cancerului cu ajutorul frotiului. In: Proceedings of the Bucharest Gynaecology Society, January 1927: 55.

20. Daniel C, Babes A. Diagnosticul cancerului colului uterin prin frotiu. In: Proceedings of the Bucharest Gynaecology Society, April 1927: 23.

21. Papanicolaou GN. Atlas of Exfoliative Cytology. New York: Commonwealth Fund; 1954.

22. Koss LG, George N. Papanicolaou – some reminiscences. Acta Cytol 1977;17:1–2.

23. Koss LG. Diagnostic Cytology and Its Histopathologic Bases. 1st edn Philadelphia: JB Lippincott; 1961.

24. ICRF Coordinating Committee on Cervical Screening. Organisation of a programme for cervical cancer screening. BMJ 1984;289:894–95.

25. McKelvey JL. Carcinoma in situ of the cervix: a general consideration. Am J Obstet Gynecol 1952;64:816–32.

26. Boyes DA, Fidler HK, Lock DR. Significance of in situ carcinoma of the uterine cervix. BMJ 1962;I:203–4.

27. Kaiser RF, Erickson CC, Everett BE, et al. Initial effect of community-wide cytologic screening on clinical stage of cervical cancer detected in an entire community. Results of Memphis-Shelby County, Tennessee, Study J Natl Cancer Inst 1960;25:863–81.

28. Knox EG. Cervical cytology: a scrutiny of the evidence. In: McLachlan G, editor. Problems and Progress in Medical Care, Essays on Current Research, 2nd series. London: Oxford University Press; 1966. p. 277–307.

29. Peterson O. Precancerous changes in the cervical epithelium in relation to manifest cervical carcinoma. Acta Radiol 1955;27(Suppl).

30. Macgregor JE, Baird D. Detection of carcinoma in situ in the general population. BMJ 1963:1631–36.

31. Editorial. Sending a whale to catch a sprat. Lancet 1960;ii:1239–40.

32. Way S. Cytological service and the ministry. BMJ 1967:296–97.

33. Laara E, Day NE, Hakama M. Trends in mortality from cervical cancer in the Nordic countries: association with organised screening programmes. Lancet 1987;i:1247–49.

34. IARC working group on evaluation of screening programmes. Screening for cervical cancer: duration of low risk after negative results of cervical cytology and its implication for screening policies. BMJ 1986;293:659–64.

35. Franzen S, Zajicek J. Aspiration biopsy in the diagnosis of palpable lesions of the breast. Acta Radiol 1968;7:241–62.

36. Soderstrom N. Fine Needle Aspiration Biopsy. Stockholm: Almqvist and Wiksell; 1966.

37. Fox CH. Innovation in medical diagnosis – the Scandinavian curiosity. Lancet 1979;i:1387–88.

38. Von Haam E. A comparative study of the accuracy of cancer cell detection by cytological methods. Acta Cytol 1962;6:508–18.

39. Hauptmann E, Crepinko I, Skrabalo Z. Aspiration cytology of the thyroid gland. Verh Dtsch Ges Inn Med 1972;78:249–53.

40. Cardoso PL. Atlas of Cytology. London: William Heinemann Medical Books; 1979.

41. Webb AJ. Aspects of aspiration cytology. In: Russel RCG, editor. Recent Advances in Surgery. Edinburgh: Churchill Livingstone; 1982.

42. Lever JV, Trott PA, Webb AJ. Fine needle aspiration cytology. J Clin Pathol 1985;38:1–11.

43. Koss LG. Aspiration biopsy – a tool in surgical pathology. Am J Surg Pathol 1988;12:43–53.

44. Santos JE, Leiman G. Nonaspiration fine needle aspiration cytology. Application of a new technique to nodular thyroid disease. Acta Cytol 1988;32:353–56.

45. Brown LA, Coghill SB. Cost effectiveness of a fine needle aspiration clinic. Cytopathology 1992;3:275–80.

46. Editorial. Cancer of the cervix: death by incompetence. Lancet 1985;2:363–64.

47. Draper GJ, Cook GA. Changing patterns of cervical cancer rates. BMJ 1983;287:510–12.

48. McIndoe WA, McLean MR, Jones RW, Mullins PR. The invasive potential of carcinoma in situ of the cervix. Obstet Gynecol 1984;64:451–58.

49. Bogdanich W. Lax laboratories: Hurried screening of Pap smears elevates error rate of the test for cervical cancer. The Wall Street Journal 1987;November 2:1.

50. Peto J, Gilham C, Fletcher O, Matthews FE. The cervical cancer epidemic that screening has prevented in the UK. Lancet 2004;364:249–56.

51. Arbyn M, Anttila A, Jordan J, editors, EU European Commission, et al. European Guidelines for Quality Assurance in Cervical Cancer Screening. Luxembourg: Office of Official Publications of the EU; 2008.

52. Solomon D, Nayar R. The Bethesda System for Reporting Cervical Cytology: Definitions, Criteria and Explanatory Notes. 2nd edn New York: Springer; 2003.

53. Herbert A, Bergeron C, Wiener H, et al. European guidelines for quality assurance in cervical cancer screening: recommendations for cervical cytology terminology. Cytopathology 2007;18:213–19.

54. Denton KJ, Herbert A, Turnbull LS, et al. The revised BSCC terminology for abnormal cervical cytology. Cytopathology 2008;19:137–57.

55. Mellors RC, Glassman A, Papanicolaou GN. A microfluorometric scanning method for the detection of cancer cells in smears of exfoliated cells. Cancer 1952;5:458–68.

56. Mellors RC, Keane JF, Papanicolaou GN. Nucleic acid content of the squamous cancer cell. Science 1952;116:265–69.

57. Kohlberger PD, Stani J, Gitsch G, et al. Comparative evaluation of seven cell collection devices for cervical smears. Acta Cytol 1999;43:1023–26.

58. Tao LC. Cytopathology of the Endometrium. Direct Intrauterine Sampling. Chicago: ASCP Press; 1993 1–55.

59. Gress F, Gottlieb K, Sherman S, et al. Endoscopic ultrasonography-guided fine-needle aspiration biopsy of pancreatic cancer. Ann Intern Med 2001;134:459–64.

60. Manfrin E, Mariotto R, Remo A, et al. Is there still a role for fine-needle aspiration cytology in breast cancer screening?. Cancer Cytopathol 2008;114:74–82.

61. Andreas H, Diacon AH, Schuurmans MM, et al. Utility of rapid on-site evaluation of transbronchial needle aspirates. Respiration 2005;72:182–88.

62. Editorial Office, International Academy of Cytology. Specifications for automated systems as submitted by their developers. Analyt Quant Cytol Histol 1991;13:300–6.

63. Intersociety Working Group for Cytology Technologies. Proposed guidelines for primary screening instruments for gynecologic cytology. Am J Clin Pathol 1998;109:10–15.

64. Intersociety Working Group for Cytology Technologies. Proposed guidelines for secondary screening (rescreening) instruments for gynecologic cytology. Acta Cytol 1998;42:273–76.

65. McGoogen E, Colgan TJ, Ramzy I. Cell preparation methods and criteria for sample adequacy. International Academy of Cytology Task Force summary. Acta Cytol 1998;42:25–32.

66. Austin RM, Ramzy I. Increased detection of epithelial cell abnormalities by liquid-based

gynecologic cytology preparations: A review of accumulated data. Acta Cytol 1998;42:178–84.

67. Hutchinson ML, Cassin CM, Ball HG. The efficacy of an automated preparation device for cervical cytology. Am J Clin Pathol 1991;96:300–5.

68. Bishop JW, Bigner SH, Colgan TJ, et al. Multicentre masked evaluation of Autocyte PREP thin layers with matched conventional smears. Acta Cytol 1998;42:189–97.

69. Payne N, Chilcott J, McGoogan E. Liquid-based cytology in cervical screening: a rapid and systematic review. Health Techn Assess 2000;4:1–73.

70. Arbyn M, Bergeron C, Klinkhamer P, et al. Liquid compared with conventional cervical cytology: a systematic review and meta-analysis. Obstet Gynecol 2008;111:167–77.

71. Tolles WE. The cytoanalyser: An example of physics in medical research. Trans NY Acad Sci 1995;17:250–56.

72. Data on automated cytology systems as submitted by their developers. Editorial Office, International Academy of Cytology. Analyt Quant Cytol Histol 1991;13:300–6.

73. Koss LG. Cervical (Pap) smear. New directions. Cancer 1993;71(Suppl):1406–12.

74. Parker EM, Foti JA, Wilbur DC. FocalPoint slide classification algorithms show robust performance in classification of high-grade lesions on SurePath liquid-based cervical cytology slides. Diagnostic Cytopathology 2004;30:107–10.

75. Davey E, d'Assuncao J, Irwig L, et al. Accuracy of reading liquid based cytology slides using the ThinPrep Imager compared with conventional cytology: prospective study. BMJ 2007;335:1–2.

76. Williams C, Rosenthal DL. Cytopathology in the 21st century. Am J Clin Pathol 1993;99:S31–3.

77. Patterson B, Domanik R, Wernke P. Molecular biomarker-based screening for early detection of cervical cancer. Acta Cytol 2001;45:36–47.

78. Anton RC, Ramzy I, Schwartz MR, et al. Should ASCUS be qualified? An assessment including comparison between conventional and liquid-based technologies. Cancer (Cancer Cytopathol) 2001;93:93–99.

79. Rimm DL. Impact of microarray technologies on cytopathology. Acta Cytol 2001;45:111–14.

80. Moch H, Kononen T, Kallioniemi OP, et al. Tissue microarrays: what will they bring to molecular and anatomic pathology? Adv Anat Pathol 2001;8:14–20.

81. Rambout L, Hopkins L, Hutton B, et al. Prophylactic vaccination against human papillomavirus infection and disease in women: as systematic review of randomised trials. Can Med Assoc J 2007;177:469–79.

82. Stanley M. Prophylactic HPV vaccines. J Clin Pathol 2007;60:961–65.

83. Franco EL, Harper DM. Vaccination against human papillomavirus infection: a new paradigm in cervical cancer control. Vaccine 2005;23:2388–94.

84. Kulasingam SL, Pagliusi S, Myers E. Potential effects of decreased cervical cancer screening participation after HPV vaccination: an example from the US. Vaccine 2007;25:8110–13.

85. Peto J. Costs and benefits of cervical screening and HPV vaccination. J Pathol 2009;217(Suppl S1–S27):S25.

86. Goodman JC. Central nervous system, pituitary gland and pineal gland. In: Ramzy I, editor. Clinical Cytopathology and Aspiration Biopsy: Fundamental Principles and Practice. 2nd edn. New York: McGraw-Hill; 2000.

# Section 2

## Respiratory System

# Respiratory tract

Thomas E. Giles, Julie McCarthy and Winifred Gray

## Chapter contents

## Introduction

The importance of cytological techniques for investigation of respiratory conditions has been recognised since the earliest days of clinical cytology,[1] as described in the Introduction to this book. The rise in incidence of bronchogenic carcinoma throughout the twentieth century, related to smoking, ensured that examination of sputum and bronchial secretions for malignant cells became a major part of the workload of all routine cytology laboratories.[2]

Developments in sampling techniques, in particular the advent of fibreoptic endoscopic techniques in the 1960s and the more recent use of fine needle aspiration (FNA) for obtaining material, have changed the practice of respiratory tract cytology, although not completely supplanting more traditional methods. Bronchial brushings and lavage procedures usually yield better diagnostic material than simple exfoliative sampling and can be used for sequential studies.[3,4] FNA cytology of the lung in many ways paralleled exfoliative cytology of the respiratory tract, initial reports of detection of lung cancer occurring as early as 1886.[5] Radiological imaging allows FNA sampling of lesions at virtually any site within the thorax and has improved the safety of these procedures.[6,7] The British Society for Clinical Cytology (BSCC) has issued guidelines on the procurement, assessment for adequacy and examination of exfoliative samples and endoscopic specimens[8] as has the Papanicolaou Society of Cytopathology in the United States.[9] The last few decades have seen ample demonstration of the sensitivity and predictive value of cytodiagnosis of lung tumours, an acceptance of all cytological modalities as a basis for management, and gradual extension of the range of diagnoses to virtually all neoplastic, and some of the non-neoplastic, processes affecting the lung and mediastinum.[10–15]

## Preparatory techniques and diagnostic applications

### Upper respiratory tract

Spontaneous nasal secretions may be collected on a moistened swab, or with a gently abrasive rhinobrush,[16] or simply by nose blowing. May-Grünwald Giemsa (MGG) staining of air-dried preparations is used to assess eosinophil levels in cases of allergic rhinitis, challenging with inhaled allergens to identify the underlying cause.[17] Increased exfoliation of epithelial cells has also been noted in cases of nasal hyper-reactivity.[18]

*The authors are pleased to acknowledge their indebtedness to Dr G. Sterrett, Dr F. Frost and the late Dr Darrel Whitaker, authors of the lung tumour section in the two previous editions of Diagnostic Cytopathology. Their work forms a substantial proportion of the current chapter and it is an honour to have been able to use their material. We are also indebted to Dr G. Kocjan for her additional help in the completion of the chapter.*

Nasopharyngeal sampling by swab has been used for rapid diagnosis of nasopharyngeal carcinoma, and has been proposed as an effective screening method in areas with a high incidence of this tumour.[19] Pharyngeal and laryngeal samples are usually collected under direct vision by direct scraping of the lesion. FNA is appropriate if there is an intact mucosa covering a tumour such as lymphoma. Imprint cytology of biopsies from laryngeal and pharyngeal biopsies has proved useful, providing a rapid accurate diagnosis for clinical management and excellent correlation with histology.[20]

## Sputum

Sputum is a complex mucoid product resulting from disease or damage within the airways. Microscopic examination of this material may yield information about both benign and malignant conditions, with the advantage that sputum cytology is non-invasive, relatively inexpensive and can detect between 60% and 90% of malignancies if 3–5 specimens are examined. However, sputum has the disadvantages of not localising the lesion, of being much less sensitive for peripheral than for central lung lesions and of resulting in delays in diagnosis for hospital inpatients if multiple samples are needed. With the widespread use of fibreoptic bronchoscopy (FOB) today, the clinical value and cost-effectiveness of examining this material is limited.[3] Sputum cytological examination combined with other screening examinations may play an important role in the early detection of lung cancer or in the selection of the optimal target population for more intensive lung cancer screening.[21] This aspect of sputum examination is discussed later in the chapter under the heading screening for squamous cell carcinoma (see p. 62).

Sputum can be processed in a variety of ways but all specimens must be regarded as potentially infective. The traditional 'pick and smear' method, using alcohol fixation and Papanicolaou (PAP) staining is optimal for routine sputum examination. A variety of other preparation and storage methods for sputum have been tried and are still evolving. Mechanical liquefaction and concentration as well as cell block technique have been used successfully in some centres.[22,23]

Recent advances in liquid-based cytology have led to a revolution in cytological specimen preparation. Thin layer preparation methods yield well-preserved, clearly displayed cells without background debris, excellent for diagnosis of malignancy. The sample is placed directly into a preservative solution available commercially from the manufacturers of the various processing devices now available, as described in Chapters 1 and 36. These liquid-based samples have the added advantage of providing spare material for special stains and other adjunctive techniques, including immunocytochemistry.[24]

Sputum cytology using the liquid-based cytology method improves the diagnostic accuracy for evaluating lung cancer by reducing the unsatisfactory and false negative rates.[25]

## Induced sputum

Where sputum production is poor, it can be increased artificially by inhalation of an aerosolised irritant solution. Induced sputum is a useful non-invasive method for the assessment of airway and parenchymal lung diseases. The procedure has proved particularly effective for obtaining adequate sputum samples in non-smokers and has a role in the investigation of opportunistic infections. It has a role and is an additional technology for the diagnosis of interstitial lung diseases, especially when there are clinical contraindications for performing bronchoscopy or when tissue confirmation is absent for any reason.[26]

## Bronchial aspirates and washings

The flexible fibreoptic bronchoscope, developed in Japan in the 1960s, has provided a greatly improved technique for aspirating secretions directly from the lumen of the bronchus or trachea compared with the rigid bronchoscope previously used. Bronchial washings obtained by FOB can reach and sample up to 90% of malignant lesions with a low rate of complications, although very peripheral lesions, pleural lesions, and submucosal and mediastinal masses cannot be directly sampled. The washings are obtained by instilling normal saline into the bronchus and withdrawing the fluid by suction to collect washings from a large area of mucosa. Direct preparations can be made, or concentration procedures by liquid-based cytology or membrane filtration may be employed.[22]

## Bronchial brushings

Using a flexible bronchoscope, the bronchoscopist can obtain a brush sample from the surface of a tumour under direct vision. Material from the brush can either be wiped onto microscope slides, then fixed in alcohol and stained by the Papanicolaou method or washed into appropriate collection fluid for specimen preparation using thin layer methods. This procedure is frequently combined with bronchial washing.

## Bronchoalveolar lavage (BAL)

BAL samples the cellular exudate in the peripheral airways and alveolar spaces by instillation and aspiration of aliquots of normal saline into a bronchoscope trap.

Elucidation of pulmonary infiltrates and identification of opportunistic infections in immunocompromised patients are important applications of this procedure as described in Chapter 16. Part of the sample should be submitted for microbiological culture. Papanicolaou staining is combined with other stains for opportunistic infections. Thin layer methods are less suitable as both organisms and inflammatory cells may be selectively lost in the preparation, a risk that can be circumvented by dividing the sample between the commercial cell fixative and saline. This will then allow MGG staining for cell differential counts.

BAL fluid examination is one of the initial procedures in the diagnosis of interstitial lung disease.[27] Differential counts on the inflammatory cell population in lavage fluid have been shown to reflect the histological findings in cases of pulmonary fibrosis and non-infectious granulomatous lung disease and serial lavage has found a place in monitoring progress of these conditions.[28] BAL also has a limited role in diagnosis of peripheral lung cancer.

## Fine needle aspiration (FNA)

FNA material may be obtained either by a transbronchial or transthoracic approach. The procedure is of particular value for tumour diagnosis and staging if bronchoscopy has failed to achieve a diagnosis or is inappropriate. The introduction of ultrasound guided imaging has improved the accuracy of sampling, while use of a fine gauge needle (19–22G) makes the procedure safe and well-tolerated.[7] Aspiration is performed at bronchoscopy using a flexible metal needle to which suction is applied.[7]

Recent advances in technology have led to the development of the combined endoscope/ultrasound probe which allows direct, real-time visualisation of the needle during aspiration (EBUS-FNA). This is particularly useful in the transcarinal aspiration of mediastinal structures but is of less value for certain pulmonary lesions due to intervening air within the lung tissue.[29–31,571]

The advantages and limitations of FNA in lung tumour diagnosis have been highlighted[31–33] and the BSCC has issued general guidelines for optimising its use.[34] Air-dried and wet-fixed slides can be prepared; spare material obtained by rinsing the needle in normal saline or tissue culture medium can be processed as a cell block or by cytospin for other stains and for immunocytochemistry.[35] Alternatively, the entire sample may be processed for liquid-based cytology. Electron microscopy, tumour proliferation studies and cytogenetic analysis are among the additional procedures that can be performed on FNA material.

Pneumothorax is a potential complication of FNA, although only 4–10% of these patients require a chest drain.[36,37] Patients with emphysema are at greater risk.[38] Because of the risk of complications, FNA is contraindicated in unconscious or unco-operative patients and in those with respiratory failure, haemorrhagic diathesis or intractable coughing.

## General respiratory tract findings

The respiratory system includes the nasal passages, sinuses and nasopharynx, the oropharynx and larynx, trachea, bronchi and bronchioles, and the air spaces beyond. Transportation of gases is the primary function of the upper respiratory tract and airways, but there is also an important role in warming and moistening inspired air, removing particulate material and providing an initial immunological defence against inhaled microorganisms. Gaseous exchange is carried out within the alveoli and other complex activities take place in the lung parenchyma, including further pulmonary defence mechanisms, some endocrine functions and maintenance of homeostasis.

Not surprisingly, there are many variations in cell structure throughout the respiratory system, and their delicate balance is frequently disturbed by disease. A comprehensive knowledge of the normal findings is therefore necessary to understand the pathological changes encountered in cytological specimens.[39]

## Normal histology of the respiratory tract

Two different types of epithelium form the mucosa of the respiratory tract, their exact distribution varying with age. Stratified squamous epithelium covers areas liable to abrasion, such as the nasal vestibule, nasopharynx, lingual surface of the epiglottis and the vocal cords. Elsewhere a complex layer of glandular cells is found. Squamous mucosa is composed of basal, parabasal, intermediate and superficial cells, and is not keratinised in health. Beneath the basement membrane of this epithelium lies a fibrocollagenous stroma containing blood vessels, lymphatics, nerves and seromucinous glands (Fig. 2.1). Inflammatory cells of the immune system, mainly lymphocytes, plasma cells and macrophages, are also seen migrating into the overlying epithelium. In strategic areas lymphoid cells aggregate into organised tissue masses forming the tonsils and adenoids.

The bronchial tree and remainder of the upper airways are lined by specialised respiratory epithelium (Fig. 2.2). This consists of a pseudostratified layer of ciliated tall columnar cells interspersed with mucin secreting goblet cells, which have microvilli on their luminal surfaces. There are approximately five ciliated cells for each goblet cell. Mucin from the goblet cells coats the airways with a sticky layer within which inhaled particles, organisms and cell debris are trapped. The cilia have a metachronous beat which sweeps this material upwards, to be expectorated or swallowed.

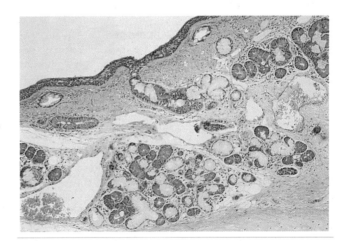

**Fig. 2.1** Normal bronchial wall showing the lining mucosa resting on fibrocollagenous submucosa containing seromucinous glands, blood vessels and lymphatic channels (H&E).

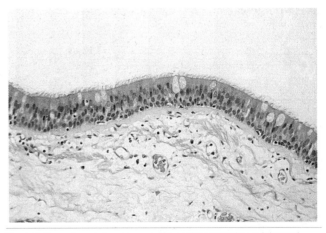

**Fig. 2.2** Normal respiratory mucosa of bronchus. Note the multilayered pseudostratified columnar epithelium composed mainly of ciliated cells with occasional goblet cells. A distinct single layer of reserve cells can be seen resting on the basement membrane. Deep to this the submucosa includes a few capillaries, lymphatics and inflammatory cells (H&E).

Two further cell types are present in respiratory epithelium. Small reserve cells rest on the basement membrane, forming an undifferentiated stem cell population from which regeneration of bronchial mucosa takes place after injury. Inconspicuous round cells with neuroendocrine properties are also found situated towards the basement membrane. Known as Feyrter or K (Kultschitzsky) cells, they are most numerous in the smaller bronchi where they are grouped around capillaries and nerve fibres forming neuroepithelial bodies. They contain neurosecretory granules producing locally active polypeptide hormones, and belong to the APUD (amine precursor uptake and decarboxylation) cell system.

Bronchioles, the first branches of bronchi without cartilaginous support in their walls, are lined by a single layer of nonciliated columnar cells interspersed with a few goblet cells. In addition there are tall columnar cells, the Clara cells, producing surfactant. Terminal bronchioles are lined by low columnar epithelium and are involved solely in air conduction. They are continuous with respiratory bronchioles, which mark the commencement of gaseous exchange. Here the lining becomes cuboidal, merging with flattened epithelial cells in the alveolar ducts. These lead into rotunda-like spaces called alveolar sacs. The periphery of each sac is partitioned into alveoli, the main site of gaseous exchange.

The principal cells lining alveoli are known as type I and type II pneumocytes. In addition, there are many macrophages of bone marrow derivation, forming an important component of cytology samples from the lower airways. They adhere to the walls of alveoli, ingesting cellular debris and foreign material, which is then transported to the bronchial tree or to lymphatic channels arising at the level of the terminal bronchioles.

It has been estimated that type I pneumocytes cover approximately 90% of the alveolar wall area, but form only about 40% of the lining cell population. Their cytoplasm is thinly spread out to allow maximal exchange of gas between the alveolar space and the underlying capillaries. Type II pneumocytes comprise 60% of the lining cells numerically, but are bulky and rounded, occupying less than 10% of the alveolar surface area. Their cytoplasm is dense, containing spherical laminated osmiophilic bodies when examined by electron microscopy, composed of the precursors of pulmonary surfactant. These cells are also the progenitors of type I pneumocytes.

## General cytological findings in respiratory samples

### Cell population

Only a few of the many different cells lining the respiratory tract are seen with any regularity in cytological preparations. The distribution of cells varies considerably with the nature of the sample, but is of importance in assessing specimen adequacy. The appearances to be described for normal and abnormal cells are those seen with Papanicolaou staining unless otherwise specified.

- *Squamous cells* (Fig. 2.3) are numerically the most common cells in sputum, but are less frequent in other specimens and usually absent from FNA samples. Superficial and intermediate cells predominate. They have small central

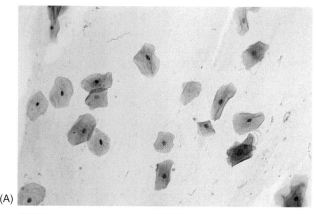

(A)

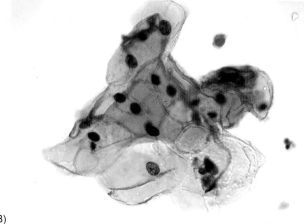

(B)

**Fig. 2.3** (A) Normal oral squamous cells in a sputum sample consisting mainly of saliva. The cells are of superficial and intermediate type but there is no keratinisation (PAP). (B) Normal mature squames in a liquid based preparation showing nuclear detail (PAP, LBC).

pyknotic or vesicular nuclei, as seen in squames from other sites

- *Bronchial epithelial cells* (Fig. 2.4) are profuse in brushings, but less common in sputum as they do not exfoliate readily. Columnar or triangular in shape, the cells lie singly, in short ribbons or in flat sheets which often have a straight 'anatomical' edge. They have delicate cyanophilic cytoplasm, bluish grey with MGG stains, tapering at the point of previous anchorage. Nuclei vary considerably in size and shape but are usually basal and rounded or oval (Fig. 2.5A), with open granular or condensed chromatin and a single small nucleolus. Multinucleation may be seen. Cilia are often preserved, arising from a dark stained terminal bar at the broader end of the cell
- *Goblet cells* are inconspicuous in sputum unless hyperplastic, but are quite often seen in brushings and increase in number with chronic bronchial irritation. They are columnar but are distended centrally by globules of mucin, which overlie or displace the nucleus (Fig. 2.5B)
- *Reserve cells* (Fig. 2.6) are rarely present in sputum but are sometimes seen in brushings and lavage specimens, mainly in reactive states. They form sheets of small regular cells slightly larger than lymphocytes, with a high nuclear/cytoplasmic ratio, coarse chromatin and a narrow rim of green cytoplasm

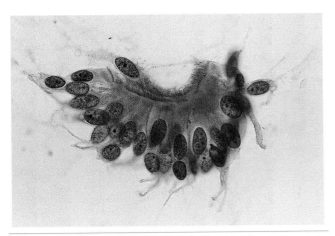

**Fig. 2.4** Bronchial epithelial cells in a bronchial brushing sample. These tall columnar cells show the tapering point of anchorage at one end and dark terminal bar, bearing pink cilia at the opposite end of the cell. Nuclei are regular, ovoid in shape and basal in position. Chromatin is finely divided and small nucleoli are visible (PAP).

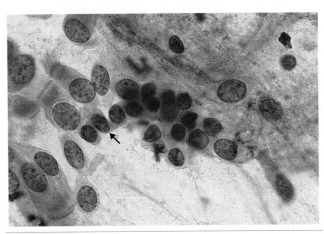

**Fig. 2.6** Reserve cells in a crowded group of small cells with dark nuclei and very little cytoplasm, surrounded by columnar epithelial cells. There is a suggestion of nuclear moulding at the right edge of the group. Bronchial brushing (PAP).

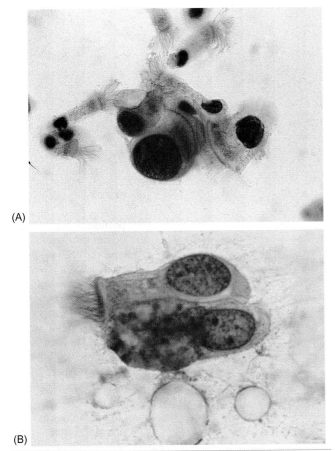

(A)

(B)

**Fig. 2.5** (A) Bronchial cells with nuclei of variable size and shape, but still within the normal range. Bronchial brushing. (B) Single bronchial epithelial cell and goblet cell, the latter showing distension centrally due to the presence of greenish grey mucin. Bronchial brushing (PAP).

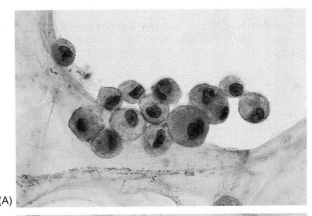

(A)

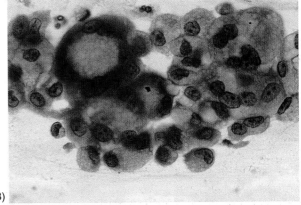

(B)

**Fig. 2.7** (A) Macrophages forming a streak of dissociated cells in sputum. Note the variation in cell size and finely vacuolated cytoplasm with a few particles of ingested carbon. Most of the nuclei are eccentrically placed, varying in shape and size. Nucleoli are visible and several cells show binucleation. (B) Sputum. Multinucleated macrophages aggregated with mononuclear forms (PAP).

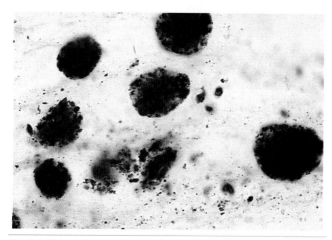

**Fig. 2.8** Carbon pigment in macrophages varies greatly in amount, but may obscure the nucleus entirely, as in this sputum sample (PAP).

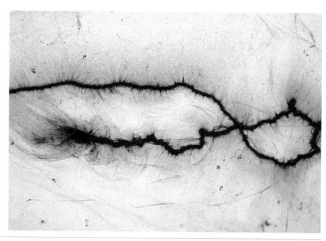

**Fig. 2.9** Curschmann's spiral composed of a compressed cast of mucus from a small bronchiole. The form, size and staining of these structures are extremely variable. Sputum (PAP).

- *Macrophages* (Figs 2.7, 2.8) are the hallmark of a satisfactory sputum sample and are found in the majority of pulmonary specimens. In sputum, the adequacy of a sample is claimed to be directly proportional to the number of alveolar macrophages it contains. Round or oval dissociated cells, they are usually over 10 μm in diameter but vary greatly in size and shape. Their cytoplasm is poorly defined, cyanophilic and often vacuolated. Phagocytosed material, usually carbon, may be present. They have central or eccentric nuclei, rounded or bean-shaped, with coarse chromatin and visible nucleoli. Binucleation is common and the cells may form giant cells with numerous nuclei
- *Inflammatory cells,* mainly polymorphonuclear leucocytes and lymphocytes, are invariably present in low numbers and are only of diagnostic significance if markedly increased. A preponderance of one inflammatory cell type may, however, be significant, for example, when eosinophils are conspicuous
- *Clara cells, Feyrter cells and types I and II pneumocytes* are prone to rapid degenerative changes and are not recognisable in respiratory samples unless hyperplastic or neoplastic.

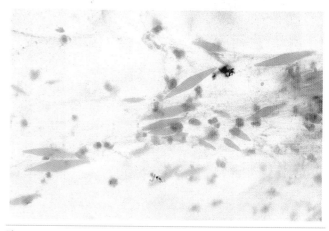

**Fig. 2.10** Charcot–Leyden crystals are bright orange or yellow and needle shaped. Eosinophils are often present since the crystals form from breakdown products of their granules. Sputum (PAP).

## Other components of respiratory samples

Non-cellular material and extraneous elements are seen in many specimens, and should be firmly identified to avoid misinterpretation. The possibilities are virtually unlimited.

- Mucus is almost invariably present in specimens obtained via the airways unless mucolytic agents have been used. It forms a pale translucent background material staining variably, and may be smooth or stringy in texture, usually with streaks of enmeshed inflammatory cells. Densely stained inspissated mucus may obscure cell detail, or give a false impression of cytological abnormality on low magnification. Coils of compressed mucus known as Curschmann's spirals (Fig. 2.9) are frequently seen in sputum from smokers or patients with obstructive airways disease, especially asthmatics. The spirals are casts of the small bronchioles and vary considerably in structure.[40]
- Inorganic material of various types may be seen and can have diagnostic significance. Charcot–Leyden crystals (Fig. 2.10), derived from the breakdown products of eosinophil granules, appear in conditions evoking pulmonary eosinophilia as orange, yellow or pinkish stained diamond- or needle-shaped crystals.[41] Calcific blue bodies and corpora amylacea are similar in routine preparations. The former consist largely of calcium carbonate and show central birefringence (Fig. 2.11).[42] Corpora amylacea are non-calcified rounded structures composed of glycoproteins including amyloid. They stain pale pink, are Congo-red positive and exhibit birefringence. Both of these are seen in various chronic lung diseases. Psammoma bodies (calcospherites) are laminated non-refractile calcified concretions sometimes found in the presence of malignancy, although not necessarily closely associated with tumour cells.[42] Isolated psammoma bodies

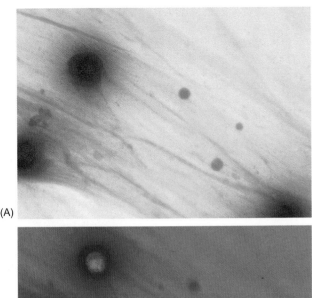

(A)

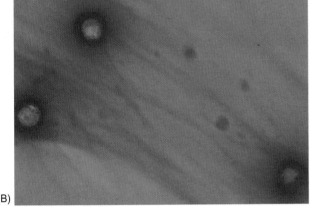

(B)

**Fig. 2.11** Calcified blue bodies are birefringent inorganic concretions seen here on (A) routine light microscopy and by (B) polarised light. Sputum (PAP).

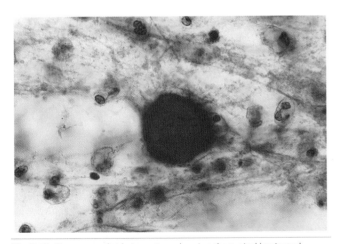

**Fig. 2.12** Psammoma body in sputum showing the typical laminated structure. No evidence of malignancy was found in this patient (PAP).

may be seen in the absence of any tumour formation (Fig. 2.12). Ferruginous bodies (see Fig. 2.64) are formed when filamentous dust particles such as asbestos become coated with protein and iron in the lung parenchyma. They vary from 5 to 200 μm in length, are light brown in colour and stain blue with Perl's stain for iron.[43]

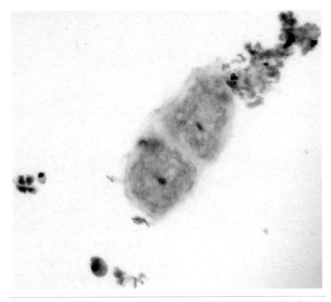

**Fig. 2.13** A pair of vegetable cells with thick cellulose walls and lack of nuclei (PAP).

## Contaminants

These may be added to respiratory samples at any stage from collection to microscopy. Following this time sequence, they include:

- Food particles, seen in association with saliva, especially in samples from elderly patients. Meat fibres are elongated and may show cross-striations. Vegetable cells usually have thick straight cellulose walls although of variable appearance. They can be confused with benign or malignant respiratory tract cells,[44] but have refractile cell walls and a repetitive structure, lacking the pleomorphism of tumour cells and the true nuclear features of malignancy (Fig. 2.13)
- Colonial growth of normal oral flora, including bacteria and yeasts, frequently occurs when there is delay in preparation of samples. The organisms obviously do not elicit any inflammatory reaction. Parasitic or saprophytic flora from the mouth, such as non-pathogenic entamoebae, have been described (see Fig. 2.46).[45] Mites have been found in respiratory specimens and are occasionally significant clinically, since they may be associated with an actual infestation of diseased airways[45]
- Aerial contaminants are acquired during specimen collection, in transit, or at the time of preparation in the laboratory. Pollen is an obvious external contaminant and must be distinguished from fungal spores. Fungal species may be seen, originating from air, soil or water. The water-borne plant pathogen Alternaria is not uncommon, forming light brown conidia 30 μm in length, with an internal segmented structure (Fig. 2.14). Although potentially pathogenic in immunosuppressed patients, they are present only in small numbers when contaminants[46]
- Carryover of cells from another sample can occur during processing, usually leaving the cells 'out of context', often in a slightly different plane of focus or at one edge of the slide.[47] Cross-contamination by tumour cells is a potential source of false positive diagnosis of malignancy.

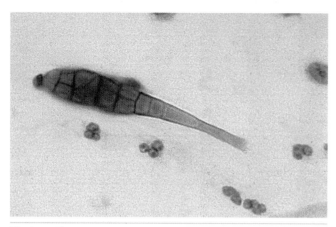

**Fig. 2.14** *Alternaria* sp. organism in sputum, probably an aerial contaminant (PAP).

## Criteria for assessing adequacy of samples

A sample providing enough cells for confident accurate diagnosis can be regarded as adequate. However, misleading reports are sometimes given if the specimen does not include appropriate material confirming the origin of the sample, or if there is insufficient abnormal material to ensure correct interpretation. Hence, it is one of the prime tasks of the cytologist to assess whether a specimen is suitable for diagnosis or whether the test should be repeated. Furthermore, when tumour cells are found, localisation of their site of origin may not always be possible. This question mainly arises with sputum samples where cells from upper or lower respiratory tract tumours may exfoliate into the sputum.

Sputum specimens are judged adequate when plentiful pulmonary macrophages can be identified.[48] The presence of columnar cells is ambiguous since they may be from the nasal passages or upper airways. Macrophage counts have been used to quantify the adequacy of sputum specimens,[49] and to relate these findings to smoking status,[50] but the procedures are too time-consuming for routine laboratory work. All samples irrespective of their apparent quality should always be screened fully as malignant cells are occasionally found.

Bronchial brushings usually show a profusion of epithelial cells or tumour cells since the material is obtained under direct vision. Poor fixation and air-drying of the cells lead to swelling of nuclei and loss of chromatin detail. Bronchial washings are generally less cellular than brushings, but are usually well-fixed, since preparation is undertaken in the laboratory. Alveolar macrophages provide unequivocal evidence of appropriate sampling.

Bronchoalveolar lavages contain many macrophages and, provided the first aliquot is discarded, should be virtually free from any cells from the upper airways. In a study of over 1500 lavage samples prepared by filtration and cytocentrifugation, however, Chamberlain et al. reported an unsatisfactory rate of 30% as judged by: fewer than 10 alveolar macrophages/high-power field; fewer macrophages than cells from the airways; a mucopurulent exudate; cellular changes due to degeneration; or the presence of laboratory artefacts.[51] These criteria are important when inflammatory cells are to be quantified as in the investigation of interstitial lung diseases.[52] Adequate sampling is also essential in evaluating specimens for opportunistic infections as discussed in Chapter 16.

FNA samples from solid lung nodules pose no problem for assessment of quality when the cells obtained are interpretable and in keeping with the site aspirated. Scanty preparations with a few normal lung parenchymal cells, macrophages and occasional fragments of bronchial epithelium are all that will be seen if the needle misses the lesion. Mesothelial cells in pavemented sheets are sometimes aspirated on traversing the pleural cavity.

Heavily blood-stained aspirates with rather scanty cells are often poorly fixed due to the presence of blood. Even in these smears, however, diagnostic fields may be found. Blood staining is not usually a problem in liquid-based cytology preparations. Inadequate sampling can be minimised by immediate assessment of the specimen by a cytologist and repeating the procedure if necessary.

## NON-NEOPLASTIC PULMONARY CONDITIONS

## Non-specific reactive changes in cytological preparations

The majority of respiratory specimens from patients with conditions other than tumours show findings reflecting non-specific host responses. These include the effects of damage by environmental agents, as well as changes seen in many of the more common respiratory infections and chronic chest diseases. Appropriate clinical details and judicious use of special stains may enable the cytologist to confirm the diagnosis in some cases.

- *Reactive squamous cells from the upper respiratory tract* are seen particularly in sputum. They have slightly enlarged hyperchromatic nuclei and have come to be known as 'Pap cells' since according to legend they were noted by Dr George Papanicolaou in his own sputum following laryngitis. They have little diagnostic significance

- *Anucleate keratinised squamous cells* are only noteworthy in sputum if present in large numbers, when they suggest an area of hyperkeratosis due to a focus of chronic irritation. The surface cells from keratotic lesions exfoliate readily, whether the underlying process is benign or malignant. The specimen must be assessed carefully to determine whether it is of upper or lower respiratory tract origin, and whether there are any cells with nuclear features suspicious of malignancy. Cells from an area of benign hyperkeratosis are usually mature anucleate squames compared with the bizarre-shaped deep orange cells shed from the keratinised surface of a well-differentiated squamous carcinoma

- *Hyperplasia of bronchial epithelial cells* can be induced by many different noxious agents. In simple repair processes, sheets of actively regenerating cuboidal to columnar cells are seen, with enlarged nuclei, vesicular chromatin and prominent nucleoli (Fig. 2.15).[53] Multinucleation is a frequent finding and has been described in cells adjacent to malignant neoplasms.[54] Papillary clusters of epithelial cells are sometimes shed, mimicking clumps of adenocarcinoma cells. Their nuclei are difficult to examine when the clusters are dense, but they should retain a normal chromatin pattern (Fig. 2.16). Nevertheless, these cell groups are a classical diagnostic pitfall in respiratory tract cytology

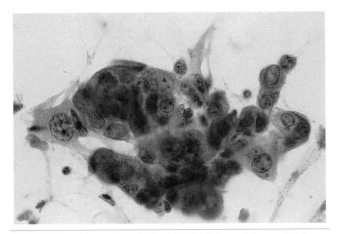

**Fig. 2.15** Hyperplasia of bronchial epithelial cells in repair is associated with disorganisation of cells, nuclear enlargement and pleomorphism and prominent nucleoli, as seen in this group of cells in BAL fluid from a transplant patient (PAP).

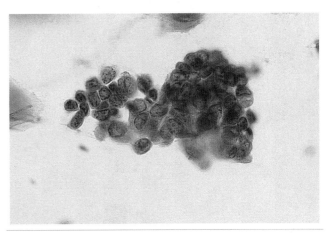

**Fig. 2.17** Reserve cell hyperplasia in bronchial brushings from a patient with a squamous carcinoma of bronchus. Note the enlarged active nuclei in this disorganised group of small crowded cells, the high nuclear/cytoplasmic ratio and the narrow rim of cytoplasm (PAP).

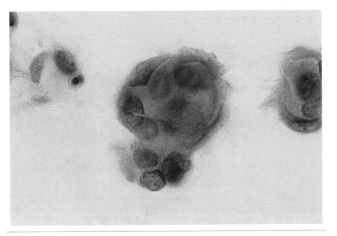

**Fig. 2.16** Hyperplastic bronchial epithelial cells forming a papillary cluster, with cilia visible on the surface of the group. The nuclei are enlarged but bland-looking. Their depth of focus requires careful examination at high magnification. Bronchial brushing (PAP).

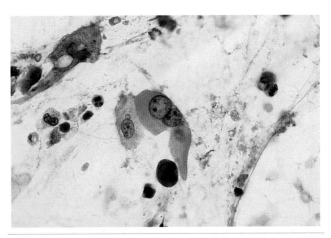

**Fig. 2.18** Alveolar cell damage and hyperplasia in BAL from a leukaemic patient receiving cyclosporin treatment. The cells at the centre are enlarged and rectangular with dense green cytoplasm, swollen nuclei and prominent nucleoli. Note lack of cilia. A damaged epithelial cell is present at top left (PAP).

- *Reserve cell hyperplasia* (Fig. 2.17) is less easily recognised in cytology specimens. Groups of small cohesive crowded cells with a high nuclear/cytoplasmic ratio and dense chromatin are typical. Nuclear moulding may be seen, hence the cells can be confused with a small cell carcinoma, as described later in this chapter (see p. 67). Absence of necrosis and cell dissociation, and the uniformity of nuclear size and shape are helpful features

- *Hyperplasia of type II pneumocytes and bronchiolar cells* (Fig. 2.18) usually occurs as a result of specific toxic effects on the lung and the regeneration that follows. The cells are polygonal or rectangular, occurring singly or in twos and threes or sometimes in larger clusters, and they may show cytoplasmic vacuolation. The nuclei are swollen, with prominent nucleoli and pale or dense chromatin. Such cells are not easy to identify with confidence unless an accurate history is available to alert the cytologist to their origin. They differ from hyperplastic bronchial cells in lacking cilia and in their dissociated cell pattern,

with no associated columnar or goblet cells. Distinction from bronchioloalveolar cell carcinoma may be virtually impossible.[55] There is usually less profuse shedding of cells in reactive hyperplasia than in neoplasia and the cells are in flatter groups, without such a striking depth of focus as is required to inspect the nuclei of malignant cells

- *Squamous metaplasia* (Fig. 2.19) is one of the commonest responses of bronchial epithelium to persistent injury.[56] It is preceded by reserve cell hyperplasia and is a frequent finding in smokers.[57] Small fragmented groups of polygonal cells of parabasal size, with regular large bland looking nuclei are found in the early stages. Dissociation increases as the metaplasia progresses to become atypical or dysplastic, and keratinisation develops in longstanding atypical metaplasia. A more detailed description of atypical metaplasia is given on p. 62 and Figures 2.83 and 2.84.

- *Ciliocytophthoria* (Fig. 2.20) is a degenerative process affecting bronchial epithelium, whereby columnar cells fragment into rounded cytoplasmic remnants, some

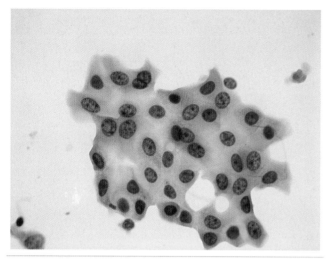

**Fig. 2.19** Squamous metaplasia in sputum from a middle-aged smoker. The group is composed of cohesive small polygonal cells with regular darkly stained nuclei. Cytoplasmic staining is variable but there is no keratinisation (PAP, LBC).

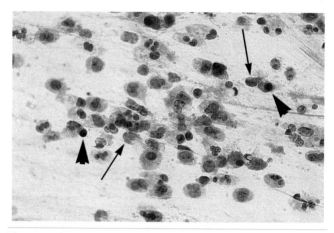

**Fig. 2.20** Ciliocytophthoria in sputum from a patient with squamous carcinoma. Scattered fragments of cytoplasmic remnants present, some ciliated (arrows), others with pyknotic nuclei (arrowheads) (PAP).

of which still show tufts of cilia, while others contain pyknotic nuclear material. The change was first observed by Papanicolaou in 1956 in association with viral infections, but can be seen in a range of acute and chronic pulmonary diseases, and in the presence of bronchial carcinoma.[58]

## Bacterial infective diseases

Infection by microorganisms is the most common cause of inflammation in the lung. In the majority of such cases, cytology has little to offer in the investigative sequence, since the findings are very often non-specific, the diagnosis depending on firm identification of the organism, usually bacterial, by culture. Certain types of infection, however, can be recognised cytologically: fungal elements may be seen, and some viral infections produce diagnostic cytopathic effects. An important additional role for the cytologist lies in helping to exclude an underlying tumour in cases of unexplained or recurrent chest infection.

## Bacterial pneumonia

The term pneumonia generally denotes acute inflammation of lung parenchyma due to invasion by microorganisms. This is in contradistinction to pneumonitis where physical agents are involved, or alveolitis, which is due to allergic or fibrosing inflammatory reactions within the alveoli.[59] Although the incidence of pneumonia and its mortality have fallen substantially with the advent of antibiotics, the disease remains an important cause of morbidity and death, especially at the extremes of life and in debilitated or immunosuppressed patients.

The usual sequence of events once organisms have lodged in the alveoli or distal airways is an immediate acute inflammatory response, with outpouring of oedema fluid, fibrin, neutrophil polymorphs and red blood cells (Fig. 2.21A). Some organisms produce a rapidly spreading infection, involving the entire lobe in a process of consolidation. Other organisms are

subject to host defence mechanisms limiting spread to a more patchy distribution. These two processes are known as lobar pneumonia and bronchopneumonia, respectively. The distinction is by no means absolute, but remains valid in many cases. Certain viruses and mycoplasma organisms induce interstitial pneumonia involving inflammation of alveolar walls rather than alveolar spaces.

Appropriate treatment and adequate host responses lead to complete resolution of inflammation in many cases, but other outcomes such as abscess formation or fibrosis may supervene in adverse circumstances. The nature of the infectious agent influences the type of inflammatory reaction, creating a more indolent chest infection in some cases. In other cases, the immune system may contribute to progression of the disease, as happens in tuberculosis.

There are marked variations in incidence of different types of pulmonary infection throughout the world, but the increasing number of patients with impaired immunity and the comparative ease of international travel have led to changes in traditional epidemiological patterns. It is, therefore, important to have a full history when assessing cases of respiratory infection.

### Cytological findings: bacterial pneumonia

- Grossly purulent or bloodstained sputum
- Predominance of neutrophil polymorphs
- Cell debris and degenerate epithelial cells
- Exfoliation of epithelial cell groups
- Causative organisms are sometimes identified.

Sputum samples are the commonest specimens to be submitted for cytology in cases of pneumonia, often prompted by the need to exclude a bronchial carcinoma rather than to establish the diagnosis of chest infection. Sputum production may be poor, especially in immunosuppressed patients; induced sputum or bronchoalveolar lavage is then more appropriate. FNA is unlikely to be attempted unless an abscess has developed, which may necessitate exclusion of malignancy.

Macroscopically, sputum is often purulent or noted to be rusty due to the presence of blood. Neutrophil polymorphs dominate the microscopic picture (Fig. 2.21B), often at the expense of pulmonary macrophages, obscuring all other cells

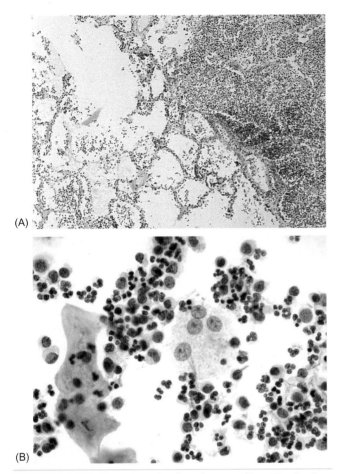

(A)

(B)

**Fig. 2.21** (A) Lobar pneumonia in histological section of lung. The alveoli are filled with a dense exudate of neutrophil polymorphs producing consolidation of the parenchyma, most marked on the right (H&E). (B) Sputum from a patient with bronchopneumonia, showing many polymorphs and other inflammatory cella (PAP, LBC).

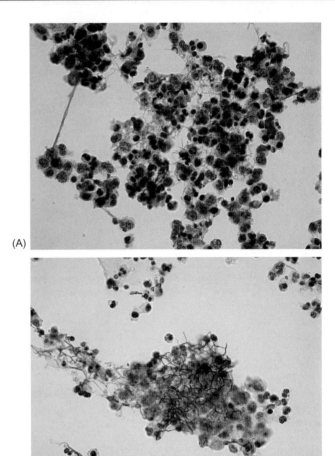

(A)

(B)

**Fig. 2.23** (A) BAL fluid from a transplant patient with respiratory collapse. Filamentous organisms tangled amongst numerous polymorphs are seen (PAP, LBC). (B) Gram staining of the same material highlights strands of *Nocardia asteroides*. This was confirmed on culture (Gram stain, LBC).

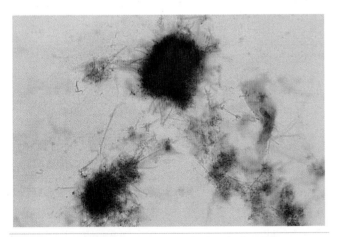

**Fig. 2.22** Actinomycotic organisms presenting in colonies of filamentous organisms in sputum with no significant inflammation. The patient was immunosuppressed and had evidence of chest infection but the colonies may represent overgrowth from the oropharynx in this setting (PAP).

in some cases. The specimen may be deemed unsatisfactory for cytological assessment if epithelial cells are totally obscured.

Cell debris is prominent in the early stages, whatever sampling method has been used, and degenerative changes such as

cytoplasmic vacuolation or ciliocytophthoria may be seen. Clusters of bronchial epithelial cells often show hyperplastic or atypical changes, such as enlarged hyperchromatic nuclei and prominent nucleoli. These features can result from pre-existing lung disease, such as chronic bronchitis or bronchiectasis.

In most cases of pneumonia, the causative organisms cannot be identified cytologically. In cases of immunosuppression, special stains including Gram, Ziehl Neelsen, PAS and Grocott should be performed.

Higher bacteria, such as *Actinomyces* organisms (Fig. 2.22) have a more defined appearance, forming colonies of radiating filamentous Gram-positive bacteria which may be visible in macroscopic samples as 'sulphur granules'.[60] The related organism, *Nocardia* (Fig. 2.23) stains faintly pink by the PAP method, exhibits negative staining with MGG and is well demonstrated by Grocott's silver stain. *Nocardia* pneumonia is a recognised cause of infection after cardiac transplantation, often producing a solitary nodule, which may be subjected to FNA.[61]

*Legionella* organisms, the bacteria causing Legionnaires' disease, have been described in sputum, bronchial samples and FNA material.[62] They are tiny Gram-negative bacilli which can be demonstrated by silver stains and by immunofluorescence.

### Diagnostic pitfalls: bacterial pneumonia

In some circumstances epithelial atypia may be extreme and difficult to distinguish from malignancy. Close liaison with clinical staff is needed in these cases, with judicious use of other investigations, and where necessary, the adoption of a wait-and-see policy.

Stains for organisms must be interpreted with care so that overgrowth of commensals from the oropharynx is not mistaken for an infection. It is important to note the context of the organisms. They are unlikely to be significant if mixed in type and found mainly in areas of saliva without accompanying inflammatory cells.

## Pulmonary tuberculosis

The incidence of infection by *Mycobacterium tuberculosis* fell dramatically in developed countries during the twentieth century, due to improvements in public health and the advent of effective chemotherapy. Nevertheless, tuberculosis remains one of the major causes of morbidity and mortality throughout the world,[63] and is again occurring more frequently in Western countries. This is partly attributable to the increasing numbers of disadvantaged groups within affluent societies but also due to the emergence of resistant strains of the organism and because conditions associated with immunosuppression are becoming more common.[64] The latter group of patients are also susceptible to infection with atypical mycobacteria such as *M. avium-intracellulare, M. kansasii* and *M. fortuitum* (see Ch. 16).

The natural history and pathogenesis of pulmonary tuberculosis were expounded by Rich, in 1951.[65] The causative organism was isolated in 1852 by Koch, and antibiotic treatment has been available from the 1940s. Awareness of the pathology and cytological findings is important to ensure early diagnosis and treatment.

Primary infection usually occurs in childhood by droplet spread. The organisms are localised in the lung parenchyma and the draining hilar lymph nodes, forming a primary tuberculous complex. Macrophages and lymphocytes mount a defence reaction; with persistence of organisms and their breakdown products macrophages take on an epithelioid appearance. After about 1 week, some of the epithelioid cells fuse to form Langhans giant cells, with many nuclei arranged in an arc at one pole of the cell. Lymphocytes accumulate and the whole circumscribed focus of inflammation is known as a granuloma (see Box 2.1). Within about 2 weeks, the centre of the granuloma starts to undergo caseation necrosis of a characteristic soft cheesy consistency (Fig. 2.24). Epithelioid histiocytes and Langhans giant cells tend to form palisades around the edge of the caseous material and it is in this area that acid-fast tubercle bacilli are most often found.

As immunity develops, resolution occurs, leaving a peripheral lung scar and calcified draining lymph nodes. If the number of infecting organisms is large, however, or the patient is debilitated, infection may spread elsewhere in the lung or via the bloodstream to other organs. Tuberculous bronchopneumonia and miliary tuberculosis develop in this way. Healing may take place but infection may occur at any time, usually by reactivation of a dormant focus of organisms in the lung. This secondary or adult infection takes the form of progressive granulomatous bronchopneumonia with caseation, cavitation and extensive lung destruction.

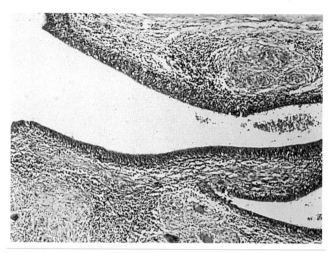

**Fig. 2.24** Section of bronchial wall with discrete epithelioid giant cell granulomata in the submucosa, a less common site for these lesions than in the lung parenchyma. Note the intact mucosa over the surface, impeding direct sampling by cytology. (H&E) (Courtesy of Dr MS Dunnill, Oxford, UK.)

Awareness of this stage of the disease is important in cytology. The patient has a cough productive of sputum. Bronchoscopy may be undertaken for the collection of washings and brushings to exclude malignancy and to obtain material for culture. Effusions are common. Localised pulmonary lesions occur, simulating malignancy radiologically and inviting FNA sampling. Thus, a variety of methods of cytological investigation may be employed. The findings are well-documented in sputum and bronchial secretions.[66] The characteristic features of granuloma formation are best seen in FNA material.[67]

### Cytological findings: pulmonary tuberculosis

- A mixed inflammatory exudate
- Epithelioid histiocytes
- Langhans giant cells are infrequently found
- Fragmented granulomas may be seen in FNA material
- Caseation is inconspicuous
- Organisms may be demonstrated, mainly in FNA samples.

An analysis undertaken in Brazil by Tani et al.[68] in 1987 of over 100 tuberculous cytology samples other than FNAs revealed increased numbers of macrophages in 100%, excess neutrophils in 98% and increased lymphocytes in 85% of the specimens. Epithelioid cells were present in 56% and giant cells in only 40% of the samples.

Epithelioid histiocytes are elongated macrophages with pale cytoplasm devoid of any tingible ingested material such as carbon pigment. Their nuclei are drawn out and indented or folded, producing a variety of footprint-like shapes. The chromatin is finely divided and nucleoli are usually inconspicuous. The cells are arranged in loose aggregates in sputum or washings, but may be aspirated in ragged clumps by FNA (Fig. 2.25). Macrophages of more usual type can also be seen.

Langhans giant cells are characteristic of the disease but are not often seen in cytology samples, apart from FNA material. They are 2–10 times the size of mononuclear macrophages and may contain up to 100 or so ovoid nuclei, typically distributed at one pole of the cell (Fig. 2.26). This feature and absence of ingested

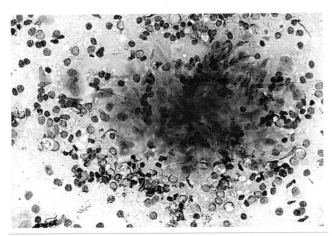

**Fig. 2.25** Ragged fragment from an epithelioid granuloma in FNA sample from a patient with pulmonary tuberculosis. Pale histiocytic cells with elongated nuclei can be seen forming the granuloma; lymphocytes and other inflammatory cells are present in the debris at the periphery (MGG).

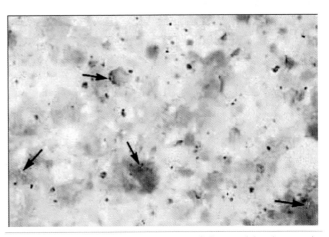

**Fig. 2.27** Caseous material obtained on FNA of a lung nodule subsequently confirmed as tuberculous. Within the amorphous debris negative images of the tubercle bacillus can be made out (arrows) (H&E). (Courtesy of Dr G. Sterrett, Perth, Western Australia.)

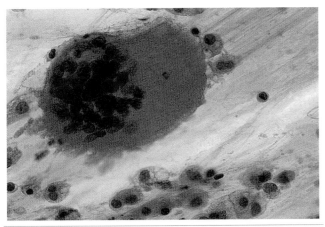

**Fig. 2.26** Langhans giant cell with abundant amphophilic cytoplasm containing many rounded or oval nuclei grouped at one pole. Note absence of any ingested material. Bronchial washing (PAP).

carbon help to distinguish them from other multinucleated pulmonary macrophages. The cytoplasm is amphophilic with Papanicolaou staining or pale blue with MGG.

Caseation necrosis is suggested by the presence of pale amorphous material, not easily seen in PAP-stained sputum or bronchial secretions unless liquid-based methods of preparation are used, but recognisable in FNA samples as faintly granular light blue stained debris in MGG or H&E preparations, sometimes speckled darker blue if calcification has occurred. It is within the caseous material that tubercle bacilli are most likely to be found.

Lavage fluid from patients with AIDS who have tuberculosis typically contains many lymphocytes and enlarged foamy macrophages, but it is unusual to find a definite granulomatous picture in these samples. A thin purulent background may be seen.

*Mycobacterium tuberculosis* may be demonstrated, especially in FNA material using Ziehl Neelsen stain, which reveals a beaded magenta pink straight or slightly curved slender bacillus 1–4 μm in length. Fluorescent methods, such as Rhodamine-auramine staining are quicker to screen if there

are large amounts of material. The organisms are sometimes visible as negative staining images within caseous material in FNA preparations stained by MGG (Fig. 2.27) or in sputum when there is a high load of acid fast bacilli.

Atypical mycobacteria differ slightly in morphology, but cannot be firmly distinguished without culture. When no spare material is available, slides can be decolourised and re-stained successfully. Nevertheless, culture is essential in all cases, submitting as much material as possible.

## Diagnostic pitfalls: pulmonary tuberculosis

The combination of epithelioid histiocytes and Langhans' giant cells is highly suggestive of tuberculosis but is not pathognomonic since either or both cell types can be seen in other conditions with granulomatous inflammation (Box 2.1).

Caseation necrosis may closely resemble tumour necrosis. A careful search for evidence of granuloma formation or for remnants of malignant nuclei should resolve this problem.

Atypical strains of mycobacteria causing lung infections are morphologically similar to *M. tuberculosis* and can only be distinguished by culture.

## Viral infections

In contrast to pneumonia due to bacteria, viral infections frequently induce specific cytopathic changes in epithelial cells and alveolar macrophages, enabling the pathologist to give an indication as to the causative agent. This is particularly important since other methods of diagnosis may take longer to complete, may not be available, or may not be as accurate. It is important, however, to obtain confirmation by culture whenever possible if a viral origin is suspected on cytology.

The cytopathic effects are noted mainly in sputum and bronchial secretions and can be seen on PAP staining. Immunostaining will provide firm identification of the virus. Non-specific inflammatory, reactive and degenerative changes are also often present, providing a background to the diagnosis.

## Box 2.1  Some conditions associated with pulmonary granulomata

### Infections

Bacteria

- *Mycobacterium tuberculosis* and other mycobacteria
- *Nocardia asteroides*

Fungi

- *Aspergillus fumigatus, niger, flavus*
- *Blastomyces dermatitidis*
- *Candida albicans*
- *Coccidioides immitis*
- *Cryptococcus neoformans*
- *Histoplasma capsulatum, duboisii*
- *Paracoccidioides brasiliensis*
- *Rhinosporidium seeberi*
- *Sporothrix schenkii*
- *Torulopsis glabrata*
- *Trichosporon capitatum*
- *Zygomycetes*

Parasites

- Arthropods
- Cestodes
- Nematodes
- Protozoa
- Trematodes

### Occupational exposure

- Asbestosis
- Silicosis
- Heavy metals
- Aluminium
- Beryllium
- Organic dusts (extrinsic allergic alveolitis)

### Idiopathic lung diseases

- Sarcoidosis
- Rheumatoid disease
- Wegener's granulomatosis
- Allergic angiitis and granulomatosis
- Necrotising sarcoid granulomatosis
- Lymphomatoid granulomatosis
- Bronchocentric granulomatosis
- Granulomatous disease of childhood

### Iatrogenic causes

- Drug toxicity
- Radiation exposure
- Oxygen therapy

### Other conditions

- Foreign body reaction
- Tumour-related granulomas

## Non-specific cytological findings: viral infections

- Necrosis and inflammation
- Ciliocytophthoria
- Bronchial and alveolar cell hyperplasia.

Inflammatory cells and necrotic debris are a frequent finding in the early stages, especially in those infections caused by influenza and parainfluenza viruses.[69] Ciliocytophthoria with fragmented ciliated and pyknotic nucleated remnants is a variable feature. The phenomenon was first described in adenovirus infections, but is not specific, occurring in other infections and also in association with neoplasia and radiotherapy.[58]

Bronchial and alveolar cell hyperplasia may be seen, producing clusters of enlarged epithelial cells with swollen hyperchromatic nuclei and prominent nucleoli, as found in a variety of inflammatory states. These changes are easily confused with malignancy but the cohesiveness of the groups in only small numbers and absence of single dissociated abnormal cells favour a reactive process.[70]

## Specific cytological findings: viral cytopathic effects

- Intranuclear inclusion bodies
- Loss of nuclear chromatin pattern
- Multinucleation
- Cytoplasmic inclusions.

Herpes simplex virus causes tracheobronchitis initially, but this may progress to necrotising bronchopneumonia in debilitated or immunodeficient patients. Varicella-zoster and cytomegalovirus (CMV) also induce cytopathic effects in the respiratory tract, usually as part of a more generalised systemic infection. Others less often encountered, although common causes of respiratory disease, include respiratory syncytial virus, measles and adenovirus.

## Herpes simplex virus (Fig. 2.28)

Bronchial epithelial cells and macrophages become multinucleated, with swollen nuclei clustered tightly together, leading to

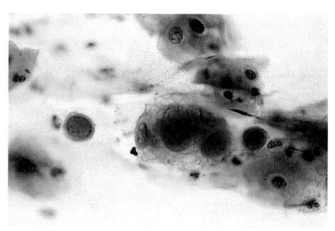

**Fig. 2.28** Herpes simplex virus cytopathic effects in bronchial columnar epithelium in sputum from a patient on immunosuppressive therapy. The cells are swollen and degenerate with enlarged nuclei, which have a 'ground glass' appearance (see single cell on left). Note the multinucleation and nuclear moulding (PAP).

characteristic moulding of nuclear contours. Loss of chromatin pattern follows, due to the presence of viral inclusions. Nuclei take on an empty homogenised 'ground glass' appearance, with a prominent surrounding nuclear membrane.[71]

As the condition progresses, brightly stained eosinophilic Cowdry type A inclusions develop in the nucleus. These are often triangular or wedge-shaped and may appear refractile. Immunocytochemical methods can be used for definitive identification of herpetic inclusions.

The cell changes often occur in a clean background, although if necrotising pneumonia has supervened acute inflammatory cells and necrotic debris are seen. Herpetic infections may be associated with atypical changes in bronchial epithelium as described above;[70] conversely, patients with treated lung cancer are predisposed to herpetic infections if treatment involves immunosuppression.[72]

## Varicella-zoster

Cytologically, the changes in the respiratory tract induced by the Varicella-zoster virus are virtually identical to those of Herpes simplex infection. The most helpful distinction is the presence of typical skin manifestations. Where necessary, the diagnosis can be confirmed by immunofluorescence or immunocytochemical methods.

## Cytomegalovirus (CMV)

In CMV infection (Fig. 2.29) characteristic large inclusion bodies appear in the nuclei of macrophages and other cells of the respiratory tract. They are surrounded by a halo and the nuclear membrane is thickened giving an 'owl's eye' appearance. The number of inclusions is said to reflect the intensity of the infection.[73]

Small basophilic cytoplasmic inclusions develop as the disease progresses. These consist of protein-coated viral particles, which impart a finely granular texture to the cytoplasm. The inclusions are difficult to identify in routine preparations. Infected cells swell and undergo degeneration or necrosis, but multinucleation and nuclear moulding are usually not conspicuous features.

Combined infections can occur, especially in immunosuppressed patients. *Pneumocystis jiroveci* may be seen, or there may be evidence of a second virus such as herpes simplex, inducing multinucleation and moulding. Bronchoalveolar lavage fluid has been used for rapid detection of CMV by direct *in situ* hybridisation.[74]

## Respiratory syncytial virus

Multinucleated giant cells are the hallmark of respiratory syncytial virus infection, as seen histologically. Basophilic inclusions have been described in the cytoplasm of multinucleated and mononuclear cells and in type II pneumocytes during the course of the illness.[75]

## Measles virus (Fig. 2.30)

Multinucleation of epithelial cells is the characteristic feature of measles pneumonia,[76] producing tightly clustered hyperchromatic nuclei at the centre of the cell cytoplasm. Eosinophilic inclusions in both nucleus and cytoplasm may be seen in these multinucleated cells, referred to as Warthin-Finkeldey cells.

## Adenovirus

In adenovirus infection,[77] small eosinophilic inclusions in infected nuclei appear early and these have been described as rosette cells because of the radiating pattern of the chromatin. Some cells have been noted to have a larger basophilic inclusion with loss of the chromatin pattern, being referred to as smudge cells. Ciliocytophthoria is a striking accompaniment to adenovirus infection, although not specific. Much acute inflammatory exudate will be seen during the stage of active infection.

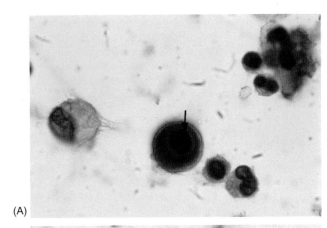

(A)

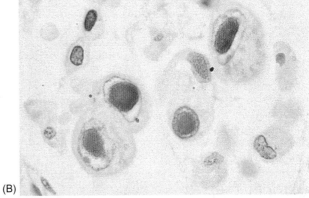

(B)

**Fig. 2.29** Cytomegalovirus inclusion bodies in bronchoalveolar lavage sample from a transplant patient (arrow). (A) PAP, (B) Immunoperoxidase.

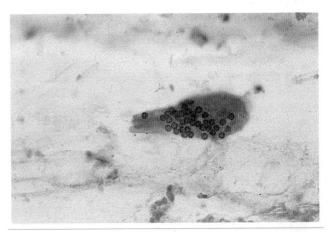

**Fig. 2.30** Multinucleation due to measles virus infection. Warthin-Finkeldey with closely packed small dark nuclei in sputum from a child with measles pneumonia (PAP).

### Diagnostic pitfalls: specific viral infections

In viral infections, clumps of hyperplastic epithelial cells may lead to a false diagnosis of adenocarcinoma, particularly bronchioloalveolar cell carcinoma (see p. 74).[70] A diagnosis of tumour should only be made if individual cells showing the nuclear changes of malignancy are identified and if there is appropriate correlation between the cytological and clinical findings.

The specific changes in different viral infections produce overlapping pictures, hence the need to confirm the identity of the virus by methods such as culture, immunocytochemistry or by serology. Furthermore, several viruses may be present, especially in immunosuppressed patients, and this may not be apparent on routine cytology. In transplant patients, identification of a virus such as CMV does not necessarily signify active infection unless associated with tissue damage. Lung biopsy may be necessary to establish the presence of viral pneumonia in these patients.

## Fungal infections

Fungus cells are generally composed of septate or non-septate hyphae that branch and twine to form a tangled mass known as a mycelium. The hyphae show expansions distally (conidiophores), from which chains of spores (conidia) emerge under aerobic conditions, producing a so-called fruiting head. Some fungi exhibit dimorphism, appearing either as hyphae or as round or oval yeast forms. The yeasts may be arranged in chains resembling hyphae and these are known as pseudohyphae.[78]

Infection and allergy are the two most important pathological effects produced in the lung by fungi. Those causing infection are either true pathogens or opportunistic organisms. The latter are saprophytic fungi, only causing disease if the host defences are lowered. They evoke a different range of clinical and pathological responses compared with infections in immunocompetent people, sometimes with very little inflammatory reaction or granuloma formation.

The presence of fungi in respiratory specimens raises one of three possibilities: they may be contaminants from the mouth or atmosphere or there may be saprophytic colonisation of an area of pre-existing diseased lung, such as a cavity or bronchus, without any invasion of live tissue. There could be an active infection (mycosis), with growth of fungi in the lung parenchyma. Which of these applies to a given cytological sample requires access to clinical details, including any history of immunosuppression, and to the radiological findings. Salivary specimens contaminated by bacterial and fungal overgrowth contrast clearly with the presence of pure fungus in a deep cough sample of sputum or a lavage specimen from a patient with a genuine infection. Inflammatory debris is usually present when there is invasion of tissues by fungi or if a fungal ball (mycetoma) has formed in cavitated lung.

Unlike the bacterial and viral infections already discussed, fungi can often be identified with some precision in respiratory samples because of their characteristic morphology. Culture of the organism is nevertheless necessary for confirmation.

## Aspergillosis

Fungi of the *Aspergillus* genus are worldwide in distribution and are present in soil and atmosphere. There are about 600 species

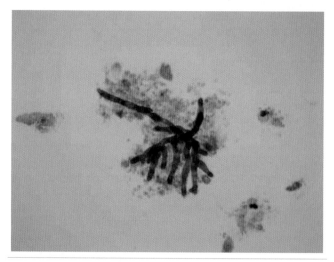

**Fig. 2.31** *Aspergillus* hyphae in a 'sunburst' pattern in lavage fluid from a patient receiving cytotoxic therapy for non-Hodgkin lymphoma. The hyphae are septate with dichotomous branching (PAP).

of *Aspergillus* organisms, but fewer than 10 are pathogenic to humans. Of these *A. fumigatus* is the most common, *A. niger* and *A. flavus* being much less frequent pathogens.[79] The different species cannot be distinguished by morphology alone.

### Cytological findings: *Aspergillus* infection

- Septate hyphae 3–4 μm in width
- Dichotomous branching at 45° angles
- Fruiting heads form in aerobic conditions
- Oxalate crystals present in some cases
- Potentially a contaminant but should always be reported.

Narrow septate hyphae showing dichotomous branching into two equal divisions at a regular angle of 45° are typical of this organism. Unless disrupted by the preparation, the hyphae appear to radiate outwards in a 'sunburst' pattern (Fig. 2.31).

The hyphae stain variably with PAP and are very pale on H&E staining, but are well shown by the periodic acid Schiff (PAS) stain. Grocott's methenamine silver method (Fig. 2.32A) shows the branching structure as stark black hyphae but their septation may not be obvious. They are refractile under polarised light.

Fruiting heads develop at the ends of hyphae in aerobic conditions. They consist of pale flask-shaped vesicles from which a projecting crown of stalks bearing chains of conidia can be seen (Fig. 2.32B). This structure resembles a brush, hence the name of the genus, derived from the brush known as an 'aspergillum', used for sprinkling holy water.

Pulmonary involvement by *Aspergillus* may take the following forms.[74]

### Superficial saprophytic colonisation of the airways

This is not uncommon in cases of bronchial mucosal damage such as in cystic fibrosis or bronchiectasis, and is usually not associated with tissue invasion.

### Allergic bronchopulmonary aspergillosis

In this condition, there is a type III hypersensitivity reaction to the presence of the fungus in the airways, with damage to

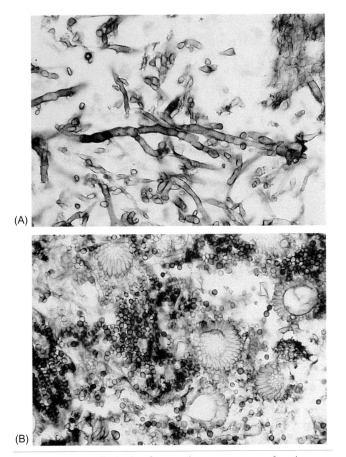

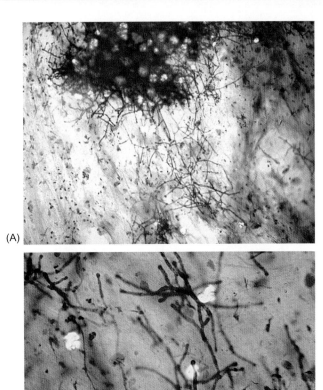

**Fig. 2.32** (A) *Aspergillus* hyphae from a pulmonary mycetoma found at post mortem in an elderly man treated for a bronchial carcinoma. (Grocott's methenamine silver) (B) *Aspergillus* fruiting heads and conidiophores from the same mycetoma. (Grocott stain) (Courtesy of Dr A. Padel, Stoke Mandeville, UK.)

**Fig. 2.33** (A,B) Oxalate crystals are seen on medium and high magnification in this aspiration sample from a patient with a mycetoma of lung. Their presence is confirmed by the use of polarised light and should prompt a thorough search for the accompanying hyphae (PAP). (Courtesy of Dr G. Sterrett, Perth, Western Australia.)

the bronchial mucosa and lung parenchyma. There may be a long-standing history of asthma, the main cytological features of which are described later in this chapter.

Cases of allergic bronchopulmonary fungal disease develop severe mucoid plugging of the airways, and it is in these plugs with their associated necrotic debris that the hyphae are seen. They may be difficult to identify on PAP staining but samples can be destained and re-stained with methenamine silver or cell blocks of the mucoid plugs may be helpful (see Fig. 2.57). The diagnosis is significant and should be borne in mind when sputum or lavage samples include large amounts of eosinophilic debris.[80]

## Pulmonary aspergilloma

Any cavitating lung disease can provide a setting for this form of saprophytic colonisation of the lung. Tuberculosis, bronchiectasis, pulmonary infarcts and necrotic carcinomas are among the pre-existing conditions that have been documented. There is no invasion of the lung parenchyma unless cavitation has arisen in lung destroyed by invasive aspergillosis, as can happen in severely immunocompromised patients.

The cytological findings in sputum, lavage and FNA material include necrotic and inflammatory debris with fragments of fungal hyphae, some of which may show fruiting heads (Fig. 2.32). Fan-shaped crystals of calcium oxalate are deposited in the

fungal ball, especially when *A. niger* is the organism involved (Fig. 2.33). These refractile crystals may be expectorated or aspirated, and may even be found in pleural fluid from an associated effusion, providing a useful clue to the presence of the fungus.[81]

The fungus goes through phases of growth and death, during which calcification may occur. Haemoptysis is a common presenting symptom in long-standing cases, due to erosion of small vessels in the cavity wall. Atypical hyperplastic or metaplastic epithelial cells are sometimes seen and must be distinguished from malignancy, while remembering that necrotic carcinoma can also be the seat of an aspergilloma.

Ultimately the diagnosis rests on a combination of the characteristic radiological appearances of an opacity capped by a meniscus of air, the opacity moving as the patient changes position, together with identification of the organism by morphology, serology and culture.

## Invasive pulmonary aspergillosis

Invasion of the lung parenchyma is seen only in debilitated patients with immunosuppression, whether iatrogenic or due to a disorder of the immune system. The nature of the immunological deficit determines the pattern of damage to the lung. Various classifications of the disease have emerged, not distinguishable

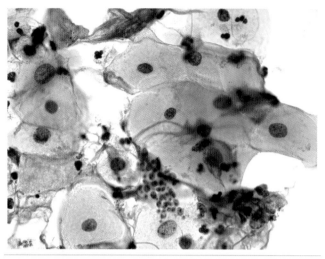

**Fig. 2.34** *Candida* spores and chains of pseudohyphae are abundant in this sputum sample which included many salivary squamous cells and few inflammatory cells. This suggests overgrowth of fungal elements from oral contamination rather than genuine fungal infection.

by cytological methods; the reader is, therefore, referred to more detailed accounts for further information.[78] Necrotising bronchopneumonia, haemorrhagic pulmonary infarction, granulomatous inflammation, abscess formation and lobar pneumonia are among the different pathological reactions found. The cytological findings relate to the pathological process that has evolved, and are not specific unless the fungus itself is seen.

Fungal identification in bronchoalveolar lavage fluid from immunocompromised patients has been reported to have a sensitivity of 64% compared with 40% sensitivity on culture[82] but published results vary considerably. Estimation of *Aspergillus* antigen levels in lavage fluid has also been reported.[76] Oxalic acid levels in lavage fluid are raised but this is not specific as it occurs in CMV infection and in other conditions.[83]

### Diagnostic pitfalls: *Aspergillus* infection

Certain other fungi resemble *Aspergillus* closely. *Candida* hyphae are thinner but are prone to swell if degenerate and may then be wrongly identified. Zygomycetes, particularly *Mucor* sp. are also similar, although their hyphae are broader with no or very few septa. Culture is necessary for firm identification.

## *Candida* infection

The ubiquitous *Candida* fungus is dimorphic, occurring both in budding yeast form and as hyphae. Healthy individuals harbour the organism as a harmless oral mucosal saprophyte, but in the presence of immunosuppression, disseminated infection may involve the respiratory tract. *Candida* is said to be the most frequent of all causes of opportunistic infection and although several potentially pathogenic species exist, *Candida albicans* is by far the most common. Individual species can only be distinguished by culture.

### Cytological findings: *Candida* infection

- Septate hyphae 3–5 μm in diameter (Fig. 2.34A)
- Yeast cells 2–4 μm in size (Fig. 2.34B)

- Chains of yeasts forming pseudohyphae.

Yeast forms and hyphae usually occur together in human infections. The hyphae have a delicate branching septate structure. They are found radiating in a disorganised fashion from a mycelial clump or as single hyphal strands separated in the process of preparing the sample. The yeast cells may elongate into budding chains to form pseudohyphae. Both yeasts and hyphae stain pale pink by the PAP method but are inconspicuous in MGG-stained material. They are well shown by PAS and methenamine silver stains.

## Types of pulmonary involvement by *Candida* spp.[78]

The patients are virtually always immunosuppressed or have an underlying predisposing condition such as diabetes mellitus, recent surgery or severe burns. Infection follows aspiration of organisms into the lungs or is by haematogenous dissemination. Bronchopneumonia results from the former mode of spread, while the latter causes tiny miliary abscesses in adults. Infants with indwelling venous catheters colonised by the fungus have been found to develop multiple infected pulmonary infarcts. This rarely happens in adults with haematogenous lesions, although other fungi such as *Aspergillus* do cause haemorrhagic infarction in severely immunocompromised adults.

The significance of *Candida* may be difficult to ascertain in sputum, washings, brushings and lavages, since the organism is such a frequent contaminant. When present in acute inflammatory debris in samples from a patient with an appropriate history, the finding should be reported to ensure that material is sent for culture, although a positive culture may not signify actual lung infection. Raised levels of *Candida* antigen in bronchoalveolar lavage fluid have been reported by Ness et al. as evidence of significant pulmonary infection. Over 90% of their patients with *Candida* pneumonia gave positive results by latex agglutination.[84]

FNA specimens, especially transthoracic aspirations, can provide definitive evidence of infection. The yeasts and hyphae are found in a non-specific inflammatory background, which includes neutrophil polymorphs unless the patient has agranulocytosis. Sometimes a picture of granulomatous inflammation is present. As with other samples, culture is essential for confirmation.

### Diagnostic pitfalls: *Candida* infection

These apply to all fungal infections and fall into two categories: the need to identify the fungus accurately with confirmation by culture, and the need to establish whether the presence of the organism is of any clinical significance. The clinical history is important, but so also is the cytological setting, since *Candida* is part of the normal oral flora and is a frequent coincidental finding in sputum. It is also a common contaminant from water baths, stain solutions and other laboratory sources and may be seen in many different specimens.

A genuine infection is suspected when hyphae and pseudohyphae are intimately related to inflammatory debris in a sample that is clearly of lower respiratory tract origin. Open lung biopsy may be necessary to establish that fungal hyphae are invading tissues. There is less of a problem with FNA material, especially when collected by the transthoracic route.

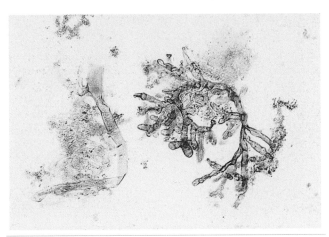

**Fig. 2.35** Mucor species found in a bronchial washing from a diabetic patient. Note the broad non-septate hyphae branching at irregularly spaced variable angles (Toluidine blue). (Courtesy of Professor B. Naylor, Michigan.)

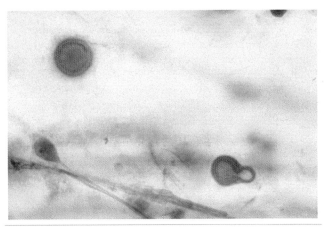

**Fig. 2.36** *Cryptococcus neoformans* in sputum stained by mucicarmine to demonstrate the thick mucoid capsule. Note the single budding by a narrow neck, characteristic of this fungus.

*Candida* spp. must be distinguished from other mycelial fungi such as *Aspergillus* spp., which branch at 45° and do not form budding yeast cells, and from the fungi with yeast-like forms, for example *Cryptococcus, Histoplasma, Torulopsis* spp. and others. These organisms do not produce budding pseudohyphae or mycelia. Thus the dimorphism of *Candida* species can be helpful in identification.

## Phycomycosis (mucormycosis)

This group of opportunistic fungal infections, also known as zygomycosis or hyphomycosis, occurs in individuals predisposed by leukaemia, lymphoma and other tumours, in cases of severe burns, renal failure or malnutrition, and as a complication of chemotherapy, diabetes mellitus and drug addiction. The fungi are widespread in nature but only a few, such as *Rhizopus, Mucor* and *Absidia*, are likely to be encountered in human infections. The disease runs a fulminant course, with haemorrhagic infarction of the lung due to the ability of the fungal hyphae to invade blood vessel walls, inducing thrombosis.[78]

### Cytological findings: phycomycosis

- Non-septate hyphae of variable width (5–50 μm)
- Irregular branching at up to 90° angles (Fig. 2.35).

All of the fungi of this group appear similar in cytological preparations. The hyphae are thick-walled and non-septate, with a ribbon-like structure averaging 10–15 μm in width. They divide at angles of up to 90°, with irregular spacing between divisions. Papanicolaou stain shows light green or pink hyphae which appear broader than *Aspergillus* or *Candida* spp.; they stain less strongly with silver impregnation, H&E and by PAS. They have been likened to a tangled mass of folded cellophane ribbons.

### Diagnostic pitfalls: phycomycosis

Problems in diagnosis of mucormycosis are similar to those already described for fungal infections in general. The organisms are common contaminants. They must therefore be seen in the appropriate context, although cellular reaction is sometimes slight in opportunistic infections. The thick-walled hyphae can be taken for plant cells, and when folded they may appear septate, resembling *Aspergillus*. Culture is necessary for identification.

## Cryptococcosis

*Cryptococcus neoformans* is the causative agent of this worldwide disease, the natural habitat of the fungus being the detritus of birds' nests and pigeon roosts. The birds are not affected but the fungus is pathogenic to humans, colonising the airways after inhalation or producing outright infection of the lung if the strain is virulent. Healthy individuals are able to confine the organism to a single focus, which often resolves but may recur or spread further in the lung parenchyma. If dissemination occurs, the fungus exhibits neurotropism, leading to central nervous system involvement and meningitis. Debilitated patients have a rapidly progressive infection with early haematogenous spread in lungs and brain.[78]

Early in lung infection, a bronchopneumonic process is seen and the affected area has a slimy surface due to the thick gelatinous capsule, a feature of this organism. At a later stage, a more defined focus of firm fibrotic tissue is seen, with very few fungi in the lesion. Extensive lung destruction, cavitation and calcification are rare but the radiological findings can simulate a lung tumour. Because of this, cytology plays a considerable part in diagnosis in sputum, lavage fluid, bronchial secretions and by FNA.

### Cytological findings: cryptococcosis

- Yeast cells 5–20 μm in size
- Thick mucoid capsule
- Single narrow-necked budding.

The fungal cells are rounded yeasts with a thick mucoid capsule of variable width surrounding each organism, holding them apart from one another and any other cytological material present (Fig. 2.36). They reproduce readily by single budding from the parent cell via a thin isthmus, leaving a slight pointed protrusion, which imparts a teardrop shape to the parent organism. Pseudohyphae are rarely seen.

With PAP staining, the central fungus is dark green or grey and the capsule is clear or only faintly stained. The organisms stain black with Grocott's methenamine silver, but again the capsule is clear. The mucopolysaccharide capsule stains bright pink with Mayer's mucicarmine and PAS stains. Indian ink preparations highlight the dark organism within its clear halo.

Cryptococcal infection may evoke very little inflammation, or there may be an intense acute inflammatory reaction. A granulomatous response with epithelioid histiocytes and giant cells can also occur.

### Diagnostic pitfalls: cryptococcosis

Problems arise from failure to identify the rather inconspicuous smaller forms of the organism unless familiar with their appearance. They may be mistaken for starch granules or artefacts by the unwary.

## Coccidioidomycosis

The causative agent of this disease is a dimorphic fungus found in desert soils of certain geographical areas, notably in the southern USA, and in Central and Southern America. It produces asymptomatic or indolent granulomatous chest infections by inhalation of air-borne arthrospores, which have ruptured from mycelia in the soil. Infection is usually self-limiting, but may be chronic and progressive in immunocompromised patients.

Productive cough, fever, chest pain, night sweats and weakness are among the presenting symptoms. In persistent disease, miliary granulomas, fibrosis and cavitation occur. The pathology is similar to that of tuberculosis, but with the presence of endospores lying within large spherules. Radiologically, there may be confusion with carcinoma or tuberculosis.[78]

The fungus has been described in all types of cytological samples. Awareness of the disease outside endemic areas is necessary today, with increasing travel and the rise in numbers of immunocompromised patients.

### Cytological findings: coccidioidomycosis

- Intact or collapsed spherules 20–60 μm in diameter
- Nucleated endospores 1–5 μm in size.

Intact spherules containing endospores, collapsed spherules and their released endospores are all found. They can be seen in any type of cytological preparation, but are best demonstrated in FNA material. Hyphae are not usually seen. Spherules show a thick cyst wall, eosinophilic or variable by PAP staining, but staining strongly with methenamine silver (Fig. 2.37). They may be packed with endospores or empty. Endospores are nucleated and are 1–5 μm in size, but larger yeast cells and deformed degenerate spores may also be seen. A variable amount of inflammatory debris is found, more pronounced if bronchopneumonia or miliary disease is present. Neutrophil polymorphs or evidence of granulomatous inflammation may be seen.

### Diagnostic pitfalls: coccidioidomycosis

The endospores are easily confused with other small yeasts, particularly *Histoplasma* and *Candida*. The endospores of *Coccidioides* organisms do not bud. Spherules resemble the large cyst-like cells of *Rhinosporidium,* and when empty

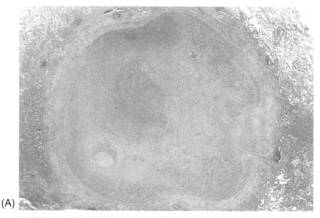

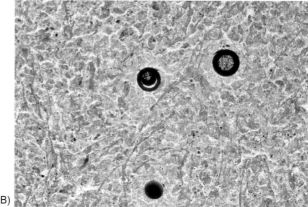

(A)

(B)

**Fig. 2.37** *Coccidioides immitis* was found to be the cause of this solitary granulomatous lung lesion in an engineer who had worked briefly in Texas where it is assumed he contracted the infection. The histological section shows an indolent caseating granuloma within which fungal spherules are demonstrated by Grocott staining (Courtesy of Dr MS Dunnill, Oxford, UK.)

they can be mistaken for the large yeast cells of *Blastomyces dermatitidis*, which shows broad-necked budding. These are problems of differential diagnosis, which can be resolved by experience in identification of fungi, and ultimately by culture.

## Histoplasmosis

This lung infection is caused by the widely distributed dimorphic fungus *Histoplasma capsulatum var. capsulatum*, but a related fungus *H. capsulatum var. duboisii*, confined to Africa, can, on occasion, cause similar lung as well as systemic disease. The more common condition due to *H. capsulatum var. capsulatum* arises by inhalation of spores from soil contaminated by bird droppings. Although occurring worldwide, it is an endemic infection in some areas of southern USA, Central America and the north of South America.[78]

The organism is an obligatory pathogen, but causes only a subclinical or minor illness in most cases. After inhalation, the yeasts are taken up by pulmonary macrophages and are rapidly disseminated to many organs without causing significant pathology. In the lung, a solitary lesion or sometimes multiple localised lesions may develop, producing respiratory symptoms and radiological shadows. Severe systemic disease is only seen in patients with impaired immunity. The diagnosis has been

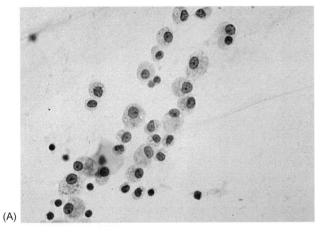

(A)

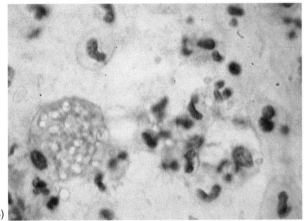

(B)

**Fig. 2.38** (A) *Histoplasma capsulatum* in sputum showing finely vacuolated macrophages which, on higher magnification (B), are seen to contain unstained organisms typical of histoplasmosis (PAP).

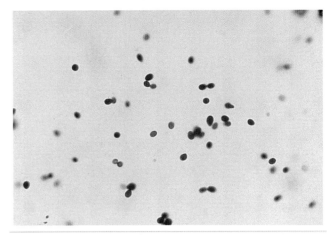

**Fig. 2.39** *Histoplasma* organisms in FNA material dispersed in a background of inflammatory cells. Grocott staining reveals scattered yeast cells, which have been released from their intracellular position within histiocytes.

The standard counterstains used with methenamine silver, such as light green, do not always allow the intracellular position of the fungus to be established with certainty. Counterstaining with H&E will help in identifying the location of the organisms, and not infrequently reveals a mixed infection in immunosuppressed patients. Immunocytochemical staining can be used to confirm the diagnosis.

## Blastomycosis

Infection caused by the dimorphic soil fungus *Blastomyces dermatitidis* occurs mainly in some southern states of North America and in parts of Central America, although occasional cases have been reported elsewhere. Inhalation of *Conidia* from the soil is followed by an acute or chronic pneumonic process, the latter mimicking tuberculosis or carcinoma in its course. Many other organs may also be involved.[78]

Histologically, the lungs show either microabscesses or a granulomatous reaction, followed by fibrosis and cavitation. A striking host response is sometimes seen in this and other fungal infections, producing a dense eosinophilic rim radiating around an individual organism. This material consists of antigen-antibody complexes formed in a hypersensitised individual and is known as the Hoeppli–Splendore phenomenon.

A cytological diagnosis can be made from any respiratory tract sample including FNA material. The presence of organisms is evidence of active infection. Confirmation of the diagnosis is obtained by culture or by direct immunofluorescence, which can be performed on smears as well as histological sections.

### Cytological findings: blastomycosis

- Yeast cells 8–15 μm in diameter
- Refractile cell wall
- Single broad-based budding (Fig. 2.40).

The round yeast form shows a dense refractile poorly stained wall, forming a halo around the cell. This may give the impression of a capsule, but the halo is mucicarmine negative and stains strongly with Grocott's technique. The cytoplasm may show a few brown granules with PAP stain, but most of the cells have shrunken central blue grey cytoplasm. Single

made in a variety of specimens, including bronchial washings and lavage fluid[85] and in FNA material. Coin lesions seen radiologically are an appropriate target for FNA sampling, but in patients with AIDS diffuse bilateral pulmonary infiltrates are more usually seen, and may require bronchoalveolar lavage for diagnosis.[86]

### Cytological findings: histoplasmosis

- Intracellular yeasts 2–5 μm in size
- Poorly visualised on PAP staining
- Strongly stained by the Grocott method.

The yeast forms are minute, rounded, single budding organisms best stained by methenamine silver and are characteristically intracellular, having been ingested by macrophages and polymorphs (Fig. 2.38). A small halo can usually be made out surrounding the yeast cells, emphasising their presence.

Their intracellular position is a helpful point of distinction from other small yeasts such as *Candida* spp., which are not usually phagocytosed in this way. This raises the possibility of other intracellular organisms, however, including *Toxoplasma gondii* and *Leishmania* spp. The latter two protozoans do not take up silver stains.[78] Free forms of *Histoplasma* are inconspicuous in routine preparations and difficult to identify confidently in Grocott-stained material (Fig. 2.39).

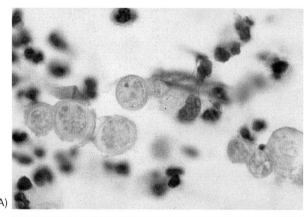

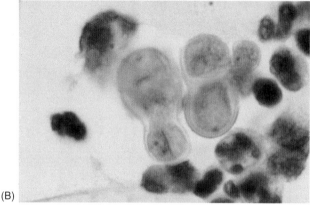

(A)

(B)

**Fig. 2.40** *Blastomyces dermatitidis* seen in a bronchoalveolar lavage specimen. The yeast has a thick clear zone peripherally with greyish-blue staining of cytoplasm centrally. Broad-based budding can be seen in (B) (PAP).

budding is seen, the daughter cell remaining closely applied to the parent, creating the appearance of a broad-based attachment. Hyphae are not formed.

Inflammatory cells reflect tissue changes, consisting either of polymorphs or chronic inflammatory cells of granulomatous type. Sometimes organisms are visible in the giant cells as well as lying free. The Hoeppli–Splendore phenomenon may be seen in cytological samples.

### Diagnostic pitfalls: blastomycosis

Organisms can be mistaken for host cells in PAP-stained preparations, assuming the core of cytoplasm to be the nucleus. Positive silver staining resolves this problem.

Confusion with other large yeasts can occur, particularly *Histoplasma capsulatum var. duboisii* in cases from Africa. The latter has a different pattern of budding, said to have an hourglass appearance, and is often intracellular. Other organisms such as *Cryptococcus* or *Paracoccidioides* have a different structure and a different geographical distribution.

## Paracoccidioidomycosis

This disease occurs in Central and South America, the habitat of the dimorphic pathogenic soil fungus *Paracoccidioides brasiliensis*. Systemic infection develops after inhalation of hyphae and a bronchopneumonic illness may ensue, progressing to fibrosis, granulomatous inflammation and cavitation.[78]

### Cytological findings: paracoccidioidomycosis

- Variable sized yeasts 6–60 μm in diameter
- Stains with Papanicolaou and Grocott methods
- Multiple budding.

The yeast form is a round organism reproducing by a highly characteristic process of multiple budding. The daughter cells remain attached around the periphery of the parent cell. This appearance, which has been likened to a steering wheel, enables accurate morphological identification of the infection in sputum, bronchial secretions, lavages and FNA samples.

A type of alveolar proteinosis (lipoproteinosis) develops in some patients with paracoccidioidomycosis and may also occur in association with histoplasmosis. Evidence of this may be found in cytological specimens, as described in Chapter 16.

## *Penicillium* spp.

Several members of this group are known to cause lung infections in healthy or immunosuppressed individuals,[87] although they are much less common as a source of opportunistic infection than the fungi already described. *P. marneffei* is a dimorphic member of the group known to cause endemic mycosis in South-east Asia and southern China.[88] The yeast form must be distinguished from *Pneumocystis* infection, which requires different treatment.

### Cytological findings: *Penicillium* spp.

- Yeast cells 2–6 μm in size
- Well stained by Grocott's method.

The organism is dimorphic, unlike other species of *Penicillium*. The yeasts are inconspicuous on PAP staining but Grocott's technique reveals rounded, oval, elongated or cup-shaped cells, some with a thickened dot on the capsule.

### Diagnostic pitfalls: *Penicillium* spp.

The differential diagnosis includes *Pneumocystis* organisms, which are less variable in shape and do not include elongated forms. They have paired dots on the capsule and are grouped in plaques of alveolar exudate, whereas *P. marneffei* is either intracellular or randomly distributed extracellularly.

## *Pneumocystis jiroveci*

This organism, which became increasingly important as a cause of opportunistic infection (see Ch. 16), was initially regarded as a protozoan, but is now classified within the order of fungi.[88,89] It is widespread in nature, being present in soil and atmosphere. The human form of this organism was renamed from *Pneumocystis carinii* to *P. jiroveci* in 2002, although the acronym PCP is still used to refer to *Pneumocystis* pneumonia.[90] Infection occurs by inhalation, causing a treatable form of pneumonia in patients with immunosuppression from any cause, particularly in transplant cases and patients with AIDS. Patients develop

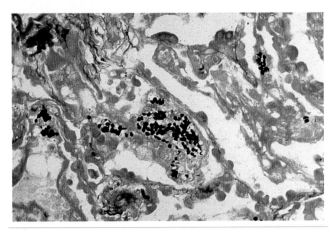

**Fig. 2.41** *Pneumocystis jiroveci* pneumonia in section of lung stained by Grocott's method to demonstrate the silver positive organisms lying in casts of amorphous debris which fill the alveolar spaces.

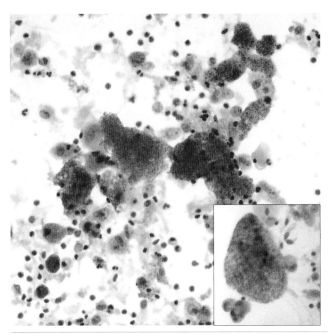

**Fig. 2.42** High-power view of the cluster of cysts that can sometimes be diagnosed even without silver staining. Inset: Alveolar cast forming a plaque of amphophilic material with a honeycomb pattern due to the presence of unstained *Pneumocystis jiroveci* cysts. Bronchoalveolar lavage sample from an HIV positive haemophiliac patient (PAP).

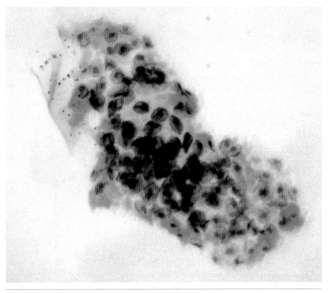

**Fig. 2.43** *Pneumocystis jiroveci* cysts seen within an alveolar plaque stained by Grocott's methenamine silver method. Trophozoites cannot be seen.

patchy or confluent consolidation of the lungs, producing radiological opacities. The presentation is often insidious, with fever, cough and shortness of breath. Histology shows foamy pale pink exudates filling alveolar spaces, and within these exudates the cyst wall of the organism can be demonstrated by methenamine silver staining. There is often little inflammatory reaction to the presence of the infection.

The organism exists as a nucleated trophozoite 1–5 μm in size, which is capable of amoeboid movement and attaches to type I pneumocytes by means of *filopodia*. It develops into a cyst 5–8 μm in diameter, the wall of which is focally thickened, giving an appearance of paired inclusions on light microscopy. The cyst contains merozoites, which mature into trophozoites on release from the cyst, thus completing the life cycle.[91]

Cytology has an established role in the diagnosis of *Pneumocystis* infection using all specimen types but particularly induced sputum and bronchoalveolar lavage fluid.[92]

### Cytological findings: *Pneumocystis jiroveci*

- Amphophilic proteinaceous alveolar casts (Figs 2.41–2.43)
- Honeycomb appearance of unstained cysts on PAP staining
- Cysts 5–8 μm outlined within casts by Grocott's stain
- Trophozoites outside the cysts are not usually visible.

Diagnosis is made by recognition of cystic forms of the organism in clusters within proteinaceous alveolar casts.[93] The latter are sometimes disrupted by specimen preparation, scattering the cysts widely. Intact alveolar casts are recognisable in PAP-stained material as vaguely rounded amphophilic three-dimensional structures up to 100 μm across. They tend to be eosinophilic centrally and more cyanophilic at the periphery, with a honeycomb texture due to the presence of the unstained cysts. Finding these casts in PAP-stained samples is strongly predictive of *Pneumocystis jiroveci* infection, with a sensitivity of up to 83% and a specificity of 100%.[94]

Traditionally, definitive cytological diagnosis rests on staining the cysts and this can be achieved in various ways, listed in Box 2.2. Grocott's modification of the Gomori methenamine silver stain is in common use, revealing cysts with several dot- or comma-shaped internal structures due to areas of thickening of the cyst wall. These cannot be seen in every cyst and are obscured if silver staining is heavy. Collapsed empty cysts are often present, assuming crescent or cup-like shapes. Degenerate cysts stain faintly and may be difficult to recognise.

Other histochemical stains advocated for demonstrating the cysts have the advantage of a shorter preparation time than the Grocott method. For example, a modified toluidine blue method has been shown to have equivalent sensitivity to methenamine silver staining, but is easier and quicker to perform as the reagents do not need fresh preparation for each specimen (Fig. 2.44). Fluorescent microscopy using monoclonal antibodies to cyst wall protein is a sensitive diagnostic technique, although more elaborate than the simpler staining procedures described earlier.[95] Pneumocystis

### Box 2.2  Methods for identification of *Pneumocystis jiroveci*

- Grocott's modification of Gomori's methenamine silver stain
- Papanicolaou stain
- Toluidine blue stain
- MGG or Diff-Quik stain
- Cresyl violet stain
- Haematoxylin and eosin stain
- Gram and Gram-Weigert stain
- Acridine orange stain
- Immunofluorescence methods
- Immunocytochemistry
- DNA hybridisation
- Polymerase chain reaction
- Electron microscopy

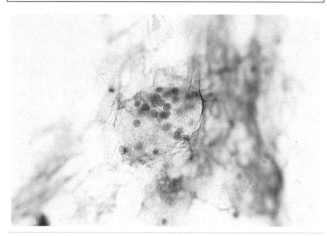

**Fig. 2.44** *Pneumocystis jiroveci* in a plaque stained with modified toluidine blue method, a more rapid technique than the traditional Grocott stain. Bronchoalveolar lavage.

detection kits are now available.[96] Immunocytochemical methods can also be used but are relatively expensive and time-consuming.[97]

Wakefield and associates have used the polymerase chain reaction to amplify specific segments of DNA from respiratory samples for diagnosis of *Pneumocystis jiroveci* infection. They found that amplification of DNA with ethidium bromide enhanced the diagnostic yield in lavage fluid[98] and in induced sputum.[99] The pick-up rate in the latter series was increased from 35% using silver stains to 90% with DNA amplification, including several positive samples that were deemed inadequate on silver staining. The authors suggest it might therefore be possible to use DNA amplification on saliva alone for identification of *Pneumocystis jiroveci*.

Trophozoites can be demonstrated by MGG or Diff-Quik stains, but are inconspicuous unless oil immersion magnification is used. Electron microscopy reveals the detailed structure of these organisms[89] but this procedure does not contribute to routine cytological diagnosis.

### Diagnostic pitfalls: *Pneumocystis jiroveci*

A reliable rapid method of diagnosis is essential in patient management in order to initiate effective treatment at the earliest possible opportunity. Exclusion of *Pneumocystis jiroveci* infection is also important in these immunosuppressed patients to hasten investigation of other treatable conditions.

Despite claims that a definitive diagnosis can be made on PAP-stained preparations alone, recognition can be difficult when only a few casts are present. There are notable variations in the numbers of organisms present in different conditions. Thus, patients with AIDS with an extremely heavy load of organisms give a higher diagnostic yield than post-transplant cases. The findings on routine stained samples may be tentative without further confirmation by special stains.[100]

Studies on the significance of the number of cysts found in cytological specimens are of interest. Pitchenk et al. have pointed out that only very small numbers of silver stained cysts may be found in induced sputum samples from patients who are found to have large numbers on transbronchial lung biopsy.[101] A separate study by Carmichael et al., however, suggested that fewer than five cysts in induced sputum may not represent a significant finding, as such cases did not develop evidence of infection on follow-up.[102]

Other fungi with budding yeasts such as *Histoplasma capsulatum*, *Candida* and *Cryptococcus neoformans* may be mistaken for *Pneumocystis jiroveci*. This risk can be avoided by the use of immunofluorescent staining.[95]

Other conditions associated with alveolar casts and amorphous exudate include pulmonary alveolar proteinosis, tracheobronchial amyloidosis and aggregates of degenerate red blood cells adherent to mucus.[93] These structures can usually be distinguished in PAP-stained preparations if appropriate criteria are applied, since there are no cysts within the plaques.

Grocott's or other staining procedures should always be performed with appropriate positive control material. Ideally a cytological preparation should be used as a control since the cysts stain more readily in histological sections than in cytology samples, which may therefore be understained.

Papanicolaou-stained preparations should always accompany the special stains and should be fully screened even if *Pneumocystis jiroveci* has already been confirmed. This is necessary to ensure recognition of multiple opportunistic infections or other conditions to which immunocompromised patients are predisposed, such as pulmonary haemorrhage or lymphoma. Cytomegalovirus may be found in association with *Pneumocystis* pneumonia and other dual infections also occur.

A further reason for screening PAP-stained preparations is to compare the amount of material present with different staining methods so as to detect artefactual loss of deposit from the slide. This can be a problem with Grocott preparations. Further slides should be stained if significant loss has occurred.

In samples from patients with treated *Pneumocystis jiroveci* infection, cysts may fail to take up the silver stain, even in the presence of recognisable foamy casts in PAP-stained preparations. Additional Grocott staining may reveal a few empty cysts (Fig. 2.45) but eventually the casts take on a hyalinised appearance and then the cysts can no longer be identified.[103] There is evidence that size of cysts relates to response to treatment, suggesting that smaller forms have a thinner cyst wall.[104]

## Other fungal infections

Many other fungal infections have been detected by cytological methods, notably *Sporothrix schenkii*,[105] *Petriellidium boydii*, previously known as *Allescheria boydii*,[106] and *Alternaria*.[46]

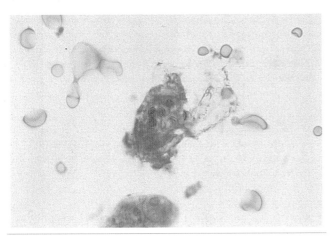

**Fig. 2.45** Poorly stained *Pneumocystis* in Grocott stained induced sputum from an immunosuppressed patient treated with sulphonamide for 5 days prior to the collection of this sample. Only occasional cysts were found, with variable staining of the residual structures and no honeycomb casts were identified in the PAP-stained material.

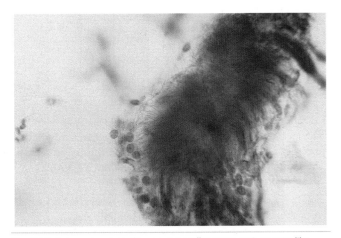

**Fig. 2.46** *Entamoeba gingivalis* organisms adherent to actinomyces-like organisms in sputum. Their presence may not signify infection in this setting, as they are saprophytic in the mouth especially if there is poor dental hygiene (PAP).

## Parasitic infections

Parasitic disease of the lung is much less common than fungal, bacterial or viral infection in developed countries. A few parasites infect the human lung as part of their regular life cycle, but the majority have a different animal host. Infection may be caused by protozoa, nematodes, trematodes, cestodes, arthropods and leeches. Cytological findings have only been described for some of these. The reader is referred to more specialised textbooks of parasitology for detailed descriptions of parasites not documented in the cytological literature.[107,108]

The protozoa that have been recognised by cytology in respiratory specimens include *Entamoeba gingivalis*[45] (Fig. 2.46) and *Entamoeba histolytica*,[109,110] *Giardia lamblia*,[111] and *Trichomonas* organisms.[112] The cytological findings in many of the protozoal infections that are recognised pulmonary pathogens in AIDS have not yet been documented,[113] but the cytological features of *Toxoplasma gondii* pneumonia in cardiac transplant recipients have been described in bronchoalveolar lavage fluid. The trophozoites were best shown by H&E or MGG stains.[114]

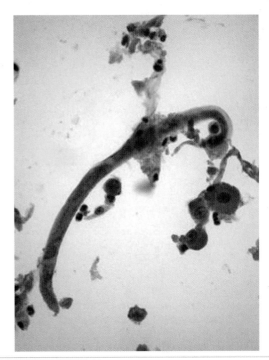

**Fig. 2.47** *Strongyloides stercoralis* larva in a BAL sample from an immunosuppressed HTLV-1 positive patient. The coiled shape is a characteristic feature but the indentation at the tail cannot be made out (LBC, PAP).

Among the nematodes or roundworms found in cytological samples, *Strongyloides stercoralis* is important as a cause of haemorrhagic pneumonia in patients receiving high doses of steroids or with impaired immune responses from other causes. Loosely coiled worm-like larvae are expectorated in the sputum, measuring 400–500 μm in length (Fig. 2.47).[115] They are thickened at one end and have a notch near the end of the tail, features which are helpful in identification.

Filariasis due to *Wucheria bancrofti* has been diagnosed in a variety of specimens including FNA material.[116] The related worm *Dirofilaria immitis* has also been described in man on FNA[117] although the natural host is the dog. *Schistosoma mansoni* has been described in bronchoalveolar lavage fluid.[118]

Trematodes identified in sputum and FNA samples include the lung flukes *Paragonimus westermani*[119] and *P. kellicotti*,[120] which are recognised by finding the golden coloured birefringent ova. They lie in a necrotic inflammatory background with many eosinophils and Charcot–Leyden crystals.

Of the cestodes that have been described, *Echinococcus granulosus*, the causative agent of hydatid disease, can be identified by finding hooklets and scolices in inflamed necrotic debris in sputum or bronchial secretions.[120] FNA is generally regarded as contraindicated in hydatid disease, since leakage of cyst contents leads to wide dissemination of the infection. Leakage has been reported in 25% of pulmonary hydatid cysts after FNA in one series.[122]

## Non-specific inflammatory lung conditions

### Chronic obstructive airways disease

Chronic bronchitis and emphysema are linked by having a common aetiological agent, namely inhaled tobacco smoke, and together form a spectrum of lung disease associated with

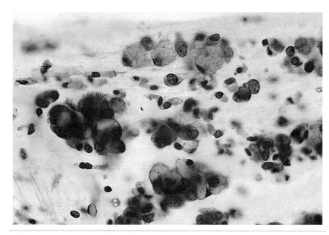

**Fig. 2.48** Clusters of hyperplastic bronchial epithelium and goblet cells in a bronchial washing from a patient with severe chronic obstructive airways disease (PAP).

recurrent chest infections. Chronic bronchitis is defined by the presence of hypertrophy of the bronchial mucous glands with increased sputum production. Emphysema results from irreversible destruction of the respiratory portion of the lung parenchyma, causing breathlessness.[123] Clinically, both conditions are frequently present together, although one or other usually predominates. Sufferers from chronic obstructive airways disease (COAD) are at risk of developing bronchial carcinoma due to the carcinogenic effects of tobacco smoke.

## Cytological findings: chronic obstructive airways disease

- Clusters of hyperplastic bronchial epithelial cells (Fig. 2.48)
- Goblet cell and reserve cell hyperplasia
- Ciliocytophthoria and other degenerative cell changes
- Squamous metaplasia, initially regular, later atypical
- Increased neutrophil polymorphs and macrophages
- Curschmann's spirals
- Any or all of these may be present but the findings are non-specific.

## Diagnostic pitfalls: chronic obstructive airways disease

Hyperplastic epithelial clusters and goblet cells must be distinguished from adenocarcinoma, bronchoalveolar carcinoma and metastatic carcinoma cells.[55] The presence of a few cilia around the border of some of the groups is evidence of reactive change. Nuclear features may not be clearly discernible for evaluation of malignancy, but macronucleoli are suspicious of malignancy. Adenocarcinoma cells tend to exfoliate more profusely than benign cells.

Reserve cell hyperplasia may resemble small cell carcinoma on low-power magnification, but closer inspection reveals more uniform nuclei with regular chromatin and little or no nuclear moulding between the reserve cells. Absence of necrosis is also a helpful feature.

Squamous metaplasia in chronic bronchitis mimics squamous carcinoma as the cells become increasingly atypical.[124] In early metaplasia nuclear changes do not suggest malignancy, the

cells retain their cohesiveness and lack the bizarre shapes and abnormal keratinisation of their malignant counterparts. Progressive nuclear and cytoplasmic abnormalities develop, accompanied by loss of cohesion. Differentiation between these cells and invasive or *in situ* carcinoma is discussed fully on p. 61.

## Bronchiectasis

Irreversible damage by severe respiratory infection may result in permanent dilatation of bronchi associated with production of foul-smelling sputum. Less common than in the past, due to effective use of antibiotics in childhood infections, bronchiectasis is now associated mainly with congenital bronchial abnormalities, cystic fibrosis, asthma, allergic bronchopulmonary aspergillosis and lung tumours. Stagnation of mucus in dilated bronchi predisposes to episodes of infection with further damage to the bronchial tree. Ultimately pulmonary fibrosis and altered vasculature complicate the clinical course of the disease.

### Cytological findings: bronchiectasis

- Sputum may be purulent, mucoid or blood stained
- Neutrophil polymorphs are increased
- In follicular bronchiectasis, lymphocytes predominate
- Hyperplasia of epithelial cells
- Regular or atypical squamous metaplasia.

### Diagnostic pitfalls: bronchiectasis

Hyperplastic bronchial epithelial clusters may be confused with adenocarcinoma cells as in chronic bronchitis. The same criteria can be used to distinguish benign from malignant clusters, but guarded reporting is necessary.

Atypical metaplastic cells (Fig. 2.49) must be distinguished from squamous carcinoma cells, relying on the presence of numerous cells fulfilling the nuclear criteria of malignancy for a diagnosis of carcinoma to be made. Isolated bizarre keratinised cells may be seen in sputum in long-standing bronchiectasis.

## Allergic bronchopulmonary disease

This group of disorders includes extrinsic and intrinsic asthma, allergic bronchopulmonary aspergillosis, eosinophilic pneumonia and extrinsic allergic alveolitis or hypersensitivity pneumonitis. Cytology plays an important role in assessment of asthmatic patients but is less helpful in diagnosing eosinophilic pneumonia and extrinsic allergic alveolitis. The latter two conditions may in time progress to pulmonary fibrosis. There is an overlap in the pathogenesis of these overtly allergic disorders and some fibrosing or granulomatous lung diseases associated with complicated immunological disturbances.

## Bronchial asthma

Although the exact definition is still debated,[123] bronchial asthma is characterised by widespread narrowing of airways, fluctuating over short periods of time, but largely reversible. The underlying mechanism is a type I allergic response to a variety of external or intrinsic allergens which are not always firmly identifiable.

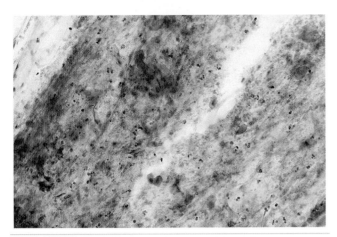

**Fig. 2.49** Bronchiectasis showing inflammatory debris with many degenerate keratinised squamous metaplastic cells arising from the wall of a large bronchiectatic cavity. The nuclei are irregular but do not appear frankly malignant. Sputum (PAP).

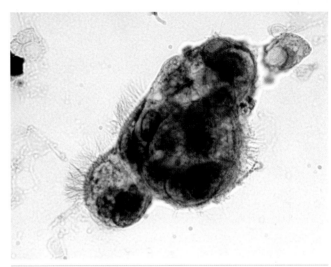

**Fig. 2.51** A large Creola body in the sputum of an asthmatic patient showing the characteristic bunched-up cell grouping, with some cilia visible around the border of the group. Liquid-based preparation (PAP).

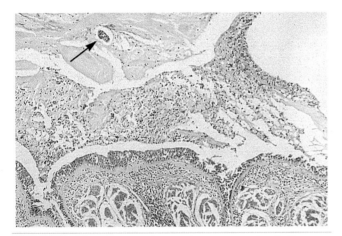

**Fig. 2.50** Bronchus in histological section from a patient who died in status asthmaticus. There is a large plug of mucus in the lumen surrounded by a serous exudate containing inflammatory cells, mainly eosinophils. Fragmentation of mucosa is present and an ovoid cluster of epithelial cells can be seen lying at the upper border (arrow) (H&E).

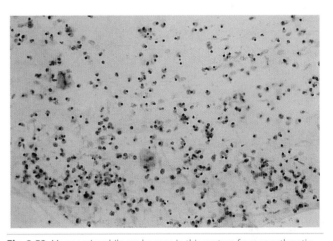

**Fig. 2.52** Many eosinophils can be seen in this sputum from an asthmatic child. They have bilobed or, if degenerate, single-lobed nuclei and the cytoplasm is filled with eosinophilic granules stained by Papanicolaou.

During an acute attack of asthma there is extensive loss of bronchial epithelium, associated with an outpouring of mucus and serous fluid into the bronchial lumen. Many eosinophils are present in this exudate, which forms viscous obstructive mucoid plugs in the airways (Fig. 2.50). The wall of the bronchus is thickened due to oedema; spasm of the smooth muscle also occurs, increasing bronchial obstruction still further.

The changes usually resolve spontaneously or with treatment, although areas of squamous metaplasia may persist, and in some patients collapse and consolidation of the lung parenchyma occurs. Fungal infection may supervene, leading to a type III allergic reaction, with damage to the bronchi and adjacent lung tissue. In Great Britain, *Aspergillus* spp. is the organism most commonly found when this complication occurs.

Characteristic changes in sputum or lavage fluid contribute to the diagnosis of asthma in many cases. However, it should be noted that other allergic diseases such as Churg–Strauss syndrome and polyarteritis nodosa can be associated with an asthmatic presentation both clinically and cytologically.[125]

## Cytological findings: bronchial asthma

- Visible mucus plugs present in lavage fluid
- Many bronchial epithelial cell clusters in sputum (Fig. 2.51)
- Eosinophils and Charcot–Leyden crystals (Figs 2.52, 2.53)
- Curschmann's spirals
- Inflammatory debris may contain fungal hyphae.

Clusters of ciliated bronchial epithelial cells may be papillary or reniform in shape and have well-defined borders due to preservation of the terminal plates. They have come to be known as Creola bodies after a young girl in whom they were reported mistakenly as adenocarcinoma cells.[126]

Eosinophils are usually present. Larger than neutrophil polymorphs, with pink cytoplasmic granules and bilobed nuclei, they are best shown by H&E or MGG stains. Mononuclear or degranulated forms occur, but are not readily identified. Charcot–Leyden crystals may be found in all types of cytological material from asthmatic patients.

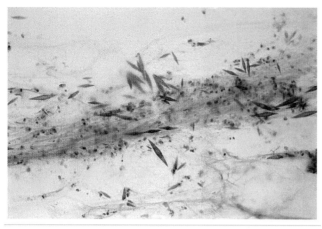

**Fig. 2.53** Charcot–Leyden crystals in sputum from an asthmatic patient showing the characteristic acicular form and bright orange staining (PAP).

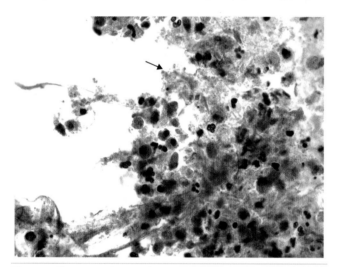

**Fig. 2.54** Charcot–Leyden crystals, eosinophils and poorly stained *Aspergillus* hyphae (arrow) seen (LBC preparation of bronchial washings, PAP stain) from a patient with allergic bronchopulmonary aspergillosis.

They are formed from breakdown of granules of eosinophils. Their acicular octahedral form and bright orange colouration with PAP staining are characteristic and eye-catching. A combination of these findings provides a cytological picture, which is strongly suggestive of bronchial asthma in an appropriate clinical setting.

Amorphous inflammatory debris is sometimes the only finding in the sputum of asthmatics. Careful searching may reveal fragments of Charcot–Leyden crystals in the debris, or fungal elements may occasionally be found (Fig. 2.54). Needle-shaped oxalate crystals arranged in rosettes or wheatsheaf patterns have been noted in sputum and FNA material from cases of aspergillosis associated with asthma. They result from precipitation of oxalic acid, which is produced by the fungus (see Fig. 2.33). They have been regarded as evidence of the presence of *Aspergillus*, even when the fungus itself cannot be identified.[81]

### Diagnostic pitfalls: bronchial asthma

Profuse exfoliation of epithelial clusters always raises the possibility of bronchioloalveolar carcinoma.[126] The presence of cilia at the borders of groups or the terminal bar are helpful benign features. There is generally more nuclear abnormality

in carcinomatous clumps, but the three-dimensional nature of the groups may impair assessment of nuclear detail. As a working principle, it is inadvisable to make a definite diagnosis of this tumour in the presence of a history of asthma. Radiology may help and FNA can provide diagnostic evidence of fungal infection or tumour if a localised lesion is present.

Increased numbers of eosinophils in sputum do not simply equate with a diagnosis of asthma. Increases are also found in conditions such as chronic bronchitis, eosinophilic pneumonia, lung tumours and parasitic infestations.[127]

Fungal elements may be overlooked unless anticipated (Fig. 2.54). They can be sparse and degenerate, or hidden beneath inflammatory debris. Destaining a PAP preparation and re-staining with methenamine silver or making use of cell blocks may reveal the hyphae.

## Non-infective granulomatous lung disease

Infections such as tuberculosis are responsible for most of the treatable granulomatous diseases of lung but there are many other disorders associated with granuloma formation. The common causes are listed in Box 2.1 (p. 30).

Granulomata can sometimes be firmly identified in FNA material whereas in sputum and bronchial brushings the findings are often non-specific. Open lung biopsy, for so long the traditional method of diagnosis, is still often employed to elucidate the nature of granulomatous lung disease. However, FNA combined with microbiological culture has proved valuable in establishing the aetiology of infective granulomata. Bronchoalveolar lavage is, however, useful for monitoring disease progress.

## Sarcoidosis

This is one of the most common of non-infective granulomatous disorders, exemplifying the changes seen in many other idiopathic granulomatous lung conditions.[128] It is a systemic disease of unknown aetiology affecting mainly young or middle-aged patients, especially women. The respiratory tract is involved in over 90% of cases. Cellular immunity is depressed systemically, but there are increased numbers of activated T lymphocytes, especially T helper cells, at sites of granuloma formation. Cytological findings have been documented in sputum,[129] lavage fluid[130] and FNA samples.[131]

### Cytological findings: sarcoidosis

- Epithelioid histiocytes
- Small and large giant cells, some of Langhans type
- Increased lymphocytes, especially T helper cells
- There is no necrosis.

Epithelioid histiocytes are the most characteristic feature, either dissociated or in clusters of spindle-shaped cells with pale cytoplasm and elongated footprint-shaped nuclei (Fig. 2.55). Single cells are more often seen in sputum and washings, whereas in FNA smears, ragged fragments of intact granulomata may be found.

Large and small multinucleated giant cells of histiocytic origin accompany the mononuclear cells. They are often of Langhans giant cell type, with nuclei orientated at one pole of the cell,

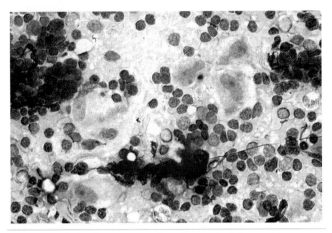

**Fig. 2.55** Epithelioid histiocytes and lymphocytes in FNA material from a middle-aged woman with a lung shadowing due to pulmonary and hilar lymph node sarcoidosis. Note the elongated pale footprint-shaped nuclei of the epithelioid cells and their poorly stained cytoplasm (MGG).

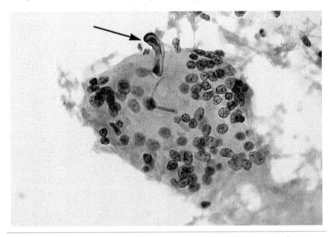

**Fig. 2.56** Multinucleated giant cell in a bronchial brushing sample from a patient with sarcoidosis. The cytoplasm contains a partly dislodged Schaumann body, seen at the upper border of the cell (arrow) (PAP). (Courtesy of Professor B. Naylor, Michigan.)

their cytoplasm devoid of any ingested carbon particles. Occasionally crystalline cytoplasmic inclusions are visible, either in the form of large conchoidal structures known as Schaumann bodies (Fig. 2.56), or smaller star-shaped asteroids. Inclusions are more readily seen in cell blocks prepared from FNA material than in direct spreads, but they have also been noted in sputum.

Lymphocytes may be found in abundance, especially in lavage fluid, reflecting a profuse lymphocytic exudate into the alveoli while the disease is active. The lymphocytes are predominantly of T cell type, constituting 10–70% of the inflammatory cell population, and are mainly T helper cells. Healthy non-smokers have levels below 7%.[132] The ratio of lymphocytes to neutrophil polymorphs, macrophages and other inflammatory cells in lavage fluid is helpful in supporting the diagnosis of sarcoidosis and in monitoring response to treatment or progression of the disease.[133] There is no necrosis.

### Diagnostic pitfalls: sarcoidosis

- Polarised light for foreign material
- Epithelioid cells mimic connective tissue cells on FNA
- Abundant necrotic material is unlikely to be due to sarcoidosis.

A diagnosis of sarcoidosis can only be made in the appropriate clinical setting since other granulomatous disorders may produce an identical picture cytologically. Infective causes of granulomatous lung disease must always be excluded by stains for acid fast bacilli, fungi and other organisms, and culture of the sample is essential. Lavage and FNA specimens may have to be divided to provide material for culture.

Foreign body reactions should be excluded by examination of the material under polarised light. Granuloma formation due to substances such as beryllium or aluminium can be excluded in this way, as can silicosis. Carbon pigment in the giant cells suggests they are not derived from a granulomatous process.

Elongated epithelioid histiocytes may be confused with connective tissue cells in FNA material. Microarchitecture may still be discernible in granulomas, in contrast to the dispersed pattern of connective tissue cells. Moreover, the footprint nuclei of epithelioid cells are unlike the elliptical and spindle-shaped nuclei of fibroblasts or smooth muscle cells.

FNA samples containing significant amounts of necrotic debris accompanying granulomatous material are unlikely to have originated from sarcoidosis. Tuberculosis and necrotic tumour tissue are more usual sources and keratinising squamous carcinomas frequently evoke a foreign body giant cell response.

## Other granulomatous diseases

Several other less common granulomatous lung conditions have yielded cytological material enabling the correct diagnosis to be proposed. These include connective tissue diseases such as rheumatoid arthritis, systemic lupus erythematosus and scleroderma, and inflammatory disorders of blood vessels in which vasculitis is the primary lesion.

The connective tissue diseases, thought to be due to autoimmune and immune complex mediated injury to collagen, are associated with a variety of pulmonary manifestations including granulomatous inflammation, pulmonary fibrosis and pleural effusions.[134] Cytological findings are variable and are only of use in diagnosis in the light of the clinical features.

Localised granuloma formation in rheumatoid arthritis can be mistaken for malignancy radiologically when there is central necrosis and cavitation. Atypical metaplasia has been found in samples from rheumatoid patients and this, together with background necrosis, may suggest a carcinoma. Strict criteria of malignancy must be sought.

Vasculitis may be a component of many different lung disorders including collagen diseases. However, there are several conditions in which vasculitis, necrosis and a granulomatous pulmonary infiltrate are the main features. Wegener's granulomatosis is the most common, producing multiple fluctuating lesions in lungs, nasal passages and kidneys. The Churg–Strauss syndrome also forms part of this spectrum.

Wegener's granulomatosis has been suggested on FNA findings by the presence of fragmented eosinophilic granular necrotic collagen, aggregates of palisaded histiocytes including some giant cells, and an acute inflammatory cell infiltrate.[135] Specific confirmation of the diagnosis can be made serologically using the ANCA test, based on the recognition of an antineutrophil cytoplasmic antibody. Confirmatory ANCA testing should be prompted by the above cytological findings when the clinical setting is appropriate.

## Diffuse parenchymal lung disease (DPLD)

DPLD, also known as interstitial lung disease, is a heterogeneous group of non-neoplastic lung disorders characterised by variable patterns of inflammation and fibrosis which result in varying degrees of restrictive ventilatory impairment.[136] As a general principle, persistent inflammation in any organ is accompanied by fibrosis, and in the lung, 25% of which is composed of fibrous tissue, pulmonary fibrosis is the common end result of many different disease processes, some of which are listed in Box 2.3.

The classification of pulmonary fibrosis (Box 2.4) has evolved over time as new information about the pathogenesis of the differing patterns has emerged.[137] The most recent classification has moved away from regarding histopathology as the 'gold standard' of diagnosis for most cases, instead emphasising that diagnosis is a dynamic process which may change with time as clinical progression becomes apparent. Diagnosis is therefore dependent on a multidisciplinary assessment incorporating in particular the clinical history, physical examination findings and a high-resolution CT scan.[138]

Fibrosis of the lung develops either within alveolar spaces following active inflammation, resulting in fibrosing alveolitis (Fig. 2.57), or in the alveolar walls leading to interstitial fibrosis (Fig. 2.58). In many patients both processes occur simultaneously. The onset may be acute and severe as in the Hamman–Rich syndrome, or insidious with gradual progression, the common course in idiopathic pulmonary fibrosis. An important subgroup includes patients with cryptogenic organising pneumonia in whom low-grade inflammation and tongues or nodules of loose fibrosis affect the small airways. These cases respond to steroid therapy, as do some patients with idiopathic fibrosing alveolitis (usual interstitial pneumonia).

Bronchoalveolar lavage (BAL) may be performed as part of the initial diagnostic work-up but this is not always the case. Lung biopsy is now only performed in a minority of cases where the findings are atypical or inconclusive. In most cases cytology cannot determine the cause of the disease process but some indication as to prognosis and effectiveness of treatment may be obtained by monitoring inflammatory cell ratios in bronchoalveolar lavage fluid.

---

### Box 2.3  Conditions associated with pulmonary fibrosis

Industrial diseases
- Silicosis
- Coal worker's pneumoconiosis (massive pulmonary fibrosis)
- Asbestosis
- Heavy metal exposure
- Organic dusts exposure

Immune disorders
- Rheumatoid disease
- Systemic sclerosis
- Dermatomyositis
- Sjögren's syndrome
- Coeliac disease

End-stage granulomatous disease
- Sarcoidosis
- Fungal infections
- Mycobacterial infections
- Viral infections
- Mycoplasma pneumonia

Iatrogenic causes
- Cytotoxic antibiotics
- Alkylating agents
- Antimetabolites
- Antirheumatic drugs
- Radiation therapy
- Oxygen toxicity

Direct lung injury
- Adult respiratory distress syndrome
- Paraquat poisoning

Idiopathic conditions
- Fibrosing alveolitis
- Bronchiolitis obliterans
- Organising pneumonia
- Pulmonary haemosiderosis
- Histiocytosis X
- Alveolar proteinosis

---

### Box 2.4  Classification of diffuse parenchymal lung disease (DPLD)

1. DPLD of known cause, e.g. drugs, collagen-vascular disease
2. Idiopathic interstitial pneumonia, e.g. idiopathic pulmonary fibrosis and histological variants
3. Granulomatous, e.g. sarcoidosis
4. Environmental/occupational, e.g. mineral pneumoconioses
5. Others, e.g. lymphangioleiomyomatosis, Langerhans cell histiocytosis

(Modified from Corrin and Nicholson: Pathology of the Lungs. 2nd ed. Churchill Livingstone; 2006: 264, with permission of Elsevier.)

---

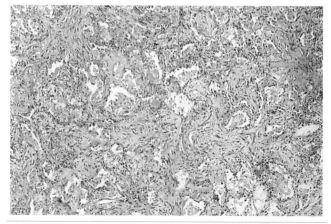

**Fig. 2.57** Fibrosing alveolitis and cryptogenic organising pneumonitis in a section of lung. Most of the alveolar spaces are filled with loose nodular connective tissue, which can be seen extending along alveolar ducts (H&E).

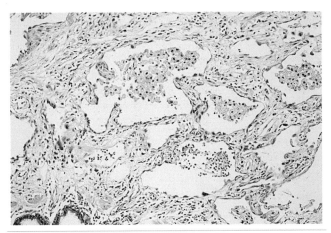

**Fig. 2.58** Section of lung with idiopathic interstitial fibrosis. The alveolar walls are thickened by fibrous tissue and alveolar epithelium is prominent. A few inflammatory cells and macrophages can be seen in the distorted alveolar spaces (H&E).

## Role of BAL in diffuse interstitial pulmonary disease (DIPD)

In most cases, BAL is no more than supportive when classifying the cause of idiopathic interstitial pneumonia (IIP). However, it is often performed during the initial diagnostic work-up when the diagnosis of IIP is being established. At this point, other important diagnoses such as infections, sarcoidosis, pulmonary alveola proteinosis and diffuse malignancy require consideration. Details of the relevant features of these conditions are covered in separate sections of this chapter. Accurate quantification of cells requires meticulous attention to detail. The first aliquot of fluid is discarded as it is contaminated with bronchial content. Subsequent material is prepared by cytocentrifugation or membrane filtration. Liquid-based techniques are not appropriate because of selective loss of cells and also because MGG staining is necessary for accurate inflammatory cell differential counts.

### Cytological findings: DIPD

#### Inflammatory cell changes

- Predominance of polymorphs with associated mononuclear cell increase
- Predominance of lymphocytes with no polymorphs
- Predominance of macrophages, often containing golden, brown or black pigment
- Eosinophilia.

There is an extensive historical literature on the analysis of inflammatory cell content following descriptions of techniques in the early 1980s, relating changes to the two broad groups seen on histology.[138] Of the four broad groups of inflammatory cell components described above, neutrophil predominance, often with a lesser increase in macrophages and lymphocytes, is typical of usual interstitial pneumonia, diffuse alveolar damage, occupational dust disease and collagen-vascular disorders. Lymphocyte predominance is typical of non-specific interstitia; pneumonia, cryptogenic organising pneumonia, lymphoid interstitial pneumonia, sarcoidosis and extrinsic allergic alveolitis. Macrophage predominance is seen in respiratory bronchiolitis and desquamative interstitial pneumonia, while eosinophilia may occur in asthma, eosinophilic pneumonia and allergic bronchopulmonary aspergillosis.

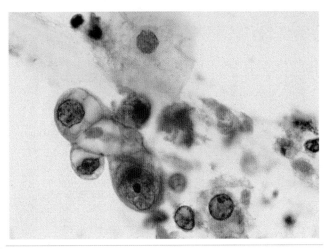

**Fig. 2.59** Hyperplasia of type II pneumocytes. These cells are from a BAL specimen in a patient with idiopathic pulmonary fibrosis. There were moderate numbers of single and paired enlarged rectangular, rounded or polygonal cells with nuclear changes regarded at the time of reporting as suspicious of malignancy. Subsequent post-mortem examination showed atypical alveolar cell hyperplasia accompanying the fibrosis, but no tumour was found (PAP).

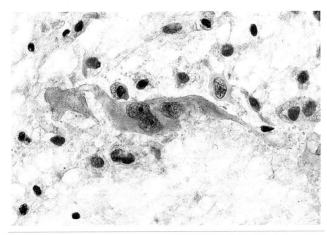

**Fig. 2.60** Fibrosing alveolitis. This imprint smear was prepared from the lung section of fibrosing alveolitis shown in Figure 2.57. Solitary bizarre cells with atypical nuclei such as shown here, reflect the alveolar cell hyperplasia seen on histology (Toluidine blue).

#### Epithelial cell changes

- Hyperplasia with atypia of bronchial epithelium (Figs 2.59–2.61)
- Atypia and degenerative changes in type II pneumocytes.

Longstanding pulmonary fibrosis is frequently associated with abnormalities of bronchial and alveolar epithelial cells regardless of the underlying cause. Type I pneumocytes undergo necrosis at an early stage, to be replaced by type II pneumocytes which enlarge, become cuboidal and eventually atypical. Bronchiolar epithelium also undergoes reactive and hyperplastic changes, and may extend to line the fibrosed alveolar spaces.

These epithelial cells sometimes show striking nuclear changes, with enlargement, hyperchromasia, prominent nucleoli and heavily stained nuclear membranes (Figs 2.59, 2.60). Multinucleation may be seen. Bronchial cells are shed in larger clusters (Fig. 2.61) than alveolar cells, which are generally in twos and threes or present as single cells. The

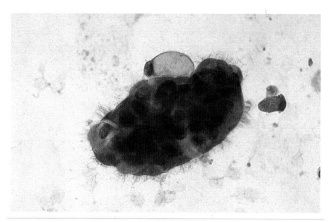

**Fig. 2.61** Fibrosing alveolitis. A clump of hyperplastic epithelial cells with a fringe of cilia visible along the outer border. Although the group is too dense for assessment of nuclear detail, the presence of cilia indicates that it is benign (PAP).

distinction may, however, not always be obvious, especially when cytoplasmic degeneration has occurred.

The appearances may bear a close resemblance to the cytology of malignancy as described more fully later in this chapter (see p. 72), and these changes form a well-recognised source of false positive diagnosis. To complicate the situation, peripheral lung tumours are prone to develop in longstanding pulmonary fibrosis. The problem of differentiating hyperplasia from malignancy is more likely to arise with sputum and bronchial secretions than in FNA material, where a pure population of tumour cells gives a diagnostic picture.

### Diagnostic pitfalls: DIPD

A profusion of epithelial cell clusters in respiratory tract samples from patients with diffuse radiological shadowing or a known diagnosis of pulmonary fibrosis should be reported with caution. In general, numerous clusters containing many cells are more suggestive of malignancy, whereas smaller groupings and single cells are more typical of alveolar cell hyperplasia.

The presence of cilia around the periphery of cell clumps indicates a reactive rather than a neoplastic process (Fig. 2.61). Swollen cells with enlarged nuclei found in cases of pulmonary fibrosis usually still maintain a fairly normal nuclear/cytoplasmic ratio compared with adenocarcinoma cells. A marked inflammatory cell component in this setting should raise the possibility of a reactive condition, although the finding by no means excludes tumour. Where the findings are highly suspicious of malignancy but the diagnosis is not confirmed, monitoring the patient over time may reveal a bronchioloalveolar cell carcinoma in a few cases, an example of a false 'false positive' diagnosis.[139]

## Specific types of pulmonary fibrosis

Certain types of lung damage eventually leading to pulmonary fibrosis will be described in further detail since the onset of fibrosis is preceded or accompanied by important cytological findings. These conditions include drug-induced toxicity, radiotherapy, other iatrogenic changes and industrial lung disease due to toxic chemicals or dusts.

---

### Box 2.5  Some drugs associated with pulmonary toxicity

| Non-cytotoxic drugs | Cytotoxic drugs |
|---|---|
| **Antibacterial agents** | **Cytotoxic antibiotics** |
| • Nitrofurantoin | • Bleomycin |
| • Sulphalazine | • Mitomycin |
| | • Cyclosporin A |
| **Analgesics** | **Nitrosoureas** |
| • Aspirin | • Carmustine |
| **Anticonvulsants** | |
| | **Alkylating agents** |
| **Antiarrhythmic agents** | • Busulphan |
| • Amiodarone | • Cyclophosphamide |
| | • Chlorambucil |
| **Antirheumatic drugs** | • Melphalan |
| • Penicillamine | |
| • Gold salts | **Antimetabolites** |
| • Colchicine | • Methotrexate |
| | • Azathioprine |
| **Diuretics** | • Cytosine arabinoside |
| **Opiates** | |
| | **Other cytotoxic drugs** |
| **Sympathomimetics** | • Procarbazine |
| **Tranquillisers** | • Vinca alkaloids |

---

## Drug-induced pulmonary toxicity

Therapeutic agents may injure the lung directly by cytotoxic effects or a hypersensitivity reaction, or may induce systemic conditions which in turn are associated with damage to the lung.[140] An example of the latter type of iatrogenic disease is the systemic lupus erythematosus syndrome induced by drugs such as hydralazine, procainamide or phenytoin.[141]

Direct toxic effects exerted on bronchiolar or alveolar cells by various compounds and hypersensitivity drug reactions causing alveolitis form an important group for cytologists since early recognition of these treatment complications can be life-saving. Some of the earliest accounts of these effects related to the use of bleomycin and busulphan in such patients.[142] The most severe lung damage is due to cytotoxic drugs used as chemotherapy for tumours, particularly haematological malignancies.[143] Many other drugs have also been found to cause diffuse lung damage or pulmonary fibrosis as a side effect of their therapeutic action (Box 2.5). Assessment of specimens for drug-induced lung disease is often complicated by the use of multiple drug therapy.

### Cytological findings: drug-induced pulmonary toxicity

- Atypical alveolar and bronchiolar cells (Figs 2.62, 2.63)
- Inflammatory debris
- Regenerative epithelium in sheets
- Lymphocytes and eosinophils in hypersensitivity pneumonitis.

A clear history of drug exposure is necessary for diagnosis. In multiple drug therapy, identification of the responsible agent

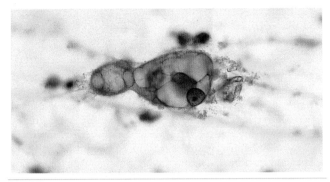

**Fig. 2.62** Atypical type II pneumocytes in bronchoalveolar lavage fluid from a young man with acute lymphoblastic leukaemia. He was receiving *Cyclosporin* therapy and had developed breathlessness with diffuse lung shadowing. Note the degenerative vacuolation of cytoplasm and the enlarged abnormal nuclei with prominent nucleoli (PAP).

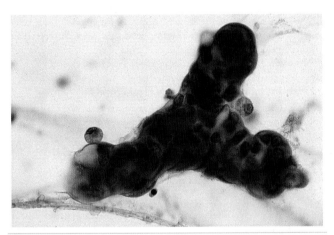

**Fig. 2.63** Hyperplastic epithelial cells from the case shown in Figure 2.62. This is a large three-dimensional group of cells and is therefore likely to be bronchial in origin. Nuclei are difficult to examine but appear enlarged and hyperchromatic (PAP).

is not usually possible from the cytological findings alone, but requires accurate clinical correlation.

Swollen polygonal or rectangular epithelial cells are present in modest numbers, scattered singly, paired or in small groups (Fig. 2.62 and see Fig. 2.80). They have dense greenish grey cytoplasm, often showing degenerative vacuolation. The nuclei are enlarged and have prominent nucleoli, with condensation of chromatin on the nuclear membrane. They may be hyperchromatic or depleted of chromatin. Cell groups are flat and often acinar in arrangement. A spectrum of changes is seen, including complete disintegration of the nucleus, leaving anucleate cytoplasmic remnants.

The origin of these cells has been investigated by electron microscopy, revealing type II pneumocytes with degeneration of lamellar bodies and cytoplasmic degranulation.[144] Type I pneumocytes undergo necrosis at an early stage of exposure, accompanied by oedema and haemorrhage. Other evidence of damage to the epithelium of the airways is sometimes present in the early stages, consisting of inflammatory and necrotic debris, with ragged sheets of regenerative inflamed bronchial epithelium composed of swollen cells with enlarged nuclei and prominent nucleoli (Fig. 2.63).

The inflammatory cell component in lavage fluid is variable, depending on the nature of the damage and the drug. In cases of drug-induced hypersensitivity pneumonitis, there are many lymphocytes and eosinophils. Increased neutrophils are seen in lavage fluid in reactions to a variety of drugs, including gold therapy.[145]

An unusual cytological picture has been documented with the antiarrhythmic drug amiodorone[146] which, in addition to causing damage to pneumocytes and pulmonary fibrosis, also produces changes in alveolar macrophages. In lavage fluid the macrophages comprise up to 85% of the cell population and develop pale lacy cytoplasm due to the presence of numerous osmiophilic inclusion bodies, derived from damaged lysosomes. A recent study of multivesiculated macrophages in FNA material from lung masses found a case of Amiodorone exposure in which 95% of macrophages showed multivesiculation and this was also present in other cells in the sample.[147] This toxic effect is seen in 6% of patients receiving the drug and may be associated with pleural effusions containing similar macrophages.

## Oxygen toxicity

Therapeutic use of oxygen for patients, including neonates, needing artificial ventilation results in alveolar damage proportionate to the concentration of oxygen rather than the duration of exposure. There is initial oedema, haemorrhage and hyaline membrane formation in the alveoli, with necrosis of type I pneumocytes. Pulmonary fibrosis may ensue.[144]

### Cytological findings: oxygen toxicity

- Atypical type II pneumocytes
- Groups of hyperplastic bronchial and bronchiolar cells
- Squamous metaplastic cells.

Shedding of atypical type II pneumocytes, arranged singly, in pairs and in small groups, is similar to the pattern found in other toxic lung reactions. Hyperplasia of bronchial and bronchiolar cells leads to exfoliation of cell clusters which may be ciliated. These are found in many reactive conditions due to chronic benign lung disease. Squamous metaplasia of bronchial mucosa is seen and samples may include atypical metaplastic cells as the changes progress.

## Radiation effects

Despite recent refinements in radiological techniques, the use of radiotherapy in the treatment of intrathoracic tumours is still associated with the risk of cytotoxic effects on the epithelial cells of airways and alveoli. The changes cause diagnostic problems, particularly when monitoring for tumour recurrence. Radiotherapy for tumours outside the thorax, such as breast or head and neck cancers, is less likely to injure the lungs, but it should be noted that cell damage is not necessarily confined to the area directly irradiated.

Histologically, within a day or two of irradiation the bronchial epithelial cells and type I pneumocytes undergo necrosis; there is an outpouring of haemorrhagic oedema fluid with hyaline membrane formation. Type II pneumocytes undergo hyperplasia and subsequently may transform into type I cells. They may also become increasingly atypical in cases of severe damage, with progression to fibrosis.[148]

### Cytological findings: radiation effects

- All epithelial cell types affected
- Swelling of cytoplasm, bizarre shapes, enlarged nuclei
- Cytoplasmic vacuolation and amphophilia
- Multinucleation and macronucleoli
- Metaplasia and dysplasia in later stages.

Squamous, columnar and alveolar epithelial cells are affected and the changes are of a similar nature in each cell type. Cytomegaly and nuclear enlargement go hand-in-hand, maintaining a nuclear/cytoplasmic ratio that is either normal or only slightly raised. Multinucleation is a frequent finding, with coarse but uniform chromatin and multiple irregular nucleoli or macronucleoli. Cytoplasmic degenerative changes consist of fine or gross vacuolation of cell cytoplasm and variable staining (see Fig. 2.86, p. 63).

Squamous metaplasia is seen in the healing phase and may persist for many years. Atypical features in metaplastic or alveolar cells can regress or become more pronounced with time.

### Diagnostic pitfalls: radiation effects

- A false positive diagnosis of malignancy may be made.
- Tumour recurrence may be masked.

The presence of nuclear and cytoplasmic changes in many different cell types is a pointer to the correct diagnosis, as is the relatively normal nuclear:cytoplasmic ratio. Knowledge of the patient's treatment and of the histology of the tumour treated by radiotherapy are clearly also important.

Radiation changes may camouflage malignant cells from a tumour recurrence. A high nuclear:cytoplasmic ratio and irregular distribution of preserved chromatin are features of malignancy and are not part of the usual spectrum of radiation changes.

## Diffuse alveolar damage (acute respiratory distress syndrome)

This serious form of lung damage was first described by Ashbaugh and associates in 1967 at which time it carried a mortality rate of nearly 70%.[149] The mortality remains over 50% despite progress in understanding the underlying mechanisms.[150] The syndrome follows conditions such as severe trauma, pancreatitis or septicaemia, developing within 1–3 days of these catastrophic states, with the onset of acute pulmonary oedema and inflammation, accompanied by proliferation of type II pneumocytes and fibroblasts. Local release of highly reactive free oxygen radicals and of enzymes such as proteases from neutrophils are postulated to cause direct damage to the lung parenchyma. Rapidly progressive pulmonary fibrosis may follow.

The cytological findings in adult respiratory distress syndrome have been recorded by Grotte et al.[151] who describe exfoliation of clusters of hyperplastic bronchoalveolar cells as seen in many other types of lung damage. It is important to distinguish such groups from adenocarcinoma cells, given the

clinical setting. Occasionally fragments of hyaline membrane can be seen, providing an important diagnostic clue.

## Organ transplantation

The lung is the seat of many of the complications arising in patients who have had organ transplantation, regardless of the nature of the transplant. The risks have been reviewed by Ettinger and Trulock[152] and the findings in bronchoalveolar lavage fluid have been documented by Selvaggi (see Ch. 15).[153]

Infectious complications generally relate to the degree of immunosuppression required to prevent rejection of the graft, whereas non-infectious conditions arise either from mechanical problems due to surgery or result from the direct toxic effects of the treatment regime. Graft versus host disease or transplant rejection may supervene. Opportunistic infections, of which the most common are CMV and *Pneumocystis carinii* pneumonia, herpes simplex virus infection and aspergillosis, have been considered earlier in this chapter and are also discussed in Chapter 16.

Non-infectious complications such as adult respiratory distress syndrome, cyclosporin A toxicity, bronchiolitis obliterans and, in the longer term, pulmonary fibrosis, may all have cytological manifestations. These are mainly seen in bronchoalveolar lavage fluid and the findings, frequently non-specific, have already been described in this chapter. Accurate clinical details are necessary to interpret the findings correctly.

## Occupational lung disease

## Industrial exposure to chemicals

Toxic chemicals such as insecticides have been implicated in the pathogenesis of pulmonary fibrosis. Damage to the alveolar lining cells is followed by changes similar to those seen in oxygen toxicity described above, posing the same diagnostic problems for the cytologist.

## Exposure to organic dusts

Organic dusts can induce pulmonary fibrosis in susceptible individuals. Originally described in 1958 as farmer's lung, the underlying mechanism is a hypersensitivity pneumonitis, also known as extrinsic allergic alveolitis. It is an industrial hazard in a wide range of occupations in which there is exposure to moulds or animal proteins. The condition may resolve on treatment or progress to pulmonary fibrosis. Histologically, lymphocytic alveolitis and chronic interstitial inflammation are seen, with the formation of small non-caseating granulomata.[154] The cytological findings vary with the stage of the disease. Lavage specimens show a raised lymphocyte count with an excess of T suppressor cells and sometimes of cytotoxic T cells.[155] Specific antibodies, immune complexes and complement components are also detectable in lavage fluid. Later, hyperplastic or atypical type II pneumocytes may appear as pulmonary fibrosis supervenes. The changes are non-specific and a firm diagnosis can only be achieved by clinicopathological correlation.

## Mineral pneumoconioses

Various pneumoconioses result from inhalation of dusts, gases or mineral fibres. This is an important group of occupational lung diseases, not least because there is often a question of industrial compensation. A range of pathological changes are known to occur, including fibrosis, cavitation, granulomatous inflammation, progressive massive fibrosis, asthma, emphysema, alveolar proteinosis and an increased risk of neoplasia.[156] These diverse responses vary with the nature of the exposure, its duration and the interplay with other factors such as cigarette smoking. A comprehensive account of these aspects of occupational lung disease has been given by Churg and Green.[157]

Cytology can be used to monitor the inflammatory cell ratios in lavage fluid in pneumoconiosis associated with fibrosis. In addition, refractile particulate material may be apparent in the cytoplasm of macrophages in respiratory specimens. These particles can be identified specifically using electron probes and other procedures.[156] Lavage fluid from cases of silicosis and other related pneumoconioses shows raised levels of polymorphs initially and may also have increased numbers of lymphocytes and macrophages. Type II pneumocytes appear in the fluid later in small numbers and may become atypical. Historically, Davison and associates have described lavage findings in hard-metal workers; the changes included the presence of many macrophages, with some increase in eosinophils and lymphocytes. Bizarre giant cells were seen, derived from both macrophages and type II pneumocytes, diminishing on treatment and with cessation of exposure.[28]

## Asbestosis

This is one of the few mineral-related lung diseases in which the fibres may be recognised in routine cytological preparations. Most cases result from industrial exposure but in a few patients it is difficult to establish this link; domestic exposure is known to account for a small proportion of the remainder. All types of asbestos are capable of causing pulmonary fibrosis, but the risk varies, being greater for crocidolite and amosite than for chrysotile, and also related to both duration and extent of exposure.[158] In addition to diffuse fibrosis, asbestos is associated with development of mesothelioma, pleural plaque formation and benign recurrent effusions as described in Chapter 3; there is also an increased incidence of bronchial carcinoma.

### Cytological findings: asbestosis

- Long, pointed fibres, variable sizes, may be fragmented or curved
- Dumbell or drumstick-shaped, beaded
- Golden brown coating of iron
- Other mineral fibres appear similar when coated (ferruginous bodies).

Asbestos fibres are composed of variable proportions of silica, magnesium and iron. They vary in length and shape in their natural state, chrysotile being smaller and curved in contrast to the more solid larger fibres of the amphibole group. Fibres measuring up to 5 μm are usually cleared from the lungs without causing disease, whereas longer ones are phagocytosed by alveolar macrophages. They are then coated with protein and iron to produce inactivated fibres known as ferruginous or asbestos bodies. These structures are up to 200 μm in length and are usually dumbbell, beaded or drumstick in shape, their golden brown coating concentrated on the pointed ends of the fibres (Fig. 2.64). Similar deposits may form around other mineral fibres, hence the more general term ferruginous bodies.[43,159]

Identification of large numbers of typical asbestos bodies in respiratory samples from patients with pulmonary fibrosis provides strong evidence of an aetiological association.[160] Even in small numbers, asbestos bodies should be regarded as an

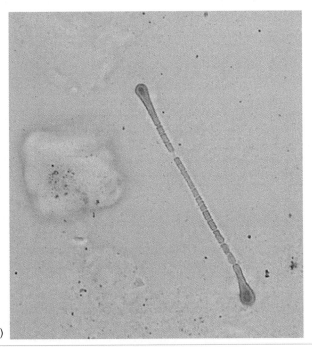

(A)

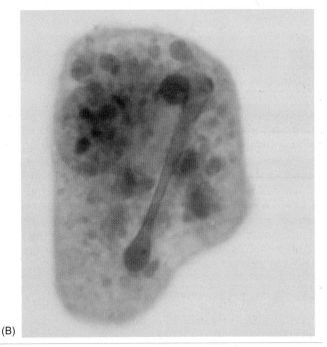

(B)

**Fig. 2.64** (A) Asbestos fibre in sputum. Note the golden brown coating with expansions at the two ends. In the second example (B) the asbestos body lies within a macrophage (PAP).

important finding in any cytological preparation, including FNA material. However, Leiman has pointed out that asbestos bodies in FNA material are commonly a marker for conditions other than asbestosis, such as carcinoma, lung abscess or tuberculosis.[161]

## Other benign pulmonary conditions

### Thromboembolism

Cytological changes in thromboembolic disease can be independent of whether or not actual infarction of the lung parenchyma has occurred. The abnormalities may be seen in sputum, washings or FNA samples and can cause problems in differentiating from malignancy.[162]

#### Cytological findings: thromboembolism

- Blood-stained sputum
- Haemosiderin laden macrophages
- Hyperplastic epithelial cell groups
- Squamous metaplasia.

Sputum may be frankly bloodstained in the early stages if infarction occurs. This is followed by the appearance of macrophages laden with brown haemosiderin pigment as the blood is broken down.

Hyperplasia of bronchoalveolar epithelium is a notable feature, although of uncertain origin. The cells are rounded and swollen and show enlarged hyperchromatic nuclei with prominent nucleoli. Clusters vary from three or four cells up to much larger collections in which cell details are difficult to visualise. Squamous metaplasia occurs as organisation proceeds and may be atypical.

#### Diagnostic pitfalls: thromboembolism

There is a risk of false positive diagnosis of malignancy if clusters of hyperplastic epithelial cells are not assessed correctly. Attention to nuclear details and the presence of other features such as iron-laden macrophages will reduce the likelihood of this mistake. This is a diagnosis that may be missed for want of consideration.

### Congestive cardiac failure

Left ventricular failure from whatever cause subjects the lungs to congestion which if persistent leads to microscopic haemorrhage into alveoli. Degradation of the blood then occurs and is associated with accumulation of haemosiderin-laden macrophages in the alveoli. These cells may be expectorated in large numbers or found in lavage or FNA material. Sputum samples are sometimes submitted specifically requesting detection of such cells for confirmation of heart failure as a cause of wheezing and shortness of breath, so-called cardiac asthma.

#### Cytological findings: congestive cardiac failure

- Watery sputum, or tinged with blood
- Haemosiderin laden macrophages (heart failure cells) (Fig. 2.65)
- Perl's stain confirms the nature of the pigment.

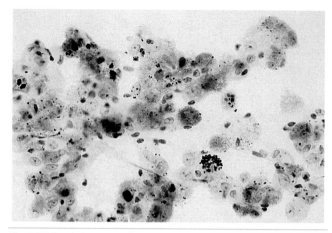

**Fig. 2.65** Iron-laden macrophages seen in sputum, stained by Perl's Prussian blue method. The sample is from a patient with congestive cardiac failure. Black carbon pigment is also visible. (Perl's stain).

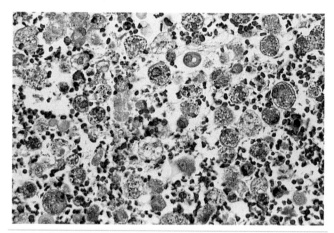

**Fig. 2.66** Many iron-laden macrophages in bronchoalveolar lavage fluid from a patient with Goodpasture's syndrome. The iron pigment is coarsely clumped and golden brown in colour (PAP). (Courtesy of Professor B. Naylor, Michigan.)

#### Diagnostic pitfalls: congestive cardiac failure

Other types of pigment must be excluded. Carbon, in black or dark brown granules, is the most common pigment in respiratory samples, obscuring iron if deposition is heavy. Iron laden macrophages identical to heart failure cells can be seen after pulmonary infarcts, in idiopathic pulmonary haemosiderosis and Goodpasture's syndrome, (Figs 2.66, 2.67) and in patients with a haemorrhagic diathesis.

### Lipoid pneumonitis

Inflammation of lung parenchyma due to the presence of lipid substances is generally the result of either local obstruction to a bronchus with accumulation of lipoidal tissue breakdown products distally, or to inhalation or aspiration of oily material.[163] These are known as endogenous and exogenous lipoid pneumonitis, respectively.

Exogenous sources include industrial oil inhalation and the risk of an iatrogenic origin from medications such as nose drops. The most common cause of endogenous lipoid pneumonia

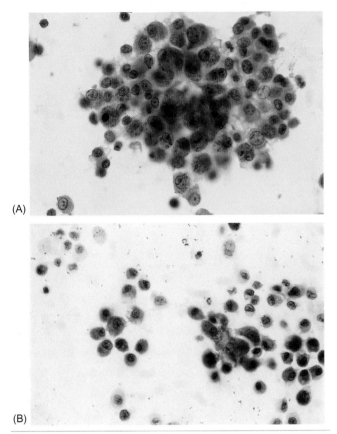

(A)

(B)

**Fig. 2.67** (A,B) Bronchoalveolar lavage fluid from a 1-year-old child with idiopathic haemosiderosis. Only the macrophages containing iron take up the Prussian blue stain. (A, PAP; B, Perl's stain).

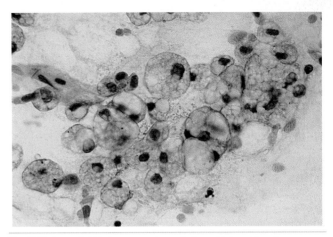

**Fig. 2.68** Large lipid-laden macrophages in bronchial washings from a patient with lipoid pneuminitis. Their cytoplasmic vacuoles show considerable variation in size and shape and some multinucleation can be seen. A few other inflammatory cells are also present (PAP). (Courtesy of Professor B. Naylor, Michigan.)

is an obstructing bronchial tumour, but there are also iatrogenic endogenous causes, for instance postoperative bronchial obstruction or due to embolisation of contrast medium to the lungs. Amiodarone toxicity is associated with accumulation of phospholipids in lung and other tissues.

The hallmark of lipoid pneumonitis, whatever the cause, is the presence of lipid-laden macrophages and pools of free lipid in the alveoli and interstitial tissues. Other inflammatory cells are almost always present, and the inflammation may become granulomatous. Cholesterol clefts from cell breakdown are seen when bronchial obstruction is present.

Multiple therapeutic BAL procedures for children with lipoid pneumonia result in significant improvement of CT findings, oxygen saturation, restoration of BAL fluid cellularity and clinical improvement.[164]

## Cytological findings: lipoid pneumonitis

- Vacuolated swollen macrophages (Fig. 2.68)
- Giant cells
- A mixed inflammatory background.

Sputum findings were originally described by Losner et al. in 1950.[165] Lavage fluid findings have also been documented.[166] Characteristically, there are numerous vacuolated fat laden macrophages, including multinucleated forms, which may have bizarre shapes and copious cytoplasm. The presence of fat can be confirmed by oil red-O staining. Other inflammatory cells may be present, in varying numbers, and in cases due to an obstructing tumour malignant cells may be seen.

## Diagnostic pitfalls: lipoid pneumonitis

Small droplets of fat in macrophages may be seen in sputum from many patients without signifying lipoid pneumonia. Cigarette smokers are especially prone to show this. The paucity of fat and absence of bizarre multinucleated cells ensure that the conditions are not usually confused. Pneumonia due to aspiration of food may include fatty material but there is usually evidence of mixed aspiration including plant products and bacterial contamination.[167]

Bizarre vacuolated cells may be mistaken for malignancy, notably adenocarcinoma or liposarcoma. The former error can be avoided by staining for fat, while the rare occurrence of liposarcoma in lung is associated with only few abnormal tumour cells and the cells show greater nuclear pleomorphism.

Fat-laden macrophages can be found transiently in sputum in some conditions without progressing to pneumonitis. An example of this is seen with fat embolism after fractures or orthopaedic surgery, when fat is released into the venous circulation and thence deposited in the lungs. Sputum examination in such patients almost invariably reveals the presence of free lipid or some fat in macrophages, which is of no consequence clinically unless massive enough to induce pulmonary oedema or allow the passage of the fat into the systemic circulation.

## Talc granuloma

Foreign material, such as particles of talc, trapped in pulmonary vessels after intravenous injection of substances mixed with talc as a base, evoke a granulomatous inflammatory reaction in the lung parenchyma, leading to diffuse or focal nodular radiological shadowing. These lesions may be investigated by FNA, yielding non-specific inflammation with or without granulomatous elements. The foreign material itself can sometimes be identified in the aspirated material with the help of polarising light (Fig. 2.69).

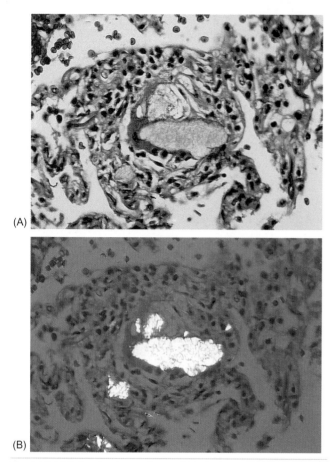

Fig. 2.69 (A) Refractile talc particles in cell block of FNA lung, with surrounding macrophage reaction. The patient was thought to be an intravenous drug user. Birefringence is apparent with polarised light (B) (H&E). (Courtesy of Professor B. Naylor, Michigan.)

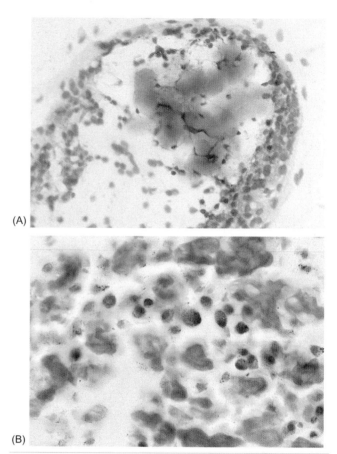

Fig. 2.70 (A) Amyloid in a lung aspirate from a patient with a plasmacytoma. There were scattered plaques of amphophilic material of variable size and shape, as shown here, with a few histiocytes and plasma cells (PAP). (B) Congo-red staining confirms the diagnosis. (Courtesy of Professor B. Naylor, Michigan.)

## Pulmonary amyloidosis

Amyloid is the term used for a group of fibrillary proteins deposited in tissues either as diffuse infiltration of organs or as localised tumorous masses. The protein itself may be derived from the light chains of immunoglobulin molecules (AL), or may be secondary to chronic infections (AA); less common types are the amyloid protein found in old age (AS) and that associated with rare endocrine tumours (AE).

Involvement of the respiratory tract may be tracheobronchial or parenchymal in distribution and at either site deposition can be localised, nodular, multifocal or diffuse. Other organs are affected in the majority of cases.

The cytology of tracheobronchial amyloid deposits has been described by Chen[168] and has been noted in bronchial brushings and in FNA material in a number of reports, as reviewed by Dundore et al. who point out that recognition of amyloid in FNA material is important as it may obviate the need for surgery.[169] Michael and Naylor have highlighted the differential diagnosis and pitfalls in the identification of amyloid in a range of cytology specimens.[170]

### Cytological findings: pulmonary amyloidosis

- Smooth amorphous eosinophilic plaques of amyloid (Fig. 2.70)
- Congo-red stain positive, with apple-green birefringence.

*Corpora amylacea* have similar staining properties but are more rounded in outline and when polarised after Congo-red staining show alternating segments of green and yellow birefringence.

Other types of amorphous plaque such as those due to alveolar proteinosis or *Pneumocystis* infection must be considered. In both of these conditions the plaques have a foamy structure. Definitive differentiation can be made with the Congo-red stain.

## Pulmonary alveolar proteinosis

This rare disease was associated with known exposure to dusts in about half of the cases originally described by Rosen et al. in 1958,[171] but the condition is probably multifactorial in origin, and there is a strong association with immunosuppression (see Ch. 16).[172] The characteristic feature is accumulation of lipid-rich proteinaceous material filling alveolar spaces but evoking little or no inflammation. This material has been shown by electron microscopy to contain large amounts of surfactant.[173] Hyperplasia of type II pneumocytes may occur and a few cases progress to pulmonary fibrosis if untreated. An underlying defect in the macrophage system of the lung has been postulated.[174] Patients present with severe shortness of breath and copious sputum production. Samples of this sputum or lavage fluid from a therapeutic lavage procedure may be received.

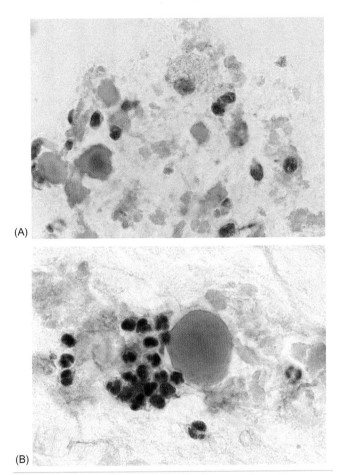

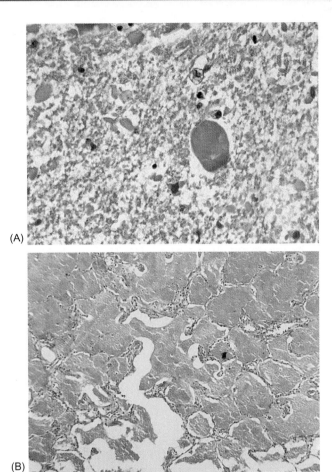

**Fig. 2.71** (A,B) Pulmonary alveolar proteinosis: plaques of granular eosinophilic and cyanophilic material seen in bronchoalveolar lavage fluid. The patient was a middle-aged man presenting with breathlessness and bilateral pulmonary infiltrates. The plaques differ in distribution, size and texture from those of *Pneumocystis* infection or amyloidosis, but both of these must be considered in the differential diagnosis. (PAP and H&E) (Courtesy of Professor B. Naylor, Michigan.)

**Fig. 2.72** Pulmonary alveolar proteinosis plaques in cell block of FNA material (A) and in histological section (B). The proteinaceous precipitate is eosinophilic and fills the alveolar spaces in the lung section. Note the virtual absence of any inflammatory reaction (H&E). (Courtesy of Professor B. Naylor, Michigan.)

### Cytological findings: pulmonary alveolar proteinosis

- Lavage specimens are opaque or milky on gross inspection
- A background of rounded amphophilic plaques and debris (Figs 2.71, 2.72)
- Osmiophilic laminated structure on electron microscopy.

Rounded fragments of amorphous material of variable size, with amphophilic or pale eosinophilic staining properties are seen on light microscopy. Cholesterol crystals may be identified.[175] Few, if any, inflammatory cells are seen. Electron microscopy is necessary for a definitive diagnosis, revealing rounded lamellated structures identical to the osmiophilic bodies of type II pneumocytes and composed of surfactant.[174] In a few cases, particulate dusts are identified.

### Diagnostic pitfalls: pulmonary alveolar proteinosis

*Pneumocystis jiroveci* casts have a honeycomb structure on PAP staining due to cysts within the plaques, as demonstrated by silver stains

Lipoproteinosis associated with *Pneumocystis* infection simulates alveolar proteinosis: the alveoli contain large amounts of lipid and careful searching usually reveals the *Pneumocystis* organisms

Other amorphous materials should be excluded, such as inspissated mucus, which stains deep blue, and amyloid which shows a positive reaction with Congo-red staining.

## Thermal injury

Severe burns from inhalation of smoke or hot gases lead to partial or complete necrosis of bronchial epithelium and the extent of damage may determine the overall prognosis. A neutrophilic response in alveoli and airways is an early event. Healing is accompanied by squamous metaplasia. Reversible atypical squamous metaplasia has been observed in firemen.[176]

A study by Clark et al.[177] of bronchoalveolar lavage cells in 42 fire victims revealed that respiratory tract damage was greatest when smoke inhalation was accompanied by cutaneous burns. Their findings suggest that there is an excessive release of chemical mediators from neutrophil polymorphs, directly damaging the lung parenchyma, and also depleting the alveolar population of mature macrophages. These combined effects then predispose to overwhelming bacterial infection.

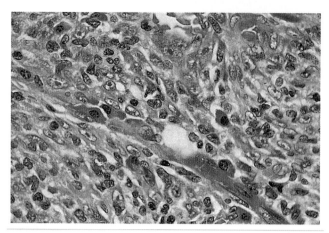

**Fig. 2.73** Plasma cell granuloma of lung (inflammatory myofibroblastoma) in histological section. A mixture of inflammatory cells including plasma cells can be seen in a background of spindle cell connective tissue. The patient was a male of 22, presenting with a lung mass 2 months after an ill-defined respiratory tract infection (H&E).

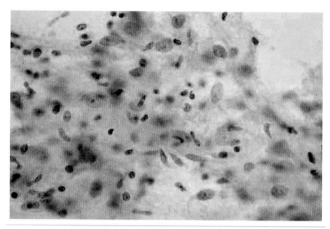

**Fig. 2.74** Plasma cell granuloma (inflammatory myofibroblastoma) of lung in FNA smear showing a mixed population of spindle cells and inflammatory cells. A few plasma cells with eccentric nuclei can be made out, together with histiocytes, lymphocytes and occasional polymorphs. Note prominent nuclei and nucleoli in the spindle cell component (PAP). (Courtesy of Dr G. Sterrett, Perth, Western Australia.)

### Cytological findings: thermal injury

- Thick mucoid sputum or bronchial aspiration samples
- Many damaged epithelial cells
- Polymorphs and macrophages increased in lavage fluid
- Squamous metaplasia occurs early.

Thick mucus is recovered by bronchial aspiration in cases of severe burns. Destruction of cilia, the terminal plate or even entire epithelial cell groups may be seen, but in less injured patients these damaged cells are mixed with exfoliated normal cells. Squamous cells may be present in abundance and may be misshapen, with hyperchromatic nuclei and multinucleation.

Secondary infection is a serious risk for the patient. Herpes simplex or CMV pneumonia, fungal infections such as candidiasis, and bacterial pneumonia, particularly due to *Pseudomonas* organisms, are the most common.

## Benign solitary pulmonary nodules (SPN)

SPN is a common radiological abnormality often detected incidentally. The majority of SPNs represent benign processes, including granulomatous inflammation, bronchogenic cysts and hamartomata. However, a solitary nodule may also potentially represent an early stage of lung cancer or a metastasis. Percutaneous FNA biopsy can exclude malignancy in a majority of cases and may eliminate the need for a more invasive surgical procedure. Correlation of the findings on FNA with radiological features is helpful in establishing benignity.[178]

Plasma cell granuloma/inflammatory myofibroblastoma is a solitary lung nodule of variable size which often follows a respiratory infection and usually occurs in young adults, although no age is exempt.[179] Previously known as 'inflammatory pseudotumour', the lesions may present clinically as a neoplasm and may therefore be investigated by FNA. The histology is diverse (Fig. 2.73), with variable numbers of foamy macrophages known as xanthoma cells, lymphocytes, plasma cells, polymorphs and sometimes also a few giant cells. There is a background of collagen with spindle-shaped fibroblastic cells, which often have a storiform pattern of growth. Some of these cells have now been shown by electron microscopy to have the characteristics of myofibroblasts and the lesion is currently classified as an inflammatory myofibroblastoma, a low-grade tumour.[180] Regression may occur with time but most of these lesions are excised, so as to exclude malignancy.

### Cytological findings: plasma cell granuloma

- Mixed inflammatory picture, including plasma cells, polymorphs, eosinophils and mast cells
- Foamy histiocytes or giant cells
- Fibroblasts and collagen.

The cytological findings have been reported by several authors.[181] Smears made from FNA material show a mixture of inflammatory cells, including plasma cells, epithelial cells and spindle-shaped stromal cells (Fig. 2.74). Xanthoma cells with finely vacuolated cytoplasm may be more numerous than plasma cells. The findings are non-specific but it is helpful to make the diagnosis since conservative management may be appropriate in certain cases.

## Role of cytology in non-neoplastic pulmonary disease

Such an array of inflammatory processes, reactive changes, hyperplasias, infective diseases and fibrosing conditions provides a great diagnostic challenge. Because the cytological findings are often non-specific they are at times more a source of frustration than reward. Good communication with clinicians is essential to ensure that the full clinical details are available at the time of interpretation and it is important that cytopathologists take part in the multidisciplinary-team meetings held regularly to discuss these cases.

Three main contributions to diagnosis can be claimed on behalf of cytopathology:

1. The most reliable of these is the confirmation of a diagnosis of infection by recognition of the causative agent or its cytopathic effects. Many of the fungal, viral and parasitic infections fall into this group. They are of increasing

importance with the rise in numbers of immunosuppressed patients. Cytology provides a relatively cheap, quick, non-invasive and dependable method of diagnosis for many of these cases. Culture of the material obtained, whether directly from the airways or by FNA, is important in cases showing acute inflammation or necrosis.

2. The next contribution lies in recognition of characteristic changes in respiratory tract samples which, when combined with clinical information, give direction or add weight to the clinical diagnosis. The cytological findings in sputum of asthmatics, in lavage fluids in cases of drug toxicity, or in FNA material that includes granuloma formation are among the many examples of this important diagnostic role.

3. Negative findings in cytology are of value clinically since they contribute to the evidence required to exclude malignancy. A study by Zakowski and associates[182] of the significance of negative FNA findings in establishing the absence of malignancy found a negative predictive value of 53.3%. Their figures included inadequate samples. The main factor contributing to false negative diagnosis was sampling error. The converse role, namely that of establishing a diagnosis of malignancy, is discussed later this chapter (see p. 100).

The diagnostic accuracy of respiratory tract cytology for non-neoplastic disease ranges from the high level of sensitivity and specificity in the recognition of fungal and some viral infections, to the entirely non-specific findings in many of the common chronic inflammatory conditions. No meaningful overall figure for accuracy can be calculated, although estimation for certain diagnoses and particular procedures has been discussed in the course of this chapter.

The accuracy of any cytological diagnosis is dependent on obtaining samples that are both appropriate and adequate. This is apparent from studies contrasting different sampling procedures. Orenstein and associates[183] reported a sensitivity of 94.4% using bronchoalveolar lavage for the diagnosis of *Pneumocystis jiroveci* pneumonia in AIDS patients. Induced sputum has generally been found to have a much lower sensitivity of 60–70%, but in a direct comparison of induced sputum and lavage for diagnosis in AIDS patients, Leigh et al.[184] achieved a sensitivity of 94.7% for induced sputum by adhering to a strict protocol for collection and handling of samples.

The advent of bronchoalveolar lavage and increasing use of FNA, especially with radiological or ultrasound guidance have undoubtedly provided new diagnostic applications and opportunities for research into benign pulmonary disease.[185] The role of cytology in this field of respiratory pathology seems likely to continue to grow.

## PULMONARY TUMOURS

*Thomas E. Giles*

## Classification and background

This section of the chapter includes tumours of bronchial and lung parenchymal origin, together with subpleural neoplasms. Box 2.6 gives a summary of the most commonly encountered lung neoplasms and tumour-like lesions, and includes an adaptation of the WHO lung tumour classification.[186,187] In the text,

the entities that are seen in cytological samples are considered in detail.

## Bronchogenic carcinoma

### Incidence and epidemiology

The number of deaths due to lung cancer in China has risen by 465% in the last 30 years and it is the leading cause of death (http://www.chinaview.cn/index.htm). Bronchogenic carcinoma is the leading cause of death from cancer in men and among the leading causes in women.[186] Environmental factors are responsible for almost all cases of lung cancer, with the vast majority of cases being related to tobacco smoking. There has been an increase in incidence of lung cancer throughout the world, such as the 465% rise in the last 30 years in China. Reduced incidence has only been shown in special subgroups such as health workers and in younger age groups accompanying reduced levels of smoking. There has been a rapid increase in mortality among women in recent years related to an increase in smoking in this group.[188]

Although precise cytological and histological typing of lung cancer is required, all subtypes of lung cancer continue to have a dismal prognosis. The 5-year survival rate is approximately 6% for squamous cell carcinoma and 2% for small cell carcinoma.[185] Operable tumours constitute only 20% of malignancies and, even in these, survival is only of the order of 20–30% at 5 years. The use of advanced chemotherapy for small cell and non-small cancer has resulted in an increase in survival time with best results in limited stage disease.

### Pathogenesis

A variety of genetic mutations have been demonstrated in lung cancer, these developing as a result of carcinogen exposure. Mutations of *k-ras*, p16, cyclin, D1, cyclin E and p53 are well described. These are accompanied by the release of autocrine growth factors including abnormal forms of gastrin releasing peptide (GRP; Bombesin), insulin-like growth factor and transferrin-like growth factor, particularly in small cell carcinomas. As well as mutation of genes, abnormal methylation has also been described, leading to aberrant gene expression. Acquisition of the invasive or malignant phenotype is associated with a large number of genetic changes including various other oncogene family mutations and chromosome deletions affecting multiple chromosomes.[189,190]

Although the sequence of accumulated genetic abnormalities is supported by a large body of molecular biological evidence, the identification of such changes has not yet been profitably applied to diagnosis.[190] Collaborative studies across Europe are being undertaken to investigate the possible use of genetic markers in blood, sputum or bronchial washings for the early detection of lung cancer.[191] Some differences between histological subtypes in terms of the frequency of different molecular abnormalities have been detected.[192] For example squamous cell carcinomas have the highest frequency of p53 mutations, but p53 is also often mutated in small cell and large cell neuroendocrine carcinomas. Rb mutations are seen in only about 15% of non-small cell carcinomas, but in 80–100% of small cell tumours. The incidence of ras oncogene mutations is very low in small cell cancer, but much higher in non-small cell cancer subtypes, particularly in adenocarcinoma, and mainly in smokers.[192] These differences are insufficiently precise to aid in tumour subtyping. The dysplasia/carcinoma *in situ*/invasive

## Box 2.6 Pulmonary tumours (adapted from WHO classification[186,187])

**Carcinoma of the lung**

- Squamous cell carcinoma (variants: papillary, clear cell, small cell, basaloid)
- Small cell carcinoma (variants: combined with other forms of carcinoma)
- Adenocarcinoma
  - Acinar adenocarcinoma
  - Papillary adenocarcinoma
  - Bronchioloalveolar carcinoma (mucinous, non-mucinous or mixed)
  - Solid adenocarcinoma with mucin
  - Other variants: well-differentiated fetal; mucinous, mucinous cystadenocarcinoma; signet ring cell; clear cell
- Large cell carcinoma
  - Large cell neuroendocrine carcinoma
  - Basaloid
  - Lymphoepithelioma-like
  - Clear cell
  - Rhabdoid phenotype
- Carcinomas with pleomorphic, sarcomatoid or sarcomatous elements
  - Spindle or giant cell
  - Carcinosarcoma
  - Pulmonary blastoma

**Other primary epithelial neoplasms**

- Carcinoid tumours
  - Typical carcinoid (variants: adenopapillary, clear cell, oncocytic, spindle, melaninogenic)
  - Atypical carcinoid
- Tumours of seromucinous gland/salivary gland type
  - Mucoepidermoid carcinoma
  - Adenoid cystic carcinoma
  - Acinic cell carcinoma
  - Mucous cell adenoma
  - Oncocytic adenoma
  - Pleomorphic adenoma
- Papillary tumours of bronchus/lung
  - Juvenile papillomatosis
  - Squamous cell papilloma and papillary carcinoma
  - Papillary adenoma and adenocarcinoma

- Mucinous cystadenoma
- Alveolar adenoma
- Sclerosing haemangioma/pneumocytoma
- Thymoma
- Malignant melanoma

**Secondary malignancies**

***Connective tissue neoplasms***

- Chondroid hamartoma/chondroma
- Granular cell tumour
- Benign clear cell ('sugar') tumour
- Localised fibrous tumour
- Inflammatory myofibroblastic tumour
- Epithelioid haemangioendothelioma
- Primary pulmonary artery sarcoma
- Leiomyosarcoma
- Malignant fibrous histiocytoma
- Neurogenic sarcoma
- Rhabdomyosarcoma

**Germ cell neoplasms**

- Teratoma mature/immature

**Lymphoproliferative disease**

- Lymphoid interstitial pneumonia
- Nodular lymphoid hyperplasia
- Low-grade marginal zone B-cell lymphoma of the mucosa-associated lymphoid tissue (MALT)
- Lymphomatoid granulomatosis (angiocentric non-Hodgkin lymphoma)
- Other non-Hodgkin lymphomas
- Hodgkin lymphoma
- Plasmacytoma
- Histiocytosis X (Langerhans histiocytosis)

**Other localised mass lesions**

- Amyloid tumour
- Hyalinising granuloma

---

carcinoma sequence for squamous cell carcinoma has been well demonstrated morphologically and epidemiologically, but precursors of large cell carcinoma and small cell carcinoma have not been established. The concept of lung scarring as an aetiopathogenetic factor for adenocarcinoma has come under attack; scars associated with cancers are most likely secondary to the neoplasm.[186] Atypical alveolar hyperplasia is a likely precursor for peripheral adenocarcinomas.[186]

## Heterogeneity of lung carcinoma

Although subclassification of lung carcinoma follows accepted guidelines,[186,187] variable differentiation in different parts of a tumour renders the subtyping of lung lesions by the use of small biopsies or cytological samples prone to some error,

and is clearly a potential cause of discrepancy when evaluating the accuracy of cytodiagnosis. Estimates of the proportion of tumours of mixed cell type by light microscopy are up to 40% of all lung carcinomas. In Roggli's series of systematically sectioned resected tumours, 10% of predominantly non-small cell tumours had a component of small cell carcinoma, and 40% of all tumours had a component of some other major subtype.[193]

Even further heterogeneity is shown if electron microscopic or immunocytochemical studies are performed. In Dunnill and Gatter's series examined in this way, only 27% of resected tumours were homogeneous in cell type.[194] Adelstein showed a non-small cell component in 10% of small cell tumours in biopsy material.[195] Autopsy studies of patients with small cell carcinoma have shown up to 25% of tumours with large cell, giant cell, squamous cell or carcinoid components, and small numbers showed pure squamous tumours, large cell or adenocarcinoma.[196] Some of this discrepancy may represent the effect of treatment or selective survival of non-small cell elements after therapy.

Immunohisto/cytochemistry is a valuable tool frequently used in the differential diagnosis of lung carcinomas whether primary or secondary to the lung. The most useful application is in distinguishing primary lung tumours from metastatic tumours to the lung from common sites (colon, breast, prostate, pancreas, stomach, kidney, bladder, ovaries, and uterus). Immunohistochemistry also aids in the separation of small cell carcinoma from non-small cell carcinoma and carcinoids particularly in small biopsy specimens limited by artifact. Although there is no 'lung-specific tumour marker,' with the help of a relatively restricted marker, thyroid transcription factor 1 (TTF-1) and napsin A, it is possible to separate a lung primary from a metastasis with a reasonable degree of certainty. Napsin A appears to complement TTF-1 in defining a lung primary (Table 2.1).[197,572]

### Lung carcinoma subtyping and interobserver agreement

Squamous cell carcinoma has been generally regarded as the most common subtype (30–50%) followed by adenocarcinoma (15–30%), small cell carcinoma (15–30%), and large cell undifferentiated tumours (5–15%) depending on the nature of the series examined.[186] Some changes in prevalence have occurred, e.g. the increase in adenocarcinomas particularly in women smokers in the USA, to the point where adenocarcinoma may now be the most common subtype overall,[198] and the increase in squamous and small cell cancer compared with adenocarcinoma in Japan.[199] Changes in types of histological or cytological samples used for diagnosis and in reporting practices for these samples may have been partly responsible.

The main role of the pathologist is to distinguish between small cell and non-small cell carcinomas, as in general the former will require chemotherapy while the latter will be managed surgically or with palliative radiotherapy or different chemotherapy regimes. When adequate material is available for study by experienced pathologists, the consistency of the distinction between small cell and non-small cell types in histological material is in the order of 90%.[200] However, high interobserver agreement for the diagnosis and subclassification of small cell carcinoma has been achieved using current simplified international classifications.[201,202] Interobserver agreement for non-small cell cancers may be less and the variation shown in reported results for cytohistological subtyping should again be assessed against this background.

Staging is the most important prognostic indicator.[186] Subdivision of squamous tumours into well, moderately and poorly differentiated tumours seems to be of prognostic value,[203] but there does not appear to be a difference between survival rates for well, moderately or poorly differentiated adenocarcinomas. Among resectable non-small cell tumours, large cell carcinoma may have a worse prognosis.

Subtyping by electron microscopy shows some differences from typing by light microscopy;[194,204] this has no proven biological or clinical significance as a routine practice but allows better subclassification of unusual tumours, and a higher rate of correlation with cytological tumour typing than with histopathology.[205,206]

### Neuroendocrine differentiation in lung carcinomas

Neuroendocrine lesions of the lung are an area of continuing debate, and the relevance of this differentiation in various

**Table 2.1** Lung-specific markers available for immunohistochemistry

| Antibody | Antigen | Sensitivity | Specificity |
|---|---|---|---|
| TTF-1 | Thyroid transcription factor 1 | For lung cancer: adenocarcinoma 75%, squamous carcinoma 11%, large cell carcinoma 50% | Lung and thyroid tissue and tumour arising in these organs stain; small cell carcinomas from other organs are positive |
| ES1 | CEACAM6 | Undifferentiated lung cancer, large cell and poorly differentiated adenocarcinoma are positive, which do not stain well with TTF-1 | Other cancers show weak immunoreactivity |
| Surfactant A and B | Surfactant protein A and B | 63% of primary lung cancers | 46% of metastatic carcinomas to lung are positive including breast carcinoma |
| Napsin A | Functional aspartic proteinase | 90% of lung adenocarcinomas express diffuse strong staining. Compared with TTF-1, napsin A appears to be superior in sensitivity and probably comparable in specificity. It is also expressed in a subset of renal cell carcinomas, particularly of the papillary type, as well as in the rare cases of papillary thyroid carcinomas | Normal lung type II pneumocytes and alveolar macrophage lysosomes; proximal renal tubules in our hands stain. Thyroid carcinomas and renal cell carcinomas express napsin A. However, the majority of the expression appears to be false positive in the latter, probably because of intrinsic biotin in these non-lung tumours |

CEACAM6, carcinoembryonic antigen-related adhesion molecule 6. (From Jagirdar J. Application of immunohistochemistry to the diagnosis of primary and metastatic carcinoma to the lung. Arch Pathol Lab Med 2008. Mar; 132(3): 384–96. Reprinted with permission from Archives of Pathology & Laboratory Medicine. Copyright 2008. College of American Pathologists.)

histological types of lung carcinoma remains uncertain. The application of ancillary techniques including electron microscopy, immunocytochemistry, cell culture and molecular biology has enhanced our understanding of the interrelationship between these lesions,[207–212] but clinical studies of various forms of therapy for them are preliminary. Some have suggested a worse prognosis overall or greater responsiveness to chemotherapy than similar tumours without neuroendocrine features[213] however this issue is controversial.[186]

Neuroendocrine differentiation in the form of dense core granules, peptide or amine hormone production and neuroendocrine cytochemical markers such as synaptophysin, chromogranin, gastrin releasing peptide (bombesin) and neural cell adhesion molecules (CD56)[214] can be demonstrated in association with a range of lung malignancies. These include small cell carcinoma, atypical carcinoid, carcinoid tumours, large cell neuroendocrine carcinoma and some examples of undifferentiated large cell carcinoma, squamous cell carcinoma and adenocarcinoma.[207–212]

A consensus has been reached on the classification of these lesions. The WHO Classification recognises carcinoid tumours, atypical carcinoids, large cell neuroendocrine carcinoma and small cell carcinoma as separate entities.[186] Studies have shown clear differences in prognosis using criteria easily applied in histological material.[215] However, mitotic rate appears to be the most important criterion and one which is not easily translated to cytological diagnosis. Cytology can usually separate lesions into carcinoid tumours, atypical carcinoids and small cell carcinomas but experience with large cell neuroendocrine tumours is less well documented. There also remains a small group of borderline tumours where a distinction between small cell carcinoma and atypical carcinoid, or small cell carcinoma and large cell neuroendocrine carcinoma is problematical despite adequate material.

## Squamous cell carcinoma

This form of lung carcinoma is usually located centrally within the lung in main bronchi or branches and is often associated with bronchial obstruction and secondary pneumonia. Central necrosis and cavitation is often seen. The defining feature is the identification of cytoplasmic keratinisation or intercellular bridges. Ultrastructurally, bundles of tonofibrils, well-formed desmosomes, concentric layering of tonofibrils around the nucleus and deposition of membrane coated granules are features of squamous differentiation.[186] The cytological findings and diagnostic pitfalls in sputum, washings and brushings (S,W,B) for each of the tumour entities will be described separately from the FNA findings in view of some differences in approach to diagnosis in these samples.

### Cytological findings (S,W,B): squamous cell carcinoma

- Abnormal squamous cells with enlarged or pyknotic nuclei of variable staining intensity
- Bizarre cell shapes, abnormal keratinisation
- Cell dissociation, especially in differentiated tumours
- Tumour diathesis.

The cytological diagnosis of squamous cell carcinoma from sputum samples, washings or brushings depends on the identification of abnormal squamous cells with malignant nuclear criteria, including enlargement, angularity and irregular chromatin distribution or 'black ink' chromatin. Large nucleoli are uncommonly seen, and are not a constant feature within a given group of cells. In well-differentiated lesions the cells may have a low nucleocytoplasmic ratio. In these cases recognition of the inappropriate immaturity of the nucleus compared to the cytoplasm and subtle abnormalities of nuclear chromatin are important in establishing the diagnosis.

Bizarre enlarged cell shapes including spindle and caudate cells, cell engulfment giving rise to 'birds-eye cells', ghost

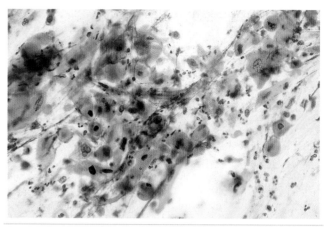

**Fig. 2.75** Sputum: keratinising squamous cell carcinoma. Irregularly shaped keratinising squamous cells in a background of necrotic debris (PAP).

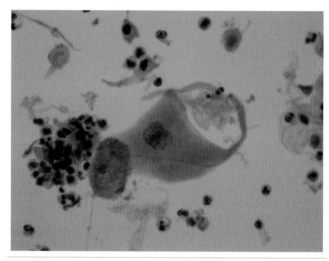

**Fig. 2.76** Bronchial washings: keratinising squamous cell carcinoma. Caudate cell with pale abnormal chromatin (PAP).

keratinised cell outlines, keratinous debris and a background of necrosis and blood help confirm invasive squamous cell carcinoma. Intense orange-yellow staining and a refractile appearance of the cytoplasm is a feature of keratinising tumours (Figs 2.75–2.80); the degree of intensity of staining is characteristic of malignancy and unlike reactive hyperkeratosis.

A dispersed or single cell pattern is usually present in well-differentiated tumours, whereas poorly differentiated tumours often present in cell groups which are disorganised. In non-keratinising tumours characteristic dense cytoplasm with well-defined cell borders allows recognition of squamous differentiation. They are less likely to be associated with necrosis.

Cavitating tumours often give rise to purulent sputum containing large amounts of necrotic debris and neutrophils (Fig. 2.75). Malignant cells are 'hyperkeratinised', shrunken, degenerate and include many ghost cells.[216] Diagnostic cells may sometimes be inconspicuous (Fig. 2.80).

In sputum, the diagnosis may occasionally be made on a few cells with sufficiently abnormal nuclei and cytoplasmic shape. Consideration of the full clinical and radiological findings is important to avoid diagnostic pitfalls. If bizarre cell shapes, ghost cells and keratinous debris are present without intact nuclei, this is also strong evidence of carcinoma, but additional

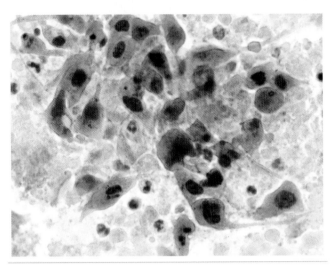

**Fig. 2.77** Sputum: keratinising squamous cell carcinoma. Aggregate of intensely orangeophilic cells with densely hyperchromatic irregular nuclei (PAP).

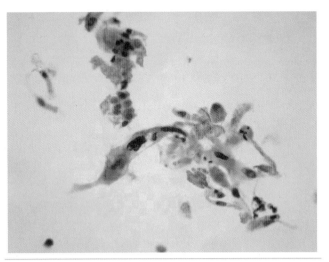

**Fig. 2.79** Bronchial brushings: keratinising squamous cell carcinoma. Inflammatory debris and a variably keratinised fibre cells (PAP).

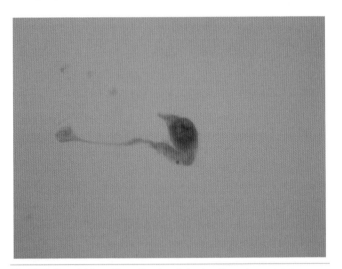

**Fig. 2.78** Bronchial washings: Non-keratinised malignant squamous cell with hypochromatic nucleus and typical dense cytoplasm in a clean background (PAP).

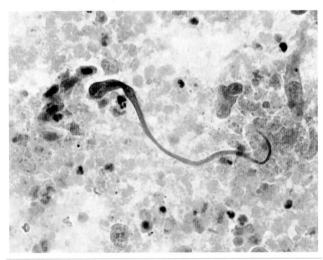

**Fig. 2.80** Sputum: necrotic debris with poorly preserved malignant squamous cells including an elongated keratinised tadpole cell showing nuclear degeneration (PAP).

samples should be requested for identification of malignant nuclear morphology.

### Diagnostic pitfalls (S,W,B): squamous cell carcinoma

Pitfalls in sputum and washings include upper respiratory tract cells with reactive changes, the dysplasia/carcinoma *in situ* sequence, reactive changes in benign pulmonary cavities, radiation effect, drug effect, instrumentation or pulmonary embolism and infarction,[217] degenerating herpesvirus affected cells, vegetable cells with bizarre morphology and contaminant abnormal cells from oropharyngeal or oesophageal carcinomas. These conditions are described and illustrated in the first part of this chapter.

Upper respiratory tract cells shed from inflammatory lesions or adjacent to ulcers present as small parakeratotic-like aggregates or sheets of eosinophilic or orangeophilic cells with pyknotic nuclei, which show some variation in nuclear size. Cell dispersal may be seen, but a combination of irregular cell shapes and

marked nuclear irregularity is not found. Epithelial repair, having essentially similar morphology to that seen in cervical smears, is occasionally seen in brushings samples, particularly in patients who undergo multiple endoscopic procedures.[218] Large cohesive sheets of cells with enlarged nuclei and prominent nucleoli, absence of dispersed abnormal cells and correlation with biopsy findings have been helpful in diagnosis (Fig. 2.81).

## Preinvasive lesions

The atypical hyperplasia/dysplasia/carcinoma *in situ* sequence in bronchial epithelium[219] is represented in sputum by a range of cytological appearances. The findings in regular squamous metaplasia are described above (see p. 25 and Fig. 2.19). Atypical squamous metaplasia/dysplasia presents as small sheets of squamous cells with nuclear pleomorphism and hyperchromasia, but without the bizarre cell configuration or fully developed nuclear criteria of carcinoma (Fig. 2.82).

Higher-grade intraepithelial abnormalities (severe dysplasia) show more advanced nuclear abnormalities and some dispersal.

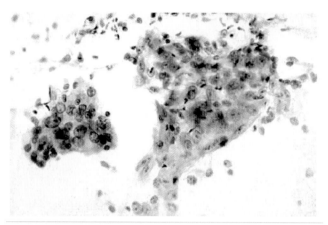

**Fig. 2.81** Bronchial brushings: reactive changes, post-bronchoscopy. Monolayered sheet of epithelial repair together with an aggregate of regenerating bronchial cells with some variation in nuclear size (PAP).

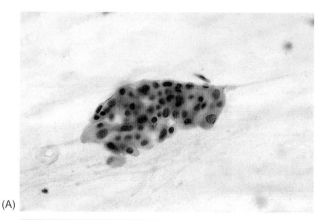

(A)

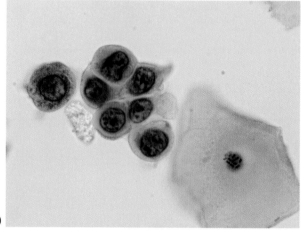

(B)

**Fig. 2.83** (A,B) Sputum: atypical squamous metaplasia. Cohesive aggregates of squamous cells showing nuclear hyperchromasia, enlargement and slight pleomorphism, but without nuclear criteria of malignancy. Clean background (PAP).

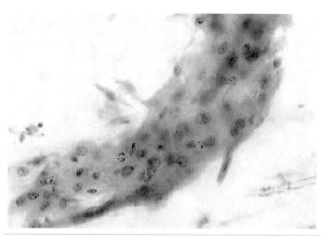

**Fig. 2.82** Sputum: upper respiratory tract squamous cells. Cohesive sheet of squamous cells with some nuclear enlargement, but with degenerative features and no significant nuclear irregularity, pleomorphism or hyperchromasia (PAP).

Carcinoma *in situ* tends to present in sputum as single cells, which are rounded, small and with central nuclei showing nuclear atypia including irregular outlines and hyperchromasia, but again without pleomorphic or bizarre cell shapes (Fig. 2.83). This appearance probably also corresponds to early invasive carcinoma and an accurate distinction between these two lesions is not possible.[220,221] Further samples should be collected if this morphological change is encountered. Subsequent investigation reveals invasive carcinoma in quite a high proportion of patients with cytological changes suggesting severe dysplasia or carcinoma *in situ*.[220]

## Screening for squamous cell carcinoma

In some centres and as part of screening programmes, clinically and radiologically inapparent *in situ* tumours or early invasive carcinomas have been detected, pursued actively, and localised by sputum cytology, endoscopy and selective brushings, washings and biopsy.[223,224] Extraordinary effort is necessary to detect these lesions in an asymptomatic population and to investigate the bronchial tree exhaustively,[223] limiting the value of this approach for screening.[225–231]

Although 5-year survival may be of the order of 65–90% for small occult carcinomas, the overall survival for screened patients is not significantly better than for non-screened groups.[232] The importance of recognising the morphological features of *in situ* or early cancers is to separate these cases from obvious invasive carcinoma and not to overdiagnose malignancy. This reinforces the importance of a multidisciplinary assessment when making a diagnosis of malignancy. When attempting the localisation of lesions using selective bronchial washings, the possibility of intrabronchial contamination should be borne in mind. In practice, malignant cells can often be identified in specimens from several lobes due to this phenomenon.

The changes described above, which suggest premalignancy or *in situ* carcinoma, but occurring in patients without clinical abnormality, may disappear from sputum and may not be followed by the detection or development of carcinoma despite careful bronchoscopic studies over a number of years. This is a further argument in favour of a cautious approach to diagnosis.[233] *In situ* carcinoma in bronchial brushings may present as large cohesive aggregates similar to the microbiopsies of cervical intraepithelial neoplasia seen in cervical smears (Fig. 2.84). The natural history of *in situ* bronchogenic carcinoma is uncertain, as is the value of local treatment for these lesions, which are often multifocal. Despite these reservations, regular repeat sputum samples and follow-up bronchoscopies have been recommended for patients with cytological findings suggesting

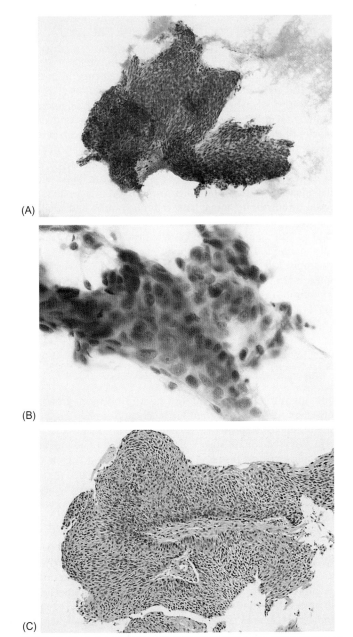

(A)

(B)

(C)

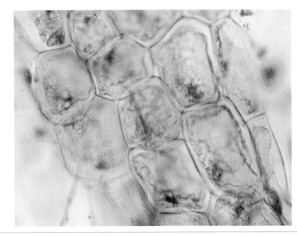

**Fig. 2.85** Vegetable matter in sputum may simulate degenerate malignant cells. The salivary nature of the specimen and the thick cellulose walls with lack of nuclear detail are helpful features.

**Fig. 2.84** Bronchial brushings: squamous cell carcinoma *in situ*. (A) Large cohesive aggregate of hyperchromatic cells (PAP). (B) Disorganised but cohesive aggregate of squamous cells with nuclear enlargement, hyperchromasia and cyanophilic cytoplasm (PAP). (C) Bronchial biopsy: histological section showing *in situ* carcinoma only (H&E).

severe dysplasia or carcinoma *in situ* in whom initial bronchoscopy reveals no abnormality.[220]

Cavities within the lung undergo squamous metaplasia and marked inflammatory changes due to associated infection.[234] These lesions can on occasions shed spindle-shaped aggregates of atypical metaplastic squamous cells, keratinised cells or reactive cells, raising the possibility of malignancy. Other infective processes such as blastomycosis and paracoccidioidomycosis[235] have been associated with highly atypical reactive/metaplastic squamous cells.

Chemotherapeutic agents such as bleomycin and busulphan may give rise to cells resembling severe atypical squamous metaplasia or even carcinoma (see Fig. 2.86A).[236,237] Pulmonary embolism is a recognised cause of atypical reactive squamous

cells which may give rise to false positive diagnoses, although few examples are recorded in the literature; Bewtra et al. describe patients with pulmonary embolism in which there were metaplastic squamous cells with marked atypia in sputum and brushings, although the most striking changes were in reactive bronchiolar cells.[238] Instrumentation of the respiratory tract can produce regenerative and degenerative changes resembling squamous cancer.[239] Patients with lung transplants often undergo BAL to detect infectious agents. Opari et al. found atypical epithelial cells in nine patients over a 7-year period, associated with diffuse alveolar damage, rejection or infection. There was significant overlap between the cytological findings and those of malignancy.

Vegetable material can usually be recognised by the birefringent structure of the cell wall, but may sometimes provide difficulties (Fig. 2.85).[240] Radiation effect has similar morphology to that in other sites (Fig. 2.86B).

Cells from oropharyngeal carcinomas or upper oesophageal cancers may shed into sputum. Matsudo et al.[241] report a surprisingly high sensitivity (60–70%) of detection of such tumours by sputum cytology; in screening programmes for lung cancer, such lesions may be detected by cytology before being symptomatic. The cells are usually present only in very small numbers and their morphology is usually that of a very well-differentiated tumour (see below).

Papillary or polypoid predominantly intraluminal carcinomas may shed squamous cells with malignant morphology into sputum or brushing samples, despite being non-invasive or minimally invasive. These lesions are rarely encountered but may provide particular difficulty in diagnosis in both cytological and small bronchial biopsy samples. They require a combined cytohistological assessment and knowledge of the bronchoscopic and chest radiographic appearances for correct management, which may involve segmental resection rather than pneumonectomy or lobectomy.

## Cytological findings (FNA): squamous cell carcinoma

These are similar to bronchial washing and brushings findings, although tumour tissue often shows greater aggregation and, in FNA material in particular, tumours often appear less-differentiated than in brushings or sputum because of a higher component of deeper tumour tissue.

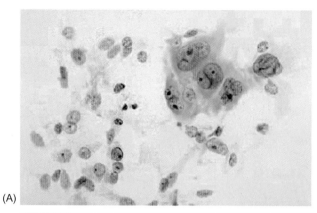

(A)

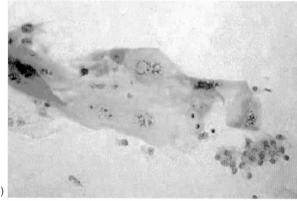

(B)

**Fig. 2.86** (A) Bronchial brushings: chemotherapy effect. Nuclei lack hyperchromasia. Cellular changes following chemotherapy for small cell carcinoma. Check bronchoscopy (PAP). (B) Bronchial brushings: radiotherapy effect. Marked nuclear and cellular enlargement with bizarre multinucleate cells, some showing nuclear vacuoles (PAP).

## Diagnostic pitfalls (FNA): squamous cell carcinoma

Contamination of transbronchial FNA samples by intrapulmonary tumour has been reported; observing lymphocytes in company with tumour cells in transtracheal or transbronchial FNA would help exclude this pitfall.[242]

In FNA, sources of error include a granulomatous reaction and the acute inflammation and suppuration accompanying central cavitation of tumours. Changes due to radiation and chemotherapy (Fig. 2.86) in brushings are found particularly in those treated for small cell carcinoma. The cells produced may be large with irregular nuclei, prominent nucleoli and abundant dense cytoplasm. They may not show any degenerative features and may have alarming nuclear morphology; however, the clinical background, prominence of multinucleation and scattered nature of the cells among normal bronchial cells helps exclude squamous or other large cell carcinoma.

Necrosis in other large cell carcinomas may simulate keratinisation[243,244] particularly in H&E preparations and more often in FNA samples; Papanicolaou staining is better at separating necrosis from the orangeophilia of keratin. In FNA samples there is a tendency to view cytoplasmic density or a sheet-like growth in other large cell carcinomas as an indicator of squamous differentiation, and this is a cause of mistyping. Rare tumours may have a pseudovascular or pseudoglandular growth.[245]

## Squamous cell carcinoma of head and neck versus primary squamous cell carcinoma of lung

The reported incidence of pulmonary malignancy in patients with head and neck cancer ranges from 4.5% to 14%.[246,247]

In the set of patients who develop a second malignancy in the lung, as many as 31% will be synchronous. Second malignancies of the lung are most frequently associated with primary laryngeal tumours, followed by pharynx. The risk of developing a metachronous second malignancy, when the larynx is the index tumour, is approximately 0.6% per year. Most second malignancies in the lung are squamous cell carcinomas, followed by adenocarcinoma, large cell lung cancer, and small cell lung cancer. Primary squamous cell carcinoma of the lung is difficult to distinguish from metastatic head and neck squamous cell carcinoma. Thyroid transcription factor 1 is negative in both squamous cell carcinomas of lung and in head and neck carcinoma so, in this instance, TTF-1 is unhelpful. Currently, there is no immunohistochemical marker that will help with this differential diagnosis, although HPV16 viral load and p16 expression could be used to express some head and neck cancers.[197]

## Small cell carcinoma

This tumour is usually central or hilar in position, grows rapidly, disseminates widely and has a very poor overall prognosis. Chemotherapy improves survival time and produces some long-term survivors. Small stage I tumours are only rarely detected cytologically[248] or histologically, and the only accepted place for surgery is for small peripheral tumours. Associated paraneoplastic syndromes such as the Eaton–Lambert myasthenic syndrome and syndromes produced by peptide hormone secretion such as ADH and ACTH are well described.

The new WHO classification[187] has abandoned subdivision of these tumours. The term used for tumours with a mixture of cell types is 'combined' carcinoma including areas of any other non-small cell morphology including large cell neuroendocrine carcinoma. These constitute up to 10% of small cell tumours.[195] All appear to behave in a similar aggressive fashion; the mixed small and large cell group has not been shown to have separate clinical significance.[249]

Ultrastructurally, most small cell carcinomas show a few intracytoplasmic dense core neurosecretory granules concentrated in small cytoplasmic processes, but these may be lacking in some tumours of classical appearance and in the small cell/large cell tumours. If neuroendocrine granules are not seen by electron microscopy in a tumour where there is diagnostic difficulty, and there is ultrastructural evidence of glandular or squamous differentiation, this would place a diagnosis of small cell carcinoma in some doubt. However, some small cell tumours, which behave aggressively, may show variable combinations of squamous, glandular or neuroendocrine differentiation ultrastructurally.

Chromogranin A and synaptophysin are neuroendocrine markers, which are demonstrable in the cytoplasm of small cell carcinomas. Antibodies to CD56 have proven to be the most reliable in confirming small cell carcinoma, however. Paranuclear dot-like positivity for keratin is also commonly seen in tumour cells.

Some other antibodies, including those to CD44,[250] preferentially react with non-small cell tumours.[251,252]

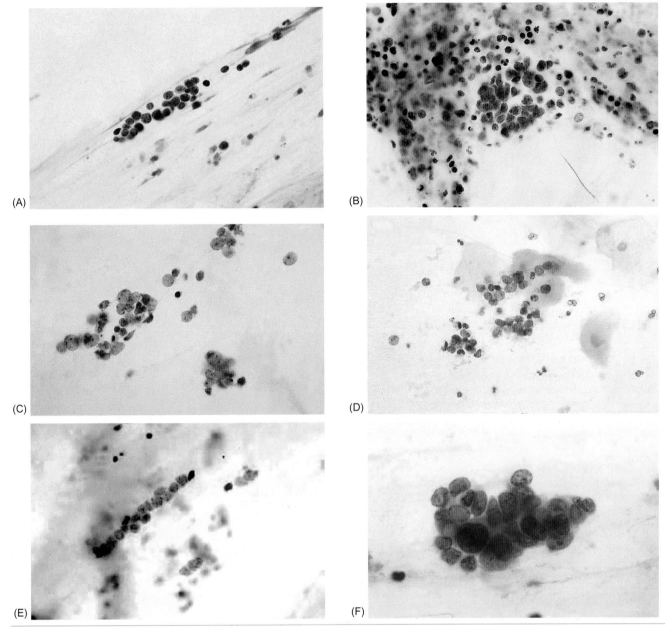

**Fig. 2.87** Sputum: small cell carcinoma. (A) Loose elongated aggregate of hyperchromatic pleomorphic small cells within a mucus streak. (B) Aggregate of preserved cells showing nuclear moulding, in a background of degenerate and necrotic cells. (C) 'Intermediate' nuclear morphology. Scattered single degenerate cells amongst larger well-preserved tumour cells. (D) Small groups of less well-preserved cells with paler nuclei, in a salivary background. (E) Well-preserved single file with nuclear compression and moulding (PAP). (F) An aggregate of tumour cells showing uniform nuclear hyperchromasia, irregular nuclear outlines and pleomorphism. Nucleoli are inconspicuous. Occasional cells show nuclear moulding (PAP).

## Cytological findings (exfoliated cells): small cell carcinoma

- Elongated groupings of small dissociating tumour cells
- Scant cytoplasm, irregular moulded nuclei
- Coarsely stippled chromatin, inconspicuous nucleoli
- Degenerative changes common.

In sputum this tumour usually presents in small rounded or elongated aggregates within streaks of mucus. The aggregates are generally loosely arranged with a complement of dissociated cells. The tumour cells are small to medium sized with minimal cytoplasm and demonstrate nuclear pleomorphism within the aggregates, together with nuclear

moulding and irregularity of nuclear outline. Nucleoli are inconspicuous. A uniformly hyperchromatic nucleus with a flat or stippled chromatin pattern is most commonly seen; distinct nuclear membranes are not a feature (Figs 2.87, 2.88).

Although cells are only 2–3 times lymphocyte size in most cases, they may be larger if better preserved and may then have a more open chromatin pattern and more easily visible nucleoli; large nucleoli would suggest some other primary or secondary carcinoma. Degenerative change may also contribute to loss of chromatin pattern and often the nuclei are pale-staining with haematoxylin. Nuclear pyknosis may render assessment difficult. Mitotic figures are seldom found in sputum samples; however, single cell necrosis within

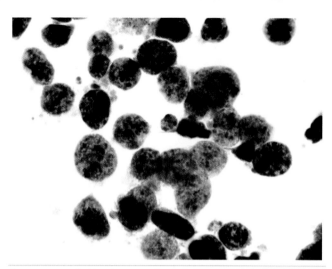

**Fig. 2.88** Bronchial brushings: small cell carcinoma. Small group of tumour cells showing uniform nuclear hyperchromasia, pleomorphism and irregularity of nuclear outline, inconspicuous nucleoli and nuclear moulding. Nuclear membranes are ill-defined (PAP).

aggregates and abundant apoptotic cell breakdown all indicate a high mitotic rate and cell turnover.

The close apposition of tumour cells in a rapidly growing tumour with minimal cytoplasm and fragile nuclei leads to the helpful feature of nuclear moulding, rarely seen in other lung carcinomas. This feature may result in single file arrangements (Fig. 2.87E) or small concentrically arranged groups. Engulfment of a single, apoptotic nuclear fragment by a tumour cell is seen in some small cell carcinomas and not in lymphomas.[253]

Small cell carcinomas are commonly accompanied by considerable necrosis; however, the background may be entirely clean and we have seen diagnostic material in paucicellular mucoid or salivary samples with no necrosis or accompanying inflammation.

Definitive diagnosis rests on finding a number of well preserved aggregates; a diagnosis should not be made on poorly preserved material or one or two abnormal cells alone.

## Diagnostic pitfalls (exfoliated cells): small cell carcinoma

The most common difficulties in diagnosis in sputum arise from degenerate bronchial cells, and in the distinction between small cell and non-small cell tumours of primary and metastatic origin.[254] Reactive lymphocytes may provide diagnostic difficulties, and, particularly when nuclear moulding is present; poorly preserved cells from lymphoma may give problems. In brushings (Fig. 2.89) the better preservation of cells leads to larger nuclei, sometimes more evident cytoplasm albeit never abundant, a more open chromatin network and more easily visible small nucleoli. Streaks of nuclear material, smeared cells, and tear-drop cells emphasise the fragility of nuclei. The fine strands of haematoxyphilic material extending from nuclei are a characteristic traumatisation artefact rarely seen in other types of malignancy.[255]

Degenerate bronchial epithelial cells can generally be easily distinguished from small cell carcinoma (Fig. 2.90). They show a similar degree of degenerative change from nucleus to nucleus within the cluster, with no well-preserved cells among the clusters; a mixture of preserved and degenerate cells within a cluster is more a feature of small cell carcinoma.

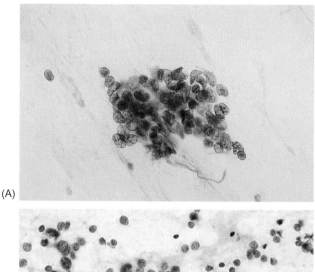

(A)

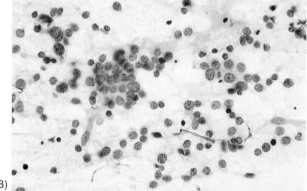

(B)

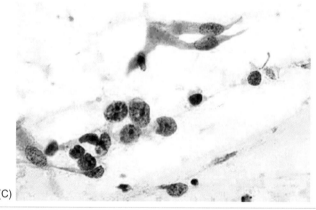

(C)

**Fig. 2.89** Bronchial brushings: small cell carcinoma. (A) Clusters of small cells with granular, stippled nuclear chromatin; nuclear moulding, absent cytoplasm (PAP). (B) More dispersed pattern with numerous single bare nuclei, but showing considerable nuclear pleomorphism (PAP). (C) Granular stippled chromatin pattern, micronucleoli, nuclear moulding and minimal cytoplasm. Compare with single bronchial cells (PAP).

Regenerating bronchial cells generally show little pleomorphism, and although they do show moulding, this usually occurs with a distinct intact rim of cytoplasm rather than the nucleus to nucleus moulding often seen in small cell carcinoma (Fig. 2.91). Observing adjacent, better preserved bronchial cells or a range of degenerative change within an area of the smear is most helpful in diagnosis.

Metastatic breast carcinoma (Fig. 2.92), prostatic carcinoma, and small celled squamous carcinomas may provide difficulties in differential diagnosis. The abundant cytoplasm usually seen in these tumours will generally be the best guide to excluding small cell cancer. More pronounced three-dimensional clustering, cohesion and prominent nucleoli are features unlike small cell carcinoma and more indicative of adenocarcinoma, either primary or secondary. Careful attention to chromatin detail also helps

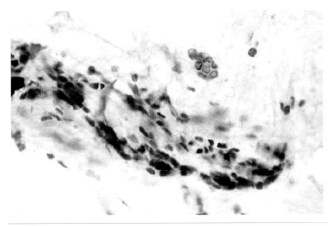

**Fig. 2.90** Sputum: degenerate bronchial epithelium. Streaks of traumatised, poorly preserved epithelial cells. One group of cells showing cell moulding but with retained cytoplasm between nuclei (PAP).

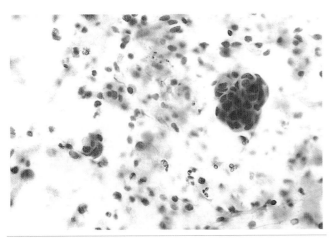

**Fig. 2.91** Sputum: post-bronchoscopy changes. Several aggregates of bronchial epithelial cells demonstrating cellular moulding, but with retained cytoplasm between nuclei (PAP).

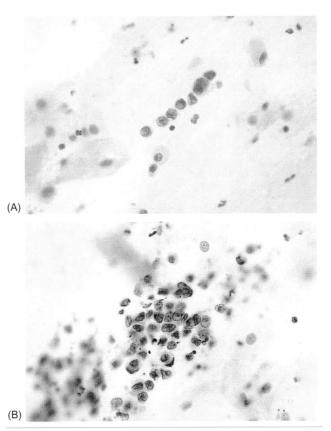

(A)

(B)

**Fig. 2.92** Sputum: metastatic breast carcinoma. (A) Single file structure of small cells closely mimicking small cell carcinoma. (B) Loose aggregate of cells showing several engulfed cells (PAP).

in avoiding this pitfall, with coarser, more irregular chromatin clumping being more typical of non-small cell tumours.

Malignant lymphoma is occasionally very difficult to distinguish from small cell carcinoma (Fig. 2.93); small cell carcinomas may occasionally be very dispersed and lymphomas may show apparent grouping of cells due to artefact. Cell engulfment or engulfment of an apoptotic body and nuclear moulding is not seen in lymphoma.[253]

One interesting non-cellular mimic of small cell carcinoma is inspissated mucus or debris (Fig. 2.94) which can collect to form moulded aggregates reminiscent of carcinoma, although without any 'nuclear' structure. Limiting diagnosis to well preserved material will prevent error.

Carcinoid tumours rarely exfoliate into sputum, but morphologically are difficult to distinguish in the occasional cases where this is seen. More uniform nuclei, greater amounts of cytoplasm and less conspicuous nuclear moulding are helpful features in distinguishing these two entities. Reserve cells or reserve cell hyperplasia may also, on occasion, resemble small cell carcinoma (see Fig. 2.6).[256]

In brushings samples a mixture with bronchial epithelium may provide difficulties as small numbers of tumour cells may be obscured by traumatised bronchial epithelium. In addition, traumatised bronchial epithelial cells stripped of cytoplasm

may artefactually aggregate and simulate carcinoma. Such cases require study either to trace a continuum between benign, well-preserved cells and traumatised cells in benign cases, or to demonstrate an unequivocal contrast between neoplastic and non-neoplastic epithelium in malignant cases.

Marchevsky et al. describe cells from a pulmonary tumorlet in a brushings sample which resembled small cell carcinoma.[257]

### Cytological findings (FNA): small cell carcinoma

- Better preserved larger cells than in sputum (see Fig. 2.95)
- Some nuclear moulding and cell clustering present
- Open chromatin pattern
- Small nucleoli may be visible
- Artefactually crushed cells and nuclei.

FNA samples show findings similar to those in brushings with well preserved cells and nuclei. The chromatin pattern and nucleoli are visible and smearing artefact is usually present, as described in brush samples above. Some cell clustering is usually maintained and moulding can usually be demonstrated. Nuclear moulding is more prominent in air dried preparations. It is important to recognise that small cell carcinoma may be formed of medium-sized to large cells. Careful assessment of nuclear features avoids the mistake of diagnosing these as non-small cell carcinoma due to the larger cell size.

### Diagnostic pitfalls (FNA): small cell carcinoma

In FNA and bronchial brushing samples, a distinction between 'intermediate' small cell carcinoma (Fig. 2.95) and other poorly differentiated tumours, particularly large cell carcinoma,

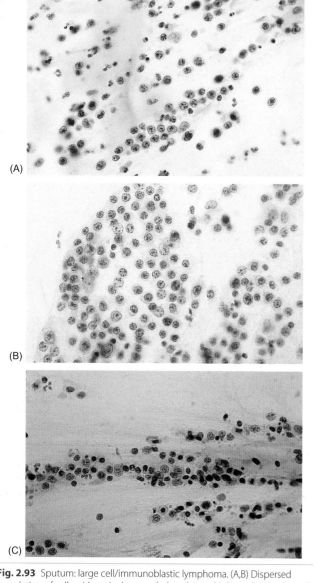

(A)

(B)

(C)

**Fig. 2.93** Sputum: large cell/immunoblastic lymphoma. (A,B) Dispersed population of cells with vesicular rounded nuclei, multiple nucleoli and small amounts of intact cytoplasm surrounding individual cells. No aggregation. (A, B, PAP). (C) Dispersal with a few apparent loose aggregates. Single cell degeneration within the abnormal cells. This pattern was not distinguishable from small cell carcinoma (PAP).

small celled or basaloid squamous carcinomas (Fig. 2.96) and secondary tumours, e.g. from breast, are among the most common diagnostic problems.

## Small cell carcinoma versus squamous cell carcinoma

Critical attention to nuclear morphology is valuable. If there are uniformly hyperchromatic nuclei with granular chromatin, inconspicuous nucleoli and minimal or no cytoplasm, the neoplasm will generally fall into the small cell group histologically; whereas vesicular nuclei and prominent nucleoli, together with well-marked nuclear membranes are generally evidence of non-small cell type. There are exceptions to this, small celled squamous carcinomas providing particular difficulty. Marked cell cohesion is a feature more often seen in squamous cell

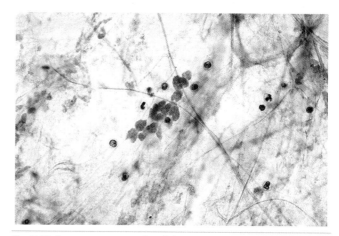

**Fig. 2.94** Sputum: aggregate of acellular material, possibly mucus. Resemblance to degenerate nuclei of small cell carcinoma. No chromatin pattern is evident (PAP).

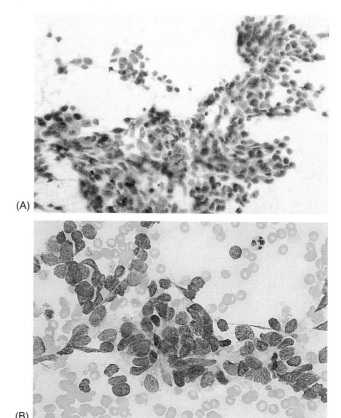

(A)

(B)

**Fig. 2.95** FNA: small cell carcinoma, 'intermediate' morphology. Larger, better preserved nuclei than usually seen in sputum and more cohesive aggregates. (A, H&E; B, MGG)

carcinomas. Electron microscopy demonstrating neuroendocrine differentiation or immunocytochemical expression of CD56 can be helpful in problematic cases.

However, in specimens with crush artefact, separating small cell carcinoma from poorly differentiated squamous cell carcinoma with or without small cell features is a problem. The markers that have been used are TTF-1 and p63 (a nuclear basal cell marker and a member of the p53 family involved in development of epithelial tissues)[258] and CK5 and CK8.[259]

Small cell carcinomas are predominantly TTF-1 positive (~90%), CD56 positive, p63 negative, CK5 negative, and CK8

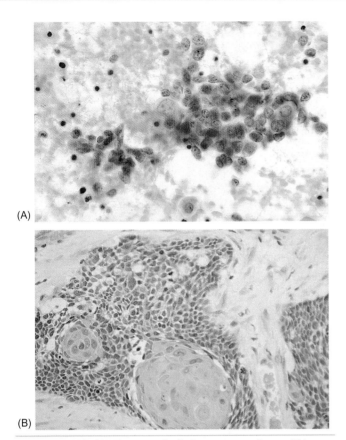

(A)

(B)

**Fig. 2.96** Bronchial brushings: small celled squamous carcinoma. (A) Loose aggregates of small cells, but including some with cyanophilic cytoplasm and vesicular nuclei with easily visible nucleoli. Some single cells with intact cytoplasm. These findings would enable a diagnosis of carcinoma, but do not permit definite tumour typing. Small cell carcinoma or a variant is difficult to exclude (PAP). (B) Bronchial biopsy: Squamous cell carcinoma with small celled and larger celled areas (H&E).

positive, and squamous cell carcinomas are typically TTF-1 negative (~90%), p63 positive, CK5 positive, and CK8 negative. In our laboratory, we use TTF-1, CD56, chromogranin, and CK5. For practical purposes if the tumour is TTF-1, CD56, chromogranin, and CK8 negative but CK5 positive, in all likelihood it is a squamous cell carcinoma.

Combined tumours with components of small cell and squamous cell or glandular carcinoma are occasionally diagnosed by cytology;[260] Zaharopoulos et al.[261] discuss the cytology of small cell variants in detail. This is, however, a rare finding in routine cytological material; Stuart-Harris et al.[202] describe less than 2% of such tumours in routine diagnostic material from small cell cancers. We have seen a few cases of small cell carcinoma in brushings where an accompanying component of atypical but not overtly malignant squamous cells had arisen from overlying intraepithelial change rather than representing evidence of a combined tumour.

Mixed small and large cell carcinomas are diagnosed with less frequency in cytological or endoscopic biopsy samples than autopsy studies.[195,202] In FNA sampling, a few large cells are quite commonly seen in association with an otherwise typical small cell pattern and these do not alter the diagnosis; however, the presence of aggregates of larger cells with prominent nucleoli should lead to some caution. Yang et al. suggested that a mixed morphology could result from degenerative changes.[262]

Cytological material from small celled areas of squamous carcinoma or basaloid carcinoma (Fig. 2.96) may closely mimic small cell anaplastic carcinoma.[263,264]

## Small cell carcinoma versus primary basaloid carcinoma of lung

Basaloid carcinomas are rare and composed of small undifferentiated round cells and may be confused with high-grade NE carcinoma. They are presumed to arise from the bronchial basal cell. However, basaloid carcinomas, whether primary or metastatic to the lung, do not have NE features. Primary basaloid carcinoma of the lung is positive for both high- and low-molecular-weight keratins, whereas small cell carcinoma is positive for the low-molecular-weight keratin only and chromogranin. The recommended panel in the differential diagnosis of small cell carcinoma of lung versus basaloid carcinoma of lung includes chromogranin, CD56, AE1 (low molecular weight) or 35β11 and AE3 (high molecular weight) separately.[197]

## Small cell carcinoma versus atypical carcinoid

In FNA material the distinction between small cell carcinoma and atypical carcinoid and large cell neuroendocrine carcinoma can be difficult (Fig. 2.97). This can be a diagnostic dilemma even on small biopsy specimens and has major prognostic and therapeutic impact on the patient. The key diagnostic features used to distinguish the two may not be present: these include number of mitoses (10 mitoses/1 high-power field for small cell carcinoma; atypical carcinoid 2–10 mitoses/10 high-power fields), presence of obvious areas of necrosis on small biopsies, and nuclear moulding with a salt and pepper chromatin pattern. However, in this differential diagnosis, morphology is still the gold standard. In ambiguous cases as recommended by Pelosi et al.,[265] Ki-67 (MIB-1) immunostaining is most helpful as most small cell carcinomas reveal more than 50% labelling.[265]

## Small cell carcinoma versus lymphoma

Follicle centre cell lymphomas with pronounced cell pleomorphism, nuclear irregularity and some cell aggregation may resemble small cell carcinoma in FNA samples. Dispersed cells of small cell carcinoma usually do not maintain cytoplasm whereas lymphoma cells usually do. Immunocytochemistry is mandatory in these cases (see Chs 13, 14).

## Adenocarcinoma

Pulmonary adenocarcinoma has become the most common and the most diverse form of primary lung carcinoma. The histological complexity of these tumours poses problems for pathologists. The current WHO classification of pulmonary adenocarcinoma does not adequately address a number of clinically relevant biological factors (Box 2.7).[266,267]

These tumours, defined histologically by the formation of acinar or papillary structures, or mucin secretion, tend to occur more peripherally within the lung than squamous cell or small cell tumours. Adenocarcinomas are ultrastructurally very variable.

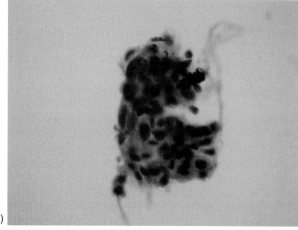

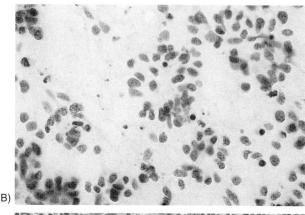

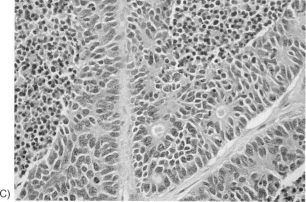

**Fig. 2.97** High-grade neuroendocrine carcinoma. (A) Bronchial brushings: A crowded group of cells with typical hyperchromatic nuclei and stippled chromatin but with more cytoplasm than is usual for small cell carcinoma (PAP). (B) FNA: Prominent rosette formation in some parts of the smear, unlike the pattern seen in small cell carcinoma (PAP). (C) Histological section showing rosettes and necrosis (H&E).

Some contain cells resembling Clara cells or type II pneumocytes or non-specific secretory cells; ultrastructural evidence of squamous or neuroendocrine differentiation may also be seen.[186]

Secretory products vary in appearance and include intracytoplasmic mucin granules, intracytoplasmic lumina or intracellular lumens containing mucus; surface morphology includes microvilli covered by fibrillar glycocalyx and junctional complexes. There are no specific light microscopic features to prove that a tumour is a primary lesion. A diagnosis of primary lung adenocarcinoma therefore requires clinicopathological correlation and reasonable efforts towards exclusion of tumours at other sites. Immunocytochemistry

---

### Box 2.7  WHO classification of lung adenocarcinoma (2004)

**Definition**

- A malignant epithelial tumor with glandular differentiation or mucin production, showing acinar, papillary, bronchioloalveolar or solid with mucin growth patterns or a mixture of the patterns

**Types**

- Adenocarcinoma, mixed subtype
- Acinar adenocarcinoma
- Papillary adenocarcinoma
- Bronchioloalveolar carcinoma
  - Non-mucinous
  - Mucinous
  - Mixed non-mucinous and mucinous or indeterminate
- Solid adenocarcinoma with mucin production

**Variants**

- Fetal adenocarcinoma
- Mucinous ('colloid') carcinoma
- Mucinous cystadenocarcinoma
- Signet ring adenocarcinoma
- Clear cell adenocarcinoma

---

(From Colby TV, Noguchi M, Henschke C, Harris CC. Adenocarcinoma. In: Travis WD, Brambilla E, Muller-Hermelink HK, Harris CC (eds) World Health Organization Classification of Tumours. Pathology and genetics of tumours of the lung, pleura, thymus and heart. Lyon: IARC Press; 2004: 35–44.)[267]

---

for thyroid transcription factor-1, cytokeratin subsets (CK 7 and 20) and other markers can help exclude metastases (Table 2.2).[197,268–270] Table 2.2A–G, shows how, by using a profile of three markers, TTF-1, CK7, and CK20, it is possible to narrow the primary site of a metastatic adenocarcinoma in the lung. The immunohistochemical profile should always be used in conjunction with the clinical presentation, distribution of the lesions, and the morphology. When the tumour has the appropriate morphology and is positive for all three markers, namely TTF-1, CK7, and CK20, primary bronchioloalveolar carcinoma either mucinous or mixed type should be considered.

### Cytological findings (exfoliative): adenocarcinoma

- Cell aggregates are a characteristic feature
- Large eccentric pleomorphic nuclei
- Prominent nucleoli
- Abundant pale or vacuolated cytoplasm.

In exfoliative samples, the hallmark of the presentation of adenocarcinoma is the cell aggregate. Cells are shed in flattened or three-dimensional clusters with enlarged eccentric nuclei showing moderate nuclear pleomorphism, irregular but well-defined nuclear membranes, nuclear hyperchromasia or hypochromasia and abundant pale or lacy cytoplasm which may be vacuolated (Fig. 2.98). Many cells demonstrate prominent rounded central nucleoli.

In poorly differentiated forms, the cell clusters are more irregular and disorganised, and a higher nuclear/cytoplasmic ratio is often seen (Fig. 2.99). Some tumours present with a

**Table 2.2** Differential expression of thyroid transcription factor 1 (TTF-1), cytokeratin (CK) 7, and CK20 in the most common primary and metastatic tumours of the lung

| Diagnosis | TTF-1 (%) | CK7 (%) | CK20 (%) |
|---|---|---|---|
| **A. TTF-1⁺CK7⁺CK20⁺ bronchioloalveolar carcinoma** | | | |
| Adenocarcinoma, bronchioloalveolar, mixed | 91 | 100 | 64 |
| Adenocarcinoma, mucinous, lung | 21 | 87 | 67 |
| **B. TTF-1⁺CK7⁺CK20⁻ tumours** | | | |
| Adenocarcinoma, bronchioloalveolar, nonmucinous | 87 | 99 | 4 |
| Adenocarcinoma, enteric differentiation, lung | 70 | 100 | 24 |
| Adenocarcinoma, follicular, papillary thyroid | 94 | 100 | 0 |
| Adenocarcinoma, lung | 77 | 97 | 9 |
| Adenocarcinoma, lung, metastatic | 77 | 98 | 9 |
| Sclerosing haemangioma of lung | 99 | 100 | 0 |
| Signet ring cell carcinoma, lung | 85 | 100 | 0 |
| **C. TTF-1⁻CK7⁺CK20⁺ tumours** | | | |
| Adenocarcinoma, ampullary | 0 | 83 | 58 |
| Adenocarcinoma, bronchioloalveolar, mucinous | 21 | 98 | 83 |
| Carcinoma, signet ring cell, stomach | 0 | 69 | 35 |
| Carcinoma, transitional cell, NOS | 0 | 91 | 403 |
| Cystadenocarcinoma, mucinous, ovarian, NOS | 0 | 93 | 70 |
| **D. TTF-1⁺CK7⁻CK20⁻ tumours** | | | |
| Carcinoma, oat cell, pulmonary | 88 | 13 | 3 |
| **E. TTF-1⁻CK7⁺CK20⁻ tumours** | | | |
| Adenocarcinoma, endometrial | 6 | 95 | 5 |
| Adenocarcinoma, gallbladder | 0 | 94 | 28 |
| Adenocarcinoma, gastric | 1 | 70 | 45 |
| Adenocarcinoma, metastatic | 0 | 100 | 0 |
| Adenocarcinoma, pancreas | 0 | 94 | 43 |
| Adenocarcinoma, peritoneal, primary | 8 | 100 | 0 |
| Carcinoma, breast | 0 | 88 | 0 |
| Carcinoma, breast, metastatic | 0 | 88 | 2 |
| Carcinoma, embryonal, NOS | 0 | 79 | 0 |
| Carcinoma, large cell, NOS | 20 | 80 | 12 |
| Carcinoma, signet ring, breast | 0 | 100 | 4 |
| Carcinoma, squamous cell, cervical | 0 | 87 | 0 |
| Cholangiocarcinoma | 0 | 95 | 44 |
| Cystadenocarcinoma, ovarian | 2 | 97 | 16 |
| Malignant mesothelioma, localised | 0 | 100 | 0 |
| Mesothelioma, NOS | 0 | 77 | 4 |
| Mucoepidermoid carcinoma, lung | 0 | 77 | 4 |
| Neuroendocrine carcinoma, high-grade, ampulla of Vater | 0 | 88 | 38 |
| Papillary cystadenocarcinoma metastatic | 0 | 100 | 0 |
| **F. Primary lung adenocarcinoma versus metastatic breast carcinoma** | | | |
| | Immunostain class | Lung adenocarcinoma (% positive) | Breast carcinoma (% positive) |
| | TTF-1 | 77 | 0 |
| | Mammaglobin | 17 | 85 |
| | ERP | 4 | 72 |
| | GCDFP-15 | 2 | 53 |
| **G. Small cell carcinoma versus Merkel cell carcinoma** | | | |
| | Immunostain class | Small cell carcinoma of lung (% positive) | Merkel cell carcinoma (% positive) |
| | CK20 | 3 | 90 |
| | TTF-1 | 87 | 0 |
| | TIMP-2 | 87 | 0 |
| | 35-H11 (keratin 903) | 75 | 0 |

NOS, not otherwise specified; ERP, oestrogen receptor protein; GCDFP-15, gross cystic disease fluid protein 15; and TIMP, tissue inhibitor of matrix metalloproteinase. (From Jagirdar J. Application of immunohistochemistry to the diagnosis of primary and metastatic carcinoma to the lung. Arch Pathol Lab Med 2008. Mar; 132(3): 384–96. Reprinted with permission from Archives of Pathology & Laboratory Medicine. Copyright 2008. College of American Pathologists.)

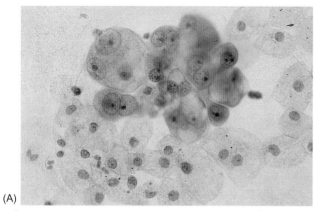

(A)

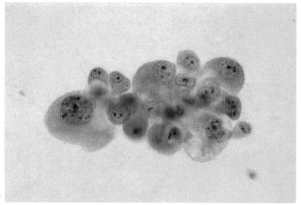

(B)

**Fig. 2.98** Sputum: adenocarcinoma – bronchogenic. (A,B) Aggregate of malignant glandular cells with marked nuclear enlargement, vesicular nuclear chromatin pattern, prominent nucleoli and some nuclear irregularity. Variable cytoplasmic vacuolation (PAP).

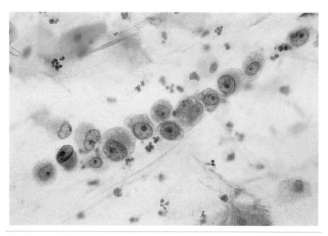

**Fig. 2.99** Sputum: adenocarcinoma – bronchogenic. Loose aggregates but showing eccentric nuclei within pale cytoplasm (PAP).

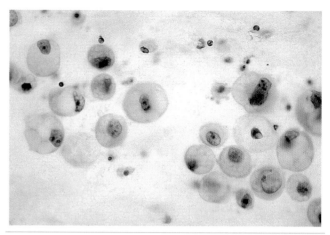

**Fig. 2.100** Sputum: adenocarcinoma – bronchogenic. Dispersed cell pattern; eccentric nuclei; vacuolated cytoplasm resembling macrophage cytoplasm, but with unequivocal nuclear features of malignancy (PAP).

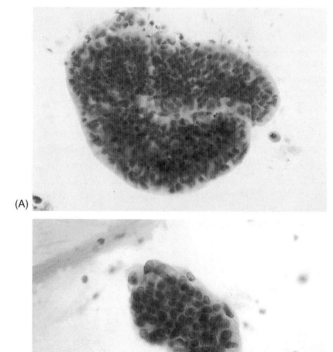

(A)

(B)

**Fig. 2.101** Sputum: reactive/shed bronchial epithelium. Post-bronchoscopy changes. (A) Large fragment of bronchial epithelium with an 'anatomical edge' (PAP). (B) More disorganised fragment of bronchial epithelium with a suggestion of an anatomical border, without obvious cilia but with some apical mucin (PAP).

largely dispersed pattern (Fig. 2.100); cell dispersal may be particularly pronounced in poorly differentiated tumours undergoing necrosis. Distortion of nuclei by large vacuoles may cause indentation of the nucleus, whereas in other cases cytoplasmic vacuolation may be fine. Papillary fragments or true acinar structures with central lumina may be seen.

Marked nuclear enlargement, anisocytosis within a cluster and nuclear irregularity and folding are the most important malignant nuclear criteria for this neoplasm.

## Diagnostic pitfalls (exfoliative): adenocarcinoma

Shed bronchial epithelial aggregates, particularly from asthmatic patients, were historically a pitfall in diagnosis. Early detailed studies of this problem[126,271] delineated criteria for distinguishing this material from adenocarcinoma. The ciliated cell surface of larger fragments with an anatomical or polarised edge of palisaded cells, and a terminal bar (as described on p. 21) are diagnostic features of benign clusters

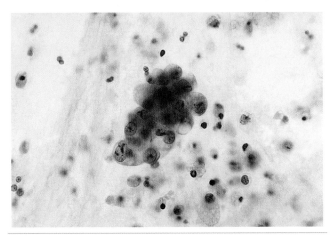

**Fig. 2.102** Sputum: reactive bronchiolar cells. Three-dimensional glandular cell cluster with considerable anisokaryosis and prominent nucleoli. Young male with pneumonia. Resolution of all symptoms while in hospital and well on follow-up (PAP).

which are generally not seen in adenocarcinoma (Fig. 2.101). A background of eosinophils and eosinophilic debris is a useful warning sign indicating allergic bronchial disease. Fragments or groups of reactive bronchiolar or bronchial epithelium as a result of pneumonitis, bronchiolitis or pulmonary infarction,[217,238] may also have markedly atypical nuclear features (Fig. 2.102).

A risk of false positive diagnosis as a result of type II pneumocyte hyperplasia or bronchiolar cell hyperplasia occurs in fibrosing alveolitis (see p. 46)[272] and diffuse alveolar damage (adult respiratory distress syndrome, ARDS) as described on p. 50. Similarly, patients receiving oxygen therapy in association with infection, e.g. in AIDS related infections, may shed abnormal cells resembling adenocarcinoma,[273] particularly in BAL samples[274] where the numbers of such cells may be higher due to the sampling process (Fig. 2.103). These groups of atypical cells may also be found in sputum but usually in small numbers. The clinical background, where there is usually no suspicion of lung carcinoma, is often helpful in preventing misdiagnosis.

### Cytological findings (FNA): adenocarcinoma

- Sheets, rosettes and acinar groupings, columnar cells and mucin production suggest adenocarcinoma
- Rounded nuclei, prominent nucleoli
- Clean or mucinous background.

In FNA and brushings, monolayered sheets, columnar cells or evidence of mucin secretion are valuable criteria in confirming glandular differentiation (Fig. 2.104). Rosettes or acinar structures may be seen. Material is, however, more likely to occur in disorganised aggregates, and rounded or three-dimensional cell aggregates are less often a feature. A combination of rounded nuclei with large central nucleoli seen in most cells within a cell aggregate which demonstrates pale, fragile cytoplasm, is most likely to indicate adenocarcinoma, although some large cell carcinomas may present in this way. The smear background is generally clean. There may be a macrophage reaction and some cell debris particularly in mucinous tumours, but necrosis is generally not a feature, particularly in the better-differentiated adenocarcinomas.

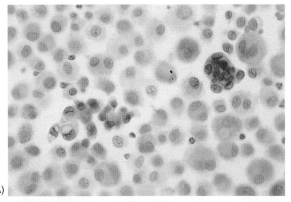

(A)

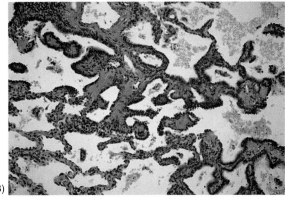

(B)

**Fig. 2.103** Bronchoalveolar lavage: reactive bronchiolar cell proliferation. (A) Aggregates of glandular cells showing quite marked variation in nuclear size including some irregular nuclear margins and psammoma body formation. Such cases are rare but pose a risk of false positive diagnosis, requiring careful clinical correlation (PAP). (B) Open lung biopsy. Interstitial pneumonitis with patchy bronchiolisation of alveolar walls. Diagnosed as extrinsic allergic alveolitis (H&E).

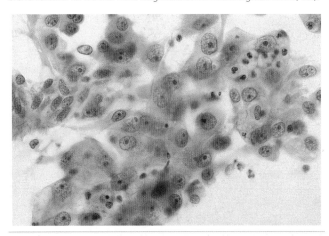

**Fig. 2.104** Bronchial brushings: adenocarcinoma. Sheet of adenocarcinoma cells contrasting with adjacent small clusters of bronchial epithelial cells. Uniform nuclear morphology with prominent cell membranes, vesicular nuclei, large nucleoli and abundant pale cytoplasm, together with some columnar cell forms, indicating glandular differentiation (PAP).

### Diagnostic pitfalls (FNA): adenocarcinoma

- Reactive or reparative changes in bronchiolar epithelium may resemble adenocarcinoma (Fig. 2.81)
- Pseudoglandular growth pattern in squamous carcinomas can mimic adenocarcinoma or vascular tumours[244]
- Rare adenocarcinoma variants such as mucinous cystadenocarcinoma have been studied in FNA samples.[275]

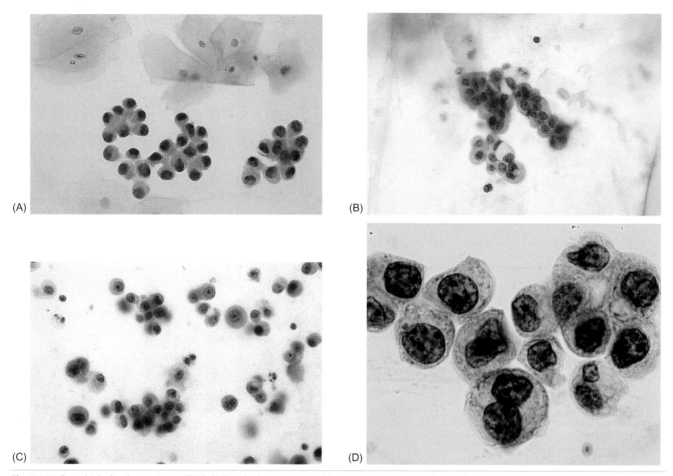

**Fig. 2.105** Bronchioloalveolar carcinoma (BAC). (A,B) Multiple aggregates with more variation in cytoplasmic density. (C) Dispersed cell pattern with some cells resembling macrophages (PAP). (D) High-power view of alveolar cell carcinoma in sputum (PAP).

In the differential diagnosis of metastatic breast carcinoma versus primary lung adenocarcinoma, TTF-1 is the most specific marker, with approximately 72% of lung adenocarcinomas being positive for TTF-1 and none of the breast tumours being positive. Oestrogen receptor is positive in 72% of breast carcinomas and far less frequently positive in lung carcinoma (~4%).[197]

## Bronchioloalveolar carcinoma (BAC)

Current WHO classification of lung adenocarcinomas includes non-invasive BAC and several patterns of invasive adenocarcinoma.[266] The most common is a mixed subtype of adenocarcinoma. This group is very heterogenous and includes a wide spectrum of tumours ranging from adenocarcinomas with a dominant BAC growth pattern (lepidic growth) to frankly invasive adenocarcinoma with no BAC component. There has been some confusion between clinicians and pathologists over the terminology. It is clear that pure BAC is an extremely rare tumour, whereas mixed subtypes of adenocarcinoma may have various clinical presentations and outcomes. Mounting evidence suggests that a subset of mixed subtype of adenocarcinomas with areas of BAC and focal invasion probably represents more indolent tumours. On the basis of the published data, there is a proposal to define a subcategory of 'minimally invasive adenocarcinoma' of the lung. Many morphological factors appear to predict the behaviour of these tumours. Depending on the results of ongoing clinical trials, their surgical management may change in the near future.[276]

These lesions are peripheral tumours with mixed patterns of histological growth including papillary and more solid forms. Several clinicopathological subtypes exist including localised or solitary lesions, those with a more diffuse spreading growth, and those with multiple foci of tumour possibly indicating either multifocal origin or aerogenous spread. The clinical concept of BAC needs to be reevaluated with careful attention to the new 2004 WHO criteria because of the major clinical implications. Existing data indicate that patients with solitary, small, peripheral BAC have a 100% 5-year survival rate.

Histologically, the pattern of growth can be mimicked by metastatic tumour from various sites, in particular pancreas, although this is uncommonly a clinical problem. Tumours of non-secretory, mucinous and pleomorphic type have been identified histologically; ultrastructurally the cells may show features in common with bronchial epithelial cells, mucin secreting cells, Clara cells, type II pneumocytes or combinations of these.[186] The diagnosis can be established on cytological preparations, provided there is a clinicopathological and radiological correlation.

### Cytological findings (exfoliative): BAC[277–283]

- Numerous cohesive glandular clusters
- Regular round cells with ample non-phagocytic cytoplasm
- Minimal increase in N:C ratio and hyperchromasia or vesicular nuclei with prominent nucleoli
- Clean mucoid background.

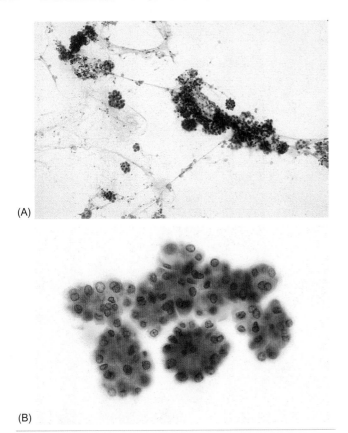

(A)

(B)

**Fig. 2.106** Bronchial washings/lavage: bronchioloalveolar carcinoma. (A) Large numbers of bronchiolar type cell aggregates of varying size (PAP). (B) Moderate variation in nuclear size with some nuclear irregularity (PAP).

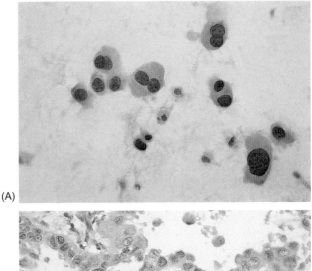

(A)

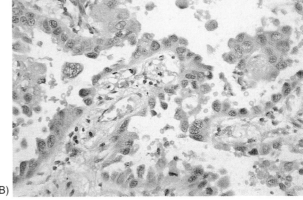

(B)

**Fig. 2.107** FNA: pleomorphic bronchioloalveolar carcinoma. (A) Dispersed pattern of pleomorphic cells showing abundant dense cytoplasm (H&E). (B) Resected tumour showing lepidic growth pattern of markedly pleomorphic cells (H&E).

This diagnosis is relatively easy if many small three-dimensional glandular cell clusters of varying size are present throughout a smear, despite the component cells being rather bland and regular (Figs 2.105, 2.106). The malignant cells usually have abundant cytoplasm, particularly in the mucinous or secretory type, and even though the nuclei may appear relatively uniform, critical evaluation often shows either hyperchromatic nuclei with some nuclear irregularity or more vesicular nuclei and prominent central nucleoli.

In sputum it is necessary to identify clusters of glandular cells as being of bronchiolar type, then to assess the numbers and size of clusters, and finally, the morphology of individual cells within the clusters. An assessment of the number of clusters is important as the likelihood of carcinoma increases with the amount of material present. The nuclear morphology of these tumours is often bland and an individual cluster indisting-uishable from reactive bronchiolar cells. The size of the clusters is also important. A large number of cells within individual clusters is more likely to occur in malignancy than in a reactive bronchiolar proliferation.

Cytoplasmic vacuoles compressing and distorting the nucleus is not a useful malignant criterion; this feature may be seen in benign or malignant bronchiolar clusters. A clean or mucoid background is common. If a prominent inflammatory background is present, caution is appropriate, although it is worth noting that prominent neutrophil ingestion by tumour cells may occasionally be seen in a clean background, a phenomenon linked to granulocyte stimulating factor production by the tumour cells.[284]

Other patterns of cytological presentation are described with this tumour, including a single cell presentation (Fig. 2.105D) closely resembling a macrophage reaction and dispersal associated with degeneration. More pleomorphic forms may shed cells indistinguishable from adenocarcinoma of bronchogenic type or large cell anaplastic carcinoma (Fig. 2.107). Some tumours are associated with psammoma bodies.[281,285]

### Diagnostic pitfalls (exfoliative): BAC

This neoplasm may be particularly difficult to diagnose if there is minimal material. In sputum, three-dimensional aggregates of reactive bronchiolar cells as a result of pneumonia, tuberculosis, infarction, bronchiolitis, bronchitis or conditions such as interstitial lung disease are an important differential diagnostic problem, as described earlier in this chapter. A few small groups of atypical bronchiolar type epithelial cells should never be used as the basis for a malignant diagnosis. The clinical background to the case may provide important additional information; some of the most atypical reactive bronchiolar cells may be seen in very young patients with pneumonia in whom there was no clinical suspicion of malignancy. This diagnosis is not often made in bronchial brushings; however, reactive bronchiolar epithelium in BAL samples may give cause for concern (Figs 2.103, 2.108).

In diagnostically difficult cases, multiple samples may eventually allow a diagnosis to be reached, although with some cases we cannot be unequivocal in reporting and rely on clinical progression of disease to help establish the diagnosis.

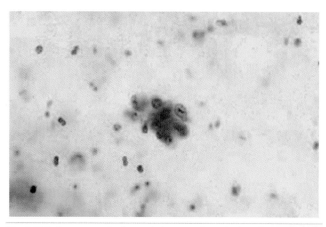

**Fig. 2.108** Sputum: markedly atypical reactive bronchiolar cells. (Same case as Fig. 2.102). There would be a risk of false-positive diagnosis of malignancy without the clinical information in this case (PAP).

This procedure is recommended by other authors.[286] Reactive bronchiolar proliferation will usually resolve within 2–3 weeks and persistence of such abnormal cells for more than 1 month or so would argue strongly in favour of neoplasia. In the series of atypical bronchiolar cells associated with pulmonary emboli reported by Bewtra et al.,[211] the cells were shed in the second and third weeks after infarction but then resolved.

Tumours with a dispersed cell presentation may be extremely difficult to recognise and distinguish from, for example, a macrophage reaction. Degenerating benign cells may show nuclear irregularity, and diagnosis should be based on well-preserved material.[282] Single cell degeneration imparts a somewhat squamous appearance to the cells; though widespread necrosis is not a feature of this tumour. Metastatic tumours such as breast and prostatic carcinoma shed small aggregates of cells with similar appearance to the ones described.

In those patients with diffuse alveolar damage (adult respiratory distress syndrome), BAL samples can contain numerous reactive glandular cell aggregates with morphological features suggesting adenocarcinoma. In the study by Grotte et al.,[274] the cells were shown by electron microscopy to be highly reactive type II pneumocytes; Linder also alludes to the many reactive bronchiolar cells seen in BAL compared with sputum.[287]

### Cytological findings (FNA): BAC[279,283,288–292]

- Best recognised in FNA samples
- Cellular aspirate, monotonous cell population
- Arrangements in cell balls, sheets and papillae
- Intranuclear cytoplasmic inclusions.

In FNA samples the material is usually diagnostic with abundant cellularity including monolayered sheets,[292] small three-dimensional cell balls resembling those seen in sputum, and papillae composed of monotonous cells with fine granular chromatin, some with intranuclear cytoplasmic inclusions, are characteristic (Fig. 2.109). Psammoma bodies may be seen in a small proportion of tumours (less than 10%).[290]

Mucinous or 'secretory' forms give rise to an appearance like that of sheets of endocervical mucosa (Fig. 2.110). Mixtures of secretory and non-secretory material are commonly seen. Mucinous tumours may show prominent nuclear grooves.[292] Pleomorphic forms with more dispersal are not identifiable

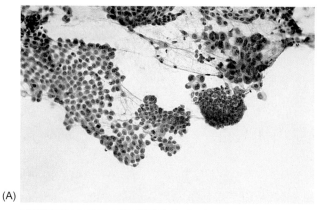

(A)

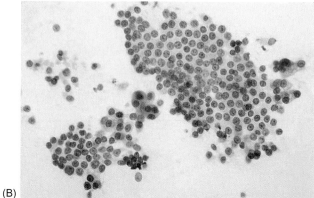

(B)

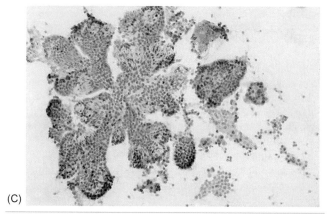

(C)

**Fig. 2.109** FNA: bronchioloalveolar carcinoma. Well-differentiated, non-mucinous type. (A,B) Monolayered sheets of very regular bronchiolar cells, together with scattered three-dimensional aggregates. (C) Papillary structures (H&E).

as having a bronchioloalveolar growth pattern (Fig. 2.107). In some FNA cases individual cells may show no malignant nuclear criteria (Fig. 2.109) and the architectural features, including cell ball and papillary formation, are most important in recognising the neoplasm.

### Diagnostic pitfalls (FNA): BAC

Such epithelium in FNA samples is usually only present in small amounts; abundant bronchiolar epithelium of non-ciliated type should raise the possibility of BAC. Reactive sheets are usually smaller; malignant ones show associated architectural three-dimensionality. Irregular nuclear outlines and large nucleolar size are helpful features in distinguishing BAC from reactive bronchiolar proliferations,[291] whereas a lack of hyperchromasia, prominence of cell borders, terminal

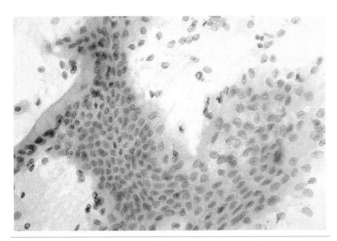

**Fig. 2.110** FNA: mucinous bronchioloalveolar carcinoma. Monolayered sheet of regular cells with abundant apical mucin (H&E).

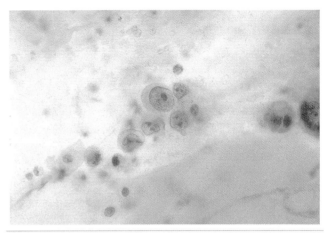

**Fig. 2.112** Sputum: poorly differentiated large cell carcinoma. Loose aggregate of malignant cells. No specific features of cell differentiation. The findings here would favour carcinoma but other anaplastic malignancies, including melanoma, could not be excluded (PAP).

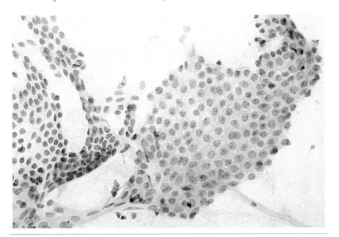

**Fig. 2.111** FNA: metastatic prostatic carcinoma. Cell pattern mimicking BAC (H&E).

plates, goblet cells and cell or nuclear moulding are more characteristic of benign reactive epithelial proliferations.[290]

In FNA samples, metastatic tumours (Fig. 2.111) and epithelial mesothelioma[293] are potential differential diagnostic problems, resolved by clinical evaluation and ancillary testing, as described above.

Intranuclear inclusions have been described as a feature of BAC; they may, however, be seen occasionally in reactive bronchiolar epithelium, in the bronchiolar epithelium of hamartomas and in papillary bronchogenic carcinoma.[294] The distinction between this last entity and BAC is arbitrary at times. Psammoma bodies also occur in other types of adenocarcinoma[295] and in mesothelioma.

Well-differentiated BAC may have a prolonged clinical course of up to 6–8 years after diagnosis before spread outside the lung occurs. The tumours are a possible source of a so-called 'false-false-positive' diagnosis of malignancy.[296] A long clinical course does not, therefore, necessarily disprove a cytological diagnosis; small tumours may be difficult to find in lobectomy specimens, may have a similar consistency to lung tissue and may require careful gross and microscopic examination of excised tissues.[296]

## Large cell carcinomas

Histologically, this subgroup is defined by exclusion as a non-small cell carcinoma without evidence of squamous or

glandular differentiation: the prognosis is similar to or slightly worse than non-small cell cancers in general.[297] Ultrastructural assessment reveals subtle features of differentiation in most cases; such subclassification does not appear to have prognostic importance.[263]

The diagnosis cannot be established by small biopsies or cytological preparations, because of an inability to sample lesions widely. Terms such as 'non-small cell carcinoma – further tumour typing not possible' or 'poorly differentiated large cell carcinoma' are generally proffered in cytological material. The WHO classification recognises basaloid, lymphoepithelioma-like, clear cell and rhabdoid variants. Pure giant cell carcinoma and spindle or sarcomatoid tumours are now described as carcinomas with pleomorphic, sarcomatoid or sarcomatous elements (Box 2.6).

### Cytological findings: large cell carcinomas

- Disorganised groups of large clearly malignant cells
- Pleomorphic single cell population
- Variable cytoplasm, high nuclear/cytoplasmic ratio
- Intracytoplasmic neutrophils and necrotic background.

In sputum, these neoplasms tend to shed disorganised aggregates of large obviously malignant pleomorphic tumour cells, often with a prominent dispersed element of single cells. They have variable amounts of cytoplasm including some tumours with a high nuclear/cytoplasmic ratio and minimal cytoplasm, others with abundant cell cytoplasm or numerous multinucleated forms (Fig. 2.112). Tumours shedding predominantly spindle-cell forms are also described.

In brushings and FNA samples, similar features are seen, including disorganised aggregates or dispersed large pleomorphic cells (Figs 2.113, 2.114). Neutrophil ingestion may be a feature of tumour cells with abundant cytoplasm (Figs 2.115, 2.116). Necrosis is a common accompaniment of large cell carcinomas in any type of cytological sample.

Broderick et al.[298] describe the cytological appearances in sputum and washings in pure giant cell tumours, in which a dispersed population of very large pleomorphic malignant cells with few aggregates was observed; phagocytosis of

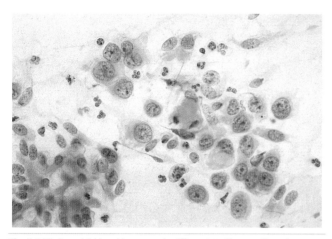

**Fig. 2.113** Bronchial brushings: poorly differentiated large cell carcinoma. Loose aggregates of pleomorphic malignant cells without specific features to indicate differentiation (PAP).

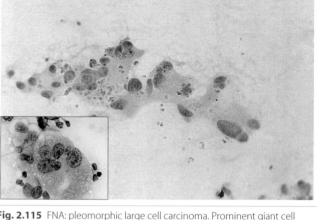

**Fig. 2.115** FNA: pleomorphic large cell carcinoma. Prominent giant cell component and neutrophil ingestion (H&E). Inset: FNA lung tumour. High magnification of tumour giant cell in a pleomorphic large cell carcinoma (MGG).

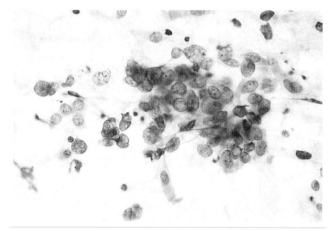

**Fig. 2.114** Bronchial brushings: poorly differentiated carcinoma. The vesicular nuclear chromatin, distinct cell membranes and preserved cytoplasm helps exclude small cell carcinoma, but further specific tumour typing cannot be suggested (PAP).

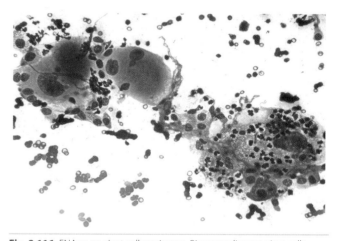

**Fig. 2.116** FNA: pure giant cell carcinoma. Bizarre malignant giant cells; prominent neutrophil ingestion (MGG).

inflammatory cells was common. Naib described similar appearances in sputum.[299] Craig et al.[300] presented a case in which brushings and FNA samples showed similar features including phagocytosis of tumour cells, and in which the tumour had probably arisen in a pre-existing bronchioloalveolar cell carcinoma. Figure 2.116 shows an example in FNA material.

### Diagnostic pitfalls: large cell carcinomas

In sputum, cell aggregates should not be mistaken for evidence of glandular differentiation when the component cells are totally disorganised. In FNA samples, necrosis causing eosinophilia is commonly mistaken for keratinisation[243] although this is a feature more of H&E than PAP staining, which distinguishes between necrosis and keratinisation more easily.

Drug and chemotherapy effect may result in highly atypical large cells, and often with multinucleation (Fig. 2.86). Radiotherapy effect usually results in cells with a low nuclear/cytoplasmic ratio, multinucleation and degenerative nuclear changes including vacuolation (Fig. 2.86). These changes are

seldom a problem in interpretation, if the clinical background is known.[301] Epithelial 'repair' similar in appearance to that seen in cervical smears (Fig. 2.81), is also occasionally found, particularly in patients with repeated bronchoscopies for diagnosis of lung cancer.[218]

Megakaryocytes[302] occasionally occur in brushings and FNA samples but in small numbers and are unlikely to be mistaken for malignant cells. Viral effect (Fig. 2.117) is seldom a problem. Other metastatic undifferentiated carcinomas, malignant melanoma and sarcoma may all give cells of similar appearance to primary large cell carcinomas.

## Adenosquamous carcinoma

Tumours with an intimate mixture of squamous and glandular growth pattern are uncommon if a significant proportion of both tumour types is required for diagnosis. Smaller foci of glandular or squamous differentiation in tumours of other types are commonly seen. Adenosquamous tumours are said to be more often peripheral in location and to be of poor prognosis (Fig. 2.118).

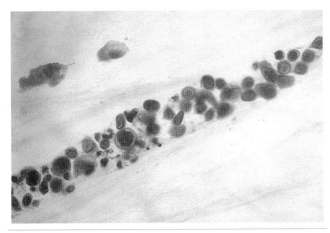

**Fig. 2.117** Sputum: herpes virus changes. Low power appearances somewhat resembling carcinoma (PAP).

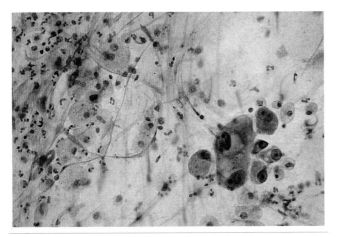

**Fig. 2.118** Sputum: adenosquamous carcinoma. Keratinising malignant cells and an aggregate of adenocarcinoma cells (PAP).

## Large cell neuroendocrine tumours

McDowell[209] in 1981 described cases which had been reported as large cell or squamous cell carcinoma or adenocarcinoma histologically and which showed cytoplasmic dense core neurosecretory granules, and demonstrated these features in 4% of 150 lung tumours. Others suggested that up to 9% of non-small cell carcinomas of the lung might contain neurosecretory granules.[210] In some studies this has not necessarily been an indicator of poor prognosis: however, others have suggested more aggressive behaviour in these tumours, and responsiveness to chemotherapy.[212]

Large cell neuroendocrine carcinoma is now recognised as an entity distinct from atypical carcinoid tumour and small cell carcinoma.[192,215] Histologically, cell nesting with palisading, rosettes or trabeculae; large cells with a low nuclear/cytoplasmic ratio; prominent nucleoli, vesicular chromatin, a high mitotic rate and abundant necrosis are suggested as features helping to identify this tumour by light microscopy.[192,215] Identification of neuroendocrine phenotype by immunocytochemistry or electron microscopy is necessary for diagnosis. A mitotic rate of >10/10 high-power fields distinguishes these lesions from atypical carcinoid tumours (2–10 mitoses/10 high-power fields).

These lesions have an extremely poor prognosis, similar to small cell carcinoma.[215] Cytological descriptions are few and diagnosis may be difficult. Nicholson and Ryan describe loose cell aggregates in a background of singly dispersed cells, tumour cells clinging to capillaries; rosette formations, delicate, granular cytoplasm, inconspicuous nucleoli, moulding in high-grade tumours and speckled or dusty chromatin patterns as general criteria useful in identifying neuroendocrine differentiation.[303]

## Carcinoid tumours

These constitute only 1% of lung tumours. They occur predominantly in earlier age groups, in the fourth and fifth decades, in contrast to patients with bronchogenic carcinoma. The tumour has an origin in a main bronchus in 85% of cases, but may be more peripheral particularly in spindle cell forms.

The classic or typical carcinoid tumour consists of uniform cells with small round to oval nuclei, few nucleoli and granular eosinophilic cytoplasm, arranged in nests, trabeculae or a mosaic pattern. Variants include clear cell tumours, papillary and oncocytic tumours and spindle cell forms. Some 5–10% of typical cases with no features of malignancy will metastasise, although superficially invasive tumours, tumours less than 3 cm in diameter and those without lymph node metastases at diagnosis generally behave in a biologically benign fashion.

### Cytological findings: carcinoid tumours[303–313]

- Best seen in brushings and FNA samples
- Uniform small cells, rounded nuclei, stippled chromatin
- Marked cell dissociation, some palisades or trabeculae
- Bare nuclei are common but necrosis is rare
- Plexiform vascular fragments in FNA samples.

## Typical/classical carcinoid

In typical/classical carcinoids, tumour cells are uncommonly seen in sputum as these neoplasms are usually submucosal, even when they assume an intrabronchial polypoid growth. In brushings or FNA samples, a dispersed cell population with some trabecula or palisading of small cell clusters, a uniform population of small cells with small amounts of intact cytoplasm and monotonous rounded or oval nuclei with a finely granular or stippled nuclear chromatin are diagnostic features (Figs 2.119–2.121).

The 'neuroendocrine nucleus' with its round or oval shape, regular outline and coarsely stippled nuclear chromatin is a useful diagnostic criterion to keep in mind. Tumour cell nuclei are usually robust, and traumatised cells, cell debris or streaks of nuclear material are not a feature, although bare nuclei are prominent in some cases. Necrosis or inflammatory changes are not usually seen but these lesions are highly vascular and may yield haemorrhagic samples.

In brushings, a contrast with bronchial epithelial cells may be a useful feature, although stripped bronchial cell nuclei and carcinoid tumour nuclei may be very similar[306] and small amounts of tumour tissue may be overlooked.[304] Traumatisation of cells by the procedure may very rarely lead to an appearance resembling small cell carcinoma.[311]

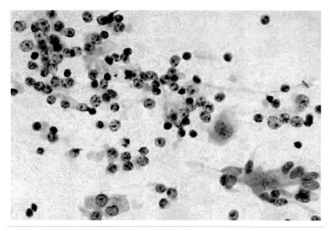

**Fig. 2.119** Bronchial brushings: carcinoid tumour. Dispersed cells including many bare nuclei with coarsely clumped 'neuroendocrine' chromatin pattern. Absence of mitotic activity, necrosis or cell traumatisation (PAP).

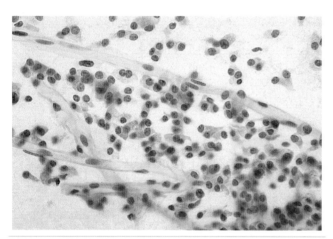

**Fig. 2.120** FNA: carcinoid tumour. Dispersed population of regular small neuroendocrine cells. Background of plexiform capillaries (PAP).

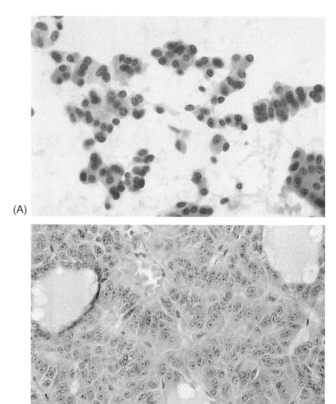

(A)

(B)

**Fig. 2.121** FNA: carcinoid tumour. (A) Clumps, cords and trabeculae of tumour cells (H&E). (B) Histological section showing 'neuroendocrine nuclei' (H&E).

to exclude small cell carcinoma.[314,315] A background of capillary blood vessels is unlike small cell carcinoma.

In FNA samples, a plexiform background of small blood vessels and adherence of cells to vascular cores is a striking feature in most cases (Fig. 2.120) and is an important additional diagnostic criterion. Anderson et al.[304] found this feature in 21 of 23 cases, including spindle and atypical tumours; Mitchell et al.[312] also draw attention to this finding.

Bronchioloalveolar carcinoma cells are usually larger, have more abundant cytoplasm, evidence of sheet-like growth and lack a vascular component. Strong positive staining for synaptophysin or chromogranin would favour carcinoid.[304] Intranuclear cytoplasmic inclusions are seen occasionally in carcinoids[304] as well as in BAC. Sclerosing haemangioma/pneumocytoma can produce similar cytological appearances to carcinoid, but is a very rare neoplasm.[304]

## Spindle cell carcinoid

Spindle cell carcinoid tumours are usually more peripheral and only seen in FNA material. They may show a closer resemblance to small cell carcinoma, or more rarely mesenchymal tumours (Fig. 2.122), but uniformity of nuclear size, absence of moulding, nuclear smearing and background debris all help

## Adenocarcinoid

Adenocarcinoid is a term used in some cytological descriptions for tumours confirmed to be neuroendocrine ultrastructurally and with histological features of carcinoid tumours but showing glandular differentiation with or without mucin secretion. They are not recognised in the WHO classification but may be a useful concept to keep in mind when low grade or columnar cell lesions are encountered. Cytologically, they may show columnar cells with round or oval nuclei in sheets, syncytia or stratified groups[316,317] and may be difficult to diagnose by cytology alone. Pilotti et al.[317] advise that carcinoids with glandular features should be considered when FNA material from asymptomatic patients with coin lesions suggests a glandular neoplasm, with an orderly structure of clusters and relatively uniform nuclei.

## Atypical carcinoid tumours

This subgroup constitutes about 10% of carcinoid tumours but may provide great diagnostic difficulty. Arrigoni et al.[318] suggested that nuclear pleomorphism, mitoses and necrosis in tumours of carcinoid architecture predicted more aggressive behaviour. In

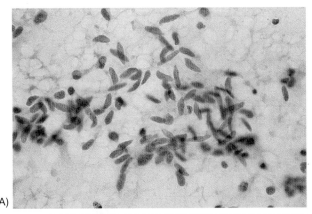

(A)

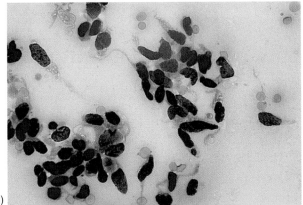

(B)

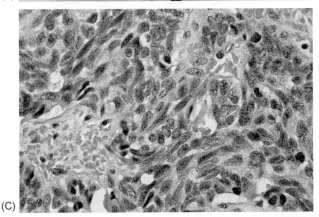

(C)

**Fig. 2.122** Imprint from resected lung specimen: carcinoid tumour, spindle cell type. Unusually elongated cells with a mesenchymal appearance (A, H&E; B, MGG; C, histological section H&E).

or abundant mitotic activity, and the presence of cohesive acinar, rosette or sheet-like groups with palisading helps exclude small cell carcinoma. Nevertheless, it is accepted that there is an overlap in cytological appearances between this lesion and small cell carcinoma or large cell neuroendocrine carcinoma, (Fig. 2.97) and that even on bronchial biopsy such a distinction may be very difficult[303,313,319–321] with major prognostic and therapeutic impact on the patient. The key diagnostic features used to distinguish the two may not be present, such as number of mitoses (>10 mitoses/high-power field for small cell carcinoma; atypical carcinoid 2–10 mitoses/10 high-power fields), presence of obvious areas of necrosis on small biopsies, and nuclear moulding with salt and pepper chromatin pattern. However, in this differential diagnosis, morphology is still the gold standard. In ambiguous cases as recommended by Pelosi et al.,[265] Ki-67 (MIB-1) immunostaining is most helpful in which most small cell carcinomas reveal more than 50% labelling.[265] Carcinoids including atypical carcinoids do show more frequent staining for NE markers such as chromogranin and synaptophysin than small cell carcinomas. However, this finding may not be helpful in small specimens suffering from sampling errors.[322] In this differential diagnosis, TTF-1 cannot be used as carcinoids, like small cell carcinomas, show TTF-1 staining, which can be quite variable in the carcinoids (0%–95%).[323]

Markers such as chromogranin and synaptophysin may be unequivocally positive in neuroendocrine tumours, but are less valuable in subtyping.

## Other carcinomas

### Adenoid cystic carcinoma

These tumours occur as primary lesions, generally of major bronchi,[324–327] or as metastatic spread to the lung from other sites.[328–330] If the large acellular basement membrane spheres and fingers so characteristic of this tumour are evident in a background of small cells with uniform nuclei, the diagnosis can be made cytologically (Fig. 2.123). Such spheres are more easily seen in MGG- than in PAP-stained preparations. They may not be present in FNA samples from the peripheral infiltrating areas of the tumour (Fig. 2.124), nor in brush samples, and distinction from other small cell neoplasms is then very difficult. Tumour shedding into brushings may not occur until after biopsy.[326] Radhika et al.[328] describe tight branching tubular clusters of malignant cells giving a cylindroid appearance as an additional criterion for diagnosis.

### Mucoepidermoid carcinoma

In current practice this term is restricted to low-grade tumours of bronchial gland origin. Nguyen[327] describes FNA material from two low-grade bronchial tumours as showing features similar to salivary gland lesions, including groups of only moderately pleomorphic squamous cells with intracytoplasmic mucus. Brooks and Baandrup[331] found a mixture of intermediate cells, squamous and mucinous cells in an FNA sample from a peripheral tumour. Tao[332] describes clusters of uniform squamous cells, mucus secreting cells associated with squamous cells and spindle cells. Segletes et al. were able to suggest the diagnosis in three cases based on combinations of mucinous, squamous and intermediate cells.[333] The cytomorphology of

his series, regional or distant metastases were evident in up to 70% of patients and were associated with a death rate of 30%. More recent studies have verified these findings[215] and suggest that a mitotic rate of 2–10/10 high-power fields or coagulative necrosis defines a subgroup of neuroendocrine tumours with a biological behaviour between typical carcinoid and large cell neuroendocrine carcinoma or small cell carcinoma.

These neoplasms usually possess neuroendocrine cytological characteristics including rounded or oval nuclei, uniform stippled chromatin and some dispersed cells with intact cytoplasm.[303,319–321] In FNA samples, increased pleomorphism and identification of any mitotic activity or necrosis helps distinguish these from typical carcinoids. The absence of widespread moulding, smeared fragile nuclei, abundant single cell necrosis

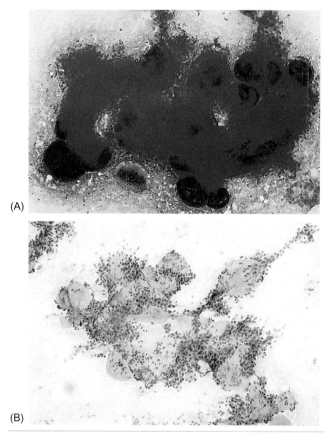

(A)

(B)

**Fig. 2.123** FNA: metastatic adenoid-cystic carcinoma. Primary tumour in the oral cavity. (A,B) Numerous hyaline globules of basement membrane material with intervening small hyperchromatic tumour cells (A, MGG; B, H&E).

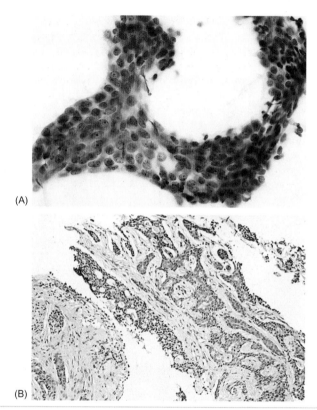

(A)

(B)

**Fig. 2.124** Transbronchial FNA: recurrent adenoid-cystic carcinoma. (A) Irregular cord of poorly differentiated carcinoma cells, not diagnosable as adenoid-cystic in type without reference to previous histology (PAP). (B) Bronchial biopsy sample at the time of transbronchial FNA showing recurrent adenoid-cystic carcinoma (H&E).

high-grade tumours is indistinguishable from adenosquamous carcinoma.[332]

## Metastatic carcinoma

Metastatic tumours to the thorax constitute up to 15–20% of lesions diagnosed by cytology in some series.[10] The principles of cytological diagnosis of metastatic tumour of lung are the same as those of the surgical pathologist in assessing tissue: detailed knowledge of the clinical history must be available, together with earlier cytological and histological preparations for review and comparison with current material.[9,10,334] Using this approach, a cytological diagnosis is highly reliable, although metastatic tumour may occasionally be misinterpreted as primary, and primary lung cancer may, on occasions, be misinterpreted as a metastasis or may mimic other unusual tumours, including sarcomas (Figs 2.125, 2.126).

Immunohistochemistry is a valuable guide,[268,335–337] although a careful clinicopathological approach is still necessary because of an overlap in immunophenotype between primary and metastatic tumours. Mucinous tumours are particularly difficult to characterise.

Attention has been drawn to the common occurrence of new primary tumours when metastases are suspected clinically,[338] and double primaries may also be encountered.[339] Metastatic tumour, particularly renal cell and colonic carcinomas,[340] may mimic

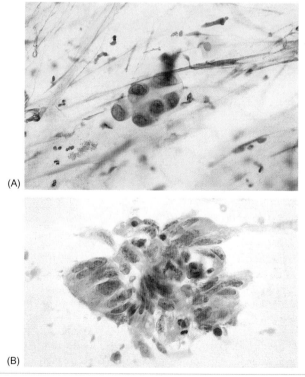

(A)

(B)

**Fig. 2.125** (A) Sputum: metastatic breast carcinoma. This cohesive group of small malignant cells includes one cell with a visible intracytoplasmic lumen (PAP). (B) Brushings: metastatic colonic adenocarcinoma. The columnar form of the malignant cells is apparent, with elongated nuclei and apical cytoplasm (PAP).

primary tumours clinically either by growing as an endobronchial lesion or because of a bronchioloalveolar growth pattern.

In more recent cytological literature, unusual metastatic lesions such as breast carcinoma with osteoclastic giant cells,[341] metaplastic breast carcinoma with prominent squamous cell components,[342] or chondroid elements,[343] adrenal carcinoma,[344] choriocarcinoma,[345] meningioma,[346,347] mesothelioma,[348,349] medullary carcinoma of thyroid,[350] adamantinoma of tibia,[351] ameloblastoma,[352] pleomorphic adenoma of salivary glands[353] and granulosa cell tumour[354] have all been confirmed cytologically. Occasional examples of unusual lesions such as leiomyosarcoma continue to be described in sputum.[355]

## Other rare tumours

Juvenile papillomatosis is most frequently an upper respiratory tract lesion associated with human papilloma virus that may occasionally involve distal bronchi. Solitary papillomas of bronchi show a range of epithelial types, including some with simple or keratinising metaplastic epithelium and others with a more transitional appearance; tumours of purely glandular type are also rarely seen. Multifocal lesions are extremely difficult to treat and may extend into lung parenchyma, although they are histologically benign. Occasionally, examples of malignant change are described. Bronchial brushings typically reveal keratinous material and mature squamous cells, but a diagnosis is not usually possible without biopsy.[356] Features similar to human papilloma virus effect in other sites may be seen.[357]

Brightman et al.[358] reported a rare case of a combined squamous cell papilloma and mucous gland adenoma in which large squamous cells, smaller polygonal cells and papillary groups of cylindrical cells were present in FNA smears.

FNA samples of a benign clear cell ('sugar') tumour of lung were described as showing large irregular clusters of benign polygonal and spindle-shaped cells with vacuolated granular PAS positive cytoplasm.[359] A distinction from inflammatory pseudotumour, renal cell carcinoma, clear cell carcinoid or carcinoma was difficult without ultrastructural assessment. The neoplastic cell is thought to be a perivascular cell related to smooth muscle.

Cwierzyk et al. describe the appearances of pulmonary oncocytoma in bronchial brushings.[360] Syncytial clusters of monotonous epithelial cells with abundant, rather dense, amphophilic cytoplasm were observed within mucus. Granular staining in PAS preparations was seen. Nuclei were round or oval with minimal variation, and had finely stippled chromatin. The tumour was 1.5 cm in diameter, polypoid and projected into the bronchial lumen; the mitochondrion-rich nature of the cytoplasm was observed ultrastructurally. There were no neurosecretory granules, although the cells resembled carcinoid tumour cells. Multicentric oncocytoma has also been diagnosed by FNA by demonstrating PTAH staining of tumour cell granules and absence of neuroendocrine markers in cell blocks.[361]

## Benign mesenchymal tumours

## Chondroid hamartoma

These lesions constitute 5–10% of small solitary rounded peripheral lung masses and are important because they may

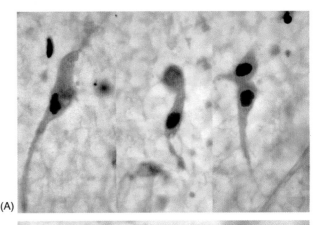

(A)

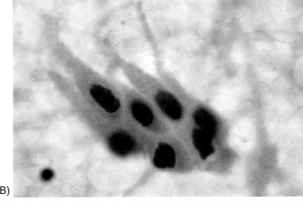

(B)

**Fig. 2.126** FNA: metastatic transitional cell carcinoma. (A) Cercariform cells with bulbous ends and long cytoplasmic processes. (B) Sheet of squamoid cells with long cytoplasmic processes (PAP).

be easily recognised cytologically, definitively diagnosed and require no further diagnostic or therapeutic procedures.

### Cytological findings: chondroid hamartoma

- Myxoid connective tissue and cartilage
- Sheets of epithelial cells
- Fat and macrophages in the background.

In FNA samples, the combination of fibrillar myxoid connective tissue, hyaline cartilage (Fig. 2.127), bronchiolar epithelium and fat is diagnostic.[362–369] In some cases, macrophages may be present in abundance in the background. The fibrillar myxoid material is the most distinctive element of the tumour, and the single most useful diagnostic indicator. It is magenta or purple in MGG preparations and pale orange or grey in PAP-stained material, where it can be more easily overlooked (Fig. 2.127). Positive staining for S100 helps distinguish this material from collagenous fibrous tissue.[369]

### Diagnostic pitfalls: chondroid hamartoma

Bronchiolar epithelium presents in sheets, may be abundant, and often shows some nuclear enlargement and intranuclear cytoplasmic inclusions, which may lead to an incorrect suspicion of epithelial malignancy. Chondrocytes may also be misinterpreted.[363] For this reason the lesion is a quite

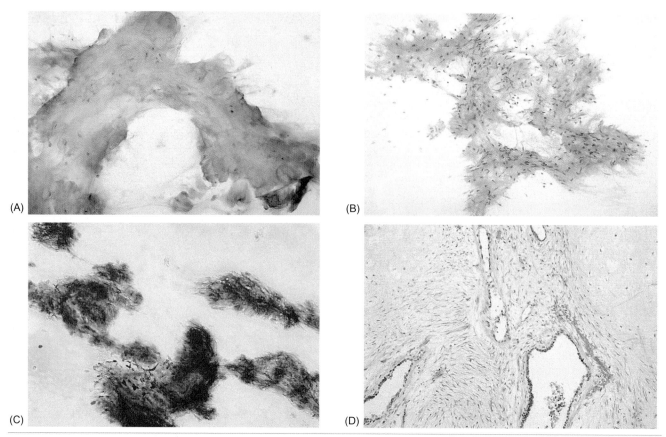

**Fig. 2.127** FNA: chondroid hamartoma. (A) Core of hyaline cartilage showing lacunae and background matrix (H&E). (B) Myxoid fibrosis tissue (H&E). (C) Fibromyxoid tissue showing striking magenta metachromasia (MGG). (D) A resected specimen showing fibromyxoid tissue, mature cartilage and trapped bronchiolar epithelium (H&E).

common source of false positive diagnosis of malignancy. Mature cartilage is sparsely cellular, containing chondrocytes in lacunae. Contamination from chest wall costal cartilage or tracheal or bronchial cartilage might lead to a false diagnosis if reliance is placed on cartilage alone.

## Sclerosing haemangioma (pneumocytoma)

This lesion is a rare benign tumour generally presenting as an incidental finding on chest X-ray, and occurring as a solitary rounded mass, mainly in women. Many of the patients are of Asian descent. The range of histological patterns is diverse. It is uncertain which cellular component is neoplastic, although the epithelial cell element is currently favoured.[186]

### Cytological findings: pneumocytoma

- Diagnosis possible in FNA material
- Bronchiolar epithelial-type around blood spaces
- Eosinophilic cytoplasm, rounded nuclei, small nucleoli.

FNA sampling in one reported case showed aggregates of epithelial-like tumour cells surrounding blood spaces. The neoplastic cells were of medium size with round or oval folded nuclei, finely reticular chromatin, small nucleoli and moderate amounts of eosinophilic cytoplasm.[370] Arrangements of cells along septa probably represented detached larger blood vessel walls. Tao[371] refers to a similar case with a proliferating network of blood vessels and adherent, irritated alveolar cells.

In several case reports, papillary or sheet-like groups of epithelial cells are described[372] having a resemblance to bronchioloalveolar carcinoma.[372,373] Kaw and Nayak[374] reported on a case presenting cytologically with a combination of bland spindle cells and epithelial cells, either bronchiolar or type II pneumocytes. Wojcik et al.[375] diagnosed a case in which regular epithelial-like cells were arranged in loose fragments containing sclerotic stromal cores; cell block preparations revealed a papillary pattern together with angiomatous areas. Haemosiderin-laden macrophages were also seen. Intranuclear inclusions were evident in the epithelial-like cells. Our single case was a young Asian male with a long history of haemoptysis and a 10 cm rounded opacity in the lung. Aspiration showed highly cellular smears composed mainly of epithelial-like cells and some macrophages (Fig. 2.128). The abundance of material and the sheet-like presentation in smears resembled BAC. A definite diagnosis of malignancy was not given because of the unusual clinical findings and absence of nuclear criteria of malignancy. The diagnosis was made on the excised specimen. Carcinoid tumour might also provide differential diagnostic problems.[304]

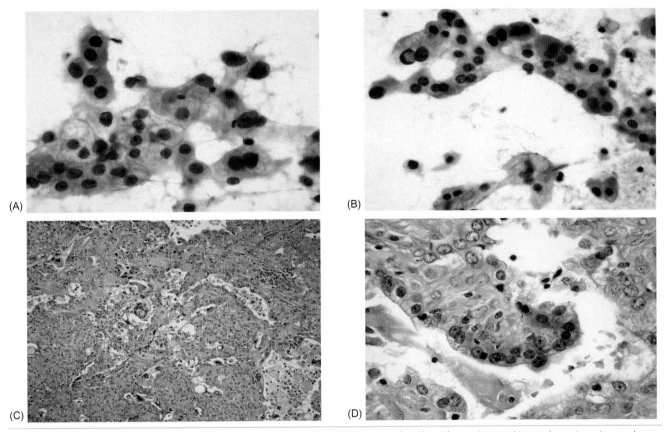

**Fig. 2.128** FNA: sclerosing haemangioma/pneumocytoma. (A,B) Sheets of bronchiolar type cells with moderate pleomorphism and prominent intranuclear cytoplasmic inclusions (H&E). (C,D) Resected specimen (C and D, H&E).

## Granular cell tumour

Bronchial tumours constitute only 5–10% of the total incidence of these tumours. They are now accepted as being of Schwann cell derivation. In the lung they usually present as endobronchial nodules, although they may sometimes grossly mimic infiltrative malignancy (see Ch. 29, p. 771).

### Cytological findings: granular cell tumour

- Single or grouped cells, abundant granular cytoplasm
- Some pleomorphism but low nuclear/cytoplasmic ratio
- Positive staining with S100.

Chen[376] reported a case in which brushings smears showed characteristic abundant eosinophilic granular cytoplasm, a few spindle cell forms and some binucleated cells. Fÿezesi et al.[377] studied a multicentric lesion diagnosed in cell blocks of bronchial lavage samples. Single cells and groups of tumour cells with abundant, granular cytoplasm were distinguishable from macrophages and epithelial cells. Glant et al.,[378] Mermolja et al.[379] and Thomas et al.[380] described similar cytomorphology, including components of strap-like and spindle cell forms. Smith et al. report a mediastinal case diagnosed by FNA.[381]

Positive S 100 staining helps confirm the cell type.[382] Occasionally giant or bizarre polygonal cells are described in cytological preparations,[378,379] but this appearance is still generally associated with benign biological behaviour. In our limited experience with this tumour in FNA samples of several sites, the very low nuclear/cytoplasmic ratio is distinctive and helps distinguish the cells even from macrophages; the large ill-defined cytoplasmic granules in PAP-stained samples are most helpful (Fig. 2.129). The tumour is rarely diagnosed in exfoliated material.[383]

## Solitary fibrous tumour/pleural fibroma

In the past, there was much debate about the origin of these pleural-based tumours, as indicated by their varied nomenclature, which previously included 'submesothelial fibrous tumour' and 'localised fibrous mesothelioma'. They are now generally regarded as tumours of fibroblasts with or without bronchial epithelial or mesothelial entrapment (Fig. 2.130), rather than being true mesotheliomas. These lesions are well circumscribed, often encapsulated and grow to a considerable size. They are generally unrelated to asbestos exposure. While most are benign some are histologically malignant, or eventually have a malignant clinical course.[384–386] These tumours have now been described in a wide range of tissues.

They rarely present with a serous effusion (5/60)[387] and on the few occasions where an effusion is present, cytology is unhelpful.[388,387] They are more likely to be sampled by the FNA approach.[385,386,389–394] We have seen aspirates from four cases of localised fibrous lesions of the pleura: two benign and

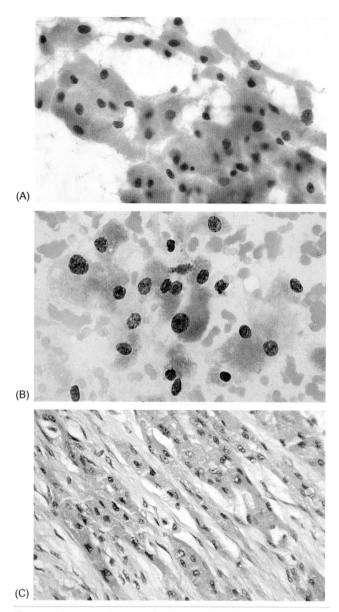

(A)

(B)

(C)

**Fig. 2.129** FNA: granular cell tumour. Malignant chest wall lesion, which metastasised to bone. (A,B) Loose aggregates and dispersed cells with abundant granular cytoplasm, rounded nuclei with some variation in shape and size and some strap shaped and spindle cell forms. (A, PAP; B, MGG) (C) Resected specimen showing cords and clumps of granular cells within a fibrous stroma (H&E).

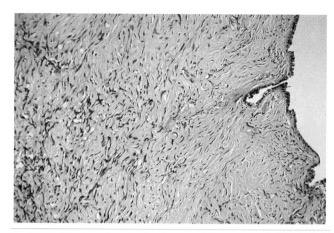

**Fig. 2.130** Histological section: benign pleural fibroma. A single layer of benign epithelial (bronchiolar) cells cover dense fibrous tumour tissue (H&E).

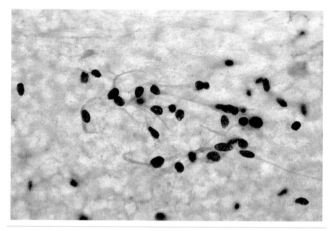

**Fig. 2.131** FNA sample: benign pleural fibroma. Several spindle-shaped cells (H&E).

fibroma do not stain with antikeratin antibodies, and most stain positively for CD34 in tumour cells.

Given the correct clinical setting and adequate cellular material, it is possible to suggest the diagnosis of localised pleural fibrous tumour by the FNA approach, although prediction of their ultimate biological behaviour as judged solely on the cytological assessment is not possible.

## Lymphoma, leukaemia and related disorders

Non-Hodgkin malignant lymphomas of extrapulmonary origin and of all histological subtypes quite frequently affect the lung during the course of the disease (see Ch. 14). Primary lymphoproliferative disorders are uncommon and are virtually confined to adults. The majority of primary tumours are low-grade B-cell lymphomas of marginal zone (MALT) type, or high-grade large cell lymphomas mainly of B cell type. An angiocentric infiltration is seen in many non-Hodgkin lymphomas of lung (so-called lymphomatoid granulomatosis pattern). This may occur in low-grade tumours with a pure small cell component as well as high-grade tumours including T-cell rich B-cell lymphomas.[186] The clinical background to primary

two having a malignant course. All were surprisingly cellular, a feature also noted by Frazer,[395] having many spindle fibroblastoid-like cells with oval nuclei (Fig. 2.131), associated with some background collagenous material; occasionally epithelial-like cells were also present. One benign case demonstrated a degree of nuclear atypia that caused a suspicion of malignancy on the FNA material.

The presence of many bare oval nuclei and collagen in the background of the smear was also observed by Dusenbery et al.[396] They also stressed the value of cell block material in making a precise diagnosis. Immunocytochemical testing for keratin is of value in the differential diagnosis of these tumours; unlike sarcomatoid malignant mesothelioma, the spindle cells of pleural

**Table 2.3** Immunohistochemical features of primary lymphomas of lung

| Type of lymphoma | CD20 | Pax-5 | CD79a | CD43 | CD5 | CD10 | CD23 | CD15 | CD30 | Cyclin DI | BCL-2 | BCL-10 | EBV | Monoclonal light chain |
|---|---|---|---|---|---|---|---|---|---|---|---|---|---|---|
| Marginal zone B cell | + | + | + | S | N | N | N | N | N | N | N | S | N | S |
| Chronic lymphocytic leukaemia/small cell lymphocytic lymphoma | + | + | + | S | S | N | N | N | N | + | S | N | N | S |
| Mantle cell lymphoma | + | + | + | S | S | N | N | N | N | S | S | N | N | S |
| Follicular lymphoma | + | + | + | N | N | S | N | N | N | N | S | N | N | S |
| Hodgkin lymphoma | S | S | S | N | N | N | N | S | S | N | S | N | S | N |
| Lymphomatoid granulomatosis | S | U | U | N | N | N | N | N | N | N | N | U | S | N |
| Intravascular lymphoma | + | + | + | R | S | U | N | N | N | S | U | U | U | U |
| Primary effusion lymphoma | N | N | N | S | N | N | N | N | S | U | U | U | S | N |
| Pyothorax-associated lymphoma | + | + | + | S | N | N | N | N | N | U | U | U | S | N |

EBV, Epstein–Barr virus; +, reactivity almost always diffuse, strong posivitity; S, sometime positive; N, almost always negative; U, uncertain; R, rare cells positive. (From Hammar SP. Immunohistology of lung and pleural neoplasms. In: Dabbs D (ed.) Diagnostic Immunohistochemistry, 2nd edn. Philadelphia: PA: Churchill Livingstone, 2006: 329–403, with permission of Elsevier.)[401]

marginal zone (MALT) lung lymphomas includes pre-existing immunopathic disorders such as Sjogren's syndrome and dysproteinaemia. AIDS patients can have interstitial lymphoid infiltrates, which progress to frank lymphoma, or present with high-grade large cell or blastic tumours.[397] The lung is not uncommonly involved in post-transplant lymphoproliferative disorders.[398] Gross patterns of lung involvement by lymphoma include masses with or without cavitation, localised areas of consolidation, multiple nodules or diffuse infiltrates.[186]

Reactive lymphoid infiltrations, including prominent germinal centre formation, may be associated with lymphoma, and representative sampling can be difficult to achieve by any cytological method. The existence of widespread benign or reactive lymphoproliferations of the lung, as expressed in the term pseudolymphoma has been disputed, mainly on the basis of frequent subsequent development of frank malignant lymphoma. However, lymphoid interstitial pneumonia appears to be a benign process[186] and cases of nodular lymphoid hyperplasia continue to be reported.[399]

Hodgkin lymphoma is rarely seen as a primary lung lesion,[400] but the lung is a common site of relapse, particularly for nodular sclerosing disease. Tumour deposits are usually nodular and may cavitate or produce endobronchial lesions.

Extramedullary plasmacytoma is occasionally seen in lung parenchyma but the lung is seldom involved in multiple myeloma.

Leukaemic infiltration of minor degree is commonly seen in the lung at post mortem, although only a small percentage of patients develop clinically significant disease leading to cytodiagnosis. The clinical background is often complex and differential diagnosis of pulmonary infiltrates will include infection and cytotoxic lung damage.

Confirmation of recurrent tumour is often possible cytologically. On the other hand, definitive diagnosis of primary lymphoma generally requires open biopsy. Respiratory samples often provide a preliminary cytological diagnosis; however, sufficient material for immunophenotyping and/or genotyping is usually considered necessary for definitive diagnosis (Table 2.3).[401] BAL samples may be useful for this purpose[402–405] and immunoelectrophoresis of lavage fluid may also prove monoclonality.[405] Flow cytometry in combination with cytology may allow diagnosis without surgical procedures.[406] Cell block preparations are useful for immunocytochemistry.[407]

## Cytological findings: lymphoma/leukaemia

- More readily diagnosed by BAL or FNA than in sputum
- Large cell lymphomas easier to diagnose than small/mixed
- Loosely aggregated lymphoid cells, intact cytoplasm
- Vesicular nuclei, no moulding, nucleoli visible
- Subtyping possible in BAL and FNA material.

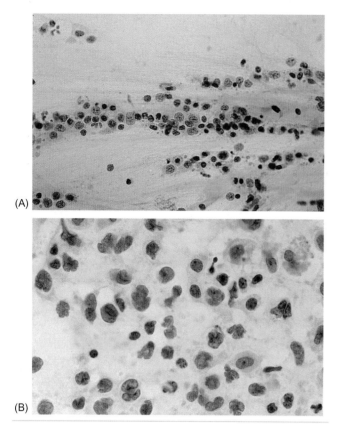

(A)

(B)

**Fig. 2.132** (A) Sputum: large cell/immunoblastic lymphoma showing streaks of dispersed cells with a few loose aggregates and degenerate forms, indistinguishable in this sample from a small cell carcinoma (PAP). (B) FNA: lung/mediastinal mass. Dispersed cells with unequivocal nuclear features of malignancy and suggesting hyperlobated malignant lymphoma cells. The diagnosis was confirmed by biopsy (H&E).

The literature on the cytodiagnosis of pulmonary involvement by non-Hodgkin lymphomas is not large. Tao[371] gives a thorough discussion of criteria for diagnosis in his monograph. Bonfiglio et al. reported on a series of 16 FNA cases.[408] Large cell lymphomas were most easily diagnosed. Small or mixed cell lesions were diagnostically difficult, although an unequivocal diagnosis was given in eight of 14 lymphomas sampled overall, and a strong suggestion of the diagnosis was made in a further five. Bardales et al.[407] report on the diagnosis of leukaemias and non-Hodgkin lymphomas in exfoliated samples from 20 patients including five presenting with pulmonary disease. In 29 of 31 specimens, a diagnosis of malignancy was made. The diagnoses of primary lung lymphoma were all confirmed histologically. A monotonous, dispersed cell population was usually seen and necrosis was often evident in washings and brushings. Gattuso et al. reported on seven cases of posttransplant lymphoproliferative disease involving lung.[398] They described two patterns, a polymorphous smear pattern with a spectrum of mature and immature lymphocytes and scattered histiocytes and plasma cells, and a monotonous pattern of large lymphoid cells.

Some cases of large B-cell lymphoma present first with groups of loosely arranged medium-sized cells with intact cytoplasm lying within mucus streaks of sputum. Nuclei are vesicular with irregular outlines and had usually prominent, often multiple, nucleoli (see Figs 2.93, 2.132). Artefactual aggregation may occur (Fig. 2.93C) and mimic epithelial clusters, but

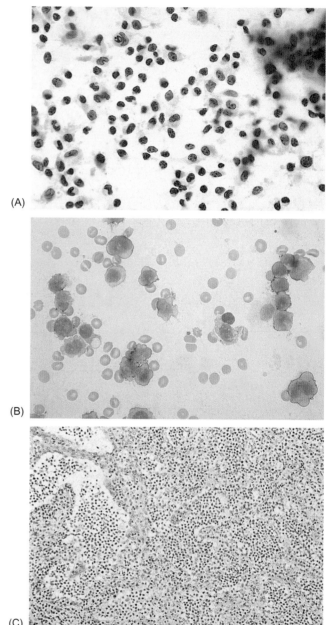

(A)

(B)

(C)

**Fig. 2.133** FNA: non-Hodgkin malignant lymphoma. Multiple nodules throughout both lung fields in a young woman. (A) Dispersed population of atypical lymphoid cells suggesting a lymphoproliferative disorder (PAP). (B) Cytocentrifuge preparation showing membrane staining for MT1 (Clonab) antigen in tumour cells, suggesting a T-cell lymphoma. (C) Open biopsy specimen showing non-Hodgkin lymphoma. The tumour was an unusual T-cell neoplasm with NK cell phenotype and large granular lymphocyte morphology on electron microscopy (H&E).

nuclear moulding is not seen nor is engulfment of apoptotic debris by tumour cells, both features of small cell carcinoma.

More abundant material is obtained by FNA and preliminary diagnoses can be made in cases of primary lymphoma later confirmed histologically (Figs 2.132, 2.133). Recurrent lymphoma of various types may be seen in sputum, and small-cleaved cell tumours in brushings and FNA samples. Several cases of lymphomatoid granulomatosis have not yielded sufficient cells for assessment. FNA samples of cases of low-grade lymphoplasmacytoid lymphoma have yielded a monotonous

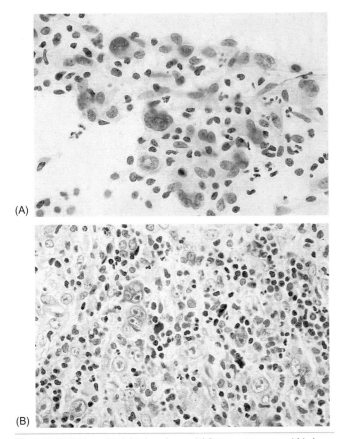

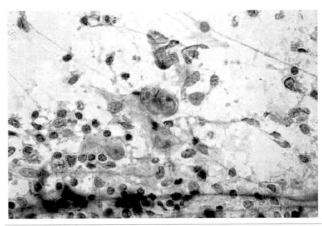

**Fig. 2.135** FNA mediastinal mass: Hodgkin lymphoma. Reed–Sternberg cell in a background of lymphoid cells and atypical mononuclear cells. Cytological findings suggesting Hodgkin lymphoma, confirmed on formal biopsy (PAP).

**Fig. 2.134** FNA lung: Hodgkin lymphoma. (A) Recurrent tumour within lung tissue. Syncytial masses of abnormal lymphoreticular cells including Reed–Sternberg cells (H&E). (B) Histology of previous lymph node biopsy (H&E).

population of small lymphocytes with plasmacytoid forms, and may be provisionally diagnosed cytologically.

Hodgkin lymphomas usually yield a mixed inflammatory cell background and variable numbers of Hodgkin mononuclear cells or Reed–Sternberg cells (Figs 2.134, 2.135). Suprun and Koss[409,410] described diagnostic Reed–Sternberg cells lying singly in sputum in a background of inflammatory cells in 10 cases of Hodgkin lymphoma. Reale et al.[411] described six patients in whom malignant cells consistent with Hodgkin lymphoma were seen in sputum. In two cases of nodular sclerosing disease, large cells with vacuolated cytoplasm and multilobated nuclei thought to correspond to lacunar cells were also evident. Flint et al.[412] reported on 13 cases of pulmonary involvement by Hodgkin disease sampled by FNA in which classic Reed–Sternberg cells and/or lacunar cells were identified in most cases and mononuclear Hodgkin cells in all, generally in a mixed cell background.

Wisecarver et al.[413] studied the appearance of Hodgkin disease in BAL samples. Unequivocal diagnoses of Hodgkin lymphoma were made in six cases; the background cell population was often a marked lymphocytosis, the lymphocytes generally being small and monotonous. Reiben et al.[414] diagnosed intrapulmonary Hodgkin disease with bronchial brush cytology and other cases have been reported from sputum,[415] washings[407] or FNA and BAL samples,[416,417] including cases in which the diagnosis had not previously been suspected.[415,418]

Dissemination of chronic lymphocytic leukaemia is occasionally diagnosed in sputum. Many dispersed cells showing the characteristic blocked nuclear chromatin pattern may allow confirmation of lung involvement in patients with a previous diagnosis and consistent clinical findings. However, large numbers of rather similar cells can be seen as a reactive process, e.g. in follicular bronchitis, and primary diagnosis by sputum is not made.

Single case examples of other lymphoid-related lesions are reported. Ludwig and Balachandran[419] described cells with characteristic nuclear grooves or folds in bronchial wash and CSF samples from a patient with a disseminated mycosis fungoides. Rosen et al.[420] and Shaheen and Oertel[421] report similar findings in sputum and aspirates. Vernon[422] describes a signet-ring cell lymphoma, in which bronchial brushings contained lymphoid cells with variable nuclear irregularity and striking cytoplasmic vacuoles, often compressing the nucleus; he warns of the possibility of confusion with epithelial malignancy, particularly adenocarcinoma.

Goldstein et al.[423] suggested that lung involvement by immunoblastic lymphadenopathy might be diagnosed by identifying large numbers of immunoblasts in sputum in a patient with a previous diagnosis on lymph node biopsy. Williams et al.[424] demonstrated the angioinvasive nature of the lymphoid infiltrate in cell blocks of an FNA specimen from lymphomatoid granulomatosis.

Multiple myeloma within brushings samples was documented by Riazmontazer et al.;[425] bronchial washings contained aggregates and dispersed cells in which the degree of clustering initially suggested an epithelial tumour. Chollet et al.[426] and Auerswald et al.[427] used immunostaining to quantitate Langerhans cells in BAL samples and suggested that >5% of Langerhan's cells strongly supported the diagnosis of Langerhan's histiocytosis. However, an increase in these cells in lung is found in smokers and in localised reactive processes and open biopsy is still often undertaken.

Bardales et al.[407] point out several pitfalls in diagnosis including the need for immunocytochemistry to distinguish Hodgkin lymphoma from anaplastic large cell lymphoma and other malignancies, the resemblance of megakaryocytes to malignant cells and the need to report only on blood free samples in leukaemic patients with lung infiltrates.

## Sarcoma in the lung

There are reports of the diagnosis of sarcoma being made in sputum[428] and several FNA series of primary or metastatic sarcomas have been published.[429,430] They suggest that many single cells and spindle-shaped cells, poorly cohesive or in flat aggregates, with fragile cytoplasm and finely granular nuclear chromatin, small nucleoli and bizarre multinucleation were general indicators of mesenchymal malignancy (see Ch. 29). A distinction between high-grade sarcoma, primary or secondary, melanoma and sarcomatoid carcinoma is usually not possible without comparison with histological material, cell block immunocytochemistry or electron microscopy. Attention has been drawn to the nuclear atypia, which may mimic malignancy, in benign neural tumours (Figs 2.136, 2.137).

Reactive processes such as inflammatory pseudotumour[431] or traumatised elements of bronchial wall may enter the differential diagnosis.[432] The use of ancillary studies, particularly immunocytochemistry, electron microscopy or cytogenetics, is essential for classification of these tumours, but even then a definitive diagnosis will often require histological assessment of biopsy or resection material.

## Pulmonary blastoma

These tumours are rare aggressive malignant neoplasms usually situated peripherally in lung and composed of epithelial and mesenchymal elements.[186] They occur at any age, but often in younger adult males. The histological appearances resemble the foetal lung. The epithelial elements consist of tubules lined by glycogen-rich columnar cells, and the mesenchymal elements are composed of small, loosely arranged spindle cells. Cartilage and smooth or striated muscles are sometimes seen. Immunocytochemistry suggests a true mixed epithelial-mesenchymal tumour. The early age at which many tumours occur supports a differencefrom carcinosarcoma or sarcomatoid carcinoma.

Cosgrove et al.[433] diagnosed a tumour in cell blocks of an FNA sample by observing a biphasic pattern of branching glands lined by multilayered columnar epithelium with subnuclear vacuoles and surrounded by a primitive stroma (Fig. 2.138). In other descriptions the epithelial component was usually evident but the mesenchymal element was more difficult to appreciate, generally leading to diagnoses of carcinoma (Fig. 2.139).[433–437] The epithelial and mesenchymal elements may merge.

Malignant teratoma, Wilm's tumour or other biphasic lesions such as synovial sarcoma are difficult to exclude without detailed clinical information or evaluation of serum markers or histological material (see Chs 29, 33). Lee and Cho[438] report on the cytological findings in a case of adenocarcinoma of foetal type which may have some relationship to blastoma.

## Pulmonary carcinosarcoma

This rare neoplasm, composed of malignant epithelial and bizarre sarcomatous components, often presents with a pedunculated mass affecting a major bronchus. It is likely that the lesion represents a form of sarcomatoid carcinoma and there

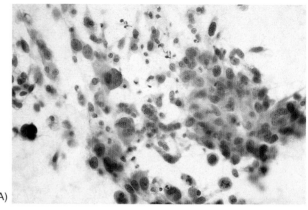

(A)

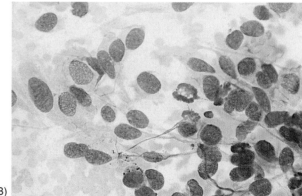

(B)

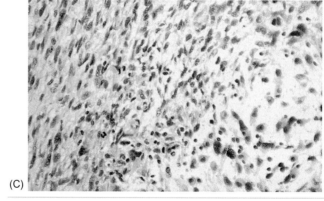

(C)

**Fig. 2.136** FNA: metastatic malignant fibrous histiocytoma. (A) Varied population of malignant cells including some epithelial-like aggregates, spindle and giant cell forms and abundant haemosiderin pigment (PAP). (B) Predominantly spindle cell forms including mitotic figures. Fragile spindle shaped cytoplasmic processes. Diagnosis made by reference to the previous resection specimen (MGG). (C) Previous resection specimen from thigh tumour (H&E).

is a similar prognosis to other poorly differentiated lung cell carcinomas. Cabarcos et al.[439] reported polygonal squamous cells and fusiform fibrosarcomatous cells in an FNA sample. In the case of Finley et al.,[440] FNA cytodiagnosis depended on identifying squamous epithelial and mesenchymal smear patterns and dual staining for keratins and vimentin. Ishizuka et al.[441] describe a case in which sputum samples showed a combination of malignant squamous and rhabdomyosarcomatous cells with cross striations allowing the diagnosis to be suggested.

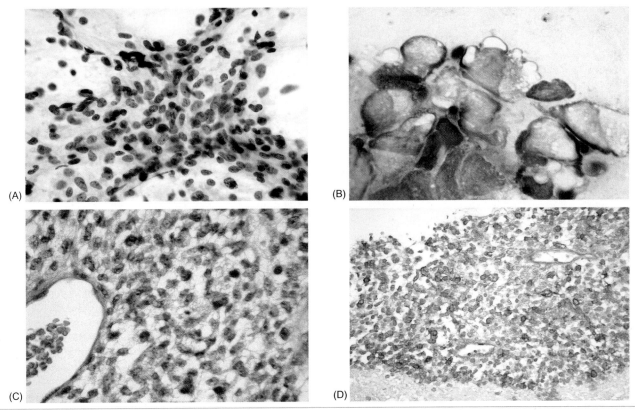

**Fig. 2.137** FNA: primitive neuroectodermal tumour (PNET). Apparent primary tumour within lung in a 35-year-old woman. (A) Loosely aggregated small round cell tumour (PAP). (B) Lakes of glycogen within tumour cells (MGG). (C) Cell block preparation (H&E). (D) CD 99 staining in tumour cells (IPOX).

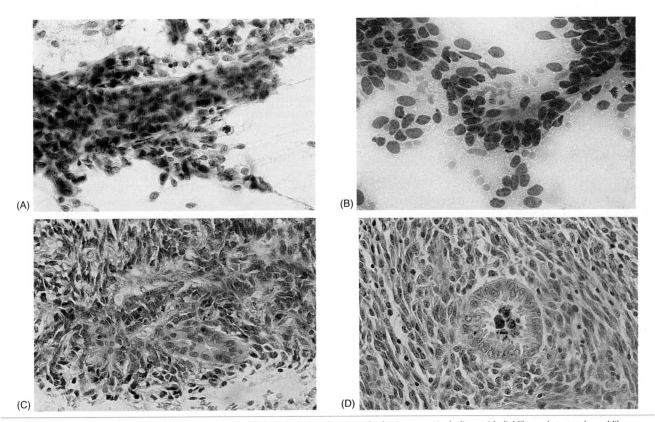

**Fig. 2.138** FNA: pulmonary blastoma. (A) Aspirated material from lung lesion showing a biphasic pattern including epithelial-like and mesenchymal-like cells (PAP). (B) Predominantly spindle cell morphology (MGG). (C) Cell block from metastasis within abdomen showing biphasic glandular and primitive mesenchymal pattern (H&E). (D) Lung resection specimen showing biphasic glandular and primitive stromal pattern (H&E). The diagnosis in this case was made following the aspiration of the abdominal metastasis.

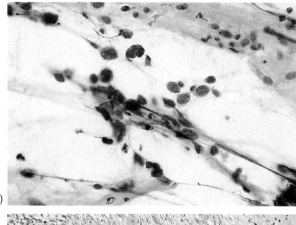

(A)

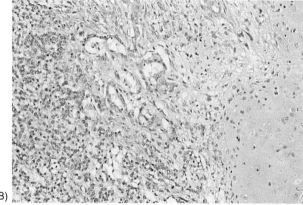

(B)

**Fig. 2.139** Bronchial brushings: pulmonary blastoma. (A) Recurrent tumour. Small cell malignancy of indeterminate type but compatible with recurrent blastoma (PAP). (B) Resected specimen showing biphasic glandular and primitive stromal pattern, together with cartilage (H&E).

# MEDIASTINAL TUMOURS

*Julie McCarthy*

A broad range of neoplasms is encountered in this site. The frequency of different neoplasms depends greatly on the patient's age and to some extent on the 'anatomical' site within the mediastinum (anterior, superior or posterior mediastinum). This arbitrary division into compartments is useful, although some overlap exists (Fig. 2.140). In adults, the most common lesions are metastases, cysts of thymic, pericardial or enteric origin, followed by thymomas, neurogenic tumours and lymphomas, with lesser numbers of germ cell tumours. Powers et al.,[442] in a multi-institutional analysis, report metastatic carcinoma in 60% of lesions sampled by FNA; malignant lymphoma and thymoma were the most frequent primary tumours. Shabb et al.[443] gave a correct diagnosis in 86% of lesions sampled. A total of 57% of their cases were primary neoplasms, 24% were metastases and 12% were other benign conditions. In the paediatric population, the most common neoplasms are malignant lymphomas, followed by neurigenic malignancies, germ cell tumours and sarcomas.[444] A meta-analysis of endobronchial ultrasound-guided transbronchial needle aspiration (EU-BNA) for staging of lung cancer showed sensitivity of 93% and specificity of 100%.[445-449]

FNA of this site has a low rate of complication and can be performed safely even when superior vena caval obstruction is present.[450] Mediastinal cystography is useful in the diagnosis of cysts or in cyst drainage. Fluoroscopy and CT are generally necessary for needle guidance and the latter has the advantage of localising the needle tip to within millimetres, thus avoiding such rare complications as cardiac puncture. CT scanning also can exclude aneurysm and delineate relationships with adjacent structures, including large vessels.

FNA material may be submitted entirely as a fluid sample to facilitate immunocytochemistry and supplemented by preparing some direct spreads of air dried material to allow rapid on site evaluation of specimen adequacy. Obtaining

| Superior |
| --- |
| • Thymoma and thymic cyst |
| • Malignant lymphoma |
| • Thyroid lesions |
| • Parathyroid adenoma |

| Anterior |
| --- |
| • Thymoma and thymic cyst |
| • Germ cell tumors |
| • Thyroid lesions |
| • Parathyroid adenoma |
| • Malignant lymphoma |
| • Paraganglioma |
| • Hemangioma |
| • Lipoma |

**Fig. 2.140** Location of most common lesions of mediastinum. (From Rosai J (ed.) Rosai and Ackerman's Surgical Pathology, 9th edn, Mosby 2004, with permission of Elsevier.)

Superior

Anterior

Posterior

Middle

| Posterior |
| --- |
| • Neurogenic tumours |
| Schwannoma |
| Neurofibroma |
| Ganglioneuroma |
| Ganglioneuroblastoma |
| MPNST |
| Neuroblastoma |
| Paraganglioma |
| • Gastroenteric cyst |

| Middle |
| --- |
| • Pericardial cyst |
| • Bronchial cyst |
| • Malignant lymphoma |

material for ancillary techniques is imperative for lesions in the mediastinum.

## Thymoma

Tumours of the thymus are among the rarest neoplasms in humans, accounting for less than 1% of adult cancers. Thymomas are the most common thymic tumours in adults but are rare in children, in whom malignant lymphoma within the thymus is more common. Thymic epithelial neoplasms are a common primary neoplasm of the anterior mediastinum. Most cases are biologically benign encapsulated lesions, although in up to 20% of cases, invasion of adjacent tissues including pleura, pericardium and/or lung may occur. This pattern of invasive growth may be seen in lesions of quite benign cytological appearance, without significant nuclear pleomorphism or mitotic activity.

The WHO classification of thymic epithelial tumours (Box 2.8) is histogenetically based, and reflects a body of evidence to suggest that thymoma subgroups form distinct entities both in clinical and morphological terms. Although the classification provides easy comparison for clinical, histological and immunological features, it may not be easily applied to cytological or small biopsy samples.[451] Other classifications recognise a spectrum of differentiation from thymoma through atypical thymoma to thymic carcinoma.[452]

Typically, type A thymomas are epithelial cell rich lesions with scanty lymphoid cells that mark with CD3 and CD5. Epithelial cells are oval or spindled and appear cytologically bland, marking with acidic cytokeratins (low molecular weight, i.e. CK 19) with the exception of CK 20 which is negative.[453] This type of thymoma is relatively uncommon (4–19%),[454]

and occurs in a slightly older age group (mean age 61 years).[455] These tumours are generally regarded as benign without risk of recurrence if completely excised.[456]

Type B thymomas are neoplasms with polygonal or round epithelial cell nuclei. This group is subdivided into types B1, B2 and B3, depending on the extent of lymphocyte infiltration and the degree of atypia of the neoplastic epithelial cells. B1 tumours recapitulate the normal thymic tissue and are lymphocyte rich, B2 are organotypic neoplasms with prominently nucleolated, polygonal epithelial cells and many immature T cells. B3 tumours are composed predominantly of slightly atypical round or polygonal epithelial cells with few lymphocytes and a sheet like growth pattern.

Mixed type AB tumours contain areas typical of both types A and B and these are one of the most common histological subtypes (15–43%).[454]

### Cytological findings: thymoma[447,457–465]

- Cohesive aggregates of epithelial cells
- Variable lymphocytic infiltration; may obscure fragments
- Epithelial cells have pale cytoplasm, regular nuclei
- Spindle cell types show granular chromatin.

Benign thymomas give rise to cohesive fragments with virtually no free epithelial cells Lymphocytic infiltration may almost completely obscure epithelial cells and it requires close scrutiny to detect epithelial cells within aggregates The component epithelial cells usually have oval or rounded pale vesicular nuclei with small nucleoli and minimal mitotic activity (Fig. 2.141). Cytoplasm is moderate in amount, pale and with indistinct borders. Spindle cell tumours show a more homogeneous

---

### Box 2.8 Mediastinal tumours (adapted from WHO classification[451])

- Thymoma
  - Spindle/medullary (A); lymphocyte rich/predominantly cortical (B1); cortical (B2); mixed (AB); epithelial/atypical (B3)
  - Encapsulated; minimally invasive; widely invasive
- Thymic carcinoma
  - Squamous cell carcinoma (keratinising; non-keratinising)
  - Lymphoepithelioma-like
  - Sarcomatoid
  - Clear cell
  - Basaloid
  - Mucoepidermoid
  - Papillary
  - Undifferentiated
- Neuroendocrine neoplasms
  - Carcinoid tumour (typical, atypical; spindle, pigmented)
  - Small cell carcinoma and variants
  - Large cell neuroendocrine carcinoma
- Lymphoproliferative disease
  - Castleman's disease (angiofollicular lymphoid hyperplasia)
  - Non-Hodgkin lymphoma
  - Large cell lymphoma, B cell, with sclerosis
  - Lymphoblastic
  - Marginal zone lymphoma of mucosa associated lymphoid tissue (MALT)
  - Hodgkin lymphoma
- Neural neoplasms
  - Schwannoma
- Neurofibroma
- Ganglioneuroma/ganglioneuroblastoma
- Neuroblastoma
- Paraganglioma
- Neurogenic sarcoma
- Germ cell neoplasms
  - Seminoma (germinoma)
  - Non-seminomatous germ cell tumours
    - Teratoma: mature; immature
    - Embryonal carcinoma
    - Endodermal sinus/yolk sac tumour
    - Choriocarcinoma
    - Mixed tumours
- Non-neoplastic cystic lesions
  - Bronchogenic cyst
  - Oesophageal and gastroenteric cyst
  - Thymic cyst unilocular/multilocular (associated with Hodgkin lymphoma, germinoma; AIDS)
  - Pericardial cyst
  - Lymphangioma
- Other mediastinal mass lesions
  - Thymic hyperplasia
  - Thyroid enlargement: retrosternal or ectopic
    - Multinodular goitre
    - Thyroid neoplasms
  - Parathyroid adenoma

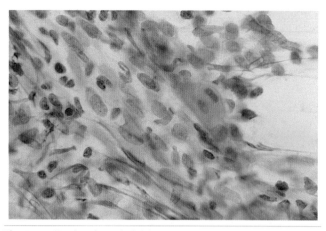

**Fig. 2.141** FNA lymphoepithelial thymoma. Metastatic tumour within lung tissue. Hassall's corpuscles are present, with surrounding oval epithelial cells and a smaller component of lymphoid cells (PAP).

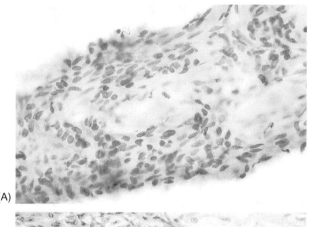

(A)

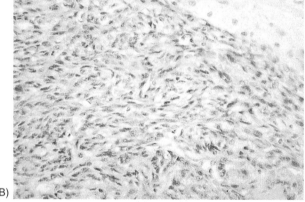

(B)

**Fig. 2.142** FNA: spindle cell thymoma. (A) Cohesive fragment of spindle cells (H&E). (B) Resection specimen (H&E).

granular chromatin and less conspicuous nucleoli (Fig. 2.142). Lymphoepithelial tumours may be diagnosed on cytological findings alone, but confirmation of the epithelial nature of the tumour cells by immunohistochemistry is now routine (see Fig. 2.144) and is essential for spindle cell tumours without a lymphoid component, when mesenchymal tumours enter the differential diagnosis.

### Diagnostic pitfalls: thymoma

FNA of thymoma is a demanding diagnostic exercise for the cytopathologist because of an overwhelming, often obscuring population of benign lymphocytes in many cases. Diagnosis requires the presence of a dual population of unequivocal epithelial cells and lymphocytes in the correct clinical-radiological context. Cytological examination alone is not sufficient to discriminate among the various subtypes of thymoma, nor can capsular invasion or invasion of adjacent structures be determined using FNA.

In tumours with a high lymphoid content, Hodgkin disease or non-Hodgkin lymphoma and angiofollicular lymphoid hyperplasia are all considerations. The degree of cohesiveness of the tissue in thymoma is generally unlike that in Hodgkin or non-Hodgkin lymphoma. However, attention has been drawn to the sclerosing large cell non-Hodgkin lymphoma as a source of error in this regard.[466] These tumours present with large fragments of cohesive cells consisting of a mixture of lymphoid cells and a background of connective tissue. The light microscopic pattern may mimic epithelial thymoma or carcinoma. Cell block sections demonstrating keratin or EMA staining in thymomas,[458] and lymphoid markers in large cell lymphomas, are the most useful ancillary tests.

Spindle cell tumours, including connective tissue neoplasms of various types, mesothelioma, or submesothelial fibromas may all be difficult to distinguish from spindle cell thymoma without ancillary investigations. Electron microscopy often proves valuable. Slagel et al. describe a range of lesions presenting with spindle cells in FNA samples. Some 11% of their series of mediastinal lesions had a significant component of spindle cells, including examples of inflammatory lesions, lymphomas of Hodgkin and non-Hodgkin type, connective tissue neoplasms, melanoma, squamous carcinoma and thymoma.[467]

Some tumours may be predominantly cystic and misinterpreted as non-neoplastic unless care is taken to sample the wall of the lesion.[468]

In general, immunocytochemistry for cytokeratins such as CK19 and AE1 highlight the epithelial cells (see Fig. 2.144), while the lymphocytic component of these tumours may express CD3, CD5 (mature T cells) or immature T-cell markers such as CD1a, CD99 and TdT.[469]

## Thymic carcinoma

Thymic epithelial tumours show a gradient in terms of malignancy. Thymoma types A and AB behave in a benign manner. Type B1 to B3 have increasing degrees of malignant behaviour and B3 is synonymous with well-differentiated thymic carcinoma. Thymic carcinoma is a term used for a number of malignant epithelial neoplasms that show unequivocal cytological atypia. This diverse group includes squamous carcinoma, basaloid carcinoma, mucoepidermoid carcinoma, lymphoepithelioma like carcinoma, sarcomatoid carcinoma, clear cell carcinoma, adenocarcinoma and poorly/undifferentiated carcinomas.

While a cytological diagnosis of carcinoma is possible from such lesions, a specific origin from thymus should only be accepted after clinical and biopsy evidence excludes other primary sites (Fig. 2.143). Some biologically aggressive cases with less obvious malignant cytological features may also be encountered.

The cytopathology of various thymic carcinomas (including neuroendocrine carcinoma) imitate their appearance in extra-thymic sites, and are generally recognisable using FNA. Separation of moderately differentiated neuroendocrine carcinoma from

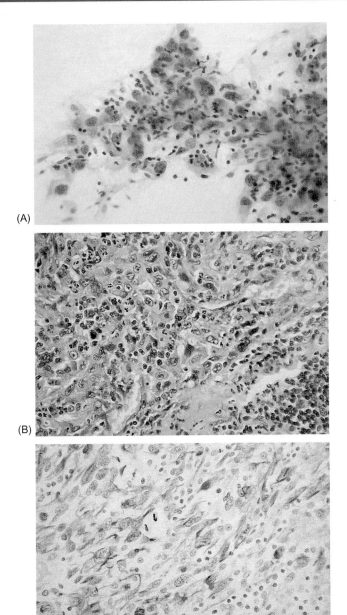

(A)

(B)

(C)

**Fig. 2.143** FNA: malignant thymoma (thymic carcinoma) (A) Disorganised aggregate of large malignant cells. The degree of cohesion suggests an epithelial origin. Background of lymphocytes. Thymic carcinoma was suggested when clinical evaluation revealed no other primary lesion (H&E) (B,C) Resected specimen. Anaplastic malignancy with epithelial features confirmed on staining for cytokeratins. (B, H&E; C, cytokeratin stain AE1–AE3).

poorly differentiated small cell neuroendocrine carcinomas is generally not possible.[470]

## Thymic carcinoma and thymoma versus primary lung carcinoma

This is rarely a problem when there is an infiltrative mediastinal mass with a lesion in the lung. CD5, a 67-kD surface glycoprotein receptor and a T-cell marker, is aberrantly expressed in thymic carcinoma.[471] CD5 is also aberrantly expressed by neoplastic B cells in lymphoproliferative disorders, small lymphocytic lymphoma/chronic lymphocytic leukaemia, and mantle cell lymphoma,

which are thought to arise from CD5[+] perifollicular centre lymphocytes. Borderline thymic tumours, with features intermediate between those of thymoma and thymic carcinoma, weakly express immunoreactivity for CD5 similar to that observed for lymphoepithelioma-like carcinomas. Benign and invasive thymomas studied for CD5 immunoreactivity are uniformly negative; NE tumours, including carcinoids and small cell carcinomas, are uniformly negative for CD5. Sixty-one other malignant neoplasms (lung, cervix, thyroid, prostate, mixed germ cell tumours, melanoma and mesothelioma) likely to occur as primary in or to metastasise to the anterior mediastinum are negative for CD5 immunoreactivity. CD99 is positive in immature lymphocytes of the thymus in benign and some borderline thymic lesions and is negative in thymic carcinomas. Thymomas are CK7 negative, whereas lung adenocarcinomas are CK7 positive. Thymomas including thymic carcinomas are TTF-1 negative.

A recommended panel of thymic carcinoma versus primary lung carcinoma includes CD5, CD99, TTF-1, and CK7.[195]

## Neuroendocrine tumours

The majority of neuroendocrine tumours arising within the mediastinum originate within the thymus. Rarely have primary mediastinal neuroendocrine tumours been documented.[472] Within the thymus, tumours that are predominantly or exclusively composed of neuroendocrine cells are classified as neuroendocrine carcinomas (NEC). They should be distinguished from conventional thymic carcinomas which may contain scattered neuroendocrine cells.[473] The spectrum of these tumours includes well-differentiated NECs (typical and atypical carcinoid) and poorly differentiated NECs (small cell carcinoma and large cell neuroendocrine carcinoma). Virtually all thymic carcinoids are atypical (necrosis present and or 2–10 mitoses per 10HPF), however their behaviour appears to be less aggressive than their pulmonary counterparts.[474,475] Primary mediastinal neuroendocrine carcinomas tend to behave aggressively.[472] Diagnosis by FNA, cell block immunocytochemistry (using markers including synaptophysin, chromogranin, CD56 and NSE) and electron microscopy demonstrating neurosecretory granules is well-described.[476–478]

## Lymphoma

Lymphoma within the mediastinum occurs either within mediastinal lymph nodes or within the thymus. Lymphomas at this site are diverse and generally speaking behave aggressively and present with symptoms of mediastinal mass effect or with pleural or pericardial effusions.

Lymphomas within the thymus reflect the function of the thymic gland as an organ of T-cell generation and differentiation.[479] As such, T-cell lymphoblastic/lymphoma is the most common. B-cell neoplasms are more infrequent and the most common entity of these is primary mediastinal large B-cell lymphoma (PMLCL) with a postulated origin in specialised thymic medullary B lymphocytes.[480] Nodular sclerosis type classical Hodgkin disease can also arise in the thymus and this shares a common epidemiology with PMLCL in that they occur most commonly in young adult females as localised disease. There are theories that these entities share a common cell of origin.[481,482] Other B lymphomas such as MALT lymphoma are relatively rare. Other entities such as natural killer (NK) tumours[479] histiocytic[483] and dendritic cell tumours

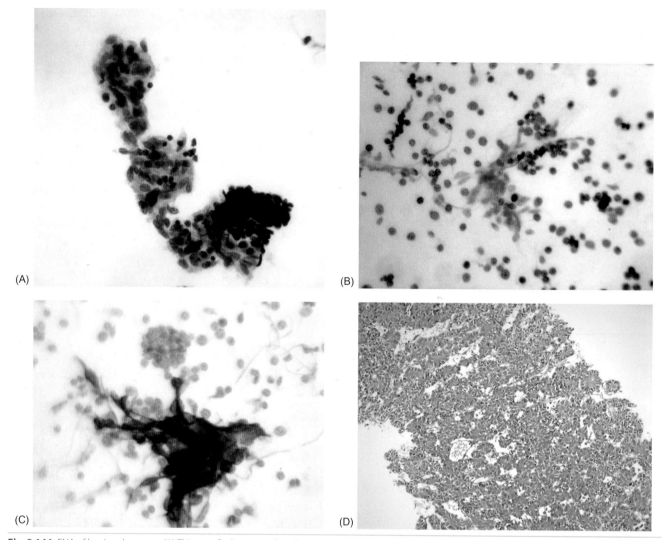

**Fig. 2.144** FNA of benign thymoma: (A) Thinprep findings: spindle cells appear bland and in cohesive fragments, with lymphocytes scattered in the background (PAP). (B) Immunocytochemistry of benign thymoma showing CD3 positive lymphocytes. (C) Immunocytochemistry of benign thymome: AE1–AE3 positive epithelial cells. (D) Histological section: benign thymoma, type A, bland spindle cells and scanty lymphocytes (H&E).

have been described. Histiocytic and myeloid neoplasms arising at this site are thought to be related to differentiation with teratomaous germ cell tumours.[484]

Lymphomas involving the mediastinal lymph nodes reflect the spectrum systemic nodal diseases and the diagnosis is usually made from sampling more accessible sites. The diagnosis of lymphoma at this site, as elsewhere, is reliant on material for immunocytochemistry or flow cytometry (see Chs 13, 14). Cytospun material is suitable for some genetic studies (such as t(2;5) ALK + translocation in anaplastic large cell lymphoma) but histopathological sampling is required prior to treatment of new cases. In residual or recurrent lymphomas, FNA alone can provide a working diagnosis, if supported by ancillary studies, as well as clinical and radiological impression discussed by the multidisciplinary team (Fig. 2.145).

## Germ cell tumours

Mediastinal germ cell tumours (GCTs) account for approximately 15% of mediastinal tumours in adults and up to 25% of mediastinal neoplasms in children.[485,486] The mediastinum is the most common site for the development of extragonal germ cell tumours and like their gonadal counterparts, can be classified into seminomas, non-seminomatous germ cell tumours (including embryonal carcinoma, yolk sac tumour, choriocarcinoma and mixed GCTs) and teratomas. The explanation for mediastinal GCTs relates to the embryonological migration of primordial germ cells from the yolk sac to the germinal ridges during early development.[487] There is a bimodal age distribution with a peak in infancy.[485] In adults, mature teratomas and malignant mediastinal GCTS are restricted to males with very rare exceptions.[488]

The majority of mediastinal GCTs occur within or adjacent to the thymus, but occasionally teratomas and yolk sac tumours arise in the posterior mediastinum[489] and more rarely in the pericardium or myocardium.[490,491]

Mature teratomas may be incidental findings in both children and adults; however, malignant GCTs are rarely asymptomatic. Patients present with symptoms relating to mediastinal mass effect and occasionally fever secondary to local inflammatory responses. Patients may present with metastatic disease: bone, liver, brain,[492] retroperitoneum and heart[493] are the most common sites. Precocious puberty due to βHCG increases with NSGCT

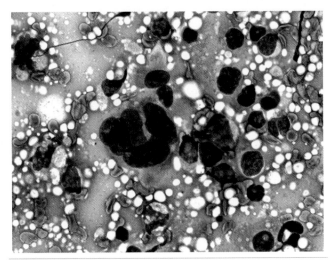

**Fig. 2.145** Intraoperative touch preparation of a mediastinal lymphoma in a 20-year-old male. There is marked pleomorphism. Histology confirmed a high-grade B-cell non-Hodgkin lymphoma (MGG).

and mixed GCTs has also been described.[494] The development of haematological malignancy clonally related to GCTs is unique to germ cell tumours arising in the mediastinum. Most commonly, these are acute leukaemias (AML M4, M5 and M7),[495] which may infiltrate locally or present as bone marrow infiltration.

Pure seminomas tend to be homogenous, non-calcified masses similar to lymphomas on imaging.[496] NSGCTs are generally heterogeneous lesions radiographically.[496] The appearance of multilocular cystic spaces is not unique to teratomas, however, as the thymus develops multilocular cysts in response to any inflammatory stimulus. Multiloculated cystic lesions may therefore be encountered in seminomas, thymomas, thymic carcinomas, Hodgkin and non-Hodgkin lymphoma and metastatic deposits. Seminomas with prominent cystic change have been described.[497] Sampling of cystic lesions may yield fluid including many mixed inflammatory cells: a careful search for atypical cells together with a panel of immunocytochemical markers should be performed. One such case of primary mediastinal seminoma in a young adult male is shown (Fig. 2.146) The typical prominent, often elongated nucleoli and delicate cytoplasm of seminomas are well demonstrated.[498]

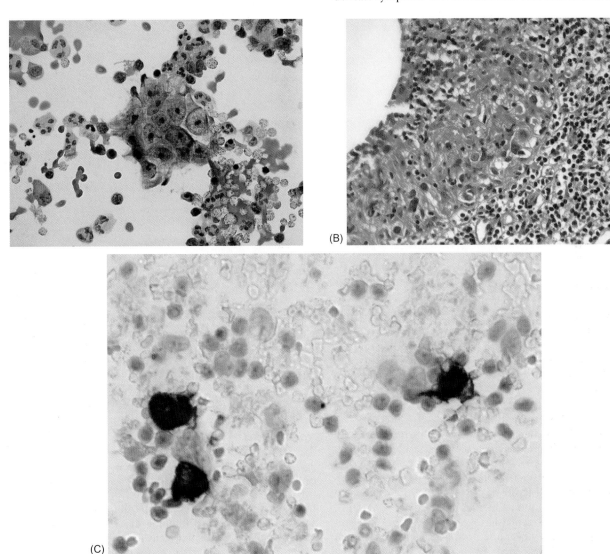

**Fig. 2.146** (A) Primary mediastinal seminoma in a young male. The mass was cystic on aspiration. Mixed inflammatory cells and cyst macrophages surround cohesive malignant cells with delicate cytoplasm and prominent nucleoli (PAP). (B) Histological section of the same tumour (H&E). (C) Pancytokeratin marker performed on the cytology sample demonstrates malignant cells.

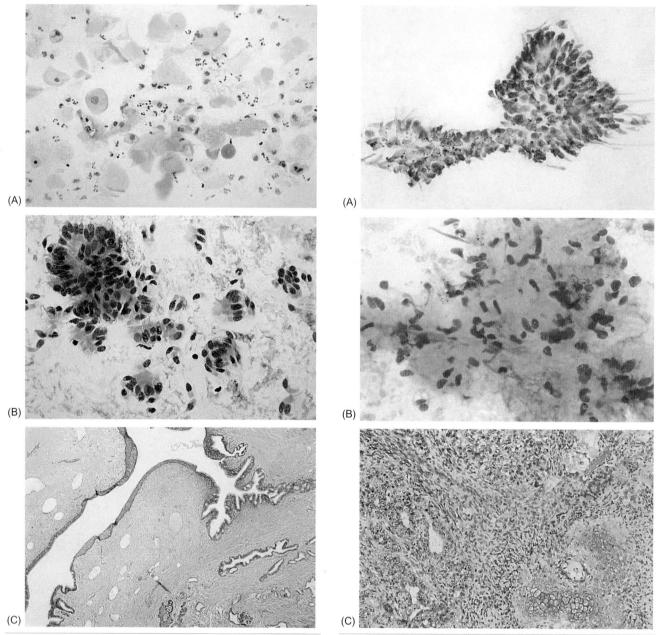

**Fig. 2.147** FNA: cystic mature teratoma of mediastinum. (A) Anucleate squamous cells, keratinous debris and mature squamous cells together with an inflammatory cell component (PAP). (B) Ciliated columnar epithelium in a background of mucoid debris (MGG). (C) Resected tumour showing mature endodermal and ectodermal elements (H&E).

**Fig. 2.148** FNA: primary malignant teratoma involving lung and mediastinum. (A) Cohesive epithelial elements with malignant nuclear features and abundant apoptotic debris (PAP). (B) Fibromyxoid mesenchymal tissue (MGG). (C) Resected tumour showing glandular and mesenchymal elements together with areas of cartilage formation (H&E). On the FNA findings, consideration was given to diagnoses of pulmonary blastoma or metastatic Wilm's tumour as well as teratoma. The patient was treated as teratoma on the basis of the cytological findings and markedly elevated serum markers prior to resection of the mass.

The immunocytochemical panel should include PLAP (80–90% cases of seminoma are positive), CD117 (commonly positive in seminomas) and CD30 (85–100% embryonal carcinomas are positive. This should be interpreted in conjunction with CD15 (negativity), alpha fetoprotein (variable reaction in yolk sac tumours but strong positivity is helpful), βHCG andzhuman placental lactogen (choriocarcinoma variable positivity). Pancytokeratin, lymphoma and melanoma markers should also be used depending on the amount of material available and the clinical context. FNA findings from a cystic teratoma are illustrated in Figure 2.147, and those of a malignant teratoma in Figure 2.148.

## Neural tumours

Dahlgren and Ovenfors[499] describe the findings in a series of Schwannian tumours. Palombini and Vetrani[500,501] outline the FNA pattern in mediastinal ganglioneuroblastoma and ganglioneuroma; in one case there was a mixture of polyhedral cells including binucleate forms with abundant eosinophilic cytoplasm and smaller cells with an oval or spindle shape. Some of the larger cells closely resembled neurons, with axonal projections.

The findings suggested ganglioneuroblastoma and were confirmed by elevated VMA and HVA estimations. In other cases, the fibrillar material between tumour cells, especially evident in MGG preparations and thought to correspond to collections of neurites emanating from tumour cells, was an important diagnostic feature.

## Soft tissue tumours

A variety of mesenchymal and neurogenic tumours arise with the mediastinum and the thymus gland. These lesions are very rare and account for less than 10% of mediastinal neoplasms. They may be incidentally found asymptomatic lesions or present with local compressive symptoms.

Heimann et al.[502] describe a case of thymolipoma where lymphoid cells, mature adipose tissue and groups of epithelial cells were found in FNA samples and included a few Hassall's corpuscles. Immunostaining of lymphocytes for pan-T and antithymocyte markers was positive and cytokeratin was demonstrated in the epithelial cells. The large size of the lesion and fat density on CT scanning were features in support of the diagnosis. Thymolipoma may arise at any age and is composed of a well circumscribed lobulated mass of cytologically bland adipose tissue and thymic elements. As this lesion can reach sizes of up to 30 cm, careful sampling is required to rule out foci of malignancy.

Liposarcoma is the most common sarcoma arising in the anterior mediastinum and is one of differential diagnoses of thymolipoma. Well-differentiated liposarcoma is the most common subtype,[503] arising usually in adults (see Ch. 29). Attal et al. diagnosed myxoid liposarcoma based on the distinctive arborising vascular pattern and myxoid background.[504] Solitary fibrous tumour (SFT) can occur in the mediastinum and may reach a large size in this site. It is morphologically and immunocytochemically identical to pleural SFT, being CD34, CD99 and bcl2 positive, cytokeratin negative.[505] Cases of synovial sarcoma, vascular tumours and leiomyomatous tumours arise within the mediastinum.

Mishriki et al.[506] diagnosed a Hurthle cell neoplasm arising in mediastinal ectopic thyroid in a FNA sample in conjunction with electron microscopy, and De Las Casas et al. report a similar case diagnosed on intraoperative cytology.[507] Cytological findings in mediastinal melanotic schwannomas were described by Marco et al.[508] and Prieto-Rodriguez et al.[509]

Neurogenic tumours occur almost exclusively in the middle and posterior mediastinum, where they are the most common neoplasms. Paragangliomas occur within the anterior, middle and posterior compartments.

## Metastatic and locally invasive tumours

Certain tumours metastasise to the mediastinum and primary tumours arising locally may involve the mediastinum by direct invasion. The most common malignancies in this category are from the lung, thyroid, breast and prostate.[510] Less commonly, the mediastinum is involved by melanoma, liposarcoma, osteosarcoma, rhabdomyosarcoma, Kaposi's sarcoma and malignant fibrous histiocytoma.[511–515]

The distinction between primary squamous carcinoma and neuroendocrine carcinomas of the thymus and metastases to the mediastinum may be difficult. There are some

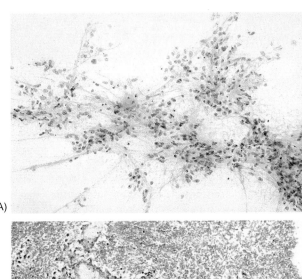

(A)

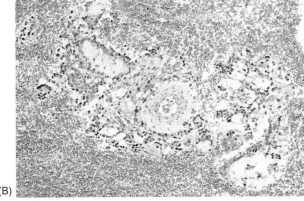

(B)

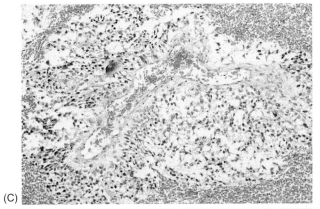

(C)

**Fig. 2.149** (A–C) FNA: metastatic endodermal sinus tumour within lung and mediastinum. Cell block preparation with histological pattern in keeping with metastatic endodermal sinus tumour (H&E).

morphological differences described, however these are unlikely to prove useful in cytological samples. Immunocytochemisty may be of some value, otherwise the distinction must rely on clinical and radiological information. The most relevant antibodies are CD5 which is positive in 50% of thymic squamous, basaloid and lymphoepithelioma-like carcinomas and negative in metastases from lung or head and neck. CD70 shows a similar profile. CD117 is positive in 40–100% of these thymic carcinomas and is not expressed in lung nor head and neck primary cancers.

For neuroendocrine malignancies, TTF-1 expression is absent in primary thymic tumours whereas it is frequent positive in lung neuroendocrine carcinoma.[516] An example of a metastatic endodermal sinus tumour invading lung and mediastinum is shown in Figure 2.149.

# ACCURACY OF CYTOLOGY FOR TUMOUR DIAGNOSIS AND MANAGEMENT

*Thomas Giles*

## Sensitivity of diagnosis of malignancy

For sputum cytology, sensitivity ranges from around 50–60% for peripheral lesions and metastases, to 70–85% for central lesions when five or six specimens can be examined.[9,11,13,14,517,518–521] Sensitivity may be as low as 40% in routine practice.[522] Blood-stained specimens and larger tumours are associated with a higher yield.[523] A tabular literature review by Bocking[524] gives a useful summary of the range of results. Bronchoscopic brushings and washings achieve 90% sensitivity for central lesions and 70% for peripheral lesions.[513,519,521,525–530] By adding transbronchial FNA, this accuracy can be extended.[531–536] Bronchoalveolar lavage gives similar sensitivity in some authors' hands.[537–540] The sensitivity of fibreoptic bronchoscopic biopsy (for histology) is similar, around 90% for central and up to 70–80% for more peripheral lesions; brushings and biopsy are complementary. Multiple sampling often increases the yield.[541]

FNA sensitivity is usually over 80% and up to 95% in selected series,[10,243,542–544] varying according to the size and depth of the lesion, the approach taken and the experience of the radiologist.[545] A negative result by any single diagnostic method cannot exclude malignancy; however, using a selection or combination of these diagnostic methods up to 98% of central lesions and 94% of peripheral lung tumours may be diagnosed pretherapeutically.[546] In special sites such as the EUS-TBNA of mediastinum, a cytological diagnosis may be reached in 93% of cases.[442,446,547,548,549]

The diagnostic accuracy of cytological samples obtained by EBUS–TBNA at Thomas Jefferson University Hospital in the USA has recently been reviewed.[549]

Comparisons of the accuracy of the various techniques used to obtain cytological material suggest that these are complementary and that the physician can select which may be most effective based on the clinical features of the lesion for individual patients. Considerations such as the economics of hospital stay may also enter into such assessment.

## Predictive value of malignant diagnosis

A 100% predictive value of malignant diagnosis is the aim, because cytological diagnosis is to be used for definitive management decisions.[550,551] The positive predictive value of malignancy has been near this level for experienced workers for many years. Regular attendance at multidisciplinary-team meetings for discussion of cases acts as a safeguard against false positive diagnosis, ensuring as it does that both the pathologist and the clinician can correlate their separate findings so as to achieve optimal patient management.

The previous authors of this chapter recorded that in their own practice, they had rare false positive diagnoses of malignancy over a 15-year period. For example, a case of highly atypical reactive bronchial epithelial proliferation in sputum was interpreted as metastatic adenocarcinoma in a patient with a previous history of colonic carcinoma. In FNA material they misdiagnosed malignancy in an atypical mesothelial cell reaction, the epithelial proliferation in chondroid hamartoma, pleomorphic fibroblastic cells in benign pleural fibroma, and a mediastinal ectopic multinodular thyroid tissue. However, the false positive rate overall was less than 0.1% of malignant diagnoses and this is of a similar order to most recent reports for sputum, brushings and FNA diagnoses.

A diagnosis of 'markedly atypical' cells may even be associated with over 99.9% specificity for malignancy.[552] Recent reviews highlight the most likely non-neoplastic cytological mimics of malignancy.[553–555] Kern[556,557] and Cagle[558] allude to the difficulty of obtaining cytohistological correlation after a marked decline in autopsy rates, pointing out that there is a tendency to overestimate false positive rates if cytohistological correlation is based on subsequent biopsy, particularly endoscopic, without adequate clinical follow-up. Caya et al.[559] suggest that only open lung biopsy, autopsy or the results of long-term clinical follow-up should be used in evaluating accuracy.

## Tumour typing

Sputum cytology provides extremely accurate tumour subtyping; for small cell carcinoma, sputum may be the most accurate modality.[11] Definitive typing of squamous cell and adenocarcinoma is also extremely accurate in sputum.[11,517,518] The accuracy of tumour typing for FNA and brushings is high, with over 90% sensitivity and predictive value.[10,243]

For small cell carcinoma FNA gives over 90% sensitivity of diagnosis and most workers show a very high predictive value/specificity.[10,243,560,561] However, in some workers' experience only 90% of diagnoses are confirmed,[562] and there is thus room for conservatism and a cautious approach to small cell carcinoma diagnosis by FNA. In problematic cases, repeat cytology or biopsy specimens are of most value.

In brushings and FNA samples, subtyping of large cell carcinomas is more difficult than in sputum, although approximately 80% of large cell tumours may be typed accurately and up to 80–90% of predictions of type are correct.[10,243]

Hess et al.[205] reviewed cytological criteria for tumour typing and suggested that revised data based on objective cytoplasmic features of functional differentiation allowed a more reliable diagnosis. Their categories had more in common with ultrastructural characterisation of lung tumours than conventional histological diagnosis and led to a high proportion of diagnosis of combined squamous and glandular tumours and few cases of large cell anaplastic carcinoma. Similar views were expressed by Mennemeyer.[206] Such studies have further emphasised the heterogeneity of lung cancer and the high frequency of ultrastructural evidence of both glandular and squamous differentiation in tumours from non-small cell categories.

A recent re-evaluation of the clinical significance of subtyping of non-small cell lung carcinoma takes account of personalised treatment as practised today.[563]

## Diagnosis of benign neoplasms

Dahlgren et al.[459] diagnosed eight of 13 thymomas by FNA; schwannoma, lymphoma and carcinoid tumours provided some diagnostic difficulty. Tao et al.[457] were able to diagnose all of the 37 FNA cases they encountered and, in most of our cases, FNA material with or without ancillary testing allowed diagnosis. Dahlgren et al.[499] diagnosed most benign neurogenic tumours, although 18 gauge needles were used; diagnostic material is difficult to obtain with 23 or 22 gauge needles in deep neural neoplasms and thin core sampling is of value if clinically feasible. Over 90% of chondroid hamartomas can be recognised by FNA.[364-366] Reports of most other benign neoplasms involve only small numbers of cases.

## Select prognostic markers for targeted chemotherapy

Select prognostic markers and markers for targeted chemotherapy that show promise are epidermal growth factor receptor (EGFR), c-Erb-B2, cell cycle markers p16, Ki-67, p53, Bcl-2, vascular endothelial growth factor C, and CD44. These markers can be applied to cell block material obtained at FNA. Identification of prognostic markers that add value beyond the TNM staging system is a priority in lung cancer, particularly in stage I. Survival for patients with stage I disease is 70% despite curative surgical resection, implying that our current staging criteria are imperfect. The use of molecular markers as a strategy to refine risk stratification beyond staging has been validated in retrospective studies and is under evaluation prospectively.[564-570]

## REFERENCES

1. Finlayson R. The vicissitudes of sputum cytology. Med Hist 1958;2:24–35.

2. Papanicolaou GN, Cromwell HA. Diagnosis of cancer of the lung by the cytological method. Dis. Chest 1949;15:412–18.

3. The Royal College of Pathologists. Histopathology and Cytopathology of Limited or No Clinical Value. London: The Royal College of Pathologists; 2005.

4. Walters EH, Gardiner PV. Bronchoalveolar lavage as a research tool. Thorax 1991;46:613–18.

5. Menetrier P. Cancer primitif du poumon. Bull Soc Anat 1886;61:643–47.

6. Nordenstrom BE. Technical aspects of obtaining cellular material from lesions deep in the lung. A radiologist's view and description of screw-needle sampling technique. Acta Cytol 1984;28:233–42.

7. Siddiqui MT, Saboorian MH, Gokaslan ST, et al. The utility of transbronchial (Wang) fine needle aspiration in lung cancer diagnosis. Cytopathology 2001;12:7–14.

8. Chandra A, Cross P, Denton K, et al. The BSCC Code of Practice – exfoliative cytopathology (excluding gynaecological cytopathology). Cytopathology 2009; 20:211–223.

9. Papanicolaou Society of Cytopathology Taskforce and Standards of Practice. Guidelines of the Papanicolaou Society of Cytopathology for the examination of cytologic specimens obtained from the respiratory tract. Diagn Cytopathol 1999; 21:61–69.

10. Johnson WW, Bossen EH. Ten years of respiratory cytopathology at Duke University Medical Centre. I. The cytopathologic diagnosis of lung cancer during the years 1970 to 1974, noting the significance of specimen number and type. Acta Cytol 1981;25:103–7.

11. Johnson WW. Percutaneous fine needle aspiration biopsy of the lung. A study of 1015 patients. Acta Cytol 1984;28:218–24.

12. Johnson WW, Bossen EH. Ten years of respiratory cytopathology at Duke University Medical Center. II. A comparison between cytopathology and histopathology in typing of lung cancer between the years 1970–1974. Acta Cytol 1981;25:499–505.

13. Johnson WW, Bossen EH. Ten years experience of respiratory cytopathology at Duke University Medical Center. III. The significance of inconclusive cytopathologic diagnosis during the years 1970 to 1974. Acta Cytol 1982;26:759–66.

14. Johnson WW. Fine needle aspiration biopsy versus sputum and bronchial material in the diagnosis of lung cancer. A comparative study of 168 patients. Acta Cytol 1988;32:641–46.

15. Johnson WW. Histologic and cytologic patterns of lung cancer in 2580 men and women over a 15 year period. Acta Cytol 1988;32:163–68.

16. Person CGA, Svensson C, Grieff L, et al. The use of the nose to study the inflammatory response of the respiratory tract. Thorax 1992;47:993–1000. Editorial.

17. Jean , Lellouch-Tubiana A, Brunet-Langot D, et al. Nasal eosinophilia in children: its use in the nasal allergen provocation test. Diagn Cytopathol 1988;4:23–27.

18. Rivasi F, Bergamini G. Nasal cytology in allergic processes and other syndromes caused by hyperreactivity. Diagn Cytopathol 1988;4:99–105.

19. Lau SK, Hsu CS, Sham JST, Wei W/I. The cytological diagnosis of nasopharyngeal carcinoma using a silk swab stick. Cytopathology 1991;2:239–46.

20. Loncar B, Pajtler M, Milicic-Juhas V, et al. Imprint cytology in laryngeal and pharyngeal tumours. Cytopathology 2007;18:40–43.

21. Fan YG, Hu P, Jiang Y, et al. Association between sputum atypia and lung cancer risk in an occupational cohort in Yunnan, China. Chest 2009;135:778–85.

22. British Thoracic Society bronchoscopy guidelines committee. British Thoracic Society Guidelines for Diagnostic Flexible Bronchoscopy. Thorax 2001; 56:11–21.

23. Erkiliç S, Ozsaraç C, Küllü S. Sputum cytology for the diagnosis of lung cancer. Comparison of smear and modified cell block methods. Acta Cytol 2003;47:1023–27.

24. Astall E, Atkinson C, Morton N, et al. The evaluation of liquid-based 'Cyto-SED' cytology of bronchoalveolar lavage specimens in the diagnosis of pulmonary neoplasia against conventional direct smears. Cytopathology 2003;14:143–49.

25. Choi YD, Han CW, Kim JH, et al. Effectiveness of sputum cytology using ThinPrep method for evaluation of lung cancer. Diagn Cytopathol 2008;36:167–71.

26. Fireman E, Lerman Y. Induced sputum in interstitial lung diseases. Curr Opin Pulm Med 2006;12:318–22.

27. Domagała-Kulawik J. BAL in the diagnosis of smoking-related interstitial lung diseases: review of literature and analysis of our experience. Diagn Cytopathol 2008; 36:909–15.

28. Davison AG, Haslam PL, Gorrin B, et al. Interstitial lung disease and asthma in hard-metal workers: bronchoalveolar lavage, ultrastructural, and analytical findings and results of bronchial provocation tests. Thorax 1983;38:119–28.

29. Cameron SEH, Andracle RS, Pambuccian SF. Endobronchial ultrasound-guided transbronchial needle aspiration cytology: a state of the art review. Cytopathology 2010;21:6–26.

30. Silvestri GA, Hoffman BJ, Hutanimi B, et al. Endoscopic ultrasound with fine needle aspiration in the diagnosis and staging of lung cancer. Ann Thorac Surg 1996;61:1441–45.

31. Rintoul RC, Tournoy KG, El Daly H, et al. EBUS-TBNA for the clarification of PET positive intra-thoracic lymph nodes-an international multi-centre experience. J Thorac Oncol 2009;4:44–48.

32. Buley ID, Roskell DE. Fine needle aspiration cytology in tumour diagnosis: uses and limitations. Clin Oncol 2000;12:166–71.

33. Annema JT, Rabe KF. State of the art lecture: EUS and EBUS in pulmonary medicine. Endoscopy 2000;38:118–22.

34. Kocjan G, Chandra A, Cross P, et al. BSCC Code of Practice – fine needle aspiration cytology. Cytopathology 2009; 20:283–96.

35. Buley ID. Update on special techniques in routine cytopathology. J Clin Pathol 1993;46:881–85.

36. Sterret GF, Whitaker D, Glancy J. Fine needle aspiration of lung mediastinum and chest wall. Pathol Annu 1982;17(Part 2):197–228.

37. Halloush RA, Khasawneh FA, Saleh HA, et al. Fine needle aspiration cytology of lung lesions: a clinicopathological and cytopathological review of 150 cases with emphasis on the relation between the number of passes and the incidence of pneumothorax. Cytopathology 2007;18:44–51.

38. Fish GD, Stanley JH, Miller KS, et al. Post biopsy pneumothorax: estimating the risk by chest radiography and pulmonary function tests. Am J Roentol 1988;150:71–74.

39. Corrin B, Nicholson AG. Pathology of the Lungs. 2nd ed. London: Churchill Livingstone/Elsevier; 2006 pp. 1–35.

40. Antonakopoulos GN, Lambrinaki E, Kyrkou KA. Curschmann's spirals in sputum: histochemical evidence of bronchial gland ductal origin. Diagn Cytopathol 1987;3:291–94.

41. Gleich G. The eosinophils: new aspects of structure and function. J Allergy Clin Immunol 1977;60:73–82.

42. Schmitz B, Pfitzer P. Acellular bodies in sputum. Acta Cytol 1984;28:136–38.

43. Wheeler TM, Johnson EH, Coughlin D, Greenberg SD. The sensitivity of detection of asbestos bodies in sputa and bronchial washings. Acta Cytol 1988;32:647–50.

44. Weaver KM, Kovak PM, Naylor B. Vegetable cell contaminants in cytologic specimens: their resemblance to cells associated with various normal and pathologic states. Acta Cytol 1981;25:210–14.

45. Dao AH. Entamoeba gingivalis in sputum smears. Acta Cytol 1985;29:632–33.

46. Radio S, Rennard SI, Ghafouri MA, Lindner JA. Cytomorphology of alternaria in bronchoalveolar lavage specimens. Acta Cytol 1987;31:243–48.

47. Hussain OAN, Grainger JM, Sims J. Cross contamination of cytological smears with automated staining machines and bulk manual staining procedures. J Clin Pathol 1978;31:63–68.

48. Johnston WW, et al. Cytopathology of the lung: diagnostic applications of sputum, bronchial brushings and fine needle aspiration biopsy. In: Wied GL, Keebler CM, Koss LG, editors Compendium on Diagnostic Cytology. Chicago: Tutorials of Cytology; 1988. p. 321–22.

49. Roby TJ, Swan GE, Schumann GB, Enkena LC, Jr. Reliability of a quantitative interpretation of sputum cytology slides. Acta Cytol 1990;34:140–46.

50. Roby TJ, Swan GE, Sorensen KW, et al. Discriminant analysis of lower respiratory components associated with cigarette smoking, based on quantitative sputum cytology. Acta Cytol 1990;34:147–54.

51. Chamberlain DW, Braude AC, Rebuck AS. A critical evaluation of bronchoalveolar lavage: criteria for identifying unsatisfactory specimens. Acta Cytol 1987;31:599–605.

52. Davis G, Giancola M, Costanza M, et al. Analyses of sequential bronchoalveolar lavage samples from healthy human volunteers. Am Rev Respir Dis 1982;126:611–16.

53. Saito Y, Imai T, Sato M, et al. Cytologic study of tissue repair in human bronchial epithelium. Acta Cytol 1988;32:622–28.

54. Chalon J, Tang C-K, Gorstein F, et al. Diagnostic and prognostic significance of tracheobronchial epithelial multinucleation. Acta Cytol 1978;22:316–20.

55. Scoggins WG, Smith RH, Frable WJ, et al. False-positive diagnosis of lung carcinoma in patients with pulmonary infarcts. Ann Thorac Surg 1977;24:474–80.

56. Nasiell M. Metaplasia and atypical metaplasia in the bronchial epithelium: a histopathologic and cytopathologic study. Acta Cytol 1966;10:421–27.

57. Saccomanno G, Saunders RP, Klein MG, et al. Cytology of the lung in reference to irritant, individual sensitivity and healing. Acta Cytol 1970;14:377–81.

58. Papanicolaou GN, Bridges EL, Railey C. Degeneration of the ciliated cells of the bronchial epithelium (ciliocytophthoria) in its relation to pulmonary disease. Am Rev Resp Dis 1961;83:641–59.

59. Corrin B, Nicholson AG. Pathology of the Lungs. 2nd edn. London: Churchill Livingstone/Elsevier; 2006 pp. 173–193.

60. Lazzari G, Vineis C, Cugini A. Cytologic diagnosis of primary pulmonary actinomycosis: a report of two cases. Acta Cytol 1981;25:299–301.

61. Ettinger NA, Trulock EP. Pulmonary considerations in organ transplantation: state of the art. Part 3. Am Rev Resp Dis 1991;144:433–51.

62. Roig J, Domingo C, Morera J. Legionnaires' disease. Chest 1994;105:1817–25.

63. WHO. Online. Available at: http://w3whosea.org/ (accessed 28 March 2006).

64. Janet DA. Tuberculosis out of control. J R Coll Physicians Lond 1996;30:352–58.

65. Rich AR. The Pathogenesis of Tuberculosis. 2nd edn. Oxford: Blackwell; 1951.

66. Nasiell M, Roger V, Nasiell K, et al. Cytologic findings indicating pulmonary tuberculosis. I The diagnostic significance of epithelioid cells and Langhans giant cells found in sputum or bronchial secretions. Acta Cytol 1972;16:146–51.

67. Orell SR, Sterret GF, Walters MN, editors, et al. Manual and Atlas of Fine Needle Aspiration Cytology. 2nd edn. London: Churchill Livingstone; 1992. p. 178–80.

68. Tani EM, Schmitt FCL, Oliviera ML, et al. Pulmonary cytology in tuberculosis. Acta Cytol 1987;31:460–63.

69. Corrin B, Nicholson AG. Pathology of the Lungs. 2nd edn. London: Churchill Livingstone/Elsevier; 2006 pp. 149–172.

70. Greenberg SB. Respiratory herpesvirus infections: an overview. Chest 1994;106:1–2.

71. Graham BS, Snell JD. Herpes simplex virus infection of the adult lower respiratory tract. Medicine 1983;62:384–93.

72. Selvaggi SM, Gerber M. Pulmonary cytology in patients with the acquired immunodeficiency syndrome. Diagn Cytopathol 1986;2:187–93.

73. Buchanan AJ, Gupta RK. Cytomegalovirus infection of the lung: cytomorphologic diagnosis by fine needle aspiration cytology. Diagn Cytopathol 1986;2:341–42.

74. Hilborne LH, Nieberg RK, Cheng L, et al. Direct in situ hybridisation for rapid detection of cytomegalovirus in bronchoalveolar lavage. Am J Clin Pathol 1987;87:766–69.

75. Zaman SS, Seykora JT, Hodinka RL, et al. Cytological manifestations of respiratory syncytial virus pneumonia in bronchoalveolar lavage fluid: a case report. Acta Cytol 1996;40:546–51.

76. Beale AJ, Campbell W. A rapid cytological method method for the diagnosis of measles. J Clin Pathol 1959;12:335–37.

77. Bayon MN, Drut R. Cytologic diagnosis of adenovirus infection. Acta Cytol 1991;35:181–82.

78. Corrin B, Nicholson AG. Pathology of the Lungs. 2nd edn. London: Churchill Livingstone/Elsevier; 2006 pp. 219–247.

79. Corrin B, Nicholson AG. Pathology of the Lungs. 2nd edn. London: Churchill Livingstone/Elsevier; 2006 pp. 224–231.

80. Aubry MC, Fraser R. The role of bronchial biopsy and washig in the diagnosis of allergic bronchopulmonary aspergillosis. Modern Pathol 1998;11:607–11.

81. Lee SH, Barnes WG, Schaetzel WP. Pulmonary aspergillosis and the importance of oxalate crystal recognition in cytology specimens. Arch Pathol Lab Med 1986;110:1176–79.

82. Levy H, Horak DA, Tegtmeier BR, et al. The value of bronchoalveolar lavage and bronchial washings in the diagnosis of invasive pulmonary aspergillosis. Resp Med 1992;86:243–48.

83. Benoit G, de Chauvin MF, Cordonnier C, et al. Oxalic acid levels in bronchoalveolar lavage fluid from patients with invasive pulmonary aspergillosis. Am Rev Resp Dis 1985;132:748–51.

84. Ness MJ, Rennard SI, Vaughn WP, et al. Detection of Candida antigen in bronchoalveolar lavage fluid. Acta Cytol 1988;32:347–52.

85. Wheat LJ, Slama TG, Zeckel ML. Histoplasmosis in the acquired immune deficiency syndrome. Am J Med 1985;78:203–10.

86. Remali S, Lofti C, Ismael A, et al. Penicillium marneffei infection in patients with the human immunodeficiency virus. Acta Cytol 1995;39:798–802.

87. Tsui WM, Ma KF, Tsang DNC. Disseminated Penicillium marneffei infection in HIV-infected subject. Histopathology 1992;20:287–93.

88. Corrin B, Nicholson AG. Pathology of the Lungs, 2nd edn. London: Churchill Livingstone/Elsevier; 2006 pp. 220–224.

89. Sidhu GS, Cassa ND, Pei ZH. Pneumocystis carinii: an update. Ultrastruct Pathol 2003;27:115–22.

90. Stringer JR, Beard CB, Miller RF, et al. A new name (Pneumocystis jiroveci) for Pneumocystis from humans. Emerg Infect Dis 2002;8:891–96.

91. Miller RF, Mitchell DM. Pneumocystis carinii pneumonia. AIDS and the lung: up date 1992. 1. Thorax 1992;47:305–14.

92. Young JA, Stone JW, McGonigle RJ, et al. Diagnosing Pneumocystis carinii pneumonia by cytological examination of bronchoalveolar lavage fluid: report of 15 cases. J Clin Pathol 1986;39:945–49.

93. Greaves TS, Strigle SM. The recognition of Pneumocystis carinii in routine Papanicolaou-stained smears. Acta Cytol 1985;29:714–20.

94. Stanley MW, Henry MJ, Iber C. Foamy alveolar casts: diagnostic specificity for Pneumocystis pneumonia in bronchoalveolar lavage fluid cytology. Diagn Cytopathol 1988;4:113–15.

95. Elvin KM, Bjorkman A, Linder E, et al. Pneumocystis carinii pneumonia: detection of parasites in sputum and bronchoalveolar fluid by monoclonal antibodies. BMJ 1988;297:381–84.

96. Wehle K, Blanke M, Koenig G, Pfitzer P. The cytological diagnosis of Pneumocystis carinii by fluorescence microscopy of Papanicolaou stained bronchoalveolar lavage specimens. Cytopathology 1991;2:113–20.

97. Wazir JF, Macrorie SG, Coleman DV. Evaluation of the sensitivity, specificity and predictive value of monoclonal antibody 3F6 for the detection of Pneumocystis carinii pneumonia in bronchoalveolar lavage specimens and induced sputum. Cytopathology 1994;5:82–89.

98. Wakefield AE, Pixley FJ, Banerji S, et al. Detection of Pneumocystis carinii with DNA amplification. Lancet 1990;336:451–53.

99. Wakefield AE, Guiver L, Miller RF, et al. DNA amplification of induced sputum samples for diagnosis of Pneumocystis carinii pneumonia. Lancet 1991;337:1378–79.

100. Naryshkin S, Daniels J, Freno E, et al. Cytology of treated and minimal Pneumocystis carinii pneumonia and a pitfall of the Grocott methenamine silver stain. Diagn Cytopathol 1991;7:41–47.

101. Pitchenk Gangei P, Torres A, et al. Sputum examination for Pneumocystis carinii in the acquired immunodeficiency syndrome. Am Rev Respir Dis 1986;133:226–29.

102. Carmichael A, Bateman N, Nayagam M. Examination of induced sputum in the diagnosis of Pneumocystis carinii pneumonia. Cytopathology 1991;2:61–66.

103. Cregan P, Yamamoto A, Lum A, et al. Comparison of four methods for rapid detection of Pneumocystis carinii in respiratory specimens. J Clin Microbiol 1990;28:2432–36.

104. Wazir JF, Wodsworth J, Coleman DV. Pneumocystis carinii pneumonia: relationship between cyst size and response to treatment. Cytopathology 1994;5:90–92.

105. Farley MI, Fagan MP, Mabry I, et al. Presentation of Sporothrix schenckii in pulmonary cytology specimens. Acta Cytol 1991;35:389–95.

106. Louria DB, Liebermnan PH, Collins HS, et al. Pulmonary mycetoma due to Allescheria boydii. Arch Intern Med 1966;748–751.

107. Corrin B, Nicholson AG. Pathology of the Lungs, 2nd edn. London: Churchill Livingstone/Elsevier; 2006 pp. 249–261.

108. Salfender K. Atlas of Parasitic Pathology. Dordrecht: Kluwer Academic; 1992.

109. Rosenberg M, Rachman R. Entamoeba gingivalis in sputum: its distinction from Entamoeba histolytica. Acta Cytol 1970;14:361–62.

110. Kenney M, Eveland LK, Yermakov V. Amoebiasis: unusual location in lung. NY State J Med 1975;75:1542–43.

111. Stevens WJ, Vermiere PA. Giardia lamblia in bronchoalveolar lavage fluid. Thorax 1981;26:875.

112. Osborne PT, Giltman LI, Ulhman EO. Trichomonads in the respiratory tract: a case report and review of the literature. Acta Cytol 1984;28:218–24.

113. Kiriazis AP, Kiriazis AA. Incidence and distribution of opportunistic lung infections in AIDS patients related to intravenous drug use: a study of bronchoalveolar lavage cytology by the Diff-Quik stain. Diagn Cytopathol 1993;9:487–91.

114. Gordon SM, Gal AA, Hertzler GL, et al. Diagnosis of pulmonary toxoplasmosis by bronchoalveolar lavage in cardiac transplant recipients. Diagn Cytopathol 1993;9:650–54.

115. Chaydhuri B, Nanos S, Soco JN, et al. Disseminated Strongyloides stercoralis infestation detected by sputum cytology. Acta Cytol 1980;24:360–62.

116. Avasthi R, Jain AP, Swaroop K, et al. Bancroftian microfilariasis in association with pulmonary tuberculois. Acta Cytol 1991;35:717–18.

117. Ro JY, Tsakalalis PJ, White VA, et al. Pulmonary dirofilariasis: the great imitator of primary or metastatic lung tumor. A clinicopathologic analysis of seven cases and a review of the literature. Hum Pathol 1989;20:69–76.

118. Abdulla MA, Hombre SM, Al-Juwaiser A. Detection of Schistosoma mansoni in bronchoalveolar lavage fluid: a case report. Acta Cytol 1999;43:856–58.

119. Rangdaeng S, Alpert LC, Khiyami A, et al. Pulmonary paragonimiasis: report of a case with diagnosis by fine needle aspiration cytology. Acta Cytol 1992;36:31–36.

120. McCallum SM. Ova of the lung fluke Paragonimus kellicotti in fluid from a cyst. Acta Cytol 1975;19:279–80.

121. Frydman CP, Raissi S, Watson CW. An unusual pulmonary and renal presentation of echinococcosis: report of a case. Acta Cytol 1989;33:655–58.

122. Lewall DB, McCorkell SJ. Rupture of echinococcal cysts: diagnosis, classification and clinical implications. Am J Roentgenol 1986;146:391–94.

123. Fletcher CM, Pride NB. Definitions of emphysema, chronic bronchitis, asthma and airflow obstruction: 25 years on from Ciba Symposium. Thorax 1984;39:81–85. (Editorial).

124. Nasiell M, Vogel B. Cytomorphology of benign changes and early carcinoma of the lung. In: Wied GL, Keebler CM, Koss LG, Reagan JW, editors. Compendium on Diagnostic Cytology. 6th edn. Chicago: Tutorials of Cytology; 1990. p. 305–13.

125. Leavitt R, Fauci AS. State of the art: pulmonary vasculitis. Am Rev Respir Dis 1986;134:149–66.

126. Naylor B. Creola bodies: their 'discovery' and significance. Cytotechnol Bull 1985;22:33–34.

127. Vieira VG, Prolla JC. Clinical evaluation of eosinophils in the sputum. J Clin Pathol 1979;32:1054–57.

128. American Thoracic Society. Statement on sarcoidosis. Am J Respir CRIT Care Med 1999;160:736–55.

129. Aisner SC, Gupta PK, Frost JK. Sputum cytology in pulmonary sarcoidosis. Acta Cytol 1997;21:394–98.

130. Costabel U, Guzman J. Bronchoalveolar lavage in interstitial lung disease. Curr Opin Pulm Med 2001;7:255–61.

131. Smojver-Jezek S, Peros-Golubicic T, Tekaved-Traniec J, et al. Transbronchial fine needle aspiration cytology in the diagnosis of mediastinal sarcoidosis. Cytopathology 2006;18:3–7.

132. Keogh BA, Crystal RG. Alveolitis: the key to interstitial lung disorders. Thorax 1982;37:1–10. (Editorial).

133. Danila E, Jurganskiene L, Norkuniene J, et al. BAL fluid in newly diagnosed pulmonary sarcoidosis with different clinical activity.

134. Corrin B, Nicholson AG. Pathology of the Lungs. 2nd edn. London: Churchill Livingstone/Elsevier; 2006 pp. 471–474.

135. Awastri A, Malhotra P, Gupta N, et al. Pitfalls in the diagnosis of Wegener's granulomatosis on fine needle aspiration cytology. Cytopathology 2007;18:8–12.

136. Corrin B, Nicholson AG. Pathology of the Lungs. 2nd edn. London: Churchill Livingstone/Elsevier; 2006 pp. 267–328.

137. Nicholson A. The pathology and terminology of fibrosing alveolitis and the interstitial pneumonias. Imaging 1999;11:1–12.

138. American Thoracic Society/European Respiratory Society. International Multidisciplinary Consensus Classification of the idiopathic interstitial pneumonias. Am J Respir Crit Care Med 2002;165:277–304.

139. Tao LC, Sanders DE, Weisbrod GL. Value and limitations of transthoracic and transabdominal fine needle aspiration cytology in clinical practice. Diagn Cytopathol 1986;2:271–76.

140. Akoun GM, Mayoud CM, Milleron BJ, et al. Drug-induced pneumonitis and drug-induced hypersensitivity pneumonitis. Lancet 1984;i:136.

141. Walker T, Muckerjee D, Levine TS. Cytopathology 2002;13:329–32.

142. Bedrossian CW, Corey BJ. Abnormal sputum cytopathology during chemotherapy with bleomycin. Acta Cytol 1978;22:202–7.

143. Huang MS, Colby TV, Goellner JR, et al. Utility of bronchoalveolar lavage in the diagnosis of drug-induced pulmonary toxicity. Acta Cytol 1989;33:533–38.

144. Corrin B, Nicholson AG. Pathology of the Lungs. 2nd edn. London: Churchill Livingstone/Elsevier; 2006 pp. 383–389.

145. Ettensohn DB, Roberts NB, Condemi JJ. Bronchoalveolar lavage in gold lung. Chest 1984;85:569–70.

146. Mermolja M, Rott T, Debeljak A. Cytology of bronchoalveolar lavage in some rare pulmonary disorders: pulmonary alveolar proteinosis and amiodorone pulmonary toxicity. Cytopathology 1994;5:9–16.

147. Reyes CV, Thompson KS, Jensen J. Multivesiculated macrophages: their implications in fine needle aspiration cytology of lung mass lesions. Diagn Cytopathol 1998;19:98–101.

148. Movsas B, Raffin TA, Bostein AH, et al. Pulmonary radiation injury. Chest 1997;111:1060–76.

149. Ashbaugh DG, Bigelow DB, Petty TL, et al. Acute respiratory distress in adults. Lancet 1967;ii:319–23.

150. Donnelly SC, Haslett C. Cellular mechanisms of acute lung injury: implications for future treatment in the adult respiratory distress syndrome. Thorax 1992;47:260–63 (Editorial).

151. Grotte D, Stanley MW, Swanson PE, et al. Reactive type II pneumocytes in bronchoalveolar lavage fluid from adult respiratory distress syndrome can be mistaken for cells of adenocarcinoma. Diagn Cytopathol 1990;6:317–22.

152. Ettinger NA, Trulock EP. Pulmonary considerations of organ transplantation: state of the art. Part 1. Am Resp Dis 1991;143:1386–405. Part 2. 1991; 144:213–223; Part 3. 1991; 144:433–451.

153. Selvaggi SM. Bronchoalveolar lavage in lung transplant patients. Acta Cytol 1992;36:674–79.

154. Corrin B, Nicholson AG. Pathology of the Lungs. 2nd edn. London: Churchill Livingstone/Elsevier; 2006. pp. 329–361.

155. Reynolds HY State of art: bronchoalveolar lavage. Am Rev Resp Dis 1987;135:250–63.

156. Fink GM, De Shatzo R. Immunological aspects of granulomatous and interstitial lung diseases. JAMA 1987;258:2938–44.

157. Churg A, Green FHY, editors. Pathology of Occupational Lung Disease. New York: Igaku Shoin; 1988.

158. Corrin B, Nicholson AG. Pathology of the Lungs. 2nd edn. London: Churchill Livingstone/Elsevier; 2006 pp. 345–353.

159. Mazzucchelli L, Radelfinger H, Kraft R. Nonasbestos ferruginous bodies in sputum from a patient with graphite pneumoconiosis. Acta Cytol 1996;40:552–54.

160. Paris C, Galateau Salle F, Creveuil C, et al. Asbestos bodies in sputum of asbestos workers: correlation with industrial exposure. Eur Respir J 2002;20:1167–73.

161. Leiman G. Asbestos bodies in fine needle aspirates of lung masses: markers of underlying pathology. Acta Cytol 1991;35:171–74.

162. Bewtra C, Dewan N, O'Donahue WJ. Exfoliative sputum cytology in pulmonary embolism. Acta Cytol 1983;27:489–499168.

163. Corrin B, Nicholson AG. Pathology of the Lungs. 2nd edn. London: Churchill Livingstone/Elsevier; 2006 pp. 387–389.

164. Sias SM, Daltro PA, Marchiori E, et al. Clinical and radiological improvement of lipoid pneumonia with multiple bronchoalveolar lavages. Pediatr Pulmonol 2009;44:309–15.

165. Losner S, Volk BW, Slade WR, et al. Diagnosis of lipid pneumonia by examination of sputum. Am J Clin Pathol 1950;20:539–45.

166. Silverman JF, Turner RC, West RL, et al. Bronchoalveolar lavage in the diagnosis of lipoid pneumonia. Diagn Cytopathol 1989;5:3–8.

167. Cowell JL, Feldman PS. Fine needle aspiration diagnosis of aspiration pneumonia (phytopneumonitis). Acta Cytol 1984;28:77–80.

168. Chen KTK. Cytology of tracheobronchial amyloidosis. Acta Cytol 1984;28:133–35.

169. Dundore PA, Aisner SC, Templeton PA, et al. Nodular pulmonary amyloidosis: diagnosis by fine-needle aspiration cytology and a review of the literature. Diagn Cytopathol 1993;9:562–64.

170. Michael CW, Naylor B. Amyloid in cytologic specimens: differential diagnosis and pitfalls. Acta Cytol 1999;43:746–55.

171. Rosen SH, Castleman B, Liebow AA. Pulmonary alveolar proteinosis. N Engl J Med 1958;258:1123–42.

172. Bedrossian CW, Luna MA, Conklin RH, et al. Alveolar proteinosis as a consequence of immunosuppression: a hypothesis based on clinical and pathologic observations. Hum Pathol 1980;11:527–35.

173. Hook GE, Bell DY, Gilmor DB, et al. Composition of bronchoalveolar lavage effluents from patients with pulmonary alveolar proteinosis. Lab Invest 1978;39:342–57.

174. Corrin B, Nicholson AG. Pathology of the Lungs. 2nd edn. London: Churchill Livingstone/Elsevier; 2006.

175. Gammon RR, Julius CJ, et al. Pulmonary alveolar proteinosis: a report of two cases with diagnostic features in bronchoalveolar lavage specimens. Acta Cytol 1998;42:377–83.

176. Koss LG. Respiratory tract cytology in the evaluation of thermal injury. In: Koss LG, editor. Diagnostic Cytopathology and its Histopathologic Bases. 6th edn London: JB Lippincott & Co; 2007.

177. Clark CJ, Reid WH, Pollock AJ, et al. Role of pulmonary alveolar macrophage activation in acute lung injury after burns and smoke inhalation. Lancet 1988;872–874.

178. Islam S, Roustan Delatour NL, Salahdeen SR, et al. Cytologic features of benign solitary pulmonary nodules with radiologic correlation and diagnostic pitfalls: a report of six cases. Acta Cytol 2009;53:201–10.

179. Corrin B. Inflammatory myofibroblastic tumour. In: Corrin B, editor. Pathology of the Lungs. London: Churchill Livingstone; 2000. p. 587–90.

180. Pettinato G, Manival JC, de Rosa N, et al. Inflammatory myofibroblastic tumours (plasma cell granuloma) – clinicopathologic study of 20 cases with immunohistochemical and ultrastructural observations. Am J Clin Pathol 1990;94:538–46.

181. Thunnissen FB, Arends JW, Buchholtz RTF, et al. Fine needle aspiration cytology of inflammatory pseudotumor of the lung (plasma cell granuloma): report of four cases. Acta Cytol 1989;33:917–92.

182. Zakowski MF, Gatscha RM, Zaman MB. Negative predictive value of fine needle aspiration cytology. Acta Cytol 1992;36:283–86.

183. Orenstein M, Webber CA, Neurich AE. Cytologic diagnosis of Pneumocystis infection by bronchoalveolar lavage in acquired immunodeficiency syndrome. Acta Cytol 1985;29:727–31.

184. Leigh TR, Hume C, Gazzard B, et al. Sputum induction for diagnosis of Pneumocystis carinii pneumonia. Lancet 1989;205–206.

185. Afify A, Davila RM. Pulmonary fine needle aspiration biopsy: assessing the negative diagnosis. Acta Cytol 1999;43:601–4.

186. Corrin B. Pathology of the Lungs. Edinburgh: Churchill Livingstone; 2000.

187. WHO. Histological typing of lung and pleural tumours. World Health Organization International Classification of Tumours. Berlin: Springer; 1999.

188. Parkin DM, Bray F, Ferlay J, et al. Global cancer statistics. CA Cancer J Clin 2002;55:74–108.

189. Leng S, Stidley CA, Willink R, et al. Double-strand break damage and associated DNA repair genes predispose smokers to gene methylation. Cancer Res 2008; 68(8): 3049–56.

190. Minna JD, Sekido Y, Fong KM, et al. Molecular biology of lung cancer. In: de Vita VT, Hellman S, Rosenberg SA, editors Cancer: Principles and Practice of Oncology. 5th edn Philadelphia: Lippincott-Raven; 1997. p. 849–57.

191. Field JK, Liloglou T, Niaz A, et al. European Early Lung Cancer (EUELC) Project: A multi-centre, multipurpose study to investigate early stage non-small cell lung cancer, and to establish a biobank for ongoing collaboration. (In press.)

192. Slebos RJC, Wagenaar SS, Meijer CJLM, et al. Frequency and significance of ras oncogene alterations in human lung tumours. Proc Am Assoc Cancer Res 1990;31:310–15.

193. Roggli VL, Vollmer RT, Greenberg SD, et al. Lung cancer heterogeneity: a blinded and randomized study of 100 consecutive cases. Hum Pathol 1985;16:569–79.

194. Dunnill MS, Gatter KC. Cellular heterogeneity in lung cancer. Histopathology 1986;10:461–75.

195. Adelstein DJ, Tomashefski JF, Snow NJ, et al. Mixed small cell and non-small cell lung cancer. Chest 1986;89:699–704.

196. Matthews MJ. Effects of therapy on the morphology and behaviour of small cell carcinoma of the lung – a clinicopathologic study. Prog Cancer Res Ther 1979;11:155–65.

197. Jagirdar J. Application of immunohistochemistry to the diagnosis of primary and metastatic carcinoma to the lung. Arch Pathol Lab Med 2008;132:384–96.

198. Auerbach O, Garfinkel L. The changing pattern of lung carcinoma. Cancer 1991;68:1973–77.

199. Tanaka I, Matsubara O, Kasuga T, et al. Increasing incidence and changing histopathology of primary lung cancer in Japan. A review of 282 autopsied cases. Cancer 1988;62:1035–39.

200. Rilke F, Carbone A, Clemente L, et al. Surgical pathology of resectable lung cancer. Prog Cancer Res Ther 1979;11:129–42.

201. Hirsch FR, Matthews MJ, Aisner S, et al. Histopathologic classification of small cell lung cancer. Changing concepts and terminology. Cancer 1988;62:973–77.

202. Stuart-Harris R, Boyer M, Greenberg M, et al. The histopathological classification of small cell lung cancer: application of the IASLC classification in 124 cases. Lung Cancer 1992;8:63–70.

203. Katlic M, Carter D. Prognostic implications of histology; size and location of primary tumours. Prog Cancer Res Ther 1979;11:143–50.

204. Leong AS-Y. The relevance of ultrastructural examination in the classification of primary lung tumours. Pathology 1982;14:37–46.

205. Hess FG, McDowell EM, Trump BF. Pulmonary cytology. Current status of cytologic typing of respiratory tract tumours. Am J Pathol 1981;103:323–33.

206. Mennemeyer R, Hammar SP, Bauermeister DE, et al. Cytologic, histologic and electron microscopic correlations in poorly differentiated primary lung carcinoma. A study of 43 cases. Acta Cytol 1979;23:297–302.

207. Gould VE, Linnoila RI, Memoli VA, et al. Neuro-endocrine cells and neuro-endocrine neoplasms of the lung. Pathol Annu (Part I) 1983;18:287–330.

208. Hammond ME, Sause WT. Large cell neuro-endocrine tumours of the lung. Clinical significance and histopathologic definition. Cancer 1985;56:1624–29.

209. McDowell EM, Wilson TS, Trump BF. Atypical endocrine tumours of the lung. Arch Pathol Lab Med 1981;105:20–28.

210. Mooi WT, Dewar A, Springall DR, et al. Non small cell lung carcinomas with neuro-endocrine features. A light microscopic, immunohistochemical and ultrastructural study of 11 cases. Histopathol 1988;13:329–37.

211. Neal MH, Kosinski R, Cohen P, et al. Atypical endocrine tumours of the lung. A histologic, ultrastructural and clinical study of 19 cases. Hum Pathol 1986;17:1264–77.

212. Warren WH, Penfield Faber,L,Gould,VE. Neuro-endocrine neoplasms of the lung. A clinicopathologic update. J Thorac Cardiovasc Surg, 1989;98:321–23.

213. Graziano SL, Tatum AH, Newman NB, et al. The prognostic significance of neuroendocrine markers and carcinoembryonic antigen in patients with resected stage I and II non-small cell lung cancer. Cancer Res 1994;54:2908–13.

214. Souhami RL. The antigens of lung cancer. Thorax 1992;47:53–56.

215. Travis WD, Rush W, Flieder DB, et al. Survival analysis of 200 pulmonary neuroendocrine tumors with clarification of criteria for atypical carcinoid and its separation from typical carcinoid. Am J Surg Pathol 1998;22:934–44.

216. Lavoie RR, McDonald JR, Kling GA. Cavitation in squamous carcinoma of the lung. Acta Cytol 1977;21:210–14.

217. Kern WH. Cytology of hyperplastic and neoplastic lesions of terminal bronchioles and alveoli. Acta Cytol 1965;9:372–79.

218. Saito Y, Imai T, Sato M, et al. Cytologic study of tissue repair in human bronchial epithelium. Acta Cytol 1988;32:622–28.

219. Brambilla E, Travis WD, Colby TV, et al. The new World Health Organization Classification of lung tumours. Eur Respir J 2001; 18:1059–68.

220. Risse EKJ, Vooijs GP, van't Hof MA. Diagnostic significance of 'severe dysplasia' in sputum cytology. Acta Cytol 1988;32:629–34.

221. Saito Y, Imai T, Nagamoto N, et al. A quantitative cytologic study of sputum in early squamous cell bronchogenic carcinoma. Analyt Quant Cytol Histol 1988;10:365–70.

222. Saccomanno G, Archer VE, Auerbach O, et al. Development of carcinoma of the lung as reflected in exfoliated cells. Cancer 1974;33:256–70.

223. Sato M, Saito Y, Nagamoto N, et al. Diagnostic value of differential brushing of all branches of the bronchi in patients with sputum positive or suspected positive for lung cancer. Acta Cytol 1993;37:879–83.

224. Woolner LB. Recent advances in pulmonary cytology: early detection and localization of occult lung cancer in symptomless males. In: Koss LG, Coleman DV, editors. Advances in Clinical Cytology, Vol. 1. London: Butterworths; 1981.

225. Humphrey LL, Teutsch S, Johnson M. Lung cancer screening with sputum cytologic examination, chest radiography, and computed tomography: an update for the U.S. Preventive Services Task Force. Ann Intern Med 2004;140:740–53.

226. Jett JR, Midthun DE. Screening for lung cancer: current status and future directions: Thomas A. Neff lecture. Chest 2004;125:158–62.

227. Kennedy T, Proudfoot S, Franklin W, et al. Cytopathological analysis of sputum in patients with airflow obstruction and significant smoking histories. Cancer Res 1996;56:4673–78.

228. Kennedy TC, Miller Y, Prindiville S. Screening for lung cancer revisited and the role of sputum cytology and fluorescence bronchoscopy in a high-risk group. Chest 2000;117:72–79.

229. Melamed MR. Lung cancer screening results in the National Cancer Institute New York study. Cancer 2000;89:2356–62.

230. Sato M, Sakurada A, Sagawa M, et al. Diagnostic results before and after introduction of autofluorescence bronchoscopy in patients suspected of having lung cancer detected by sputum cytology in lung cancer mass screening. Lung Cancer 2001;32:247–53.

231. Thunnissen FB. Sputum examination for early detection of lung cancer. J Clin Pathol 2003;56:805–10.

232. Fontana RS. Screening for lung cancer: recent experience in the United States. Cancer Treat Res 1986;28:91–111.

233. Band PR, Feldstein M, Saccomanno G. Reversibility of bronchial marked atypia: implication for chemoprevention. Cancer Detect Prevent 1986;9:157–60.

234. Garret M. Cellular atypias in sputum and bronchial secretions associated with tuberculosis and bronchiectasis. Am J Clin Pathol 1960;34:237–46.

235. deMattos MCFI, de Oliveira MLS. Pseudoepitheliomatous proliferation, a pitfall in sputum cytology. Diagn Cytopathol 1991;7:656–57.

236. Bedrossian CWM, Corey BJ. Abnormal sputum cytopathology during chemotherapy with bleomycin. Acta Cytol 1978;22:202–7.

237. Koss LG, Melamed MR, Mayer K. The effect of busulphan on human epithelia. Am J Clin Pathol 1965;44:385–97.

238. Bewtra C, Dewan N, O'Donahue WJ, Jr. Exfoliative sputum cytology in pulmonary embolism. Acta Cytol 1983;27:489–96.

239. Berman JJ, Murray RJ, Lopez-Plaza IM. Widespread posttracheostomy atypia simulating squamous cell carcinoma. Acta Cytol 1991;35:713–16.

240. Weaver KM, Novak PM, Naylor B. Vegetable cell contaminants in cytologic specimens. Their resemblance to cells associated with various normal and pathologic states. Acta Cytol 1981;25:210–14.

241. Matsuda M, Nagumo S, Horai T, et al. Cytologic diagnosis of laryngeal and hypopharyngeal squamous cell carcinoma in sputum. Acta Cytol 1988;32:655–57.

242. Baker JJ, Solanki PH, Schenk DA, et al. Transbronchial fine needle aspiration of the mediastinum. Importance of lymphocytes as an indicator of specimen adequacy. Acta Cytol 1990;34:517–23.

243. Mitchell ML, King DE, Bonfiglio TA, et al. Pulmonary fine needle aspiration cytopathology. A five year correlation study. Acta Cytol 1984;28:72–76.

244. Suprun H, Pedio G, Ruttner JR. The diagnostic reliability of cytologic typing in primary lung cancer with a review of the literature. Acta Cytol 1980;24:494–500.

245. Smith AR, Raab SS, Landreneau RJ, et al. Fine-needle aspiration cytologic features of pseudovascular adenoid squamous-cell carcinoma of the lung. Diagn Cytopathol 1999;21:265–70.

246. Shaha AR, Hoover E, Mitrani Metal. Synchronicity, multicentricity, and meta chronicity of head and neck cancer. Head Neck Surg 1988;10:225–28.

247. Kuriakose MA, Loree TR, Rubenfeld A, et al. Simultaneously presenting head and neck and lung cancer: a diagnostic and treatment dilemma. Laryngoscope 2002;112:120–23.

248. Bell WR, Jr., Johnston WW, Bigner SH. The cytologic diagnosis of occult small-cell undifferentiated carcinoma of the lung. Acta Cytol 1982;26:73–77.

249. Ronai Z, Yabubovskaya MS, Zhang E, et al. K-ras mutation in sputum of patients with or without lung cancer. J Cell Biochem Suppl 1996;25:172–76.

250. Ariza A, Mate JL, Isamat M, et al. Standard and variant CD44 isoforms are commonly expressed in lung cancer of the non-small cell type but not of the small cell type. J Pathol 1995;177:363–68.

251. Koprowska I, Zipfel SA. The potential usefulness of monoclonal antibodies in the determination of histologic types of lung cancer in cytologic preparations. Acta Cytol 1988;32:675–79.

252. Tabatowski K, Vollmer RT, Tello JW, et al. The use of a panel of monoclonal antibodies in ultrastructurally characterised small cell carcinomas of the lung. Acta Cytol 1988;32:667–74.

253. Walker WP, Wittchow RJ, Bottles K, et al. Paranuclear blue inclusions in small cell undifferentiated carcinoma: a diagnostically useful finding demonstrated in fine-needle aspiration biopsy smears. Diagn Cytopathol 1994;10:212–15.

254. Naib ZM. Pitfalls in the cytologic diagnosis of oat cell carcinoma of the lung. Acta Cytol 1964;8:34–38.

255. Davenport RD. Diagnostic value of crush artefact in cytologic specimens. Occurrence in small cell carcinoma of the lung. Acta Cytol 1990;34:502–4.

256. Johnston WW, Frable WJ. Diagnostic Respiratory Cytopathology. New York: Masson; 1979.

257. Marchevsky A, Nieburgs HE, Olenko E, et al. Pulmonary tumourlets in cases of 'tuberculoma' of the lung with malignant cells in brush biopsy. Acta Cytol 1982;26:491–94.

258. Kalhor N, Zander DS, Liu J. TTF-1 and p63 for distinguishing pulmonary small-cell carcinoma from poorly differentiated squamous cell carcinoma in previously Pap stained cytologic material. Mod Pathol 2006;19:1117–23.

259. Johansson L. Histopathologic classification of lung cancer: relevance of cytokeratin and TTF-1 immunophenotyping. Ann Diagn Pathol 2004;8:259–67.

260. Rollins SD, Genack LJ, Schumann GB. Primary cytodiagnosis of dually differentiated lung cancer by transthoracic fine needle aspiration. Acta Cytol 1988;32:231–34.

261. Zaharopoulos P, Wong JY, Stewart GD. Cytomorphology of the variants of small cell carcinoma of the lung. Acta Cytol 1982;26:800–8.

262. Yang GC. Mixed small cell/large cell carcinoma of the lung. Report of a case with cytologic features and ultrastructural correlation. Acta Cytol 1995;39:1175–81.

263. Dugan JM. Cytologic diagnosis of basal cell (basaloid) carcinoma of the lung. A report of two cases. Acta Cytol 1995;39:539–42.

264. Vesoulis Z. Metastatic laryngeal basaloid squamous cell carcinoma simulating primary small cell carcinoma of the lung on fine needle aspiration lung biopsy. A case report. Acta Cytol 1998;42:783–87.

265. Pelosi G, Rodriguez J, Viale G, Rosai J. Typical and atypical pulmonary carcinoid tumors overdiagnosed as small-cell carcinoma on biopsy specimens: a major pitfall in the management of lung cancer patients. Am J Surg Pathol 2005;29:179–87.

266. Kerr KM. Pulmonary adenocarcinomas: classification and reporting. Histopathology 2009;54:12–27.

267. Colby TV, Noguchi M, Henschke C, editors, et al. World Health Organization Classification of tumours. Pathology and genetics of tumours of the lung, pleura, thymus and heart. Lyon: IARC Press; 2004. p. 35–44.

268. Blumenfeld W, Turi GK, Harrison G, et al. Utility of cytokeratin 7 and 20 subset analysis as an aid in the identification of primary site of origin of malignancy in cytologic specimens. Diagn Cytopathol 1999;20:63–66.

269. Kaufmann O, Dietel M. Expression of thyroid transcription factor-1 in pulmonary and extrapulmonary small cell carcinomas and other neuroendocrine carcinomas of various primary sites. Histopathology 2000;36:415–20.

270. Fetsch PA, Marincola FM, Filie A, et al. Melanoma-associated antigen recognized by T cells (MART-1): the advent of a preferred immunocytochemical antibody for the diagnosis of metastatic malignant melanoma with fine-needle aspiration. Cancer 1999;87:37–42.

271. Naylor B, Bailey C. A pitfall in the cytodiagnosis of sputum of asthmatics. J Clin Pathol 1964;17:87–89.

272. McKee G, Parums DV. False-positive cytodiagnosis in fibrosing alveolitis. Acta Cytol 1990;34:105–7.

273. Selvaggi SM, Rerber M. Pulmonary cytology in patients with the acquired immunodeficiency syndrome (AIDS). Diagn Cytopathol 1986;2:187–93.

274. Grotte D, Stanley MW, Swanson PE, et al. Reactive type II pneumocytes in

bronchoalveolar lavage fluid from adult respiratory distress syndrome can be mistaken for cells of adenocarcinoma. Diagn Cytopathol 1990;6:317–22.

275. Cohen J-M, Kreitzer R, Dicpinigaitis P. Mucinous cystadenocarcinoma of the lung; correlation of intraoperative cytology with histology. Acta Cytol 1991;35:626.

276. Dacic S. Minimally invasive adenocarcinomas of the lung. Adv Anat Pathol 2009;16:166–71.

277. Elson CE, Moore SP, Johnston WW. Morphologic and immunocytochemical studies of bronchiolo-alveolar carcinoma at Duke University Medical Centre 1968–1986. Analyt Quant Cytol Histol. 1989;11:261–74.

278. Gupta RK. Value of sputum cytology in the differential diagnosis of alveolar cell carcinoma from bronchogenic carcinoma. Acta Cytol 1981;25:255–58.

279. Lozowski W, Hajdu SI. Cytology and immunocytochemistry of bronchioloalveolar carcinoma. Acta Cytol 1987;31:717–25.

280. Roger V, Nasiell M, Linden M, et al. Cytologic differential diagnosis of bronchioloalveolar carcinoma and bronchogenic adenocarcinoma. Acta Cytol 1976;20:303–7.

281. Smith JH, Frable WJ. Adenocarcinoma of the lung. Cytologic correlation with histologic types. Acta Cytol 1974;18:316–20.

282. Spriggs AI, Cole M, Dunnill MS. Alveolar-cell carcinoma: a problem in sputum cytodiagnosis. J Clin Pathol 1982;35:1370–79.

283. Tao L-C, Delarue NC, Sanders D, et al. Bronchioloalveolar carcinoma: a correlative clinical and cytologic study. Cancer 1978;42:2759–67.

284. Kimura M, Hiruma S, Hara S, et al. Cytopathology of granulocyte colony-stimulating factor-producing lung adenocarcinoma. Acta Cytol 1997;41:952–53.

285. Gupta PK, Verma K. Calcified (psammoma) bodies in alveolar cell carcinoma of the lung. Acta Cytol 1972;16:59–61.

286. Hirsch FR, Matthews MJ, Aisner S, et al. Histopathologic classification of small cell lung cancer: changing concepts and terminology. Cancer 1988;62:973–77.

287. Linder J, Rennard S. Bronchoalveolar Lavage. Chicago: American Society of Clinical Pathologists Press; 1988.

288. Tao L-C, Weisbrod GL, Pearson FG, et al. Cytologic diagnosis of bronchioloalveolar carcinoma by fine needle aspiration biopsy. Cancer 1986;57:1565–70.

289. Silverman JF, Finley JL, Park HK, et al. Fine needle aspiration cytology of bronchioloalveolar-cell carcinoma of the lung. Acta Cytol 1985;29:887–94.

290. Silverman JF, Finley JL, Park HK, et al. Psammoma bodies and optically clear nuclei in bronchiolo-alveolar cell carcinoma. Diagnosis by fine needle aspiration biopsy with histologic and ultrastructural confirmation. Diagn Cytopathol 1985;1:205–15.

291. Jarrett DD, Betsill WL. A problem-orientated approach regarding the fine needle aspiration cytologic diagnosis of bronchioloalveolar carcinoma of the lung: a comparison of diagnostic criteria with benign lesions mimicking carcinoma. Acta Cytol 1987;31:684–85.

292. Auger M, Katz RL, Johnston DA. Differentiating cytological features of bronchioloalveolar carcinoma from adenocarcinoma of the lung in fine-needle aspirations: a statistical analysis of 27 cases. Diagn Cytopathol 1997;16:253–57.

293. Broghamer WL, Collins WM, Mojsejenko IK. The cytohistopathology of a pseudomesotheliomatous carcinoma of the lung. Acta Cytol 1978;22:239–42.

294. Tsumuraya M, Kodama T, Kameya T, et al. Light and electron microscopic analysis of intranuclear inclusions in papillary adenocarcinoma of the lung. Acta Cytol 1981;25:523–32.

295. Chen KTK. Psammoma bodies in fine needle aspiration cytology of papillary adenocarcinoma of the lung. Diagn Cytopathol 1990;6:271–74.

296. Tao L-C, Weisbrod G, Ritcey EL, et al. False 'false positive' results in diagnostic cytology. Acta Cytol 1984;28:450–55.

297. Albain KS, True LD, Golomb HM, et al. Large cell carcinoma of the lung. Ultrastructural differentiation and clinical pathologic correlations. Cancer 1985;56:1618–23.

298. Broderick PA, Corvese NL, Lachance T, et al. Giant cell carcinoma of the lung: a cytologic evaluation. Acta Cytol 1975;19:225–30.

299. Naib ZM. Giant cell carcinoma of the lung: cytologic study of the exfoliated cells in sputa and bronchial washings. Chest 1961;40:69–73.

300. Craig ID, Desrosiers P, Lefcoe MS. Giant cell carcinoma of the lung. A cytologic study. Acta Cytol 1983;27:293–98.

301. Albright CD, Hafiz MA. Cytomorphologic changes in split course radiation treated bronchogenic carcinomas. Diagn Cytopathol 1988;4:9–13.

302. Chess Q. Megakaryocytes in bronchial brushings. Acta Cytol 1988;23:130.

303. Nicholson SA, Ryan MR. A review of cytologic findings in neuroendocrine carcinomas including carcinoid tumors with histologic correlation. Cancer 2000;90:148–61.

304. Anderson C, Ludwig ME, O'Donnell M, et al. Fine needle aspiration cytology of pulmonary carcinoid tumours. Acta Cytol 1990;34:505–10.

305. Collins BT, Cramer HM. Fine needle aspiration cytology of carcinoid tumors. Acta Cytol 1996;40:695–707.

306. Gephardt GN, Belovich DM. Cytology of pulmonary carcinoid tumours. Acta Cytol 1982;26:434–38.

307. Givens CD Jr., Marini JJ. Transbronchial needle aspiration of a bronchial carcinoid tumour. Chest 1985;88:152–53.

308. Horan DC, Bonfiglio TA, Patten SF Jr. The needle aspiration cytopathology of bronchial carcinoid tumours. An analytical study of the cells. Analyt Quant Cytol 1982;4:105–9.

309. Kim K, Mah C, Dominquez J. Carcinoid tumours of the lung: cytologic differential diagnosis in fine-needle aspirates. Diagn Cytopathol 1986;2:343–46.

310. Lozowski W, Hajdu SI, Melamed MR. Cytomorphology of carcinoid tumours. Acta Cytol 1979;23:360–65.

311. Kyriakos M, Rockoff SD. Brush biopsy of bronchial carcinoid – a source of cytologic error. Acta Cytol 1972;16:261–68.

312. Mitchell ML, Parker FP. Capillaries. A cytologic feature of pulmonary carcinoid tumours. Acta Cytol 1991;35:183–85.

313. Nguyen GK. Cytopathology of pulmonary carcinoid tumors in sputum and bronchial brushings. Acta Cytol 1995;39:1152–60.

314. Craig JD, Finley RJ. Spindle cell carcinoid of lung. Cytologic, histopathologic and ultrastructural features. Acta Cytol 1982;26:495–98.

315. Fekete PS, Cohen C, DeRose PB. Pulmonary spindle cell carcinoid. Needle aspiration biopsy, histologic and immunohistochemical findings. Acta Cytol 1990;34:50–56.

316. Nguyen G-K, Shnitka TK. Aspiration biopsy cytology of adenocarcinoid tumour of the bronchial tree. Acta Cytol 1987;31:726–30.

317. Pilotti S, Rilke F, Lombardi L. Pulmonary carcinoid with glandular features. Report of 2 cases with positive fine needle aspiration cytology. Acta Cytol 1983;27:511–14.

318. Arrigoni MG, Woolner LB, Bernatz PE. Atypical carcinoid tumour of lung. J Thorac Cardiovasc Surg 1972;64:413–21.

319. Szyfelbein WM, Ross JS. Carcinoids, atypical carcinoids and small cell carcinoma of the lung: differential diagnosis of fine needle aspiration biopsy specimens. Diagn Cytopathol 1988;4:1–8.

320. Frierson FHF Jr., Covell JL, Mills SE. Fine needle aspiration cytology of atypical carcinoid of the lung. Acta Cytol 1987;31:471–75.

321. Jordan AG, Predmore L, Sullivan MM, et al. The cytodiagnosis of well differentiated neuro-endocrine carcinoma. A distinct clinicopathologic entity. Acta Cytol 1987;31:464–70.

322. Pelosi G, Rodriguez J, Viale G, et al. Typical and atypical pulmonary carcinoid tumor overdiagnosed as small-cell carcinoma on biopsy specimens: a major pitfall in the management of lung cancer patients. Am J Surg Pathol 2005;29:179–87.

323. Lau SK, Luthringer DJ, Eisen RN. Thyroid transcription factor-1: a review. Appl Immunohistochem Mol Morphol 2002;10:97–102.

324. Buchanan AT, Fauck R, Gupta RK. Cytologic diagnosis of adenoid cystic carcinoma in tracheal wash specimens. Diagn Cytopathol 1988;4:130–32.

325. Gupta RK, McHutchison AG. Cytologic findings of adenoid cystic carcinoma in a tracheal wash specimen. Diagn Cytopathol 1992;8:196–97.

326. Lozowski MS, Mishriki Y, Solitaire GB. Cytopathologic features of adenoid cystic carcinoma. Case report and literature review. Acta Cytol 1983;27:317–22.

327. Nguyen G-K. Cytology of bronchial gland carcinoma. Acta Cytol 1988;32:235–39.

328. Radhika S, Dey P, et al. Adenoid cystic carcinoma in a bronchial washing. A case report. Acta Cytol 1993;37:97–99.

329. Anderson RJ, Johnston WW, Szpak CA. Fine needle aspiration of adenoid cystic carcinoma metastatic to the lung. Cytologic features and differential diagnosis. Acta Cytol 1985;29:527–32.

330. Smith RC, Amy RW. Adenoid cystic carcinoma metastatic to the lung. Report of a case diagnosed by fine needle aspiration biopsy cytology. Acta Cytol 1985;29:535–36.

331. Brooks B, Baandrup U. Peripheral low grade mucoepidermoid carcinoma of the lung – needle aspiration cytodiagnosis and histology. Cytopathol 1992;3:259–65.

332. Tao LC, Robertson DI. Cytologic diagnosis of bronchial mucoepidermoid carcinoma by fine needle aspiration biopsy. Acta Cytol 1978;22:221–24.

333. Segletes LA, Steffee CH, Geisinger KR. Cytology of primary pulmonary mucoepidermoid and adenoid cystic carcinoma. A report of four cases. Acta Cytol 1999;43:1091–97.

334. Burke MD, Melamed MR. Exfoliative cytology of metastatic cancer in lung. Acta Cytol 1968;12:61–74.

335. Chu P, Wu E, Weiss LM. Cytokeratin 7 and cytokeratin 20 expression in epithelial neoplasms: a survey of 435 cases. Mod Pathol 2000;13:962–72.

336. Saleh H, Masood S. Value of ancillary studies in fine-needle aspiration biopsy. Diagn Cytopathol 1995;13:310–15.

337. O'Reilly PE, Brueckner J, Silverman JF. Value of ancillary studies in fine needle aspiration cytology of the lung. Acta Cytol 1994;38:144–50.

338. Korfhage L, Broghamer WL, Richardson ME, et al. Pulmonary cytology in the post-therapeutic monitoring of patients with bronchogenic carcinoma. Acta Cytol 1986;30:351–55.

339. Ebihara Y, Fukushima N, Asakuma Y. Double primary lung cancers; with special reference to their exfoliative cytology and to the rare malignant 'mixed' tumour of the salivary-gland type. Acta Cytol 1980;24:212–23.

340. Braman SS, Whitcomb ME. Endobronchial metastasis. Arch Intern Med 1975;135:543–47.

341. Ludwig RA, Gero M. Bronchoscopic cytology of metastatic breast carcinoma with osteoclast like giant cells. Acta Cytol 1987;31:365–68.

342. Selvaggi S, Kissner D, Qureshi F. Metastatic metaplastic carcinoma of the breast. Diagnosis by bronchial brush cytology. Diagn Cytopathol 1989;3:396–99.

343. Chell SE, Nayar R, De Frias DV, et al. Metaplastic breast carcinoma metastatic to the lung mimicking a primary chondroid lesion: report of a case with cytohistologic correlation. Ann Diagn Pathol 1998;2:173–80.

344. Varma S, Amy RW. Adrenal cortical carcinoma metastatic to the lung. Report of a case diagnosed by fine needle aspiration biopsy. Acta Cytol 1990;34:104–5.

345. Craig ID, Shum DT, Desrosiers P, et al. Choriocarcinoma metastatic to the lung: a cytologic study with identification of human choriogonadotrophin with an immunoperoxidase technique. Acta Cytol 1983;27:647–50.

346. Tao LC. Pulmonary metastases from intracranial meningioma diagnosed by aspiration biopsy cytology. Acta Cytol 1991;35:524–28.

347. Baisden BL, Hamper UM, Ali SZ. Metastatic meningioma in fine-needle aspiration (FNA) of the lung: cytomorphologic finding. Diagn Cytopathol 1999;20:291–94.

348. Ehya H. Cytology of mesothelioma of the tunica vaginalis metastatic to the lung. Acta Cytol 1985;29:79–84.

349. Whitaker D, Sterrett GF, Shilkin KB, et al. Malignant mesothelioma cells in sputum. Diagn Cytopathol 1986;2:21–24.

350. Hamilton C, Bigner SH, Wells S, et al. Metastatic medullary carcinoma of the thyroid in sputum – a light and electron microscopic study. Acta Cytol 1983;27:49–53.

351. Tabei SZ, Abdollahi B, Nili F. Diagnosis of metastatic adamantinoma of the tibia by pulmonary brushing cytology. Acta Cytol 1988;32:579–81.

352. Levine SE, Mossler JA, Johnston WW. The cytopathology of metastatic ameloblastoma. Acta Cytol 1981;25:295–98.

353. Landolt U. Pleomorphic adenoma of the salivary glands metastatic to the lung: diagnosis by FNA cytology. Acta Cytol 1990;34:101–2.

354. Liu K, Layfield LJ, Coogan AC. Cytologic features of pulmonary metastasis from a granulosa cell tumor diagnosed by fine-needle aspiration: a case report. Diagn Cytopathol 1997;16:341–44.

355. Ali SZ, Kronz JD, Plowden KM, et al. Metastatic pulmonary leiomyosarcoma: cytopathologic diagnosis on sputum examination. Diagn Cytopathol 1998;18:280–83.

356. Roglic M, Jukic S, Damjanov I. Cytology of the solitary papilloma of the bronchus. Acta Cytol 1975;19:11–13.

357. Rubel LR, Reynolds RE. Cytologic description of squamous cell papilloma of the respiratory tract. Acta Cytol 1979;23:227–30.

358. Brightman I, Morgan JA, Zwehl D, et al. Cytological appearances of a solitary squamous cell papilloma with associated mucous cell adenoma in the lung. Cytopathology 1992;3:253–57.

359. Nguyen G-K. Aspiration biopsy cytology of benign clear cell ('sugar') tumour of the lung. Acta Cytol 1989;33:511–15.

360. Cwierzyk TA, Glasberg SS, Virshup MA, et al. Pulmonary oncocytoma: report of a case with cytologic, histologic and electron microscopic study. Acta Cytol 1985;29:620–23.

361. Laforga JB, Aranda FI. Multicentric oncocytoma of the lung diagnosed by fine-needle aspiration. Diagn Cytopathol 1999;21:51–54.

362. Hamper UM, Khouri NF, Stitik FP, et al. Pulmonary hamartoma: diagnosis by transthoracic needle-aspiration biopsy. Radiology 1985;155:15–18.

363. Curtin CT, Proux J, Davis E. Cartilaginous hamartoma of the lung: a potential pitfall in pulmonary fine needle aspiration. Acta Cytol 1988;32:764.

364. Dahlgren SE. Needle biopsy of intrapulmonary hamartoma. Scand J Respir Dis 1966;47:187–94.

365. de Rooij PD, Meijer S, Calame J, et al. Solitary hamartoma of the lung; is thoracotomy still mandatory? Neth J Surg 1988;40:145–48.

366. Dunbar F, Leiman G. The aspiration cytology of pulmonary hamartomas. Diagn Cytopathol 1989;5:174–80.

367. Ramzy I. Pulmonary hamartomas: cytologic appearances of fine needle aspiration biopsy. Acta Cytol 1976;20:15–19.

368. Sinner WN. Fine needle biopsy of hamartomas of the lung. Am J Roent 1982;138:65–69.

369. Wiatrowska BA, Yazdi HM, Matzinger FR, et al. Fine needle aspiration biopsy of pulmonary hamartomas. Radiologic, cytologic and immunocytochemical study of 15 cases. Acta Cytol 1995;39:1167–74.

370. Chow LT-C, Chan S-K, Chow W-H, et al. Pulmonary sclerosing haemangioma. Report of a case with diagnosis by FNA. Acta Cytol 1992;36:287–92.

37.1 Tao LC. Guides to Clinical Aspiration Biopsy. Lung, Pleura and Mediastinum. Tokyo: Igaku-Shoin; 1988.

37.2 Wang SE, Nieberk RK. Fine needle aspiration cytology of sclerosing haemangioma of the lung, a mimicker of bronchioloalveolar carcinoma. Acta Cytol 1985;30:51–54.

373. Gottschalk-Sabag S, Hadas-Halpern I, Glick T. Sclerosing haemangioma of lung mimicking carcinoma diagnosed by fine needle aspiration (FNA) cytology. Cytopathology 1995;6:115–20.

374. Kaw YT, Nayak RN. Fine needle biopsy cytology of sclerosing haemangioma of the lung. A case report. Acta Cytol 1993;37:933–37.

375. Wojcik EM, Sneige N, Lawrence DD, et al. Fine needle aspiration cytology of sclerosing haemangioma of the lung: case report with immunohistochemical study. Diagn Cytopathol 1993;9:304–9.

376. Chen K. Cytology of bronchial benign granular cell tumour. Acta Cytol 1991;35:381–84.

377. Fÿezesi L, Hšer P-W, Schmidt W. Exfoliative cytology of multiple endobronchial granular cell tumour. Acta Cytol 1989;33:516–18.

378. Glant MD, Wall RW, Ransburg G. Endobronchial granular cell tumour: cytology of a new case and review of the literature. Acta Cytol 1979;23:477–82.

379. Mermolja M, Rott T. Cytology of endobronchial granular cell tumour. Diagn Cytopathol 1991;7:524–26.

380. Thomas L, Risbud M, Gabriel JB, et al. Cytomorphology of granular cell tumour of the bronchus. A case report. Acta Cytol 1984;28:129–32.

381. Smith AR, Gilbert CF, Strausbauch P, et al. Fine needle aspiration cytology of a mediastinal granular cell tumor with histologic confirmation and ancillary studies. A case report. Acta Cytol. 1998;42:1011–16.

382. Guillou L, Gloor E, Anani P, et al. Bronchial granular cell tumour – report of a case with preoperative cytologic diagnosis on bronchial brushings and immunohistochemical studies. Acta Cytol 1991;35:375–80.

383. Naib ZM, Goldstein HG. Exfoliative cytology of a case of bronchial granular cell myoblastoma. Dis Chest 1962;42:645–47.

384. Henderson DW, Shilkin KB, Whitaker D, et al. The pathology of malignant mesothelioma, including immunohistology and ultrastructure. In: Henderson DW, Shilkin KB, Langlois S, Le P, Whitaker D, editors. Malignant Mesothelioma. New York: Hemisphere; 1992. p. 69–139.

385. Okike N, Bernatz PE, Woolner LB. Localized mesothelioma of the pleura. Benign and malignant variants. J Thorac Cardiovasc Surg 1978;75:363–72.

386. England DM, Hochholzer L, McCarthy MJ. Localized benign and malignant fibrous tumors of the pleura. Am J Surg Pathol 1989;13:640–58.

387. Burrig KF, Pfitzer P, Hort W. Well differentiated papillary mesothelioma of the peritoneum: a borderline mesothelioma. Report of two cases and a review of the literature. Virchow Arch (A) 1990;417:443–47.

388. Tao LC. The cytopathology of mesothelioma. Acta Cytol 1979;23:209–13.

389. Orell SR, Sterrett GF, Walters MN, et al. Manual and Atlas of Fine Needle Aspiration Cytology. 2nd edn. Edinburgh: Churchill Livingstone; 1992.

390. Obers VJ, Leiman G, Girdwood RW, et al. Primary Chest wall and pleura, malignant pleural tumors (mesotheliomas) presenting as localised masses. Fine needle aspiration cytologic findings, clinical and radiologic features and review of the literature. Acta Cytol 1988;32:567–75.

391. Tao LC. Aspiration biopsy cytology of mesothelioma. Diagn Cytopathol 1989;5:14–21.

392. Jayaram G, Ashok S. Fine needle aspiration cytology of well-differentiated papillary peritoneal mesothelioma: report of a case. Acta Cytol 1988;32:563–66.

393. Bonfiglio T. Cytopathologic interpretation of transthoracic fine-needle biopsies. In: Johnston WW, editor. Masson Monographs in

Diagnostic Cytopathology, Vol. 4. New York: Masson; 1983.

394. Conces DJ, Schwenk GR, Doering PR, et al. Thoracic needle biopsy: improved results utilizing a team approach. Chest 1987;91:813–16.

395. Fraser RS. Transthoracic needle aspiration. The benign diagnosis. Arch Pathol Lab Med 1991;115:751–61.

396. Dusenbery D, Grimes MM, Frable WJ. Fine needle aspiration cytology of localized fibrous tumor of pleura. Diagn Cytopathol 1992;8:444–50.

397. Strigle SM, Gal AA. A review of pulmonary cytopathology in the acquired immunodeficiency syndrome. Diagn Cytopathol 1989;5:44–54.

398. Gattuso P, Castelli MJ, Peng Y, et al. Posttransplant lymphoproliferative disorders: a fine-needle aspiration biopsy study. Diagn Cytopathol 1997;16:392–95.

399. Abbondanzo SL, Rush W, Bijwaard KE, et al. Nodular lymphoid hyperplasia of the lung: a clinicopathologic study of 14 cases. Am J Surg Pathol 2000;24:587–97.

400. Yousem SA, Weiss LM, Colby TV. Primary pulmonary Hodgkin's disease. A clinicopathologic study of 15 cases. Cancer 1986;57:1217–24.

401. Hammar SP. Immunohistology of lung and pleural neoplasms. In: Dabbs D, editor. Diagnostic Immunohistochemistry. 2nd edn. Philadelphia: Churchill Livingstone/Elsevier; 2006. p. 329–403.

402. Davis WB, Gadek JE. Detection of pulmonary lymphoma by bronchoalveolar lavage. Chest 1987;91:787–89.

403. Gouldesbrough DR, McGoogan E. Primary pulmonary lymphoma: a case diagnosed by bronchial cytology and immunocytochemistry. Histopathol 1988;13:465–67.

404. Myers JL, Fulmer JD. Bronchoalveolar lavage in the diagnosis of pulmonary lymphomas. Chest 1989;91:642–43.

405. Oka M, Kawano K, Kanda T, et al. Bronchoalveolar lavage in primary pulmonary lymphoma with monoclonal gammopathy. Am Rev Resp Dis 1988;137:957–59.

406. Zaer FS, Braylan RC, Zander DS, et al. Multiparametric flow cytometry in the diagnosis and characterization of low-grade pulmonary mucosa-associated lymphoid tissue lymphomas. Mod Pathol 1998;11:525–32.

407. Bardales RH Jr., Powers CN, Frierson HF, et al. Exfoliative respiratory cytology in the diagnosis of leukemias and lymphomas in the lung. Diagn Cytopathol 1996;14:108–18.

408. Bonfiglio TA, Dvoretsky PM, Piscioli F, et al. Fine needle aspiration biopsy in the evaluation of lymphoreticular tumours of the thorax. Acta Cytol 1985;29:548–53.

409. Suprun H, Koss LG. The cytological study of sputum and bronchial washings in Hodgkin's disease with pulmonary involvement. Cancer 1964;17:674–80.

410. Suprun HZ. Cytodiagnosis of Hodgkin's disease in sputum specimens. Acta Cytol 1984;28:190–91.

411. Reale FR, Variakojis D, Compton J, et al. Cytodiagnosis of Hodgkin's disease in sputum specimens. Acta Cytol 1983;27:258–61.

412. Flint A, Kumar NB, Naylor B. Pulmonary Hodgkin's disease. Diagnosis by fine needle aspiration. Acta Cytol 1989;32:221–25.

413. Wisecarver J, Ness M, Rennard S, et al. Bronchoalveolar lavage in the assessment of pulmonary Hodgkin's disease. Acta Cytol 1988;32:766–67.

414. Reiben AE, Ben-Shachar M, Malberger E. Cytologic diagnosis of pulmonary Hodgkin's disease via endobronchial brush preparation. Chest 1989;96:948–49.

415. Fullmer CD, Morris RP. Primary cytodiagnosis of unsuspected mediastinal Hodgkin's disease. Report of a case. Acta Cytol 1972;16:77–81.

416. Levij IS. A case of primary cavitary Hodgkin's disease of the lungs, diagnosed cytologically. Acta Cytol 1972;16:546–49.

417. Morales FM, Matthews JI. Diagnosis of parenchymal Hodgkin's disease using bronchoalveolar lavage. Chest 1991;5:785–86.

418. Eisenberg RS, Dunton BL. Hodgkin's disease first suggested by sputum cytology. Chest 1974;65:218–19.

419. Ludwig RA, Balachandran I. Mycosis fungoides: the importance of pulmonary cytology in the diagnosis of a case with systemic involvement. Acta Cytol 1983;27:198–201.

420. Rosen SE, Vonderheid EC, Koprowski I. Mycosis fungoides with pulmonary involvement: cytopathologic findings. Acta Cytol 1984;28:51–57.

421. Shaheen K, Oertel YC. Mycosis fungoides cells in sputum. A case report. Acta Cytol 1984;28:483–86.

422. Vernon SE. Cytodiagnosis of 'signet-ring'-cell lymphoma. Acta Cytol 1981;25:291–94.

423. Goldstein J, Leslie H. Immunoblastic lymphadenopathy with pulmonary lesions and positive sputum cytology. Acta Cytol 1978;22:165–67.

424. Williams WL, Clark DA, Saiers JH. Fine needle aspiration diagnosis of lymphomatoid granulomatosis. A case report. Acta Cytol 1992;36:91–94.

425. Riazmontazer N, Bedayat G. Cytology of plasma cell myeloma in bronchial washing. Acta Cytol 1989;33:519–22.

426. Chollet S, Soler P, Dournovo P, et al. Diagnosis of pulmonary histiocytosis X by immunodetection of Langerhans' cells in bronchoalveolar lavage fluid. Am J Pathol 1984;115:225–32.

427. Auerswald U, Barth J, Magnussen H. Value of CD-1 positive cells in bronchiolar lavage fluid for the diagnosis of pulmonary histiocytosis X. Lung 1991;169:305–9.

428. Fleming WH, Jove DF. Primary leiomyosarcoma of the lung with positive sputum cytology. Acta Cytol 1975;19:14–20.

429. Crosby JH, Hoeg K, Hager B. Transthoracic fine needle aspiration of primary and metastatic sarcoma. Chest 1984;85:696–97.

430. Kim G, Naylor B, Han IH. Fine needle aspiration cytology of sarcomas metastatic to the lung. Acta Cytol 1986;30:688–94.

431. Michacao CN, Sorensen K, Abdul-Karim FW, et al. Transthoracic needle aspiration in inflammatory pseudotumours of the lung. Diagn Cytopathol 1989;5:400–3.

432. Takeda M, Burechailo FA. Smooth muscle cells in sputum. Acta Cytol 1969;13:696–99.

433. Cosgrove M, Chandrasoma PT, Martin SE. Diagnosis of pulmonary blastoma by fine needle aspiration biopsy: cytologic and immunocytochemical findings. Diagn Cytopathol 1991;7:83–87.

434. Francis D, Jacobsen M. Pulmonary blastoma: preoperative cytologic and histologic findings. Acta Cytol 1979;23:437–42.

435. Non DP Jr., Lang WR, Patchefsky A, et al. Pulmonary blastoma. Cytopathologic and histopathologic findings, Acta Cytol 1976;20:381–86.

436. Spahr J, Draffin R, Johnston WW. Cytopathologic findings in pulmonary blastoma. Acta Cytol 1979;23:454–59.

437. Yokoyama S, Hayashida Y, Nagahama J, et al. Pulmonary blastoma: a case report. Acta Cytol 1992;36:293–97.

438. Lee KG, Cho NH. Fine needle aspiration cytology of pulmonary adenocarcinoma of fetal type. Report of a case with immunohistochemical and ultrastructural studies. Diagn Cytopathol 1991;7:408–14.

439. Cabarcos A, Dorronsoro MG, Beristain J. Pulmonary carcinosarcoma: a case study and review of the literature. Br J Dis Chest 1985;79:83–94.

440. Finley JL, Silverman JF, Dabbs DJ. Fine needle aspiration cytology of pulmonary carcinosarcoma with immunocytochemical and ultrastructural observations. Diagn Cytopathol 1988;4:239–43.

441. Ishizuka T, Yoshitake J, Yamada T, et al. Diagnosis of a case of pulmonary carcinosarcoma by detection of rhabdomyosarcoma cells in sputum. Acta Cytol 1988;32:658–62.

442. Powers CN, Silverman JF, Geisinger KR, et al. Fine-needle aspiration biopsy of the mediastinum. A multi-institutional analysis. Am J Clin Pathol 1996;105:168–73.

443. Shabb NS, Fahl M, Shabb B, et al. Fine-needle aspiration of the mediastinum: a clinical, radiologic, cytologic, and histologic study of 42 cases. Diagn Cytopathol 1998;19:428–36.

444. Temes R, Allen N, Chavez T, et al. Primary mediastinal malignancies in children; report of 22 patients and comparison to 197 adults. Oncologist 2000;5:179–84.

445. Das DK, Pant CS, Rath B, et al. Fine needle aspiration diagnosis of intrathoracic and intra-abdominal lesions: review of experience in the paediatric age group. Diagn Cytopathol 1993;9:383–93.

446. Gu P, Zhao YZ, Jiang LY, et al. Endobronchial ultrasound-guided transbronchial needle aspiration for staging of lung cancer: a systematic review and meta-analysis. Eur J Cancer 2009;45:1389–96.

447. Sterrett GF, Whitaker D, Shilkin KB, et al. Fine needle aspiration cytology of mediastinal lesions. Cancer 1983;51:127–35.

448. Weisbrod GL. Percutaneous fine needle aspiration biopsy of the mediastinum. Clin Chest Med 1987;8:27–41.

449. Weisbrod GL, Lyons DJ, Tao L-C, et al. Percutaneous fine needle aspiration biopsy of mediastinal lesions. Am J Roent 1984;143:525–29.

450. Reyes CV, Thompson KS, Massarani-Wafai R, et al. Utilization of fine-needle aspiration cytology in the diagnosis of neoplastic superior vena caval syndrome. Diagn Cytopathol 1998;19:84–88.

451. WHO. Histological typing of tumours of the thymus. World Health Organization International Classification of Tumours. Berlin: Springer; 1999.

452. Suster S, Moran CA. Primary thymic epithelial neoplasms: spectrum of differentiation and histological features. Semin Diagn Pathol 1999;16:2–17.

453. Kuo T. Cytokeratin profiles of the thymus and thymomas; histogenetic correlations and proposal for a histological classification of thymomas. Histopathology 2000;36:403–14.

454. Okamura M, Ohta M, Tateyama H, et al. The World Health Organization histological classification system reflects the oncologic behavior of thymoma: a clinical study of 273 patients. Cancer 2002;94:624–32.

455. Pan CC, Chen WY, Chiang H. Spindle cell and mixed spindle/lymphocytic thymomas: an integrated clinicopathologic and immunohistochemical study of 81 cases. Am J Surg Pathol 2001;25:111–20.

456. Muller-Hermelink HK, Marx A. Thymoma. Curr Opin Oncol 2000;12:426–33.

457. Tao LC, Griffith Pearson F, Coper JD, et al. Cytopathology of thymoma. Acta Cytol 1984;28:165–70.

458. Ali SZ, Erozan YS. Thymoma. Cytopathologic features and differential diagnosis on fine needle aspiration. Acta Cytol 1998;42:845–54.

459. Dahlgren SE, Sandstedt B, Sunstrom C. Fine needle aspiration cytology of thymic tumours. Acta Cytol 1983;27:1–6.

460. Miller J, Allen R, Wakefield JSL. Diagnosis of thymoma by fine needle aspiration cytology: light and electron microscopic study of a case. Diagn Cytopathol 1987;3:166–69.

461. Pak HY, Yokota SB, Friedberg HA. Thymoma diagnosed by transthoracic fine needle aspiration. Acta Cytol 1982;26:210–16.

462. Sajjad SM, Lukeman JM, Llamas L, et al. Needle biopsy diagnosis of thymoma. Acta Cytol 1982;26:503–6.

463. Shin HJ, Katz RL. Thymic neoplasia as represented by fine needle aspiration biopsy of anterior mediastinal masses. A practical approach to the differential diagnosis. Acta Cytol 1998;42:855–64.

464. Sherman ME, Black-Schaffer S. Diagnosis of thymoma by needle biopsy. Acta Cytol 1990;34:63–68.

465. Suen K, Quenville N. Fine needle aspiration cytology of uncommon thoracic lesions. Am J Clin Pathol 1981;75:803–9.

466. Silverman JF, Raab SS, Park HK. Fine needle aspiration cytology of primary large cell lymphoma of the mediastinum. Cytomorphological features with potential pitfalls in diagnosis. Diagn Cytopathol 1993;9:209–15.

467. Slagel DD, Powers CN, Melaragno MJ, et al. Spindle-cell lesions of the mediastinum: diagnosis by fine-needle aspiration biopsy. Diagn Cytopathol 1997;17:167–76.

468. Pinto MM, Dovgan D, Kaye AD, et al. Fine needle aspiration for diagnosing a thymoma producing CA-125. A case report. Acta Cytol 1993;37:929–32.

469. Chilosi M, Doglioni C, Yan Z, et al. Differential expression of cyclin-dependent kinase 6 in cortical thymocytes and T-cell lymphoblastic lymphoma/leukaemia. Am J Pathol 1998;152:209–17.

470. Wakely PE Jr. Fine needle aspiration in the diagnosis of thymic epithelial neoplasms Hematol Oncol Clin North Am 2008;22:433–42.

471. Dorfman DM, Shahsafaei Aliakbar MS, Chan John KC. Thymic carcinomas, but not thymomas and carcinomas of other sites, show CD5 immunoreactivity. Am J Surg Pathol 1997;21:936–40.

472. Macchiarini P, Ostertag H. Uncommon primary mediastinal tumours. Lancet Oncol 2004;5:107–18.

473. Lauriola L, Erlandson RA, Rosai J. Neuroendocrine differentiation is a common feature of thymic carcinoma. Am J Surg Pathol 1998;22:1059–66.

474. Travis WD, Rush W, Flieder DB, et al. Survival analysis of 200 pulmonary neuroendocrine tumours with clarification of criteria for atypical carcinoid and its separation from typical carcinoid. Am J Surg Pathol 1998;22:934–44.

475. Kondo K, Monden Y. A questionnaire about thymic epithelial tumours as compared to pulmonary typical carcinoids. Nihon Kokyuki Geka Gakkai Zasshi 2001;15:633–42.

476. Gherardi G, Marveggio C, Placidi A. Neuroendocrine carcinoma of the thymus: aspiration biopsy, immunocytochemistry, and clinicopathologic correlates. Diagn Cytopathol 1995;12:158–64.

477. Nichols GL Jr., Hopkins MB 3rd., Geisinger KR. Thymic carcinoid. Report of a case with diagnosis by fine needle aspiration biopsy. Acta Cytol 1997;41:1839–44.

478. Wang DY, Kuo SH, Chang DB, et al. Fine needle aspiration cytology of thymic carcinoid tumor. Acta Cytol 1995;39:423–27.

479. Spits H, Blom B, Jaleco AC, et al. Early stages in the development of human T, natural killer and thymic dendritic cells. Immunol Rev 1998;165:75–86.

480. Isaacson P, Norton AJ, Addis BJ. The human thymus contains a novel population of B lymphocytes. Lancet 1987;2:1488–91.

481. Gonzalez CL, Medeiros LJ, Jaffe ES. Composite lymphoma. A clinicopathologic analysis of nine patients with Hodgkin disease and B cell non-Hodgkin lymphoma. Am J Clin Pathol 1991;96:81–89.

482. Perrone T, Frizzera G, Rosai J. Mediastinal diffuse large-cell lymphoma with sclerosis. A clinicopathologic study of 60 cases. Am J Surg Pathol 1986;10:176–91.

483. Koo CH, Reifel J, Kogut N, et al. True histiocytic malignancy associated with a malignant teratoma in a patient with 46XY gonadal dysgenesis. Am J Surg Pathol 1992;16:175–83.

484. Orazi A, Neiman RS, Ulbright TM, et al. Haemopoietic precursor cells within the yolk sac tumour component are the source of secondary haemopoietic malignancies in patients with mediastinal germ cell tumours. Cancer 1993;71:3873–81.

485. Moran CA, Suster S. Primary germ cell tumours of the mediastinum: 1. Analysis of 322 cases with special emphasis on teratomatous lesions and a proposal for histopathologic classification and clinical staging. Cancer 1997;80:681–90.

486. Takeda S, Miyoshi S, Akashi A, et al. Clinical spectrum of primary mediastinal tumours: a comparison of adult and pediatric populations at a single Japanese institution. J Surg Oncol 2003;83:24–30.

487. Looijenga LH, Oosterhuis JW. Pathobiology of testicular germ cell tumours; views and news. Anal Quant Cytol Histol 2002;24:263–79.

488. Coskun U, Gunel N, Yildirim Y, et al. Primary mediastinal yolk sac tumour in a 66-year-old woman. Med Princ Pract 2002;11:218–20.

489. Takeda S, Miyoshi S, Ohta M, et al. Primary mediastinal germ cell tumours in the mediastinum: a 50 year experience at a single Japanese institution. Cancer 2003;97:367–76.

490. Meissner A, Kirsch W, Regensburger D, et al. Intrapericardial teratoma in an adult. Am J Med 1988;84:1089–90.

491. Schneider DT, Calaminus G, Reinhard H, et al. Primary mediastinal germ cell tumours in children and adolescents: results of the German cooperative protocols MAKEI 83/86, 89 and 96. J Clin Oncol 2000;18:832–39.

492. Dueland S, Stenwig AE, Heilo A, et al. Treatment and outcome of patients with extragonadal germ cell tumours- the Norwegian Radium Hospital's experience 1979–1994. Cancer 1998;77:329–35.

493. Alliota PJ, Castillo J, Englander LS, et al. Primary mediastinal germ cell tumours. Histologic patterns and treatment failures at autopsy. Cancer 1988;62:982–84.

494. Schwabe J, Calaminus G, Vorhoff W, et al. Sexual precocity and recurrent beta-human chorionic gonadotrophin upsurges preceding the diagnosis of a malignant mediastinal germ cell tumour in a 9-year-old boy. Ann Oncol 2002;13:975–77.

495. Nichols CR, Roth BJ, Heerema N, et al. Haematologic neoplasia associated with primary mediastinal germ cell tumours. New Engl J Med 1990;322:1425–29.

496. Strollo DC, Rosado-de-Christenson ML. Primary mediastinal malignant germ cell neoplasms: imaging features. Chest Surg Clin N Am 2002;12:645–58.

497. Moran CA, Suster S. Mediastinal seminomas with prominent cystic changes: a clinicopathologic study of 10 cases. Am J Surg Pathol 1995;19:1047–53.

498. Caraway NP, Fanning CV, Amato RJ, et al. Fine needle aspiration cytology of seminoma: a review of 16 cases. Diagn Cytopathol 1995;12:327–33.

499. Dahlgren SE, Ovenfors C-O. Aspiration biopsy diagnosis of neurogenous mediastinal tumours. Acta Radiol Diagn (Stockh) 1970;10:289–98.

500. Palombini L, Vetrani A. Cytologic diagnosis of ganglioneuroblastoma. Acta Cytol 1976;20:286–87.

501. Palombini L, Vetrani A, Veccione R, et al. The cytology of ganglioneuroma on fine needle aspiration smear. Acta Cytol 1982;26:259–60.

502. Heimann A, Sneige N, Shirkhoda A, et al. Fine needle aspiration cytology of thymolipoma. A case report. Acta Cytol 1987;31:335–59.

503. Klimstra DS, Moran CA, Perino G, et al. Liposarcoma of the anterior mediastinum and thymus. A clinicopathologic study of 28 cases. Am J Surg Pathol 1995;19:782–91.

504. Attal H, Jensen J, Reyes CV. Myxoid liposarcoma of the anterior mediastinum. Diagnosis by fine needle aspiration biopsy. Acta Cytol 1995;39:511–13.

505. Morimitsu Y, Nakajima M, Hisaoka M, et al. Extrapleural solitary fibrous tumour: clinicopathologic study of 17 cases with molecular analysis of the p53 pathway. APMIS 2000;108:617–25.

506. Mishriki YY, Lane BP, Lozowski MS, et al. Hurthle cell tumour arising in the mediastinal ectopic thyroid and diagnosed by fine needle aspiration. Light microscopic and ultrastructural features. Acta Cytol 1983;27:188–92.

507. De Las Casas LE, Williams HJ, Strausbauch PH, et al. Hurthle cell adenoma of the mediastinum: intraoperative cytology and differential diagnosis with correlative gross, histology, and ancillary studies. Diagn Cytopathol 2000;22:16–20.

508. Marco V, Sirvent J, Alvarez Moro J, et al. Malignant melanotic schwannoma fine-needle aspiration biopsy findings. Diagn Cytopathol 1998;18:284–86.

509. Prieto-Rodriguez M, Camanas-Sanz A, Bas T, et al. Psammomatous melanotic schwannoma localized in the mediastinum: diagnosis by fine-needle aspiration cytology. Diagn Cytopathol 1998;19:298–302.

510. McLoud TC, Kalisher L, Stark P, et al. Intrathoracic lymph node metastases from extrathoracic neoplasms. Am J Roentgenol 1978;131:403–7.

511. Akman ES, Ertem U, Tankal V, et al. Aggressive Kaposi's sarcoma in children, a case report. Turk J Pediatr 1989;31:297–303.

512. Goldstein LS, Kavuru MS, Meli Y, et al. Uterine rhabdomyosarcoma metastatic to mediastinal lymph nodes: diagnosis by transbronchial needle aspiration. South Med J 1999;92:84–87.

513. Hitota T, Konno K, Fujimoto T, et al. Unusual late extrapulmonary metastasis in ostersarcoma. Pediatr Hematol Oncol 1999;16:545–49.

514. Souma T, Oguma F, Ueno M, et al. A case report of pulmonary metastasis of malignant fibrous histiocytoma (MFH) accompanied by mediastinal lymph node metastasis. Kyobu Geka 1993;46:1149–51.

515. Springfield D. Liposarcoma. Clin Orthop 1993:50–57.

516. Oliveira AM, Tazelaar HD, Myers JL, et al. Thyroid transcription factor-1 distinguishes metastatic pulmonary from well differentiated neuroendocrine tumours of other sites. Am J Surg Pathol 2001;25:815–19.

517. Koss LG, Melamed MR, Goodner JT. Pulmonary cytology – a brief survey of diagnostic results from 1 July 1952 until 31 December 1960. Acta Cytol 1964;8:104–13.

518. Ng AB, Horak GC. Factors significant in the diagnostic accuracy of lung cytology in bronchial washing and sputum samples. II. Sputum samples. Acta Cytol 1983;27:397–402.

519. Bender BL, Cherock M, Sotos SN. Effective use of bronchoscopy and sputa in the diagnosis of lung cancer. Diagn Cytopathol 1985;1:183–87.

520. Castella J, de la Heras P, Puzo C, et al. Cytology of postbronchoscopically collected sputum samples and its diagnostic value. Respiration 1981;42:116–21.

521. Chopra SK, Genovesi MG, Simmons DH, et al. Fiberoptic bronchoscopy in the diagnosis of lung cancer. Comparison of pre- and post-bronchoscopy sputa, washings, brushings and biopsies. Acta Cytol 1977;21:524–27.

522. Gledhill A, Bates C, Henderson D, et al. Sputum cytology: a limited role. J Clin Pathol 1997;50:566–68.

523. Risse EKJ, Vooijs GP, van't Hof MA. Relationship between the cellular composition of sputum and the cytologic diagnosis of lung cancer. Acta Cytol 1987;31:170–76.

524. Bocking A, Biesterfeld S, Chatelain R, et al. Diagnosis of bronchial carcinoma on sections of paraffin-embedded sputum. Sensitivity and specificity of an alternative to routine cytology. Acta Cytol 1992;36:37–47.

525. Bibbo M, Fennessy JJ, Lu C-T, et al. Bronchial brushing technique for the cytologic diagnosis of peripheral lung lesions. A review of 693 cases. Acta Cytol 1973;17:245–51.

526. Ng ABP, Horak GC. Factors significant in the diagnostic accuracy of lung cytology in bronchial washing and sputum samples. I. Bronchial washings. Acta Cytol 1983;27:391–96.

527. Naryshkin S, Daniels J, Young NA. Diagnostic correlation of fiberoptic bronchoscopic biopsy and bronchoscopic cytology performed simultaneously. Diagn Cytopathol 1992;8:119–23.

528. Nowels KW, Burford-Foggs A, et al. Epithelioid haemangioendothelioma. Cytomorphology and histological features of a case. Diagn Cytopathol 1989;5:75–78.

529. Hsu C. Cytologic diagnosis of lung tumours from bronchial brushings of Chinese patients in Hong Kong. Acta Cytol 1983;27:641–96.

530. Lachman MF, Schofield K, Cellura K. Bronchoscopic diagnosis of malignancy in the lower airway. A cytologic review. Acta Cytol 1995;39:1148–51.

531. Bhat N, Bhagat P, Pearlman E, et al. Transbronchial needle aspiration biopsy in the diagnosis of pulmonary neoplasms. Diagn Cytopathol 1990;6:14–17.

532. Horsley JR, Miller RE, Amy RWM, et al. Bronchial submucosal needle aspiration performed through the fiberoptic bronchoscope. Acta Cytol 1984;28:211–17.

533. Rosenthal DL, Wallace JM. Fine needle aspiration of pulmonary lesions via fiberoptic bronchoscopy. Acta Cytol 1984;28:203–10.

534. Schenk DA, Bower JH, Bryan CL, et al. Transbronchial needle aspiration staging of bronchogenic carcinoma. Am Rev Respir Dis 1986;134:246–48.

535. Wang KP. Flexible transbronchial needle aspiration biopsy for histologic specimens. Chest 1985;88:860–63.

536. Reichenberger F, Weber J, Tamm M, et al. The value of transbronchial needle aspiration in the diagnosis of peripheral pulmonary lesions. Chest 1999;116:704–8.

537. Levy H, Horak DA, Lewis MI. The value of bronchial washings and bronchoalveolar lavage in the diagnosis of lymphangitic carcinomatosis. Chest 1988;94:1028–30.

538. Linder J, Radio SJ, Robbins RA, et al. Bronchoalveolar lavage in the cytologic diagnosis of carcinoma of the lung. Acta Cytol 1987;31:796–801.

539. Sestini P, Rottoli L, Gotti C, et al. Bronchoalveolar lavage diagnosis of bronchioloalveolar carcinoma. Eur J Resp Dis 1985;66:55–58.

540. Springmeyer SC, Hackman R, Carlson JJ, et al. Bronchioloalveolar cell carcinoma diagnosed by bronchoalveolar lavage. Chest 1983;83:278–79.

541. Popp W, Merkle M, Schreiber B, et al. How much brushing is enough for the diagnosis of lung tumours? Cancer 1992;70:2278–80.

542. Levine MS, Weiss JM, Harrell JH, et al. Transthoracic needle aspiration biopsy following negative fiberoptic bronchoscopy in solitary pulmonary nodules. Chest 1988;93:1152–55.

543. Dahlgren SE. Aspiration biopsy of intrathoracic tumours. Acta Pathol Microbiol Scand (B) 1967;70:566–76.

544. Young JA. Colour Atlas of Pulmonary Cytopathology. Oxford: Harvey Miller Press; 1985.

545. Layfield LJ, Coogan A, Johnston WW, et al. Transthoracic fine needle aspiration biopsy. Sensitivity in relation to guidance technique and lesion size and location. Acta Cytol 1996;40:687–90.

546. Rosenthal DL. Cytopathology of pulmonary disease. In: Wied GL, editor. Monographs in Clinical Cytology, Vol. 11. Basel: Karger; 1988.

547. Adler OB, Rosenberger A, Peleg H. Fine needle aspiration biopsy of mediastinal masses: evaluation of 136 experiences. Am J Roent 1983;140:893–96.

548. Bartholdy NJ, Anderson MJ, Thommesen P. Clinical value of percutaneous fine needle aspiration biopsy of mediastinal masses. Analysis of 132 cases. Scand J Thor Cardiovasc Surg 1984;18:81–83.

549. Rossi G, Pelosi G, Graziano P, et al. A re-evaluation of the clinical significance of histological subtyping of non-small-cell lung carcinoma: diagnostic algorithms in the era of personalized treatments. Int J Surg Pathol 2009;17:206–18.

550. Caya JG, Gilles L, Tieu TM, et al. Lung cancer treated on the basis of cytologic findings: an analysis of 112 patients. Diagn Cytopathol 1990;6:313–16.

551. Caya JG, Wollenberg NJ, Clowry LJ, et al. The diagnosis of pulmonary small cell anaplastic carcinoma by cytologic smears: a 13 year experience. Diagn Cytopathol 1988;4:202–5.

552. Benbasset J, Regev A, Slater P. Predictive value of sputum cytology. Thorax 1987;42:165–72.

553. Naryshkin S, Young NA. Respiratory cytology: a review of non-neoplastic mimics of malignancy. Diagn Cytopathol 1993;9:89–97.

554. Ritter JH, Wick MR, Reyes A, et al. False-positive interpretations of carcinoma in exfoliative respiratory cytology. Report of two cases and a review of underlying disorders. Am J Clin Pathol 1995;104:133–40.

555. Silverman JF. Inflammatory and neoplastic processes of the lung: differential diagnosis and pitfalls in FNA biopsies. Diagn Cytopathol 1995;13:448–62.

556. Kern WH. The diagnostic accuracy of sputum and urine cytology. Acta Cytol 1988;32:651–54.

557. Kern WH. The elusive 'false positive' sputum and urine cytology. Acta Cytol 1990;34:587–88.

558. Cagle PT, Kovach M, Ramzy I. Causes of false results in transthoracic fine needle lung aspirates. Acta Cytol 1993;37:16–20.

559. Caya JG, Clowry LT, Wollenberg NJ, et al. Transthoracic fine needle aspiration cytology. Analysis of 82 patients with detailed verification criteria and evaluation of false negative cases. Am J Clin Pathol 1984;82:100–3.

560. Stewart CJ, Stewart IS. Immediate assessment of fine needle aspiration cytology of lung. J Clin Pathol 1996;49:839–43.

561. Delgado PI, Jorda M, Ganjei-Azar P. Small cell carcinoma versus other lung malignancies. Diagnosis by fine-needle aspiration cytology. Cancer (Cancer Cytopathol) 2000;90:279–85.

562. Weisbrod GL, Cunningham I, Tao LC, et al. Small cell anaplastic carcinoma: cytological histological correlations from percutaneous fine needle aspiration biopsy. J Can Assoc Radiol 1987;38:204–8.

563. Jacob-Ambuero MP, Haas AR, Ciocca V, et al. Cytologic accuracy of samples obtained by EBUS-TBNA at Thomas Jefferson University Hospital. Acta Cytol 2008;52:687–90.

564. Jagirdar J. Application of immunohistochemistry to the diagnosis of primary and metastatic carcinoma to the lung. Arch Pathol Lab Med 2008;132:384–96.

565. Harpole DH Jr., Herndon JE II., Young WG, et al. Stage I non-small cell lung cancer: a multivariate analysis of treatment methods and patterns. Cancer 1995;76:787–96.

566. Harpole DH Jr, Herndon JE II, Wolfe WG. et al. A prognostic model of recurrence and death in stage I non-small cell lung cancer utilizing presentation, histopathology, and oncoprotein expression. Cancer Res 1995;55:51–56.

567. Harpole DH Jr., Richards WG, Herndon JE II., et al. Angiogenesis and molecular biologic substaging in patients with stage I non-small cell lung cancer. Ann Thorac Surg 1996;61:1470–76.

568. Strauss GM, Kwiatkowski DJ, Harpole DH, et al. Molecular and pathologic markers in stage I non-small cell carcinoma of the lung. J Clin Oncol 1995;13:1265–79.

569. Kwiatkowski DJ, Harpole DH Jr., Godleski J, et al. Molecular pathologicsubstaging in 244 stage I non-small cell lung cancer patients: clinical implications. J Clin Oncol 1998;16:2468–77.

570. Pastorino U, Andreola S, Tagliabue E, et al. Immunocytochemical markers in stage I lung cancer: relevance to prognosis. J Clin Oncol 1997;15:2858–65.

571. Herbert A, Santis G. EBUS-TBNA: an opportunity for clinicians, cytopathologists and patients to gain from multidisciplinary collaboration. Cytopathology 2010;21:3–6.

572. Bishop JA, Sharma R, Illei PB. Napsin A and thyroid transcription factor-1 expression in carcinomas of the lung, breast, pancreas, colon, kidney, thyroid and malignant mesothelioma. Hum Pathol 2010;41(1):20–5.

# Section 3

## Serous Cavities

# Serous effusions

Vinod B. Shidham and Mary Falzon[1]

## Chapter contents

## Introduction

Serous cavity effusions are relatively simple to drain and collect for therapeutic and diagnostic purposes. For this reason, they comprise a significant proportion of general laboratory specimens. Paradoxically, the cytopathological evaluation of these specimens is relatively complex. Proper handling of specimens from the initial stage of collection to final interpretation is important. For optimal results with effusions, all the personnel involved, including clinicians, cytotechnologists and pathologists, should be familiar with the intricacies of specimen collecting, processing and interpreting.[1]

## Anatomy, histology and cytology

### Anatomy

The major serous cavities include the two pleural cavities, the peritoneal cavity and the pericardial sac (Fig. 3.1). These cavities are lined by parietal and visceral mesothelium. The visceral mesothelium is reflected over the organs therein. The serous cavity histology and serous fluid cytology of individual cavities are significantly identical without any site specific differences.

## Histology

The serous cavities are lined by a flat monolayer of mesothelial cells, which have a tendency to undergo reactive changes to various stimuli leading to a somewhat cuboidal appearance (Fig. 3.2). Serous cavity effusions contain these 'reactive' mesothelial cells as one of the major components. Although mesothelial cells are derived from mesoderm, they demonstrate many morphological and biological features of epithelial cells (Fig. 3.2).

A thin layer of fibrous connective tissue with a varying amount of adipose tissue, small blood vessels and lymphatics supports the mesothelial cells. The lymphatic vessels open through gaps (stoma) between the mesothelial cells on to the surface of the serous cavities[2,3] and are a significant component of the system for absorption of fluid in serous cavities.

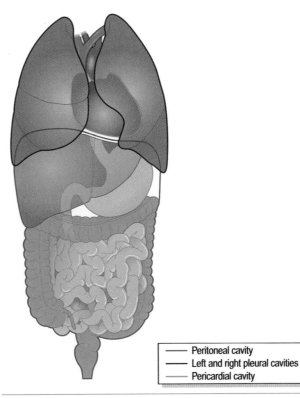

Peritoneal cavity
Left and right pleural cavities
Pericardial cavity

**Fig. 3.1** Four major serous cavities. (Reproduced from Shidham and Atkinson 2007.[1])

[1]We would like to acknowledge the many faculty members, staff members, residents and fellows at the Medical College of Wisconsin, Milwaukee, WI. We thank Bryan Hunt, Cytopathology Fellow at the Medical College of Wisconsin for scrutinising the proofs of this chapter. We also thank Anjani Shidham for proofreading the entire chapter. Our thanks to Horatiu Olteanu for providing images for lymphoproliferative conditions in effusion fluids.

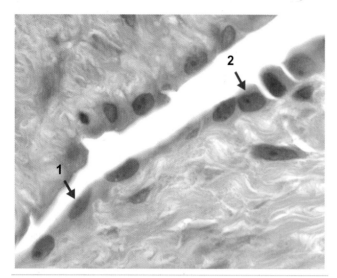

**Fig. 3.2** Histology of serous lining (inguinal hernia sac). The flat mesothelial cells (arrow 1) line the fibrous tissue. They assume a focal cuboidal contour (arrow 2) as they undergo reactive changes (H&E).

Imbalance of homeostatic forces in this system results in accumulation of fluid in serous cavities, leading to effusions.

## General cytology of serous fluids

In addition to mesothelial cells, effusion fluids contain a variety of non-neoplastic cells, including macrophages and other blood-derived cells. Other components may include psammoma bodies and various incidental cellular/non-cellular elements.

### Mesothelial cells

Mesothelial cells round-up and appear polyhedral after exfoliation due to the surface tension of the surrounding fluid. The morphology of mesothelial cells (Box 3.1) can be evaluated in Papanicolaou (PAP) and Diff-Quik (DQ)-stained smears. In general, the PAP stain allows better evaluation of nuclear details, while the DQ stain highlights cytoplasmic details.

### Cytological findings: mesothelial cells

In cytological preparations, mesothelial cells are usually about 15–30 µm in diameter (1.5 to 2 times the size of neutrophils), but they may vary significantly, ranging up to 50 m in diameter. They may be present as solitary cells (Fig. 3.3) or in small cohesive clusters (Figs 3.4, 3.5). They appear larger in Diff-Quik-stained air-dried smears than the wet-fixed shrunken cells in Papanicolaou-stained smears (Fig. 3.6).

The cytoplasm of mesothelial cells usually shows two zones. In PAP-stained smears, a narrow zone of pale ectoplasm associated with microvilli surrounds the endoplasm of the dense staining perinuclear zone, with its higher density of intermediate filaments. In DQ–stained smears, the endoplasm is lightly-stained with peripheral darker ectoplasm. The round cell borders with smooth contours show blebs along the ruffled surface. In general, DQ-staining highlights the two-zone staining pattern of mesothelial cells more distinctly than the PAP stain.

**Box 3.1  Cytomorphological spectrum of mesothelial cells**

- Uniform cell population
- Monotonous, oval to round nuclei
- Mononucleated cells with mostly centrally placed nuclei
- Evenly distributed fine powdery chromatin
- Inconspicuous to prominent nucleoli
- Multinucleation with anisonucleosis
- Moderate amount of translucent cytoplasm
- Two zone cytoplasm
- Peripheral vacuoles containing glycogen
- A faint staining thin halo along the edge (microvilli)
- Fuzzy cell border (due to microvilli)
- Peripheral blebs in DQ-stained smears (microvilli related)
- Monolayer cell aggregates
- Doublets or triplets with clasp-like articulation
- Mesothelial windows between the cells (microvilli related)
- Nuclear hyperchromasia
- Coarse chromatin clumping
- Prominent macronucleoli
- Nuclear pleomorphism
- Irregular nuclear membrane
- Numerous mitotic figures
- Mesothelial cells in large groups
- Cell groups with scalloped borders
- Cellular moulding
- Multi-nucleation
- Mitotic figures
- Cell-to-cell apposition
- Cell-in-cell configuration
- Proliferative cell balls
- True papillary aggregates
- Acini-like structures
- Degeneration of cytoplasm
- Signet-ring change
- Spheres with collagenous cores
- Psammoma bodies
- Occasional papillary groups
- Ballooning of cytoplasm with signet ring-like vacuolation
- Extensive morphologic variation
- High nucleocytoplasmic ratio

The nuclear details are better seen in PAP-stained smears. The nuclei are usually central or slightly off centre, but may be distinctly eccentric (Figs 3.7, 3.8). When eccentric, the nuclear membrane does not touch the cell border. Careful examination shows this narrow rim is due to microvilli on the surface adjacent to the eccentric nucleus (Fig. 3.8). This feature may be applied to distinguish mesothelial cells from histiocytic macrophages and adenocarcinoma cells, which characteristically show peripherally located nuclei touching the cell membrane (Fig. 3.9). They are best appreciated in DQ-stained preparations (Fig. 3.10). The nuclei are typically round to oval with smooth contours. Even malignant mesothelial cells may have a perfectly round nucleus with smooth contours.

Mesothelial cell cytoplasm does not always show two zones in DQ-stained preparations (Fig 3.11). In some cells it may be finely granular with a variable degree of basophilia, without

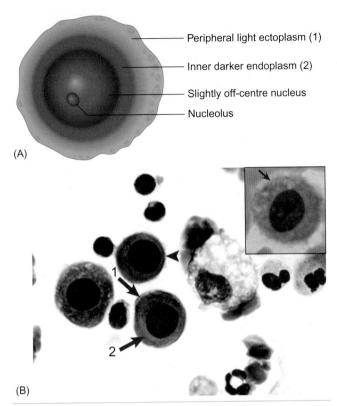

Peripheral light ectoplasm (1)

Inner darker endoplasm (2)

Slightly off-centre nucleus

Nucleolus

(A)

(B)

**Fig. 3.3** Mesothelial cell (pleural fluid). Two zone cytoplasmic staining with outer paler ectoplasm (1) with the inner denser endoplasm (2). The nucleus is central to slightly eccentric and does not touch the cell periphery (arrowhead). The peripheral cell border ruffled with blebs (arrow in insert) (DQ cytospin).

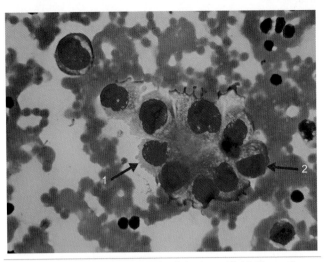

**Fig. 3.4** Group of reactive mesothelial cells (peritoneal fluid). The swollen microvilli impart ruffled borders with peripheral blebs (arrow 1) and a rim (arrow 2) separating the nuclei from cell borders. The margins formed predominantly by cytoplasm are knobbly as compared to the smooth borders of adenocarcinoma cell groups which are mainly comprised of nucleus (DQ Cytospin).

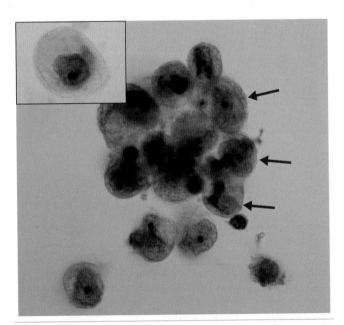

**Fig. 3.5** Mesothelial cell group (peritoneal fluid). A rim (arrows) separates the nuclei from the cell borders. Unlike adenocarcinoma cell groups, the outline is knobbly and is formed predominantly by the cytoplasm (PAP Cytospin). Inset: Mesothelial cell (peritoneal fluid). Outer faintly stained ectoplasm with inner denser (rich in intermediate filaments) endoplasm. The nucleus is near centre. Nucleoli are readily observed. The vacuolation begins at the periphery in the ectoplasm (PAP SurePath).

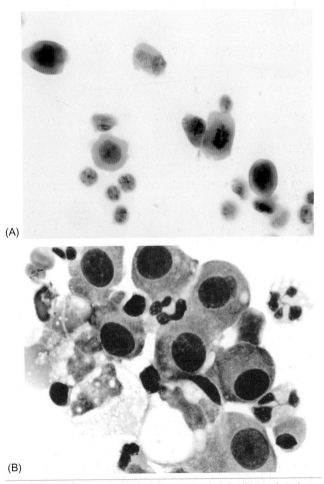

(A)

(B)

**Fig. 3.6** Mesothelial cells (peritoneal fluid). Mesothelial cells are relatively smaller in PAP-stained liquid-based cytology preparations (A); compare with the Diff-Quik-stained air-dried Cytospin preparations (B) of the same specimen at the same magnification (A: PAP SurePath) (B: DQ Cytospin).

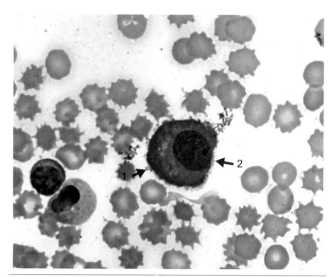

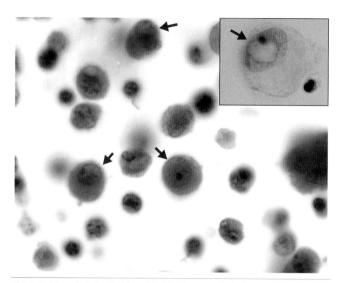

**Fig. 3.7** Mesothelial cell (pleural fluid). This mesothelial cell shows a relatively eccentric nucleus. The swollen microvilli are obvious as ruffled borders with peripheral blebs (arrow 1). Although subtle and difficult to perceive, there is a rim (arrow 2) separating the nuclei from the cell border. This feature helps to distinguish eccentric cells in adenocarcinoma, which may lack this rim (compare with Figure 3.9A) (DQ Cytospin).

**Fig. 3.8** Mesothelial cells (pleural fluid). The mesothelial cells show relatively eccentric nuclei (arrows). The microvilli and a rim may be difficult to perceive when PAP-stained due to its tendency to make the cytoplasm more transparent (arrow in inset). This may compromise evaluation of adenocarcinoma cells with a tendency to show eccentric nuclei without a cytoplasmic rim adjacent to the nuclei (PAP SurePath).

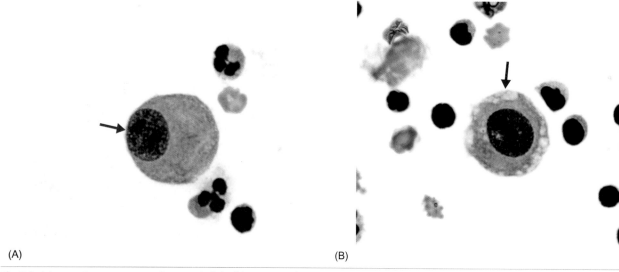

(A)                                                                                            (B)

**Fig. 3.9** Adenocarcinoma versus reactive mesothelial cell (metastatic adenocarcinoma in pleural fluid). (A) The adenocarcinoma cell has no distinct two zone cytoplasmic staining and has an eccentric nucleus which touches the cell border without a cytoplasmic rim (arrow). (B) Note the tendency for peripheral vacuolation in the reactive mesothelial cell (arrow) (DQ Cytospin).

the two-zone pattern. As the mesothelial cells imbibe water from the surrounding fluid, their cytoplasm may acquire a foamy macrophage phenotype with pale vacuolated cytoplasm. The degree of vacuolation is directly proportional to the duration for which the cells were in the fluid. When the effusion becomes chronic, the cytoplasmic vacuoles become larger but the vacuoles of mesothelial cells are usually small. They occur at the periphery of the cells (Fig. 3.11), but may be randomly distributed (Fig. 3.13) or even central with nuclear overlap. The nuclei in some mesothelial cells may be displaced to the periphery by the vacuolated cytoplasm secondary to phagocytic activity or degenerative changes. A single, large cytoplasmic vacuole displacing the nucleus may resemble that in signet ring cells of adenocarcinoma.

Differences between macrophage-like mesothelial cells and histiocytic macrophages, although difficult to identify by morphology alone, are not of diagnostic significance. Mesothelial cells have round to oval nuclei with smooth contours, whereas histiocytic macrophages typically show kidney-shaped nuclei with slightly irregular contours.

The microvilli of mesothelial cells may prevent adjacent cells from completely opposing each other, thereby creating a gap between two cells. This space between two adjacent mesothelial cells is referred to as a mesothelial window (Fig. 3.14), which may be subtle or very wide in cytology smears. Such spaces between adjacent cells in effusions are not specific for mesothelial cells and may be seen in other types of cell groups including those of metastatic cancers.[4]

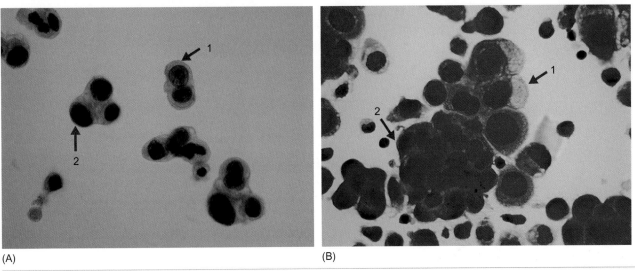

**Fig. 3.10** Metastatic adenocarcinoma with a two-cell population (ascitic fluid). (A) Reactive mesothelial cells (arrow 1) with central nuclei, peripheral vacuolation, and knobby borders formed by the cell membrane, contrast better in Diff-Quik-stained preparation (B) from adenocarcinoma cells (arrow 2) with eccentric nuclei touching the cell membranes without any rim of cytoplasm between the nucleus and cell membrane. Compare the community border of adenocarcinoma cell groups formed mostly by nuclear contours. (A, PAP ThinPrep; B, DQ Cytospin). (A, from Shidham and Atkinson 2007.[1])

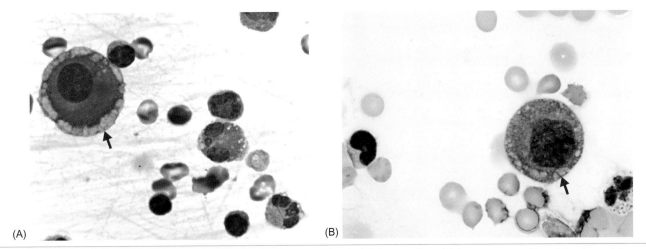

**Fig. 3.11** Mesothelial cells (ascitic fluid). Reactive mesothelial cells (arrows in A,B) with slightly eccentric nuclei show two zones with peripheral vacuolation (DQ Cytospin).

In PAP-stained preparations, the cytoplasm stains light green with a variable degree of intensity and vacuolation. The cytoplasmic details are less distinct and more transparent. They are relatively lost due to cellular shrinkage by wet fixation. Mesothelial windows and cytoplasmic vacuoles, although less distinct, may still be evident in PAP-stained smears.

The surface of mesothelial cells has numerous long slender microvilli, which impart a peripheral rim of pallor in PAP-stained preparations. This characteristic feature of mesothelial cells has been applied to distinguish them from other cells such as carcinoma cells.[5–7] Although the microvilli cannot be seen directly under the light microscope, their presence may be inferred by a thin rim of cytoplasm along the side of the eccentric nucleus in some mesothelial cells (Figs 3.7, 3.8). This feature, although observed in both types of staining, is more easily recognised with DQ stain (Fig. 3.7). The swollen microvilli

impart ruffled borders and peripheral blebs in DQ smears (Fig. 3.7). Microvilli are best seen by electron microscopy (EM).

Although mesothelial cells do not proliferate in effusions after exfoliation, they may complete an already started mitotic division. The presence of mitotic figures (Fig. 3.15) in effusion cytology suggests a process that is capable of causing significant proliferative activity in response to whatever is causing the effusion. As with cytopathological evaluations in general, the presence of nucleoli and mitotic figures should not lead to a false interpretation of malignancy.[1] Other general morphological features of malignancy should be applied to arrive at such conclusion. Once a specimen is correctly interpreted as malignant, nucleoli and mitotic figures may then be considered for further categorisation and grading of a neoplasm.

Mesothelial cells produce hyaluronic acid, which, if present, may be seen as magenta coloured intracytoplasmic or extracellular

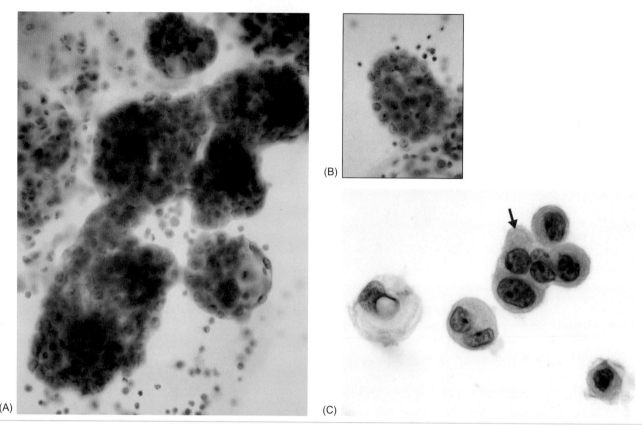

(A)

(B)

(C)

**Fig. 3.12** Malignant epithelioid mesothelioma (pleural fluid). The mesothelioma cells are numerous with more mesothelial cells in individual groups than in reactive conditions and with three-dimensional, papillary-like groups (B), showing knobbly borders formed predominantly by cytoplasm. Individual mesothelioma cells do not show significant variation from reactive mesothelial cells and lack overt features of malignancy. As with reactive mesothelial cells, the mesothelioma cells show two-zone staining with peripheral vacuolation (arrow in C) (PAP ThinPrep). (Shidham and Atkinson 2007.[1])

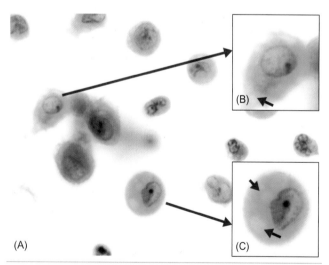

(A)

(B)

(C)

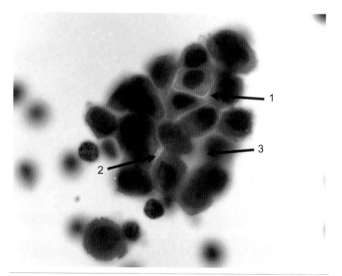

**Fig. 3.13** (A) Mesothelial cells (ascitic fluid). Reactive mesothelial cells (B,C insets) show peripherally (arrow in B) or randomly (arrows in C) placed cytoplasmic vacuoles. Compared with Diff-Quik-stained preparations, the cytoplasmic vacuoles are less distinct in this PAP-stained preparation (PAP SurePath).

**Fig. 3.14** Mesothelial cell group (ascitic fluid). Monolayered flat sheet of mesothelial cells. Microvilli prevent the adjacent mesothelial cells from apposing their cell borders, creating mesothelial windows which may be subtle (arrow 1), wide (arrow 2), or so wide that they may resemble acini (arrow 3). (PAP SurePath).

material in DQ-stained smears. Although less distinct, this may be seen as light grey streaks in the background in PAP-stained smears. Hyaluronic acid in the centre of small groups of mesothelial cells may be misleading as it superficially resembles mucin in adenocarcinoma acini. Hyaluronic acid is positive with

periodic acid-Schiff (PAS) and Alcian blue stains. This is lost if the sections are treated with hyaluronidase prior to staining. Hyaluronic acid is not a substrate for diastase, and is not digested by it.

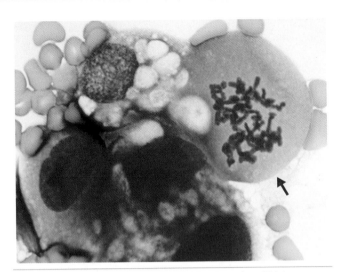

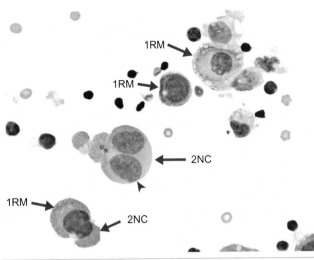

**Fig. 3.15** Mitotic figures. Ovarian carcinoma (peritoneal wash). It is not uncommon to find mitotic figures (arrow) in serous cavity specimens in association with malignancy and reactive processes. Its role in interpreting malignancy is limited. Although an impressive finding, it may be distracting and lead to false positive reporting (DQ Cytospin).

**Fig. 3.16** Metastatic mammary carcinoma (pleural fluid). A second population of neoplastic cells (arrows 2NC) superficially resemble reactive mesothelial cells (arrows 1RM). Careful scrutiny shows peripheral vacuoles (arrows 1RM) and a thin rim of cytoplasm separating the nucleus from periphery (arrow 1RM). Compare this with the nucleus of the neoplastic cells touching the cell periphery (arrowhead) (DQ Cytospin).

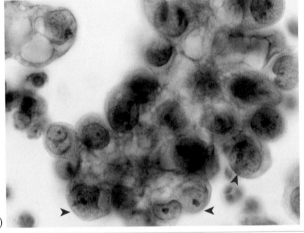

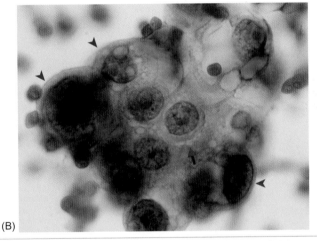

(A)

(B)

**Fig. 3.17** Metastatic ovarian carcinoma (peritoneal wash). Second population of neoplastic cells (A) superficially resembles reactive mesothelial cells (B). Careful examination reveals peripheral cytoplasmic vacuolation (arrow in B) in mesothelial cells. Most of the mesothelial cells show a cytoplasmic rim of variable thickness separating the nucleus from the cell border (arrowheads in (B)). As compared to this the nuclei in some of the adenocarcinoma cells touch the cell periphery (arrowheads in A) (PAP Cytospin).

Although these typical features are not specific for mesothelial cells, they help to distinguish them from other cells in effusions including metastatic malignant cells. Some mesothelial cells may show a morphological spectrum overlapping with that of certain neoplasms, including malignant melanoma and adenocarcinoma, especially of the breast and ovary (Figs 3.16, 3.17).

## Reactive mesothelial cells

Various pathological processes such as inflammation, neoplasia, and trauma lead to reactive changes in the extremely sensitive mesothelial cells lining the serosal cavities. Mesothelial cell hypertrophy and proliferation in response to an altered environment may lead to a remarkably wide morphological spectrum, which may even overlap with malignant cells (Figs 3.18, 3.19).[2,8,9] Such exfoliated mesothelial cells with a wide range

of appearances are usually referred to as 'reactive mesothelial cells'. The resolution of the underlying pathological process may reverse these changes.

### Cytological findings: reactive mesothelial cells

*Reactive mesothelial cells* range in size from 15 to 30 μm but may be larger than 50 μm in diameter with variable amounts of cytoplasm (Figs 3.3, 3.18, 3.19). The enlarged nuclei show some variation in their size and shape, usually with conspicuous nucleoli. Binucleation and multinucleation are frequent (Fig. 3.20). They may be present as cohesive clusters including papillary configurations. Some cells may show high nuclear/cytoplasmic ratios with scant cytoplasm and slightly hyperchromatic nuclei with prominent nucleoli (Fig. 3.19). This astonishingly wide morphological spectrum may overlap

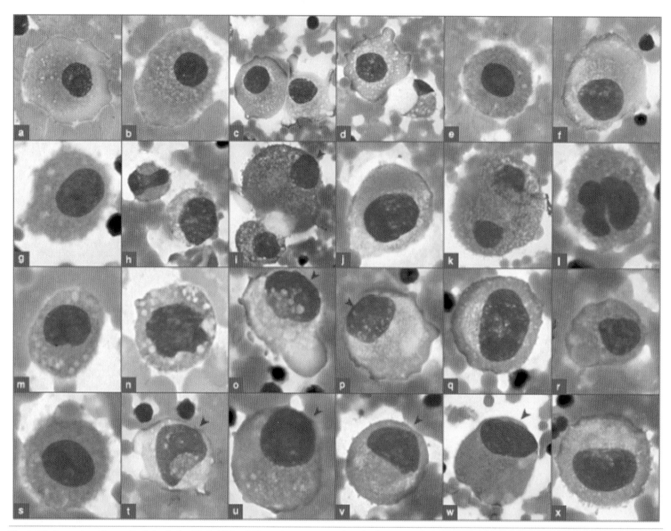

**Fig. 3.18** Panorama of mesothelial cells (ascitic fluid) (a–x). Central to near central nuclei. Rare mesothelial cells may show eccentric nuclei touching the cell membrane, but usually there is a narrow rim of cytoplasm separating the nucleus from the cell border (arrowheads). (DQ Cytospin). (Reproduced from Shidham and Atkinson 2007.[1])

remarkably with that of some malignant cells in effusions (Figs 3.18, 3.19) and may lead to diagnostic pitfalls.

*Binucleation and multinucleation*: Two or more nuclei may be present in reactive mesothelial cells as *in vivo* change within the serous cavity (Fig. 3.20) and are frequent in peritoneal dialysis fluids.[10] However, this may also be due to *in vitro* changes. Formation of small aggregates secondary to processing such as filtration, Cytospin® preparation, centrifugation, or liquid-based cytology preparations may lead to fusion of the cytoplasmic borders of the 'sticky' reactive mesothelial cells with degenerative change and may appear multinucleated. This is not uncommon in specimens left at room temperature for several hours.

*Gigantic nuclei*: Nuclear membranes may also fuse in degenerate cells, with formation of mesothelial cells having one or more gigantic nuclei. These nuclei have fine, powdery, smudged chromatin with evenly distributed, small nucleoli. They are not observed in biopsy specimens. Cells with such degenerate gigantic nuclei may be misinterpreted as 'atypical' cells.

*Phagocytic activity*: Phagocytic activity of reactive mesothelial cells transforms them into foamy macrophages (Figs 3.11, 3.13)

with pale vacuolated cytoplasm as they imbibe water from the effusion fluid. Distinguishing foamy reactive mesothelial cells from foamy histiocytic macrophages is usually of little clinical significance. But morphological features of some mesothelial cells with vacuoles may overlap with malignant cells and mislead one to interpret these cells as adenocarcinoma.

The extent of vacuolation depends on the duration the cells are in the effusion fluid after exfoliation. The cytoplasmic vacuoles increase in number and size as the effusion becomes chronic. They are usually small and peripheral, but may be randomly distributed and even central with nuclear overlap. A large cytoplasmic vacuole pushing the nucleus to the cell margin in a mesothelial cell may resemble the signet ring observed in some adenocarcinoma cells. If indicated this may be differentiated objectively by immunocytochemistry and in some cases by mucicarmine staining.

Although of little clinical significance, morphological differentiation between macrophage-like mesothelial cells and histiocytic macrophages is difficult. Some nuclear features may assist. A round to oval nucleus with smooth contours favours

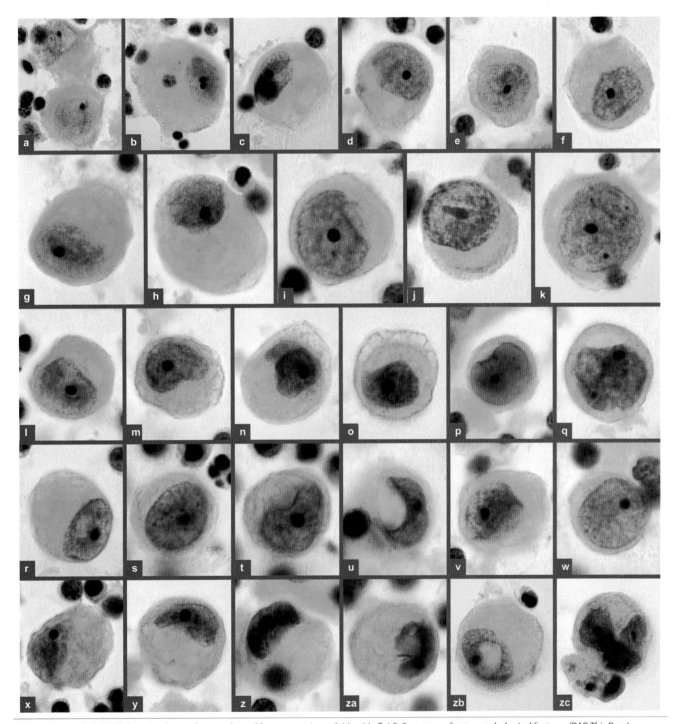

**Fig. 3.19** Mesothelial cells (a–zc) with mostly central to seldom eccentric nuclei (ascitic fluid). Spectrum of cytomorphological features (PAP ThinPrep). (Reproduced from Shidham and Atkinson 2007.[1])

a mesothelial cell origin and a bean-shaped (kidney-shaped, reniform) nucleus with slightly irregular contours favours a histiocytic macrophage.

*Cell-in-cell configuration*: One cell may wrap around an adjacent cell, leading to the appearance of a cell-in-cell arrangement. Although this is commonly associated with reactive mesothelial cells, it is highly non-specific and may also be seen in malignant cells in serous fluids.[9]

*Cohesive clusters and/or papillary structures*: Reactive changes in the mesothelial lining of serous cavities may exfoliate some cohesive cell groups. Some of these may demonstrate papillary configurations (Fig. 3.21). As a quantitative feature, there are fewer cohesive clusters but more solitary mesothelial cells in reactive effusions (Fig. 3.22) than those associated with mesothelioma, which show a cellular specimen with relatively more and larger cohesive groups and/or papillary clusters (Fig. 3.12).

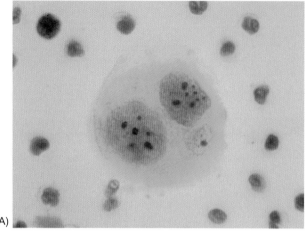

(A)

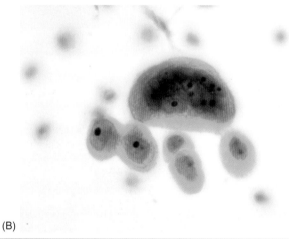

(B)

**Fig. 3.20** Mesothelial cells (A,B) with multinucleation (dialysis fluid) (PAP SurePath).

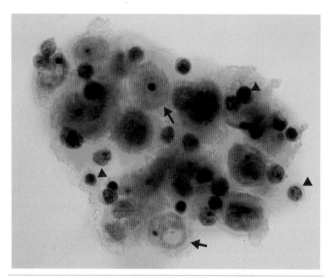

**Fig. 3.21** Reactive mesothelial cells (ascitic fluid). A small group in an ill-defined papillary configuration with reactive mesothelial cells (arrows) and some chronic inflammatory cells (arrowheads) (PAP Cytospin).

*Mesothelial cell clusters with scalloped (knobbly) contours* generally have fewer cells than those found in mesotheliomas. Scalloped contours may also resemble clusters of cells from other neoplasms (Fig. 3.23). However, the individual mesothelial cells at the periphery show the recognisable

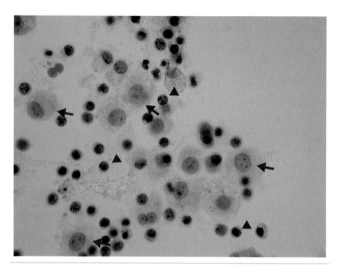

**Fig. 3.22** Reactive mesothelial cells (ascitic fluid). Less cohesive reactive mesothelial cells (arrows) admixed with some chronic inflammatory cells (arrowheads) (PAP Cytospin).

two-zone cytoplasmic features of mesothelial cells, and the nuclei do not touch the cell borders of the cells along the periphery of the reactive mesothelial cell groups. The cytoplasmic rim of individual cells in the group forms the outline of such clusters (Fig. 3.12). In contrast, usually the nuclear border forms a significant proportion of this peripheral outline of the groups in adenocarcinoma cell clusters (Fig. 3.24).

## Diagnostic pitfalls: reactive mesothelial cells

Reactive mesothelial cells (Fig. 3.25) in effusions, especially those associated with some of the conditions mentioned below, may lead to potential pitfalls.

*Hepatomegaly associated with congestive heart failure:* Peritoneal effusions associated with congestive heart failure and hepatomegaly show exfoliated sheets of mesothelial cells with marked reactive changes.

*Hepatocellular carcinoma:* Cases of hepatocellular carcinoma associated with effusion are usually negative for malignant cells, but frequently show atypia within the reactive mesothelial cells.[11]

*Ischaemic processes* associated with occlusion of pulmonary or mesenteric blood vessels frequently induce florid reactive changes in the serosal covering overlying the ischaemic organs. Exfoliation of th``e reactive mesothelial cells into the effusions from these areas may be in sheets. They may show intracytoplasmic haemosiderin granules, red blood cells or both.

*Trauma* to organs covered with mesothelium such as spleen, liver and lung.

*Large retroperitoneal masses:* Slowly growing retroperitoneal masses, such as benign retroperitoneal neoplasms close to the serosal surface, may generate reactive changes in the overlying mesothelium. Peritoneal effusions in such cases may exfoliate mesothelium in sheets.

*Pelvic inflammatory diseases:* Mesothelial cell clusters (Fig. 3.26) frequently observed in benign reactive conditions such as pelvic inflammatory diseases may lead to a diagnostic pitfall, with erroneous interpretation as ovarian adenocarcinoma. This

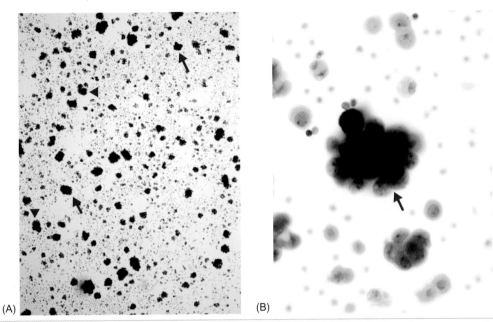

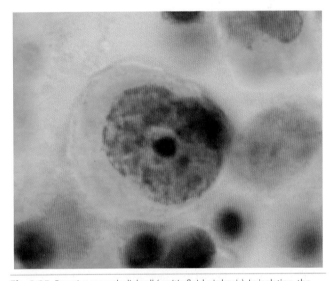

**Fig. 3.23** Metastatic mammary carcinoma (pleural fluid). Cohesive cell pattern in longstanding/recurrent malignant effusions. Many proliferation spheres (arrows) are present due to continued division of carcinoma cells in nutrient rich effusions. Conglomerations of several proliferation spheres may generate papillary configurations (arrowheads) with superficial resemblance to papillary carcinoma (PAP SurePath).

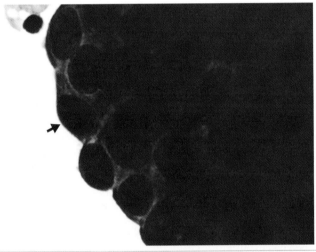

**Fig. 3.24** Metastatic mammary carcinoma (pleural fluid). The periphery of the group is formed predominantly by the areas where the nucleus touches the cell borders (arrow) without any rim of cytoplasm. Compare this with groups of mesothelial cells- both reactive (Fig. 3.5) and neoplastic (Fig. 3.17). (DQ Cytospin smears).

**Fig. 3.25** Reactive mesothelial cell (ascitic fluid, cirrhosis). In isolation, the cell changes could be misinterpreted as malignant but, because of the cirrhosis, the findings fall within the spectrum of reactive mesothelial cells without cytomorphological or immunocytochemical evidence of a second foreign population (PAP; SurePath (Autocyte) preparation).

is significant especially in aspirates of the cul-de-sac, which often contain some clusters in a papillary-like configuration.[12]

*Postoperative, following laparotomy and thoracotomy.* Surgical trauma may desquamate sheets of mesothelial cells mechanically.

*Pelvic or peritoneal washings:* Sheets of mesothelial cells are rare in effusions, but they are usual features in pelvic or peritoneal washings. They are the result of forcible mechanical detachment from the serosal membrane during operative incision or intra-operative lavages, or both. Although superficially they may resemble the clusters of squamous cells, they usually are not a diagnostic challenge.[13]

*'Atypical' mesothelial cells:* Reactive effusions, especially those associated with some clinical conditions may elicit marked changes in mesothelial cells. Some of these reactive mesothelial cells may resemble malignant cells. However, the morphological features and other criteria discussed in this chapter are not sufficient to be interpreted definitively as malignant. Such cells may be categorised as 'atypical'.[14] Such reactive mesothelial cells with atypia may demonstrate: high nuclear/cytoplasmic ratios, nuclear enlargement, nuclear hyperchromasia, coarse clumped chromatin, and prominent macronucleoli. They may be seen as large cohesive groups with scalloped edges and moulding of cells, with extensive morphological variation. The

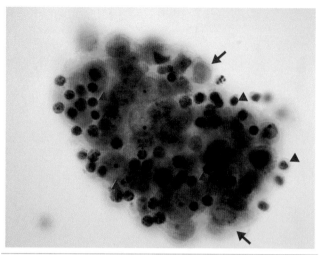

**Fig. 3.26** Reactive mesothelial cell group (ascitic fluid). This consultation case was initially interpreted as malignant. However, search for a primary did not show any neoplasm. The constituent cells have features of reactive mesothelial cells (arrows) and are admixed with chronic inflammatory cells (arrowheads) (PAP Cytospin).

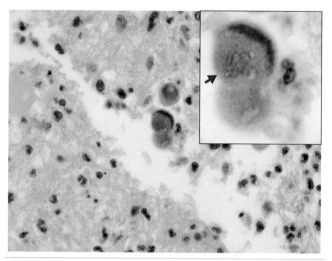

**Fig. 3.27** Mucin stain in mucinous type cholangiocarcinoma (ascitic fluid). The neoplastic cell with a cytoplasmic vacuole shows mucicarmine positivity, consistent with mucin in adenocarcinoma cell. (Cell block section, mucicarmine stain).

terminology of 'atypical mesothelial cells' (Fig. 3.25) should be discouraged strongly and should not be used without an explanatory note/comment in the report.[8]

Such cells are not uncommon in effusions associated with cirrhosis of the liver, pulmonary infarction, congestive heart failure, collagen vascular diseases, renal failure with uraemia, pancreatitis,[15] bile peritonitis, therapeutic radiation, chemotherapy, and large benign intra-abdominal masses with florid reactive mesothelial hyperplasia of the overlying serosa.[14]

## Macrophages

Cells with macrophage activity in effusions may be of either mesothelial or histiocytic cell origin. Some effusions may show such cells as the predominant cell population.

### Cytological findings: macrophages

*Histiocytic macrophages* are generally non-cohesive and singly scattered, with well to ill-defined cell borders. They may, however, be seen in small, ill-defined, loose groups with irregular peripheral contours. The kidney shaped (reniform) nuclei are usually eccentric and the nuclear margin may be closely approximated to the cell membrane. This feature overlaps with that of adenocarcinoma cells. The nucleoli are indistinct.

*Mesothelial cell macrophages* have overlapping morphological features but show some subtle differences such as round to oval nuclei in contrast to reniform nuclei in histiocytic macrophages, and centrally placed nuclei rather than peripheral or eccentric nuclei in histiocytic macrophages (Figs 3.11, 3.13). Some cells may show eccentric nuclei, but the nuclear margin is usually not in close approximation to the cell border. Usually there is a narrow rim of cytoplasm due to numerous long slender microvilli in mesothelial macrophages (Figs 3.7, 3.8, 3.9). In contrast to the ill-defined cell borders in histiocytic macrophages, those in mesothelial cell

macrophages are well defined with blebs. They may exfoliate as cohesive groups with distinct knobbly contours, in contrast to the ill-defined loosely cohesive groups with irregular outlines of histiocytic macrophages.

*Extensive vacuolation* with peripheral displacement of nuclei in some macrophages resembles the secretory vacuoles of adenocarcinoma cells. The mucicarmine stain for mucin performed on cell block sections or direct cytology smears may help. Positive mucin staining favours adenocarcinoma (Fig. 3.27); however, negative staining does not confirm a reactive macrophage nature. Using a histochemical stain such as mucicarmine to confirm adenocarcinoma is a relatively simple approach. It is economical, but variation in inter-laboratory reproducibility and improper quality control may compromise the sensitivity and specificity of this test.

## Blood-derived cells

Other cells present in effusions include red blood cells, lymphocytes, neutrophils, eosinophils, basophils and megakaryocytes.[16] Their proportion depends on the extent of peripheral blood contamination and the cause of the effusion.

### Cytological findings and diagnostic pitfalls: blood-derived cells

Red blood cells, lymphocytes, neutrophils, eosinophils, and basophils are morphologically similar to those in DQ-stained peripheral blood and bone marrow smears. Their morphology is interpreted more easily in DQ rather than PAP-stained preparations.

Megakaryocytes (Fig. 3.28) in effusions are rare. They may be associated with a myeloproliferative disorder or with extramedullary haemopoiesis, secondary to conditions such as extensive bone marrow replacement by metastatic carcinoma. Their interpretation is relatively easy in DQ-stained preparations. They are seen as large cells with a variable amount of cytoplasm and multilobed nuclei. Multilobation

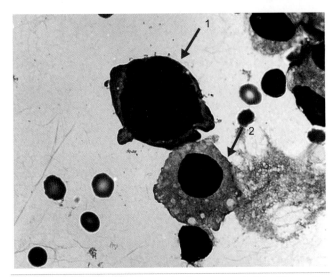

**Fig. 3.28** Megakaryocyte (arrow 1) with adjacent mesothelial cell (arrow 2) in haemorrhagic pleural fluid (DQ Cytospin). (Reproduced from Shidham and Atkinson 2007.[1])

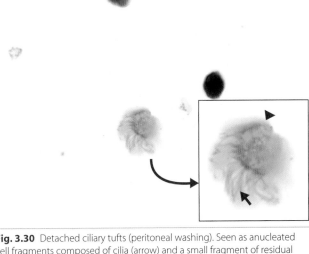

**Fig. 3.30** Detached ciliary tufts (peritoneal washing). Seen as anucleated cell fragments composed of cilia (arrow) and a small fragment of residual cytoplasm (arrowhead) (PAP SurePath).

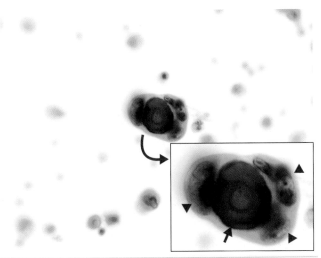

**Fig. 3.29** Metastatic ovarian carcinoma (peritoneal fluid). Psammoma body (arrow): round, acellular, calcific structures with concentric lamellation in association with abnormal tumour cells (arrowheads) (PAP SurePath).

may not be distinctly visible in all cells. Their presence in a pleural effusion may be secondary to haemorrhaging pulmonary microvasculature.[17] They may be misinterpreted as neoplastic or as a viral cytopathic effect especially in PAP-stained preparations.

## Other intrinsic entities[16]

In addition to mesothelial and peripheral blood-derived cells, other cells and some non-neoplastic entities including psammoma bodies, collagen balls, and detached ciliary tufts may be present in effusions, washings and cul-de-sac fluids .

### Cytological findings and diagnostic pitfalls: other intrinsic entities

#### Psammoma bodies

These concentrically lamellated calcific spherules (Fig. 3.29) are encountered in up to 3.7% of effusions.[18] The acellular

structures have a tendency to crack in smears. They may be surrounded by benign or malignant cells. In PAP-stained preparations, they appear cyanophilic (blue-green) to acidophilic (pink).

In pleural and pericardial effusions, psammoma bodies are usually associated with malignancies including papillary thyroid carcinoma, ovarian papillary serous carcinoma and others (Fig. 3.29). However, in peritoneal effusions and washings, they may also be associated with benign conditions. One-third of cases with psammoma bodies in peritoneal specimens may be associated with benign processes such as ovarian cystadenoma/cystadenofibroma, endometriosis, endosalpingiosis and papillary mesothelial hyperplasia.[18]

#### Collagen balls

These mesothelial cell covered fragments of collagen have been reported in 4–29% of peritoneal washings.[13] Their prevalence is relatively higher in specimens submitted as pelvic washings (5.8%) than those submitted as peritoneal washings (1.6%).[19,20] They should not to be misinterpreted as a component of a papillary or mucinous gynaecological neoplasm.[21] They probably originate from the surface of the ovaries, and are usually restricted to specimens from females,[16] but collagen balls have been reported in ascitic fluid from a male with encapsulating peritonitis.[22]

#### Detached ciliary tufts

Fluid from the pouch of Douglas and peritoneal washings[1] may show detached ciliary tufts from the ciliated epithelium lining the fallopian tubes. They are seen as non-nucleated fragments of cells with cilia (Fig. 3.30). They may demonstrate linear, rotating, jerky motility in wet preparations of fresh specimens, and may be misinterpreted as parasites.[23] In PAP-stained smears they are relatively difficult to find. They do not have any pathological significance and probably represent cyclical physiological shedding from the tips of ciliated cells in the fallopian tubes during the luteal phase of the menstrual cycle.[24]

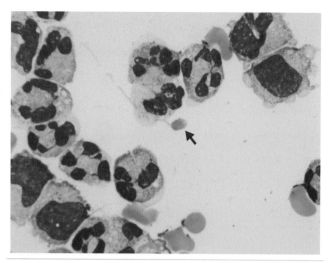

**Fig. 3.31** Sperm with inflammatory reaction (ascitic fluid). Mixed inflammatory cells with predominance of neutrophils. A few sperm (arrow) are present (along with some degenerate forms, mostly sperm heads not seen in this field) (DQ Cytospin).

### Curschmann's spirals

Curschmann's spirals are similar to those seen in sputum and bronchial washings, although generally smaller in effusions. They have been reported in spontaneous pleural and peritoneal effusions. They are hypothesised to be formed from mucus secreted by mucus-producing adenocarcinoma cells in neoplastic conditions. In non-neoplastic conditions, they are formed from submesothelial connective tissue mucosubstance released into the effusion fluid through the inflamed serosal lining, which has increased permeability.[25]

### Sperm

Rarely sperm may be observed unexpectedly. The possibility of contamination during collection, transportation, and processing should be ruled out. However, the authors recently observed spermatozoa in an effusion with mixed inflammation, mostly acute inflammatory cells and histiocytes. The number of sperm was low, with degenerative changes in many. Some neutrophils showed phagocytosed heads of sperms (personal experience) (Fig. 3.31).

## Extraneous entities and non-cellular material

A variety of extraneous structures may be present in effusion specimens.[16] Physiological mechanisms may result in spontaneous exfoliation of cells from such structures in some effusions. Depending on the path of the needle through neighbouring structures while aspirating the specimen, these can be a challenge, especially for the inexperienced interpreter and in cases with inadequate clinical details.

### Cytological findings and diagnostic pitfalls: extraneous entities

Fragments of fibro-adipose tissue may be present as contaminants either during the washings procedure or as fragments of tissue dislodged by the needle aspirating the effusion.

Normal hepatocytes can be present in peritoneal and pleural effusions. They may resemble mesothelial cells or well-differentiated cells of hepatocellular carcinoma. Some of these hepatocytes so-called dysplastic hepatocytes (hepatocytes with atypia) may be misinterpreted as neoplastic cells. Isolated hepatocytes with lipofuscin resemble haemosiderin laden macrophages and steatohepatocytes with lipid vacuoles may resemble vacuolated macrophages or adenocarcinoma cells with secretory vacuoles.

Cells from the female genital tract with degenerative changes may accumulate in the cul-de-sac in longstanding effusions as a result of reflux via the fallopian tubes secondary to menstruation. This phenomenon occurs particularly in the presence of an intrauterine contraceptive device. Peritoneal effusions may show implants of endometriosis and endosalpingiosis. Some may demonstrate degenerative nuclear atypia with hyperchromasia and may lead to the pitfall of malignant misinterpretation. The latter pitfall is also applicable to müllerian inclusions encountered in peritoneal washings.[26,27]

Ectopic pancreas has been misinterpreted as malignant in a patient with a history of ovarian adenocarcinoma, the cells having been aspirated from the small bowel wall.[28]

Ascitic fluid or cul-de-sac aspirates may contain vegetable matter secondary to bowel perforation or penetration of the gastrointestinal tract by the aspirating needle.

Longstanding effusions may show cholesterol crystals, especially in rheumatoid pleuritis.

Serosanguinous effusions may show haematoidin crystals with haemosiderin-laden macrophages.

## Specimen types, collection and processing

## Effusions

The narrow gap of 5–10 μm that separates the parietal and visceral layers of the serosa under physiological conditions is widened in the presence of an effusion of fluid into the serous cavity. Irrespective of their cellular composition, all effusions are pathological. The causative factors include increased vascular permeability, vasodilatation, blockage of lymphatics, breakdown of small blood vessels and haemodynamic imbalance of the microcirculation. An association between vascular endothelial growth factor (VEGF) and malignant effusions due to increased vascular permeability has been reported.[29]

The peritoneal cavity can accumulate up to 15–20 L and the pleural cavities can hold up to 3 L of fluid in each cavity. In comparison, the pericardial cavity cannot hold more than 0.6 L without leading to cardiac tamponade and adversely affecting heart function.

Even in tertiary care institutions reactive effusions are more common than malignant effusions. Malignant effusions usually show diagnostic malignant cells on cytological evaluation. Some benign effusions, however, may also show diagnostic cytomorphological features.[30]

## Types of effusions

With reference to diagnostic cytopathology, effusions may be reactive (secondary to conditions such as collagen diseases,

**Table 3.1** Types of effusions

| | Transudate | Exudate | Chylous |
|---|---|---|---|
| Biochemical features | Accumulation of fluid as an ultra-filtrate of plasma<br>a. Total protein <3.0 g/dL (30 g/L)<br>b. Specific gravity <1.015<br>c. Ratio of fluid lactic dehydrogenase to serum lactic dehydrogenase <0.6<br>d. Does not coagulate | Associated with increased permeability of the capillaries leading to exudation of protein rich fluid<br>a. Total protein >3.0 g/dL (30 g/L)<br>b. Specific gravity >1.015<br>c. Ratio of fluid lactic dehydrogenase to serum lactic dehydrogenase >0.6<br>d. May coagulate on standing | Leakage of lymphatic fluid secondary to trauma or the obstructed thoracic duct or cisterna chyli, caused by malignant neoplasms including lymphomas and carcinomas<br>a. Milky white fluid<br>b. Wet preparations usually show small free fat droplets |
| Cytological features | Hypocellular smears<br>Mostly mesothelial cells | Hypercellular smears<br>Predominantly inflammatory cells with reactive mesothelial cells with or without malignant cells | The smears are rich in lymphocytes and some lipid-laden macrophages |
| Causes | 1. Congestive heart failure<br>2. Pulmonary atelectasis<br>3. Nephrotic syndrome<br>4. Postpartum effusion<br>5. Peritoneal dialysis<br>6. Superior vena cava obstruction<br>7. Portal hypertension secondary to cirrhosis, schistosomiasis and diffuse metastatic neoplasm in liver<br>8. Postoperative abdominal surgery<br>9. Meig's syndrome<br>10. Chronic renal diseases with impaired renal function<br>11. Inferior vena cava hypertension<br>12. Coagulation disorder and anticoagulant therapy | 1. Malignant neoplasms<br>2. Infections, including bacterial pneumonia, lung abscess, tuberculosis, fungal infections, viral infections and parasitic diseases<br>3. Collagen vascular diseases including systemic lupus erythematosus and rheumatoid pleuritis<br>4. Pulmonary embolism/infarction<br>5. Some abdominal diseases including pancreatitis, subphrenic abscess, oesophageal rupture and hepatic abscess<br>6. Radiotherapy<br>7. Bile peritonitis<br>8. Trauma<br>9. Myocardial infarction and post-myocardial infarction syndrome<br>10. Aortic dissection<br>11. Cardiac rupture | 1. Metastatic cancer<br>2. Trauma, including blunt trauma and operative trauma<br>3. Retroperitoneal cancers and lymphoma<br>4. Tuberculosis<br>5. Congenital lymphatic anomalies |

circulatory system disorders, trauma, inflammation and infection) or malignant (that is, positive for malignant cells).[1]

Pathophysiologically, effusions may be: transudates, exudates, or chylous (Table 3.1). Although transudative effusions usually do not require diagnostic evaluation for malignant cells, exudative effusions generally need cytological evaluation to determine their cause.

In adults, most effusions are due to benign conditions such as congestive heart failure, cirrhosis of the liver or pericarditis. Malignant effusions are usually secondary to adenocarcinoma from breast, lung, gastrointestinal, or genitourinary tract. Additional malignant causes include lymphoma/leukaemia and other neoplasms.

### Reactive effusions

Cytomorphological features of floridly reactive mesothelial cells overlap significantly with malignant cells and may be misinterpreted as malignant. Some non-malignant effusions, such as those associated with hepatic cirrhosis, pulmonary infarction, and acute pericarditis are a potential pitfall for misinterpretation more frequently than other reactive effusions. A cautious and conservative approach is recommended when interpreting effusion cytology with such a clinical history.

### Malignant effusions

Effusions secondary to cancer are usually recurrent and haemorrhagic. Non-traumatic massive haemorrhagic effusions are almost always due to cancer. Perhaps with the exception of central nervous system tumours, malignant neoplasms from almost any site can metastasise to serous cavities and present as an effusion. However, a rare case of diffuse leptomeningeal gliomatosis involving the peritoneal cavity has been reported in a patient with a ventriculo-peritoneal shunt.[31]

For malignant pleural effusions, carcinoma of lung is the most common cause in men, followed by gastrointestinal tract and pancreatic carcinomas. Carcinoma of the breast is followed by lung and ovary in women. In the peritoneal cavity, cancers of the gastrointestinal tract, ovary and pancreas predominate.

A malignant effusion re-accumulates rapidly in comparison to reactive effusions. With this information in mind, it is prudent to recommend a repeat specimen if the initial specimen is suspicious but not conclusive for malignancy as it is easy to obtain a repeat sample when it re-accumulates. This can lead to a definitive diagnosis without the danger of false positive interpretation.[1]

The predominant cause of an initially indeterminate interpretation is artefact secondary to degenerative changes both *in vivo* and *in vitro*. A repeat specimen should be recommended to be submitted immediately after collection, to avoid *in vitro* degenerative artefacts.[32] The significance of relevant clinical details cannot be overstated. The cytological interpretation of a repeat specimen is usually easier, because the number of neoplastic cells in recurrent malignant effusions often increases, with many cohesive clusters and cell balls.

Both epithelial and non-epithelial neoplasms may cause malignant effusions. Epithelial neoplasms include metastatic carcinoma[4] and malignant mesothelioma.[33] Haematological neoplasms,[34] melanoma and sarcomas[35] are the non-epithelial neoplasms and, apart from the haematological malignancies such as lymphoma, these are rare cause of effusions.

### Paediatric malignant effusions[36,37]

Salient features related to paediatric effusions:

- Most paediatric effusions are benign
- Malignant paediatric effusions are usually secondary to small round blue cell neoplasms, mostly lymphoma and leukaemia
- Distinguishing neoplasms of small cell type from mononuclear inflammatory cells is the major diagnostic difficulty
- The role of peritoneal washings in the paediatric group is similar to that in adults.

## Washings, lavages, brushings, scrapings and touch imprints[13]

Involvement of serous cavities by cancer cells correlates with a poor prognosis, even in the absence of an obvious effusion. Cases positive for malignant cells in serous cavity samples are upstaged clinically.[38–40]

In the absence of an effusion at the time of presentation, the method used for evaluating cancer cells in this subset of cancer patients involves procurement of irrigated physiological saline as washings and lavages. Peritoneal washings (peritoneal lavage, pelvic washing) are a component of gynaecological cancer staging.[21] Cul-de-sac (pouch of Douglas) specimens may be collected intraoperatively or aspirated transvaginally.[1,41]

The morphological features and interpretation criteria, although similar to those of effusions, have to be slightly modified to avoid misinterpretation. In contrast to effusions, many cells in washings may not be exfoliated. These mechanically dislodged cells are seen as monolayered flat sheets which may resemble squamous metaplastic cells (Fig. 3.32). The individual mesothelial cells have well-defined cytoplasmic borders and show a jigsaw puzzle pattern, with distinct slits between some cells. Contrary to naturally exfoliated cells in effusions, the mechanically dislodged cells in washings may not be round and may show angulated rhomboidal/trapezoidal shapes with centrally placed, bland nuclei. Curling of some mesothelial sheets onto themselves may impart a three-dimensional appearance. They usually have straight margins and should be distinguished from the three-dimensional proliferation spheres of neoplastic cell groups which have round contours. Careful scrutiny of the morphology especially along the periphery, helps to interpret the true nature of these monolayered sheets. In addition, washings may dislodge other contaminants such as Mullerian inclusions[26] and atypical papillary proliferations[17] and may lead to serious errors in cytological interpretation.[13,27]

In some centres, the cytological findings in pleural lavages are included in the staging of lung[38–40,42] and oesophageal cancers.[43] Other methods such as pleural brushings[44] and intraoperative touch imprint cytology of visceral serosa[45] have been evaluated. Scrapings and brushings from serous cavities such as diaphragmatic scrapings have also been evaluated.[46] Rarely, peritoneal dialysis fluids, which have a higher frequency of cytological atypia, may be submitted for cytopathological evaluation (Fig. 3.20).[10]

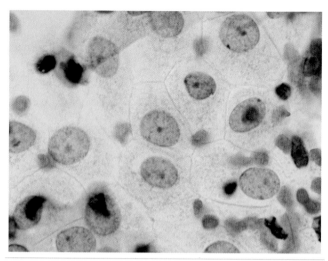

**Fig. 3.32** Mechanically dislodged monolayer of mesothelial cells (peritoneal washing) (PAP Cytospin).

A cautious approach is recommended to avoid malignant misinterpretation of peritoneal dialysis fluid specimens.

### Interpretive problems for washings

Artificial contamination from tumours during procedures is a distinct and disturbing possibility. However, the prognostic value of peritoneal washings in tumour management is based on the assumption that the finding of tumour cells in the specimen reflects the natural history of disease. This artefact, however, can be prevented by routinely collecting the washings as the initial step during the procedure, with extra care to avoid contamination.

Although washings are expected to yield a cell sample comparable to effusion fluids, these samples have crucial differences, and have to be evaluated with a slightly modified approach for optimum interpretation. Compared to the spontaneously exfoliated cells in effusions, washings contain many cells that have been mechanically dislodged from the underlying connective tissue during the procedure. This is further complicated by an increased tendency to show rare cell types (e.g. müllerian rests) and some unusual structures, such as psammoma bodies, in larger numbers and in higher frequency in washings than effusions. These are otherwise not commonly seen in effusions, probably because they shed in very low numbers under *in vivo* mechanically undisturbed conditions.[13,47]

In contrast to effusions, a second foreign population in a washing specimen is not equivalent to metastatic disease. Similarly, immunocytochemistry is also a less useful ancillary tool for interpretation of peritoneal washings, due to a significant overlap in the immunoreactivity patterns of gynaecological tumours and mesothelium. Comparative review, evaluating the histomorphology in cell block sections from washings with that of the primary tumour, which is usually resected concurrently, with the washing procedure as the initial step, is a simple but reliable interpretive approach.

### Cytological examination of effusions versus biopsy of the serous lining

Although challenging, in experienced hands cytological examination of effusions is better than biopsy of the serous cavity lining for the diagnosis of malignancy affecting any of the cavities.[48–52]

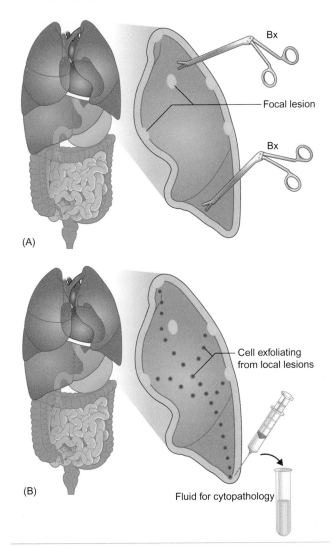

(A)

(B)

Bx

Focal lesion

Bx

Cell exfoliating
from local lesions

Fluid for cytopathology

**Fig. 3.33** Sampling of pleural lesions: biopsy (A) versus effusion cytology (B). Focal lesions may be missed by biopsy. However, cells exfoliated from any of these focal lesions are pooled in the fluid and should be present in a related effusion or washing. (Reproduced from Shidham and Atkinson 2007.[1])

Focal lesions on a serous surface may be missed by biopsy, potentially leading to false negative results. In contrast, malignant cells exfoliate and accumulate in an effusion from all surfaces lining that cavity, providing representation of the entire serous cavity (Fig. 3.33). In addition, effusions are relatively simple to collect. The rate of detection of cancer cells is increased further if multiple effusion specimens are evaluated consecutively.[53]

## Collection and processing of effusion fluids for cytopathological evaluation[32]

### Sampling of serous effusions

Removal of peritoneal fluid is by abdominal paracentesis (paracentesis abdominis), pleural fluid by thoracentesis and pericardial fluid is by pericardiocentesis. Collection is performed with a wide-bore needle, such as an 18-gauge needle, inserted under local anaesthesia and sterile conditions through the body wall into the serous cavity in its most dependent location.[52] The specimen is collected in a clean, dry, large container with or without anticoagulant.[32] For microbiological culture, the container should be sterile.

### Sampling of other specimens

Peritoneal or pelvic washing/lavage[13] for staging of gynaecological cancers or evaluating the spread of pancreatic and gastric cancers[54–56] is performed by instilling physiological saline solution into the peritoneal cavity, then withdrawing the fluid for cytopathological evaluation. Although these specimens are processed just like serous effusions, their interpretation criteria need to be modified.[13] Preparation of cell blocks is routinely recommended.

Peritoneal dialysate from patients undergoing long-term peritoneal dialysis for renal failure is processed just like serous effusions; however, the reactive mesothelial cells demonstrate atypia more significantly than in routine effusions.[10]

Pleural lavage cytology may be performed for staging of lung and oesophageal cancers.[38,39,42,43] Collection, processing and evaluation are similar to that for peritoneal washing,[38,39,42,43] including cell block preparation.

Other related specimens, such as intraoperative touch cytology,[45] pleural brushings[44] and diaphragmatic scrapings[46] may also be performed for evaluation of serosal involvement by cancer.

### Transporting effusion specimens

Freshly collected fluid, up to 1000 mL, should be transported to the laboratory. If a delay is expected, the specimen may be stored in a refrigerator at 4°C with the precaution of not allowing the specimen to freeze.[32]

Selection and use of anticoagulants and/or fixatives varies between laboratories.[32] Use of fixatives to ensure integrity of effusion specimens during prolonged transportation, under non-refrigerated conditions, may be indicated but routine use of fixatives is strongly discouraged, because it prevents ideal processing of effusions, with loss of the ability to prepare Diff-Quik-stained preparations.

### Anticoagulants/fixatives

Heparin (3 U/mL of fluid) is widely used because of its easy availability in clinical settings. Although it does not interfere with cytological details,[2,32,57] it may interfere by introducing background staining with Diff-Quik. Di-sodium EDTA and acid-citrate-dextrose[2,32] also do not interfere with cellular morphology and do not cause background staining, making them preferable to heparin.

As mentioned above, fixatives should be avoided for collecting and transporting effusion specimens. Simple refrigeration, even for several days, preserves the specimen for evaluation.[32,52] If the specimen is to have prolonged transportation at a high ambient temperature, a variety of fixatives or cellular preservative can be used including 10% buffered formalin, alcohol (ethanol, methanol, isopropanol), or others.

Formalin fixed cells do not adhere to the slide and the staining quality is severely compromised for both PAP and Diff-Quik stains. Similarly, alcohol denatures protein which prevents adherence of cells to the slide. Specimens may be mixed in a 1:1 proportion with various fixatives such as preservatives for liquid-based cytology (CytoLyt® for ThinPrep™ and CytoRich® Red, Yellow, or Blue for SurePath™) or 50% ethanol.[32] However, such specimens are not suitable for Diff-Quik staining.

Critically, the exposure of effusion specimens to these fixatives during the initial stages may affect the results of immunophenotyping, even if processed later with a protocol for formalin-fixed paraffin-embedded cell block sections. Exposure to other fixatives during the initial collection phase should be identified in the record for awareness during interpretation of immunocytochemistry results. This is an important note of caution, because the results may not be accurate or comparable with the published data.

## Processing of effusion fluids

### Gross examination

Gross findings such as volume, colour, clarity, opalescence, unusual odour and high viscosity are additional pieces of information that may contribute to cytopathological interpretation.

#### The colour

- Blood-stained haemorrhagic effusions: the majority of malignant effusions are haemorrhagic, with colour ranging from orange to deep red. Approximately half (46%) of the blood-stained effusions are positive for malignant cells[52,58]
- Light brown: effusions with many haemosiderophages due to chronic haemorrhage
- Chocolate brown: effusions with numerous melanoma cells with melanin
- Brown-orange or even greenish: effusions in cases with jaundice or associated with leakage of bile into the peritoneal cavity. After centrifugation, the discolouration persists in the supernatant.

#### Sediment

- Thick greyish-white to yellow sediments settle spontaneously at the bottom of hypercellular effusions if allowed to stand for a while. Malodour suggests a cellular purulent effusion with numerous neutrophils and high bacterial content. Heavy whitish and flocculent sediment suggests rheumatoid pleuritis or pericarditis. Grossly visible spheroids, ellipsoids, or similar shapes up to 2 mm in size resembling small sesame seeds represent proliferation spheres and individual groups of cancer cells. Such specimens yield excellent diagnostic material in cell block sections.

#### Other features

- Turbid yellow effusions with shimmers are due to cholesterol crystals, which can be seen in stained wet films and in Diff-Quik-stained, air-dried Cytospin smears. They are dissolved and not seen easily in PAP-stained preparations. Chylous effusions are milky white, with a top layer of emulsified lipid, and are due to rupture or blockage of lymphatics
- Viscous effusions may be related to diffuse malignant mesothelioma of epithelial type, and are typically associated with a high concentration of hyaluronic acid (HA). This has also been reported in a pleural fluid from a child with metastatic Wilms tumour.[32,59] Pseudomyxoma peritonei show a markedly viscous specimen because of heavy mucoid content, which may be extremely difficult to aspirate. Processing of a viscous specimen may be difficult because the cells in it do not sediment during centrifugation. Viscous specimens may be thinned with a suitable mucolytic agent such as dithiothreitol (in 50 µg/mL final concentration).

### Cytopreparation[32]

For semiquantitative evaluation of cellularity, a direct smear of the unconcentrated effusion specimen-stained with Diff-Quik is recommended.[32] In addition, the concentrated sediment is processed for Diff-Quik-stained Cytospin smears, PAP-stained smears, and haematoxylin and eosin (H&E)-stained cell block sections.

Availability of cell blocks is important for performing elective immunocytochemistry and other ancillary tests such as histochemical studies including mucicarmine, PAS and various other stains including stains for microorganisms. They are especially crucial in cases with a clinical history or suspicion of cancer, or when initial examination of the smears suggests malignancy. Preparation of cell blocks should be performed routinely for peritoneal washings. Although not ideal for many reasons, immunocytochemistry can be performed technically on cytological smears,[60–62] including PAP-stained smears without or after de-staining. However, cell blocks are preferred for immunocytochemical evaluation for both technical and quality control measures.[37,60]

Electron microscopy was performed in the past in the pre-immunohistochemistry era for distinguishing mesotheliomas from adenocarcinomas. However, with refinements in immunocytochemistry, the traditional role of electron microscopy in the cytopathology of effusions has diminished.

Stained wet films have been advocated[2,32,52] for initial evaluation to triage effusion specimens for various tests including immunocytochemistry, flow cytometry, cytogenetics, microbiology and cell biology. A study by Filie et al.[63] concluded that individual specimen triage does not offer any practical advantage over non-triaged, routinely processed effusion specimens.

Thus, depending on laboratory preferences and experience, effusions may be processed for various types of cytology preparations:[32]

- *Wet-fixed smear*: The direct smear is immersed quickly in fixative prior to drying of the smeared material; 95% ethanol is the commonly used, time-tested fixative but other alcohols such as 95% methanol, 95% isopropanol, or a commercially available spray fixative with carbowax (polyethylene glycol) may also be used. 'Pooling' artefact may be created especially in bloody specimens by spray fixatives. This artefact forms small round 'pools' throughout the smear. Although visually annoying, it does not interfere with interpretation. Carbowax residue on spray fixed smears must be removed with absolute alcohol prior to staining. For the PAP stain wet-fixed smears are preferred but these cannot be used for Romanowsky stains
- *Air-dried smear*: The cellular material on the slide is allowed to dry completely. The drying should be hastened by gently moving the smear in the air, or with a hair-dryer, or hand-held battery-operated fan.[64,32] Air-dried smears are fixed in 95% methanol and stained with Romanowsky stains. However, recently reported studies describe benefits of using air-dried smears for PAP staining after saline rehydration followed by fixatives such as 95% ethanol or 95% ethanol with 5% acetic acid[65,32]
- *Preparation of other smears*:[32] A variety of techniques may be used such as Cytospin smears and proprietary liquid-based

cytology smears (SurePath or ThinPrep or others). Non-proprietary methods for liquid-based cytology preparations have also been reported.[66,67] Cytospin smears may be air-dried or wet-fixed and may be stained with a Romanowsky or the PAP stain. Smears prepared by liquid-based cytology methods cannot be stained with Romanowsky stains.

The cells in the direct smears prepared from concentrated fresh unfixed effusion specimens are generally flat, with better cytomorphology. However, mechanical spreading may introduce artefacts especially in specimens with fragile cells, as in small cell carcinoma and high-grade lymphoma. In addition, homogeneous distribution of the cells may not be achieved with mechanical spreading. Cytospin smears, in comparison,[68] concentrate cells from fresh unfixed effusion specimens, and show a thinly dispersed layer of cells with good morphology. However, the cellularity of Cytospin smears may not be reproducible.

- *Filters* were used in the past. They achieve good concentration and retrieval of cells from effusions; however, the cellular details may not be as clear because of optical interference by the filter
- *Liquid-based cytology* preparations concentrate and distribute all cells in the specimen.[32] Their benefits and limitations depend on the method chosen, and the pathologist should consider associated morphological variations inherent with any selected method. Non-proprietary liquid-based cytology methods[67,69] may require standardisation by each laboratory with variable results. SurePath smears[70] are relatively cellular with well-preserved cells. However, the cytomorphological details are not crisp due the lesser transparency of the plump, partially fixed shrunken cells. Similarly, these smears are also difficult to photograph as the cells in the groups are difficult to focus in the same plane.[71] ThinPrep smears[72] have relatively flat cells with good cellular details, similar to those in direct smears and Cytospin smears.

## Interpretation of serous effusion cytopathology

### General approach[71]

With the exception of high-grade neoplasms with obvious cytomorphological features, one cannot apply basic cytological criteria of malignancy to a few cells in serous fluid specimens for interpreting them as positive for malignancy.[71] Because of surface tension, cells in effusions 'round-up', and the native shapes of cancer cells seen in traditional fine needle aspiration (FNA) cytology specimens cannot be applied to effusions when deciphering the primary origin of the malignant cells. Cancer cells with the potential to proliferate may continue to divide and form proliferation spheres in nutrient-rich effusion fluids. Apart from detection of cancer cells, cytopathological examination of serous effusions may reveal inflammatory conditions, parasitic infestations, bacterial, fungal, or viral infections, and certain other non-neoplastic conditions.[30]

Application of a 'two cell population approach' for making a final interpretation of malignancy in effusion specimens is simple and effective (Fig. 3.34).[71] Although mesothelial cells in effusions show a wide morphological spectrum, all cells are seemingly of one type and demonstrate a subtle morphological continuum (Figs 3.18, 3.19). In contrast, malignant effusions with metastatic tumour cells usually show a morphologically alien population (Fig. 3.10). However, as explained previously, the second alien population is relatively easy to differentiate in Diff-Quik-stained preparations, even under low magnification, as compared to PAP-stained slides (Fig. 3.10). In some cases, especially with metastatic carcinomas of the breast and ovary, this distinction, although suggestive, may be difficult. In such cases, further evaluation with ancillary tools such as immunocytochemistry may be used for objective demonstration of a second population (Fig. 3.35).[71]

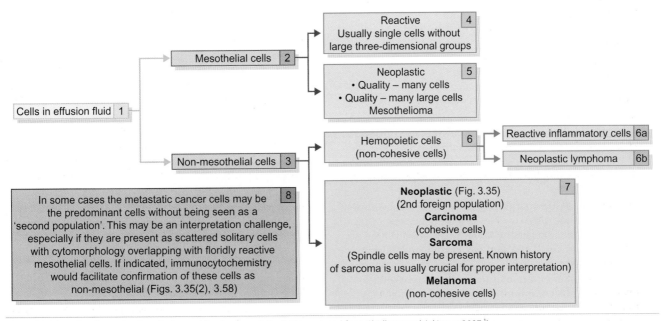

**Fig. 3.34** Algorithm for evaluation of a 'second foreign population'. (Reproduced from Shidham and Atkinson 2007.[1])

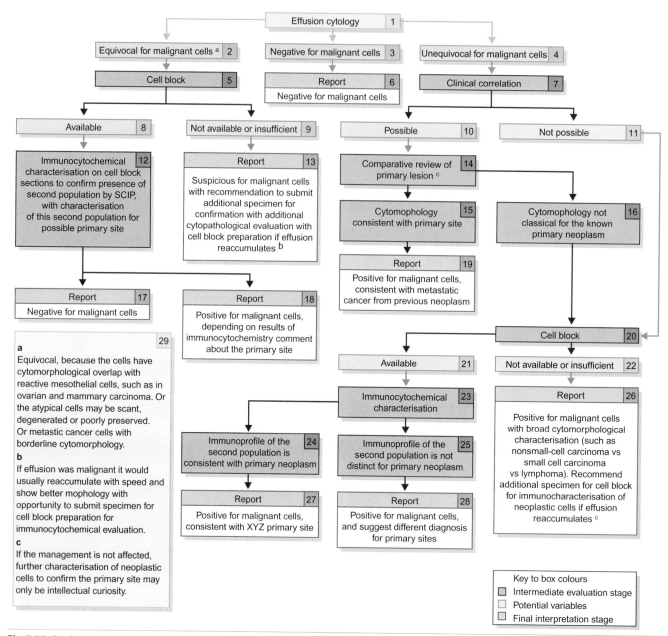

**Fig. 3.35** Cytological evaluation of effusion fluids for primary sites. (Reproduced from Shidham and Atkinson 2007.[1])

Although any type of cancer, including carcinoma, melanoma, haemopoietic neoplasms, sarcomas and mesothelioma could spread to the serous cavities, adenocarcinomas are the most common neoplasm to do so. In general, sarcomas metastatic to serous cavities are rare. Compared with other cytology specimens, the morphological features of most cancer cells in effusions are different. This is mainly because of morphological alterations related to surface tension and preservation related factors associated with the dynamics of effusions.

As reactive mesothelial cells are a universal component of effusion fluids, and their cytomorphology overlaps significantly with malignant cells, the interpreter should be familiar with the wide spectrum of cytomorphological appearances of these cells in effusions (Figs 3.18, 3.19, also see Box 3.1)[16,17] and should

consider all these multifactorial nuances unique to effusion fluids. This increases the diagnostic accuracy by avoiding various diagnostic pitfalls. Careful consideration of the uniqueness of the cytomorphological features of effusions and related pitfalls would achieve diagnostic expertise in this field, even without using ancillary tests (Figs 3.34, 3.35).[1] Pitfalls that arise from the various factors related to processing and interpretation of effusions are summarised in Table 3.2.

## Processing approach

Proper specimen collection and processing of serous fluids is an extremely important component for effective cytopathological

**Table 3.2** Potential pitfalls in effusion cytology

| | Categories and subcategories | | Misintrp. FP | Misintrp. FN | Remarks |
|---|---|---|:---:|:---:|---|
| a | Surface tension related alterations in cytomorphology | | | X | Frequent with sarcoma |
| b | Improper specimen processing | | | | |
| | i | Improper collection in fixative | X | X | |
| | ii | Improper storage with excessive degenerative changes | X | | |
| | iii | Lack of Diff-Quik-stained smears | X | X | |
| | iv | Lack of cell block | X | X | |
| | v | Improper orientation of immunostained sections may compromise SCIP | X | X | |
| c | Many faces of RM | | | | |
| | | Positive bias in cases with history of cancer, e.g. hepatocellular carcinoma with higher incidence of atypia in mesothelial cells | X | | Frequent with some clinical situations |
| d | Proliferation related features | | | | |
| | i | Proliferation spheres | | | Potential misinterpretation of cancer subtype |
| | ii | Increased number of mitotic figures | X | | |
| | iii | Prominent nucleoli | X | | |
| e | Degenerative changes | | | | |
| | i | Nuclear hyperchromasia | X | | |
| | ii | Cytoplasmic vacuolation | X | | Potential misinterpretation of cancer subtype as adenocarcinoma |
| f | Presence of some unexpected patterns and unusual entities | | | | |
| | i | Reactive lymphoid population | X | | May be misinterpreted as positive for polymorphic lymphomas such as low-grade follicular lymphoma |
| | ii | Polymorphic lymphoma cells | | X | |
| | iii | Tumour cells as single population | | X | In metastatic mammary and ovarian carcinoma |
| | iv | Psammoma bodies | X | | Seen in 30% peritoneal effusions, washings and culdocenteses. Benign associations in peritoneal specimens include: papillary mesothelial hyperplasia, endometriosis, endosalpingiosis, ovarian cystadenoma/cystadenofibroma |
| | v Three-dimensional benign cell groups | | X | | Potential misinterpretation of cancer subtype |
| | | Benign papillary inclusions, | | | |
| | | Gland-like epithelial structures | | | |
| | | Mullerian inclusions | | | |
| | vi | Megakaryocytes | X | | May be misinterpreted as atypical cells or cells with viral cytopathic effect |
| | vii | Rheumatoid effusions | X | | Spindle cells with background debris may be misinterpreted as sarcoma or squamous cell carcinoma |

FN, false negative; FP, false positive; Misintrp., misinterpretation; RM, reactive mesothelial cells; X, Usually responsible for this type of misinterpretation, SCIP, subtractive coordinate immunoreactivity pattern. (Modified from Shidham and Atkinson 2007.[71])

evaluation. An approach for accomplishing the following objectives is recommended:

1.  Highlight the differences between various cellular components to detect a 'second population of foreign cells' (Fig. 3.10)

2.  Facilitate evaluation of the nuclear details of the 'second population'

3.  Semiquantitative evaluation of effusion cellularity (Fig. 3.34(5))

4.  Evaluate the cells of haematolymphoid lesions

5.  Application of immunocytochemistry for detecting a 'second foreign population' objectively and for evaluation of their primary site as indicated.[74,60]

If these objectives are not considered from the start, and are not applied during the entire collection-processing stages there is a risk of misinterpretation and suboptimal results. Approaches to fulfil the objectives are suggested below.[71]

*1st objective*: Diff-Quik stain (Romanowsky-stained air-dried Cytospin smears or an air-dried direct smear prepared from the cell pellet) highlights the differences between reactive mesothelial cells and cancer cells more distinctly.

*2nd objective*: PAP stain (such as wet-fixed direct smears from the cell pellet, liquid-based cytology preparations: SurePath®, ThinPrep®, Cytospin smears, or filters) demonstrates the nuclear details more vividly.

*3rd objective*: Evaluation of direct smear (Diff-Quik stain or other) prepared from effusion fluid prior to concentration.

*4th objective*: Romanowsky stain (Diff-Quik) is traditionally used for evaluation of haematolymphoid cells.

*5th objective*: Cell block allows evaluation of various effusion cells by ancillary tests, including immunocytochemistry, as indicated.

Blood contaminated effusions with an excess of erythrocytes obscuring cellular detail may be processed by removing erythrocytes prior to the preparation of smears.[32] However, liquid-based cytology preparations such as SurePath remove/lyse erythrocytes during processing, so they are not a significant distraction unless the specimen is mostly blood from haemorrhage.

Proper clinical details are a critical component and should be available with the request form. As highlighted above, optimum interpretation of effusion fluid cytology begins with specimen processing. In cases with a clinical suspicion or history suggestive of cancer, immunocytochemistry is an important ancillary tool and may be indicated. For this reason, the technical staff handling the specimen at initial stages should have the proper clinical information to initiate the preparation of cell blocks in such cases.

Diff-Quik and PAP-stained preparations, even at low magnification, provide initial evaluation. Examination at a higher magnification allows for evaluation of cytomorphological features of cellular components and narrows the differential diagnosis. Ancillary tests such as histochemical stains, immunostains, flow cytometry, or other ancillary studies may provide objective confirmation. Depending on the clinical scenario and level of cytomorphological experience, ancillary tests may not be required in straightforward cases, without sacrificing accuracy of the final interpretation (Fig. 3.36).

## Interpretation approach (Fig. 3.34)[48,71,75–79]

As mentioned previously, with the exception of specimens with high-grade neoplasms with obvious overt features of malignancy,

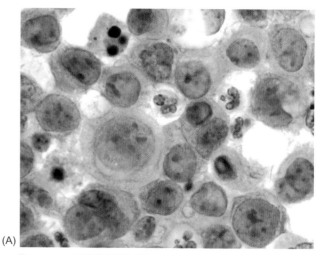

(A)

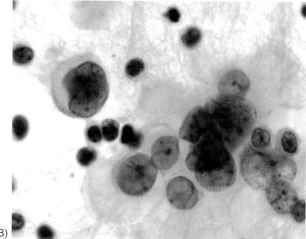

(B)

**Fig. 3.36** Metastatic mammary carcinoma (peritoneal fluid). The tumour cells (A,B) show obvious features of malignancy (PAP Cytospin).

standard diagnostic criteria of malignancy are not applicable to a few single cells in effusion cytology.[1] As compared to other types of specimen, the evaluation and final interpretation of serous fluid cytology should to be based on collective information deduced after considering the following issues unique for effusion cytology:[9,71]

1.  Reactive mesothelial cells demonstrate a wide cytomorphological spectrum overlapping significantly with neoplastic cells (Fig. 3.25).[9] Some clinical conditions may induce significantly florid reactive changes in mesothelial cells. This may lead to false positive interpretation of these cells as malignant cells.[80]

2.  Interpretation of reactive mesothelial cells or mesothelioma cells is favoured in effusions with a single population of cells with a cytomorphological spectrum demonstrating a continuum between all cells, with features of reactive mesothelial cells and without any evidence of a 'second foreign' population of cells. This feature, however, needs to be considered with the important caveat that in rare cases metastatic cancer cells may outnumber the mesothelial cells and present as a single predominant population of neoplastic cells with the potential for a false negative misinterpretation. This is mainly but not exclusively seen with metastases from breast carcinoma of lobular subtype.

3. The presence of a 'second foreign population' of non-mesothelial and non-inflammatory cells in effusion specimens is consistent with a metastatic neoplasm (Fig. 3.10).

4. A 'second foreign population' may be obvious in cases with sarcoma cells, and is usually easy to interpret. Availability of the previous history is helpful as sarcomas usually do not present as an effusion of unknown primary.[81,82]

5. The 'second population' of cells is highlighted with significant ease in Diff-Quik-stained preparations as compared to PAP-stained preparations (Fig. 3.10).[71]

6. Confirmation of a 'second population' with ancillary tests such as immunocytochemistry using a selective method known as the Subtractive Coordinate Immunoreactivity Pattern (SCIP) approach (see pp. 142, 144) facilitates objective interpretation.

7. Identical orientation of serial sections of cell blocks on all slides is crucial for precise evaluation by the SCIP approach (Fig. 3.47).[37,60]

8. Mesothelioma cells usually lack overt atypia and may easily be overlooked. The significant clues are:

   a. *Quantitative* with relatively hypercellular smears showing many isolated, scattered cells of mesothelial lineage

   b. *Qualitative* with increased numbers of large groups of three-dimensional cells of mesothelial lineage (Figs 3.12, 3.37). Diff-Quik stain facilitates easy evaluation of these clues.

9. The presence of apoptosis in unequivocally non-inflammatory cells, especially in association with mitotic figures, correlates with malignancy.[4] However, apoptosis may be difficult to evaluate unequivocally, especially in specimens with many apoptotic inflammatory cells and in some specimens with solitary small scant cells with apoptosis.

10. Many of these features have to be modified further for serous cavity specimens associated with mechanical dislodgement of constituent cells, in contrast to naturally exfoliated cells in effusions.[13]

## Cytological approach[1,48,75–79]

Effusion cytology demonstrates relatively unique cytomorphological features summarised below.

### Cell groups and intercellular cohesion

Malignant lymphomas and melanomas show non-cohesive, individual, solitary neoplastic cells, scattered throughout the smears or present as loose ill-defined aggregates (Figs 3.34(7), 3.56, 3.85). Lack of cohesiveness of cells is helpful, but other reactive and neoplastic cells may also show this feature with variable frequency, dependent on methods of cytopreparation.

Most carcinoma cells demonstrate good intercellular cohesion, but in effusions some metastatic carcinomas may show a tendency towards single scattered cells as a potential pitfall. Examples include linitis plastica type anaplastic gastric adenocarcinoma (see Fig. 3.77), non-cohesive cell type adenocarcinoma of the lung (Fig. 3.58), pleomorphic giant cell carcinoma of the pancreas, keratinising squamous cell carcinoma, giant cell carcinoma of the lung, and epithelioid mesotheliomas with a non-cohesive cell pattern (Fig. 3.34(7,8)). Carcinoma cells in poorly differentiated small cell carcinoma of the lung are usually

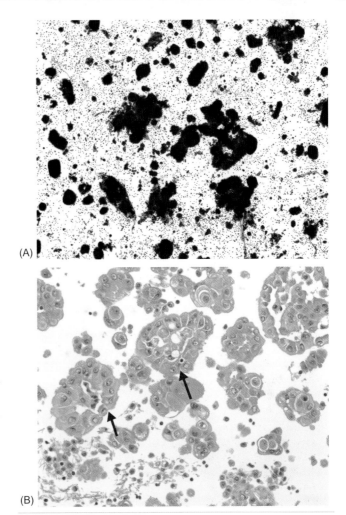

(A)

(B)

**Fig. 3.37** Malignant epithelioid mesothelioma (pleural fluid). Note the hypercellularity with many large groups of mesothelial cells that include numerous cells. Some papillary configuration is present. Most of the groups are solid and some have central stromal cores (arrows in B) in contrast to hollow proliferation spheres in carcinoma; (A, PAP SurePath (compare with Figure 3.39) B, H&E stained cell block section).

seen as solitary cells in newly developed malignant effusions, but they show cohesive clusters or proliferation spheres in effusions of longer duration or recurrent effusions.

### Proliferation spheres

*Proliferation spheres* (Figs 3.40, 3.41, 3.73) is a term initially used by Dr Nathan Chandler Foot. These round, to irregular groups of cells without stromal cores are solid or hollow in comparison to those observed in mesothelioma, which may show cores (Fig. 3.39). Some experts use the term 'tissue fragments' to highlight the fact that they are true fragments formed *in vivo* and are not physical aggregations secondary to *in vitro* processing factors. The neoplastic cells of adenocarcinoma in the proliferation spheres may show ill-defined gland formations (Fig. 3.40). They are observed typically in metastatic carcinoma such as metastatic mammary carcinoma (Fig. 3.40). The cytomorphological details are best observed in the cells along the periphery of such groups by adjusting the fine focus (Fig. 3.41) with additional details from the solitary neoplastic cells present in the background.

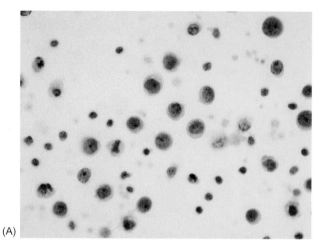

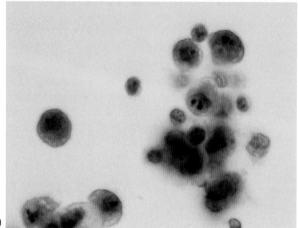

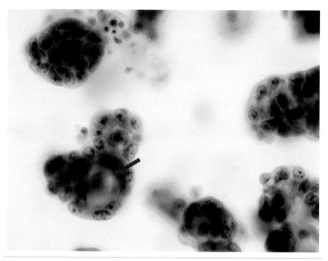

**Fig. 3.40** Metastatic mammary carcinoma (pleural fluid). A hollow proliferation sphere without any stromal core (arrow). This may be an attempt to form acini. Compare this with the three-dimensional groups of mesothelioma cells, which are solid with stromal cores (Fig. 3.53) (PAP SurePath).

**Fig. 3.38** Metastatic gastric carcinoma (peritoneal fluid). The tumour cells (A,B) are predominantly non-cohesive, solitary cells with eccentric nuclei without the rim of cytoplasm along the nuclear margin. Such cells may be difficult to differentiate from reactive mesothelial cells and lymphoma-leukaemia cells. However, cytomorphology in the Diff-Quik stain was not consistent with lymphoma and the typical two zone pattern of reactive mesothelial cells was absent. Rather, they showed randomly distributed vacuoles. Immunocytochemistry and flow cytometry would contribute to diagnosis (A,B, PAP SurePath).

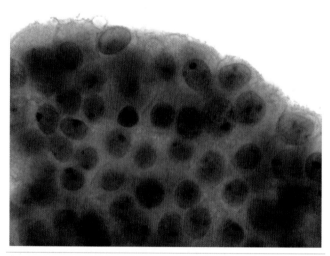

**Fig. 3.41** Metastatic mammary carcinoma (pleural fluid). Proliferation sphere shows radial polarity at the periphery of the proliferating neoplastic cells (PAP ThinPrep).

## Arrangement of neoplastic cells

Apart from proliferation spheres, the neoplastic cells may be seen in papillary configurations. Such papillary-like formations in effusion specimens may be the result of cytopreparation secondary to conglomeration of cell clusters or fusion of multiple proliferation spheres (see Fig. 3.73). This warrants caution, in that cell groups with papillary arrangements in effusions may not represent true papillary tumours. In addition, peritoneal washings may show benign papillary inclusions and müllerian inclusions, which may lead to misinterpretation as malignant.[17]

## Cytoplasm of neoplastic cells

Lack of typical two-zone cytoplasmic pattern in non-mesothelial metastatic cells is evaluated more easily in Diff-Quik than PAP-stained preparations and Romanovsky staining is

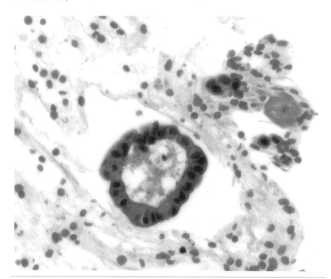

**Fig. 3.39** Metastatic mammary carcinoma (pleural fluid). Hollow proliferation sphere without any stromal core. In contrast to this, the three-dimensional groups of mesothelioma cells may be solid with stromal cores (see Figure 3.37) (H&E-stained cell block section).

**Table 3.3** Comparison of degenerative intracytoplasmic vacuoles versus secretory vacuoles

| Degenerative intracytoplasmic vacuoles | Secretory intracytoplasmic vacuoles |
|---|---|
| Do not occupy the entire cytoplasm of a cell and do not show ballooning | Secretory vacuoles with mucin and other material such as colloid in the vacuoles, usually balloon the entire cell and occupy most of the cytoplasm |
| Borders of vacuoles: usually ill-defined | Borders of vacuoles: well-defined |
| Does not show secretion in the lumen | May show secretion in the lumen (targetoid vacuole) |
| PAS stain after diastase digestion, and mucicarmine stain: negative | PAS stain after diastase digestion and a mucicarmine stain: may show positive secretion |
| May show other associated degenerative features such as nuclei with hyperchromatic smudgy chromatin | Hyperchromatic nuclei show features of malignancy with clumped crisp chromatin |

therefore strongly recommended.[71] The vacuolated cytoplasm of mucin-producing carcinoma cells may show mucicarmine and PAS stain positivity (Table 3.3, Fig. 3.27). Some non-cohesive solitary cells from epithelioid type mesotheliomas may have an abundance of dense granular or vacuolated cytoplasm, which may overlap morphologically with different types of carcinoma, such as renal cell carcinoma.

### Special structures and cytological features

Some morphological features with typical arrangements and characteristics may suggest a certain primary neoplasm. Examples include colonic adenocarcinoma demonstrating a palisading arrangement of elongated nuclei with apoptotic bodies and squamous cell carcinoma with keratinisation. Psammoma bodies favour papillary carcinoma of the thyroid, serous adenocarcinoma of the ovary (Fig. 3.29), bronchioloalveolar cell carcinoma of the non-secretory cell type and papillary type mesothelioma of epithelial type. However, free-floating psammoma bodies in some serous cavity specimens such as peritoneal fluids, cul de sac aspirates, and pelvic washings in women may be secondary to benign processes. Psammoma bodies under these situations are non-specific, without diagnostic significance, and may be observed in patients with pelvic inflammatory disease.[18]

### Other features

The wide morphological spectrum of reactive mesothelial cells is responsible for many 'look-alikes' in effusion cytology (Figs 3.18, 3.19, 3.25). Although the morphological features of various neoplasms are different in effusions from those in other types of specimens, metastatic cancers observed in usual practice may show typical cytological appearances that are recognisable with experience.[4,83,84]

The presence of 'lacunae' surrounding individual cells or groups of cells in cell block sections is reported more frequently in malignant effusions (75%) than reactive effusions (32%). Although it is a non-specific feature,[9] lacunae are useful for locating atypical cells, especially for evaluation of non-immunoreactive cells in immunostained sections under lower magnification.

The above features, with proper perspective, are effective for the final cytomorphological interpretation of effusion specimens with or without ancillary tests.

## Immunocytochemical approach

Diff-Quik and PAP-stained preparations may be suggestive but not unequivocal for a 'second foreign population'. Ancillary tests such as immunostaining of cell block sections (Fig. 3.35(2)) may be applied for objective confirmation of a second foreign population or for immunocharacterisation of this second population to confirm or suggest the primary site. Multiple limiting factors related to effusion fluids may compromise such evaluations unless properly analysed with the SCIP approach (see pp. 142, 144).[37,60]

## Ancillary techniques

Ancillary techniques including cell block preparation for histochemical staining and immunocytochemistry[37,60] introduce objectivity to the interpretation of effusions. Immunocytochemistry is an extremely valuable adjunct for objective interpretation. It may be used along with other ancillary techniques as indicated. Ongoing refinement in immunostaining technology with ever-increasing numbers of immunomarkers is pushing it further to the forefront.

## Cell block preparation[32]

Although cell blocks are not routinely prepared in all laboratories, most experts in this field strongly recommend the practice.[1,63,85] The residual sediment and/or any spontaneously formed clot may be processed for a cell block after preparation of the smears. Various methods are described.[32]

HistoGel™ or other non-proprietary gels such as gelatin,[86] albumin, or agar may be used for cell blocks on fresh or fixed samples. The plasma-thrombin method is another choice,[69,87] but it cannot be used if the specimen is submitted in fixative. Some experts have observed background staining in immunostained sections of cell blocks prepared with plasma-thrombin (or albumin) due to the high protein content. In our laboratory, immunostained cell block sections prepared with HistoGel do not show significant background staining.[32]

A large clot may be present in effusions without anticoagulant. Such a clot, especially if it has formed very soon after collection, may trap virtually all of the cells, including neoplastic cells, and lead to negative results. This can be pre-empted by the routine preparation of a cell block. If the effusion fluid is collected in anticoagulant, then any neoplastic and other cells remain in the fluid and are not lost.

Recently, we standardised a protocol for preparing a cell block from specimen containing solitary cells and loosely scattered cell groups, usually observed in serous cytology specimens.[247] This protocol involves centrifugation steps to concentrate the cells along the cutting plane of the cell block. A beacon-like dark AV-marker assists in monitoring the depth while cutting the paraffin block in order to appreciate cells in it. This decision assists the technologist from cutting too superficial or too deep into the paraffin block, beyond the level with most of the cells. This marker also serves as a reference point in the immunostained sections for applying the SCIP approach while interpreting the immunostaining pattern to detect a second population.

Cell block sections may demonstrate certain histological features helpful for final interpretation of a particular neoplasm such as papillary, acinar or duct-like formations, and psammoma bodies.[1,52] This is particularly helpful when evaluating peritoneal washings. It provides an opportunity to compare with the histomorphology in tissue sections of the corresponding known primary neoplasm. Some of these structures in washings may not be sampled or may be difficult or impossible to interpret in cytology smears alone.

## Biochemical analysis

Some of the following tests may help to evaluate the underlying cause of a particular effusion.

*Glucose level*: Tuberculosis and rheumatoid arthritis related effusions show low glucose levels.

*Amylase level*: Chronic pancreatitis associated effusions show a high amylase level.

*Adenosine deaminase level*: Tuberculous effusions show adenosine deaminase levels higher than 45 IU/L.

## Microbiological methods

If an infectious aetiology is suspected, special stains and microbiological culture detect and characterise the causative organisms. Bacteria, parasites and fungal organisms can be identified by appropriately selected special stains such as silver stains, PAS, Ziehl–Neelsen or other special stains on cytology smears or cell block sections.

Microbiology culture provides final identification and sensitivity of organisms.

## Other ancillary techniques including flow cytometry, molecular techniques[88]

A variety of other ancillary techniques may be applied for evaluation of effusion fluids. A partial list includes: electron microscopy (EM), flow cytometry, cytochemistry, immunocytochemistry on smears, fluorescent *in situ* hybridisation (FISH) and chromogenic *in situ* hybridisation (CISH), cytogenetics, DNA cytometry,[89,73] digitised imaging,[90] genetic molecular tests such as polymerase chain reaction (PCR) including reverse transcriptase-PCR (RT-PCR), and other tests such as suppressive subtractive hybridisation, laser capture micro-dissection, proteomics with surface-enhanced laser desorption ionisation mass spectrometry (SELDI-MS), matrix-assisted laser desorption/ionisation mass spectrometry (MALDI-MS). Currently many of these are not used clinically, but at least a few may be applied routinely in the future.[88]

## Electron microscopy

Electron microscopy (EM) demonstrates the characteristic long, slender, numerous microvilli in epithelioid mesothelioma.[91]

The microvilli vary in number and slenderness from one case to another and also in the same tumour from cell to cell.[5–7,92,93] With advances in immunocytochemistry, the role of electron microscopy has been shrinking due to its many limitations, including difficulty in actual objective localisation of cells of interest with certainty in EM sections. EM is rarely used in the current era of effusion fluid evaluation.

## Immunocytochemistry of effusions

### General discussion

Many variables from the time of collection of the specimen to its final immunostaining contribute to the quality of immunocytochemistry results.[37,60] Although interpretation criteria are taken for granted, they are difficult to reproduce in relation to many immunomarkers. The duration and ambient conditions in which paraffin-blocks are archived are also significant factors especially in regard to retrospective study.

However, the most significant challenge associated with immunocytochemistry of effusions is intricacy of finding and locating the cells of interest in cell block sections. This requires a careful special approach for reproducible interpretation of immunocytochemical results. Although not exclusive to serous fluid cytology, small cell groups and solitary cells in cell block sections introduce a unique challenge in interpreting the coordinate immunoreactivity patterns of the various components in effusion specimens. The parameters to be considered in effusion fluid immunocytochemistry for objective interpretation include:

1. Cancer cells in effusions may be present as solitary scattered cells or small cohesive groups, which are difficult to follow in different sections without a proper methodical approach. Most of the cells will be present in at least a few 4 μm thick serial sections (Figs 3.43, 3.44). If all the sections are identically orientated, these cells can be followed in different serial sections with relative precision (see Fig. 3.47). All serial sections should be orientated identically and identified sequentially. Routine application of this practice expedites and simplifies effusion fluid immunocytochemistry.

2. Confirmation of a second, foreign, non-inflammatory, non-mesothelial cell population is the most effective approach for diagnosis of metastatic disease in effusions. The so-called 'Subtractive Coordinate Immunoreactivity Pattern' (SCIP) approach identifies the 'second-foreign' population by applying the relevant immunopanel which highlights most of the mesothelial and inflammatory cells, creating a topographic map of the specimen.[37,60]

3. Epithelioid mesothelioma cells and reactive mesothelial cells cannot be differentiated currently by immunohistochemistry. They are distinguished by their quantitative (numerous versus a few) and qualitative (numerous large groups versus a few small groups) features, together with proper clinical and radiological correlation. If the cytological features favour mesothelioma over reactive mesothelial cells, exclusion of adenocarcinoma is relatively simple with immunocytochemistry.[37]

4. The final step in interpretation of the observed immunoprofile is comparison with published data from various studies performed predominantly on formalin-fixed

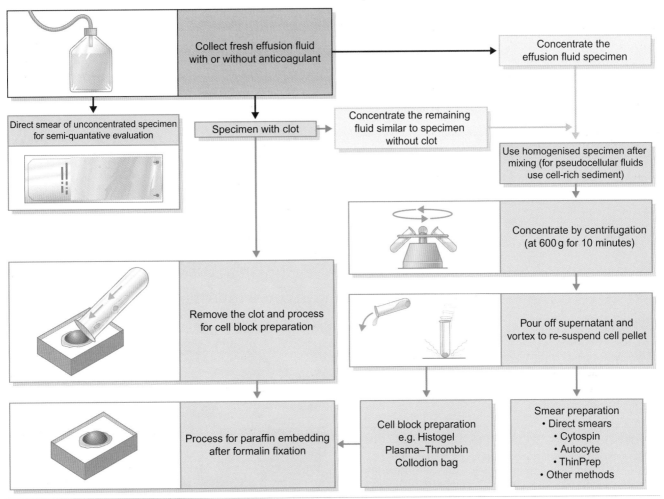

**Fig. 3.42** Processing effusion fluid for cytopathologic evaluation. (Reproduced from Shidham and Atkinson 2007.[1])

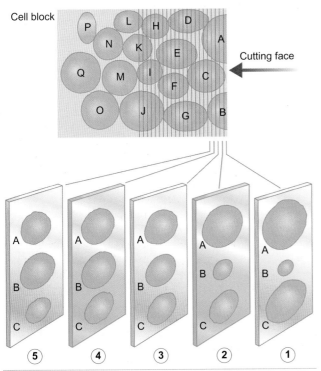

**Fig. 3.43** Serial numbering and orientation of cell block sections. (Reproduced from Shidham and Atkinson 2007.[1])

paraffin-embedded tissue sections. Variation in fixation and processing protocols is known to alter the immunoreactivity pattern.[94] Thus, it is critical to apply immunocytochemistry protocols matching with routine formalin-fixed paraffin-embedded tissue sections. Other protocols that include the use of cytology smears, whether direct smears wet-fixed in alcohol or acetone, air-dried fixed with alcohol, air-dried smears rehydrated and post-fixed in formol alcohol, liquid-based cytology smears or Cytospin smears, are not recommended as a routine choice.[85,61]

5. Evaluation of coordinate immunoreactivity patterns in the same cells in different serial sections (see Fig. 3.46) is one of the crucial components of immunohistochemical interpretation. Since the same unique cells cannot be seen on more than one slide, cytology smears are less suitable for routine immunocytochemical evaluation of effusion fluids.[95,96]

6. Effusion cells are suspended in a proteinaceous background. This may introduce unexpected, nonspecific immunoreactivity. For example, nonspecific staining of adjacent inflammatory cells may interfere with evaluation of membranous immunostaining patterns in some cases.

7. Immunocytochemistry of effusion fluids on cell block sections may show discrepant results in comparison to tissue sections from surgical pathology specimens. The potential causes include selection of fixatives, sample size

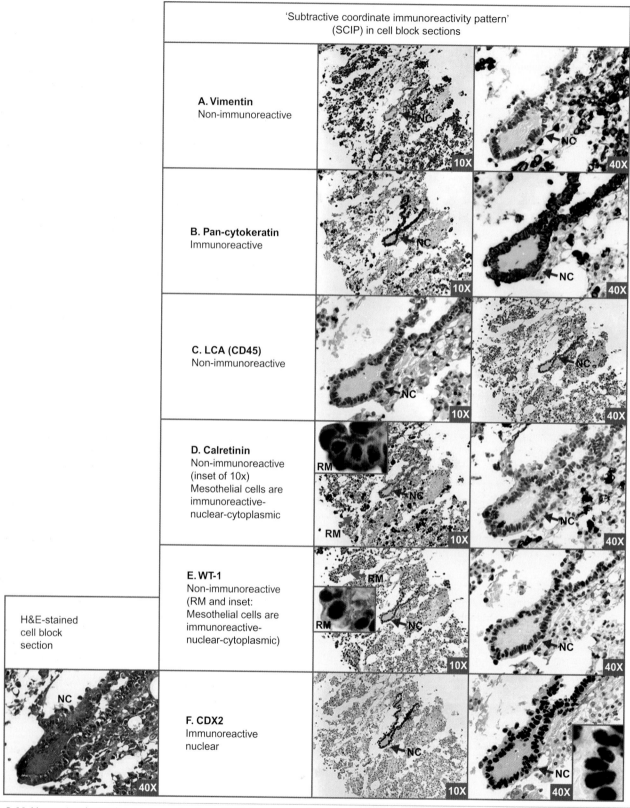

**Fig. 3.44** Metastatic colonic adenocarcinoma (peritoneal fluid). Immunocytochemical evaluation by SCIP approach. The neoplastic cells (arrow NC) are immunoreactive for pan-cytokeratin (B) and non-immunoreactive for vimentin (A), CD45 (C), calretinin (D), and WT-1 (E). They have nuclear immunoreactivity for CDX2 (F), which is consistent with a colonic primary. The reactive mesothelial cells (RM) [with immunoreactivity for calretinin (nuclear-cytoplasmic) (D), WT-1 (nuclear-cytoplasmic) (E), vimentin (A)] and inflammatory cells [with immunoreactivity for vimentin (A) and LCA (C)] in the background can be subtracted from neoplastic cells to deduce a diagnostic coordinate immunoreactivity pattern. LCA, leucocyte common antigen; NC, neoplastic cell; RM, reactive mesothelial cell; WT-1, Wilms' tumour-1. (A–F, immunostained cell block sections). (Reproduced from Shidham and Atkinson 2007.[1])

(tiny cell groups or single cells), antigen retrieval methods (i.e. heat-induced epitope retrieval, enzyme digestion, etc.), antibody clones used, antibody titre, and other variations in immunostaining protocols.[92,97] Other variables are qualitative, such as the pattern of immunostaining (membranous, cytoplasmic, nuclear, etc.)[37] and quantitative interpretation criteria.[98]

## Perspective on immunocytochemistry of effusions

Cell blocks allow morphological interpretation, relative comparability of immunoreactivity results with formalin-fixed paraffin-embedded tissue sections, evaluation of many immunomarkers simultaneously, and an archival benefit with availability of material for other types of testing in the future.[37,60,94,99]

If material is insufficient for cell block preparation, it is advisable to recommend resubmission cof adequate additional specimen for cell block preparation. Because malignant effusions usually re-accumulate quickly, acquiring a new sample is generally not a challenge. To ensure sufficient material it is worth requesting submission of most of the drained effusion fluid (up to 1000 mL).

Heat-induced epitope retrieval techniques have improved the quality of immunostaining of cytology smears significantly. The use of cytology smears in general for immunocytochemical evaluation has increased for different reasons[100,101] and this also applies to effusion smears.[60-62,94] Most experts, however, do not recommend it.[94] It may be justified with caution in rare instances; for example for a scanty specimen from a case with a known primary neoplasm which has a specific immunoreactivity pattern and when the cell blocks are not available. Examples include situations where a single immunomarker such as PSA in prostatic adenocarcinoma and CDX-2 in colonic adenocarcinoma are applicable.

Evaluation of effusion immunocytochemistry on cell block sections should be performed after considering many variables which may not be applicable to other specimens. Some of these variables are:

- Reactive mesothelial cells, as the predominant background cells in cell block sections of most effusion fluids, demonstrate a wide morphological spectrum overlapping with some malignant cells. Because of this, the cells to be scrutinised may not be obvious
- A variety of inflammatory cells intricately intermingle, enhancing the complexity further
- Scattered solitary cells and small groups of cells in effusion fluid cell block sections are difficult to follow in sections on different slides. This makes proper evaluation of coordinate immunoreactivity difficult (see Fig. 3.46)
- Non-specific immunoreactivity, related to a protein rich background in cell block sections which is not observed in surgical pathology tissue specimens
- Variations in cell block preparation protocols at different steps, such as:
  - Use of fixative instead of submission as a fresh, unfixed specimen
  - Variation in fixatives, such as ethanol or proprietary fixatives, without data on the exact composition
  - Time and temperature variation during specimen transportation

- Delayed processing of an unfixed specimen
- Variation in methods of cell block preparation, for example agar gel method, picric acid method, thrombin clot and others.

Some variables interfere more significantly than others. Collection of effusions in fixatives, specimen processing after delayed transportation/storage at room temperature, and application of some cell block preparation protocols such as picric acid method are the most deleterious for immunocytochemistry.

As with H&E-stained sections, numerous qualitative and quantitative morphological features (Fig. 3.45) should be considered during immunocytochemical evaluation of effusion fluids to reach a final interpretation. A reflexive positive-negative binary approach for immunocytochemical interpretation, although usually applied in other situations, is less effective in effusion fluid immunocytochemistry. Different aspects of individual and complementary immunomarkers are considered collectively (Figs 3.44, 3.46). An alphabetical list of immunomarkers routinely used for effusion immunocytochemistry is given in Table 3.4.

## Categorisation of effusion immunomarkers[74,60]

Various immunomarkers are used in effusion fluid immunocytochemistry, and may be categorised as follows:

### 'Positive' mesothelial markers

Currently, calretinin (Fig. 3.45), D2–40 (podoplanin), cytokeratin 5/6,[174] and WT1 appear to be the best immunomarkers for reactive and neoplastic mesothelial cells. Although calretinin and D2–40 are more sensitive than cytokeratin 5/6 and WT1, a minority of carcinomas may rarely show immunoreactivity for all of these immunomarkers. WT1 is not expressed in lung adenocarcinomas and most other adenocarcinomas. It may be expressed in ovarian/peritoneal carcinoma and desmoplastic small round cell tumour,[122] thus decreasing the specificity of WT-1 in peritoneal fluid. It may be considered more specific in the non-peritoneal setting.

Other immunomarkers reported initially as mesothelial markers, but less effective in this role, include thrombomodulin, mesothelin, HBME-1, N-cadherin, OV632 and CD44S. They are less sensitive and less specific, with overlapping immunoreactivity patterns for mesothelial and non-mesothelial cells. Further refinement and standardisation may allow some of these to be used as reliable 'positive' immunomarkers for mesothelial cells in the future.

Vimentin and cytokeratin 7 are additional mesothelial immunomarkers with high sensitivity but lower specificity. However, they are effective immunomarkers in this category, subject to proper evaluation with the SCIP approach.

### 'Negative' mesothelial markers

An immunomarker which is negative in reactive and/or neoplastic mesothelial cells is an ideal 'negative' mesothelial marker. Although not absolute, Ber-EP4, mCEA, MOC-31, BG-8, and B72.3 are among those in this group. They are relatively sensitive and specific for distinguishing malignant mesotheliomas from adenocarcinomas, but rarely mesothelial cells may show unexpected immunoreactivity. In specific clinical settings, additional immunomarkers that are less sensitive but relatively specific 'negative' mesothelial immunomarkers are TTF-1, prostate

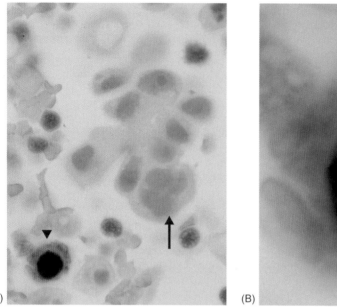
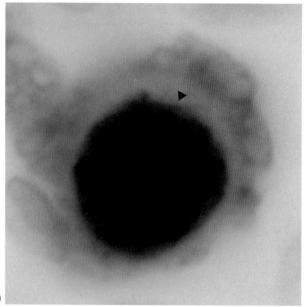

**Fig. 3.45** Calretinin immunoreactivity in mesothelial cells (metastatic ovarian carcinoma, ascitic fluid). (A) The neoplastic cells (arrow) are non-immunoreactive for calretinin. Rare mesothelial cells (arrowhead), which are an inbuilt positive control, show characteristic nuclear immunoreactivity (arrowhead in B). Associated variable cytoplasmic immunostaining may be present, but cytoplasmic immunoreactivity without nuclear immunoreactivity is not definitive for mesothelial cells and may be observed in many other cells including adenocarcinomas (cell block section immunostained for calretinin).

specific antigen (PSA), calcitonin, estrogen receptor, CDX-2 and a few others.[60,74]

## Other adjunct immunomarkers

1. Typical of the immunostaining with some antibodies is the thick membranous staining that highlights microvilli, favouring mesothelial cells. Adenocarcinoma cells may demonstrate diffuse, coarse, cytoplasmic or flimsy, membranous immunostaining patterns.[74] The markers in this group are epithelial membrane antigen (EMA) and HBME-1. If their immunostaining patterns are not considered, they would otherwise be categorised as non-specific.

2. Immunomarkers highlighting various components of effusion fluids:
   - Non-epithelial (and mesothelial) component by vimentin
   - Epithelial component by pan-cytokeratin (e.g. mixture of AE1/AE3 & CAM5.2) or other cytokeratins including cytokeratin 7
   - Inflammatory cell component by the leucocyte common antigen, (LCA CD45) or PGM1 (CD68) or mixture of LCA & PGM1. For selection of a CD68 antibody, in our experience PGM1 usually lacks non-specific immunoreactivity frequently observed with KP1.[60] Recently, CD163 has shown superior specificity for histiocytes.[244,246] This group of immunomarkers is especially effective for establishing a topographic map of various components in a particular effusion specimen facilitating evaluation, localisation, and identification of neoplastic cells (Figs 3.44, 3.46) by the SCIP approach (see below).

Various combinations of these immunomarkers distinguish reactive and neoplastic mesothelial cells from cells of metastatic neoplasms. More details about immunomarkers related to the evaluation of neoplasms associated with serous cavities may be found in specific reviews.[37,60,85,143,175] With continuous advances in immunocytochemistry frequently updated, the basic principles including the SCIP approach to be described in this chapter may be applied to contemporary immunomarkers after relevant adjustments.

## Subtractive coordinate immunoreactivity pattern (SCIP) approach

Immunohistochemical evaluation of tissue specimens from serous cavities is relatively straightforward and an immuno-panel with four immunomarkers (two positive and two negative mesothelial markers) may be enough for distinguishing mesothelial cells and adenocarcinoma cells. However, the challenge with effusion specimens is more complex and commands a special approach. In some cases, neoplastic cells may not even be identifiable for specific interpretation of immunoreactivity. Sequential serial sections are oriented identically (Fig. 3.47) for reproducible tracking of the relative position of different cells and cell groups in all serial sections. This allows evaluation of coordinate immunoreactivity patterns of various cellular components in effusion specimens (Figs 3.43, 3.44, 3.46, 3.47).[74]

A topographic map of all the components in a particular specimen is achieved by evaluating serial sections immunostained with vimentin, pan-cytokeratin (such as a mixture of AE1/AE3 and CAM5.2), and LCA (CD45) or PGM1 (CD68) or a mixture of LCA and PGM1. The next step is the evaluation of coordinate immunoreactivity in different components of that specimen. Immunoreactivity and non-immunoreactivity in various constituents, in concert with calretinin and vimentin, helps to characterise different cells and detect a second foreign population. Additional immunomarkers may be added

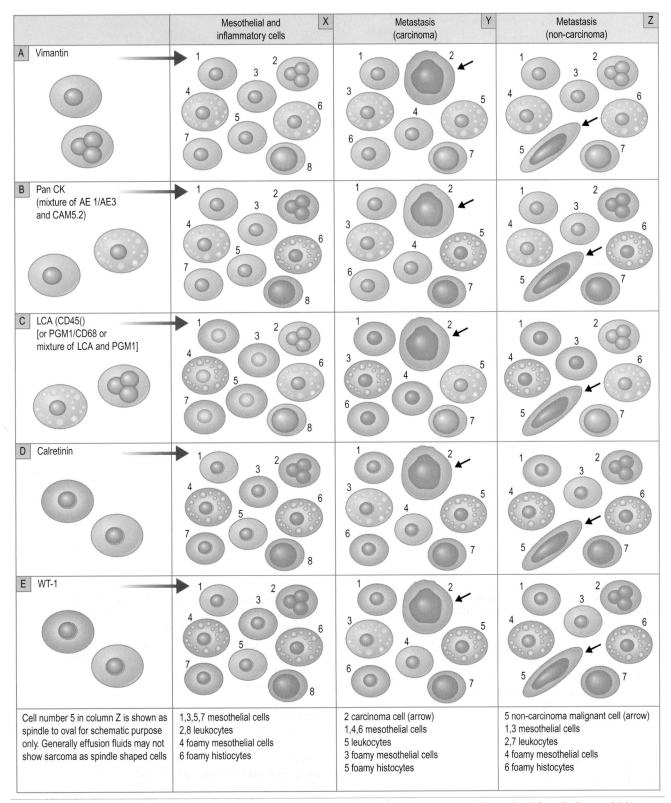

| | Mesothelial and inflammatory cells X | Metastasis (carcinoma) Y | Metastasis (non-carcinoma) Z |
|---|---|---|---|
| **A** Vimantin | | | |
| **B** Pan CK (mixture of AE 1/AE3 and CAM5.2) | | | |
| **C** LCA (CD45() [or PGM1/CD68 or mixture of LCA and PGM1] | | | |
| **D** Calretinin | | | |
| **E** WT-1 | | | |
| Cell number 5 in column Z is shown as spindle to oval for schematic purpose only. Generally effusion fluids may not show sarcoma as spindle shaped cells | 1,3,5,7 mesothelial cells 2,8 leukocytes 4 foamy mesothelial cells 6 foamy histiocytes | 2 carcinoma cell (arrow) 1,4,6 mesothelial cells 5 leukocytes 3 foamy mesothelial cells 5 foamy histocytes | 5 non-carcinoma malignant cell (arrow) 1,3 mesothelial cells 2,7 leukocytes 4 foamy mesothelial cells 6 foamy histocytes |

**Fig. 3.46** Basic immunopanel for evaluation by subtractive coordinate immunoreactivity pattern (SCIP) approach. (Reproduced from Shidham and Atkinson 2007.[1])

to evaluate the second population further, depending on the specific clinical situation. This approach, to locate, identify and characterise the foreign cell population in cell block sections by immunocytochemistry, is designated 'Subtractive coordinate immunoreactivity pattern' (SCIP) evaluation.[74]

## SCIP with dual colour immunostaining[150,247]

Based on the various immunomarkers discussed above, two colour immunocytochemistry can be applied to effusion fluids by selecting a proper combination of two complementary

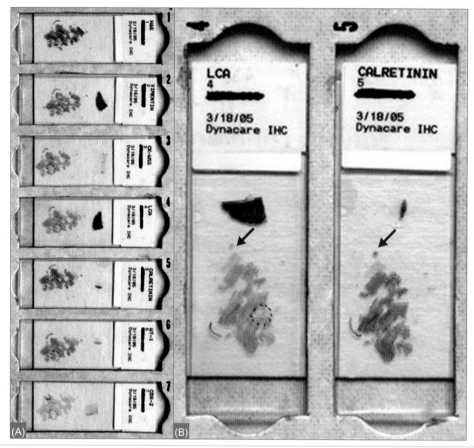

**Fig. 3.47** (A,B) Identical orientation of serial sections on different slides. A crucial component of SCIP approach. (Reproduced from Shidham and Atkinson 2007.[1])

immunomarkers (Fig. 3.48). However, not all combinations may be effective and the immunostaining protocol for each combination should be standardised prior to clinical application.[150,247] In our study, the following two combinations:

1. Vimentin (brown) followed by cytokeratin 7 (red) and
2. Calretinin (brown) followed by BerEP4 (red)

showed good results. However, calretinin and BerEP4 was less effective. The major benefit of dual colour immunostaining of effusion specimens is that evaluation by the SCIP approach is simplified for objective identification of foreign populations of malignant cells in fewer sections.

## The immunopanel for effusions[60,74]

It is advisable to select more than one immunomarker, as the pattern of immunoexpression may be heterogeneous. Because different neoplasms may have significantly overlapping immuno-profiles, evaluation with an optimum number of immunomarkers is recommended for appropriate interpretation. *Use of a suboptimal, restricted immunopanel may result in spurious interpretation.*

Different immunomarkers may be evaluated sequentially (to economise) or simultaneously (for rapid turnaround time). The choice depends on the institutional preferences and cost considerations. However, for proper application of the SCIP approach, the sections should be cut and serially numbered from the same ribbon, at one time. The unstained, serially numbered sections

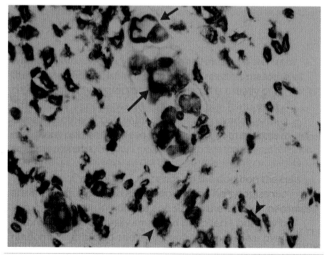

**Fig. 3.48** Dual colour immunostaining. Metastatic mammary carcinoma (pleural fluid). Metastatic carcinoma cells (arrows) are immunoreactive only for cytokeratin 7 (red) without vimentin (brown) immunostaining. For additional confirmation, these cells were weakly immunoreactive for BerEP3 in other serial sections. The background inflammatory cells (arrowheads) are highlighted by vimentin (brown) only. There were very few reactive mesothelial cells (not present in the figure), which showed simultaneous red (cytokeratin 7 immunoreactivity) and brown (vimentin immunoreactivity) [Dual colour immunostained cell block section, vimentin (brown) followed by cytokeratin 7 (red)].

may be used later for sequential immunostaining, as indicated by the results of an initial broad immunopanel. Once the neoplastic cells are confirmed as a foreign population with the SCIP approach,[74] they may be characterised with immunocytochemistry to determine the primary site, in concert with clinical details (Fig. 3.49).

- Vimentin, pan-cytokeratin (a mixture of AE1/AE3 & CAM5.2), and LCA [CD45] (or PGM1 [CD68] or preferably a combination of LCA & PGM1) helps to create the basic map for the SCIP approach, in identifying a second cell population
- The addition of calretinin and D2–40 as positive mesothelial markers locates mesothelial cells
- Microscopic assessment of immunostaining by subtractive evaluation of all serial sections allows confirmation of non-mesothelial/non-inflammatory cells, and if present, this 'foreign cell population' is usually consistent with a metastatic neoplasm
- A cytokeratin (rarely also vimentin) immunoreactive second foreign population is consistent with carcinoma. The cells are usually immunoreactive for most of the 'negative' mesothelial markers such as Ber-EP4, mCEA, B72.3, and/or MOC-31 (Table 3.4)
- A vimentin immunoreactive second population, which is non-immunoreactive for cytokeratin, may represent sarcoma, melanoma (immunoreactive for melanoma markers), or lymphoma (immunoreactive for LCA and other lymphoma markers with flow cytometry or immunocytochemistry as indicated). All these, except for lymphoma, are relatively rare causes of malignant effusions.

In summary, an optimal immunopanel includes pan-cytokeratin, such as cocktail of AE1/AE3 and CAM5.2, vimentin, LCA [CD45] or PGM1 [CD68] or preferably mixture of LCA & PGM1, calretinin, D2–40, BerEP4, and B72.3 for evaluation with the SCIP approach.[74] The initial immunopanel is modified according to the clinical situation:

- *If the primary neoplasm is known*: A brief panel such as TTF-1 for lung, PSA for prostate, CK7/ER/mammaglobin/CRxA-01 for breast, CK20/CDX2 for colon, appropriate lymphoma panel for lymphoma, S-100 protein and other melanoma markers for melanoma, may be added
- *If the primary neoplasm is unknown*: Extend the immunopanel by adding other broad categories including CK7 with CK20.[96,176,177]

In some cases the population of foreign cells may be numerous. They may be solitary and scattered with negligible numbers of mesothelial cells predominantly with a non-mesothelial population showing relevant immunoprofile (calretinin [nuclear]- non-immunoreactive, vimentin- non-immunoreactive) and consistent with a metastatic neoplasm (Fig. 3.34(8) and see Fig. 3.46). The immunoprofile of these cells, corresponding cytomorphology, and relevant clinical history may be consistent with a carcinoma (cytokeratin+) (Fig. 3.44), lymphoma (CD45+), sarcoma (vimentin +, cytokeratin−), or melanoma (S-100+ with one of the melanoma markers).[37,60,96,177]

However, even if the absence of a 'second foreign' population is confirmed, mesothelioma cannot be excluded by immunocytochemistry alone. This interpretation is based on qualitative and quantitative cytological features, in correlation with clinical and radiological findings.[33] A 'magic' immunomarker distinguishing mesothelioma cells from reactive mesothelial cells does not exist,[168,178,179] but rare reports have suggested that p53 and OV632 may be applied. Evaluation of clones E29

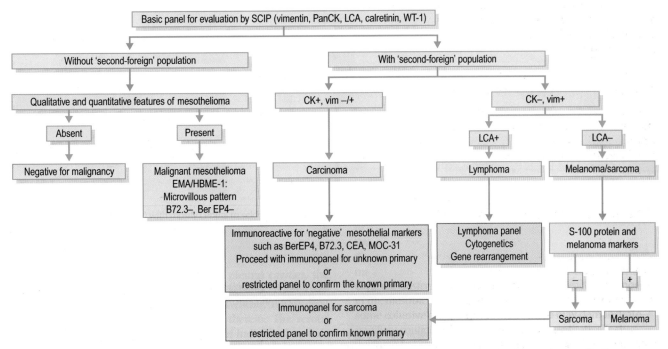

\* Effusions containing numerous lymphocytes and suspicious for lymphoma (even if lymphoid population is polymorphic) should be immunophenotyped by flow cytometry (or by immunocytochemistry on cell block sections). In high-grade large cell lymphoma the atypical cells seen as 'second-foreign' population will be LCA (CD45) immunoreactive at the initial SCIP approach.

**Fig. 3.49** Algorithm for immunocytochemical evaluation of effusions. (Reproduced from Shidham and Atkinson 2007.[1])

**Table 3.4** Immunomarkers (in alphabetical order) for immunocytochemical evaluation of effusions

| Immunomarker | Pattern | Immunoreactivity in | Remarks | References |
|---|---|---|---|---|
| Anti-mesothelial cell antibody | Cytoplasmic | Mesothelioma | Not evaluated and reported by a study other than Donna et al. 1992[103] | 103 |
| B72.3 | Membranous | AdCa | Good general immunomarker for adenocarcinoma. Slightly weaker than BerEP4 | 103–110 |
| BerEP4 | Membranous | AdCa | Good general immunomarker for adenocarcinoma. Relatively better than B72.3 | 106–108, 110–113 |
| CA19–9 | Cytoplasmic; luminal | AdCa | Most pancreatic, gastric, colonic and gall bladder adenocarcinomas 50% of ovarian carcinomas and 35% of mucoepidermoid carcinomas of salivary gland | 108, 114–119 |
| E-Cadherin (HECD-1) | Membranous; cytoplasmic | AdCa and reactive/neoplastic meso in some cases | Not a significantly useful immunomarker in effusion immunocytochemistry | 110, 118, 120, 121, 123, 124 |
| N-Cadherin | Membranous; cytoplasmic | AdCa and reactive/neoplastic meso in some cases | Not a significantly useful immunomarker in effusion immunocytochemistry | 106, 110, 112, 120, 121 |
| Calretinin | Nuclear (with or without cytoplasmic) | Mesothelioma; mesothelial cells | Relatively specific mesothelial immunomarker in effusion immunocytochemistry | 110, 125–134, 144, 158 |
| CD15 (LeuM1) | Membranous; cytoplasmic | AdCa; haemopoietic cells | Weaker immunomarker for adenocarcinoma. Overlaps with mesothelioma. Less useful immunomarker for effusion immunocytochemistry | 105–107, 108–110, 126, 127, 135, 136 |
| CD44S (CD44H) | Membranous | Mesothelial cells; AdCa | Not a useful immunomarker in effusion immunocytochemistry | 128, 137 |
| CD45 (LCA) | Cytoplasmic | Inflammatory cells and lymphoma cells | Useful immunomarker in effusion immunocytochemistry. Distinguishes the inflammatory cells from mesothelial cells and metastatic carcinoma | 60 |
| CD68 (Preferably PGM1, not KP1) | Cytoplasmic | Inflammatory cells and lymphoma cells | Useful immunomarker in effusion immunocytochemistry. Distinguishes the inflammatory cells from mesothelial cells and metastatic carcinoma | 60 |
| CDX2 | Nuclear | Colon (and gastric) AdCa | Useful immunomarker for differential diagnosis of specific primary site | 140–142, 145 |
| mCEA (monoclonal CEA) | Cytoplasmic | AdCa | Good immunomarker for adenocarcinoma, but less sensitive than BerEP4 | 103, 105–108, 117, 146, 148 |
| CRxA-01 | Membranous | Breast Ca | Useful immunomarker in the differential diagnosis of specific primary site. Slightly more non-specific than Mammaglobin | 60, 139 |
| Cytokeratin | Cytoplasmic | Carcinoma; mesothelioma (with concentric pattern) | Useful immunomarker for differential diagnosis from non-mesothelial/non-carcinoma neoplasms | 106, 110, 128, 149, 151 |
| Cytokeratin 5/6 | Cytoplasmic | Carcinoma (rare); mesothelial cells | Useful immunomarker to distinguish mesothelial cells from carcinoma cells. Less effective than calretinin and D2–40, but popular with some groups | 174 |
| Cytokeratin 7 | Cytoplasmic | Carcinoma (some); mesothelial cells | Useful immunomarker to distinguish mesothelial cells from some carcinoma cells | 139 |
| Cytokeratin 20 | Cytoplasmic | Carcinoma (some) | Useful immunomarker to distinguish some carcinoma cells from mesothelial cells | 139 |
| Cytokeratin 19 | Cytoplasmic | Carcinoma; mesothelial cells (rarely) | Useful immunomarker to distinguish lung carcinoma cells from mesothelial cells | 99 |
| D2–40 (Podoplanin) | Membranous (microvillous) | Mesothelioma; lymphatic endothelium; testicular germ cell tumours | Specific mesothelial immunomarker in effusion setting. Approaches that for calretinin | 152–157, 159, 160 |
| EMA (epithelial membrane antigen) | Membranous (microvillous); cytoplasmic | Mesothelioma; AdCa, Large cell anaplastic lymphoma | Not a useful immunomarker in effusion immunocytochemistry | 106, 108, 112, 127, 135 |

(Continued)

**Table 3.4** Continued

| Immunomarker | Pattern | Immunoreactivity in | Remarks | References |
|---|---|---|---|---|
| HBME-1 | Membranous (thick microvillous) | Epithelioid mesothelioma; thyroid Ca; sarcoma; lymphoma | Not a useful immunomarker in effusion immunocytochemistry (but popular with some groups) | 99, 116, 127, 161, 162 |
| HMFG-2 (human milk fat globule) | Cytoplasmic | AdCa; some mesothelioma | Not useful immunomarker in effusion immunocytochemistry | 106 |
| Mammaglobin | Cytoplasmic | Breast Ca | Useful immunomarker for differential diagnosis of specific primary site. | 139 |
| Mesothelin | Membranous | Mesothelioma; many AdCa | Not useful immunomarker in effusion immunocytochemistry | 163 |
| MOC-31 | Cytoplasmic | AdCa | Good immunomarker for adenocarcinoma, but is less sensitive and specific than BerEP4 | 164, 165, 170 |
| OV632 |  | Ovarian ca; mesothelioma | May be useful immunomarker for differential diagnosis of specific primary site | 167, 169 |
| Thrombomodulin | Membranous | Mesothelial cells; AdCa | Not useful immunomarker in effusion immunocytochemistry | 43, 45, 51, 56, 116, 128, 161, 163 |
| TTF-1 | Nuclear | AdCa; lung and thyroid | Useful immunomarker for differential diagnosis of specific primary site | 137, 165, 171, 172 |
| Vimentin | Cytoplasmic | Mesothelioma; sarcoma; lymphoma | Useful immunomarker in effusion immunocytochemistry. Distinguishes most metastatic carcinomas by negative immunostaining | 138, 146, 166, 173 |
| WT-1 | Nuclear (with or without cytoplasmic) | Mesothelioma; ovarian Ca; DSRCT | May be specific mesothelial immunomarker in pleural and pericardial effusion setting, but less useful than calretinin and D2–40 | 110, 118, 122, 127 |

AdCa, adenocarcinoma; Ca, carcinoma; DSRCT, desmoplastic small round cell tumour; EMA, epithelial membrane antigen; meso, mesothelial cells; TTF-1, thyroid transcription factor-1; WT-1, Wilms tumour-1. (Modified from Shidham 2007.[60])

and Mc5 of EMA reportedly can distinguish between reactive mesothelial cells and neoplastic mesothelial cells.[179]

The availability of clinical details, especially when there is a history of cancer, is crucial for proper selection of the initial immunopanel. In cases with an unknown primary, the challenge is relatively complex, and a wider range of site specific immunomarkers is needed. The approach is comparable to that of other metastatic neoplasms.[37,60,96,176,177]

In SCIP evaluation, the combination of immunomarkers can be modified depending on the individual pathologist's experience with a particular immunomarkers, the quality of immunostaining, the availability of resources and additional availability of improved immunomarkers in the future.[62,94,101,174,180] Common immunomarkers applicable to effusion fluid immunocytochemistry are summarised in Table 3.4.[60]

## Reactive conditions causing effusions

### Reactive conditions[30] showing features overlapping with carcinoma

A diagnosis of malignancy should be made with extreme caution in patients in this category.

The atypical cells usually demonstrate a 'morphological continuum' with mesothelial cells. Immunophenotyping by the SCIP approach introduces objectivity in distinguishing reactive mesothelial cells from metastatic tumour cells.[74]

### Cirrhosis with activity, uraemia and acute pancreatitis

Reactive mesothelial cells may be present singly, in groups (Figs 3.3–3.5), may form pseudopapillary structures or may form small gland-like structures. Reactive atypia may be extreme with multinucleation, enlarged nuclei, nuclear membrane irregularities, nuclear hyperchromasia, prominent nucleoli (Fig. 3.25) and mitoses.

### Pulmonary embolism and Infarction

Reactive mesothelial cells may resemble adenocarcinoma cells. The effusions usually also have increased haemosiderin laden macrophages, neutrophils and eosinophils.[30]

### Systemic lupus erythematosus (SLE)[37,181]

SLE effusions usually involve the pleural cavities, followed in frequency by the pericardial cavity. Effusions characteristically

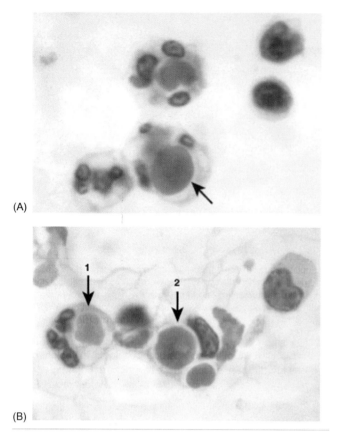

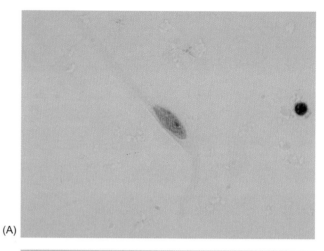

(A)

(B)

**Fig. 3.50** LE bodies (arrows) in this pleural effusion from a patient with a history of systemic lupus erythematosus (SLE) (ThinPrep), LE bodies in neutrophils (arrow 1 in B), LE bodies in macrophage (arrow 2 in B), (A, DQ cytospin; B, PAP). (Reproduced from Shidham and Atkinson 2007.[1])

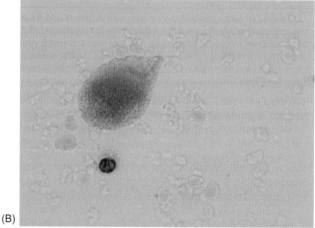

(A)

(B)

**Fig. 3.51** Rheumatoid effusion (pleural fluid). This turbid specimen showed significant amorphous debris in the background of a relatively hypocellular specimen with scanty inflammatory cells and a few spindle cells (A), and with scanty degenerate mesothelial cells (B). This could be a potential pitfall leading to a false positive interpretation as squamous cell carcinoma, sarcomatoid carcinoma, or sarcoma with extensive necrosis especially in the absence of a clinical history or in patients with a concomitant mass lesion (PAP SurePath (Autocyte) preparation).

are exudative and show a predominance of inflammatory cells (neutrophils, rarely eosinophils or lymphocytes) with the presence of LE cells.

LE cells are usually neutrophils, but can be macrophages, filled with homogeneous, basophilic nuclear material known as a *haematoxylin body* (Fig. 3.50). Their number in any SLE effusion is variable, and they may not be present consistently in all cases. Although characteristic of SLE, they are not pathognomonic, and may also be associated with various drug toxicities.

## Rheumatoid effusions[37,182]

Pleural effusion is a rare complication of rheumatoid arthritis, concurrently or after the development of joint manifestations. The effusions are exudative with a low glucose level and affect males more frequently than females. The cytological features include many degenerate cells, much necrotic debris, and some bland spindle cells. The inflammatory cells include histiocytes, multinucleated giant cells (Fig. 3.51) and many lymphoplasmacytic cells. However, not all rheumatoid effusions show these characteristic features, and some effusions may only show increased inflammatory cells with neutrophils, lymphocytes and mononuclear cells. Reactive mesothelial cells are either absent or rare.

Necrosis in an effusion is considered characteristic of a rheumatoid nodule. Spindle cells with varying degrees of degeneration may raise the differential diagnosis of squamous cell

carcinoma with potential false positive interpretation as cancer and sarcomatoid mesothelioma.

## Other causes

Depending on geographic and other factors further causes of reactive effusions include: parasites, other infections such as tuberculosis, asbestos exposure associated effusions, talc associated effusions, effusions due to fistulous tract and endometriosis.

### Parasitic causes

In any effusion of unclear cause parasitic infections should be considered. The causative parasites vary depending on the geographic situation, occupational background of the patient and also on the type of serous cavity specimen. The effusion may be reactive to parasitosis or by direct involvement of the serous cavity.[183] The evidence of parasitic cause ranges from direct demonstration of parasites to one of the stages such as cyst, ova, larvae, etc. Various parasites that have been reported to cause effusions include amoebiasis, cystic hydatid disease,

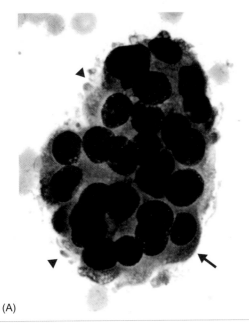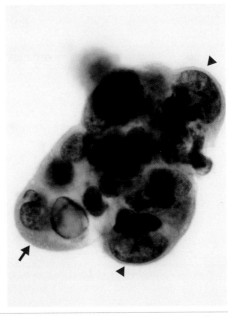

(A)                                                           (B)

**Fig. 3.52** Malignant epithelioid mesothelioma (pleural fluid). Large groups of mesothelial cells with many cells in each group in a papillary configuration. The neoplastic mesothelial cells show a knobbly outline mostly formed by cytoplasm (arrows in A,B). Diff-Quik-stained preparation highlights the blebs to further confirm their mesothelial nature (arrowheads in (A). Although not common, sometimes the overt features of malignancy may be seen. They are better appreciated in PAP-stained preparations (B). Note thin rim of cytoplasm separating the nuclei from cell borders (arrowheads in B) in neoplastic mesothelial cells (A, DQ Cytospin; B, PAP SurePath).

paragonimiasis, pneumocystosis, Loeffler's syndrome, micro-filaria, tropical pulmonary eosinophilia, toxocariasis, anisakiasis, hypodermiasis, strongyloidiasis, schistosomiasis, pentastomids, *Mansonella* sp. and others.[183–187]

## Mesothelioma

### General discussion

Malignant mesotheliomas[33] arise from mesothelial cells lining the pleural, peritoneal and pericardial cavities. Pleural mesotheliomas are the commonest (~90%) (Fig. 3.52), followed by peritoneal and pericardial mesotheliomas (6–10%). Other sites such as the tunica vaginalis are extremely rare.

During the 1960s the first definite link between mesothelioma and asbestos exposure was made. Asbestos is a natural mineral which is mined from rock and is found in many countries. The majority of mesothelioma cases are associated with asbestos exposure. In many patients diagnosed with mesothelioma, the exposure would have happened 20–40 years previously and, in some cases, it may be longer. In the UK, there is financial help through government benefits and compensation from employers. The Child Maintenance & Other Payments Act 2008 is new legislation in the UK which allows an up-front lump sum payment to be made within 6 weeks of presenting a claim to the Department of Works and Pensions.

Most cases present with breathlessness and pleuritic pain associated with recurrent, unilateral, bloody pleural effusions. As collection of effusions is relatively simple, cytopathological evaluation is of great clinical significance in the diagnosis of mesothelioma but cytological interpretation of effusions of unknown aetiology is generally not straightforward, with relatively high false-negative rates mostly related to sampling

**Table 3.5** Working classification of mesothelial-related neoplasms

| Malignant mesothelioma | Epithelial |
| --- | --- |
| | Biphasic |
| | Sarcomatous |
| Unusual or rare variants[33] | Clear cell, decimoid, lymphohistiocytoid, signet ring and small cell type |
| Other neoplasms of mesothelial origin or differentiation | Well-differentiated papillary mesothelioma of peritoneum |
| | Cystic mesothelioma |
| | Adenomatoid tumour of male and female genital tract |
| Neoplasms likely to be of subserosal origin | Benign fibrous tumour of pleura (so-called localised fibrous mesothelioma, benign pleural fibroma) |
| | Localised malignant fibrous tumours of pleura |

artefact. This is further affected by the widely acknowledged challenge of distinguishing reactive and neoplastic mesothelial cells, and of separating mesothelioma cells from adenocarcinoma cells. Application of various ancillary tests including immunocyto/histochemistry is therefore highly recommended. They are routinely performed in most centres.[60,74,188]

The main histological types of mesothelioma are listed in Table 3.5. Epithelial (epithelioid) and mixed (biphasic) types are the commonest, while the sarcomatoid type is rarely seen in effusion cytology. *In situ* mesothelioma is a recognised entity histologically. Rare types of mesothelioma, not related to asbestos exposure include the cystic mesothelioma of peritoneum and mesothelioma of the tunica vaginalia testis.

**Table 3.6** Comparison of reactive mesothelial cells and mesothelioma in effusions

| | Feature | Reactive mesothelial cells | Mesothelioma |
|---|---|---|---|
| **Quantitative features** | | | |
| 1 | Specimens cellularity | Moderate to low | Hypercellular |
| 2 | Size of cell groups | Relatively smaller | Relatively larger |
| 3 | Number of cells in each group | Usually few | Usually more |
| **Qualitative features** | | | |
| 1 | Morphology of cell groups | Mainly mono-layered with knobbly outlines | 2- and 3-dimensional cell groups with knobbly outlines |
| 2 | Cell size variability | Mild variation | Greater variation |
| 3 | Giant mesothelial cells and multinucleate cells | Usually absent | May be present |
| 4 | Peripheral cytoplasmic blebs and microvilli | Present, but not very prominent | Usually prominent |
| 5 | Nuclear features of malignancy – pleomorphic enlarged nuclei, prominent nucleoli, atypical mitoses | Not a feature | May be present |

**Table 3.7** Comparative cytomorphology of mesothelioma versus adenocarcinoma in effusions

| Feature | Mesothelioma | Adenocarcinoma |
|---|---|---|
| Specimen celluarity | Hypercellular | Hypercellular |
| Cell groups | Two- and three-dimensional | Two- and three-dimensional |
| Outlines to groups | Knobbly | Smooth ('community borders') |
| Acinar formations | Usually absent | Usually present |
| Cellular variability | Present | Usually present |
| Abnormal cells | Giant mesothelial cells present | Bizarre malignant cells present |
| Overt features of malignancy – pleomorphic enlarged nuclei, prominent nucleoli, and atypical mitoses | Present, but usually subtle | Are usually present |
| Two-zone cytoplasmic appearance | Present | Absent |
| Intercellular windows | Present: large windows may resemble acini | Absent: narrow acini may resemble windows |
| Cytoplasmic blebs with microvilli | Present | Absent |
| Distinct 'foreign' second population | Absent | Present |

## Cytological features of mesothelioma

Classical descriptions of mesothelioma cells were published in 1957 by Dr. A.I. Spriggs in his textbook *The Cytology of Effusions*,[189] and in subsequent publications, culminating in the *Atlas of Serous Fluid Cytopathology*.[190] The morphology of cells in effusions has never been better displayed.

Due to the significant overlap between benign and malignant mesothelial cells, and between mesothelioma and adenocarcinoma cells, cytological diagnosis of mesothelioma is difficult. However, an approach evaluating quantitative and qualitative aspects of effusions simplifies interpretation (Tables 3.6, 3.7).[191,192] Evaluation of both nuclear (PAP) and cytoplasmic (Romanowsky) characteristics is necessary for identifying discriminatory features of mesothelial cells and adenocarcinoma cells.[71] Cell blocks allow proper immunocytochemical evaluation along with the additional benefit of a secondary cytomorphological perspective.[37]

### Cytological findings: mesothelioma

- Hypercellular smears
- Single enlarged cells of mesothelial type and in sheets
- Three-dimensional groups with scalloped contours, sometimes papillary with stromal core
- Wide intercellular windows
- Nuclei central, variable enlargement, may be multinucleated
- Nucleoli often visible
- Mitotic figures may be present
- Cytoplasmic metachromasia, vacuoles, blebs
- Cell-in-cell arrangements
- Frankly malignant nuclear changes are not common.

Epithelial mesothelioma effusions are generally hypercellular, whereas the spindle cell components in biphasic and sarcomatoid mesotheliomas do not usually exfoliate well.[193] Quantitatively, epithelial mesothelioma effusions have many monolayered sheets and three-dimensional cell groups (Fig. 3.37). Qualitatively, these groups may show a variety of features, but the characteristic description is irregular knobbly outlines (Fig. 3.54). Some cases have a papillary architecture (Fig. 3.53). Acini associated with adenocarcinoma are not seen in mesotheliomas, but wide intercellular windows may be misinterpreted as acini (Fig. 3.54). The cytological features include the presence of a single malignant mesothelial cell population, multinucleation, intercellular windows, cell-in-cell arrangements, cytoplasmic vacuoles, peripheral blebs, groups with knobbly outlines (scalloped borders), variable nuclear enlargement, prominent nucleoli and cytoplasmic metachromasia.

In comparison, benign effusions with reactive, non-neoplastic mesothelial cells are usually hypocellular with smaller cell groups that are mostly two-dimensional (Figs 3.21, Table 3.6). Individual mesothelial cells may show considerable reactive changes approaching atypia in some clinical conditions, but the two-dimensional nature of the cell groups is retained in most benign effusions. Adenocarcinomas do show three-dimensional and complex cell groups, but they generally have smooth contours (community borders) (Fig. 3.24) in contrast to the knobbly outlines of mesothelioma cell groups (Figs 3.12, 3.52).

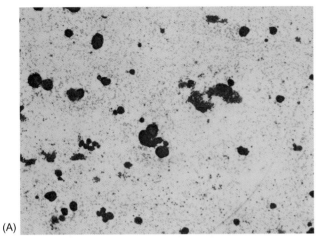

(A)

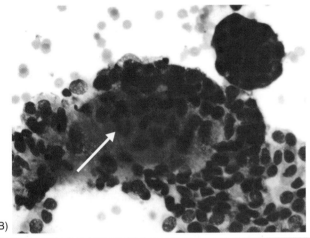

(B)

**Fig. 3.53** Malignant epithelioid mesothelioma (pleural fluid). Large groups of mesothelial cells (A) with many cells in each group in a papillary configuration (B). Some papillary groups show stromal cores (arrow), which are not observed in proliferation spheres of carcinoma (Figs 3.39, 3.40) (DQ Cytospin smear).

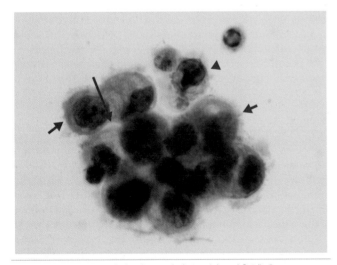

**Fig. 3.54** Malignant epithelioid mesothelioma (pleural fluid). Groups of atypical mesothelial cells with mesothelial windows are seen (long arrow) due to microvilli between the cells. The knobbly outline formed predominantly by cytoplasm with microvillous fuzzy outlines (short arrows) also favours mesothelioma. Rare malignant mesothelial cells show apoptosis (arrowhead). Immunocytochemistry with SCIP approach confirmed these cells as mesothelial without a second population of foreign cells. The clinical and cytomorphological (both quantitative and qualitative) features were consistent with mesothelioma (PAP SurePath).

Individual mesothelioma cells are larger with frequent variation in cell size. However, they still resemble mesothelial cells, fitting in the wide morphological spectrum of mesothelial cells, and do not suggest a second population. Giant mesothelial cells may be present.[33] Such cells are usually absent in benign effusions and adenocarcinoma. However, bizarre malignant cells are rare and generally suggest another neoplasm.

Cytoplasmic vacuoles are a non-specific finding, and glycogen- or lipid-containing vacuoles may be seen in mesothelial cells. Lipid vacuoles are centrally located. Glycogen vacuoles seen as golden yellow colour on the PAP stain, are periodic–acid Schiff positive and are peripheral. Mucin vacuoles of adenocarcinoma are usually irregular and push the nucleus eccentrically. However, they may resemble degenerative vacuoles, which usually have indistinct margins in contrast to the sharp distinct margins of mucin vacuoles containing targetoid mucin in the centre. A mucin stain may help to identify adenocarcinoma.

In some cases of mesothelioma the general cytological features of malignancy also apply. The nuclei may be irregular, pleomorphic and enlarged with prominent nucleoli including macronucleoli. Bi- and multinucleation can be seen, and rarely, there are atypical mitoses. These features are usually subtle and require careful scrutiny.

An additional useful feature is stromal hyaluronic acid[33] seen as a metachromatic background in Romanowsky-stained direct smears, and as a fluffy pale green/blue background in PAP-stained direct smears. Stromal cores may be seen within papillary clusters (Fig. 3.53B).

Spindle cells exfoliate sparingly in effusions. They become polyhedral secondary to the surface tension phenomenon and may be difficult to appreciate. Scattered atypical spindle cells are suspicious for mesothelioma.[33]

## Rare variants

Morphological variants of mesothelioma are reported mostly as retrospective case reports recognised in the light of a subsequent histological diagnosis. It is important to be conversant with their morphology to avoid misinterpretation. Clinical history, radiological findings and ancillary studies are significant for differentiating mesothelioma from other conditions. Some rare variants with their cytological features are described below:[33]

### Clear cell pattern

The mesothelioma cells predominantly show clear cytoplasm. However, epithelioid mesothelial cells with conventional morphology are usually admixed in varying proportions. The main cytological differential diagnosis includes tumours with clear cell features, including renal cell carcinoma of clear cell type and clear cell carcinoma of the lung metastasising to the pleura. Immunoreactivity for mesothelial immunohistochemical markers in neoplastic cells with clear cytoplasm is an excellent ancillary test for confirming their mesothelial nature.[60,74]

### Deciduoid pattern[194]

The mesothelioma cells are large, round to polygonal, with abundant glassy eosinophilic cytoplasm and regular cell borders (Fig. 3.55). The cytoplasm may still show a two-zone pattern with a paler outer and glassy inner zone. The nuclei with

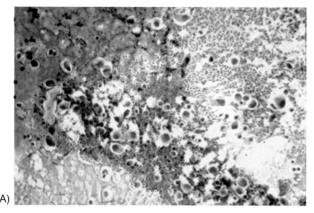

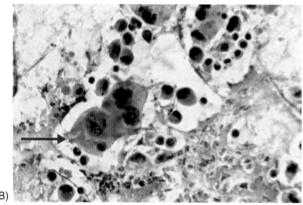

**Fig. 3.55** Peritoneal fluid with deciduoid mesothelioma. (A) Discohesive, scattered, single, atypical, enlarged mesothelial cells. (B) Enlarged malignant cells with a binucleate form and glassy cytoplasm (arrow). Scattered smaller atypical mesothelial cells are present in the background (PAP direct smear). (Courtesy of Dr Bernard Naylor). (Reproduced from Shidham and Atkinson 2007.[1])

prominent nucleoli have vesicular chromatin. Pleomorphism with binucleation and multinucleation may be present, but mitotic figures are infrequent.

## Lymphohistiocytoid pattern[195]

The mesothelioma cells show histiocytoid morphology with inflammatory mononuclear cells in the background. Histologically, this variant is associated with an unequivocal sarcomatous component, but as highlighted previously the spindle cells may not exfoliate well. All these features impede correct interpretation. Atypical mesothelial cells with histiocytoid morphology, admixed with a rich inflammatory infiltrate, should raise suspicion of this entity in the proper clinical scenario. Ancillary immunohistochemical studies would be decisive in most of these cases.[60,74,195]

## Signet-ring pattern

The mesothelioma cells with cytoplasmic lipid-rich vacuoles push the nucleus eccentrically and resemble signet-ring cells associated with signet-ring cell adenocarcinoma. However, the cells do not contain mucin and are negative for mucicarmine stain.[196]

## Small cell pattern

The mesothelioma cells of this type are small, uniform, round cells with bland nuclei and high nuclear/cytoplasmic ratios.[188]

They may resemble small round cell tumours metastatic to the pleura but the cells are not reactive for neuroendocrine immunomarkers.

### Diagnostic pitfalls: mesothelioma

Factors responsible for false negative results include coexistent fibrinous pleuritis preventing exfoliation of diagnostic cells into the effusion, inadequate samples (quantitative), presence of excess blood, and the basic challenge due to the cytologically bland appearance of mesothelioma cells. Large aggregates of disorganised reactive mesothelial cells may lead to false positive results.

As highlighted previously, quantitative and qualitative clues simplify the interpretation in concert with ancillary tests such as immunocytochemistry on cell block sections with the SCIP approach in correlation with clinico-radiological data. Quantitative clues include hypercellularity with numerous solitary mesothelial cells and large groups of mesothelial cells. Qualitative clues are increased numbers of cells in individual three-dimensional large groups of mesothelial cells. Most of these features are more easily evaluated in Romanowsky-stained preparations. Comparison of various cytological features of reactive mesothelial cells, malignant mesothelial cells, and adenocarcinoma cells are summarised in Tables 3.6, 3.7.

## Special stains in mesothelioma

Although less sensitive than immunocytochemistry, histochemistry performed on cell block sections is a simple approach for distinguishing mesothelioma from adenocarcinoma.

Hyaluronic acid, an acidic mucin, is associated with mesothelioma and is seen in the background[33] of direct smears of effusion fluids. It is positive for acidic mucin stains such as Alcian blue, disappearing after hyaluronidase predigestion.

Adenocarcinoma cells produce neutral (epithelial) mucin seen as intracytoplasmic staining with mucicarmine stain. It is also PAS-positive (diastase-resistant). Glycogen, which is present in mesothelial cells, disappears with diastase digestion.

A positive mucicarmine stain for epithelial mucin is diagnostic of adenocarcinoma, but a negative result does not rule it out.

## Mesothelioma and immunocytochemistry

Morphology alone may be insufficient to distinguish mesothelioma and adenocarcinoma in effusion fluids. Currently, immunocytochemistry on effusion fluid cell block sections is an excellent ancillary test for objective interpretation. However, performance and interpretation of immunocytochemistry in effusion fluids is tricky and challenging without proper evaluation by the SCIP approach.[60,74] The antibodies most helpful in diagnosing mesothelioma are shown in Table 3.4.

## Other ancillary methods

Electron microscopy may be performed on cells in effusions to distinguish adenocarcinoma cells from mesothelial cells,[197,198] but microvilli do not distinguish reactive from malignant mesothelial cells. It is also difficult to decide if the cells under scrutiny are actually reactive mesothelial cells from the effusion, or the population of abnormal cells that are to be evaluated.[33] With progressive refinements in immunocytochemical techniques, including the introduction of newer immunomarkers, the role of electron microscopy in evaluating effusion fluids for mesothelioma has regressed considerably.

## Metastatic carcinoma in effusion fluids

## General discussion[4]

Any neoplasm, including rare examples of central nervous system tumours,[31] may involve serous cavities and manifest as a malignant effusion. Adenocarcinoma metastatic to serous cavities is the most common cause.[199] The spread may be direct to the serous cavities by extension of a primary malignancy of a serosa-lined organ such as lung, intestine, liver or ovary. Carcinomas from most of the sites metastasise via the lymphatics. The serosal lining is rich in lymphatic channels which open through stoma (narrow gaps) into the serous cavities.[3] The carcinoma cells spread through these and lead to an effusion.[4]

### Cytological findings and diagnostic pitfalls: metastatic carcinoma

The cytomorphology of reactive mesothelial cells, forming a major or minor component of malignant effusions, may overlap significantly with cancer cells from some sites such as the breast and ovary.[9] The most important issue is avoidance of a false positive interpretation, which may subject the patient to improper management decisions and emotional distress. Reciprocally, well-differentiated and low-grade adenocarcinoma cells may resemble reactive mesothelial cells and lead to false negative interpretation (Table 3.8).[4,16,200]

An aspect complicating this process further is the possibility of changes associated with radiation and other therapy effects. Radiotherapy effects include bizarre cells in effusions with: cytomegaly, degenerative hyperchromasia and two-tone staining (cyanophilia – blue/green and acidophilia – pink). Vacuolation of cytoplasm due to degeneration may deform the nucleus, the chromatin is often smudgy and mitotic figures are present.[201] Although usually associated with irradiation, these are not specific. They may lead to false-positive interpretation, suggesting recurrence of the initial disease. Additional potential pitfalls include: poorly preserved, degenerate or scanty cells in improperly processed specimens. In such cases resubmission of a properly preserved effusion specimen with revaluation after optimum processing should be recommended. Malignant effusions usually re-accumulate and contain unequivocal cancer cells, with improved morphology.[71]

In addition to detecting metastatic carcinoma cells in effusions, cytomorphological evaluation can also suggest or confirm the primary site of origin (Table 3.8, Fig. 3.35) with help of the clinical history, radiological findings, and ancillary tests such as immunocytochemistry.[60,74] However, if it does not change the clinical management, this exercise of identifying the primary site may just be an intellectual curiosity.[74] Although there is a significant overlap amongst different neoplasms, many show characteristic cytomorphological features such as intercellular windows, papillary configurations, Indian file pattern, etc.[202]

A summary of the characteristic features favouring some metastatic carcinomas from specific primary sites is shown in Table 3.8 and Figs 3.57–3.71, 3.73, 3.76–3.82.[4]

## Haematolymphoid disorders

## General discussion

Usually discohesive cells in cytology specimens favour a haematolymphoid process (Figs 3.74, 3.75, 3.83–3.87),[1,203] whereas the presence of cohesive groups rules it out but this is not absolute and exceptions are not unusual, either, as a natural *in vivo* phenomenon or due to *in vitro* artefact.[34,88] A few examples are lymphocytes in tuberculous effusions[203,204] and serosal lymphoma simulating carcinoma (anaplastic large cell lymphoma) showing apparent 'glands', 'papillary' structures, and cytoplasmic vacuoles.[205]

On the other hand, the cells of melanoma and desmoplastic small round cell tumour (Fig. 3.88) may be seen as solitary cells or as loose clusters resembling a haematolymphoid process.[37] In contrast to FNA material from solid specimens, classic lymphoglandular bodies (representing remnants of lymphocyte cytoplasm) are typically inconspicuous or absent in effusions secondary to haematolymphoid disorders.

In addition to deducing the lymphoid nature of cells, the major challenge in cytological evaluation of haematolymphoid effusions is distinguishing between low-grade lymphoma and reactive lymphocytosis. This may be impossible by morphology alone, since cellular atypia is often minimal or absent.[34,88] However, with high-grade lymphomas, the challenge is different and involves a differential diagnosis of undifferentiated sarcoma and carcinoma. Integration of cytological findings (Figs 3.74, 3.75, 3.83–3.87) with the clinical history and immunophenotype data (immunostains and/or flow cytometry) with or without molecular studies[88] provides accurate diagnosis and classification in most cases.

In *adults*, lymphoma is the third most common cause of a malignant pleural effusion after lung and breast carcinoma,[206–209] leading to approximately 10% of all malignant *pleural effusions*. It also ranks third after ovary (32%) and breast (13%) carcinoma, leading to 7% of malignant *peritoneal effusions*.[204,205] In *children*, haemopoietic neoplasms are the most common cause of malignant effusions.[36] Usually there is a clinical history with a prior tissue diagnosis of lymphoma/leukaemia.

Haematolymphoid disorders affecting the serous cavities may be categorised in different ways. They may be divided based on the predominant cells in the effusion – lymphocytic and non-lymphocytic effusions. Each may be reactive or malignant (Fig 3.56).[34,88]

## Lymphocytic effusions

Effusions with a lymphocyte differential cell count of more than 50% are defined as lymphocytic effusions.[208–210] They may be either transudative or exudative and reactive or neoplastic depending on the aetiology of the effusion and the patient population.[34,88,210]

**Table 3.8** Cytomorphological features suggestive of different primary sites in metastatic effusions

| Cytomorphology | Possible primary carcinoma | Cytomorphology | Possible primary carcinoma |
|---|---|---|---|
| **Architecture-based features** | | **Individual cellular features** | |
| Predominantly scattered isolated malignant cells | Gastric adenocarcinoma | Extensive cytoplasmic vacuolation | Renal cell carcinoma (glycogen, fat) |
| | Non-cohesive variant of lung adenocarcinoma | | Adrenocortical carcinoma (fat) |
| | Breast lobular carcinoma | | Benign mesothelial cells |
| | Adrenocortical carcinoma | | Pancreatic adenocarcinoma (mucin) |
| | Also lymphoma, melanoma and sarcoma) | | Ovarian adenocarcinoma (mucin) |
| | | | Lung adenocarcinoma |
| | | | Clear cell carcinoma endometrium |
| Three-dimensional round cell groups – proliferation spheres or 'cannonballs' | Breast adenocarcinoma | Targetoid intracytoplasmic vacuole containing secretion | Breast adenocarcinoma (especially lobular) |
| | Ovarian adenocarcinoma | | Thyroid carcinoma (colloid) |
| | Mesothelioma of epithelioid type | | Ovarian carcinoma |
| | Reactive mesothelial proliferations | | Pancreatic carcinoma |
| Acini/glands | Adenocarcinoma of breast, lung, colorectum, stomach, ovary, endometrium, etc. | Prominent nucleoli | Hepatocellular carcinoma |
| | | | Renal cell carcinoma |
| | Mesothelioma of epithelioid type | | Prostatic adenocarcinoma |
| Three-dimensional groups in papillary configurations | Bronchioloalveolar carcinoma | Signet ring cells | Gastric adenocarcinoma |
| | | | Colorectal adenocarcinoma |
| | Colonic adenocarcinoma | Cytoplasmic pigment | Hepatocellular carcinoma (bile pigmento) |
| | Endometrial adenocarcinoma | | Melanoma (melanin) |
| | Breast adenocarcinoma | | |
| Three-dimensional papillary groups containing psammoma bodies | Ovarian carcinoma – serous papillary | Small cells | Small cell carcinoma of lung |
| | | | Carcinoma of breast (lobular) |
| | | | Non-Hodgkin lymphoma (low grade) |
| | Thyroid papillary carcinoma | Giant tumour cells | Lung large cell carcinoma (giant cell type) |
| | Pancreatic papillary carcinoma | | Pancreatic adenocarcinoma |
| Carcinoma cells in chains and rows ('Indian file' pattern) | Breast – lobular and ductal carcinoma | | Thyroid anaplastic carcinoma |
| | | | Squamous cell carcinoma |
| | Poorly differentiated small cell carcinoma | | Melanoma and pleomorphic sarcoma |
| | Gastric adenocarcinoma | Cellular pleomorphism | Poorly differentiated carcinomas of lung, pancreas, ovary, thyroid, urothelium |
| | Ovarian adenocarcinoma | Sharp angulated cell borders with keratinisation | Keratinising squamous cell carcinoma |
| *Pseudomyxoma peritonei* | Mucinous neoplasms of ovary and appendix | Squamous cells | Squamous cell carcinomas |
| | Carcinoma of pancreas, endocervix and breast | Spindle cells | Sarcomas |
| | | | Spindle cell carcinoma |
| Cell groups of tall columnar cells with a picket fence pattern | Colonic adenocarcinoma | | Melanoma |
| | | | Mesothelioma |
| | Pancreato-biliary carcinoma | Large polyhedral cells | Hepatocellular carcinoma |
| | | | Transitional cell carcinoma |
| (Modified from Shidham 2007.[4]) | | | Large cell type squamous cell carcinoma |

Lymphomatous and leukaemic pleural effusions are classically exudative. Effusions with negative cytology in cases with lymphoma/leukaemia may be due to blockage of lymphatic drainage or the presence of a concurrent unrelated condition causing effusion.[211] Transudative lymphocytic effusions may be present in cases with renal failure or heart failure.[212]

About 20% of pleural effusions in cases with Hodgkin lymphoma are due to obstruction of mediastinal or pulmonary lymphatic drainage.[213] Chylothorax is produced by accumulation of lymphatic fluid in the pleural spaces. It is associated with increased levels of triglyceride in effusion fluids: a level over 110 mg/dL is highly suggestive of a chylous effusion.[214] Of malignant effusions with chylothorax 50% are secondary to lymphoma.[206]

## Non-lymphocytic effusions

These effusions are either reactive or neoplastic. The haemopoietic cells present may comprise eosinophils, neutrophil polymorphs or histiocytes.[34]

## Metastatic sarcomas, melanoma and other neoplastic effusions

### General discussion

Some examples of non-epithelial neoplasms leading to malignant effusions include malignant melanoma, sarcomas, germ cell tumours and some paediatric malignant tumours. In these associations there usually is history of a known primary tumour. These effusions are relatively more frequent in children than in adults. In fact in paediatric population, the commonest causes of malignant effusions include lymphoma and leukaemia, followed by other non-epithelial neoplasms such as Wilms' tumour, neuroblastoma, Ewing sarcoma and embryonal rhabdomyosarcoma.[35]

Sarcomas are rare cause of malignant effusions and account for only 3–6%. Identifying the primary of these non-epithelial malignancies based on cytomorphology alone is difficult, because they often exhibit variable morphological features in effusions different from the initial primary tumour. However, with proper clinical history, the diagnosis is generally straightforward and simple comparison of the tumour morphology in cell block sections of effusion preparations with the original primary tumour may be sufficient. However, depending on the clinical scenario, ancillary studies may be performed to help the interpretation (Fig. 3.88).[35,88,122]

Studies reporting cytological features of sarcomas in effusions are relatively uncommon.[35] Surface tension related interference and alterations due to the surrounding fluid alter the cells in to polyhedral configuration with loss of architectural features which usually are obvious in the fine-needle aspiration specimens. Most of these specimens are sparsely cellular with a few solitary cells or loose clusters. The sarcoma cells may show indistinct cytoplasmic borders with bipolar cytoplasmic processes. The neoplastic cells may be binucleated or multinucleated with round, oval and sometimes fusiform or spindle-shaped nuclei. The nuclei usually demonstrate obvious features of malignancy with irregular outlines and frequent nuclear membrane infolding. The chromatin is clumped with parachromatin clearing.

The nuclei are usually prominent. The high-grade sarcomas usually show a significant number of mitotic figures. These nuclear features can be evaluated better in PAP-stained preparations than in DQ-stained preparations.[1] Background is an additional feature to support interpretation of sarcoma, because most the effusions secondary to metastatic sarcoma have proteinaceous background with altered blood and a few inflammatory cells.[35]

## Malignant effusions: evaluation of unknown primary

### General discussion[83,84,176]

Despite the grave prognosis imparted by a diagnosis of malignant effusion, it is clinically important to determine the primary site of origin (Fig. 3.35)[4,176]. Malignant effusions caused by lymphomas, breast cancer, ovarian cancer and small cell lung carcinoma may respond to systemic chemotherapy or hormonal therapy, as compared with effusions secondary to therapy-resistant cancers, such as non-small cell lung carcinoma, which are approached with palliative measures, such as pleurodesis or a pleuroperitoneal shunt.[215,216]

Paradoxically, malignant mesothelioma as a primary tumour of serous cavities needs to be confirmed, especially in patients with a history of asbestos exposure with potential medico-legal implications (see p. 151).[1] Evaluating the primary site of origin includes proper correlation of various findings at different levels mentioned below.

### Clinical findings

Correlation with clinical history is the simplest and most dependable factor, as in most cases there is history of a malignant neoplasm. The cytomorphology of the malignant cells in the current fluid specimen should correspond to that of the primary neoplasm. Review of any prior surgical and/or cytological materials may help in some cases, but not all, due to effusion related secondary morphological alterations.[217] In addition, the cytomorphology of some primary sites may overlap significantly and objective confirmation of the origin of the malignant cells may not be straightforward without ancillary tests.

Depending on the clinical scenario and the cytological picture, clinical details can be misleading, resulting in a false positive interpretation. However the availability of clinical history on the request form plays a critical role in directing proper triaging and processing of effusion specimens, in order to avoid suboptimal cytopathological interpretation.

A clinical history of a previous malignancy may not be available in all cases and in some patients a malignant effusion may be the initial presentation.[218] This has been reported in 7–14% of patients with pleural and ascitic effusions.[219] The location of the effusion along with age and sex of the patient narrow the differential diagnosis: An ovarian primary is an important differential in an elderly female,[220] and gastrointestinal tract is a favoured primary in adult males with malignant ascites.[221] Lung cancer is a frequent primary site in both males and females with malignant pleural effusions in the adult group. In females, breast cancer is an additional possible primary.

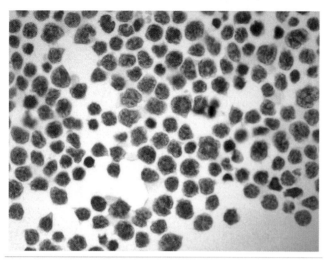

**Fig. 3.56** Single-cell pattern in a malignant lymphoma. The specimen consists of a monotonous population of discohesive atypical lymphocytes with irregular nuclear contours and hyperchromasia (DQ Cytospin preparation, PAP). (Reproduced from Shidham and Atkinson 2007.[1])

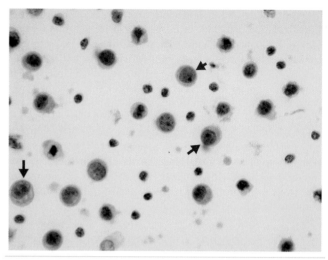

**Fig. 3.57** Single-cell population of malignant cells (gastric carcinoma, ascitic fluid). Most of the cells are neoplastic cells (arrows) which are relatively difficult to distinguish from reactive mesothelial cells (not present in this field). Such cells may be interpreted as reactive mesothelial cells in the absence of a second foreign population (PAP SurePath).

Malignant effusions are relatively uncommon in children and most are secondary to malignant lymphomas and leukaemias. Other primaries include the so-called small blue cell tumours of childhood such as neuroblastoma, Wilms tumour, and rhabdomyosarcoma.[37,222] Additional rare examples include germ cell tumour and osteosarcoma.

## Cytology[4]

Primary tumours from various sites usually have characteristic cytomorphology, and often the cytomorphology of metastases resembles that of the primary tumour, but in the case of effusions, resemblance may be remote. However, some cytomorphological features may still be applicable in the differential diagnosis, at least in broad sense. These are broadly categorised into architecture and cell morphology (Table 3.8).

### Architecture (Table 3.8)

#### Single cell pattern
*Haematolymphoid malignancies*: Typically these present with a single cell pattern without any 'tissue' aggregates (Fig. 3.56). It is important to recognise haematological malignancies for instituting effective management. Lymphoma or leukaemia seldom present as an effusion without a known history,[34] except in cases with an initial effusion presentation of systemic disease or in cases of primary effusion lymphoma.[223,224]

Generally, there is a monomorphic lymphoid population with or without reactive mesothelial cells. In Hodgkin lymphoma Reed–Sternberg cells may be seen in a background of mixed lymphocytes, eosinophils and plasma cells. Although chronic inflammation is polymorphic, florid processes such as tuberculosis may be difficult to distinguish from lymphoma on morphology alone. Immunophenotyping with techniques such as flow cytometry is indicated to evaluate the reactive nature of the cells. Additionally flow cytometry can sub-classify non-Hodgkin lymphomas and leukaemias (see Ch. 33).[34]

*Epithelial malignancies*: Some cases may show a solitary, non-cohesive cell population. The usual primary sites are breast,

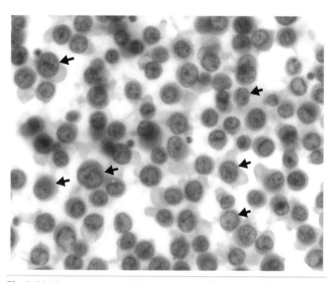

**Fig. 3.58** Metastatic non-small cell carcinoma of lung (pleural fluid). Singly scattered, numerous, medium sized, pleomorphic carcinoma cells (arrows) show features overlapping with other anaplastic carcinomas. They constitute a predominant population. (Pitfall: this may be misinterpreted as other tumours with tendency for numerous isolated cells, e.g. large cell lymphomas, germ cell tumours and melanoma.) (PAP Cytospin).

stomach (Figs 3.38, 3.57), kidney, lung (Fig. 3.58) and prostate. Squamous cell carcinomas can also shed single cells into body cavity fluids and may resemble reactive mesothelial cells, potentially a false negative pitfall.

*Other malignancies*: Melanoma cells are mostly solitary in effusions. With cytoplasmic melanin pigment, the diagnosis is often straightforward, however, the vast majority of melanomas are amelanotic. The clinical history and immunocytochemistry help.[35]

*Small blue round cell tumours* (such as Ewing's sarcoma, neuroblastoma, etc.) often show non-cohesive, solitary, small, round to oval cells (see Ch. 33).[37,222]

### Solid cell ball pattern

These are also called a cannonball pattern or proliferation spheres (Fig. 3.39, 3.40) and consist of three-dimensional balls with smooth community borders (Fig. 3.41).

- Usually large enough to be seen at low power and rarely even to the naked eye
- The cohesive, tightly packed cells within the cell balls range from a few to several hundred
- They are typically seen in carcinomas of breast and ovary and very large cell balls in elderly women favour the ductal variant of infiltrating mammary carcinoma (Fig. 3.23)
- Other carcinomas with this pattern include lung, stomach and prostate.

Malignant mesothelioma cell balls and rarely, mesothelial hyperplasia, typically demonstrate a scalloped border.[2,33] Fusion of multiple spheres may resemble a papillary configuration which can be misinterpreted as a papillary neoplasm, potentially a pitfall (Fig. 3.61).

### Acini/glands

These may be relatively difficult to appreciate in cytology smears (Fig. 3.40), but are better seen in cell block sections (Fig. 3.39). Larger mesothelial windows may be misinterpreted as acini and artefactual clustering may entrap spaces resembling acini. The differential diagnosis also includes rosettes in blue cell tumours. When present and unequivocal (Fig. 3.59) their presence is consistent with adenocarcinoma.

### Papillary formation and psammoma bodies

- *Papillae* are three-dimensional, cohesive structures derived from papillary neoplasms. They may show fibrovascular cores and have one axis longer than the others (Figs 3.60–3.62). Individual cells in the clusters are usually polarised with nuclei arranged perpendicular to the long axis or to the fibrovascular cores. Possible primary sites include ovary (Fig. 3.61), thyroid gland, kidney and lung. Intranuclear cytoplasmic inclusions are seen in papillary carcinoma of the thyroid and bronchioloalveolar carcinoma. However, other non-papillary neoplasms with tendency for proliferation spheres may show papillary-like structures and may be misinterpreted as a papillary neoplasm (potential pitfall).
- *Psammoma bodies* are round to oval calcified structures with concentric lamellations (Fig. 3.61B) usually in association with papillary clusters. They represent degeneration and calcification of the cells within the papillae. In ascitic fluid from an elderly female patient they are highly suggestive of a metastatic ovarian carcinoma (Fig. 3.61). Other malignancies associated with psammoma bodies include primary peritoneal serous tumour, papillary carcinoma of the thyroid, bronchogenic carcinoma, malignant mesothelioma and, less frequently, breast and gastric carcinomas.[2,33]

Caution must be exercised not to misinterpret psammoma bodies and/or papillary formation in fluid specimens as unequivocal evidence of malignancy, especially in peritoneal fluid. Benign conditions such as: ovarian cystadenoma/cystadenofibroma, papillary mesothelial hyperplasia, endosalpingiosis, endometriosis and other miscellaneous benign diagnoses may

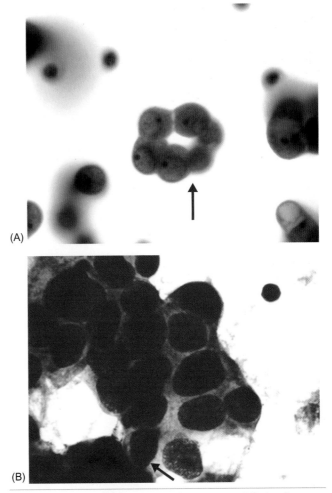

(A)

(B)

**Fig. 3.59** Glandular acini in metastatic adenocarcinoma (effusions from different cases). (A) Metastatic duodenal adenocarcinoma (ascitic fluid). (B) Metastatic breast adenocarcinoma (ascitic fluid). Formation of glandular acini (arrows) in both cases are clearly seen consistent with features of adenocarcinoma (A, PAP SurePath (Autocyte) preparation; B, DQ Cytospin).

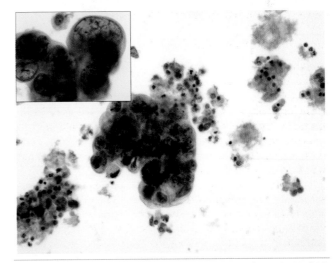

**Fig. 3.60** Metastatic papillary serous cystadenocarcinoma of ovary (ascitic fluid). Cohesive clusters showing papillary configurations under lower magnification. Higher magnification of other field (inset), highlights the features of malignancy in medium to large neoplastic cells. The overt features of malignancy with hyperchromatic nuclei, variation in nuclear sizes, irregularities in nuclear margins, and coarse clumped irregularly distributed chromatin with parachromatin clearing were distinctly seen in PAP-stained preparations (PAP ThinPrep).

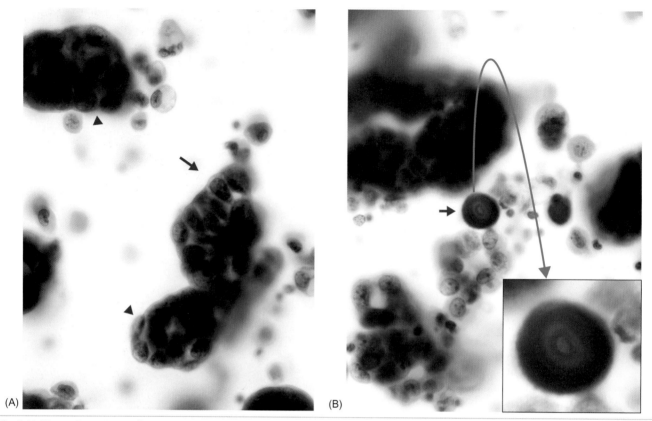

(A)

(B)

**Fig. 3.61** Metastatic ovarian papillary serous cystadenocarcinoma with psammoma bodies (ascitic fluid). Cohesive clusters or papillary structures (arrowheads in (A)) of medium to large cells with palisading along their periphery (arrow in (A)). A few Psammoma bodies (arrow in (B)) were present (PAP SurePath).

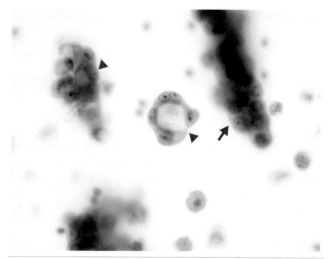

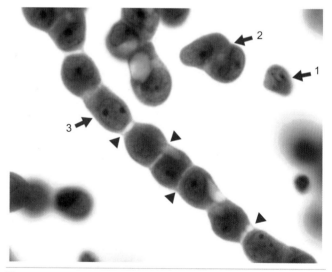

**Fig. 3.62** Metastatic mucinous papillary cystadenocarcinoma of the ovary (ascitic fluid). Cohesive clusters may show ill-defined papillary structures (arrow) without peripheral palisading. Some cells show cytoplasmic vacuoles (arrowheads). Psammoma bodies were absent (PAP SurePath).

**Fig. 3.63** Metastatic ovarian carcinoma (ascitic fluid). Solitary cells (1), small groups (2), or loosely cohesive groups in single cell file (3). They may be difficult to identify as a second population due to cytomorphologic overlap with reactive mesothelial cells. However, generally in higher grade tumours the morphologic differences are relatively overt to be identified as second population. Spaces between individual tumour cells may resemble 'mesothelial windows' and further mislead the interpretation (arrowheads) (PAP SurePath).

show psammoma bodies as found in one-third of the serous cavity fluid specimens.[18,27,217]

### Single file arrangement

This refers to alignment of tumour cells in a single row. Intercellular connections are noted in electron microscopy between the individual cells within the file. Long chains of small, bland-appearing cells favour infiltrating lobular mammary carcinoma. However, other neoplasms including infiltrating ductal carcinoma and ovarian carcinoma (Fig. 3.63) may show cells arranged in single file, but the cells are larger and more pleomorphic. Small cell carcinoma of the lung can also

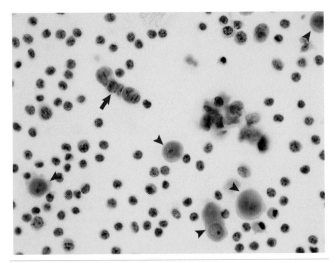

**Fig. 3.64** Metastatic small cell carcinoma of the lung (pleural fluid). The neoplastic cells (arrow) are arranged in a single cell file pattern (stack of coin pattern, Indian file pattern). Although common with lobular carcinoma and small cell carcinoma, this pattern is non-specific and may be observed with other tumours in effusions (see also Fig. 3.63). The background shows many chronic inflammatory cells with a few reactive mesothelial cells (arrowheads) (PAP SurePath).

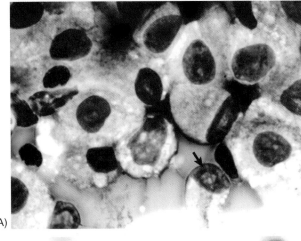

(A)

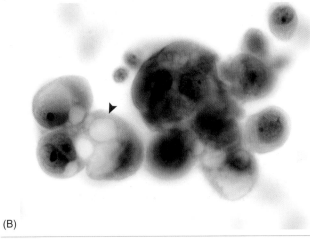

(B)

**Fig. 3.65** (A,B) Adenocarcinoma cells in group (ascitic fluid). Eccentric nucleus touches the cell periphery without a cytoplasmic rim in a few cells (arrow in (A)). Presence of multiple vacuoles (arrow head in (B)) may be due to degenerative changes and may not reflect true adenocarcinoma (A, DQ Cytospin smears; B, PAP SurePath).

show single file pattern with prominent nuclear moulding (Fig. 3.64). These have been described as 'stacks of dishes', 'piles of coins', or 'vertebral column'.[226] Individual cells show high N:C ratio with scant cytoplasm and 'salt and pepper' chromatin.

### Pseudomyxoma peritonei

This refers to the presence of a high content of mucin in ascitic fluid.[229,230] The mucin appears as light blue to magenta amorphous material with Diff-Quik stains. Solitary cells or small clusters of epithelial cells are scattered within the mucin. The individual cells often appear bland, with or without cytoplasmic mucinous vacuoles. In males, the appendix is the most common primary site. In females the ovary is most likely primary (mucinous cystadenoma and cystadenocarcinoma), while the appendix is the second most common primary site.[230] Other possible primaries include gastrointestinal and pancreatic cancers, endocervical adenocarcinoma and mucinous carcinomas, such as those occurring in the breast.[1,2]

## Cell morphology

### Extensive cytoplasmic vacuolation

This feature is seen in clear cell tumours. Many tumours show clear cell changes with a long differential diagnosis but the commonest in this category is renal cell carcinoma. The vacuolation is better seen in Diff-Quik-stained preparations, and is less clear with PAP stains. However, degenerative vacuolation is frequent in effusion specimens (Fig. 3.65) (potential pitfall).

### Targetoid intracytoplasmic vacuole containing secretion

True secretory vacuoles have sharp outlines (Fig. 3.69) with secretions, usually mucin, but other material such as colloid within the vacuole, may give a targetoid appearance. This is commonly seen in breast adenocarcinoma (especially lobular), thyroid carcinoma with colloid, ovarian and pancreatic carcinoma. Special stains such as mucicarmine highlight the mucin secretion in adenocarcinoma (Fig. 3.27).

### Prominent nucleoli

Prominent nucleoli on their own cannot be used for diagnosing malignancy. However, the finding can be critical for subtyping the neoplasm. The lack or inconspicuousness of nucleoli with the characteristic chromatin and other details is an important feature of small cell carcinoma. In addition to melanoma, prominent nucleoli raise the possibility of hepatocellular carcinoma, renal cell carcinoma, germ cell format, and prostatic adenocarcinoma.

### Signet ring cells

These are isolated neoplastic cells with a single large cytoplasmic vacuole pushing the nucleus to the cell periphery (Figs 3.67–3.69). The vacuole content is most likely to be mucin followed by lipid in renal cell carcinoma and, occasionally, immunoglobulin in plasma cells.[1,229,230] Individual cell nuclei show moderate to marked atypia. The most likely primary sites are stomach followed by breast, which is usually an infiltrating lobular carcinoma, having smaller cells than those of gastric carcinoma. Other malignancies include carcinomas of gall bladder, colon, pancreas and ovary. Degenerative changes in mesothelial cells may lead to a single large cytoplasmic vacuole. The lack of nuclear atypia is an important clue, as are features suggestive of a second population, especially seen in Diff-Quik-stained preparations.

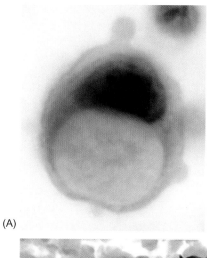

(A)

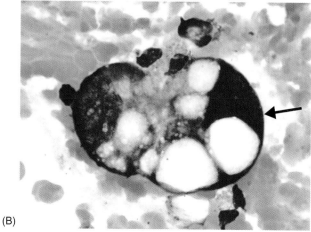

(B)

**Fig. 3.66** Secretory vacuoles. (A) Ovarian carcinoma, ascitic fluid; (B) gastric carcinoma, ascitic fluid. In contrast to degenerative vacuoles, the secretory vacuoles have a sharp outline and may show secretions (see Table 3.3). They usually indent the nucleus (arrows in (B)). They are seen more distinctly and easily in Diff-Quik-stained preparations (B). (A, PAP SurePath (Autocyte) preparation; B, DQ Cytospin smears).

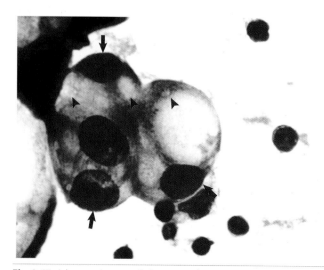

**Fig. 3.67** Adenocarcinoma cells (metastatic breast carcinoma, pleural fluid). The eccentric nucleus touches the cell periphery without a cytoplasmic rim (arrows). Presence of multiple vacuoles with ill-defined, indistinct margins are degenerative changes and do not reflect true secretory vacuoles of adenocarcinoma (arrowheads) (DQ Cytospin).

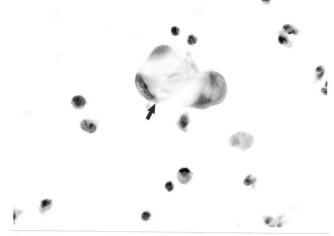

**Fig. 3.68** Metastatic cholangiocarcinoma (ascitic fluid). Features significantly overlap with pancreatic ductal adenocarcinoma. This case shows mucin producing adenocarcinoma cells (arrow). Only proper clinical correlation with imaging can demonstrate the actual primary site of these neoplasms (intrahepatic cholangiocarcinoma versus extrahepatic cholangiocarcinoma versus pancreatic ductal carcinoma) (PAP SurePath preparation).

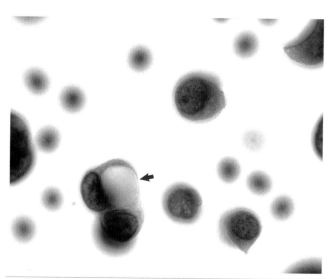

**Fig. 3.69** Signet ring adenocarcinoma cells with vacuole (ascitic fluid). The neoplastic cells show a single, large cytoplasmic vacuole (arrow) pushing the nucleus to the cell periphery. The vacuole content may be mucin, lipid (renal cell carcinoma), colloid (thyroid carcinoma), or occasionally, immunoglobulin (plasma cells). Individual cell nuclei show moderate to marked atypia. Most likely sites include gastric adenocarcinoma, followed by breast (usually infiltrating lobular carcinoma), then carcinomas of gall bladder, colon, pancreas and ovary. Potential pitfall: The vacuoles must be distinguished from degenerative vacuoles in mesothelial cells or other non-adenocarcinoma neoplastic cells (see Table 3.3) (PAP SurePath).

### Pigmented cells

Pigmented neoplastic cells are diagnostic of malignant melanoma.[176] However, melanomas are more commonly amelanotic. Other cytological features of melanoma include solitary non-cohesive cells with eccentric nuclei giving a plasmacytoid appearance, prominent nucleoli, intranuclear cytoplasmic inclusions and frequent binucleation.[35] Other cells with other brown pigments include inspissated intracytoplasmic bile within tumour cells (hepatocellular carcinoma) or

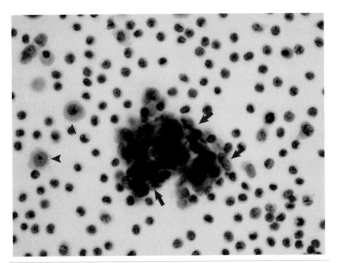

**Fig. 3.70** Metastatic small cell carcinoma of lung (pleural fluid). Second population of neoplastic cells (arrows) with a few reactive mesothelial cells (arrowheads) and many chronic inflammatory cells in the background. Loosely cohesive groups of fragile cells with high nucleocytoplasmic ratios and scant cytoplasm. This scant rim of cytoplasm is highlighted better with Diff-Quik-stained smears. The hyperchromatic nuclei have 'salt and pepper' chromatin without nucleoli. However, as compared to conventional cytology of small cell carcinomas in other specimens, effusion cytology may exhibit small insignificant nucleoli in some nuclei (PAP SurePath).

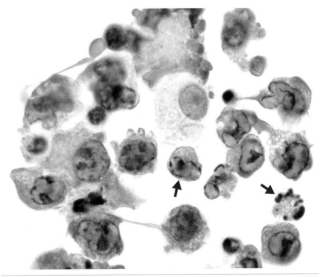

**Fig. 3.71** Metastatic non-small cell carcinoma of lung (pleural fluid). A predominant population with pleomorphic, overtly malignant, loosely cohesive cells showing tendency to be scattered as isolated cells can be interpreted easily as malignant cells. A few neoplastic cells show apoptosis (arrows) (PAP SurePath).

haemosiderin within macrophages in conditions with chronic haemorrhage such as endometriosis.

### Small cells

This refers to cells ranging from slightly larger than or about 2–3 times the small round lymphocyte. The differential diagnosis includes epithelial and non-epithelial malignancies, especially breast carcinoma, both ductal and lobular types, and especially the latter. Small cell lung carcinoma (Fig. 3.70) is a additional example. When the neoplastic small cells are discohesive[34] low grade non-Hodgkin lymphoma such as small lymphocytic lymphoma/chronic lymphocytic leukaemia (SLL/CLL), grade I follicle centre lymphoma and mantle cell lymphoma are possibilities. In children and young adults all small blue cell tumours should be considered.[189,222]

### Pleomorphic and multinucleated giant cells

The list of diagnostic possibilities is extensive (Fig. 3.71) as these cells may be associated with carcinomas of: lung, pancreas, kidney, or thyroid, melanomas, sarcomas, malignant lymphomas, and germ cell tumours, among others. Based on morphology alone it may be impossible to identify the origin without the history of a known primary tumour. Ancillary studies such as immunocytochemistry are often required to aid in the differential diagnosis. Some histiocytic-type cells as seen in rheumatoid effusions (Fig. 3.51) and mesothelial cells as well as megakaryocytes may be multinucleated but should not be mistaken for malignant multinucleated giant cells (potential pitfall).[205]

### Squamous cells

These cells are rarely shed into effusions. They are seen in only about 5% of pleural fluids, fewer than 2% of ascites[205] and even less often in pericardial effusions.[231] A diagnosis of keratinising squamous cell carcinoma is usually straightforward.[35] The cells have abnormal shapes with squamous pearl formation and dense orange cytoplasm. However, the non-keratinising variant is relatively more common in fluids than the keratinising type. Ruptured dermoid cyst[232] and incidental needle pick ups from skin can be confusing. In the absence of keratinisation, the cells may be mistaken for adenocarcinoma or reactive mesothelial cells.

### Spindle cells

These cells are primarily associated with sarcomas.[176] Features suggestive of metastatic sarcoma in fluid specimens include sparsely cellular specimens, loosely cohesive arrangements, binucleation and/or multinucleation, and irregular nuclear contours.[233] In general, sarcomas almost never present as effusions without a history of a known primary. Sarcomatous spindle cells have a tendency to become oval or round in body cavity fluids.[233] Morphology based sub-classification is less reliable in fluids. Ancillary tools such as electron microscopy and immunocytochemistry are useful, especially in cases without clinical data. Other non-mesenchymal malignancies with a spindle cell component in effusions: include spindle cell carcinomas, melanomas and mesotheliomas.

### Large polyhedral cells

These are a non-specific feature, but may suggest: hepatocellular carcinoma, transitional cell carcinoma or large cell type squamous cell carcinoma The rare deciduoid variant of mesothelioma (Figs 3.55, 3.72) also shows overlapping features.

### Cell groups of tall columnar cells with a picket fence pattern

Typically these suggest adenocarcinoma, most commonly colonic adenocarcinoma or pancreato-biliary carcinoma. The presence of apoptosis with extensive single cell necrosis favours a colonic primary.

## Ancillary studies

Different ancillary studies may be applied to cytopathological evaluation of effusion fluids for malignancy.[88] They facilitate a

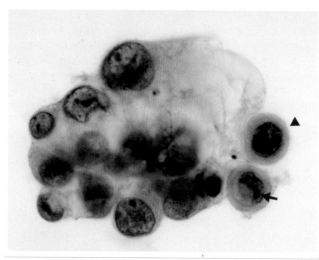

**Fig. 3.72** Mesothelioma (pleural fluid). This case shows some of the general cytological features of malignancy, including irregular, pleomorphic, and enlarged nuclei with prominent nucleoli and macronucleoli (arrow). These features are usually subtle and require careful examination (arrowhead) in most of mesothelioma (PAP ThinPrep).

definitive interpretation and assist in distinguishing mesothelioma/reactive mesothelial cells from metastatic adenocarcinoma and other tumours. In addition, they may provide clues to the possible primary site. Useful ancillary studies that have been commonly used for effusion specimens include immunocharacterisation with immunocytochemistry and flow cytometry, cytochemistry-histochemistry (so-called special stains), and rarely electron microscopy.

### Immunocytochemistry

This is the most common ancillary technique applied during interpretation of effusion cytology. Proper processing is crucial for optimal immunocytochemical evaluation. In addition to distinguishing mesothelioma from metastatic adenocarcinoma, immunocytochemistry of cell block sections of effusions with the 'Subtractive coordinate immunoreactivity pattern' (SCIP) approach is an important ancillary tool for determination of the primary tumour site (Figs 3.43, 3.44, 3.46, 3.47).[60,74]

### Cytochemistry-histochemistry

Cytochemistry-histochemistry may be performed on smears or on cell block sections respectively. Cytoplasmic melanin in melanoma cells may be confirmed by the Fontana–Masson method. Argentaffin and/or argyrophil stains highlight polypeptide hormones, active amines, or amine precursors in the cytoplasm and suggest neuroendocrine differentiation. Mucicarmine demonstrates mucin and favours adenocarcinoma (Fig. 3.27).[234–236] Although these stains are inexpensive and useful in the appropriate settings, they may not be as sensitive and may lack specificity depending on the stringency of quality control.

### Electron microscopy

Tumour cells from some primary sites may display distinctive ultrastructural features such as intracellular junctions, cytoplasmic organelles and secretory products.[1,2,237,238] However, electron microscopy is rarely used for tumour sub-classification in

effusion fluids. Some of the reasons for this are the higher cost, non-availability in some laboratories, the labour intensive technique, and the time-consuming process. More importantly, various cells in effusion fluids may not be identified and located for proper ultrastructural evaluation. Currently with significant advances in immunocytochemistry, electron microscopy is not a preferred ancillary tool in effusion cytology.

## Diagnostic pitfalls in cytopathology of serous cavity fluids

### Factors leading to diagnostic pitfalls

Positive cytology in effusion fluids has ominous significance. It is prudent to be conservative to avoid false positive results and prevent lost opportunity for proper treatment. Even with the most careful approach, a false-positivity rate of up to 0.5% has been reported in effusion fluid cytology.[53] However, this approach leads to false negative reporting in up to 30% of cases. Some of the factors related to effusions and responsible for diagnostic pitfalls include:

#### Alterations in primary cytomorphology due to surface tension phenomenon

The surface tension of the effusion fluid alters the cytomorphology of cells exfoliated in it. For example metastatic sarcoma cells may not show classical spindle shapes and may change to polyhedral cells. Interpreters may be familiar with the conventional morphology observed in FNA smears, but surface tension related alterations can be a diagnostic pitfall.

#### Inappropriate specimen collection-processing

Proper collection-processing of effusion specimens is extremely crucial for an appropriate interpretation. Any compromise at this stage, from improper collection/storage[32] to final processing steps, such as Diff-Quik staining and cell block preparation, may lead to suboptimal interpretation.[71] Similarly, lack of proper orientation of cell block sections for evaluation with the 'SCIP' approach as previously described may adversely affect the final interpretation of immunohistochemistry.[74]

#### Multiple faces of reactive mesothelial cells with wide morphological spectrum

A variety of reactive processes including acute pancreatitis,[15] tuberculosis,[53] ovarian fibroma,[53] pulmonary infarction,[50] chemotherapy,[239] cirrhosis[53] and hepatocellular carcinoma without metastatic disease to peritoneal cavity[11] may induce reactive changes approaching atypia in mesothelial cells, leading to misinterpretation, due to morphological appearances overlapping with malignant cells (Fig. 3.25).

#### Proliferation related morphological alterations[1]

The cytomorphological changes secondary to continued proliferation of exfoliated cells in the nutrient rich effusion fluids may lead to the potential pitfalls. The cytomorphological changes in this category include proliferation spheres or tissue fragments, mitotic figures and nucleolar prominence.

The malignant cells may continue to proliferate even after they are exfoliated into a serous cavity fluid to form proliferation spheres or tissue fragments (Figs 3.39–3.41).[71] These are cohesive groups of three-dimensional cell balls (and not passively aggregated cells during processing), that may be solid or

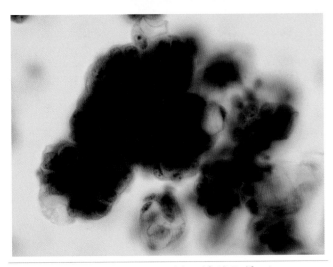

**Fig. 3.73** Metastatic breast carcinoma (pleural fluid). Proliferation spheres may join and lead to papillary configurations. Because of this, the interpretation of papillary carcinoma as primary carcinoma should be made conservatively with effusion cytology alone (PAP SurePath).

hollow. They do not have a stromal core (Fig. 3.39). The milieu in urine and cerebrospinal fluid is not favourable for proliferation of exfoliated neoplastic cells, therefore urothelial carcinoma cells in urine and metastatic cancer cells in cerebrospinal fluid do not show proliferation spheres.

The constituent cells of proliferation spheres divide and increase in number with resultant enlargement of these groups. Due to their rapid proliferation, the cells in the peripheral layer of the spheres are usually arranged radially (Fig. 3.41). At lower magnification, other structures such as acinar and glandular arrangements may show morphological features overlapping with proliferation spheres but such groups are significantly smaller and careful scrutiny at higher magnification with fine focus adjustment usually shows the central space (Fig. 3.59).

Due to the lack of sufficient time for proliferation, rapidly accumulating malignant effusions usually lack proliferation spheres. They are generally observed at a later stage. As the constituent cells divide, the proliferation spheres continue to grow up to 0.5 mm in diameter. Larger proliferation spheres may even be visible to the naked eye.

Proliferation spheres are associated with effusions secondary to many types of malignancies. Most common are ductal carcinoma of the breast, epithelioid mesothelioma and poorly differentiated small cell carcinoma of the lung. They are not formed in effusions secondary to cancers with relatively discohesive cells such as anaplastic gastric carcinoma (linitis plastica type), the non-cohesive type of adenocarcinoma of the lung, non-cohesive epithelioid mesothelioma, pleomorphic giant cell carcinoma of the pancreas, giant cell carcinoma of the lung, lobular carcinoma of the breast, adrenocortical carcinoma and lymphomas. Such effusions usually show predominantly isolated cells unrelated to the duration of effusion.

*The proliferation spheres may join each other and result in configurations resembling papillary structures* (Fig. 3.61). This is usually an *in vitro* phenomenon during specimen processing. Thus even non-papillary adenocarcinomas of the colon and pancreas may show such papillary-like structures. They should not be misinterpreted as a feature suggestive of the metastatic papillary neoplasm in effusions.

Mitotic figures may be present in proliferation spheres, especially in fresh effusions and along the periphery of spheres. They are seen when there has been no chemotherapy and also in un-refrigerated specimens. Neoplastic cells usually show apoptosis with karyorrhexis in solitary and loose groups of cells after effective chemotherapy. The presence of mitotic figures and nucleolar prominence are common in highly reactive mesothelial cells and may lead to the pitfall of malignant misinterpretation. Peritoneal dialysis fluids show mitotic figures with multinucleation at a higher frequency.[10]

### Degenerative changes, nuclear hyperchromasia and cytoplasmic vacuolation[1]

Degenerative changes may be *in vitro* secondary to improper storage/handling of specimen or *in vivo* changes in chronic effusion. It introduces atypical morphological features resulting in nuclear hyperchromasia and cytoplasmic vacuolation. Both of these features may lead to malignant misinterpretation.

In chronic effusions the mesothelial cells show many small vacuoles resembling those of foamy macrophages (Figs 3.65, 3.66) without a significant diagnostic challenge. However, these vacuoles may join and form a large single cytoplasmic vacuole which may displace the nucleus to the periphery, leading to an appearance resembling a signet-ring adenocarcinoma cell. Similar changes may also be produced *in vitro* if the specimen is left at room temperature for a longer time, such as when collected during the weekend and not processed immediately. In such situations the degenerative intracytoplasmic vacuoles may lead to misinterpretation of these reactive mesothelial cells as adenocarcinoma cells with mucin especially if the mesothelial cells also show degenerative hyperchromasia in large nuclei.

Paradoxically, neoplastic cells may also show degenerative changes with cytoplasmic vacuoles. This is relatively more frequent than the true mucin vacuoles in adenocarcinoma cells, which may lead to misinterpretation of non-mucin-producing neoplastic cells with degenerative vacuoles as mucin-producing adenocarcinoma cells.[217]

Clues to the differentiation of degenerative intracytoplasmic vacuoles from true secretory vacuoles of adenocarcinoma cells are shown in Table 3.3 (Figs. 3.65, 3.66).

## True negative results in effusions caused by cancer[1]

The above-mentioned pitfalls highlight the possible factors leading to a false positive interpretation. Awareness of these pitfalls along with a properly applied specimen processing protocol (Figs 3.42, 3.76) should minimise the chances of misinterpretation.[37,53,239] However, so-called false negative results may not be due to misinterpretation alone. Up to 5% of clinically proven malignant effusions may not show malignant cells. Possible causes for such negative results include:

- *Blockage of the lymphatics* by neoplastic cells as observed with neoplasms spreading via lymphatics. The effusion with or without inflammatory cells only shows reactive mesothelial cells and is negative for malignant cells
- *Increased capillary permeability* due to chemical mediators, such as VEGF (vascular endothelial growth factor) from malignant cells, leading to accumulation of fluid without malignant cells

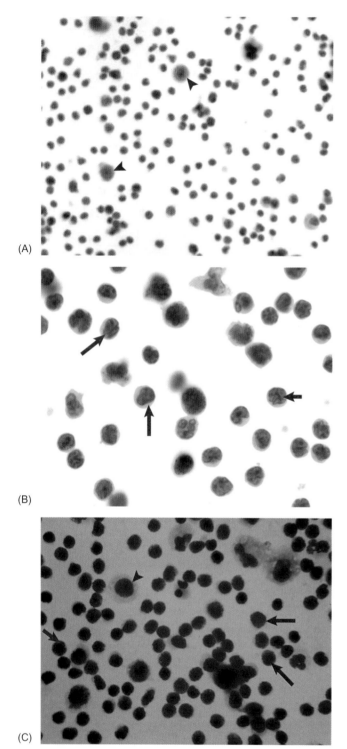

(A)

(B)

(C)

**Fig. 3.74** Reactive mesothelial cells (arrowheads) with chronic inflammatory cells (arrows) (effusions from different cases). (A,B, PAP SurePath; C, DQ Cytospin).

- *Lack of exfoliation* of the tumour cells into effusions. Some neoplasms such as low-grade sarcomas and spindle cell mesotheliomas do not exfoliate well and may have a negative result
- *Encapsulation with an organised thick layer of fibrin* covering the serosa. This type of encapsulation is seen

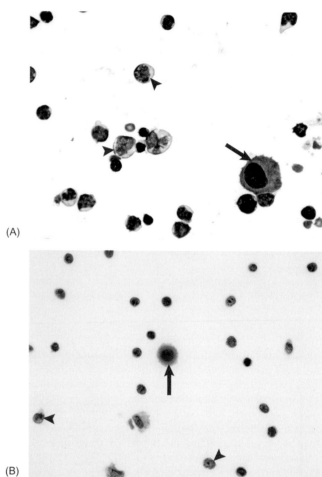

(A)

(B)

**Fig. 3.75** Colon MALT lymphoma-high-grade (ascitic fluid). The lymphoid cells (arrowheads) with rare reactive mesothelial cells (arrows) are relatively polymorphic. This polymorphic lymphoid population is difficult to distinguish on cytomorphology alone from reactive chronic inflammatory cells. Ancillary tools such as flow cytometry and immunocytochemistry to confirm the monoclonality of lymphoid population with proper clinical details is important for final interpretation. (A, DQ Cytospin; B, PAP SurePath preparation).

more commonly in pleural cavities with epithelioid mesothelioma

- *Reduction in the number of neoplastic cells* over time and eventually total disappearance. Various associated factors such as irradiation, obstructive or aspiration pneumonia, atelectasis, pleuritis and infarction may contribute to this.

If the initial cytological features are not consistent with metastatic disease, repeating the cytopathological examination is recommended, especially when the effusion recurs or persists. This is extremely important if clinical features are suspicious for malignancy. *The detection rate of malignant cells is increased if repeated specimens are examined.*[1,53,218,242]

## Management role

The role of serous cavity cytology in patient management depends on the clinical situation and on the type of specimen (effusion versus washings). Evaluation of washings

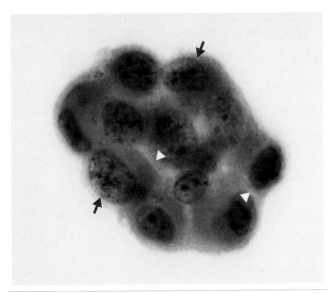

**Fig. 3.76** Metastatic endometrial carcinoma (peritoneal washing). The three-dimensional group with some areas suggesting 'mesothelial windows' (arrowheads) is difficult to distinguish from mesothelial cells. Some atypical nuclei (arrows) suggest malignancy. Comparing the cell block section with the primary tumour is a simple approach for interpreting the serous cavity washings. This case showed similar groups in the cell block. They were morphologically comparable to the histomorphology of the primary tumour (PAP ThinPrep).

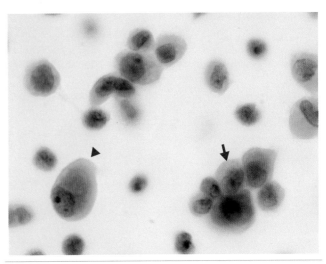

**Fig. 3.78** Metastatic duodenal adenocarcinoma (ascitic fluid). Features overlap with other well-differentiated adenocarcinomas. Loosely cohesive groups (arrow) of medium to large cells (arrowhead) with hyperchromatic, round to oval nuclei with finely to coarsely granular chromatin and variably conspicuous nucleoli (PAP SurePath).

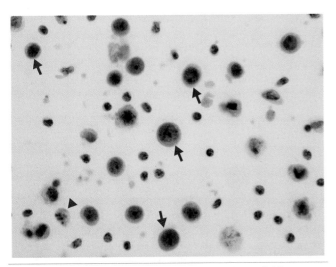

**Fig. 3.77** Metastatic gastric carcinoma, linitis plastica (ascitic fluid). Numerous single, medium-sized, pleomorphic carcinoma cells (arrows) with features overlapping with other anaplastic carcinomas. Although easily recognised as a second population, as seen in this case, they may be the predominant population and may not be perceived as a second population. Some of the neoplastic cells showed apoptosis (arrowhead). (Pitfall: Resemblance to the tumours with tendency for numerous isolated cells, e.g. large cell lymphomas, germ cell tumours, and melanoma.) (PAP SurePath preparation).

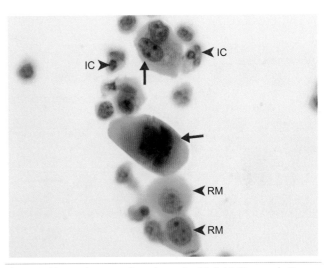

**Fig. 3.79** Metastatic pancreatic carcinoma (ascitic fluid). The neoplastic cells (arrows) are seen as a second foreign population amongst reactive mesothelial cells (arrowheads RM) and inflammatory cells (arrowheads IC) (PAP SurePath).

has been routinely included as a staging procedure of gynae-cological malignancies and has been recommended in the staging of other malignancies such as oesophageal and lung carcinomas.

Because crucial management decisions are dependent on the cytopathological opinion, the cytopathologist should be a member of the core team at the multidisciplinary meetings (MDM) that are held regularly to discuss all aspects of a case. In particular, the presence of the cytopathologist at the MDM to discuss the interpretation of serous effusions in the light of the full clinical picture is becoming ever more important.

In general, once an effusion or serous cavity specimen such as washing is positive for malignant cells, the prognosis is worse and the management is mainly palliative rather than curative.[102,241]

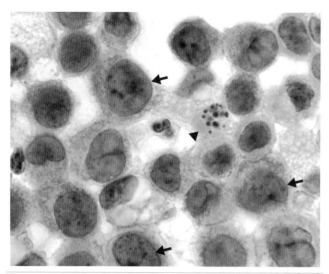

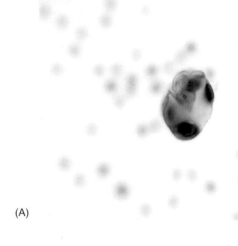

(A)

**Fig. 3.80** Metastatic poorly differentiated adenocarcinoma (pleural fluid). Many loosely cohesive high-grade tumour cells (arrows) show pleomorphism with apoptosis (arrowhead). The interpretation of these cells as malignant is obvious even though they constitute a single predominant population (PAP Cytospin).

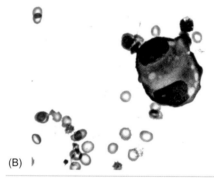

(B)

**Fig. 3.82** Metastatic adenocarcinoma of the prostate (ascitic fluid). Cohesive small groups of medium to large cells with usually eccentric nuclei and prominent nucleoli. Small degenerative vacuoles are seen more easily in Diff-Quik stain (B). (A, PAP SurePath preparation; B, DQ Cytospin).

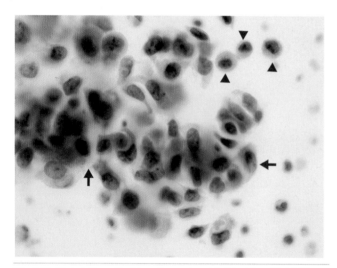

**Fig. 3.81** Metastatic urothelial carcinoma from bladder (pleural fluid). The loosely cohesive clusters (arrows) without proliferation spheres are present among rare mesothelial cells (arrowheads) as second population. These groups may resemble other poorly differentiated carcinomas including poorly differentiated non-keratinising squamous cell carcinoma. The 'cercariform' cells may help in the differential diagnosis (PAP SurePath).

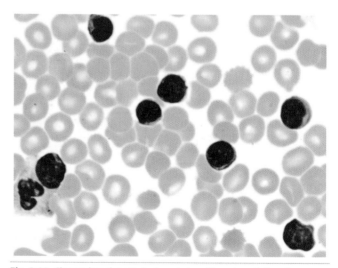

**Fig. 3.83** Chronic lymphocytic leukaemia/small lymphocytic lymphoma (CLL/SLL) (pleural fluid). Moderately clumped chromatin, inconspicuous nucleoli and scant amount of moderately basophilic cytoplasm. Note background of red blood cells. Pitfall of contamination from peripheral blood should be considered prior to final interpretation (Wright–Giemsa stain, Cytospin, courtesy of Horatiu Olteanu, MD, PhD).

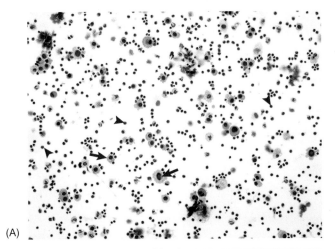

(A)

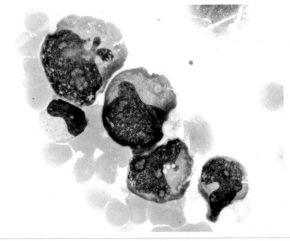

**Fig. 3.85** Diffuse large B-cell lymphoma (serous fluid). Non-cohesive groups of large lymphoid cells are present with variably irregular nuclei, multiple prominent nucleoli, and moderate amounts of deeply basophilic cytoplasm (Wright–Giemsa stain Cytospin, courtesy of Horatiu Olteanu, MD, PhD).

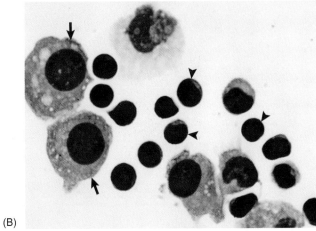

(B)

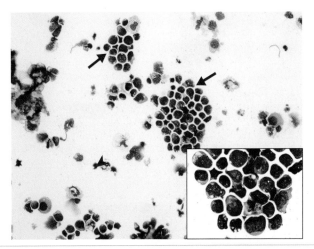

**Fig. 3.86** Diffuse large B-cell lymphoma (pleural fluid). Non-cohesive groups of medium to large-sized lymphoid cells (arrows) with irregular nuclear contours, coarse chromatin, one to several distinct nucleoli and a scant amount of deeply basophilic cytoplasm (inset). Rare reactive mesothelial cells are present in the background (arrowhead) (Wright–Giemsa stain Cytospin, courtesy of Horatiu Olteanu, MD, PhD).

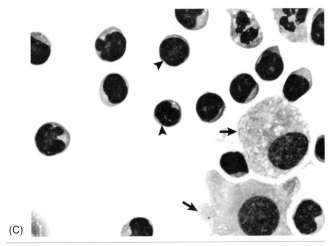

(C)

**Fig. 3.84** Follicular lymphoma (pleural fluid). (A–C) Flow cytometry demonstrated a distinct population of light chain-restricted B cells with an immunophenotype consistent with follicular lymphoma (reactive mesothelial cells – arrows, lymphoma cells – arrowheads) (Wright–Giemsa stain Cytospin, courtesy of Horatiu Olteanu, MD, PhD).

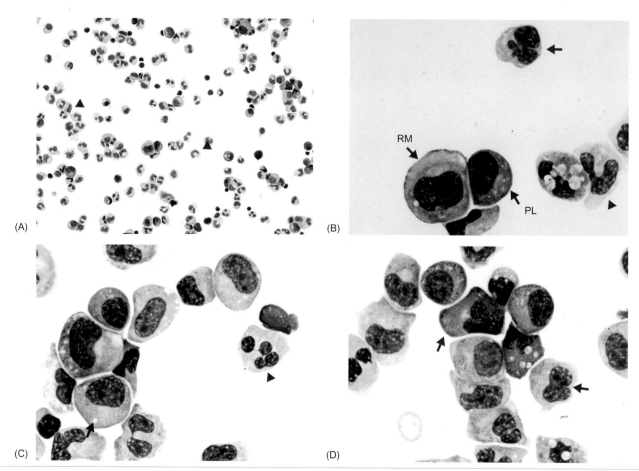

**Fig. 3.87** Primary effusion lymphoma in the patient with AIDS (Pleural fluid). (A) Large lymphoid cells with irregular nuclear contours and basophilic cytoplasm (arrows, B–D) in a background of neutrophils (arrowheads). Some of the cells show plasmacytoid/immunoblastic morphology (arrow PL), with basophilic cytoplasm and eccentric nuclei with inconspicuous nucleoli. Note rare reactive mesothelial cells (arrow RM) (Wright–Giemsa stain Cytospin, courtesy of Horatiu Olteanu, MD, PhD).

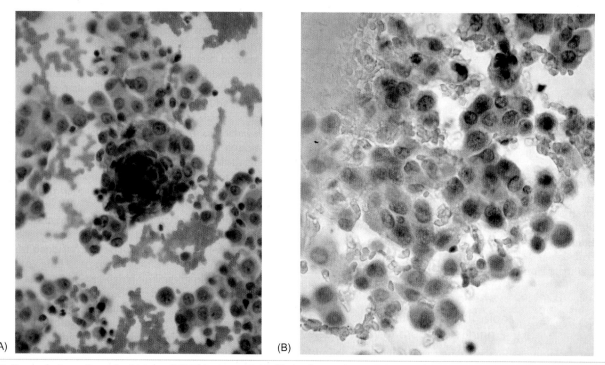

**Fig. 3.88** Desmoplastic small round cell tumour (DSRCT) (peritoneal fluid). Effusion from patient with DSRCT exhibiting high cellularity. (A) DSRCT cells; (B) The tumour cells show nuclear immunoreactivity for WT1 performed on cytology preparation (A, PAP stain; B, WT-1 immunostain). (From Granja et al. 2005.[122])

# REFERENCES

1. Shidham VB, Atkinson BF. Cytopathologic Diagnosis of Serous Fluids. 1st edn. London: Elsevier; 2007.

2. Bedrossian CW. Malignant Effusions: A Multimodal Approach to Cytologic Diagnosis. New York: Igaku-Shoin; 1994.

3. Carter D, True L, Otis CN. Serous membranes. In: Sternberg SS, editor. Histology for Pathologists. 2nd edn. Philadelphia: Lippincott-Raven; 1997. p. 223–39.

4. Shidham VB. Metastatic carcinoma in effusions. In: Shidham VB, Atkinson BF, editors. Cytopathologic Diagnosis of Serous Fluids. 1st edn. London: Elsevier; 2007. p. 115–45.

5. Ordóñez NG. Mesothelioma with clear cell features: an ultrastructural and immunohistochemical study of 20 cases. Hum Pathol 2005;36:465–73.

6. Yao DX, Shia J, Erlandson RA, et al. Lymphohistiocytoid mesothelioma: a clinical, immunohistochemical and ultrastructural study of four cases and literature review. Ultrastruct Pathol 2004;28:213–28.

7. Davidson B, Suo Z, Nesland JM. Malignant mesothelioma. Ultrastruct Pathol 2004;28:179–80.

8. Bedrossian CW. Diagnostic problems in serous effusions. Diagn Cytopathol 1998;19:131–37.

9. Shidham VB. The panorama of different faces of mesothelial cells. In: Shidham VB, Atkinson BF, editors. Cytopathologic Diagnosis of Serous Fluids. 1st edn. London: Elsevier; 2007. p. 19–30.

10. Selvaggi SM, Migdal S. Cytologic features of atypical mesothelial cells in peritoneal dialysis fluid. Diagn Cytopathol 1990;6:22–26.

11. Thrall MJ, Giampoli EJ. Routine review of ascites fluid from patients with cirrhosis or hepatocellular carcinoma is a low-yield procedure: An observational study. CytoJournal 2009;6:16.

12. Kern WH. Benign papillary structures with psammoma bodies in culdocentesis fluid. Acta Cytol 1969;13:178–80.

13. Zuna RE. Diagnostic cytopathology of peritoneal washing. In: Shidham VB, Atkinson BF, editors. Cytopathologic Diagnosis of Serous Fluids. 1st edn London: Elsevier; 2007. p. 91–105.

14. Soendergaard K. On the interpretation of atypical cells in pleural and peritoneal effusion. Acta Cytol 1977;21:413–16.

15. Kutty CP, Remeniuk E, Verkey B. Malignant-appearing cells in pleural effusion due to pancreatitis: Case report and literature review. Acta Cytol 1981;25:412–16.

16. Shidham VB. Introduction. In: Shidham VB, Atkinson BF, editors. Cytopathologic Diagnosis of Serous Fluids. 1st edn. Elsevier; 2007. p. 1–17.

17. Ventura KC, Yang GC, Levine PH. Atypical papillary proliferation in gynecologic patients: a study of 32 pelvic washes. Diagn Cytopathol 2005;32:76–81.

18. Parwani AV, Chan TY, Ali SZ. Significance of psammoma bodies in serous cavity fluid: a cytopathologic analysis. Cancer 2004;102:87–91.

19. Wojcik EM, Naylor B. 'Collagen balls' in peritoneal washings. Prevalence, morphology, origin and significance. Acta Cytol 1992;36:466–70.

20. Szporn AH, Chen X, Wu M, et al. Increase in the incidence of peritoneal collagen balls over a 10-year period. Acta Cytol 2005;49:387–90.

21. Selvaggi SM. Diagnostic pitfalls of peritoneal washing cytology and the role of cellblocks in their diagnosis. Diagn Cytopathol 2003;28:335–41.

22. Kobayashi TK, Ueda M, Nishino T, et al. Appearance of 'collagen balls' in ascitic fluid cytology with abdominal cocoon (encapsulating peritonitis). Diagn Cytopathol 1997;16:469–70.

23. Kuritzkes DR, Rein M, Horowitz S, et al. Detached ciliary tufts mistaken for peritoneal parasites: a warning. Rev Infect Dis 1988;10:1044–47.

24. Sidawy MK, Chandra P, Oertel YC. Detached ciliary tufts in female peritoneal washings. A common finding. Acta Cytol 1987;31:841–44.

25. Naylor B. Curschmann's spirals in pleural and peritoneal effusions. Acta Cytol 1990;34:474–78.

26. Sneige N, Fernandez T, Copeland LJ, et al. Mullerian inclusions in peritoneal washings. Potential source of error in cytologic diagnosis. Acta Cytol 1986;30:271–76.

27. Covell JL, Carry JB, Feldman PS. Peritoneal washings in ovarian tumors. Potential sources of error in cytologic diagnosis. Acta Cytol 1985;29:310–16.

28. Sams VR, Benjamin E, Ward RH. Ectopic pancreas. A cause of false-positive peritoneal cytology. Acta Cytol 1990;34:641–44.

29. Sherer DM, Eliakim R, Abulafia O. The role of angiogenesis in the accumulation of peritoneal fluid in benign conditions and the development of malignant ascites in the female. Gynecol Obstet Invest 2000;50:217–24.

30. Jhala NC, Jhala DN, Chhieng DC. Reactive conditions. In: Shidham VB, Atkinson BF, editors Cytopathologic Diagnosis of Serous Fluids. 1st edn: Elsevier; 2007. p. 79–89.

31. Bilic M, Welsh CT, Rumboldt Z, Hoda RS. Disseminated primary diffuse leptomeningeal gliomatosis: a case report with liquid-based and conventional smear cytology. Cyto Journal 2005;2:16. Online. Available at: www.cytojournal.com/content/2/1/16.

32. Shidham VB, Epple J. Appendix I: Collection and processing of effusion fluids for cytopathologic evaluation. In: Shidham VB, Atkinson BF, editors. Cytopathologic Diagnosis of Serous Fluids. 1st edn. Elsevier; 2007. p. 207–35.

33. Rao RN. Mesothelioma. In: Shidham VB, Atkinson BF, editors. Cytopathologic Diagnosis of Serous Fluids. 1st edn. Elsevier; 2007. p. 107–13.

34. Sanchez SR, Chang CC. Hematolymphoid disorders. In: Shidham VB, Atkinson BF, editors. Cytopathologic Diagnosis of Serous Fluids. 1st edn. Elsevier; 2007. p. 171–93.

35. Chivukula M, Saad R. Metastatic sarcomas, melanoma, and other non-epithelial neoplasms. In: Shidham VB, Atkinson BF, editors. Cytopathologic Diagnosis of Serous Fluids. 1st edn. Elsevier; 2007. p. 147–56.

36. Wong JW, Pitlik D. Abdul-Karim FWCytology of pleural, peritoneal and pericardial fluids in children. A 40-year summary. Acta Cytol 1997;41:467–73.

37. Hallman JR, Geisinger KR. Cytology of fluids from pleural, peritoneal and pericardial cavities in children. A comprehensive survey. Acta Cytol 1994;38:209–17.

38. Enatsu S, Yoshida J, Yokose T, et al. Pleural lavage cytology before and after lung resection in non-small cell lung cancer patients. Ann Thorac Surg 2006;81:298–304.

39. Mohamed KH, Mobasher AA, Yousef AI, et al. Pleural lavage: a novel diagnostic approach for diagnosing exudative pleural effusion. Lung 2000;178:371–79.

40. Buhr J, Berghauser KH, Morr H, et al. Tumor cells in intraoperative pleural lavage. An indicator for the poor prognosis of bronchogenic carcinoma. Cancer 1990;65:1801–4.

41. Kobilkova J, Kuzel D, Toth D, et al. Aspiration cytology from the pouch of Douglas at hysteroscopy. Cytopathology 2001;12:44–47.

42. Vicidomini G, Santini M, Fiorello A, et al. Intraoperative pleural lavage: is it a valid prognostic factor in lung cancer? Ann Thorac Surg 2005;79:254–57.

43. Jiao X, Zhang M, Wen Z, et al. Pleural lavage cytology in esophageal cancer without pleural effusions: clinicopathologic analysis. Eur J Cardiothorac Surg 2000;17:575–79.

44. Aksoy E, Atac G, Sevim T, et al. Diagnostic yield of closed pleural brushing. Tuberk Toraks 2005;53:238–44.

45. Saito Y, Yamakawa Y, Kiriyama M, et al. Diagnosis of visceral pleural invasion by lung cancer using intraoperative touch cytology. Ann Thorac Surg 2002;73:1552–57.

46. Eltabbakh GH, Mount SL. Comparison of diaphragmatic wash and scrape specimens in staging of women with ovarian cancer. Gynecol Oncol 2001;81:461–65.

47. Assaly M, Bongiovanni M, Kumar N, et al. Cytology of benign multicystic peritoneal mesothelioma in peritoneal washings. Cytopathology 2008;19:224–28.

48. Cibas ES. Pleural, pericardial, and peritoneal fluids. In: Cibas ES, Ducatman BS, editors. Cytology Diagnostic Principles and Clinical Correlates. 2nd edn. Philadelphia: WB Saunders; 2003. p. 119–44.

49. Prakash UBS, Reiman HM. Comparison of needle biopsy with cytologic analysis for the evaluation of pleural effusion: Analysis of 414 cases. Mayo Clin Proc 1985;60:158–64.

50. Nance KV, Shermer RW, Askin FB. Diagnostic efficacy of pleural biopsy as compared with that of pleural fluid examination. Mod Pathol 1991;4:320–24.

51. Seferovic PM, Ristic AD, Maksimovic R, et al. Diagnostic value of pericardial biopsy: improvement with extensive sampling enabled by pericardioscopy. Circulation 2003;107:978–83.

52. Naylor B. Pleural, pericardial, and pericardial fluids. In: Bibbo M, editor. Comprehensive Cytopathology. 2nd edn. Philadelphia: WB Saunders; 1997. p. 551–621.

53. Motherby H, Nadjari B, Friegel P, et al. Diagnostic accuracy of effusion cytology. Diagn Cytopathol 1999;20:350–57.

54. Cibas ES. Peritoneal washings. In: Cibas ES, Ducatman BS, editors Cytology – Diagnostic Principles and Clinical Correlates. 2nd edn. Philadelphia: Saunders; 2003. p. 145–61.

55. FIGO Cancer Committee Announcement. Gynecol Oncol 1989;35:125–27.

56. FIGO Cancer Committee Announcement. Gynecol Oncol 1986;25:383–85.

57. Roffe BD, Wagner FH, Derewicz HJ, et al. Heparinized bottles for the collection of body cavity fluids in cytopathology. Am J Hosp Pharm 1979;36:211–14.

58. Broghamer WL Jr., Richardson ME, Faurest SE. Malignancy-associated serosanguinous pleural effusions. Acta Cytol 1984;28:46–50.

59. Hajdu SI. Exfoliative cytology of primary and metastatic Wilms tumors. Acta Cytol 1971;15:339–42.

60. Shidham VB. Appendix II: Immunocytochemistry of effusions- processing and commonly used immunomarkers. In: Shidham VB, Atkinson BF, editors. Cytopathologic Diagnosis of Serous Fluids. 1st edn. Elsevier; 2007. p. 237–57.

61. Liu J, Farhood A. Thyroid transcription factor-1 immunocytochemical staining of pleural fluid cytocentrifuge preparations for detection of small cell lung carcinoma. Acta Cytol 2004;48:635–40.

62. Metzgeroth G, Kuhn C, Schultheis B, et al. Diagnostic accuracy of cytology and immunocytology in carcinomatous effusions. Cytopathology 2008;19:205–11.

63. Filie AC, Copel C, Wilder AM, et al. Individual specimen triage of effusion samples: an improvement in the standard of practice, or a waste of resources? Diagn Cytopathol 2000;22:7–10.

64. Baig MA, Fathallah L, Feng J, et al. Fast drying of fine needle aspiration slides using a hand held fan: impact on turn around time and staining quality. CytoJournal 2006;3:12.

65. Shidham V, Kampalath B, England J. Routine air drying of all the smears prepared during fine needle aspiration and intraoperative cytology studies: An opportunity to practice a unified protocol, offering the flexibility of choosing a variety of staining methods. Acta Cytol 2001;45:60–68.

66. Maksem JA, Finnemore M, Belsheim BL, et al. Manual method for liquid-based cytology: a demonstration using 1,000 gynecological cytologies collected directly to vial and prepared by a smear-slide technique. Diagn Cytopathol 2001;25:334–38.

67. Liqui-PREP™, LGM International, Inc. 4350 Oakes Road, Fort Lauderdale, FL 33314, USA. Online. Available at: www.lgmintl.com/.

68. Shandon EZ Megafunnel™ with Shandon Cytospin®. Online. Available at: www.thermo.com/com/cda/product/detail/1,1055,116770,00.html.

69. Yang GC, Wan LS, Papellas J, et al. Compact cellblocks. Use for body fluids, fine needle aspirations and endometrial brush biopsies. Acta Cytol 1998;42:703–6.

70. Tripath Imaging, SurePath™. Online. Available at: www.tripathimaging.com/us_sp.htm.

71. Shidham VB, Atkinson BF. Approach to diagnostic cytopathology of effusions. In: Shidham VB, Atkinson BF, editors Cytopathologic Diagnosis of Serous Fluids. 1st edn. Elsevier; 2007. p. 31–42.

72. Cytyc, ThinPrep™ Non-gyn. Online. Available at: www.thinprep.com/lab/lab_thinprep_nongyn_fluids.shtml.

73. Ceyhan BB, Demiralp E, Celikel T. Analysis of pleural effusions using flow cytometry. Respiration 1996;63:17–24.

74. Shidham VB, Atkinson BF. Immunocytochemistry of effusion fluids: Introduction to the SCIP approach. In: Shidham VB, Atkinson BF, editors.

Cytopathologic Diagnosis of Serous Fluids. 1st edn. Elsevier; 2007. p. 55–78.

75. Tao LC. Cytopathology of Malignant Effusions. Chicago: American Society of Clinical Pathologists, ASCP Press; 1996.

76. Geisinger KR, Stanley MW, Raab SS, editors, et al. Effusions. Modern Cytopathology. Philadelphia: Churchill Livingstone; 2004. p. 257–309.

77. DeMay RM, editor. Fluids. The art and science of cytopathology – Exfoliative cytology. 1st edn. Chicago: ASCP Press; 1996. p. 257–325.

78. Laucirica A, Schultenover SJ. Body cavity fluids. In: Ramzy I, editor. Clinical Cytopathoilogy and Aspiration Biopsy. 2nd edn. New York: McGraw-Hill; 2001. p. 205–23.

79. Kini SR. Serous effusions. In: Kini SR, Baltimore. Color Atlas of Differential Diagnosis in Exfoliative and Aspiration Cytopathology. London: Williams & Wilkins; 1999. p. 119–42.

80. Garza OT, Abati A, Sindelar WF, et al. Cytologic effects of photodynamic therapy in body fluids. Diagn Cytopathol 1996;14:356–61.

81. Ng WK, Lui PC, Ma L. Peritoneal washing cytology findings of disseminated myxoid leiomyosarcoma of uterus: report of a case with emphasis on possible differential diagnosis. Diagn Cytopathol 2002;27:47–52.

82. Chen KT. Effusion cytology of metastatic extraskeletal myxoid chondrosarcoma. Diagn Cytopathol 2003;28:222–23.

83. Murphy W, Ng ABP. Determination of primary site by examination of cancer cells in body fluids. Am J Clin Pathol 1972;58:479–88.

84. Spieler P, Gloor F. Identification of types and primary sites of malignant tumors by examination of exfoliated tumor cells in serous fluids. Acta Cytol 1985;29:753–74.

85. Fetsch PA, Simsir A, Brosky K, et al. Comparison of three commonly used cytologic preparations in effusion immunocytochemistry. Diagn Cytopathol 2002;26:61–66.

86. Mikel UV. Advanced Laboratory Methods in Histology and Pathology. Washington DC: Armed Forces Institute of Pathology, American Registry of Pathology; 1994. 217.

87. De Girolami E. Applications of plasma-thrombin cellblock in diagnostic cytology, Part II: Digestive and respiratory tracts, breast and effusions. Pathol Annu 1977;12(Pt 2):91–110.

88. Vejabhuti C, Chang CC. The flow cytometry, molecular analysis, and other special techniques. In: Shidham VB, Atkinson BF, editors. Cytopathologic Diagnosis of Serous Fluids. 1st edn. Elsevier; 2007. p. 195–205.

89. Decker D, Stratmann H, Springer W, et al. Benign and malignant cells in effusions: diagnostic value of image DNA cytometry in comparison to cytological analysis. Pathol Res Pract 1998;194:791–95.

90. da Silva VD, Prolla JC, Diehl AR, et al. Comparison of conventional microscopy and digitized imaging for diagnosis in serous effusions. Anal Quant Cytol Histol 1997;19:202–6.

91. Kobzik L, Antman KH, Warhol MJ. The distinction of mesothelioma from adenocarcinoma in malignant effusions by electron microscopy. Acta Cytol 1985;29:219–25.

92. Ordóñez NG. The immunohistochemical diagnosis of mesothelioma: differentiation of mesothelioma and lung adenocarcinoma. Am J Surg Pathol 1989;13:276–91.

93. Corson JM. Pathology of mesothelioma. Thorac Surg Clin 2004;14:447–60.

94. Fetsch PA, Abati A. Immunocytochemistry in effusion cytology: a contemporary review. Cancer Cytopathology 2001;93:293–308.

95. Wang NP, Zee S, Zarbo R, et al. Coordinate expression of cytokeratins 7 and 20 defines unique subsets of carcinomas. Appl Immunohistochem 1995;3:99–107.

96. Shidham VB, Kajdacsy-Balla AA. Immunohistochemistry: diagnostic and prognostic applications. In: Detrick B, Hamilton RG, Folds JD (eds) Manual Molecular and Clinical Laboratory Immunology, 7th edn. New York: American Society of Microbiology Press; 2009. p. 408–13.

97. Betta PG, Andrion A, Donna A, et al. Malignant mesothelioma of the pleura: the reproducibility of the immunohistological diagnosis. Pathol Res Pract 1997;193:759–65.

98. Ordóñez NG. The immunohistochemical diagnosis of epithelial mesothelioma. Hum Pathol 1999;30:313–23.

99. Politi E, Kandaraki C, Apostolopoulou C, et al. Immunocytochemical panel for distinguishing between carcinoma and reactive mesothelial cells in body cavity fluids. Diagn Cytopathol 2005;32:151–55.

100. Shidham VB, Chang CC, Rao RN, et al. Immunostaining of cytology smears: a comparative study to identify the most suitable method of smear preparation and fixation with reference to commonly used immunomarkers. Diagn Cytopathol 2003;29:217–21.

101. Shidham VB, Komorowski R, Macias V, et al. Optimisation of an immunostaining protocol for the rapid intraoperative evaluation of melanoma sentinel lymph node imprint smears with the 'MCW melanoma cocktail'. CytoJournal 2004;1:2.

102. Yoneda KY, Mathur PN, Gasparini S. The evolving role of interventional pulmonary in the interdisciplinary approach to the staging and management of lung cancer. Part III: diagnosis and management of malignant pleural effusions. Clin Lung Cancer 2007;8:535–47.

103. Donna A, Betta PG, Bellingeri D, et al. Cytologic diagnosis of malignant mesothelioma in serous effusions using an antimesothelial-cell antibody. Diagn Cytopathol 1992;8:361–65.

104. Monoclonal antibody to tumor-associated glycoprotein (TAG-72) package insert. San Ramon, CA: BioGenex; 1998.

105. Kho-Duffin J, Tao L-C, Cramer H, et al. Cytologic diagnosis of malignant mesothelioma, with particular emphasis on the epithelial noncohesive cell type. Diagn Cytopathol 1999;20:57–62.

106. Betta P-G, Andrion A, Donna A, et al. Malignant mesothelioma of the pleura: the reproducibility of the immunohistological diagnosis. Pathol Res Pract 1997;193:759–65.

107. Shield PW, Callan JJ, Devine PL. Markers for metastatic adenocarcinoma in serous effusion specimens. Diagn Cytopathol 1994;11(3):237–45.

108. Davidson B, Risberg B, Kristensen G, et al. Detection of cancer cells in effusions from patients diagnosed with gynaecological malignancies: evaluation of five epithelial markers. Virchows Arch 1999;435:43–49.

109. Koss MN, Fleming M, Przygodzki RM, et al. Adenocarcinoma simulating mesothelioma: a clinicopathologic and immunohistochemical study of 29 cases. Ann Diagn Pathol 1998;2:93–102.

110. Ordóñez NG. Role of immunohistochemistry in differentiating epithelial mesothelioma

from adenocarcinoma. Am J Clin Pathol 1999;112:75–89.

111. Monoclonal mouse anti-human epithelial antigen, clone Ber-EP4 package insert. Carpenteria, CA: Dako Corporation; 1998.

112. Dejmek A, Hjerpe A. Reactivity of six antibodies in effusions of mesothelioma, adenocarcinoma and mesotheliosis: step-wise logistic regression analysis. Cytopathology 2000;11:8–17.

113. Diaz-Arias AA, Loy TS, Bickel JT, et al. Utility of BER-EP4 in the diagnosis of adenocarcinoma in effusions: an immunocytochemical study of 232 cases. Diagn Cytopathol 1993;9:516–21.

114. Monoclonal mouse CA 19–19 package insert. Dedham, MA: Signet Pathology Systems; 1994.

115. Monoclonal mouse anti-BG-8 (murine) package insert. Dedham, MA: Signet Laboratories; 1994.

116. Fetsch PA, Abati A, Hijazi Y. Utility of the antibodies CA19–CA19, HBME-l, and thrombomodulin in the diagnosis of malignant mesothelioma and adenocarcinoma in cytology. Cancer (Cancer Cytopathol) 1998;84:101–8.

117. Miedouge M, Rouzaud P, Salama G, et al. Evaluation of seven tumour markers in pleural fluid for the diagnosis of malignant effusions. Br J Cancer 1999;81:1059–65.

118. Ordóñez N. Value of thyroid transcription factor-1, E-cadherin, BG8, WT1, and CD44S immunostaining in distinguishing epithelial pleural mesothelioma from pulmonary and nonpulmonary adenocarcinoma. Am J Surg Pathol 2000;24:598–606.

119. Carella R, Deleonardi G, D'Errico A, et al. Immunohistochemical panels for differentiating epithelial malignant mesothelioma from lung adenocarcinoma: a study with logistic regression analysis. Am J Surg Pathol 2001;25:43–50.

120. Simsir A, Fetsch PA, Mehta D, et al. E-cadherin, N-cadherin, and calretinin in pleural effusions: the good, the bad, the worthless. Diagn Cytopathol 1999;20:125–30.

121. Han A, Peralta-Soler A, Knudsen K, et al. Differential expression of N-cadherin in pleural mesotheliomas and E-cadherin in lung adenocarcinomas in formalin-fixed, paraffin-embedded tissues. Hum Pathol 1997;28:641–45.

122. Granja NM, Begnami MD, Bortolan J, et al. Desmoplastic small round cell tumour: Cytological and immunocytochemical features. CytoJournal 2005;2:6.

123. Schofield K, D'Aquila T, Rimm DL. The cell adhesion molecule, E-cadherin, distinguishes mesothelial cells from carcinoma cells in fluids. Cancer 1997;81:293–98.

124. Kitazume H, Kitamura K, Mukai K, et al. Cytologic differential diagnosis among reactive mesothelial cells, malignant mesothelioma, and adenocarcinoma: utility of combined E-cadherin and calretinin immunostaining. Cancer (Cancer Cytopathol) 2000;90:55–60.

125. Ordóñez N. Value of calretinin immunostaining in differentiating epithelial mesothelioma from lung adenocarcinoma. Mod Pathol 1998;11:929–33.

126. Ordóñez NG, Mackay B. Glycogen-rich mesothelioma. Ultrastruct Pathol 1999;23:401–6.

127. Oates J, Edwards C. HBME-l, MOC-31, WT1, and calretinin: an assessment of recently described markers for mesothelioma and adenocarcinoma. Histopathology 2000;36W:341–47.

128. Cury PM, Butcher DN, Fisher C, et al. Value of the mesothelium-associated antibodies thrombomodulin, cytokeratin 5/6, calretinin, and CD44H in distinguishing epithelioid pleural mesothelioma from adenocarcinoma metastatic to the pleura. Mod Pathol 2000;13:107–12.

129. Doglioni C, Dei Tos AP, Laurino L, et al. Calretinin: a novel immunocytochemical marker for mesothelioma. Am J Surg Pathol 1996;20:1037–46.

130. Polyclonal rabbit anti-calretinin package insert. South San Francisco, CA: Zymed Laboratories; 1999.

131. Kotov P, Chang CC, Shidham V. Calretinin for the differential diagnosis of mesothelial and non-mesothelial neoplasms: Nuclear immunostaining pattern should be considered positive. Acta Cytol 2003;47:915. Abstract no. 150.

132. Granville LA, Younes M, Churg A, et al. Comparison of monoclonal versus polyclonal calretinin antibodies for immunohistochemical diagnosis of malignant mesothelioma. Appl Immunohistochem Mol Morphol 2005;13:75–79.

133. Wieczorek TJ, Krane JF. Diagnostic utility of calretinin immunohistochemistry in cytologic cellblock preparations. Cancer 2000;90:312–19.

134. Nagel H, Hemmerlein B, Ruschenburg I, et al. The value of anti-calretinin antibody in the differential diagnosis of normal and reactive mesothelia versus metastatic tumors in effusion cytology. Pathol Res Pract 1998;194:759–64.

135. Arber DA, Weiss LM. CD15: a review. Appl Immunohistochem 1993;1:17–30.

136. CD15 (Leu-Mi) package insert. San Jose, CA: Becton-Dickinson Immunocytometry Systems; 1993.

137. Attanoos RL, Webb R, Gibbs AR. CD44H expression in reactive mesothelium, pleural mesothelioma and pulmonary adenocarcinoma. Histopathology 1997;30:260–63.

138. Riera JR, Astengo-Osuna C, Longmate JA, et al. The immunohistochemical diagnosis panel for epithelial mesothelioma: a reevaluation after heat-induced epitope retrieval. Am J Surg Pathol 1997;21:1409–19.

139. Ciampa A, Fanger G, Khan A, et al. Mammaglobin and CRxA-01 in pleural effusion cytology: potential utility of distinguishing metastatic breast carcinomas from other cytokeratin 7-positive/cytokeratin 20-negative carcinomas. Cancer 2004;102:368–72.

140. Logani S, Oliva E, Arnell PM, et al. Use of novel immunohistochemical markers expressed in colonic adenocarcinoma to distinguish primary ovarian tumors from metastatic colorectal carcinoma. Mod Pathol 2005;18:19–25.

141. Groisman GM, Bernheim J, Halpern M, et al. Expression of the intestinal marker Cdx2 in secondary adenocarcinomas of the colorectum. Arch Pathol Lab Med 2005;129:920–23.

142. Dennis JL, Hvidsten TR, Wit EC, et al. Markers of adenocarcinoma characteristic of the site of origin: development of a diagnostic algorithm. Clin Cancer Res 2005;11:3766–72.

143. Fetsch PA, Abati A. Overview of the clinical immunohistochemistry laboratory: regulations and troubleshooting guidelines. In: Javois LC, editor. Methods in Molecular Biology, Vol. 115: Immunocytochemical methods and protocols. Totowa: Humana Press; 1999. p. 405–14.

144. Simsir A, Fetsch PA, Abati A. Calretinin immunostaining in benign and malignant pleural effusions. Diagn Cytopathol 2001;24:149–52.

145. Saqi A, Alexis D, Remotti F, et al. Usefulness of CDX2 and TTF-1 in differentiating gastrointestinal from pulmonary carcinoids. Am J Clin Pathol 2005;123:394–404.

146. Brockstedt U, Gulyas M, Dobra K, et al. An optimized battery of eight antibodies that can distinguish most cases of epithelial mesothelioma from adenocarcinoma. Am J Clin Pathol 2000;114:203–9.

147. Boehringer-Mannheim. Anti-carcinoembryonic antigen package insert. Indianapolis: Boehringer-Mannheim; 1995.

148. Stoetzer OJ, Munker R, Darsow M, et al. P53-immunoreactive cells in benign and malignant effusions: diagnostic value using a panel of monoclonal antibodies and comparison with CEA-staining. Oncol Rep 1999;6:433–36.

149. Moll R, Franke W, Schiller D, et al. The catalog of human cytokeratins: patterns of expression in normal epithelia, tumors and cultured cells. Cell 1982;31:11–24.

150. Cihlar KL, Markelova N, Varsegi G, et al. Two Color Immunocytochemistry for Evaluation of Serous Cavity Fluids: United States and Canadian Academy of Pathology (USCAP). Mod Pathol 2007;20(supplement 2):[A-3804] (Abstract 285).

151. Boehringer-Mannheim. Anti-cytokeratin AE1/AE3 package insert. Indianapolis: Boehringer-Mannheim; 1998.

152. Kahn HJ, Bailey D, Marks A. Monoclonal antibody D2-40, a new marker of lymphatic endothelium, reacts with Kaposi's sarcoma and a subset of angiosarcomas. Mod Pathol 2002;15:434–40.

153. Chu AY, Litzky LA, Pasha TL, et al. Utility of D2-40, a novel mesothelial marker, in the diagnosis of malignant mesothelioma. Mod Pathol 2005;18:105–10.

154. Ordóñez NG. The diagnostic utility of immunohistochemistry and electron microscopy in distinguishing between peritoneal mesotheliomas and serous carcinomas: a comparative study. Mod Pathol 2006;19:34–48.

155. Ordóñez NG. D2-40 and podoplanin are highly specific and sensitive immunohistochemical markers of epithelioid malignant mesothelioma. Hum Pathol 2005;36:372–80.

156. Chivukula M, Kapali M. Expression of D2-40 in primary peritoneal serous carcinomas, ovarian serous carcinomas, uterine carcinomas and sex cord stromal tumors. Mod Pathol 2006; 19(Supplement 1):1A–359A. Abstract no. 794.

157. Sonne SB, Herlihy AS, Hoei-Hansen CE, et al. Identity of M2A (D2-40) antigen and gp36 (Aggrus, T1A-2, podoplanin) in human developing testis, testicular carcinoma in situ and germ-cell tumours. Virchows Arch 2006;449:200–6.

158. Chhieng DC, Yee H, Schaefer D, et al. Calretinin staining pattern aids in the differentiation of mesothelioma from adenocarcinoma in serous effusions. Cancer 2000;90:194–200.

159. Schacht V, Dadras SS, Johnson LA, et al. Up-regulation of the lymphatic marker podoplanin, a mucin-type transmembrane glycoprotein, in human squamous cell carcinomas and germ cell tumors. Am J Pathol 2005;166:913–21.

160. Ordóñez NG. Podoplanin: a novel diagnostic immunohistochemical marker. Adv Anat Pathol 2006;13:83–88.

161. Chenard-Neu MP, Kabou A, Mechine A, et al. Immunohistochemistry in the differential diagnosis of mesothelioma and adenocarcinoma. Evaluation of 5 new

antibodies and 6 traditional antibodies. Ann Pathol 1998;18:460–65.

162. Dako. Monoclonal mouse anti-human mesothelial cell (HBME-l), package insert. Carpenteria, CA: Dako Corporation; 1998.

163. Ordóñez NG. Application of mesothelin immunostaining in tumor diagnosis. Am J Surg Pathol 2003;27:1418–28.

164. Morgan RL, DeYoung BR, McGaughy VR, et al. MOC-31 aids in the differentiation between adenocarcinoma and reactive mesothelial cells. Cancer (Cancer Cytopathol) 1999;87:390–94.

165. Gonzalez-Lois C, Ballestin C, Sotelo MT, et al. Combined use of novel epithelial (MOC-31) and mesothelial (HBME-1) immunohistochemical markers for optimal first line diagnostic distinction between mesothelioma and metastatic carcinoma in pleura. Histopathology 2001;38:528–34.

166. Roberts F, Harper CM, Downie I, et al. Immunohistochemical analysis still has a limited role in the diagnosis of malignant mesothelioma. A study of thirteen antibodies. Am J Clin Pathol 2001;116:253–62.

167. Delahaye M, Hoogsteden HC, Van der Kwast TH. Immunocytochemistry of malignant mesothelioma: OV632 as a marker of malignant mesothelioma. J Pathol 1991;165:137–43.

168. Abati A, Fetsch PA. OV632 as a possible marker for malignant mesothelioma: high expectations; low specificity. Diagn Cytopathol 1995;12:81–82.

169. Ordóñez NG. Thyroid transcription factor-1 is a marker of lung and thyroid carcinomas. Adv Anat Pathol 2000;7:123–27.

170. Sosolik RC, McGaughy VR, De Young BR. Anti-MOC-31: a potential addition to the pulmonary adenocarcinoma versus mesothelioma immunohistochemistry panel. Mod Pathol 1997;10:716–19.

171. Khoor A, Whitsett JA, Stahlman MT, et al. Utility of surfactant protein B precursor and thyroid transcription factor 1 in differentiating adenocarcinoma of the lung from malignant mesothelioma. Hum Pathol 1999;30:695–700.

172. Ordóñez NG. Value of thyroid transcription factor-1, E-cadherin, BG8, WT1, and CD44S immunostaining in distinguishing epithelial pleural mesothelioma from pulmonary and nonpulmonary adenocarcinoma. Am J Surg Pathol 2000;24:598–606.

173. Garcia-Prats MD, Ballestin C, Sotelo T, et al. A comparative evaluation of immunohistochemical markers for the differential diagnosis of malignant pleural tumours. Histopathology 1998;32:462–72.

174. Shield PW, Koivurinne K. The value of calretinin and cytokeratin 5/6 as markers for mesothelioma in cellblock preparations of serous effusions. Cytopathology 2008;19:218–23.

175. Abati A, Fetsch PA, Filie A. If cells could talk: the application of new techniques to cytopathology. Clin Lab Med 1998;18:561–83.

176. Chhieng DC, Jhala N. Where do they come from? Evaluation of unknown primary site of origin. In: Shidham VB, Atkinson BF, editors. Cytopathologic Diagnosis of Serous Fluids. 1st edn. London: Elsevier; 2007. p. 157–69.

177. Shidham VB. Respiratory cytology. In: Atkinson BF, editor. Atkinson Atlas of Diagnostic Cytopathology. 2nd edn. Philadelphia: WB Saunders; 2004. p. 273–356.

178. Attanoos RL, Griffin A, Gibbs AR. The use of immunohistochemistry in distinguishing reactive from neoplastic mesothelium. A novel use for desmin and comparative evaluation with epithelial membrane antigen,

p53, platelet-derived growth factor-receptor, P-glycoprotein and Bcl-2. Histopathology 2003;43:231–38.

179. Saad RS, Cho P, Liu YL, et al. The value of epithelial membrane antigen expression in separating benign mesothelial proliferation from malignant mesothelioma: a comparative study. Diagn Cytopathol 2005;32:156–59.

180. Ordóñez NG. Immunohistochemical diagnosis of epithelioid mesothelioma: an update. Arch Pathol Lab Med 2005;129:1407–14.

181. Fazio J, Friedman HD, Swerdlow J, et al. Diagnosis of systemic lupus erythematosus in an elderly male by pericardial fluid cytology: a case report. Diagn Cytopathol 1998;18:346–48.

182. Chou CW, Chang SC. Pleuritis as a presenting manifestation of rheumatoid arthritis: diagnostic clues in pleural fluid cytology. Am J Med Sci 2002;323:158–61.

183. Roberts PP. Parasitic infections of the pleural space. Semin Respir Infect 1988;3:362–82.

184. Vercelli-Retta J, Mañana G, Reissenweber NJ. The cytologic diagnosis of hydatid disease. Acta Cytol 1982;26:159–68.

185. Kumar ND, Bhatia A, Misra K, et al. Comparison of pleural fluid cytology and pleural biopsy in the evaluation of pleural effusion. J Indian Med Assoc 1995;93:307–9.

186. Marwah N, Singh P, Singh S, et al. Filarial pleural effusion. Trop Doct 2007;37:262.

187. Marathe A, Handa V, Mehta GR, et al. Early diagnosis of filarial pleural effusion. Indian J Med Microbiol 2003;21:207–8.

188. Motherby H, Nadjari B, Friegel P, et al. Diagnostic accuracy of effusion cytology. Diagn Cytopathol 1999;20:350–57.

189. Spriggs AI. The Cytology of Effusions. London: Heinemann; 1957.

190. Spriggs AI, Boddington MM. Atlas of Serous Fluid Cytopathology. London: Kluwer; 1989.

191. Renshaw AA, Dean BR, Antman KH, et al. The role of cytologic evaluation of pleural fluid in the diagnosis of malignant mesothelioma. Chest 1997;111:106–9.

192. Whitaker D. The cytology of malignant mesothelioma. Invited review. Cytopathology 2000;11:139–51.

193. Whitaker D, Shilkin KB. Diagnosis of pleural malignant mesothelioma in life—a practical approach. J Pathol 1984;143:147–75.

194. Gillespie FR, Van der Walt JD, Derias N, et al. Deciduoid peritoneal mesothelioma. A report of the cytological appearances. Cytopathology 2001;12:57–61.

195. Khalidi HS, Medeiros JL, Battifora H. Lymphohistiocytic mesothelioma: an often misdiagnosed variant of sarcomatous malignant mesothelioma. Am J Clin Pathol 2000;113:649–54.

196. Corson J. Pathology of mesothelioma. Thorac Surg Clin 2004;14:447–60.

197. Comin C, de Klerk NH, Henderson DW. Malignant mesothelioma: current conundrums and whither electron microscopy for diagnosis? Ultrastruct Pathol 1997;21:315–20.

198. Oury TP, Hammar SP, Roggli VL. Ultrastructural features of diffuse malignant mesothelioma. Hum Pathol 1998;29:1382–92.

199. Galindo LM. Effusion cytopathology. In: Atkinson BF, Silverman JF, editors. Atlas of Difficult Diagnoses in Cytopathology. 1st edn. Philadelphia: WB Saunders; 1998. p. 165–99.

200. Yu GH, Sack MJ, Baloch ZW, et al. Occurrence of intercellular spaces (windows) in metastatic adenocarcinoma in serous fluids: a cytomorphologic, histochemical, and ultrastructural study. Diagn Cytopathol 1999;20:115–19.

201. Wojno KJ, Olson JL, Sherman ME. Cytopathology of pleural effusions after radiotherapy. Acta Cytol 1994;38:1–8.

202. Hemachandran M, Dey P. Indian file pattern of adenocarcinoma cells in effusions. Acta Cytol 2004;48:385–86.

203. DeMay RM. Practical principles of cytopathology. Chicago: ASCP Press; 1999 xi, 402.

204. Suh YK, Shabaik A, Meurer WT, et al. Lymphoid cell aggregates: a useful clue in the fine-needle aspiration diagnosis of follicular lymphomas. Diagn Cytopathol 1997;17:467–71.

205. Dunphy CH, Collins B, Ramos R, et al. Secondary pleural involvement by an AIDS-related anaplastic large cell (CD30+) lymphoma simulating metastatic adenocarcinoma. Diagn Cytopathol 1998;18:113–17.

206. Kjeldsberg CR, Knight JA, Kjeldsberg CR. Body fluids [slide]. Chicago: ASCP Press; 1993.

207. Sears D, Hajdu SI. The cytologic diagnosis of malignant neoplasms in pleural and peritoneal effusions. Acta Cytol 1987;31:85–97.

208. Travis WD. Armed Forces Institute of Pathology (US), Universities Associated for Research and Education in Pathology. Non-neoplastic disorders of the lower respiratory tract. Washington, DC: American Registry of Pathology: Armed Forces Institute of Pathology; 2002 xix, 939.

209. Valdes L, Alvarez D, Valle JM, et al. The etiology of pleural effusions in an area with high incidence of tuberculosis. Chest 1996;109:158–62.

210. Das DK, Al-Juwaiser A, George SS, et al. Cytomorphological and immunocytochemical study of non-Hodgkin lymphoma in pleural effusion and ascitic fluid. Cytopathology 2007;18:157–67.

211. Mihaescu A, Gebhard S, Chaubert P, et al. Application of molecular genetics to the diagnosis of lymphoid-rich effusions: study of 95 cases with concomitant immunophenotyping. Diagn Cytopathol 2002;27(2):90–95.

212. Das DK. Serous effusions in malignant lymphomas: a review. Diagn Cytopathol 2006;34:335–47.

213. Elis A, Blickstein D, Mulchanov I, et al. Pleural effusion in patients with non-Hodgkin lymphoma: a case-controlled study. Cancer 1998;83(8):1607–11.

214. Ashchi M, Golish J, Eng P, et al. Transudative malignant pleural effusions: prevalence and mechanisms. South Med J 1998;91:23–26.

215. Olson PR, Silverman JF, Powers CN. Pleural fluid cytology of Hodgkin disease: cytomorphologic features and the value of immunohistochemical studies. Diagn Cytopathol 2000;22:21–24.

216. Staats BA, Ellefson RD, Budahn LL, et al. The lipoprotein profile of chylous and nonchylous pleural effusions. Mayo Clin Proc 1980;55:700–4.

217. Ruckdeschel JC. Management of malignant pleural effusions. Sem Oncol 1995;22(2 Suppl 3):58–63.

218. Fenton KN, Richardson JD. Diagnosis and management of malignant pleural effusions. Am J Surg 1995;170:69–74.

219. Shidham VB. Diagnostic pitfalls in effusion fluid cytology. In: Shidham VB, Atkinson BF, editors. Cytopathologic Diagnosis of Serous Fluids. 1st edn. London: Elsevier; 2007. p. 43–54.

220. Johnston WW. The malignant pleural effusion. A review of cytopathologic diagnoses of 584 specimens from 472 consecutive patients. Cancer 1985;56:905–9.

221. Monte SA, Ehya H, Lang WR. Positive effusion cytology as the initial presentation of malignancy. Acta Cytologica 1987;31:448–52.

222. Pavlidis N, Briasoulis E, Hainsworth J, et al. Diagnostic and therapeutic management of cancer of an unknown primary [see comment]. Eur J Cancer 1990;39:1990–2005.

223. Chu DZ, Lang NP, Thompson C, et al. Peritoneal carcinomatosis in nongynecologic malignancy. A prospective study of prognostic factors. Cancer 1989;63:364–67.

224. Geisinger KR, Hajdu SI, Helson L. Exfoliative cytology of nonlymphoreticular neoplasms in children. Acta Cytologica 1984;28:16–28.

225. Ascoli V, Lo-Coco F. Body cavity lymphoma. Curr Opin Pulm Med 2002;8:317–22.

226. Walts AE. Malignant melanoma in effusions: a source of false-negative cytodiagnoses. Diagn Cytopathol 1986;2:150–53.

227. Kimura N, Kimura I. Podoplanin as a marker for mesothelioma. Pathol Int 2005;55:83–86.

228. Salhadin A, Nasiell M, Nasiell K, et al. The unique cytologic picture of oat cell carcinoma in effusions. Acta Cytol 1976;20:298–302.

229. Green N, Gancedo H, Smith R, et al. Pseudomyxoma peritonei-nonoperative management and biochemical findings. A case report. Cancer 1975;36:1834–37.

230. Rammou-Kinia R, Sirmakechian-Karra T. Pseudomyxoma peritonei and malignant mucocele of the appendix. A case report. Acta Cytologica 1986;30:169–72.

231. Young JA, Crocker J. Pleural fluid cytology in lymphoplasmacytoid lymphoma with numerous intracytoplasmic immunoglobulin inclusions. A case report with immunocytochemistry. Acta Cytologica 1984;28:419–24.

232. Spriggs AI, Jerrome DW. Intracellular mucous inclusions. A feature of malignant cells in effusions in the serous cavities, particularly due to carcinoma of the breast. J Clin Pathol 1975;28:929–36.

233. Hoda RS, Cangiarella J, Koss LG. Metastatic squamous-cell carcinoma in pericardial effusion: report of four cases, two with cardiac tamponade. Diagn Cytopathol 1998;18:422–24.

234. Cobb CJ, Wynn J, Cobb SR, et al. Cytologic findings in an effusion caused by rupture of a benign cystic teratoma of the mediastinum into a serous cavity. Acta Cytologica 1985;29:1015–20.

235. Abadi MA, Zakowski MF. Cytologic features of sarcomas in fluids. Cancer 1998;84:71–76.

236. Cibas ES, Corson JM, Pinkus GS. The distinction of adenocarcinoma from malignant mesothelioma in cellblocks of effusions: the role of routine mucin histochemistry and immunohistochemical assessment of carcinoembryonic antigen, keratin proteins, epithelial membrane antigen, and milk fat globule-derived antigen. Hum Pathol 1987;18:67–74.

237. Kannerstein M, Churg J, Magner D. Histochemistry in the diagnosis of malignant mesothelioma. Ann Clini Lab Sci 1973;3:207–11.

238. Bauer Z, Milic N, Handl S, et al. The results of some cytochemical reactions in metastatic malignant tumor cells in pleural and peritoneal effusions. Acta Cytol 1977;21:141–46.

239. Herrera GA, Reimann BE. Electron microscopy in determining origin of metastatic adenocarcinomas. South Med J 1984;77:1557–66.

240. Hanna W, Kahn HJ. Ultrastructural and immunohistochemical characteristics of mucoepidermoid carcinoma of the breast. Hum Pathol 1985;16:941–46.

241. Hsu C. Cytologic detection of malignancy in pleural effusion: a review of 5,255 samples from 3,811 patients. Diagn Cytopathol 1987;3:8–12.

242. Garcia LW, Ducatman BS, Wang HH. The value of multiple fluid specimens in the cytological diagnosis of malignancy. Mod Pathol 1994;7:665–68.

243. Zivanovic O, Barakat RR, Sabbatini PJ, et al. Prognostic factors for patients with stage IV epithelial ovarian cancer receiving intraperitoneal chemotherapy after second-look assessment: results of long-term follow-up. Cancer 2008;112:2690–97.

244. Swanson N, Mirza I, Wijesinghe N, et al. Primary percutaneous balloon pericardiotomy for malignant pericardial effusion. Catheter Cardiovasc Interv 2008;71:504–7.

245. Varsegi GM, Shidham V. Cell block preparation from cytology specimen with predominance of individually scattered cells. J Vis Exp 2009; 29: 1316. doi: 10.3791/1316. PMID: 19623160. Video article is available FREE on web as open access at http://www.jove.com/index/Details. stp?ID=1316.

246. Lau SK, Chu PG, Weiss LM. CD163: a specific marker of macrophages in paraffin-embedded tissue samples. Am J Clin Pathol 2004; 122:794–801.

247. Shidham VB, Varsegi G, D'Amore K. Two-color immunocytochemistry for evaluation of effusion fluids for metastatic adenocarcinoma. CytoJournal, 2009.

# Section 4

## Breast

# The breast

Torill Sauer and Derek Roskell

## Chapter contents

## Introduction

Fine needle aspiration (FNA) cytology is a valuable tool in the work-up of all breast abnormalities, both palpable and non-palpable. The use of FNA varies considerably in different centres. In some, its main role is to provide almost instant diagnosis in a one-stop clinic. Here the cytopathologist is a key part of the clinical team, assessing the lesion clinically, taking and interpreting a sample, and providing a rapid report so that definitive management decisions can be made straight away. In other centres, the role of FNA is essentially a less traumatic alternative to core biopsy (CB), with samples processed in the laboratory before reporting, and used for ancillary techniques such as immunohistochemical assessment of prognostic markers.

In all settings, the main goal of breast FNA is to confirm benign or probably benign clinical and/or radiological findings in order to avoid unnecessary surgery or to give an unequivocal, preoperative diagnosis of malignancy in order to allow appropriate patient counselling and definitive clinical management. Equivocal cytological diagnoses should lead to a diagnostic biopsy. For a breast FNA clinic to be successful, it is critical that the rates of inadequate and equivocal cytological diagnoses are low. The cytological findings should always be evaluated in conjunction with the clinical and radiological findings (triple assessment). Often FNA combined with radiology will determine patient management irrespective of clinical impression. Discordant FNA and radiological results usually warrant a diagnostic biopsy. In specialised centres, sensitivity and specificity of breast FNA is around 90%, somewhat higher for palpable and non-palpable ultrasound guided FNA than for stereotactic FNA.[1-8] The percentage of inadequate specimens should be less than 10%.[9] The percentage of false negative diagnoses (FN) varies in the literature, but in specialised centres is usually less than 5%.[1,5,6,8,10-18] The main cause of FN diagnoses is sampling error (SE). In about 70% of FN the target lesions is less than 1 cm in size.[18] False positive (FP) diagnoses are always interpretation errors (IE). They are highly undesirable, but in large volume institutions, they will occur from time to time in the process of evaluation of rare lesions, diagnostic pitfalls and look-alikes, such as some fibroadenomas with myoepithelial hyperplasia, complex sclerosing lesions and sclerosing adenosis. Most screening and other guidelines demand that the percentage of FP should be less than 1%.[9]

## Clinical assessment

It is helpful to note the sensation obtained when the needle enters the lesion, largely because this can help inform the operator that the lesion has been successfully targeted. Details may be included in the report for subsequent audit. The character of the lesion can be described and correlated in the following way, according to the modified United Kingdom National Health Service Breast Screening Programme (NHSBSP) guidelines.[9]

### Clinical characteristics of lesions sampled by FNA

- Soft: fibroadenoma, mucoid carcinoma, medullary carcinoma
- Rubbery: fibrocystic change, lobular carcinoma, fibroadenoma
- Variable resistance with popping sensation: fibrocystic change
- Leathery: dense fibrous change, ancient fibroadenoma
- Gritty: carcinoma, partial calcification, a few fibroadenomas
- Solid: completely calcified ancient fibroadenomas.

## Fine needle aspiration (FNA)

In order to obtain an optimal or near optimal cell yield, aspirator skill is critical for success of FNA.[4,19]

Results from the UK National Health Service Breast Screening Programme (NHSBSP) have shown that a low sensitivity to a large degree is due to a high inadequacy rate, most often due to the lack of aspirator skill.[20] Overall, results are better when cytopathologists perform their own aspirations.[21] In a rapid one-stop clinic setting, a cytopathologist can further reduce the incidence of non-diagnostic or equivocal results by taking a new sample if the initial one is suboptimal.

## Equipment

- Needles sized 0.7 mm in diameter or less (23–25G) in palpable lesions are ideal. The thinner the needle, the less resulting blood contamination. Larger needles (0.8 mm) (21G) invariably yield more blood and not necessarily more cellular material
- In stereotactic FNA larger needles may be used in order to avoid deviation of the needle in firm/sclerotic breast tissue
- 10 mL or 20 mL syringe in order to obtain negative pressure during aspiration and allow cystic lesions to be drained.

Some operators use a syringe-holder to allow one hand to operate the syringe, leaving the other to fix the lesion.

## FNA of palpable lesions

- Fix the lump between the second and the third finger of the non-dominant hand
- Insert the needle ideally at a 90° angle (Fig. 4.1), but adapting this to take account of structures that are normally avoided, such as pleura and areola. This angle will minimise missing small lesions. For central lesions, it is usually possible to sample without going through the areola either by approaching from the side, or asking the patient to pull the skin gently so that the lesion is no longer under the areola
- Apply negative pressure when the needle tip is in the lesion
- Move the needle to and fro and sample from as many parts of the lump as feasible. Sampling is then a result of both aspiration/suction and/or capillary action. Avoid holding the needle still and only applying suction, as this will result in more blood and less tissue and cells. Soft cellular lesions will tend to need fewer movements of the needle than hard sclerotic ones. The aim is to move the needle sufficiently to notice the sample or blood in the hub of the needle at which point it is best to stop
- Unless a cyst is being drained, stop when material appears in the needle hub or if there is excessive bleeding
- Release the negative pressure before the needle is withdrawn.

## FNA of non-palpable lesions

This is performed under ultrasound guidance, in conjunction with the radiologists. The FNA procedure is the same, except for the first two points.

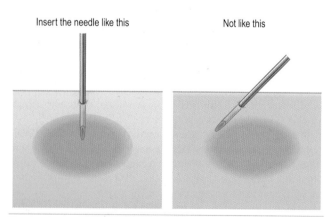

Insert the needle like this      Not like this

**Fig. 4.1** Aspiration technique: it is important to insert the needle vertically. Small lesions may be missed if the needle is inserted obliquely.

## FNA using the needle alone

The capillary method has been most widely reported in thyroid lesions but can be applied to any site, including the breast.[22–24] The main benefit of this approach is reducing patient anxiety by not using a relatively bulky instrument described above and instead using the needle alone. Another benefit is better control of the needle and the closer feel of the lesion by the aspirator. Capillary method also reduces blood contamination, particularly when sampling a very vascular site such as a tiny cutaneous tumour deposit. Moving the needle to sample multiple parts of the lesion is crucial.

## Preparation

The aspirated material can be handled in several ways, the choice depending on the setting in which cytology is being used. In a 'one-stop rapid diagnosis clinic' speed normally dictates that air dried direct smears are used. In other settings, it may be advantageous to prepare both alcohol (usually spray)-fixed and air dried smears. Alcohol fixation must be done immediately, as air drying starts within seconds after smearing.

Another option is to flush the aspirated material into a collection or transport fluid. This can be done with the whole content of the needle, but also with the remnants after the main part has been prepared as direct smears. The fluid can contain a fixative such as ethanol, methanol or a mixture of more than one fixative, or a commercially available transport fluid such as ThinPrep® Cytolyte or Autocyte®. Buffered saline without a fixative is also acceptable.

Liquid suspensions must be centrifuged and the precipitate handled according to the in-house procedures. Cytospin preparations as well as preparations from ThinPrep® or Autocyte® all give high-quality specimens for routine staining. A major advantage is the possibility of preparing additional smears for ancillary procedures.[25–30]

## Cytological evaluation of the nipple and nipple secretion

Bloodstained nipple secretion is an indication for cytological examination of the nipple fluid. However, it is recognised that cytology of nipple discharge has a low sensitivity for identifying underlying malignancy and a negative result should not preclude further investigation. Nipple discharge fluid is best prepared by placing a glass slide tangentially to the nipple in such a way as to touch the drop of secretion, making sure not to touch the surrounding skin in order to avoid contamination. After the secretion is transferred to the glass, a conventional smear is made.

Ulceration or eczematous changes on the nipple likewise warrant further investigation and scrape material may be examined. The debris covering the ulceration is carefully removed and the non-cutting edge of a scalpel blade or the edge of a clean slide is used to scrape cells from the surface. Preparation of both nipple fluid and scrape material can be handled in the same way as FNA material.

## Staining methods

Breast cytological material is usually stained with conventional cytological stains, such as Papanicolaou (PAP) for alcohol-fixed slides and May-Grünwald Giemsa (MGG) for air-dried slides. MGG is ideal as a rapid stain (Diff-Quik® or equivalent), and hence is the stain of choice in one-stop clinics. It can be done in less than 2 min on air dried direct smears. The smears can be examined without a cover glass, which is particularly useful for checking adequacy when the patient is still on the couch and the cytologist is considering whether to take a second sample. If a Diff-Quik® smear is not adequately stained, it may be restained with MGG in the laboratory.

## Artefacts

Stain precipitates may be observed in MGG. Its appearance should prompt a change of staining solutions. Starch granules from gloves may seriously impair the evaluation of MGG-stained smears. To avoid this problem the aspirator should not use starched gloves. Air drying artefact causing 'exploded nuclei' is the most serious artefact besetting MGG air-dried smears. If widespread, it may render a specimen inadequate for assessment. Furthermore, the novice may try to interpret the less affected cells that appear artificially large. The appearance, sometimes called 'the osmotic effect', is that of a cell whose nucleus has expanded and ruptured with spillage of chromatin at the cell border, forming a flare. This artefact has been attributed to the effects of saline, local anaesthetic fluid and autolysis from slow drying, as when the smear is placed directly into an airtight box. Over-heating when an electric hairdryer is used to ensure rapid drying and the use of excessive pressure when making the smear, causing the crush artefact, are also possible culprits.

Crushed nuclei (Fig. 4.2) are distinct from the phenomenon of exploded nuclei described above as the spilt chromatin is spread in the direction of the smear. It is due to the use of excessive pressure, but some types of malignant tumours are particularly prone to this problem and the artefact can be a clue to the diagnosis.

A few red blood cells provide a scale for comparison with the size of the nucleated cells. The presence of a large amount of blood, however, will obscure other cellular or extracellular material and in air-dried aspirates the stains often do not penetrate a thick film of blood.

As ultrasound localisation of breast lumps is adopted more widely, cell lysis by contamination by ultrasound transmission jelly poses a threat to cytological diagnosis.[31] The effect of the jelly on cell morphology is dramatic and, in experiments *in vitro*, varies with the length of exposure before fixation. The phenomenon is seen even in rapidly air-dried samples, presumably from the mixing of the jelly with the sample within the needle rather than on the slide. Initially, there is some swelling of the cell cytoplasm and nucleus (Fig. 4.3). This can make benign cells more worrying when compared with uncontaminated controls. Cell swelling is closely followed by leakage of nuclear chromatin, then complete dissolution of cell structure to form granular basophilic material and, eventually, a basophilic 'soup'. The jelly may be misinterpreted as necrotic material or mucin. Radiologists regard ultrasound jelly as a bland substance. If made aware of its detrimental effects on aspirated cells, they can modify their technique to lessen the risk of contamination.

## Ancillary techniques

Cytological material is well suited for immunocytochemistry (ICC), *in situ* hybridisation (ISH) and other molecular diagnostic or research procedures. Oestrogen receptor (ER) (Fig. 4.4), progesterone receptor (PgR) and HER-2/neu status are routine markers that are determined in all breast carcinomas. Although usually undertaken on histological material, with a careful technique they can be assessed using cytological specimens. ER and PgR are steroid receptors which are highly vulnerable to suboptimal handling of both cells and tissues. In cytological procedures, the critical point seems to be air drying of the smears at any point, both pre- and post-fixation. Air drying starts immediately after smearing and can be recognised on smears stained with antibodies to ER and/or PgR as a rim of negative tumour cell nuclei in the periphery of the smears. Optimal fixation of cytological material depends on the type of fixative. The most common is 4% buffered formalin, as in histology, or a three-step fixation with methanol, acetone and formalin. Some centres use 96% ethanol with acceptable

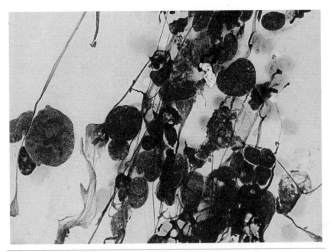

**Fig. 4.2** Crushing artefact. These breast carcinoma cells show typical crushing and spreading of the chromatin. The tendency for this artefact to develop is a function of the fragility of the cells and the pressure used to make the smear.

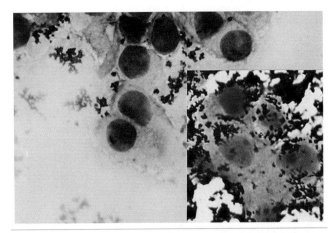

**Fig. 4.3** Ultrasound jelly artefact. These breast carcinoma cells show and intermediate degree of damage as a result of the presence of ultrasound jelly. The nuclei show loss of the chromatin detail and the constituent of the jelly is seen as a purple granular precipitate. The inset shows the cells at a slightly more advanced stage of dissolution resulting from a greater concentration of the jelly (MGG).

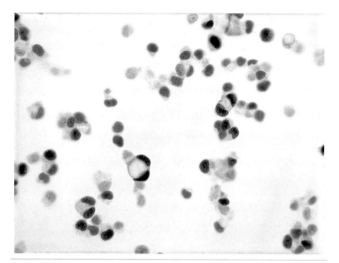

**Fig. 4.4** (ER) Liquid-based preparation. Oestrogen receptor positivity in breast carcinoma cells.

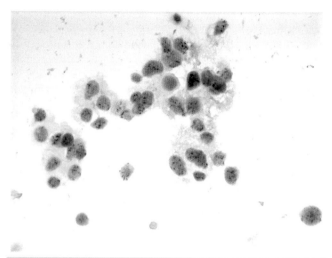

**Fig. 4.5** CISH on direct smear: HER-2 gene amplification in breast carcinoma cells (not the same case as Fig. 4.6).

results. The literature results favour liquid-based fixation.[32–37] Subject to adequate fixation and the absence of air drying, ER/PgR ICC results correlate closely with the histological findings.[38–44] Positive results should be expressed as the percentage of tumour cells showing positive nuclear staining[45] and can be used reliably in patient management, that is if >50% of cell nuclei are ER positive. If ER/PgR are either negative or weakly positive (<50% of the cells positive), the receptor status should be repeated on the histological specimen. Most institutions will perform ER/PgR primarily on the histology. However, in metastases and recurrences, resection is not always indicated and ER/PgR ICC is a valuable procedure in such cases. The advantage of using liquid-based cytology techniques is that the known positive cases can be used as controls. Cells in suspensions (stored at room temperature) and smears made from such suspensions may be stored for several months (at −20°C or −80°C) without losing their reactivity.

HER-2/neu is a transmembrane growth factor receptor. Both protein overexpression and gene amplification are associated with poor prognosis. HER-2/neu status is a routine marker and is at present being evaluated on all breast carcinomas in order to predict responsiveness to anthracycline and trastuzumab (Herceptin®). Protein expression may be determined by ICC, but all commercial kits and procedures are standardised for histological rather than cytological specimens. Reports in the literature indicate a high correlation of cytological results with histological results and *in situ* hybridisation (ISH).[46–49]

ISH, with fluorescent (FISH) chromogenic (CISH) or silver (SISH) visualisation, can be applied on cytological material,[45,50,51] both direct smears (Figs 4.5, 4.6) and preparations from liquid suspensions as well as on cell blocks (Fig. 4.7). Different fixations may require some modifications of the pre-treatment (demasking), but in general, cytological material requires little or no pre-treatment at all.[46–50,52–54]

HER-2/neu status may occasionally vary between the primary tumour and the metastases. Recurrences and metastases should therefore, as a rule, have a re-determination of their HER-2 status. If resection or biopsy is not indicated, ISH on cytological material is a valid option. ISH signal counts on cytological material will be higher than on histological sections, because the nuclei are not truncated. The HER-2/CEP17 (chromosome 17)

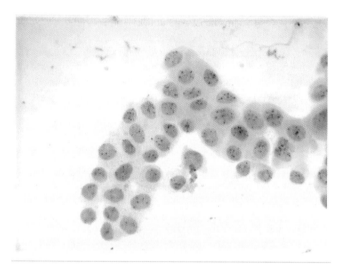

**Fig. 4.6** CISH on direct smear: Chromosome 17 centromere probe in sheet of breast carcinoma cells showing polysomy (not the same case as Fig. 4.5).

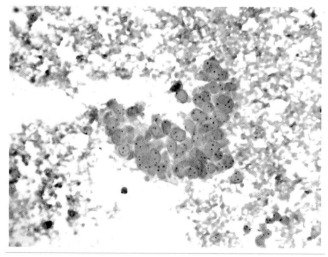

**Fig. 4.7** CISH on cell block: chromosome 17 centromere probe.

ratio will be the same and the cut-offs will be the same as for histology.[55]

A number of other prognostic markers have been investigated using cytological preparations. Proliferation markers such as Ki-67, tumour suppressor gene TP53, EGFR, topoisomerase IIα as well as ploidy/DNA measurements have all been investigated, but in most institutions, these results have no therapeutic implications at present (see Ch. 34).[46,47,56–58]

## Complications of FNA breast

Complications are few and seldom serious. The only common problem encountered clinically is the formation of a haematoma. This is unpredictable and can be minimised by prolonged pressure following aspiration, but sometimes the bleeding occurs very rapidly, even before the needle is withdrawn. This can obscure the lesion, making a second attempt difficult or impossible. Haemorrhage following FNA may cause interpretive problems for mammograms and ultrasound images, and as a rule, the radiological investigation should be completed before FNA is done.

Pneumothorax has been reported as a very rare complication,[59,60] the most risk probably being in the axillary tail of a thin patient. Strict adherence to the method outlined earlier in this chapter should minimise this risk.

Needle tract seeding after FNA has been reported in various tumours but is rare in breast cancer.[61]

## The normal breast

Under the influence of oestrogen and following menarche, progestogens, and in a complex hormonal milieu of growth hormone, thyroxine and insulin, the breast parenchyma grows by a process of duct elongation and branching. The formation of buds destined to become the lobular structures also occurs.

The parenchyma of human breast becomes fully developed at puberty and is then subjected to the waxing and waning stimuli of the menstrual cycle, interrupted only by the additional effects of pregnancy until the menopause.

The occurrence of masses in the prepubertal breast is rare. Pubertal hyperplasia occurs in both males and females and can be temporarily unbalanced or unilateral, but should not be mistaken for a pathological process when seen in the appropriate stage of development of the child. It subsides with progressing sexual maturation.

Following ovulation, rising levels of progesterone cause hyperplasia and dilation of terminal ductules. Mitotic activity appears in the lobular epithelium as does vacuolation, the morphological expression of a low level of secretion. In the secretory phase of the cycle the stroma becomes oedematous, sometimes giving the woman a sensation of fullness of the breasts. Late in the secretory and menstrual phase apoptotic activity occurs with some shedding of epithelial cell debris into the ductal lumina. Secretory products of non-lactating breast are slight and are presumably largely resorbed, only becoming obvious when part of the duct lobular system becomes obstructed by an inflammatory or neoplastic process.

In menopause, stromal and epithelial elements undergo involution with atrophy of glands. Women on hormone replacement therapy (HRT) may experience continuing oestrogen and progesterone influence on their breast tissue, not involution, and for some even hyperplasia with increased mammographic density of the breast tissue.

## The normal, mature breast

Histologically, the breast is composed of regularly arranged, radially disposed, independent glandular units forming a bush-like structure, with ducts as branches and lobules as berries. These 15–25 separate units end at the collecting ducts. The collecting ducts lead to lactiferous sinuses, distensible structures that act as a temporary reservoir for milk, which then form the lactiferous ducts that open onto the nipple. The glandular units contain the terminal duct-lobular units (TDLU). The TDLU, the most hormone sensitive part of the breast, is the main functional component, and therefore not surprisingly is the major site of origin for most of the pathological processes. There are tens of thousands of lobules in each breast. Subgross stereomicroscopy of cleared breast tissue reveals that the lobules overlap and mingle with those of adjacent segments.

All the glandular elements are surrounded by connective tissue. The undistinguished interlobular connective tissue contains a very variable amount of adipose tissue.

Accessory and ectopic breast tissue as well as intramammary lymph nodes are normal clinical variants. The breast is not a well demarcated or encapsulated organ and mammary lobules may be found beyond the normal anatomical boundaries. Most commonly, this is proved by the presentation of ectopic axillary breast tissue as a lump either in pregnancy or because of increased 'breast awareness'. Aspiration of such a lump reveals normal breast tissue components only.

Lymph nodes from the lower axillary group may be found in the upper outer quadrant or even the lower outer quadrant of the breast where they may present as a lump. The combination of the clinical features and an aspirate of normal or reactive lymphoid tissue permits diagnosis and reassurance.

### Cytological findings: the normal, mature breast

FNA from normal, adult breast tissue will contain variable amounts of ductal epithelial cell groups, small stromal fragments and fatty tissue. The epithelial cell yield is usually higher in younger age groups.

- Normal epithelial cells (Figs 4.8–4.10)
- Small cohesive groups
- Monolayer sheets
- Occasional complete TDLU
- Oval nuclei with regular outlines, 8–10 μm in diameter
- Inconspicuous nucleolus
- Evenly distributed chromatin
- Scanty cytoplasm
- Myoepithelial cells appear as ovoid, dense nuclei at the periphery of ductal sheets and groups
- Naked, bipolar (myoepithelial cell) nuclei in the background.

Fatty tissue may be the sole component of breast aspirates and is a common additional finding in both benign and malignant aspirates. Fatty aspirates contain balloon-like fat cells in clusters of variable sizes, sometimes associated with strands of fibrocollagenous tissue or occasional capillaries. The stromal fragments

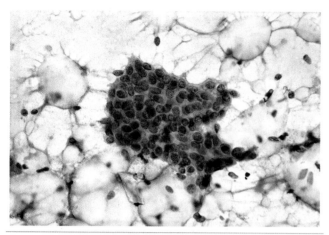

**Fig. 4.8** Normal breast. A group of benign ductal cells surrounded by single bipolar nuclei in the background (PAP). (Courtesy of Dr G McKee, Boston).

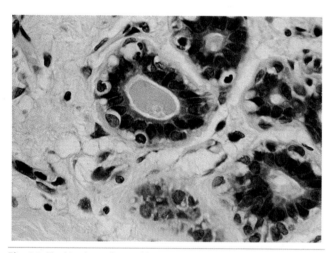

**Fig. 4.9** The histology of normal breast lobules (H&E).

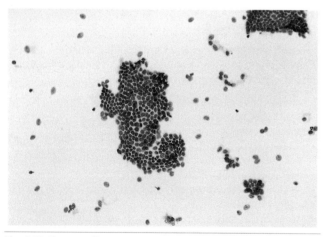

**Fig. 4.10** The typical benign pattern (C2) of a sheet of cohesive epithelial cells with bipolar nuclei in the background (H&E).

are usually small and few. Occasional naked, spindled fibrocyte nuclei may be found. The number of naked myoepithelial cell nuclei will mirror the amount of epithelial cell groups and sheets. Platelets appear as small granular amphophilic aggregates. Skeletal muscle fibres are seen rarely, particularly if the

correct aspiration technique is used. They appear as distinctive elongated cylinders with basophilic cytoplasm, on air-dried smears, orange on PAP-stained aspirates, with cross striations and peripherally located nuclei, intense blue on MGG. Organising haematoma may contain degenerate material, large spindle cells, large cells containing pigment and prominent nucleoli giving a potential for misdiagnosis as metastatic melanoma.

## The breast in pregnancy

During the 6th–20th weeks of pregnancy, the breast undergoes intensive growth. At the cellular level, there is enlargement of both the nuclei and the cytoplasm of duct and lobular epithelial cells. This growth slows dramatically in the third trimester when secretory changes become more prominent. During lactation the secretory cells become smaller and flattened with vacuolation of their cytoplasm. Following the cessation of lactation, the breast undergoes an involutionary process over several months, until the TDLUs return to their resting state. The development of a mass during pregnancy may be due to an uneven response to hormonal stimulation or enlargement of a pre-existing lesion such as a fibroadenoma. Other masses, such as *lactating adenoma* and *galactocele* arise de novo in pregnancy. Most galactoceles are so characteristic clinically that no further investigation is undertaken and the majority resolve spontaneously. The commonest cause of a mass during lactation is the development of an abscess. The accompanying pain and erythema usually make the diagnosis obvious but anxiety over the possibility of an inflammatory carcinoma may lead to a request for FNA cytology diagnosis.

Tumours and tumour-like lesions that occur during pregnancy and lactation are usually benign. However, carcinomas do occur, and tend to be high grade and oestrogen receptor negative. Some are reluctant to do mammography during pregnancy. Evaluation of mammograms during pregnancy and lactation may be difficult because the breast tissue is usually very dense. Ultrasound and FNA cytology are the two most important tools in work-up of tumours and tumour-like lesions during pregnancy and lactation.

### Cytological features of pregnancy-related changes

Acinar cells have abundant granular or vacuolated cytoplasm that is unusually fragile, frequently stripping away leaving naked nuclei in a granular 'dirty' background. The nuclei are large and round with active vesicular chromatin and a distinct large nucleolus. The nucleolus in lactating epithelial cells is larger than in most malignant breast tumours (Figs 4.11, 4.12). However, the presence of lipid-laden secretory material in the background is a helpful feature.

### Cytological findings: pregnancy-related changes

- The aspirate may be moderately or markedly cellular
- The cells are single and well dispersed in a lipid rich foamy or granular background
- The cells and their nuclei are large; there is abundant vacuolated or wispy cytoplasm
- Bare nuclei are common

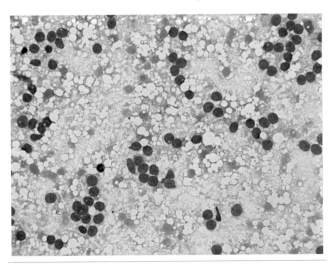

**Fig. 4.11** Typical lactation pattern with a granular-vacuolated background due to cytoplasmic rupture of the fragile epithelial cells. Loose cellular sheets. Nucleoli are large, larger than in most breast carcinomas (MGG).

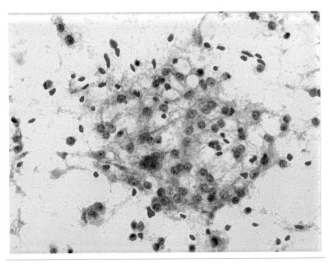

**Fig. 4.12** Typical lactation pattern with a granular-vacuolated background due to cytoplasmic rupture of the fragile epithelial cells. Loose cellular sheets. Nucleoli are large, larger than in most breast carcinomas (PAP).

- The nuclei are round and uniform with active granular or vesicular, but evenly distributed chromatin.
- Single prominent nucleoli

### Diagnostic pitfalls: pregnancy-related changes

The main risk is that the low-power impression of a cellular aspirate of single, large cells is taken as evidence of malignancy when the pathologist is not aware of the pregnant or lactational state of the patient. The distinctive granular background and critical assessment of the nuclear features should prevent this error.

It is important for the cytopathologist to be informed about pregnancy or lactation when the aspirate is performed by others, to lessen the likelihood of interpretive errors; one must also remember that foci of lactational change can occur unassociated with pregnancy and generalised lactation.

## Galactocele

Galactoceles are often easily diagnosed clinically without need for further investigation. However, occasionally a galactocele can accumulate abundant inspissated milk to form a large mass, even up to 80 mm in diameter, and this can be clinically worrying. It generally arises shortly after pregnancy, during lactation. The diagnosis may be readily made from the history, confirmed by the aspiration of milk, a procedure both diagnostic and therapeutic. The smears show abundant secretory material with scattered foamy macrophages. Epithelial cells are rarely seen. In the light of the clinical details the diagnosis should be benign, not inadequate.

### Cytological findings: galactocele

- The aspirated material is composed of milk
- Abundant granular, secretory material
- Foamy macrophages
- Calcified debris in 'old', longstanding lesions.

## Milk granuloma

Milk granuloma is thought to arise when milk leaks into the mammary stroma. The aspirates are likely to have an inflammatory appearance.[62]

## Gynaecomastia

Gynaecomastia is the enlargement of the male breast (Figs 4.13–4.15) due to hypertrophy and hyperplasia of both the glandular and stromal components. When arising before the age of 25, it is usually due to pubertal hormonal changes and commonly reverses spontaneously. In later life, the most common causes are drug therapy, androgenic steroid abuse, hormone producing tumours and cirrhosis of the liver with resulting failure to metabolise endogenous oestrogen.

Gynaecomastia may be unilateral or bilateral. The superficial nature of the mass in gynaecomastia generally makes sampling easy but it should be noted that the procedure is particularly painful in the male breast and good technique, even combined with the use of local anaesthetic, is important.

### Cytological findings: gynaecomastia

- Scanty or moderately cellular smears
- Small- to medium-sized epithelial fragments that may be hyperplastic and three-dimensional
- Small to moderate numbers of bipolar cells.

### Diagnostic pitfalls: gynaecomastia

- In florid hyperplasia there may be marked anisokaryosis that can be misinterpreted as atypia
- Fibrocystic change may rarely occur in the male breast[60] as can most benign/reactive and malignant lesions that occur in the female breast.

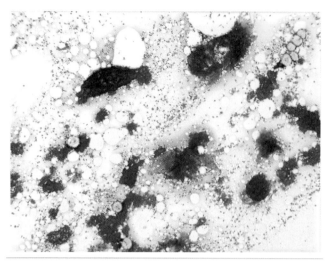

**Fig. 4.13** A typical pattern of benign (gynecomastia) ductal sheets and aggregates and stroma fragments (MGG).

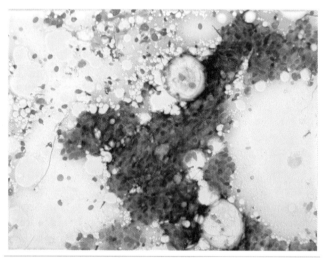

**Fig. 4.14** Gynaecomastia cohesive and complex aggregate of ductal epithelial cells and a moderate number of naked nuclei (MGG).

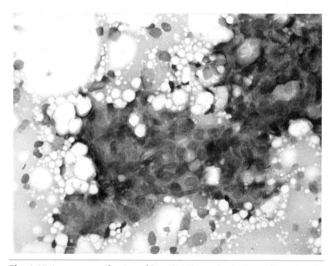

**Fig. 4.15** Larger magnification of Fig. 4.14. Hyperplastic, three-dimensional aggregate with benign ductal nuclei and scattered myoepithelial cell nuclei (MGG).

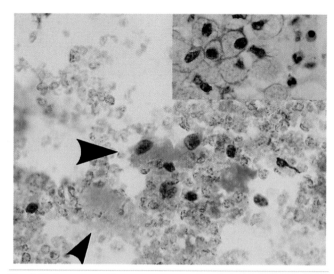

**Fig. 4.16** Duct ectasia. This aspirate contained numerous foamy macrophages (upper arrowhead) and amorphous debris (lower arrowhead). There is little if any epithelium. The appearances are typical of those seen in duct ectasia. The inset shows the histological appearances of the same case (PAP).

## Mammary duct ectasia

Histologically there is dilatation of large or intermediate ducts that are filled with secretion, and to a variable extent foamy macrophages, siderophages and cholesterol crystals that form the inspissated, pasty material seen on gross examination (Fig. 4.16). Epithelial proliferation is not a feature, but reparative changes in epithelium next to areas of inflammation may give rise to a spurious impression of atypia both histologically and cytologically. Rupture of the epithelial layer and basement membrane cause chronic inflammation, fibrosis and scarring of the surrounding stroma. It is usually an incidental finding in FNA or seen in smears of nipple discharge. Smears contain secretory debris and a variable number of foamy macrophages. Macroscopically the aspirated material often appears thick, creamy and homogeneous. Much of the material appears to dissolve in methanol fixative.

## Inflammatory conditions

The breast is susceptible to a limited range of inflammatory conditions, a few of which have a recognised infective aetiology. Trauma and extravasation of duct contents account for a proportion, but in some conditions, no obvious tissue insult is recognised. Inflammation is characteristically manifest by the presence of *dolor, calor, rubor* and *tumor*. It is the formation of a mass in the breast with or without pain that results in the patient with an inflammatory condition seeking medical assistance. Inflammatory lumps may frequently mimic malignancy both to the patient and on initial clinical assessment. FNA can usually provide a reliable generic diagnosis of inflammation and frequently a highly specific one when an organism is cultured from aspirated material.

## Fat necrosis

Fat necrosis of the breast (Fig. 4.17) may be associated with mammary duct ectasia and fibrocystic change when there is

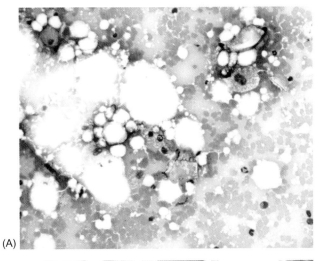

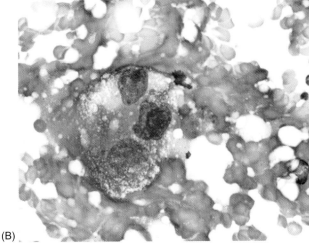

**Fig. 4.17** Fat necrosis. (A) At low power the pattern may be dominated by focal under-staining artefact due to impenetrable lipid, with foamy macrophages, lymphoid cells and sometimes lipid crystals visible in the better stained areas (MGG). (B) Occasionally histiocytes can demonstrate severe nuclear atypia which may mimic carcinoma (MGG).

rupture of a duct or cyst causing extravasation of contents with secondary necrosis of adjacent fat. It may also follow surgery and radiotherapy. Traumatic fat necrosis tends to be more superficial, often occurring in the subcutaneous fat, rather than within the breast itself. There is usually a history of injury 1–2 weeks, or even longer, before the lump is noted and there may or may not be bruising. The lesion is often tender on palpation. Clinically and/or radiologically, the lump may be suspicious, even with a hint of skin tethering in healing cases. Radiological findings may show an image that is typical of fat necrosis, but often mammography and/or ultrasound imaging is equivocal and occasionally suspicious for malignancy.

Post-surgical, or post-traumatic fat necrosis can persist for some years. Fat necrosis may be seen in old surgical sites as lumps or thickenings which become more prominent after the menopause as the surrounding breast atrophies, and may be both a clinical and a cytological mimic of recurrent cancer.

FNA of fat necrosis tend to be thick, granular and fatty when spread and contain many foamy macrophages and variable numbers of multinucleate giant cells. Other inflammatory cells may be present, but there is usually a paucity of epithelial elements.

The background contains fatty globules and fragments of fatty tissue, some showing degeneration. Occasionally, particularly in cases of old or membranous fat necrosis, an aspirate may contain only oily lipid material, with few or no cells visible.

### Cytological findings: fat necrosis

- Foamy macrophages and multinucleate giant cells with foamy cytoplasm
- Small irregular groups of (reactive) histiocytic cells
- Fragments of normal as well as degenerate fatty tissue
- Variable numbers of other inflammatory cells but usually sparse
- Few if any epithelial cells
- Free lipid droplets, seen as empty spaces that may be surrounded by blood or as empty spaces in a granular background
- Granular background debris.

### Diagnostic pitfalls: fat necrosis

- Aspirates from tuberculosis or other causes of panniculitis may be mistaken for fat necrosis
- Epithelioid cells in fat necrosis and granulation tissue can imitate carcinoma closely
- Vacuolated histiocytic cells may be mistaken for lobular carcinoma cells
- Fat necrosis is often found in the periphery of a tumour in areas where the carcinoma cells infiltrate fatty tissue. If the aspirated cells are from the periphery only, cells from the underlying tumour may not be seen.

## Plasma cell mastitis (periductal mastitis, comedo mastitis)

Clinically, this lesion may mimic carcinoma, as there can be retraction of the nipple associated with a well-defined lesion, usually centrally located. In a fifth of cases there is nipple discharge. It can be seen as part of the spectrum of duct ectasia. Mammography may reveal tubular, annular or linear calcifications. The aetiology is not clear but the basic abnormality is stagnation of secretion, possibly due to loss of elastin support in duct walls, leading to ectasia. There is an association with cigarette smoking.

Histologically, there is a spectrum of appearances reflecting the different stages of the disease process, but plasma cells are a characteristic finding. Macroscopically, the aspirated material may have the same appearance as simple duct ectasia.

Microscopically, there is amorphous debris with variable numbers of foamy macrophages and other inflammatory cells. Occasionally small numbers of reactive epithelial cells with degenerative and/or reparative changes are seen.

### Cytological findings: plasma cell mastitis

- Abundant, thick spreading pasty aspirate
- Loss of much of the material on smears because of dissolution in the methanol fixative
- Abundant amorphous debris in smears
- Foamy macrophages, occasional giant cells and plasma cells
- Scant epithelium which may show reactive atypia.

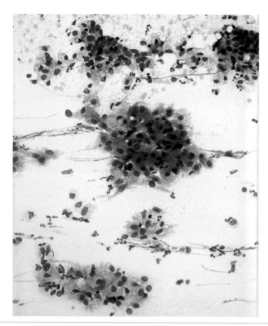

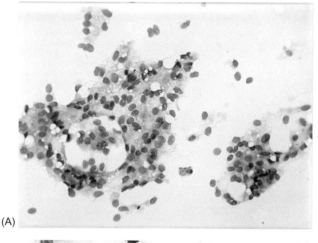

(A)

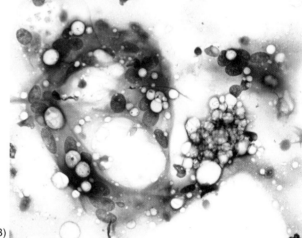

(B)

**Fig. 4.18** Irregular histiocytic aggregates in a case of granulomatous mastitis in a woman with SLE (MGG).

**Fig. 4.19** Silicone granuloma. (A) Loose histiocytic aggregates in a granulomatous reaction to silicone from an implant (MGG). (B) Foamy macrophages are associated with intracellular and extracellular globules of refractile, colourless silicone. The presence of other inflammatory cells is variable (MGG).

### Diagnostic pitfalls: plasma cell mastitis

- As with fat necrosis, the clinical features can falsely raise the index of suspicion
- If epithelium is included, it can appear atypical because of the inflammation
- Necrotic carcinomas, including comedo ductal carcinoma *in situ* can be mistaken for duct ectasia.

## Granulomatous mastitis (Figs 4.18, 4.19)

Various systemic and local conditions can give rise to the formation of a granulomatous response in the breast. Some cases of granulomatous mastitis are part of the spectrum of duct ectasia. There is a distinct group in which the granulomatous inflammation is lobulocentric[63] and associated with either recent pregnancy or another cause of high serum prolactin levels, such as phenothiazine therapy. Sarcoidosis of the breast is rare. Tuberculosis (Figs 4.20, 4.21) of the breast is more common in developing countries.[64] In the developed world, tuberculous mastitis is usually found in immigrants from countries with a high prevalence of tuberculosis.

Other entities that display granulomatous features on aspirates include granulomatous autoimmune disorders (Wegener's granulomatosis,[65] rheumatoid nodule, giant cell arteritis) as well as fungal infections, foreign body reaction to implanted silicone and tumours. Clues to the most probable aetiology of the granulomatous infiltration may be had from the gestational history, previous medical history, ethnic origin or other clinical findings, but the cytological features will rarely allow a specific diagnosis.

As few, if any, of these diseases benefit from surgical intervention, the provision of a specific diagnosis on aspirated material is particularly gratifying. Additional material for special stains (Fite, Ziehl-Neelsen, Grocott, PAS) is important to identify specific organisms.

Idiopathic granulomatous mastitis[66–72] has no known aetiology. It can be seen as a clinical mass, ranging in size from <1 cm to 8 cm and may mimic carcinoma clinically, radiologically and cytologically.[73,74] The diagnosis depends on the exclusion of other causes of granulomatous inflammation in the breast.

### Cytological findings: granulomatous mastitis

- Sheets or clusters of epithelioid cells with abundant cytoplasm and elongated nuclei
- Multinucleate giant cells associated with epithelioid cells. The giant cells often have epithelioid cell characteristics. Langhans type giant cells may be identified
- A variable number of inflammatory cells: lymphocytes, plasma cells, neutrophilic granulocytes
- In tuberculosis and fungal infections, a mixture of necrotic debris and inflammatory cells is often the dominant finding
- Admixture of ductal or lobular epithelial cells which may be reactive with enlarged nuclei and distinct nucleolus.

### Diagnostic pitfalls: granulomatous mastitis

- Nuclear features in histiocytic/epithelioid cells may give the impression of pleomorphism and these cells may be mistaken for carcinoma cells. Necrosis, as in tuberculosis, may add to this suspicion

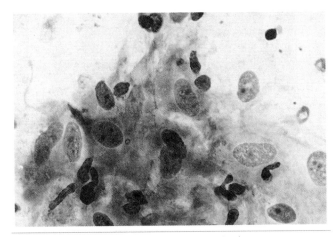

**Fig. 4.20** Tuberculous mastitis. This aspirate contained numerous groups of epithelioid histiocytes and occasional giant cells. Cultures and histology confirmed a diagnosis of tuberculous mastitis (MGG).

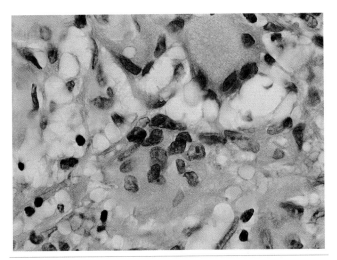

**Fig. 4.21** Tuberculous mastitis. Histological section (H&E).

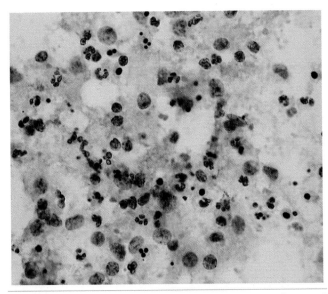

**Fig. 4.22** Breast abscess. This aspirate contains numerous macrophages and neutrophil polymorphs with little if any epithelium (PAP).

- Carcinomas or lymphomas may rarely elicit a granulomatous response which is often most pronounced in the periphery of the tumour. Sampling from both periphery and central parts of the lesion ensures a representative material for microscopic evaluation
- Carcinoma with osteoclast-type giant cells must be considered
- A largely necrotic carcinoma can occasionally give the misleading appearance of a granulomatous condition. Usually, however, there will be large numbers of degenerate or not fully necrotic epithelial cells with malignant features. In cases of doubt, a repeat aspirate from the periphery of the lesion will usually provide a more viable sample and confirm the diagnosis
- Reactive/reparative epithelial cells with additional degenerative nuclear changes may be interpreted as atypical and reported as suspicious. Cells with degenerative nuclear changes should never be the basis of an unequivocal malignant diagnosis.

## Abscess and acute mastitis

Breast abscesses and acute mastitis (Fig. 4.22) occur most commonly, but not invariably, in the puerperium. The diagnosis is usually made clinically and effective antibiotic treatment is given without need for a cytological or tissue diagnosis. Occasionally, however, resolution does not occur or is slow and surgical drainage is planned. The possibility of an inflammatory carcinoma may then be considered and an FNA diagnosis sought.

Aspirates contain neutrophil polymorphs and macrophages in considerable numbers as well as abundant cell debris. Reactive/reparative epithelial cells, derived from adjacent inflamed and possibly lactating breast tissue may also be found.

## Subareolar abscess (Fig. 4.23)

This condition is thought to have some affinity with mammary duct ectasia. There is often a history of the recurrent formation of a tender mass in the subareolar region, sinus tract formation

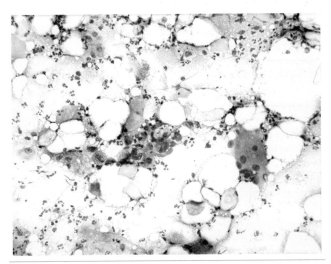

**Fig. 4.23** Subareolar abscess with a mixed inflammatory infiltrate with many neutrophilic granulocytes, anuclear squames, macrophages and multinucleated histiocytic giant cells (MGG).

and discharge with partial healing. Histologically, excised lesions are seen to consist of an inflammatory sinus tract lined by granulation tissue but often partially by squamous epithelium. FNA consists primarily of inflammatory exudate but additionally there may be anucleate squames, multinucleate giant cells and epithelium showing reactive atypia. The cytological appearance is not dissimilar to that of an infected or ruptured epidermal cyst except that these do not contain ductal cells.

### Cytological findings: subareolar abscess

- Anucleate squames
- Multinucleate giant cells
- Macrophages
- Epithelium showing reactive atypia.

### Diagnostic pitfalls: subareolar abscess

- Other inflammatory conditions including tuberculosis
- Sometimes the reactive atypia in the epithelial component of the aspirate is such that it may be confused with a more significant lesion.

## Sclerosing lymphocytic lobulitis of the breast

This lesion, also referred to as lymphocytic or diabetic mastopathy, has well-documented histopathological features of dense lobulocentric lymphoid infiltration associated with marked stromal fibrosis. There is an association with insulin-dependent diabetes mellitus, thyroiditis and arthropathy, although many cases are sporadic without known underlying disease. An overlap with fibrous disease is apparent. It can present as a lump and it might be expected to be the target of a FNA. The cytological features are not specific, merely showing a paucicellular benign pattern with lymphocytes.[75] These lesions can be clinically quite suspicious, and the condition is frequently identified in a core biopsy following scanty benign or non-diagnostic cytology in the presence of an irregular, hard mass.

## Amyloid 'tumour'

Localised collections of amyloid can occur in a variety of sites including the breast.[76] These deposits have been termed amyloid tumour and present as a solitary localised mass, rarely bilateral. It occurs in older women and can be firm or hard and discrete. It can imitate carcinoma clinically and mammographically.

Cytological preparations show amorphous translucent material similar to thick thyroid colloid. This material stains violet with May-Grünwald Giemsa and pale pink with the Papanicolaou method. Scanty bland spindle cells are seen, and more rarely, reactive giant cells are a feature. Faced with this picture, the pathologist can take further aspirates for Congo red staining to confirm the diagnosis.

## Silicone granuloma

Silicone implants quite frequently leak, which may give rise to a local mass and to axillary lymphadenopathy (Fig. 4.19).[77] Aspirates from the breast or lymph node contain numerous macrophages containing large cytoplasmic vacuoles of refringent silicone as well as giant cells of foreign body type, and often free silicone. Silicone spreads as a very sticky translucent, colourless material similar to DPX mountant. Silicone granuloma can persist for many years after removal of an implant.

Cytopathologists should be aware of the risks of sampling breast lesions adjacent to mammary prostheses. If possible, these lesions should be aspirated under ultrasound guidance to avoid penetration of the implant capsule.

## Rare inflammatory conditions

Parasitic lesions in the breast are rare. The cytological appearance of cysticercosis of the breast[78] has been described. Myospherulosis is a pseudomycotic condition that can occur following the subcutaneous injection of penicillin and presents an intriguing histological appearance. Altered erythrocytes coated with lipid are deposited in the tissues within spherules. In smears they stain brown with MGG staining, but are red in PAP preparations and are negative with PAS and silver stains.

In parts of Asia, some women have injections of foreign material to increase their breast size. This gives rise to extraordinary mammographic and ultrasound findings. Cytologically the most common finding is a foreign body reaction with multinucleated giant cells and lymphocytes. Remnants of the foreign material may be aspirated and may appear oily on the smears. Dystrophic calcified debris may be found.

## Breast cysts and fibrocystic change

Cytological examination of cyst fluid that is not blood-stained has little utility. If cyst fluid is blood-stained, it should be examined cytologically, but with the caveat that a negative result will not necessarily exclude the presence of an intracystic carcinoma.

Any residual mass following the drainage of a cyst whatever the nature of the cyst contents should be reaspirated, as a cyst may mask an adjacent carcinoma. A lesion that provides more than 1 mL of fluid has been defined as a cyst. Not infrequently, however, aspiration of a breast lump will provide a watery sample with a volume sufficiently small to allow it to be spread over one or two slides. Microscopical examination usually reveals proteinaceous granular debris, macrophages and a moderate number of benign apocrine cells (Fig. 4.24). Occasionally, the apocrine cells show degenerative changes that may be mistaken for atypia (Figs 4.25, 4.26).

## Fibrocystic change (Figs 4.27–4.31)

Clinically, the appearance of this, the most common cause of a palpable breast lump, has certain characteristic findings. The typical patient is between 30 and 50 years old, but an age range of 25–70 has been quoted. Often, there is a convincing history of change of the breast lump with the menstrual cycle and fibrocystic lesions are more commonly tender or painful than malignant ones. The palpable lesion is not always well-defined and may range in size from a few millimetres to a change occupying the whole breast.

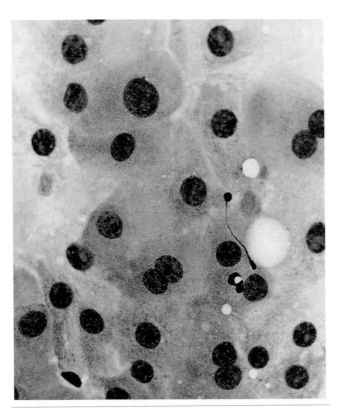

**Fig. 4.24** Benign apocrine cells from fibrocystic change (MGG).

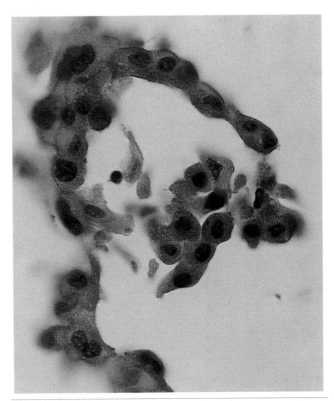

**Fig. 4.26** Apocrine cyst lining from the same case as Fig. 4.25. This section showed that the atypical apocrine epithelium showed only degenerate change with no evidence of premalignancy (H&E).

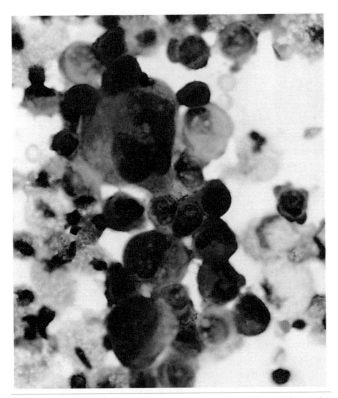

**Fig. 4.25** Cyst fluid containing atypical apocrine cells which were deemed suspicious (MGG).

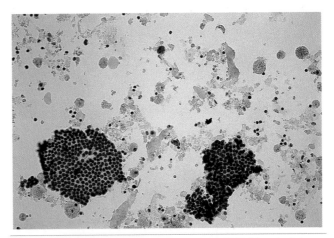

**Fig. 4.27** Fibrocystic change with a benign pattern (C2) of ductal cell sheets, bipolar nuclei, cyst debris and macrophages in the background (H&E).

The condition may be synchronously bilateral, but often the first presentation is as a solitary lesion. Patients are prone to developing multiple sequential lumps and thus may be less anxious about the appearance of further masses than women presenting with the first breast lump. Each lesion must be assessed on its own merit. Most fibrocystic lesions are radiologically benign or equivocal. Some fibrocystic lumps can present appearances that are worrying clinically, radiologically and histologically.

The spectrum of histological appearances generally included under the heading of 'fibrocystic change' is very wide. The basic histological elements are:

1. The formation of cysts
2. Apocrine metaplasia of cyst lining cells and of duct and lobular epithelium

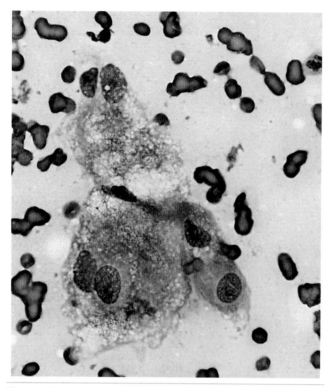

**Fig. 4.28** Foamy macrophages in benign fibrocystic change (MGG).

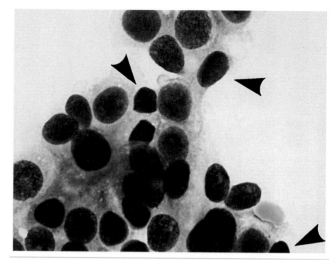

**Fig. 4.30** Benign breast epithelium. This field illustrates the typical appearance of benign breast epithelium. The apparent anisonucleosis is spurious and due to the presence of a number of interspersed myoepithelial cells (arrowheads) (MGG).

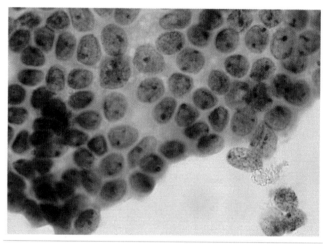

**Fig. 4.31** Hyperplasia. The typical appearances of benign hyperplastic breast epithelium. Occasional bipolar nuclei are seen, bottom right (PAP).

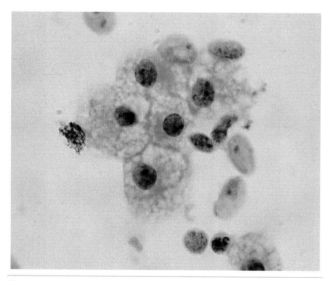

**Fig. 4.29** Foamy macrophages in benign fibrocystic change (PAP).

3. Rupture of the cyst lining with extravasation of contents and associated inflammation
4. Fibrosis of the stroma
5. Chronic inflammation of non-specific type
6. Epithelial hyperplasia of various types
7. Fibroadenomatoid change.

Following examination, the aspirator gains a further important diagnostic clue when the needle enters the lump. The fibrous elements frequently present in this condition will often have a distinctly rubbery or leathery feel to the needle. The cellularity of the sample usually bears a relation to the ease with which the specimen is obtained. When the needle is gripped by leathery fibrous tissue, a poorly cellular aspirate may be anticipated and a little more vigour can be applied in the movement of the needle. In other cases, the aspirate will often appear watery allowing it to be spread over the whole of one or two slides with ease.

The amount of material for microscopy varies considerably, depending on whether the lesion is from the fibrous or proliferative end of the spectrum seen in this condition. The basic pattern is benign, but there may be several cell types present. The most reassuring component is the presence of obviously benign apocrine cells. These may be in large cohesive sheets or dispersed singly or in small groups. The nuclei are large, round and relatively hyperchromatic. The nucleoli are large and prominent. The cytoplasm is abundant and usually granular. Cell borders should be well-defined in contrast to the cells of a low-grade apocrine carcinoma, which have wispy poorly defined cytoplasmic margins. Further reassurance is obtained from the presence of bipolar bare myoepithelial nuclei.

## Cytological findings: fibrocystic change

- Scanty, often watery smear
- Low or moderate cellularity
- Apocrine cells either dominating the cellular picture or in variable numbers
- Macrophages and granular debris form microscopical cysts
- Sheets or fragments of ductal epithelium with bland nuclei arranged in a honeycomb pattern with admixed myoepithelial cells and dispersed bipolar nuclei
- Three-dimensional epithelial aggregates representing intraductal hyperplasia
- Fat or fibrous stroma in variable quantities.

## Diagnostic pitfalls: fibrocystic change

- Benign fibrocystic change may mask an adjacent carcinoma
- A carcinoma infiltrating in an area of fibrocystic changes may be underdiagnosed as reactive/hyperplastic
- Apocrine carcinoma can occasionally be interpreted as benign if low grade
- Benign apocrine metaplasia may appear atypical when degenerate
- In florid hyperplasia there may be marked anisokaryosis that can be misinterpreted as atypia.

## Benign tumours and tumour-like lesions

### Fibroadenoma

The typical clinical presentation of fibroadenoma (Figs 4.32–4.34) is a firm, discrete and highly mobile lump in a young woman.[79] Fibroadenoma most commonly presents in women between the ages of 20 and 35 years, but can come to the attention of the patient for the first time in later life, sometimes after unrelated weight loss. The use of mammography has increased the diagnosis of longstanding fibroadenomas in older women. These lesions are often of the poorly cellular 'ancient' type. The size may vary from a few millimeters to several centimeters, but is usually within the range of 5–30 mm. On mammograms, fibroadenomas typically present as round, well-defined lesions. On ultrasonography they appear solid, round or round-oval, with a distinct margin all around. Particularly in older women, the margins may become less distinct leading to recall and biopsy in mammographic screening.

The risk of developing carcinoma within a fibroadenoma or in a breast previously treated for fibroadenoma is not significantly increased, although, as both carcinoma and fibroadenoma are relatively common lesions, they may occur together. Fibroadenomas may also be colonised by *in situ* carcinoma.

The cytological features of fibroadenoma closely reflect the histological features. When the cytopathologist has the opportunity to obtain the aspirate, the clinical features and cytological appearances allow a specific diagnosis in many cases.

Microscopically, the diagnosis is often obvious at low power with characteristic large frond-like epithelial groups with peripheral finger-like projections. These are sometimes likened to the antlers of stags. At high power, this epithelium is composed of closely packed, uniform cells with an irregular

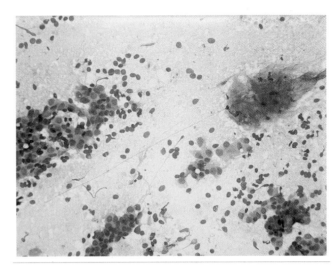

**Fig. 4.32** Fibroadenoma. Pink stromal fragment, epithelial groups and naked nuclei in the background. Typical of FA (MGG).

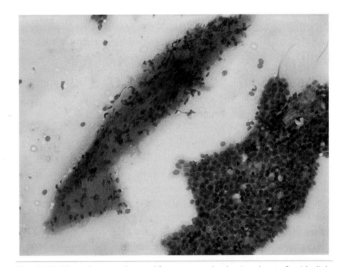

**Fig. 4.33** Fibroadenoma. Stromal fragment and cohesive sheet of epithelial cells and a few naked nuclei in the background (MGG).

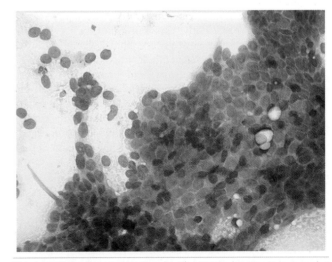

**Fig. 4.34** Fibroadenoma. Monolayer sheet with some smaller, darker myoepithelial cell nuclei and naked nuclei (MGG).

honeycomb appearance, best visualised on the Papanicolaou-stained smear. In air-dried preparations, sometimes it is only at the edge of the epithelial groups that the cells will be sufficiently flattened to allow satisfactory close examination. The nuclei are approximately the size of one or two erythrocytes and are round or slightly ovoid, having one or two small nucleoli and finely granular chromatin. Myoepithelial cells are seen scattered over the surface of the sheets of ductal epithelial cells.

The other essential feature is the presence of an often generous population of bare nuclei, which include stripped epithelial and myoepithelial nuclei, and some stromal cells. The bipolar cell nuclei have condensed chromatin packed into a small elongated nucleus. Although some of the nuclei are truly naked, probably representing myoepithelial cells, many are stromal cells displaying more spindly nuclei and a strand of pale blue cytoplasm at each pole, seen best under high power. In some fibroadenomas, a scattering of foamy macrophages or apocrine cells is seen. Classically aspirates from fibroadenomas are described as containing large fragments of stroma, coloured magenta by Giemsa stains. In clinical practice, the amount of stroma is variable, reflecting the histological spectrum of fibroadenomas. More fibrotic fibroadenomas may yield no stroma at all and have a rather non-specific benign pattern on FNA. At the other end of the spectrum fibroadenomas with abundant cellular stroma merge with phyllodes tumours both histologically and cytologically.

There are circumstances in which aspirates from fibroadenomas can pose diagnostic traps leading to false positive diagnosis of carcinoma: The very high cellularity of fibroadenoma aspirates can cause concern particularly if an aspirate is over-spread, leading to artefactual dissociation, or if a smear is poorly prepared and subject to, for example, slow drying artefact which makes the cells appear large and atypical.

A few FA smears may contain cells with cytological atypia such as enlarged nuclei with more prominent nucleolus, irregular nuclear margin, but uniform chromatin pattern. The cytoplasm is often dense. These cells may occur in small irregular groups or as single cells and may appear suspicious of malignancy. Some of these are probably myoepithelial hyperplastic cells. In histological sections, they usually appear rather inconspicuous, but in a few cases there may be intraductal hyperplasia with or without atypia. It is important that the general low power pattern is fully appreciated before looking at the aspirate at higher power when the spuriously worrying features may be apparent. The recognition of bipolar cells and stromal fragments is also particularly helpful in these cases.

Some fibroadenomas have a stroma that is so highly myxoid that on smears, the pattern can mimic mucinous carcinoma.

Histological variants that may lead to special cytological features include the occurrence of apocrine metaplasia, haemorrhagic infarction, especially during pregnancy, squamous metaplasia (although this is more common in phyllodes tumour) and stromal metaplasias, including the formation of smooth muscle, cartilage, bone or dystrophic calcification. The formation of bone and calcification is commoner in older women and is likely to become apparent on taking the aspirate, as the needle may refuse to enter the mass or may give a very gritty sensation. These lesions typically reveal scant cellularity. A few stromal fragments are usually present, but epithelial cell groups may not always be seen.

There is a histological and cytological overlap with phyllodes tumours at the benign end of the phyllodes spectrum. In aspirates from a clinical fibroadenoma showing highly cellular stromal fragments, very large numbers of plump, naked bipolar nuclei with hyperplastic duct cells, giant cells and an absence of apocrine cells, a diagnosis of phyllodes tumour should be considered. This is more likely in older women.

### Cytological findings: fibroadenoma

- Moderate or high cellularity, but may be scanty in older or fibrotic lesions
- Cohesive sheets with an antler-like appearance containing recognisable myoepithelial cell nuclei
- Many naked bipolar cell nuclei in the background
- If apocrine or foamy cells are present they are few.

### Diagnostic pitfalls: fibroadenoma

- As with all cellular benign lesions, the high cellularity should not be interpreted as suspicious
- Some fibroadenomas show reduced cellular cohesion and significant nuclear enlargement with anisonucleosis and prominent nucleoli that may risk a false positive diagnosis of carcinoma
- Occasionally, a very myxoid stroma, particularly when associated with over-spread dissociate epithelium, may mimic mucinous carcinoma
- Misdiagnosis of fibroadenoma is the commonest cause of false positive diagnoses, although these are rare
- Phyllodes tumour shares some cytological features with fibroadenoma.

## Tubular adenoma

The clinical features of this lesion are indistinguishable from fibroadenoma and occasional examples show areas resembling classical fibroadenoma.[80] This suggests some homology between these conditions. Histologically, these lesions consist of a mass of densely packed benign tubular structures with a double layer of epithelial and myoepithelial cells but with very little stroma between the tubules. They represent the part of the spectrum of fibroepithelial neoplasms where the stromal component is minimal. Tubular adenomas tend to be easy to aspirate, being softer than the average fibroadenoma.

The cytological features are similar to those of a fibroadenoma but there are fewer bipolar cells and the larger complex epithelial sheets are not a feature. The relative rarity of these lesions makes it unlikely that a specific diagnosis will be made by FNA cytology and a preoperative diagnosis of fibroadenoma, fibroadenosis or non-specific benign lesion is likely.

### Cytological findings: tubular adenoma

- Moderate to highly cellular aspirate with a basic benign pattern
- No large antler-like groups are seen
- The epithelial cells are cytologically benign and in small groups, some displaying a microacinar arrangement
- Bipolar cells are fewer than seen in fibroadenomas.

### Diagnostic pitfalls: tubular adenoma

- These are largely as for other cellular benign lesions.

## Lactating adenoma and lactational change in benign mass lesions

Lactating adenoma, contrary to what the name might suggest, occurs more commonly during rather than after pregnancy. Its origin is controversial, but many regard it as a fibroadenoma or tubular adenoma modified by the hormonal influences of pregnancy. Foci of lactational change with identical histological and cytological features may occasionally be seen within fibroadenomas and other benign breast changes outside of the context of pregnancy. It is in that unexpected setting (or indeed in the context of known pregnancy that is not included in the clinical details provided to the cytologist) that failure to appreciate lactational changes in an aspirate from a clinical mass has a serious risk of diagnostic error. Aspirates show moderate numbers of cells singly or in groups, including intact lobules and acini. Most cells, however, are dispersed. There is a characteristic granular or foamy background consisting of cell cytoplasm fragments and lipid. The intact cells show obvious cytoplasmic vacuolation and have large round or ovoid nuclei with a smooth nuclear membrane and fine chromatin with a prominent nucleolus. The appearances are thus similar to those of the pregnancy-related changes. Cytometric analysis reveals no statistically significant difference between the mean nuclear areas of lactating adenoma cells and those of well-differentiated ductal or lobular carcinoma. There is therefore the risk that these lesions will result in a false positive diagnosis.

### Cytological findings: lactating adenoma and lactational change in benign mass lesions

- Moderately cellular aspirates composed of dispersed cells singly or in small groups in a foamy background containing cell fragments and lipid droplets
- The cytoplasm is vacuolated or wispy and stripped epithelial nuclei may be present
- The nuclei are uniform and show fine, stippled chromatin and a prominent nucleolus.

### Diagnostic pitfalls: lactating adenoma and lactational change in benign mass lesions

- As for pregnancy-related changes
- Benign lumps in lactating and pregnant breasts can feel suspicious clinically
- If the secretory background and cytological features are not appreciated there is a significant risk of false positive diagnosis of malignancy or unwarranted suspicious diagnosis. When a non-pathologist is taking the aspirate, failure to supply the essential clinical information of pregnancy makes this more likely.

## Benign phyllodes tumour

Phyllodes tumours[81] (Figs 4.35, 4.36) form a spectrum of fibroepithelial tumours from benign with a strong resemblance to fibroadenomas, through borderline with notable stromal overgrowth and proliferation to malignant, in which the stroma is frankly sarcomatous. Benign phyllodes tumours have a propensity for local recurrence following surgery, and the borderline

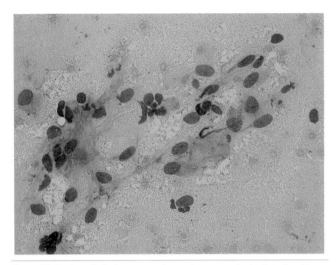

**Fig. 4.35** Benign phyllodes tumour. Loose fragment of spindle cells with small, but recognisable nucleoli. Some stromal cells are more polygonal and have ample cytoplasm (MGG).

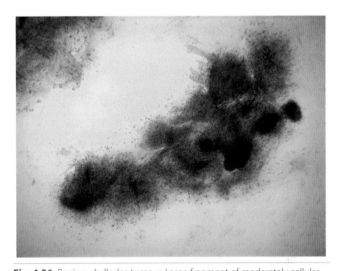

**Fig. 4.36** Benign phyllodes tumour. Large fragment of moderately cellular stroma (MGG).

or low-grade malignant ones may recur at a higher grade. Phyllodes tumour is, therefore, an important lesion to consider when assessing an aspirate from a fibroepithelial tumour.

Benign phyllodes tumour is seen in women on average 20 years older than those with fibroadenoma. There is, however, considerable overlap and, while phyllodes tumours tend to be larger on presentation, they may present at any stage of development. Conversely, fibroadenomas may reach 100 mm or more in diameter before the patient seeks help. The differentiation between giant fibroadenoma and benign phyllodes tumour depends entirely on the histological appearance of the stroma and the distinction is frequently impossible cytologically. Late presentation, particularly in a large breast, has resulted in some very large specimens of phyllodes tumour.

On examination, these tumours are softer, less mobile and less well-defined than fibroadenomas. There is usually little resistance to the needle, unless the rare occurrence of metaplastic bone or cartilage is encountered. The aspirate is generally blood free and appears glairy when spread.

The smears are usually very cellular and the differentiation from a cellular fibroadenoma can be impossible. The clinical features are of assistance in balancing the probabilities. Additionally, the cellularity of the stromal fragments and the size and possible atypia of the many dispersed stromal cells is important in suggesting the diagnosis. MGG-stained preparations may reveal pink or purple staining ground substance within the stromal fragments. In an aspirate from a probable phyllodes tumour, the most critical cytological feature in deciding whether the lesion may be benign, borderline or malignant, is the number of and the degree of atypia of the stromal cells. They may occasionally be frankly malignant cytologically; more commonly the atypia is of a lesser degree suggesting a borderline lesion (see p. 204). Numerous mitoses might be an indication of a malignant lesion, buy are usually not so prominent in cytological material as in histological sections. Even histological assessment is difficult in this regard. There is a distinct risk of making a false positive diagnosis of malignancy when assessing a benign phyllodes tumour. Occasional phyllodes tumours contain keratin cysts leading to further diagnostic problems.

Although difficult to achieve with certainty, there is considerable value in making a correct preoperative diagnosis of phyllodes tumour as the enucleation that would be adequate for a fibroadenoma may result in a local recurrence if applied to a phyllodes tumour. Most surgeons would wish to take a margin of normal tissue around a known or suspected phyllodes tumour.

### Cytological findings: benign phyllodes tumour

- Cellular smears with occasional large sheets of benign epithelium
- Numerous plump, single stromal cells with little cellular pleomorphism
- The prominence and number of bipolar cells are usually greater than in fibroadenomas
- Obvious stromal fragments, some large and with high cellularity
- Fragments composed entirely of bipolar cells containing pink or purple ground substance in MGG preparations.

### Diagnostic pitfalls: benign phyllodes tumour

- Frequently impossible to distinguish from a fibroadenoma
- Borderline lesions are difficult to differentiate from benign cytologically.

## Mammary hamartoma

The histological features of these uncommon lesions are well described, consisting of varying amounts of breast parenchyma and adipose tissue. Cytologically this lesion cannot be reliably distinguished from normal breast tissue, fibroadenoma or other cellular benign lesions.

## Epithelial hyperplasias and tumour-like lesions

## Epithelial hyperplasia (proliferative breast changes)

The clinical picture is usually benign, but can be highly suspicious.

Histologically, the basic appearances described as fibrocystic changes frequently include epithelial proliferative changes of various types. Cytologically, this may be suspected when an aspirate, otherwise typical of 'simple' fibrocystic change, is cellular with the additional cells being non-apocrine type. These proliferative changes also commonly occur without more conventional fibrocystic change. The histological changes include adenosis (sclerosing, microglandular), hyperplasias (intraductal hyperplasia, columnar cell lesions, duct papillomatosis), atypical ductal hyperplasia, adenomyoepithelial hyperplasia, adenosis tumour, apocrine adenosis with and without sclerosis, radial scar and complex sclerosing lesions.

One rare variant of benign epithelial hyperplasia that does have a distinctive cytological appearance is collagenous spherulosis. In May-Grünwald Giemsa-stained preparations the collagenous spherules are very conspicuous and appear magenta in colour. Collagenous spherulosis is of no clinical significance, but cytologically it may be confused with adenoid cystic carcinoma. It should be excluded when a diagnosis of adenoid cystic carcinoma is being considered.

Microcalcifications can be recognised in cytological preparations when present. They are of relatively little assistance in microscopic diagnosis as they look morphologically similar in both benign and malignant lesions. However, they are useful in confirming that a mammographic lesion containing microcalcifications has been sampled.

### Cytological findings: epithelial hyperplasia

- Low or moderate cellularity with small epithelial groups or high cellularity with large flat or folded sheets and three-dimensional aggregates of cohesive regular cells
- Adenosis lesions may show a microacinar appearance in smears as well as true tubular structures
- Nuclei may be enlarged, but the chromatin pattern is fine and nucleoli inconspicuous
- The epithelial groups contain the smaller darker ovoid nuclei of myoepithelial cells
- Variable numbers of bipolar nuclei between the groups
- Any separate epithelial cells present also have a fine chromatin pattern and small nucleoli
- The nuclear membrane, often difficult to see in compact groups, has a smooth profile
- Macrophages and apocrine cells may be present
- An absence of nuclear atypia, widespread loss of cell cohesion or necrotic debris.

## Microglandular adenosis

The typical clinical presentation is of a palpable mass that can vary from 3 to 30 mm in diameter. The term adenosis is something of a misnomer as these lesions are infiltrative and lack myoepithelial cells just like a well-differentiated carcinoma.[81]

Cytological findings are of an abundantly cellular aspirate with many cells in small clumps and elongated cohesive three-dimensional tubular arrays. The cells have scant cytoplasm but have round and uniform nuclei. The chromatin pattern is reassuringly fine and evenly dispersed and each nucleus has a single nucleolus. No bipolar cells or other features are seen and an atypical or suspicious diagnosis may result. There is clearly a risk of making a false diagnosis of tubular carcinoma on the aspirate.

Histologically, microglandular adenosis displays very round glandular profiles, complete absence of cellular pleomorphism and each gland is shown on staining to be invested by a complete layer of peritubular reticulin, with no myoepithelial cells. Tubular carcinoma by contrast shows slight irregularity or angulation of the tubular profiles, luminal 'snouting', frequently has an associated characteristic stroma, and should show at least mild cellular pleomorphism. Finding foci of intraduct carcinoma is obviously helpful but cannot be relied upon. Cytological differentiation is therefore even more problematic. The regular honeycomb pattern within the epithelial groups of microglandular adenosis is not found in tubular carcinoma and so the actual arrangement of the nuclei within epithelial groups is very important.

## Cytological findings: microglandular adenosis

- Abundant cellularity
- Epithelial cells in small groups and cohesive three-dimensional elongated tubular arrays
- The cells have scant cytoplasm, but round uniform nuclei with fine evenly dispersed chromatin and single nucleoli
- No bipolar cells.

## Diagnostic pitfalls: microglandular adenosis

- Possible confusion with tubular carcinoma.

## Radial sclerosing lesions: complex sclerosing lesion/radial scar

The lesions described by the terms complex sclerosing lesion and radial scar are distinguished only by their size[81,82] (Figs 4.37–4.39). They consist of a central core of elastotic fibrous tissue surrounded by a proliferation of ductal and lobular structures demonstrating a range of epithelial and myoepithelial proliferation and forming a lesion with a characteristic stellate architecture. These radial sclerosing lesions present as spiculated, and thus suspicious, mammographic lesions. On ultrasound they may be suspicious or equivocal with unsharp margins. They are usually not palpable, but may occasionally present as a palpable lump.

Radial scars may yield scanty material with a mixture of small groups and some dissociated epithelial cells and a few bipolar cells. Complex sclerosing lesions (and some of the radial scars) are usually more proliferative and often yield moderate to abundant cellular material. The smears may show cellular and nuclear pleomorphism within groups and cohesive three-dimensional epithelial aggregates with or without recognisable myoepithelial cells. In the background there may be single cells, both epithelial cells and fibroblasts, naked nuclei, stromal fragments and mucoid material. Some cells with distinct columnar or apocrine morphology may be seen.

Radial sclerosing lesions are one of the main causes of discrepancies in the preoperative work-up of suspicious breast abnormalities (radiological findings suspicious and FNA benign). On the other hand, they are also an important cause of false suspicious or malignant cytological diagnoses.[83] Epithelial hyperplasia, invasive (particularly tubular) and *in situ* carcinoma are reasonably frequently seen within radial sclerosing lesions, so there is potential for both false positive and false

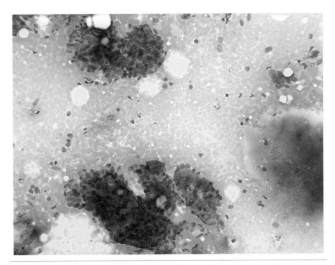

**Fig. 4.37** Complex sclerosing lesion. Epithelial cells in cohesive three-dimensional, small groups and single cells. Mucoid material and naked nuclei in the background (MGG).

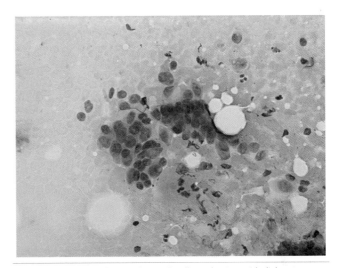

**Fig. 4.38** Complex sclerosing lesion. Smaller, cohesive epithelial groups, a few single cells and a stromal fragment (MGG).

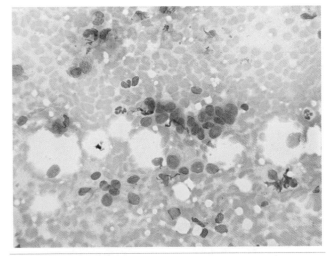

**Fig. 4.39** Complex sclerosing lesion. Small epithelial cell group, loose clusters of 4–5 cells and a few single cells. Some variation in nuclear size and shapes, but finely granulated and evenly distributed chromatin (MGG).

negative diagnosis of malignancy. For this reason they are generally excised for full assessment.

- Variable cellularity from scanty to abundant
- Cohesive three-dimensional epithelial aggregates without recognisable myoepithelial nuclei
- Small groups of uniform or slightly pleomorphic epithelial cells and dispersed bipolar cells
- Apocrine and/or columnar cells may be present, usually in small numbers
- Stromal fragments, partly as cell poor elastoid fragments
- Single fibroblasts, histiocytic cells, macrophages and mucoid material.

- Mild cell pleomorphism, single cells and absence of myoepithelial nuclei on the groups and aggregates may lead to a false positive or false suspicious cytological diagnosis.

## Adenosis tumour and duct adenoma

Adenosis tumour is the term applied to a clinically palpable mass, which histologically is composed of confluent areas of sclerosing adenosis[81] (Fig. 4.40). These lesions are quite uncommon but occur over a wide age range (22–68 with a mean of 40 years), mainly in premenopausal women. There is hyperplasia of both epithelial and myoepithelial cells with distortion of the lobular structure.

Clinically and histologically, there is a risk of misdiagnosis of carcinoma. Cytology, therefore, has a useful role in preventing such an error at an early stage in the assessment, but cannot be expected to provide a specific diagnosis as the appearances closely resemble benign hyperplastic breast disease of other types. It has been suggested, however, that cytology is less likely than frozen section to provide a false positive diagnosis. Aspirates show a biphasic pattern of groups of uniform epithelial cells and many elongated bipolar cell nuclei.

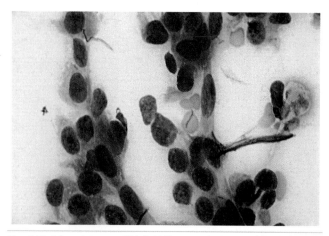

**Fig. 4.40** Adenosis tumour. This field illustrates the intimate blend of elongate bipolar ells and epithelial cells that typified this lesion (MGG).

- Moderate to high cellularity
- Small groups of uniform epithelial cells and myoepithelial cells
- The relationship of sclerosing stroma and microacinar epithelium may be preserved.

- Clinically may resemble carcinoma.

## Benign papillary lesions

### Nipple adenoma, papilloma of the nipple ducts, erosive adenosis of the nipple, subareolar papillomatosis

The condition occurs in late middle age and the appearance is that of an eroded and weeping nipple with no mass on either clinical examination or mammography. There is, therefore, a chance of an erroneous clinical diagnosis of Paget's disease of the nipple with the risk of over treatment. Before aspiration it is useful to take contact specimens from any moist eroded area directly on to a slide. Aspiration of the nipple and areola can be acutely painful and so some skill is required to obtain an adequate sample without undue discomfort for the patient. It is important to avoid the areola and to pass the needle through normal skin sampling the nipple lesion obliquely.

The histological pattern of these lesions can be variable with both papillomatous and adenomatous forms.[81] The interpretation may be complicated by the presence of adenosquamous nests that occur where the ductal epithelium interacts with that of the epidermis.

Cytologically, the described appearance is that of considerable cellularity with a profusion of epithelial cells presenting singly and in clusters. Uniform nuclei contain finely distributed chromatin and inconspicuous nucleoli. Some variation in nuclear size and occasional hyperchromatic nuclei should not exclude the diagnosis but clearly there should be no overtly suspicious feature. Small amounts of cellular debris, inflammatory cells and siderophages are also possible. The differentiation from Paget's disease of the nipple with an underlying carcinoma in or associated with the lactiferous ducts should not be a problem.

- Moderate or high cellularity with a basic benign pattern
- Dispersed epithelial cells and small groups
- Little anisonucleosis, the uniform nuclei showing finely distributed chromatin and small nucleoli
- Occasional hyperchromatic nuclei possible
- Adenosquamous nests may be apparent
- Small amount of debris, inflammatory cells and siderophages may be a feature
- Apocrine cells may be present.

**Diagnostic pitfalls: nipple adenoma, papilloma of the nipple ducts, erosive adenosis of the nipple, subareolar papillomatosis**

- Clinically, may be mistaken for Paget's disease of the nipple
- Low-grade carcinoma may be difficult to exclude except by local excision, which is in any case appropriate.

### Intraductal/intracystic/sclerosing papilloma/papillomatosis (Figs 4.41–4.44)

The clinical presentation of duct papilloma of the breast is variable, nipple discharge sometimes being the main symptom, a palpable mass in other cases.[81] It is usually soft on palpation. The mean age of presentation is 48, but the lesion can present commonly in the 6th and 7th decades. Smaller lesions may be impalpable but can still produce a bloody discharge appearing from one duct on the nipple. This may direct examination to a particular breast segment where careful palpation may reveal a target for FNA cytology. Benign papillomatous lesions

rarely exceed 30 mm in diameter and are usually soft and friable, which explains their tendency not to present as a mass. Firmer examples usually transpire to be sclerotic or are intracystic, a feature that becomes rapidly apparent on aspiration. Even where not obviously intracystic, the aspirate is frequently watery and blood-stained.

The initial cytological assessment may engender anxiety because of variable cellularity, sometimes poor cohesion of the epithelial cells and small cell groups. The fact that the aspirate is likely to have come from a woman in the peak age range for carcinoma may heighten suspicion.

Attention to the larger groups may give an impression of a papillary structure and occasional bipolar cells may be found in the background. Apocrine cells are a frequent feature and macrophages are commonly seen. Examination of the nipple discharge by gently dabbing it on to a slide, fixing and staining it, is usually helpful. The smear shows blood, abundant foamy macrophages, haemosiderin-laden macrophages and papillary clusters of ductal cells, sometimes accompanied by apocrine cells.

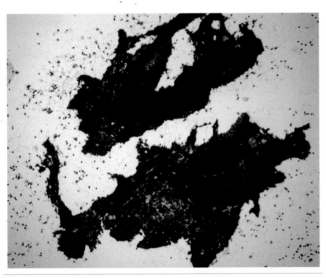

**Fig. 4.41** Benign papilloma. Overview showing complex folded sheets (MGG).

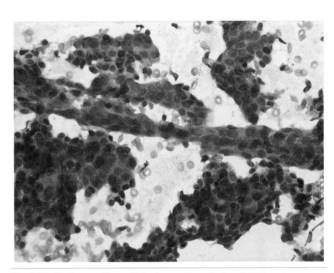

**Fig. 4.43** Benign papilloma. Cohesive papillary clusters (MGG).

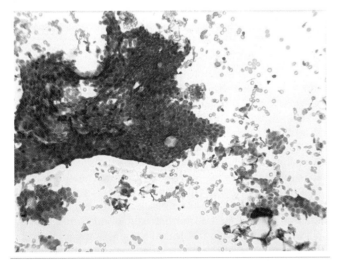

**Fig. 4.42** Benign papilloma. Large folded sheet, smaller groups, macrophages and microcalcs (MGG).

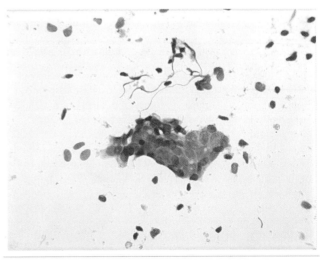

**Fig. 4.44** Benign papilloma. Micropapillary group and naked nuclei (MGG).

## Cytological findings: intraductal/intracystic/sclerosing papilloma/papillomatosis

- Variable cellularity with a basic benign pattern
- The epithelial cells are often dispersed or in small groups
- Complex, folded three-dimensional epithelial aggregates
- Papillary clusters may be preserved
- Papillary stromal fragments may be present
- Small numbers of bipolar cells
- Apocrine cells may be present
- A small amount of debris and macrophages may be present.

## Diagnostic pitfalls: intraductal/intracystic/sclerosing papilloma/papillomatosis

- When the lesions are cellular, differentiation from a well-differentiated papillary carcinoma may be difficult.

## Other benign tumours

### Adenomyoepithelioma

This is a rare tumour of the breast[81] (Figs 4.45, 4.46), which usually presents as a solitary and solid mass and with a size range of less than 10 mm to several centimeters. Median size is about 2.5 cm. Radiological findings may be of a round tumour with somewhat fuzzy margins, often resulting in an equivocal or suspicious radiological diagnosis. Histologically, it is characterised by a dual tumour population (epithelial and myoepithelial cells) and fibrous septa with hyalinisation. The cytological appearances mirror the histology; both epithelial cell groups and spindle cells are present.

## Cytological findings: adenomyoepithelioma[84–87]

- A dual cell population of both epithelial and spindled cells
- The cells may show mild to moderate nuclear pleomorphism
- Occasional intranuclear cytoplasmic vacuoles
- Naked bipolar cells
- Metachromatic, fibrillary myxoid material
- No necrosis or mitoses
- Metachromatic, basal membrane-like globules may be present.

## Diagnostic pitfalls: adenomyoepithelioma

- There may be a distinct cellular pleomorphism, especially of the myoepithelial cells which may lead to a false suspicious or false positive diagnosis. Presence of basal membrane-like globules may mimic the findings in adenoid-cystic carcinoma
- Adenomyoepithelial carcinoma does occur and can be considered a malignant variant of adenomyoepithelioma, but is usually diagnosed as ductal carcinoma on cytology, rather than mistaken for a benign lesion.

## Benign non-epithelial lesions

Benign neoplastic non-epithelial lesions also make rare appearances in FNA of breast.

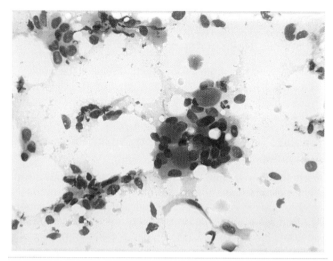

**Fig. 4.45** Adenomyoepithelioma. Stromal fragments with magenta, basal membrane-like globules, naked nuclei, a few spindle cells and an acinar epithelial group (MGG).

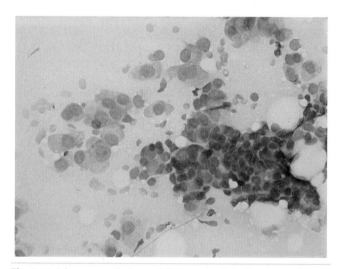

**Fig. 4.46** Adenomyoepithelioma. Cohesive epithelial cell groups and dissociated (myoepithelial) cells (MGG).

## Focal fibrosis of the breast (fibrous 'disease' of the breast, fibrous 'tumour')

The clinical features vary from a vague thickening to a craggy lump. Some argue that many cases presenting with an indurated mass show stromal changes and parenchymal atrophy that fall within the normal range histologically. Many more cases present to the surgeon than are biopsied. Aspiration is frequently difficult, with dense fibrous tissue gripping the needle, making the routine of several passes hard to accomplish. FNA usually reveals a paucicellular aspirate, perhaps with increased lymphocytes. Often, no sample can be expressed from the needle or a trace of acellular fluid is obtained. If the same result is obtained on further aspiration of a lump showing the appropriate clinical features, a presumptive diagnosis of fibrous disease of the breast may be suggested. Follow-up histology confirms that the tissue is composed of virtually acellular collagen.

## Clinical and cytological findings: focal fibrosis of the breast

- Penetration of the needle usually difficult and restricted
- Acellular or very scanty aspirate containing only bipolar nuclei, resulting in a non-diagnostic specimen.

## Diagnostic pitfalls: focal fibrosis of the breast

- Very fibrous stromal reaction in ductal, or more especially lobular, carcinomas can yield very scanty or acellular aspirates. Confusion of these lesions with benign fibrous change accounts for some false negative cytology reports.

## Lipoma

The diagnosis of lipoma on FNA cytology depends on the clinical correlation with a soft (usually subcutaneous) lump and an aspirate of mature adipose tissue.

## Nodular fasciitis

This usually occurs in young subjects and is more likely to occupy the subcutaneous plane rather than presenting as a deep mass within the breast. The lesion usually comes to the patient's attention because of localised pain but may present as a mass of up to 20–30 mm. Cytologically, the presence of moderately large numbers of active looking spindle cells may cause anxiety. Knowledge of this possibility is the best protection against overdiagnosis of this entirely benign and probably reactive process (see Ch. 29).

## Cytological findings: nodular fasciitis

- A moderately cellular aspirate may be obtained
- The cells are dispersed in a finely granular amphophilic background. Most are single but occasional small groups of two or three cells are seen
- All the cells have a pronounced spindle-shaped nucleus. Some have no cytoplasm but many are obvious spindle cells with moderately abundant basophilic cytoplasm
- The nuclei are large but uniform with no bizarre forms. Each nucleus has one fairly or very prominent nucleolus and the chromatin has a coarse texture, although is evenly distributed
- Variable number of inflammatory cells, depending on the age/duration of the age and duration of the lesion.

## Diagnostic pitfalls: nodular fasciitis

- As with histological assessment, the main danger is misdiagnosis of a sarcomatous condition. Familiarity with the clinical features of the case minimises this risk.

## Granular cell tumour

The breast is a rather common site for this tumour[81,88] (Fig. 4.47), derived from nerve sheath cells, usually presenting as a firm, painless mass. Radiologically it may present as a round tumour with not quite sharp margins. The abundant cytoplasm of the tumour cells retains its granular quality in cytological preparations. The cytoplasm may be fragile and smearing may cause a granular background due to ruptured cells as well as naked nuclei (see Ch. 29).

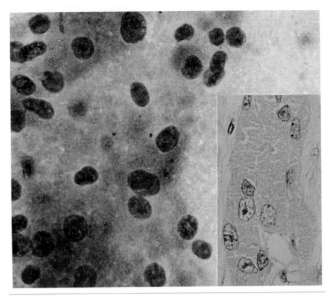

**Fig. 4.47** Granular cell tumour. This smear was obtained from a woman presenting with a mass deep within the breast, simulating carcinoma. The appearance was of a cellular smear comprised of cells with poorly defined cytoplasm with a distinctly granular texture. The nuclei showed a fairly marked degree of variation in size and the nucleoli were very prominent. Histologically, this proved to be a malignant granular cell tumour. The appearances of a benign lesion are similar but with rather less nuclear pleomorphism. The inset illustrates the H&E histological appearances of this case (MGG).

## Cytological findings: granular cell tumour

- Dispersed cells and cell clusters
- Naked nuclei common
- Abundant granular cytoplasm when preserved or as a granular background on the smear
- Round nuclei with uniform chromatin and prominent nucleoli.

## Diagnostic pitfalls: granular cell tumour

- May be misinterpreted as a ductal carcinoma.

## Neurilemmoma

Neurilemmomas[81] may occur anywhere in the breast in conjunction with a peripheral nerve. Radiologically and clinically they may present as a round, well circumscribed tumour. The cytological criteria are described in Chapter 29.

## Diagnostic pitfalls: neurilemmoma

Ancient schwannomas may present with bizarre nuclear changes that may lead to a suspicion of non-epithelial malignancy.

## Borderline epithelial and stromal lesions

## Hyperplasia with atypia

It is widely accepted that there is correlation between the degree of hyperplasia, whether usual type or atypical, and the risk of subsequent development of invasive ductal carcinoma. Recent evidence suggests that CCL (columnar cell lesions) and

**Table 4.1** The relative risk (RR) of future breast carcinoma associated with various forms of benign breast disease and *in situ* lesions

| | RR |
|---|---|
| Fibrocystic change with no hyperplasia, duct ectasia, sclerosing adenosis | 1.00 |
| Fibrocystic change with hyperplasia but no atypia, increased risk | 1.5–2.0 |
| Atypical ductal (ADH) or atypical lobular hyperplasia (ALH), increased risk | 4–5 |
| Lobular carcinoma *in situ* increased risk | 7–12 |
| DCIS (low grade) increased risk | 8–10 |
| DCIS (high grade) increased risk | 15–20 |

low-grade DCIS represent low-grade ductal neoplasia sharing identical chromosomal abnormalities. Much the same is true for atypical lobular hyperplasia and LCIS (lobular neoplasia). Risk of the future development of invasive carcinoma is related to the size of the abnormal area of lobular neoplasia. Atypical ductal hyperplasia (ADH) has been defined as being less than 3 mm in maximum diameter with low-grade cytology. Any atypical ductal proliferation with high-grade cytology must be called DCIS whatever the size. The risk of future invasive breast cancer in women showing such abnormalities is shown in Table 4.1.

It is sometimes possible to distinguish lesions carrying an increased risk of carcinoma from other benign processes.[89–91] These risk-bearing lesions must be viewed in the light of the high total life-time risk for breast cancer. This is approximately 1 in 12 for women in the industrialised world. There are problems in categorising hyperplastic, atypical and premalignant lesions of the breast, with poor interobserver agreement, even in histological assessment of atypical lesions.

The main role for cytological assessment of symptomatic and screening detected non-palpable benign breast disease is, together with imaging, to select those cases where excision biopsy and detailed histological assessment are indicated and avoid biopsy in the majority of cases. This should then allow an acceptably low benign to malignant biopsy ratio. Close liaison between surgeon, pathologist and radiologist is important in symptomatic cases as well in the assessment of breast screening cases.

### Cytological findings: hyperplasia with atypia

- Increased crowding and overlapping of cells within the groups
- Three-dimensional epithelial aggregates
- Obvious papillary groups
- Decreased cohesion of epithelial cells
- More variation in nuclear size
- More prominence of nucleoli
- Less evidence of cells of apocrine type.

The features used to differentiate atypical cases cytologically are very much a matter of degree and are therefore highly subjective. Where there is any doubt as to the presence of atypia, the triple assessment findings should be considered and excision biopsy or follow-up undertaken, as appropriate.

### Diagnostic pitfalls: hyperplasia with atypia

- ALH and LCIS cannot be differentiated cytologically or chromosomally, and can have the same FNA appearances as invasive lobular carcinoma
- CCL, ADH and low-grade DCIS cannot be differentiated cytologically or chromosomally
- Fibroepithelial neoplasms may appear atypical when the clinical and mammographic features are not available and the cytology is viewed under a high-power lens
- Low-grade and lobular carcinomas may be mistaken for a hyperplastic process
- Inflammatory lesions may cause quite marked reactive atypia
- Previous radiotherapy may cause atypia.

## Columnar cell change (columnar cell lesions (CCLs))

CCLs[81,92,93] (Fig. 4.48) of the breast comprise a group of conditions characterised by dilatation of terminal duct lobular units (TDLU) lined by columnar epithelial cells. There may be from one to several layers of thickly packed benign epithelium with or without discrete nuclear atypia. CCL can be subdivided according to the extent of cellular proliferation and atypia. In columnar cell hyperplasia, the acini are lined by more than two layers of columnar type epithelial cells. The proliferating cells may form small micropapillae. Apical snouts and luminal secretions with calcification, sometimes resembling psammoma bodies, are common. The group of lesions categorised as CCLs with cytological atypia encompass lesions also described as low-grade clinging carcinoma or flat epithelial atypia. The cytological features have not been described, but would most probably be found among cases of hyperplasia with and without atypia. They would represent a spectrum ranging from benign, monolayer sheets and crowded strips to three-dimensional aggregates resembling low-grade ductal carcinoma *in situ* (DCIS).

Columnar cell change has recently assumed a new significance due to its recognised association with mammographic calcification. There is a potential for overdiagnosis as DCIS both mammographically and cytologically.

## Cellular papillary lesions

Intracystic/intraductal papillary tumours[81] (Figs 4.49, 4.50) may have growth patterns that range from a 'simple' benign papilloma (see p. 198) to very cellular lesions with a marked epithelial proliferation and hyperplasia that resemble epithelial hyperplasia with and without atypia as well as fully diagnostic papillary intracystic carcinoma. Cytologically, these will present as cellular lesions with a moderate to distinct cellular/nuclear pleomorphism, papillary fragments and fibrovascular stalks. Usually, the epithelial fragments are rather cohesive, but a population of single cells is almost always present as well. Apocrine cells, macrophages and intracystic debris is common. As these lesions are so heterogeneous, it may be impossible to give a confident diagnosis of benign versus malignant lesion and they should all be excised. Most papillary, intracystic carcinomas are low-grade and show a discrete atypia. However, they often have

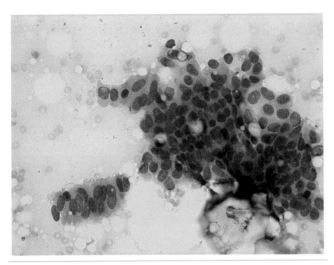

**Fig. 4.48** Columnar cell lesion. Palisading strip and monolayer sheet (MGG).

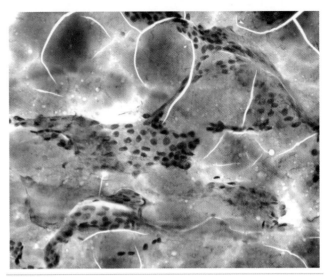

**Fig. 4.51** Mucocele-like lesion. Abundant mucin and monolayer sheets of epithelial cells without atypia.

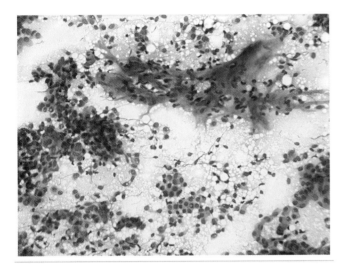

**Fig. 4.49** Cellular papillary lesion. Discohesive sheets and groups and single cells with some variation in nuclear size and shape, but with a fine, even chromatin. Apocrine differentiation in sheets on the right side. Stromal, capillary fragment (MGG).

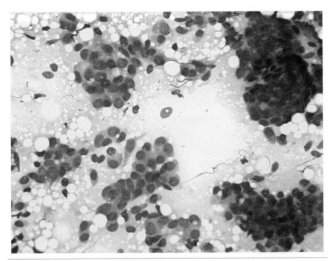

**Fig. 4.50** Cellular papillary lesion. Cohesive, micropapillary epithelial groups, a few single cells, minimal pleomorphism and fine, even chromatin (MGG).

a monotonous cell appearance ('monoclonality'), whereas the benign, cellular papillomas reveal a more polymorphic ('polyclonal') cell population as is found in epithelial hyperplasia (see p. 196).

## Mucocele-like lesions (MLLs)

MLLs[94–97] (Fig. 4.51) have been described as being associated with ductal hyperplasia, atypical ductal hyperplasia, intraductal carcinoma and invasive carcinoma. Pathological features are defined by the presence of cysts containing mucinous material that rupture, expelling secretions and epithelium into surrounding tissues. Cytologically, these lesions are characterised by abundant mucin and monolayer clusters or sheets of epithelial cells without nuclear atypia and none or few single cells. However, they may form a continuous spectrum ranging from benign to invasive mucinous carcinoma.

### Cytological findings: MLLs

- Abundant mucin
- Scant to moderate cellularity with cohesive, monolayer clusters and sheets of epithelial cells
- No or up to moderate nuclear atypia
- No or only few single cells.

### Diagnostic pitfalls: MLLs

- Risk of overdiagnosis as mucinous carcinoma.

## Lobular neoplasia/lobular carcinoma *in situ*

Lobular neoplasia[81] (Fig. 4.52) is characterised by a proliferation of small and often loosely cohesive cells originating in the TDLU. They may or may not show pagetoid involvement of the terminal ducts. These lesions are usually not palpable and have no radiologic appearance. When sampled on FNA they are an incidental finding to a radiological and/or clinical abnormality. The cytological features have been described in a few cases.[98]

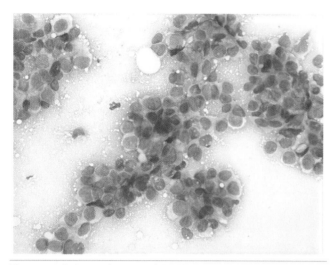

**Fig. 4.52** Lobular neoplasia. Loosely lobuloid arrangement of monomorphic epithelial cells with a discrete atypia (MGG).

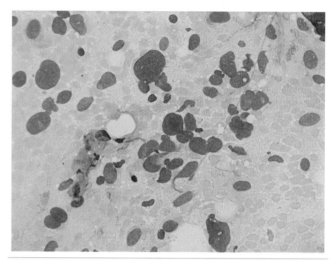

**Fig. 4.53** Borderline phyllodes tumour. Bizarre, degenerative type nuclear atypia of stromal cells (MGG).

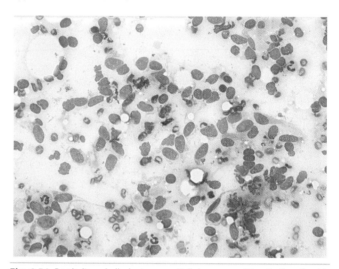

**Fig. 4.54** Borderline phyllodes tumour. Cellular smear with spindle cells with some pleomorphism and small/indistinct nucleoli (MGG).

They were characterised by loosely cohesive cell groups composed of uniform cells with occasional intracytoplasmic lumina, slightly irregular and eccentric nuclei. In addition a few cases were hypercellular with dissociated and more pleomorphic tumour cells, consistent with a pleomorphic subtype. There are no reliable cytological criteria that help in differentiating *in situ* lobular neoplasia from invasive lobular carcinoma (ILC).

### Cytological findings: lobular neoplasia

- Loosely cohesive groups
- Uniform cells with occasional intracytoplasmic lumina
- Slightly irregular and eccentric nuclei.

### Diagnostic pitfalls: lobular neoplasia

- May be mistaken for benign cells
- More pleomorphic tumour cells may be diagnosed as carcinoma.

## Borderline (low-grade malignant) (Figs 4.53, 4.54) and high-grade malignant phyllodes tumours

Women with this tumour often present with a large tumour that has grown rapidly.[81] Both mammography and ultrasound may appear suspicious. A borderline phyllodes tumour is histologically characterised by a modest stromal hypercellularity, moderate cellular pleomorphism, an intermediate number of mitoses, heterogeneous stromal expansion and rare heterologous stromal differentiation. Cytological smears usually show a mixture of stromal cells and epithelial sheets. The stromal cells may predominate. Mitoses are rare. It may be difficult or sometimes impossible to make a specific cytological diagnosis of 'borderline' phyllodes tumour. The most important thing is to recognise it as a phyllodes tumour and not as a fibroadenoma (see p. 196). Predominance of stromal cells with a moderate pleomorphism compared with epithelial sheets may favour a diagnosis of borderline tumour.

The differentiation of benign, borderline and malignant phyllodes tumours can be very difficult histologically. Distinction is based on the degree of atypia and mitotic activity of the stromal cells and the appearance of the margin of the tumour. Cases in which there is a lesser degree of atypia may be classified as borderline lesions. Malignant lesions tend to be larger than benign/borderline cases.

In frankly malignant cases, pleomorphic, high-grade spindle cells are seen, with a fibrosarcoma-type pattern. Rarely, heterologous sarcomatous elements are present in the form of lipoblasts or malignant cartilage with abundant ground substance. Even histological assessment is subjective in this regard and the extent of infiltration that is important in histological assessment is obviously not apparent on the smears.

### Cytological findings: borderline (low-grade malignant) phyllodes tumour

- Cellular smears with occasional large sheets of benign epithelium
- Numerous plump, single stromal cells with moderate cellular pleomorphism
- Occasionally bizarre, degenerative type nuclear abnormalities
- Occasional mitoses.

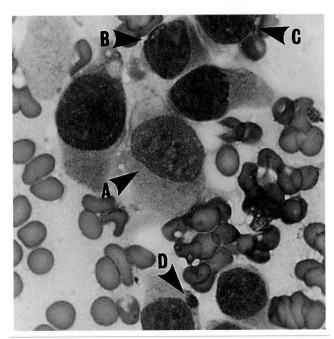

**Fig. 4.55** Classical ductal carcinoma of breast showing features of malignancy. (A) Coarse chromatin pattern and multiple nucleoli of variable size, with nuclear holes; (B) irregular nuclear membrane; (C) extrusion of chromatin from the surface of the nucleus; (D) extranuclear chromatin. There is also noticeable anisonucleosis and poor cell cohesion. Red cells serve as an index of size (MGG).

### Diagnostic pitfalls: borderline (low-grade malignant) phyllodes tumour

- May be mistaken for a fibroadenoma
- Fibroblastic proliferative entities as fibromatosis and nodular fasciitis
- Spindle cell sarcomas
- Malignant myoepithelioma
- Bizarre degenerative nuclear atypia may be interpreted as a feature of malignancy.

### Cytological findings: high-grade malignant phyllodes tumour

- Properly taken aspirates are generally abundantly cellular
- Large atypical stromal cells, often in cohesive groups
- Sometimes overtly sarcomatous elements or fragments of densely cellular stroma with obvious mitoses are seen
- The epithelial content is variable but tends to be particularly sparse in frankly malignant phyllodes tumours. It is benign but may demonstrate hyperplasia and mild atypia.

### Diagnostic pitfalls: high-grade malignant phyllodes tumour

- Obvious malignancy in a phyllodes tumour may be misdiagnosed as carcinoma, particularly metaplastic carcinoma.

## Fibromatosis (desmoid tumour)

Breast is an uncommon location for desmoid tumours.[81] The patient usually presents with a palpable breast lump, suspicious

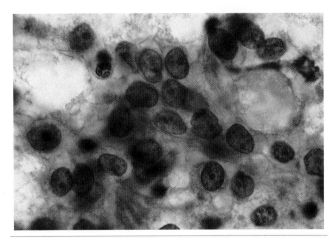

**Fig. 4.56** High-grade ductal carcinoma. Notice the poor cell cohesion, pleomorphism, and prominent nucleoli (PAP). (Courtesy of Dr G. McKee, Boston.)

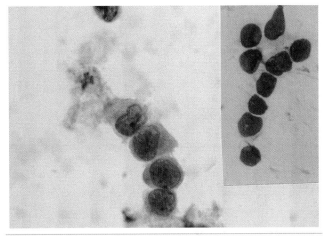

**Fig. 4.57** The classical appearance of lobular carcinoma of the breast. The inset shows the corresponding MGG appearance at a lower power (PAP).

of carcinoma on clinical and mammographic assessment. The aspirate is usually scanty, yielding bland, isolated spindle cells and small groups of benign ductal cells.

## Malignant breast tumours

### General criteria for malignancy

No single morphological feature can be relied upon to distinguish benign from malignant cells at any site. It is the complete picture with the 'pattern of the smear', the nuclear and cytoplasmic details in conjunction with the radiological and clinical findings that leads to an accurate diagnosis. The classical appearances of breast carcinomas are illustrated in Figures 4.55–4.57, the criteria of malignancy are listed in Table 4.2.

### Cellularity of the specimen

Most carcinomas produce aspirates with moderate or abundant cellularity. On the other hand, carcinomas with a scirrhous stroma, and those in which tumour density is low, notably many of the lobular carcinomas, yield a more scantily cellular

**Table 4.2**  General diagnostic criteria for the recognition of benign and malignant conditions (modified from UK NHSBSP)[9]

| Criterion | Benign | Malignant |
|---|---|---|
| Cellularity | Poor or moderate | Usually high |
| Cell-to-cell cohesion | Good, with large defined clusters of cells | Dissociated cells |
| Cell arrangement | Even, usually in flat sheets | Irregular, overlapping, often three-dimensional |
| Cell types | Mixture of epithelial, myoepithelial and other cells, e.g. stromal | Usually uniform cell population |
| Bipolar (elliptical) bare nuclei | Present | Not conspicuous |
| Background | Generally clean | Occasionally with necrosis and macrophages |
| **Nuclear characteristics** | | |
| Size (in relation to RBCs) | Small | Variable, often large, depending on tumour type and grade |
| Pleomorphism | Rare | Common |
| Nuclear membranes (PAP) | Smooth | Irregular with indentations |
| Nucleoli (PAP) | Indistinct or small and single | Variable, may be prominent |
| Chromatin | Smooth or fine | Clumped, may be irregular |
| Additional features | Apocrine metaplasia, foamy macrophages | Mucin, intracytoplasmic lumina |

specimen. Also, many benign lesions found in younger women may provide intensely cellular smears.

## Dispersal of cells

Lack of cell-to-cell cohesion is a characteristic malignant feature, but it is not diagnostic of an invasive lesion. Most *in situ* lesions yield a variable amount of single cells. Also, some benign lesions may show discohesion, either genuinely or as an artefact due to too much pressure when smearing the material. Cellular discohesion is preserved in LBC preparations.

## Absence of biphasic pattern with myoepithelial cells

In most invasive carcinomas, myoepithelial cell nuclei are missing, both in the background and in the periphery of the tumour cell groups and aggregates. Tubular carcinomas and some low-grade ductal carcinomas are an exception where a few myoepithelial cells may still be found.[99] The naked myoepithelial nuclei in the background of the smear are also missing

in *in situ* lesions. However, remnants of myoepithelial cells are found in the periphery of the cell groups and aggregates in a substantial proportion of non-high-grade ductal carcinoma *in situ* (DCIS) and even in some high-grade DCIS.[7]

Some carcinomatous aspirates contain a population of naked epithelial/tumour cell nuclei. Usually, these have obvious malignant features. However, some may be ovoid and therefore mistaken for bipolar cells. Careful attention to the quality of the chromatin and the appearance of the nucleoli should avoid this pitfall. Some malignant aspirates also contain hyperplastic but benign tissue resulting in a population of bipolar cells that distract attention from the population of malignant cells.

## Nuclear size and pleomorphism

The size of nuclei in breast carcinoma cells may vary enormously, from one and a half to two times the diameter of a red blood cell (RBC) and even up to more than five times the size (Figs 4.58–4.60). Most low-grade carcinomas have nuclear sizes

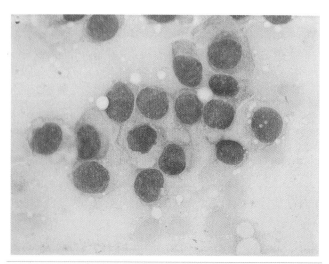

**Fig. 4.58**  Invasive ductal carcinoma, G1. Nuclear size approximately 2 × RBC, granular chromatin and small, indistinct nucleoli. Slightly irregular nuclear outlines (MGG).

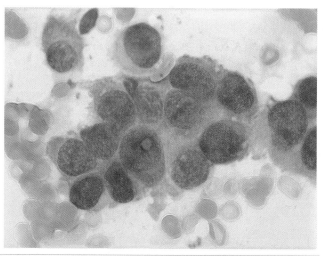

**Fig. 4.59**  Invasive ductal carcinoma, G2. Nuclear size approximately 4 × RBC, small or distinct nucleoli, granular chromatin; more irregularities in the nuclear outlines with buds and indentations (MGG).

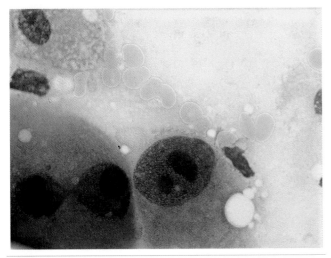

**Fig. 4.60** Invasive ductal carcinoma, G3. Nuclear size >5 × RBC, highly abnormal nucleoli and granular chromatin (MGG).

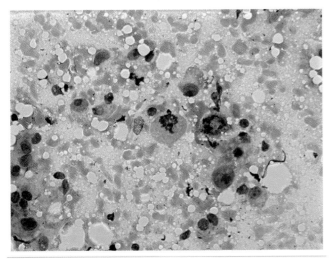

**Fig. 4.61** Atypical nucleolus. High-grade carcinoma cells with one mitotic figure. In one of the tumour cells there is a large, atypical nucleolus with bizarre shape (MGG).

### Nuclear membrane irregularity and extranuclear chromatin

Malignant nuclei almost invariably show nuclear profiles in which there are small indentations as folds, grooves and clefts or projections/buds. Box-shaped and angular nuclei are also suspicious. Extranuclear chromatin is very much a malignant feature but tends to be seen more commonly in higher grade carcinomas where diagnosis is not a problem.

### Nuclear/cytoplasmic ratio and cytoplasmic features

This is of less help than at any other site in the body as normal breast epithelial cells can have scanty cytoplasm and carcinoma cells showing apocrine differentiation may have a great abundance. Intracytoplasmic lumina are an occasional feature of both lobular and ductal carcinoma cells but are only very rarely seen in benign breast epithelium.

### Chromatin texture

In PAP-stained preparations, the appearance of a coarsely and unevenly stippled nucleus with variable but prominent chromocentres suggests malignancy. MGG-stained preparations give a more subtle, but no less characteristic appearance of a coarse 'rope-like' texture that, when marked, can give the impression of small nuclear holes.

### Nuclear fragility

Malignant nuclei show a greater tendency to rupture under the physical pressure of being smeared. This tendency is variable and is seldom marked in breast aspirates unless excessive pressure is used. Nuclear rupture may, however, be a clue that dissociation of otherwise unremarkable epithelial cells may be artefactual rather than a sign of malignancy.

### Mitotic figures

These are rarely seen in breast aspirates except those of high-grade ductal carcinomas. They can be a feature of benign lesions such as fibroepithelial neoplasms. Unless frequent and atypical, they should not be given a heavy diagnostic bias.

### Contents of the background

Abundant necrotic material in an otherwise cellular smear is usually attributable to tumour necrosis. Most high-grade DCIS[7] and a few grade 3 invasive ductal carcinomas show comedo type necrosis on the smears. Necrosis is thus not pathognomonic of invasion, and may even be more suggestive of a DCIS mass.

### Cytological grading of invasive breast carcinoma and DCIS

Histological grading is an integral part of the histopathology report on all breast carcinomas.[101] Together with a number of other parameters, it determines the treatment strategies of each individual patient. Preoperative (cytological) grading is possible, but is not commonly done. There are a number of cytological grading systems, mainly variants of nuclear grading.[102–111] All of them show a good correlation with both histological grading and ploidy. An example that has been used in several cytological studies is shown in Table 4.3 (see Figs 4.62–4.64).[112]

in the range of two to three times that of an RBC.[100] Nuclear pleomorphism with varying size within a smear is characteristically found in grade 2 and grade 3 carcinomas. Nuclear size pleomorphism is less distinct in low-grade carcinomas and a few may appear deceptively monotonous.

Except for apocrine metaplastic cells, and secretory cells as in pregnancy and lactation, it is unusual for normal benign breast epithelial cells to have prominent or multiple nucleoli. Most low-grade carcinomas have small or indistinct nucleoli.[100] Distinct or prominent/abnormal nucleoli are a feature of grade 2 and 3 carcinomas. However, a number of benign, but proliferative lesions, including fibroadenomas may present with a distinct nucleolus. In these cases the nucleus will have a uniform/smooth chromatin pattern. Some of the largest nucleoli are found in benign, lactating cells. Nucleoli, and the size of the nucleoli, are a feature of active cells. This is the case in most carcinomas, but the nucleoli as such are not a feature of malignancy. Atypical nucleoli with bizarre shapes and sharp edges in well-preserved cells (Fig. 4.61) are a feature of malignancy.

**Table 4.3** Cytological grading according to Robinson et al. 1994[112]

| Criterion | Score 1 | Score 2 | Score 3 |
|---|---|---|---|
| Cell dissociation | Mostly clusters | Single cells and clusters | Mostly single cells |
| Nuclear size | 1–2 times size of an erythrocyte | 3–4 times size of an erythrocyte | ≥5 times size of an erythrocyte |
| Cell uniformity | Monomorphic | Mildly pleomorphic | Pleomorphic |
| Nucleoli | Indistinct/small | Noticeable | Abnormal |
| Nuclear margin | Smooth | Slightly irregular/folds and grooves | Buds and clefts |
| Chromatin pattern | Vesicular | Granular | Clumping and clearing |

Score 6–11, Grade 1; Score 12–14, Grade 2; Score 15–18, Grade 3.

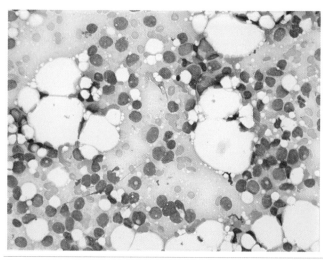

**Fig. 4.63** G2. Cell dissociation 3; nuclear size 2; cell uniformity 3; nucleoli 2; nuclear margin 2; chromatin pattern 2. Total score = 14 (MGG).

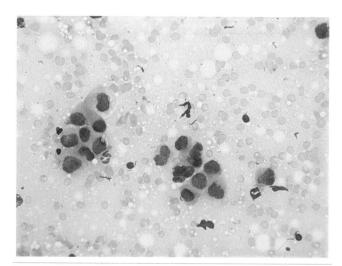

**Fig. 4.64** G3. Cell dissociation 2; nuclear size 2 (–3); cell uniformity 3; nucleoli 3; nuclear margin 3; chromatin pattern 2. Total score = 15 (–16) (MGG).

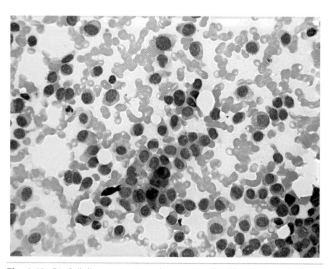

**Fig. 4.62** G1. Cell dissociation 3; nuclear size 1; cell uniformity 2; nucleoli 1; nuclear margin 2; chromatin pattern 2. Total score = 11 (MGG).

Even if the cytological grading does not have therapeutic implications in invasive carcinomas, providing it may be beneficial as the cytological grading will give an indication of the presumed aggressiveness of the tumour.

Few institutions diagnose DCIS on FNA smears, but when FNA is relied on for diagnosing DCIS, grading is feasible.[7] A modified Van Nuy[113] grading can easily be applied to FNA. High-grade DCIS may receive a more aggressive treatment than low-grade DCIS.

## Invasive carcinoma and ductal carcinoma *in situ*

Table 4.4 shows the ranges for different subtypes of invasive carcinomas. In FNA, the vast majority of samples will be from IDC, some will be from lobular carcinomas (ILC), whereas the other subtypes will appear less often. Some of them have well-defined cytological features that may be recognised on the smears. In most cases, the subtype is irrelevant for the primary surgical procedure. Most uncommon subtypes are low grade with a good prognosis, and the main problem may be in recognising them as malignant.

## Invasive ductal carcinoma (IDC)

Of all epithelial malignancies of the breast, up to 80% of breast carcinomas fall into this category.[81] The general features of malignancy pertain to these common tumours. IDC is very heterogeneous as to grade of atypia, growth pattern and stromal reaction and this heterogeneity is reflected in the smear patterns. The mammographic imaging of IDC is likewise heterogeneous, ranging from the classical spiculated lesions to rounded, deceivingly sharply demarcated tumours and non-specific

**Table 4.4** Histological subtypes of invasive breast carcinomas

|  | (%) |
| --- | --- |
| Ductal of no special type | 65–80 |
| Lobular carcinoma | 5–14 |
| Basal and medullary-like carcinoma | 5–7 |
| Tubular carcinoma | 2–8 |
| Mucinous carcinoma | 2–4 |
| Papillary carcinoma | 1–2 |
| Apocrine carcinoma | 1–4 |
| Other rare types | <1 |

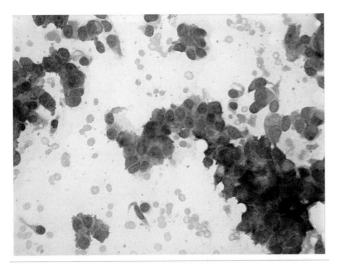

**Fig. 4.65** DCIS nuclear grade 3. Carcinoma cells with nuclear size >2 × RBC (MGG).

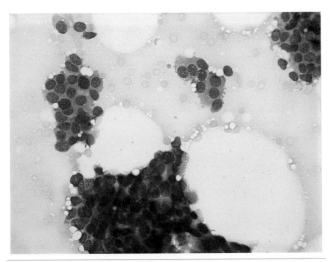

**Fig. 4.66** DCIS low nuclear grade. Cells from DCIS nuclei size up to 2 × RBC (MGG).

densities and 'spots'. The heterogeneity is reflected also in the ultrasonographic (US) findings. Most IDC will have an irregular outline on US with the largest diameter of the lesion in the vertical plane, some may be rounded lesions with indeterminate features and a few may mimic a fibroadenoma.

The cellularity of the aspirate will depend on the interplay between the skill of the aspirator, the size of the lesion and the degree of desmoplasia within the lesion. Scirrhous ductal carcinomas provide the lowest cell yield of all proliferative breast lesions while high-grade, poorly collagenous ductal carcinoma can provide even the novice with a very thick spread of aspirated cells. The cellular pattern can be very variable. There can be large three-dimensional arrays of folded epithelium interspersed with smaller groups and occasional single cells. Others show a lack of cohesion resulting in a virtual monolayer, resembling the low-power pattern of a high-grade lymphoma. Occasionally, recognisable acini and tubular structures are apparent. Mixed carcinomas are common: IDC may harbour elements of all other subtypes, including papillary, micropapillary and mucinous, and all of these may be found on the smears.

Necrosis is not common except in a few usually extremely high-grade carcinomas. However, necrosis is common in high-grade DCIS and tumours with a distinct population of DCIS will reveal material both from the invasive and the *in situ* component, including comedo type necrosis. Microcalcification is quite common and may originate both from *in situ* and invasive elements.[7,99]

Within the groups and aggregates there is loss of polarity, the nuclei can appear crowded and moulded and the general appearance may resemble a syncytium. The nucleocytoplasmic ratio may vary, but most IDC have a rather scanty amount of cytoplasm. Mitoses are not commonly found, except in high-grade carcinomas.

All these cytological features tell us that the cells are malignant, but not whether they are invasive or just part of an *in situ* lesion. In the presence of a mass lesion, invasive carcinoma is far more likely than *in situ* carcinoma, though high-grade ductal carcinoma *in situ* can form a palpable mass, often with inflamed desmoplastic stroma surrounding enlarged ducts and lobules which are filled by neoplastic cells, necrosis and calcification. Invasion criteria have been described. When applied,[114] it is only possible to diagnose about 50% of the invasive carcinomas as invasive.

### Cytological findings: invasive ductal carcinoma

- Varying cellularity from abundant to scanty
- The epithelial cells present as single cells, loose aggregates and cohesive groups often three-dimensional in appearance
- Varying cellular and nuclear atypia according to histological grade
- Cells may be vacuolated and occasional signet ring cells are seen
- Microcalcification is quite common
- Mitoses are uncommon, but may be seen in high-grade lesions
- Necrosis is not common.

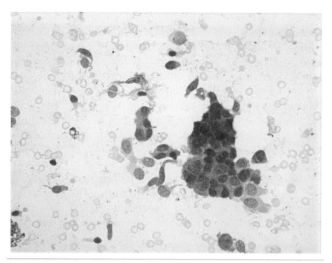

**Fig. 4.67** IDC. Single, well-preserved fibroblasts intermingled with carcinoma cells (MGG).

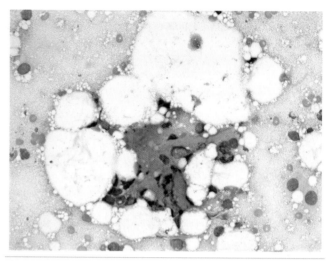

**Fig. 4.69** Invasion of single carcinoma cells in stromal fragment (MGG).

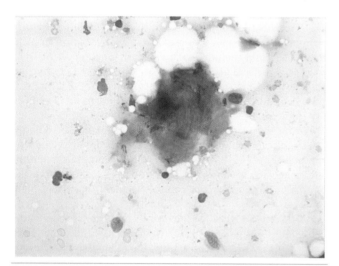

**Fig. 4.68** IDC. Pink elastoid, cell poor stromal fragment (MGG).

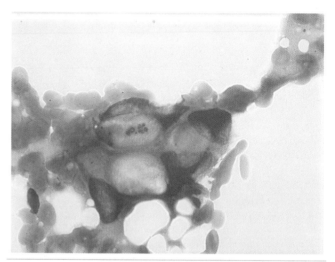

**Fig. 4.70** IDC. High magnification of signet ring cells with large intracytoplasmic vacuoles (MGG).

*Criteria suggestive of invasive lesion*[114]

- Proliferation of fibroblasts (a sign of tumour induced stromal reaction) (Fig. 4.67)
- Cell poor elastoid stromal fragments (Fig. 4.68)
- Invasion of single or small groups of 2–3 carcinoma cells in stromal tissue and fatty fragments (Fig. 4.69)
- Intracytoplasmic vacuoles (Fig. 4.70)
- Tubular structures (Fig. 4.71).

## Ductal carcinoma *in situ* (DCIS)

DCIS is characterised by enlarged ducts with proliferation of neoplastic epithelial cells. It is a heterogeneous lesion with a variety of growth patterns and a cellular/nuclear atypia that ranges from low grade with very subtle nuclear abnormality to striking high-grade atypia. This heterogeneity is reflected in the FNA material. A large majority of lesions (>75%) present with a high-grade nuclear atypia.[7]

The majority of DCIS is non-palpable and presents as mammographic microcalcification without a tumour (both

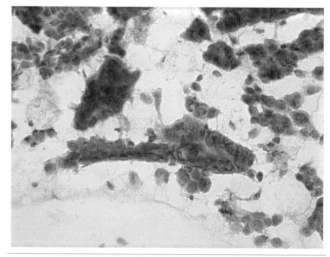

**Fig. 4.71** Tubular carcinoma. Tubular structure with a clear lumen is the equivalent of the histological tubular structure. It is the hallmark of tubular carcinomas, but may also be found in IDC and adenosis (PAP).

on mammography and ultrasonography). The lesions are less likely to be seen on ultrasound. About 2–3% of palpable carcinomas are tumour-forming DCIS.[115] About 20% of lesions with a primary FNA or CNB diagnosis of DCIS have an additional invasive tumour in the surgical specimen.[17,116,117] The larger the extent of DCIS, the higher is the risk or probability of finding an additional invasive component in the surgical specimen. The invasive lesion can be within the DCIS area, in the vicinity or anywhere else in the breast. As they have not been recognised radiologically, the vast majority of these invasive lesions have not been sampled preoperatively.

Experience with cytological material from DCIS is well described in the literature.[7,17,117–123] Most institutions have some experience with the occasional palpable, tumour-forming (and usually) high-grade DCIS. With the advent of mammography screening, some institutions have also gained experience with FNA material from non-palpable, mammographic microcalcifications. The cytological diagnosis of DCIS and the distinction of DCIS from invasive carcinoma has been the subject of much discussion and controversy. As a result, most institutions have abandoned FNA on microcalcifications and primarily investigate them by CNB or vacuum-assisted biopsy (VAB).

Where done by FNA, material from microcalcifications is best sampled by a stereotactic device. The number of passes depends on the extent of the microcalcifications, but a minimum of three is recommended. In the majority of cases this is sufficient to obtain a representative and sufficient material. Both high-grade and low-grade DCIS usually present with ample microcalcifications on the smears. The aspirator can usually both hear and feel when they are targeted and 'hit' by the needle. When smearing the material, abundant microcalcifications will feel as if smearing on sand paper. The amount of cellular material depends on how 'large' the lesion is, but with precise targeting the material is usually moderate to abundant. Microcalcifications are readily identified both in PAP- and MGG-stained specimens as well as in liquid-based preparations. They appear as small, irregular pieces resembling broken glass 'coated' with stain and appear blue/black irrespective of the staining method. They can be found within epithelial groups and aggregates, along the side/periphery of cell groups, within areas with necrosis and also free on the smears (Figs 4.72–4.75). Psammoma bodies are not a feature of DCIS, and are rare in breast lesions. If found, they should raise suspicion of a metastatic lesion, for example from an ovarian carcinoma or a papillary lung carcinoma.

## High-grade DCIS

The cytological features of high-grade DCIS (Fig. 4.76) have been described in several papers in the literature.[7,118–120,122] In a setting of mammographic microcalcifications without a tumour, the following features are characteristic of high nuclear grade DCIS: high-grade atypical carcinoma cells in three-dimensional, solid aggregates and as single cells, microcalcifications and comedo type necrotic material. An eventual additional invasive component is, for all practical purposes, not recognisable in the smears.[124] A radiological tumour with calcifications, will practically always be an invasive carcinoma which may or may not have a variable component of DCIS within it. Most high-grade DCIS will predominantly present as solid, three-dimensional epithelial aggregates. In some cases the aggregates may be cribriform. Micropapillary and true papillary

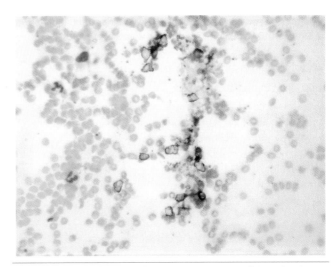

**Fig. 4.72** Microcalcifications in breast FNA appear as small, irregular pieces resembling broken glass coated with stain and appear blue/black irrespective of the staining method (MGG).

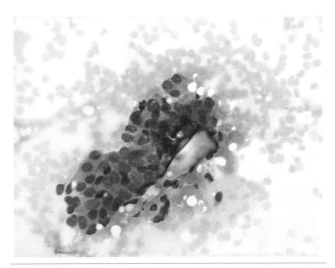

**Fig. 4.73** Microcalcifications can be found within epithelial groups and aggregates, along the side/periphery of cell groups (MGG).

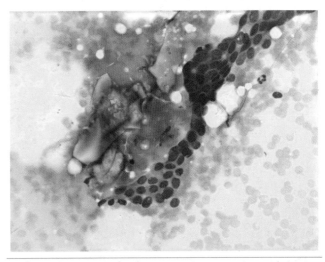

**Fig. 4.74** Microcalcifications can be found within areas of necrosis and also free on the smears (MGG).

structures are occasionally seen.[7] A few myoepithelial cells may be seen in the periphery of cell groups and aggregates.

## Cytological findings: high-grade DCIS

- Solid or cribriform, three-dimensional aggregates of epithelial cells with high-grade nuclear atypia
- Occasionally micropapillary and true papillary structures as well as monolayer sheets
- Variable number of single cells; occasional cases may present as an almost exclusively single cell population
- Microcalcifications
- Comedo type necrosis.

## Diagnostic pitfalls: high-grade DCIS

- Some cases of grade 3 IDC may present with necrosis and microcalcification, but the clinical and radiological appearance will be that of a tumour

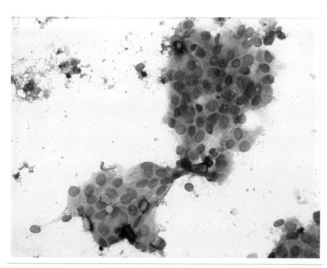

**Fig. 4.75** Microcalcification. Varying appearance of microcalcifications in breast FNA (MGG).

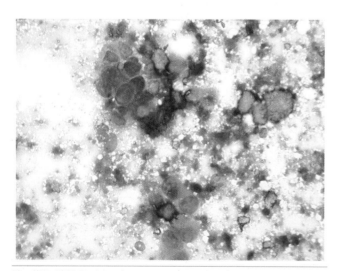

**Fig. 4.76** DCIS G3. Comedo type necrosis with high-grade carcinoma cells and microcalcifications (MGG).

- Microinvasion or invasive lesions that have not been seen radiologically will not be sampled, and about 20% of cases will have an invasive component in the surgical specimen
- A large number of single cells is not a feature of invasion.

## Low- and intermediate-grade DCIS

Low-grade and intermediate-grade (or non-high-grade DCIS) is more heterogeneous in appearance than high-grade DCIS both histologically and cytologically (Fig. 4.77). The cytological features have been described in the literature, but the number of cases that form the basis of the criteria listed below, are far less than for the high-grade DCIS.[7,120] The criteria overlap with criteria for epithelial hyperplasia both with and without atypia.[7,118,125] Typical non-high-grade DCIS presents as very large, cohesive, three-dimensional and cribriform aggregates, as well as some solid aggregates, micropapillary groups and microcalcifications. Pure subtypes are virtually non-existent. The number of single cells may vary. In most cases, there are rather few, but here also, occasional cases may present with a dominant single cell pattern. The nuclear atypia is discrete to moderate with nuclear sizes one and a half to two times that of a red blood cell. A diagnosis or suggestion of a low-grade/non-high-grade DCIS should lead to a local excision only.

## Cytological findings: low- and intermediate-grade DCIS

- Very large three-dimensional epithelial aggregates, cribriform and solid, often more cohesive than high-grade lesions
- Cell monotony
- Micropapillary groups
- True papillary structures
- Monolayer sheets
- Variable number of single cells; usually few, but occasional cases may present as an almost pure single cell population
- Microcalcifications
- Occasional comedo type necrosis
- Low to moderate nuclear atypia

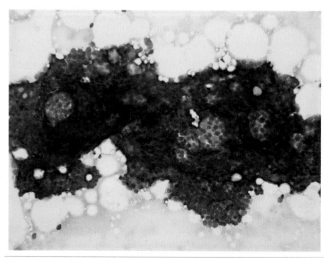

**Fig. 4.77** DCIS G1. Large, three-dimensional and cribriform aggregate with epithelial cells with discrete atypia and nuclear size not more than 2 × RBC (MGG).

- Recognisable myoepithelial cell nuclei in epithelial aggregates and sheets not rare (!).

### Diagnostic pitfalls: low- and intermediate-grade DCIS

- The cytological criteria overlap with epithelial hyperplasia with and without atypia. A diagnosis or suggestion of a non-high-grade DCIS should only result in a local excision or core biopsy confirmation of the type and extent of the lesion, never mastectomy or removal of axillary lymph nodes
- Some of the lesions may appear quite monotonous ('monomorphous') in contrast to benign, hyperplastic lesions ('polymorphous' cell pattern)
- Numerous single cells are not indicative of an invasive lesion
- Myoepithelial cell nuclei on the epithelial groups are no 'proof' of a benign lesion.

## Mucinous (colloid) carcinoma

Depending on the rigidity with which the diagnostic criteria are applied histologically, the incidence of mucinous carcinoma is quoted to be between 1% and 5% of all breast carcinomas (Fig. 4.78).[81] This is typically a tumour of older post-menopausal women occurring at an age of 60 years or more. Most mucinous carcinomas are low grade, slow growing and have a favourable prognosis with a 5-year survival of up to 86%. However, high-grade mucinous carcinomas do occur.

On examination, mucinous carcinoma tends to be well-defined, hard and mobile. Because of the smooth outline, it may be mistaken clinically and radiologically for a fibroadenoma or cyst but awareness of the typical age of presentation for each of these lesions reduces this error. Aspiration is generally easy, giving a sensation on the needle similar to or softer than that of a cellular fibroadenoma. On spreading, the aspirate is often very mucinous.

The cells tend to be in loose aggregates and small cohesive groups bathed in a mucinous background. The single cells show eccentricity of the nucleus and little variation of nuclear size or shape when compared with intraduct carcinoma (IDC) of no special type (NST). The chromatin tends to be bland but there may be recognisable hyperchromatism and coarsening. Nucleoli are not prominent. The mucinous nature of the background is usually more immediately obvious in MGG-stained smears where the mucin is a bright crimson, than in PAP-stained smears where it is usually wispy and pale grey/green in colour. With either preparation, however, a specific diagnosis is nearly always possible. The favourable prognosis of mucinous carcinoma is only maintained in pure low-grade forms of the tumour. As otherwise unremarkable ductal carcinomas of any grade can occasionally contain foci of mucin-producing carcinoma, there is the potential for overdiagnosis of this entity on cytological assessment, dependent on the area sampled.

Some mucinous carcinomas may be shown to contain endocrine cells histochemically but these are not apparent cytologically. In otherwise typical mucinous carcinomas, the occasional signet ring cell can be seen. This should not be taken as evidence of a signet ring cell carcinoma, which has a much worse prognosis.

### Cytological findings: mucinous (colloid) carcinoma

- On spreading, the aspirate is quite glairy, hinting at a high mucin content
- The smear is usually cellular
- The epithelial cells present as single cells, loose aggregates and cohesive groups often three-dimensional in appearance
- The cells are small, with small, uniform, round nuclei, smooth nuclear outlines, bland, possibly granular, chromatin and inconspicuous nucleoli
- The cells are bathed in mucin of variable density. This is more obvious in MGG preparations, where it stains violet
- Cells may be vacuolated and occasional signet ring cells are seen
- Some cases contain microcalcifications.

### Diagnostic pitfalls: mucinous (colloid) carcinoma

- These tumours are so bland cytologically that they may be misdiagnosed as benign, particularly when they occur in younger women
- Some ductal carcinomas of no special type can contain large foci of mucinous carcinoma
- Cell poor samples with ample mucin and scanty tumour cells may mimic mucocele/mucocele-like lesions.

## Signet ring cell carcinoma

These rare lesions[81] occur in a younger age group than mucinous carcinomas. In contrast to mucinous carcinomas they are invariably aggressive lesions attended by a high risk of metastatic spread. Although both lobular and ductal carcinomas may show cytoplasmic vacuoles in cytological and histological preparations, lesions showing a sufficient degree to warrant a diagnosis of signet ring cell carcinoma are rare.

With cytological assessment, there is a risk of misdiagnosis of mucinous (colloid) carcinoma with an underestimate of the aggressiveness of the lesion. A mistaken diagnosis of metastatic signet ring carcinoma of gastrointestinal origin leads to the assumption of an unduly gloomy prognosis. Awareness of the existence of this lesion should prevent these mishaps.

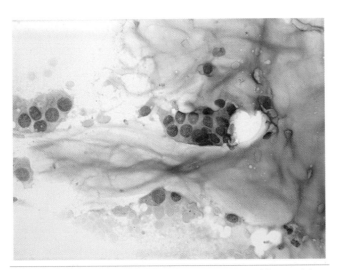

**Fig. 4.78** MCC. Abundant mucinous material with groups of (low-grade) carcinoma cells.

The cells are usually abundant and poorly cohesive with only small stringy groups. The cells are large with large eccentric, crescentic-shaped nuclei displaced to a marginal position by cytoplasmic mucin (Fig. 4.70). There is quite marked anisonucleosis and moderate to marked hyperchromasia.

### Cytological findings: signet ring cell carcinoma

- On smearing, the thick, mucinous nature of these lesions may be apparent
- Smears are cellular containing poorly cohesive, large malignant cells with moderate to marked anisonucleosis and hyperchromatism
- The cytoplasm is abundant and vacuolated
- The nucleus is typically crescentic and displaced to the edge of the cell.

### Diagnostic pitfalls: signet ring cell carcinoma

- May be confused with low-grade mucinous carcinoma
- The possibility of metastatic spread from a visceral signet ring carcinoma should be considered.

## Neuroendocrine carcinoma

Clinically, these tumours present like a ductal carcinoma (Figs 4.79–4.81).[81] They are often well circumscribed both clinically and radiologically. They express neuroendocrine markers in over 50% of the tumour cell population. Cytologically, eccentric nuclei with stippled chromatin may be noted. The cells resemble plasma cells. There is an overlap with solid invasive papillary carcinoma.

### Cytological findings: neuroendocrine carcinoma

- Cellular aspirates contain dispersed single cells and cells in small groups
- The cells are remarkably uniform with an eccentrically placed nucleus resembling plasma cells
- The chromatin is stippled and thickening of the nuclear border may be noted
- Cytoplasmic (endocrine) granules may be seen in a few tumour cells.

### Diagnostic pitfalls: neuroendocrine carcinoma

- Lymphoplasmacytoid lymphoma or plasmacytoma can form deposits in soft tissue and breast. Lymphoma usually displays complete absence of cell cohesion.

## Medullary carcinoma with lymphoid stroma

Medullary carcinoma[81] (Fig. 4.82) is part of the spectrum of basal-like carcinomas of the breast. It is diagnosed less frequently if strict criteria are applied to the diagnosis. It presents in a younger age group and typically in women under 50 years old. Histologically, it is composed of large syncytial sheets of high-grade atypical cells, no glandular structures, scant stroma and a prominent lymphoplasmacytic infiltrate. As it is a well-defined, mobile lesion there is a risk of a clinical and radiological

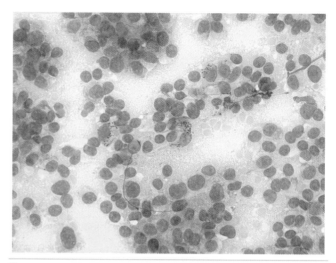
**Fig. 4.79** Neuroendocrine carcinoma cells with some of the cells showing pink endocrine cytoplasmic granules (MGG).

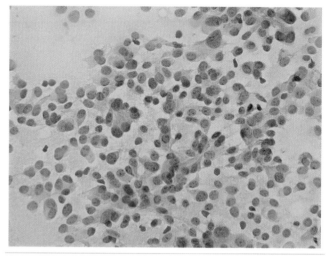
**Fig. 4.80** Neuroendocrine carcinoma cells with plasmacytoid appearance (PAP).

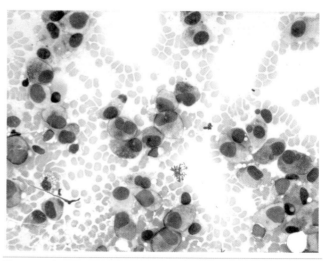
**Fig. 4.81** Plasmacytoid cells from a neuroendocrine carcinoma with abundant endocrine cytoplasmic granules (MGG).

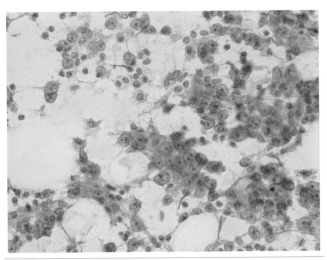

**Fig. 4.82** Medullary carcinoma. Loosely cohesive sheets of high-grade carcinoma cells intermingles with numerous lymphocytes (PAP).

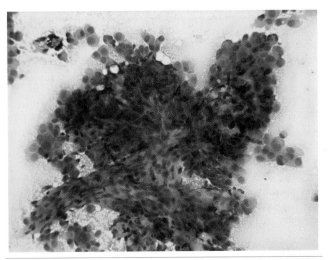

**Fig. 4.83** Papillary, intracystic/intraductal carcinoma *in situ* with papillary stromal fragment and discohesive carcinoma cells (MGG).

misdiagnosis of fibroadenoma. Even the macroscopic assessment of a histological specimen may give a similar impression. The lesion is very soft to the needle. Aspiration of these lesions is generally very easy as they are particularly cellular and contain little stroma. On smearing, the sample is frequently opaque, spreading evenly like a lymphomatous aspirate of a lymph node but usually appearing more granular. Microscopically, the appearance is that of a poorly cohesive, high-grade carcinoma. Syncytial fragments of carcinoma cells are likely to survive intact and these are infiltrated by lymphoid cells and surrounded by a background of small lymphocytes and occasional plasma cells.

### Cytological findings: medullary carcinoma with lymphoid stroma

- Very cellular smears are easily obtained
- Poorly cohesive large malignant cells with abundant pale staining cytoplasm, some forming syncytial aggregates
- Large angular nuclei with coarse chromatin and prominent nucleoli. Mitotic figures are not unusual
- The background of small lymphocytes and plasma cells is a vital feature but their number is very variable and can be so few that they are overlooked. These cells may be entirely separate from the epithelial cells or intimately mixed with the syncytial groups
- Tumour giant cells are sometimes a feature.

### Diagnostic pitfalls: medullary carcinoma with lymphoid stroma

- Although the diagnosis of carcinoma is not usually difficult, the presence of lymphoid cells and the clinical features of a circumscribed round nodule can cause difficulty in distinguishing a primary carcinoma high in the axillary tail from a lymph node metastasis.

## Papillary intracystic carcinoma

Pure papillary carcinoma (Figs 4.83, 4.84) has a better prognosis than IDC, with an 80% 5-year survival rate. This is probably

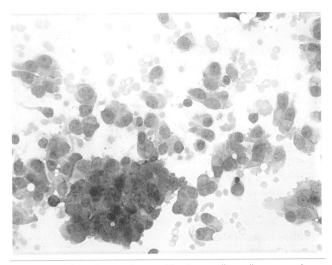

**Fig. 4.84** Solid/papillary carcinoma with micropapillary cell groups and single cells (MGG).

because papillary carcinoma is one of the breast cancers that forms a mass lesion while still *in situ*, and even when invasive the area of invasion may represent only a small part of the whole tumour. Because of the possibility of a papillary carcinoma being entirely *in situ*, this is one of the breast carcinomas in which an FNA diagnosis of the sub-type can be of benefit in deciding the extent of surgery.

There can be difficulty in distinguishing histologically between a low-grade papillary carcinoma and a benign papilloma with epithelial hyperplasia. Some lesions are heterogeneous and benign papillomas can be found in association with intraduct carcinoma of cribriform type. Papillary carcinoma may arise de novo or in or adjacent to a papilloma, further compounding the difficulties. Most papillary carcinomas are pure *in situ* lesions, typically intracystic, or represent solid, circumscribed types.[126]

Clinically, these tumours vary in presentation but they may be small, coming to the patient's attention because of associated fibrocystic change or because of the development of a mass due to the cyst around a papillary intracystic carcinoma.

Non-palpable lesions are not uncommon in mammography screening. They present radiologically as a rounded, often equivocal lesion. When palpable, they are usually small and soft on aspiration. They may be macroscopically or microscopically cystic with some debris and macrophages.

Cytologically, these lesions can be problematic as the nuclear pleomorphism is usually low-grade and bare nuclei may be present. This picture can cause confusion with fibroadenoma or benign papilloma. The smears tend to be cellular with three-dimensional papillary structures that may include a fibrovascular core. Denuded fibrovascular cores may be apparent. The cells often have a definite columnar appearance and may appear in small rows or palisades. Dissociated and clustered epithelial cells tend to have a monotonous 'clonal' appearance. Naked nuclei in the background have the same size, shape and chromatin pattern as the epithelial cells and, therefore, should not be confused with benign bipolar stromal cells. There is frequently a population of haemosiderin laden macrophages in the background.

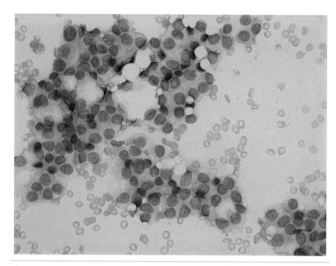

**Fig. 4.85** Loosely cohesive fragments of low-grade carcinoma cells with cribriform pattern (MGG).

### Cytological findings: papillary intracystic carcinoma

- May be cystic on aspiration
- The cell material is usually abundant
- Epithelial cells are monotonous and appear 'clonal'
- Anisonucleosis, hyperchromasia, coarse chromatin and prominent nucleoli are uncommon
- Benign bipolar cells are absent from the background and myoepithelial cells are not seen within the groups
- Large papillary cell clusters forming arborising arrays bearing overlapping, palisaded cells on a fibrovascular core may be present as with papillomas
- Cells may be dispersed and the fibrovascular cores denuded
- The cells are often distinctly columnar in appearance, although this feature is shared with papillomas.

### Diagnostic pitfalls: papillary intracystic carcinoma

- These lesions are usually low-grade and lack obvious cytological features of malignancy often leading to a suspicious diagnosis
- The diagnosis may be missed if blood stained cyst fluid is discarded rather than sent for cytological examination, although in some cases the cyst fluid is not diagnostic. If there is any residual mass after drainage of cyst fluid, re-aspiration should be undertaken
- Distinction between a benign, proliferative papilloma and a papillary carcinoma may be difficult. In general the neoplastic lesion will appear 'monoclonal' with a distinct monotony of the cells, whereas the benign lesions are 'polyclonal' with a more polymorphic cell pattern
- Most lesions are histologically *in situ*, and whether there is an invasive component is not apparent cytologically. A cytological diagnosis or suggestion of a papillary tumour or papillary carcinoma should only lead to a local excision. Core biopsy is equally likely to miss a focus of invasion, so it is common for these tumours to be excised without a certain diagnosis of invasion.

## Invasive cribriform carcinoma

When present in its pure histological form, this entity confers a very good prognosis. The cytological findings will be that of a low-grade IDC with medium-sized to large cribriform epithelial aggregates (Fig. 4.85).

## Tubular carcinoma

This low-grade variant of breast carcinoma generally has a very good prognosis. Being very slow growing lesions and having a significantly collagenous stroma, these tumours commonly present when small or on a routine screening mammogram. Clinically, they are firm and discrete and give a fibrous sensation on aspiration. Both mammography and ultrasonography appear suspicious (Figs 4.71, 4.86, 4.87).

On aspiration it can be quite difficult to obtain smears with adequate cellularity and suboptimal sampling is a major cause of not reaching a definite diagnosis of malignancy.[99] The cells usually exhibit bland nuclear features. Nuclei are often $1\frac{1}{2}$–2 × RBC with slightly irregular nuclear outlines, granular chromatin and indistinct or small nucleoli.[100] They may be cuboidal or columnar. The groups are usually very cohesive, but a few single cells may be found in most cases.

### Cytological findings: tubular carcinoma

- Aspirates may be poorly cellular, but with an optimal technique, they may yield a more cellular and diagnostic material
- Epithelial cells in cohesive clusters and sheets that have a recognisable acinar structure, but abnormal rigid finger-like groups and cell balls also may be seen
- Monolayer sheets, often folded and with part of an intact tubular structure in one end
- True tubular structures, often broken with sharp angles
- There is slight anisonucleosis and mild hyperchromasia. The chromatin is finely granular and evenly distributed
- Nucleoli are indistinct or small

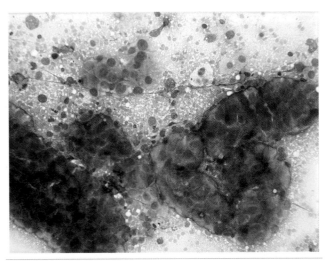

**Fig. 4.86** Overview of smear from a tubular carcinoma with numerous tubular structures, partly as broken tubuli (PAP).

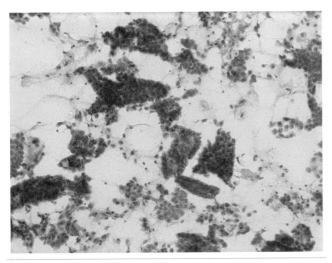

**Fig. 4.88** Cohesive, micropapillary pattern as well as single cells (MGG).

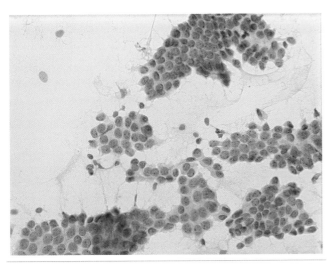

**Fig. 4.87** Monolayer sheets representing ruptured tubular structures with minimal nuclear abnormalities. No naked myoepithelial nuclei (PAP).

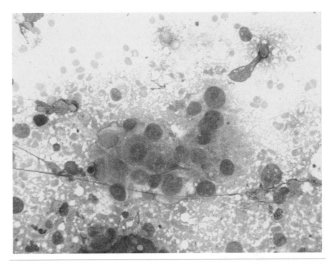

**Fig. 4.89** Micropapillary group of high-grade carcinoma cells (compare RBC size) (MGG).

- Bipolar nuclei are present in occasional cases
- 'Messy' background of cell fragments and stromal elements
- No apocrine or foam cells present
- Dissociated cells where present may have a columnar appearance.

### Diagnostic pitfalls: tubular carcinoma

- This type of carcinoma accounts for some false negative cytological diagnoses as the malignant characteristics are very subtle. Suboptimal sampling add to the diagnostic problems, and frequently the cytological category is suspicious rather a confident malignant. It is important to take the clinical and mammographic features into account when managing the patient
- There is an overlap in appearance with complex sclerosing lesions and radial scars, mammographically and cytologically.

### Invasive micropapillary carcinoma

This is a carcinoma[81] (Figs 4.88, 4.89) composed of small clusters of tumour cells lying within clear stromal spaces and resembling vascular channels. This is mirrored in the FNA smears which is dominated by well demarcated micropapillary clusters.[127,128] The nuclear atypia is usually high grade. Micropapillary carcinoma has a propensity for lymphatic invasion and metastasis.

### Apocrine carcinoma

Pure apocrine carcinoma (Fig. 4.90) is unusual, forming only 1–4% of all breast carcinomas. The tumours may present with all grades of atypia.

Apocrine carcinoma is diagnosed on an aspirate when the cells have malignant nuclei and abundant eosinophilic or amphophilic cytoplasm, which may be granular or finely vacuolated. The cell outline tends to be polygonal. Features helpful in the differentiation of benign from malignant apocrine cells

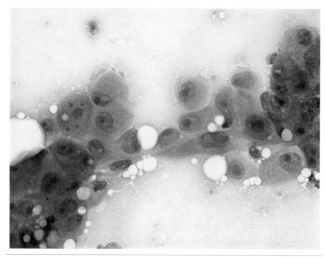

**Fig. 4.90** Cells from a high-grade carcinoma with apocrine differentiation with abundant dense cytoplasm (MGG).

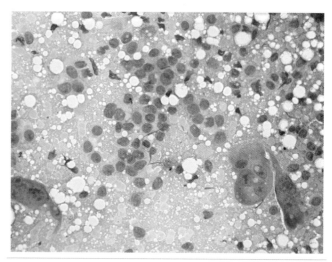

**Fig. 4.91** Loosely cohesive sheets and single carcinoma cells from IDC and large, multinucleated osteoclast-like giant cells (MGG).

are pleomorphic nuclei, poorly defined cell borders and cellular discohesion in the latter.

### Cytological findings: apocrine carcinoma

- Aspirates tend to be cellular and the cells dispersed
- The cells are large with abundant acidophilic cytoplasm that may be granular but this is less marked than in benign apocrine epithelium
- The cell borders tend to be indistinct or ragged in contrast to the well-defined borders of benign apocrine cells. This is an important feature if low-grade apocrine carcinoma is suspected
- The nucleus is also large and the chromatin coarse and unevenly distributed
- The single nucleolus is very large, sometimes spectacularly so. Multiple nucleoli are also seen in the higher-grade tumours.

### Diagnostic pitfalls: apocrine carcinoma

- The main danger is in dismissing a low-grade apocrine carcinoma as apocrine metaplasia or vice versa
- Benign apocrine epithelium can look quite atypical, particularly when the lining of a cyst has become degenerate or inflamed or in the context of apocrine adenosis.

### Secretory carcinoma

Clinically, these tumours are well circumscribed and most are less than 20 mm at presentation. The cytological features have been described in a few cases[129] and include cells with prominent, intracytoplasmic vacuoles and secretions, occasional signet ring cells and diffuse mucin positivity.

### Glycogen rich (clear cell) carcinoma

This may resemble signet ring carcinoma in sections but special stains will readily reveal the cytoplasm to be filled with glycogen and not mucin.

### Cytological findings: glycogen rich (clear cell) carcinoma[130]

- Abundantly cellular aspirate
- Tumour cells in groups, clusters and as single cells
- Large dispersed cells with plentiful clear or eosinophilic, finely granular to vacuolated cytoplasm and centrally placed nuclei
- Fragile cytoplasm that may smear out and appear as a granular background material
- Moderate to marked nuclear pleomorphism.

### Diagnostic pitfalls: glycogen rich (clear cell) carcinoma

- The cytological appearance may resemble signet ring carcinoma but the prognosis is in any case similar
- Occasionally, clear cell carcinoma of the kidney metastasises to breast or skin and may present a similar appearance.

## Carcinoma with osteoclast-like stromal giant cells

Some otherwise unremarkable ductal carcinomas are associated with osteoclast-like stromal giant cells (Fig. 4.91). The stromal cells are not malignant and are thought to be a reaction to the tumour.

### Cytological findings: carcinoma with osteoclast-like stromal giant cells

- Aspirates are cellular, containing malignant ductal epithelial cells of any grade
- The giant cells have abundant basophilic cytoplasm and variable numbers of nuclei but are not cytologically malignant.

### Diagnostic pitfalls: carcinoma with osteoclast-like stromal giant cells

- Occasional cases may be dominated by the giant cells and there is a risk that they may be diagnosed as granulomatous inflammation, fat necrosis or foreign body reaction.

## Invasive lobular carcinoma (ILC)

The prognosis for classical cases is midway between that of tubular carcinoma and IDC, but there is an increased risk of synchronous or asynchronous multifocality and bilaterality (Figs 4.92–4.95). Overall, however, the outlook is similar for each grade of lobular carcinoma to that of IDC.

Histologically, the most important features of classical invasive lobular carcinoma are the relatively small size of the cells and a tendency not to form acini or cell groups but rather to infiltrate diffusely through the tissues with little stromal reaction. Because of this they are often larger than is appreciated clinically or radiologically. These tumours have lost the adhesion molecule e-cadherin and infiltrate as individual cells, often forming lines and rings on histological sections, and to some extent this is reflected on cytological smears. Intracytoplasmic lumina are a feature of many classical invasive lobular carcinomas but are also seen in some invasive ductal carcinomas and DCIS.[124]

Lobular carcinomas are important to the cytopathologist because, with the more fibrotic ductal carcinomas, they are responsible for many false negative cytological diagnoses in palpable breast lesions.[99] This is because lobular carcinomas, particularly the classical type, tend to yield poorly cellular aspirates composed of small uniform cells with small and relatively bland nuclei. The more cellular alveolar variant is easier to sample.

A most valuable clue to the presence of lobular carcinoma is the tendency to form small chains of cells in the aspirate. The nuclear/cytoplasmic ratio is high. In PAP-stained preparations, there is a fine stippling of the chromatin but marked hyperchromasia is not a feature and the nucleolus is characteristically very small, except in the histiocytoid or pleomorphic variant in which the nuclei are pleomorphic, the nucleoli prominent and the cytoplasm abundant. The nuclear outlines are irregular with folds and grooves.

MGG-stained preparations show a small, dense and compact nucleus and usually no nucleolus is visible. The variation in nuclear size is slight but detectable. Occasional intracytoplasmic lumina with a target-like appearance may be seen. Signet-ring cells may also be seen.

The presence of moderate or sparse, small but bold and robust appearing nuclei with an absence of bipolar stromal

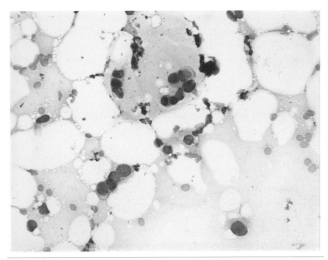

**Fig. 4.93** ILC. Scanty cellular material from a case of classical ILC. Carcinoma cells in 'indian file' as well as small irregular groups and single cells (MGG).

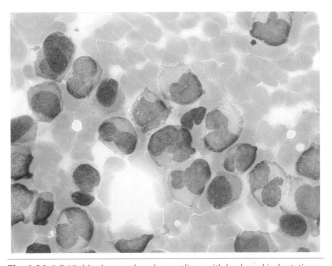

**Fig. 4.94** ILC. Highly abnormal nuclear outlines with buds and indentations, inconspicuous nucleoli and granular chromatin. Nuclear size 2–3 × RBC (MGG).

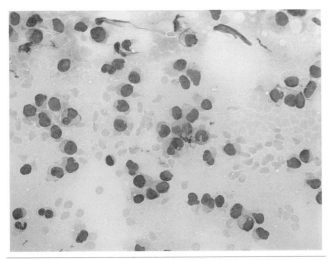

**Fig. 4.92** ILC. Moderately cellular from an alveolar type ILC. Carcinoma cells in rows, small irregular groups and as single cells (MGG).

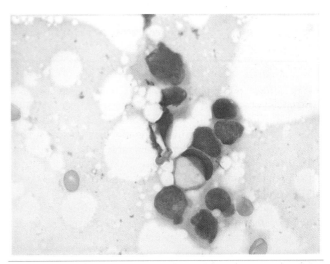

**Fig. 4.95** ILC. Carcinoma cells in a short 'indian file'. There is irregular nuclear outline with folds and buds and a signet ring cell with a large cytoplasmic vacuole (MGG).

cells from a clinically suspicious lump should alert the cytologist to the possibility of an invasive lobular carcinoma. It is not always possible to distinguish lobular carcinoma from the smaller celled varieties of ductal carcinoma but the following features may help.

### Cytological findings: invasive lobular carcinoma

- Scanty aspirates are common
- Tumour cells are well dispersed and mainly single or in small groups of two to five cells
- Cells are small, nuclei have an abnormal appearance with irregular outline
- Occasional single file 'chains', usually containing only three or four cells, may be seen
- Cytoplasm is scanty, with the nucleus eccentrically placed and some cells may contain an intracytoplasmic lumen with a signet-ring appearance
- Nuclei show slight but definite variation in size but tend to be round in shape. The chromatin is stippled but not coarse and the nucleolus inconspicuous in the classic type.

### Diagnostic pitfalls: invasive lobular carcinoma

- Lobular carcinomas account for many of the false negative cases in most series. There are also problems in categorising the tumour cytologically
- It is not always possible to distinguish lobular carcinomas from ductal carcinomas. Cases with prominent intracytoplasmic lumina may be mistaken for signet ring carcinoma
- High-grade or 'pleomorphic' lobular carcinoma resembles high-grade ductal carcinoma
- Because of the diffusely infiltrative nature of these tumours it is common for lobular carcinoma cells to be seen along with a variety of benign epithelial changes.

## Squamous carcinoma

Clinically, it appears to behave similarly to IDC. These lesions, in their pure form, are rare and tend to occur in elderly women. More commonly areas of squamous differentiation occur in otherwise unremarkable ductal carcinomas and metaplastic carcinomas (Fig. 4.96).

On clinical presentation, squamous carcinomas are similar to ductal carcinoma, although somewhat larger. An initial clue to the unusual nature of the lesion is obtained when the needle enters a central cystic cavity and thick yellow fluid is withdrawn. This phenomenon occurs most commonly in those tumours showing marked keratinisation and will be familiar to those used to taking aspirates from neck nodes involved by secondary squamous carcinoma.

When this type of sample is obtained from the breast, the possibility of fibrocystic change is quickly dispelled by the microscopic appearance of squamous cells of varying degrees of maturity. Advice that straw-coloured fluid from a breast cyst may safely be discarded should not lead to a missed diagnosis with this lesion as there is always likely to be a residual mass that will prompt immediate re-aspiration. A further possible

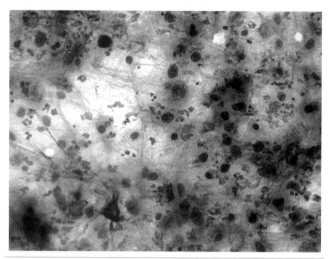

**Fig. 4.96** Squamous cell carcinoma. Debris with inflammatory cells and more or less degenerated squamous cells with the typical dense, non-transparent blue cytoplasm (MGG).

source of cytological confusion is with an epidermal cyst. Epidermal cysts are generally very superficial lesions and therefore clinically distinct; however, when an epidermal cyst occurs adjacent to the inframammary fold, its true depth may be difficult to assess. More importantly, the squamous cells in epidermal cysts do not display malignant features. Squamous cells may also be seen in aspirates from fibroadenomas and phyllodes tumours with squamous metaplasia.

Cytologically, the squamous nature of the less well-differentiated squamous carcinoma is more readily apparent in PAP-stained smears than in air-dried ones. Although mature and anucleate squames may be present, there are usually obviously malignant epithelial cells to be found. The cells tend to be single or in small groups, usually with fairly abundant cytoplasm that is keratinised. The intracytoplasmic keratin is well demonstrated as an orange, refractile hue on PAP-stained smears but stains a more subtle blue with the MGG-stain. There tends to be a dirty background because of necrotic cellular and keratinous debris. An additional feature is the presence of multinucleate giant cells as a reaction to tumour keratin.

### Cytological findings: squamous carcinoma

- No distinctive clinical features unless there has been central cystic degeneration
- The cells are usually poorly cohesive with dense angular nuclei. The squamous nature of the cells is more obvious in PAP-stained preparations but in MGG-stained smears the dense blue grey cytoplasm is quite distinctive
- Necrotic debris is common
- Anucleate cells may be present.

### Diagnostic pitfalls: squamous carcinoma

- A squamous carcinoma with a cystic centre may be mistaken clinically for fibrocystic change
- Squamous carcinoma cells may be dismissed as degenerate atypia in apocrine cells particularly if a well-differentiated area is sampled.

## Adenoid cystic carcinoma

This uncommon tumour has a very good prognosis but strict histological criteria need to be applied. It is classically an oestrogen receptor negative low-grade carcinoma with histology identical to salivary gland adenoid cystic carcinoma (Fig. 4.97). Ductal carcinoma without special features can have cribriform and papillary areas that may be misdiagnosed as adenoid cystic carcinoma. Adenoid cystic carcinoma of the breast tends to be small at presentation and is usually found in older women near the nipple.

The cytological features are distinctive and are similar to those seen in salivary gland tumours of this type. The cells do not always show obviously malignant features. The presence of globules that stain magenta with MGG was formerly said to be pathognomonic of this entity but collagenous spherulosis and adenomyoepithelioma of the breast can be identical in this respect. Diagnostic caution is therefore required.

### Cytological findings: adenoid cystic carcinoma

- The aspirate is likely to be moderately cellular with cohesive cell groups
- In MGG-stained preparations the cell groups contain very distinctive magenta/metachromatic coloured bodies which are round or cylindrical, measuring between 0.01 and 0.08 mm in diameter and up to 0.04 mm in length; they are less apparent in PAP-stained slides being pale blue
- Most cells are three-dimensional groups, many incorporating metachromatic basement membrane bodies. Smaller numbers of single cells and cells in small groups are present
- In the groups the nuclei are crowded and overlapping but where the details are more easily seen they are round or oval with slight but definite anisonucleosis and slight coarsening of the chromatin. Nucleoli are small and generally single
- No bipolar cells are present.

### Diagnostic pitfalls: adenoid cystic carcinoma

- The very distinctive basement membrane bodies are also seen in aspirates of benign breast disease with collagenous spherulosis and adenomyoepithelioma. Adenoid cystic carcinoma aspirates do not usually contain a benign component whereas the two others are likely to include abundant benign epithelial and myoepithelial cells.

## Mucoepidermoid carcinoma

Focal squamous and mucinous differentiation may be found independently in ductal carcinomas of breast. When they occur together in a moderate- or high-grade lesion there seems little merit in including such a tumour in a special category. When present in a low-grade lesion the term mucoepidermoid tumour may be invoked implying a better than average outcome. The cytological features are similar to those described in the salivary gland.

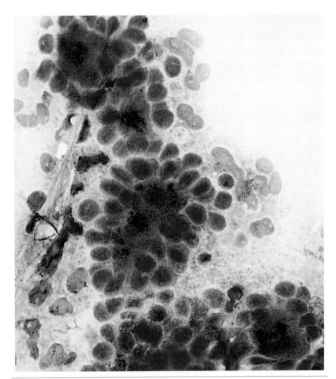

**Fig. 4.97** Adenoid cystic carcinoma. The combination of fairly bland but nonetheless malignant epithelial cells and the bright violet globules can be confused with collagenous spherulosis (MGG).

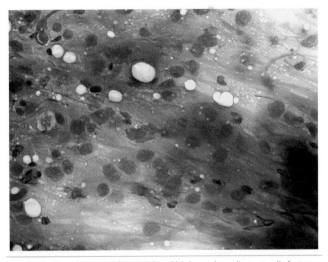

**Fig. 4.98** Chondro-myxoid material and high-grade malignant cells from a metaplastic carcinoma (MGG).

## Other malignant tumours

### Metaplastic carcinoma/carcinosarcoma

Metaplastic carcinomas[81] (Fig. 4.98) are high-grade carcinomas in which much of the tumour undergoes metaplastic change producing a sarcomatous pattern. The sarcomatous element can resemble fibrosarcoma, chondrosarcoma, osteosarcoma, rhabdomyosarcoma or anaplastic sarcoma with giant cells. These rare tumours represent around 0.2% of breast cancers. Even more rarely, a pure spindle cell variant is encountered.

The diagnosis suggests a worse prognosis than that for IDC. The greater the sarcomatous component, the worse the prognosis. Clinically, these appear as rapidly growing lesions.

The clinical presentation is not significantly different from that of ductal carcinoma and the average age is the same. Cytologically, there is seldom any difficulty in recognising the presence of malignancy and occasionally both the epithelial and heterologous elements are recognised in aspirates. If however, as often happens, either the carcinomatous or sarcomatous element predominates there is a possibility that the lesser component will not be apparent or will be overlooked.

The epithelial cell component is indistinguishable from a high-grade ductal carcinoma but there may be transitional forms providing a spectrum through to obviously spindle-shaped cells. When cartilaginous differentiation is present, magenta-coloured ground substance may be noted. Osteosarcomatous metaplasia does occur. The presence of well-mineralised malignant osteoid can provide a definite clue that a clinically obvious carcinoma has unusual features and the aspirator's needle encounters areas that are very gritty and virtually impenetrable. If osteoclast-like giant cells and malignant spindle cells are present in the aspirate the picture is complete.

### Cytological findings: metaplastic carcinoma/carcinosarcoma

- The aspirates are usually cellular
- The cells may be indistinguishable from those of a high-grade ductal carcinoma of breast depending on the area aspirated
- Additional features depending on the extent and type of the metaplastic malignancy may include:
  - Large, malignant multinucleated giant cells
  - Malignant cells associated with fragments of amorphous metachromatic material
  - Large malignant spindle cells singly or in syncytial clusters
  - Squamous cell differentiation.

### Diagnostic pitfalls: metaplastic carcinoma/carcinosarcoma

- The extent and degree of metaplasia are variable and so some cases may be diagnosed as ductal carcinoma without special features on cytological assessment
- The aspirate may contain only spindle cells and may be diagnosed as a sarcoma
- High-grade malignant phyllodes tumour has similar sarcomatous elements.

## Malignant myoepithelioma

Malignant myoepithelioma[81] (Fig. 4.99) is an infiltrating tumour composed purely of myoepithelial, predominantly spindled cells. The tumour size may range from 1 cm to over 10 cm. It usually presents as a palpable nodule, and a mammographic density without distinctive features. Histologically the tumour is clearly invasive, with spindle cells with or without atypia.

Cytologically one may find[131] cellular smears consisting mainly of single spindle or polymorphic, polygonal cells with a few admixed groups of benign ductal epithelial cells and

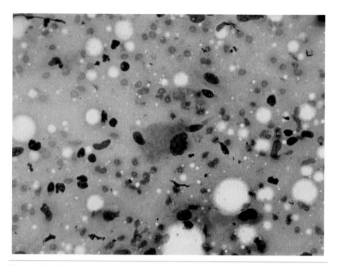

**Fig. 4.99** Pleomorphic spindle and polygonal cells from a malignant myoepithelioma (MGG).

lymphocytes. The nuclei may range in size from two to five times that of an RBC. A distinct medium-sized nucleolus may be found as well as irregular nuclear outlines with buds and folds and granular chromatin. A few cells may show intranuclear cytoplasmic vacuoles. The cytoplasm may be bluish, variable in amount and often dense. In the background abundant granular metachromatic ground substance and some metachromatic stromal fragments could be found. A few mitotic figures have been described. Necrotic debris has not been found.

### Cytological findings: malignant myoepithelioma

- Single and small groups of spindled cells which may reveal a distinct pleomorphism
- Metachromatic ground substance as well as metachromatic stromal fragments
- Admixed benign ductal epithelial cells and lymphocytes.

### Diagnostic pitfalls: malignant myoepithelioma

- May resemble metaplastic carcinoma where only the non-epithelial component has been aspirated or another non-epithelial lesion.

## Malignant phyllodes tumour

See p.204 and Fig. 4.100.[81]

## Sarcomas

Non-epithelial malignancies, other than malignant phyllodes tumours, occurring as primary lesions in the breast include the full spectrum of sarcoma types.[81] The cytological features are identical to those of such lesions presenting at their more usual sites. Angiosarcoma (Fig. 4.101) following radiation therapy is probably the most frequently encountered sarcoma seen in breast FNA.

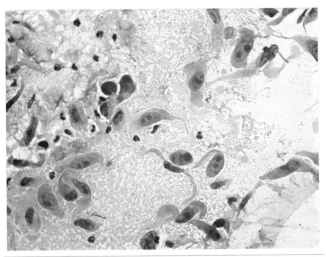

**Fig. 4.100** High-grade malignant spindle cells from a malignant phyllodes tumour. Pleomorphic nuclei with large nucleoli (MGG).

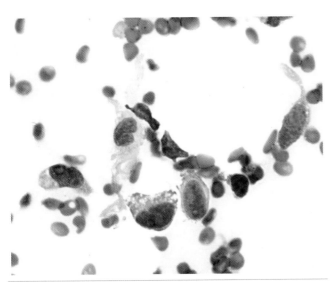

**Fig. 4.101** Postirradiation angiosarcoma. Spindle and polygonal cells with high-grade atypia and large, abnormal nucleoli (MGG).

## Metastatic malignancy

Metastatic lesions[81] in the breast are uncommon and make up about 3% of all malignant tumours in the breast. Most of them are metastases from the contralateral breast and less than 0.5% will represent metastases from a primary tumour outside the breast.[132] Malignant lymphoma/leukaemia and malignant melanomas are the most common non-epithelial metastases, whereas lung, ovaries, kidney, thyroid, cervix, stomach and prostate are the most common origins of epithelial malignancies.

They are often located superficially, but cannot be differentiated from a primary breast tumour on clinical appearance. They often occur as palpable round tumours, firm and freely movable with no fixation of the overlying skin or the underlying pectoral muscle. There is no nipple discharge. Radiologically, there may be a single or multiple nodules that tend to have the same size on palpation and mammography. Mammographically there is typically a circumscribed, round nodule with slightly irregular margins. There is usually no microcalcification or spiculation. Microcalcification may occur, but usually as psammoma bodies in metastatic ovarian carcinomas.

Bronchogenic carcinomas and lymphomas are most likely to create a mass in the breast. Both may present initially in the breast and the former may be confused with a high-grade ductal carcinoma cytologically and the latter with a low-grade ductal carcinoma or lobular carcinoma. Secondary lymphomas usually involve the breast as a late event. The aspirates are very cellular and the cells poorly cohesive, and so diagnostic difficulties should be avoidable. Amelanotic melanomas with no known primary create a risk of wrong diagnosis.

It is most important that metastatic malignancy is at least considered in all cases that are not completely typical of any of the recognised varieties of breast carcinoma so as to prevent an unnecessary mastectomy.

### Cytological findings: metastatic malignancy

- Often there will be a history of a recognised extramammary primary tumour
- Helpful features are those that are not typical of a primary breast carcinoma such as oat cell appearance, melanin pigment, clear cell differentiation.[81,132–134]

### Diagnostic pitfalls: metastatic malignancy

- Metastatic small cell carcinoma and lymphoma can imitate small celled ductal and lobular carcinoma, and amelanotic melanoma may mimic high-grade ductal carcinoma
- Renal clear cell carcinoma can imitate clear cell carcinoma of the breast, as can signet ring carcinomas of the gastrointestinal tract.

## Malignant lymphomas

Malignant lymphomas[81] (ML) may on rare occasions be primary in the breast. They will show the same morphological spectrum as ML in lymph nodes (see Ch. 13).

## Recurrent and metastatic breast lesions

The major role of aspiration cytology is in the primary diagnosis of malignancy. There is, however, an important subsidiary role in the follow-up assessment of patients after treatment is complete. Here too, there is considerable scope for reducing the need for surgery and speeding therapeutic and prognostic evaluation.

The problem of inexperienced aspirators obtaining non-representative aspirates may be increased here, possibly reflecting the smaller size of the lesions, the difficulty aspirating cutaneous rather than deep lesions, or the effect of local scar tissue.

Metastasis of breast malignancy to remote sites is commonly detected by cytology. It is usually possible to indicate that the breast is the likely source of the metastatic cells. If the previous history is available, there is seldom much doubt but occasional cases present with distant metastasis before the breast primary is clinically apparent, or if there is a history of primary carcinoma at more than one site.

Lobular carcinoma exhibits a different pattern of metastatic spread from that of ductal carcinoma and may spread widely before becoming clinically apparent. It may therefore present in specimens from unusual sites in cases where the primary tumour has not been detected or in which it has not been mentioned by the referring clinician.

Diagnostic pitfalls that a cytologist needs to consider when aspirating a possible recurrent breast carcinoma near a site of previous excision include irradiation atypia in residual breast tissue, unexpected residual normal or hyperplastic breast tissue following mastectomy, epithelioid cells in fat necrosis or silicone granuloma, and lymph nodes showing a variety of reactive patterns. Aspirates from benign tumours of the skin and subcutis, such as appendage tumours and granular cell tumour, may also risk misinterpretation as recurrent carcinoma. Post-irradiation angiosarcoma can be confused with carcinoma.

## Radiation-induced changes in the breast

In common with other tissue, breast shows characteristic histological changes following therapeutic irradiation (Fig. 4.102). These changes vary in extent and severity among patients and within individual patients. This variation is not related to the presence of residual carcinoma, radiation dose, patient age, adjuvant chemotherapy or time to post-irradiation sampling.

The most characteristic effect is the presence of atypical epithelial cells in the terminal duct lobular unit, with associated lobular sclerosis and atrophy. This atypia of the epithelium is accompanied by vascular changes and abnormal fibroblasts.

The epithelial atypia can be reflected in the aspiration cytology of lesions in patients where the index of suspicion is already very high.

### Cytological findings: radiation-induced changes in the breast

- The aspirates are usually scanty unless there is a recurrence of the neoplasm
- The cells are in small groups and do not exhibit the loss of cohesion seen in carcinoma
- Some nuclei may be very large and there is characteristically quite marked anisonucleosis

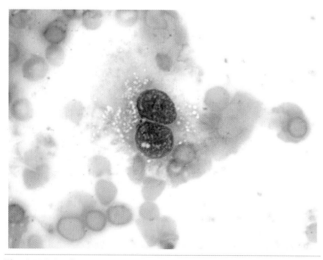

**Fig. 4.102** Irradiation atypia. Enlarged (benign) nuclei with smudged, degenerative chromatin pattern and vacuolised, fuzzy cytoplasm (MGG).

- The nuclear/cytoplasmic ratio is normal, however, and there is usually a scattering of bipolar cells
- The appearances of fat necrosis may also be present.

### Diagnostic pitfalls: radiation-induced changes in the breast

- Differentiation from recurrent carcinoma can be difficult but attention to the above usually leads to a correct assessment. The main danger is overdiagnosis due to lack of information that the patient has had radiotherapy.

## FNA in the management strategies of symptomatic and screening detected abnormalities

FNA has been extensively used for many years in the diagnosis of breast lesions, but its use has gradually been reduced in many screening programmes because of its controversial inadequacy rates and suboptimal accuracy in inexperienced hands.[135,136] In specialised centres, both sensitivity and specificity of breast FNA is ≥90%.[10,11,137] A survey of current practice in Europe[138] revealed that the use of breast FNA cytology differs. When used, cytology forms part of the triple assessment approach (clinical, imaging and pathology) to breast diagnosis and it is the first-line pathological investigation in symptomatic and some screening populations (with the exception of cases with microcalcifications). The majority of centres practice a degree of one-stop diagnosis with a cytopathologist present in the out-patient clinic. Image guidance (ultrasonography and stereotactic device) is used in most centres and is an important part of the modern approach to FNA in non-palpable lesions. Stereotactic CB is performed for microcalcifications. Centres vary as to who performs FNA – radiologists or cytopathologists. Pathologists specialised in cytopathology are best qualified to collect and interpret FNA samples, but this is not always possible or practical. When triple assessment is concordant, final treatment may proceed on the basis of FNA, without a tissue biopsy. ER and PR assessment can be done safely on FNA material, provided there is local expertise. The same applies to investigation of HER-2 status by *in situ* hybridisation.

Local (cytopathological and radiological) expertise is one of the major factors influencing the extent of FNA use. In well-trained hands, FNA is cheap, reliable and the least invasive method for obtaining a preoperative diagnosis. Whenever possible, the cytopathologists should be active participants wherever samples are taken, both in the aspiration process and in the preparation of the aspirated material. Rapid assessment of smear quality and a preliminary diagnosis should be routine practice. Cytopathologists must receive appropriate training in both sampling and interpretation. Likewise, radiologists must be fully trained in all aspects of image-guided sampling. Poor FNA practice is worse than none.

## Reporting breast FNAs

A crucial factor in the practice of breast FNA, as with all diagnostic cytology, is that there is good communication between the cytologist and the clinical teams involved in managing the patient. Written communication can be helped by the use of standardised reporting systems.[139] In Europe, the majority of centres use a C1–C5 reporting system, as recommended

**Table 4.5** Modified reporting categories in breast FNA according to NHSBSP guidelines[9]

| Reporting category | Description |
|---|---|
| C1 | *Inadequate.* Assessment is subjective and based on the presence of a sufficient number of epithelial cells to provide sample adequate for confident assessment. Aspirates from cysts, abscesses, fat necrosis and nipple discharge should not be classified as inadequate. Apart from hypocellularity, crush, air-drying, blood and thickness of smear could cause inadequate sample. It is helpful to comment on the cause of inadequate specimens. |
| C2 | *Benign.* Adequate sample without evidence of atypia, composed of regular epithelial cells, usually in monolayers; background composed of dispersed individual or paired nuclei. A specific diagnosis, such as fibroadenoma, fat necrosis, granulomatous mastitis, breast abscess or lymph node, can be given if sufficient features are present. |
| C3 | *Atypia, probably benign.* In addition to benign features, certain features not commonly seen in benign aspirates may be present: nuclear pleomorphism, loss of cell cohesion, nuclear or cytoplasmic changes (pregnancy, pill, hormone replacement therapy) and increased cellularity. |
| C4 | *Suspicious of malignancy.* This category should be used for aspirates with highly atypical features, such that the pathologist is almost certain that they come from a malignant lesion, although a confident diagnosis cannot be made due to the following: (a) specimen is scanty, (b) the sample shows some malignant features in the absence of overt malignant features, (c) the sample has an overall benign pattern with large numbers of naked nuclei and/or cohesive sheets of cells but with occasional cells showing distinct malignant features. <br><br> Definitive therapeutic surgery SHOULD NOT be undertaken on the basis of C3 or C4 report. |
| C5 | *Malignant.* Adequate sample containing cells characteristic of carcinoma. Malignancy should not be diagnosed on the basis of a single criterion. |

by the UK NHSBSP and European Guidelines for Quality Assurance.[140] In the USA, the majority of breast FNA reporting is done according to the recommendations of the NIH Consensus Development Conference,[141,142] but descriptive diagnoses are also used.[9] Specific diagnoses are made following the WHO histological classification of tumours of the breast.[143]

In the five-tier system used both in Europe and in the USA, C5 (malignant) describes a definite malignancy; C4 (suspicious/probably malignant) describes a probable (perhaps 95%) malignancy; C3 (atypical/indeterminate) a probably benign lesion with atypia implying a risk of malignancy of perhaps 20%; C2 (benign) an aspirate with clear benign features, and C1 (unsatisfactory) a non-diagnostic aspirate (Table 4.5).[9,141,142] Diagnostic codes are useful because they offer a clear indication of the degree of certainty of a cytological diagnosis, avoiding the ambiguity that can be read into phrases such as 'strongly suggestive of' or 'suspicious of'. However, the strict criteria often applied to these systems can lead to difficulty if, for example, an aspirate of an area of fibrous scar tissue is reported as C1, non-diagnostic or 'inadequate', and the patient is subjected to repeated further biopsies because the clinician is given the impression that something has gone wrong with the test, rather than that the aspirate contains exactly what would be expected from such a lesion. A written diagnosis with some explanation of whether this is likely to fit the clinical and radiological features is clearly useful, and can be given alongside a coded diagnosis.

Outside of screening programmes, there is variation between centres in how strictly diagnostic coding is applied. This need not be a problem provided the diagnosis, degree of certainty, and any implications for repeat testing or core biopsy are clearly communicated to and understood by the clinical team. Although the report should be provided in writing even

in a one-stop setting so that there is a clear contemporaneous record of the diagnosis at the time that management decisions are made, there is no substitute for talking through complicated or unusual diagnoses with the surgeons and radiologists to make sure both that the cytological diagnosis is understood and that the cytologist has a clear idea of the clinical and radiological concerns

## The role of the multidisciplinary team

In most centres the management of patients with cancer or suspected cancer is coordinated through a multidisciplinary team (MDT) of surgeons, oncologists, radiologists, pathologists, specialist nurses and other staff. In breast disease, the MDT has two key roles. The first is to provide a forum for the discussion of individual patients and deciding which options of treatment should be recommended. The second role of the MDT that particularly applies in centres offering a one-stop FNA clinic is to agree protocols for the initial management of patients diagnosed with malignancy in those clinics. The one-stop setting has the advantage for the patient that initial treatment can be discussed straight away, but the MDT will not discuss the individual patient until later when the stage, grade, receptor and margin status of the tumour have been established. The MDT therefore agrees protocols for initial surgical treatment following FNA and radiological diagnosis. For patients whose situation at diagnosis fits the protocol, there is no need for an MDT discussion at that point. For patients whose situation does not fit the protocol or who has complicating factors such as significant coexistent disease, recommendation of a treatment pathway normally requires MDT discussion before initial surgical treatment.

# REFERENCES

1. Boerner S, Fornage BD, Singletary E, et al. Ultrasound-guided fine-needle aspiration (FNA) of non-palpable breast lesions: a review of 1885 FNA cases using the National Cancer Institute-supported recommendations on the uniform approach to breast FNA. Cancer 1999;87:19–24.

2. Bofin AM, Lydersen S, Isaksen C, et al. Interpretation of fine needle aspiration cytology of the breast: a comparison of cytological, frozen section, and final histological diagnoses. Cytopathology 2004;15:297–304.

3. Leifland K, Lagerstedt U, Svane G. Comparison of stereotactic fine needle aspiration cytology and core needle biopsy in 522 non-palpable breast lesions. Acta Radiologica 2003;44:387–91.

4. Ljung BM, Drejet A, Chiampi N, et al. Diagnostic accuracy of fine-needle aspiration biopsy is determined by physician training in sampling technique. Cancer 2001;22:126–30.

5. Okamoto H, Ogawara T, Inoue S, et al. Clinical management of nonpalpable or small breast masses by fine-needle aspiration biopsy (FNAB) under ultrasound guidance. J Surg Oncol 1998;67:246–50.

6. Pisano ED, Fajardo LL, Caudry DJ, et al. Fine-needle aspiration biopsy of nonpalpable breast lesions in a multicenter clinical trial: results from the Radiologic Diagnostic Oncology Group V. Radiology 2001;219:785–92.

7. Sauer T, Lømo J, Garred Ø, et al. Cytologic features of ductal carcinoma in situ in fine-needle aspiration of the breast mirror the histopathologic growth pattern heterogeneity and grading. Cancer Cytopathol 2005;105:21–27.

8. Zanconati F, Bonifacio D, Falcioneri G, et al. Role of fine-needle aspiration cytology in nonpalpable mammary lesions: A comparative study based on 308 cases. Diagnostic Cytopathology 2000:87–91.

9. Guidelines for non-operative diagnostic procedures and reporting in breast cancer screening. Non-operative Diagnosis Subgroup of the National Coordinating Group for Breast Screening Pathology. NHSBSP Publication 2001; 50:15.

10. Arisio R, Cuccorese C, Acinelli G. Role of fine-needle aspiration biopsy in breast lesions: analysis of a series of 4,110 cases. Diagn Cytopathol 1998;18:462–67.

11. Feichter GE, Habertur F, Gobat S, et al. Breast cytology. Statistical analysis and cytohistologic correlations. Acta Cytologica 1997;41:327–32.

12. Mitnick JS, Vazquez MF, Pressman PI, et al. Stereotactic fine-needle aspiration biopsy for the evaluation of nonpalpable lesions: report of an experience based on 2988 cases. Annals of Surgical Oncology 1996;3:185–91.

13. Rubin M, Horiuchi K, Joy N, et al. Use of fine needle aspiration for solid breast lesions is accurate and cost-effective. Am J Surg 1997;174:694–96.

14. Saarela AO, Kiviniemi HO, Rissanen TJ, et al. Nonpalpable breast lesions: pathologic correlation of ultrasonographical needle aspiration biopsy. J Ultrasound Med 1996;15:549–53.

15. Saravanja S. Ultrasound-guided fine-needle aspiration of the breast. Schweiz Rundsch Med Prax 2005;94:673–79.

16. Sarfati MR, Fox KA, Warneke JA, et al. Stereotactic fine-needle aspiration cytology of nonpalpable breast lesions of 258 consecutive cases. Am J Surg 1994;168:529–31.

17. Sauer T, Young K, Thoresen S. Fine needle aspiration cytology in the work-up of mammographic and ultrasonographic findings in breast cancer screening: an attempt at differentiating in situ and invasive carcinoma. Cytopathology 2002;13:101–10.

18. Sauer T, Myrvold K, Lømo J, et al. Fine-needle aspiration cytology in nonpalpable mammographic abnormalities in breast cancer screening: results from the breast cancer screening programme in Oslo 1996–2001. The Breast 2003;12:314–19.

19. Snead DRJ, Vryenhoef P, Pinder SE, et al. Routine audit of fine needle aspiration (FNA) cytology specimens and aspirator inadequate rates. Cytopathology 1997;8:236–47.

20. Wells CA, Perera R, White FE, et al. Fine needle aspiration cytology in the UK breast screening programme: a national audit of results. The Breast 1999;8:261–66.

21. Singh N, Ryan D, Berney D. Inadequacy rates are lower when FNAC samples are taken by cytopathologists. Cytopathology 2003;14:327–31.

22. Haddadi-Nezhad S, Larijani B, Tavangar SM, et al. Comparison of fine-needle-nonaspiration with fine-needle-aspiration technique in the cytologic studies of thyroid nodules. Endocr Pathol 2003;14:369–73.

23. Kamal MM, Arjune DG, Kulkarni HR. Comparative study of fine needle aspiration and fine needle capillary sampling of thyroid lesions. Acta Cytol 2002;46:30–34.

24. Tublin ME, Martin JA, Rollin LJ, et al. Ultrasound-guided fine-needle aspiration versus fine-needle capillary sampling biopsy of thyroid nodules: does technique matter? J Ultrasound Med 2007;26:1697–701.

25. Bedard YC, Polett AF, Leung SW, et al. Assessment of thin-layer breast aspirates for immunocytochemical evaluation of HER2 status. Acta Cytol 2003;47:979–84.

26. Konofaos P, Kontzoglu K, Georgoulakis J, et al. The role of ThinPrep cytology in the evaluation of estrogen and progesterone receptor content of breast tumors. Surg Oncol 2006;15:257–66.

27. Nasuti JF, Tam D, Gupta PK. Diagnostic value of liquid-based (ThinPrep) preparations in nongynecologic cases. Diagn Cytopathol 2001;2:137–41.

28. Tabbara SO, Sidawy MK, Frost AR, et al. The stability of estrogen and progesterone receptor expression on breast carcinoma cells stored as preservCyt suspensions and as ThinPrep slides. Cancer 1998;84:355–60.

29. Veneti S, Daskalopoulou D, Zervoudis S, et al. Liquid-based cytology in breast fine needle aspiration: Comparison with the conventional smear. Acta Cytol 2003;47:188–92.

30. Vocaturo A, Novelli F, Benevolu M, et al. Chromogenic in situ hybridisation to detect HER-2/neu gene amplification in histological and ThinPrep-processed breast cancer fine-needle aspirates: A sensitive and practical method in the trastuzumab era. Oncologist 2006;11:878–86.

31. Molyneux AM, Coghill SB. Ultrasound contact jelly causes an artefact in breast aspirates. Cytopathol 1993;5:41–45.

32. Dowsett M. Estrogen receptor: methodology matters. J Clin Oncol 2006;24:5626–28.

33. Konofaos P, Kontzoglou K, Georgoulakis J, et al. The role of ThinPrep cytology in the evaluation of estrogen and progesterone receptor content of breast tumors. Surg Oncol 2006;15:257–66.

34. Leung SW, Bedard YC. Estrogen and progesterone receptor contents in ThinPrep-processed fine needle aspirates of breast. Am J Clin Pathol 1999;112:50–56.

35. Nadiji M, Gomez-fernandez C, Ganjei-Azar P, et al. Immunohistochemistry of estrogen and progesterone receptors reconsidered. Am J Clin Pathol 2005;123:21–27.

36. Petroff BK, Clark JL, Metheny T, et al. Optimisation of estrogen receptor analysis by immunocytochemistry in random periareolar fine-needle aspiration samples of breast tissue processed as thin-layer preparations. Appl Immunohistochem Mol Morphol 2006;14:360–64.

37. Sauer T, Beraki E, Jebsen PW, et al. Assessing estrogen and progesterone receptor status in fine needle aspirates from breast carcinomas. Analyt Quant Cytol Histol 1998;20:122–26.

38. Gong Y, Fraser Symmans W, Krishnamurthy S, et al. Optimal fixation conditions for immunocytochemical analysis of estrogen receptor in cytologic specimens of breast carcinoma. Cancer Cytopathol 2004;102:34–40.

39. Konofaos P, Kontzoglou K, Georgoulakis J, et al. The role of ThinPrep cytology in the evaluation of estrogen and progesterone receptor content of breast tumors. Surg Oncol 2006;15:257–66.

40. Krishnamurthy S, Dimashkieh H, Patel S. Immunocytochemical evaluation of estrogen receptor on archival Papanicolaou-stained fine-needle aspirate smears. Diagn Cytopathol 2003;29:309–14.

41. Leung SW, Bedard YC. Estrogen and progesterone receptor contents in ThinPrep-processed fine-needle aspirates of the breast. Am J Clin Pathol 1999;112:50–56.

42. Petroff BK, Clark JL, Metheny T, et al. Optimisation of estrogen receptor by analysis by immunocytochemistry in random periareolar fine-needle aspiration samples of breast tissue processed as thin-layer preparations. Appl Immunohistochem Mol Morphol 2006;14:360–64.

43. Shidham VB, Chang CC, Rao RN. Immunostaining of cytology smears: a comparative study to identify the most suitable method of smear preparation and fixation with reference to commonly used immunomarkers. Diagn Cytopathol 2003;29:217–21.

44. Tafjord S, Bøhler PJ, Risberg B. Estrogen and progesterone hormone receptor status in breast carcinoma: comparison of immunocytochemistry and immunohistochemistry. Diagn Cytopathol 2002;26:137–41.

45. Kocjan G, Bourgain C, Fassina A, et al. The role of breast FNAC in diagnosis and clinical management: a survey of current practice. Cytopathology 2008.

46. Bofin A, Ytterhus B, Hagmar BM. TOP2A and HER-2 gene amplification in fine needle aspirates from breast carcinomas. Cytopathology 2003;14:314–19.

47. Bozzetti C, Personeni N, Nizzoli R, et al. HER-2/neu amplification by fluorescence in situ hybridisation in cytologic samples from distant

metastatic sites of breast carcinoma. Cancer Cytopathol 2003;99:310–515.

48. Nizzoli R, Guazzi A, Naldi N, et al. HER-2/neu evaluation by fluorescence in situ hybridisation on destained cytologic smears from primary and metastatic breast cancer. Acta Cytol 2005;49:27–30.

49. Vocatura A, Novelli F, Benevolo M, et al. Chromogenic in situ hybridisation to detect HER-2/neu gene amplification in histological and ThinPrep-processed breast cancer fine-needle aspirates: a sensitive and practical method in the trastuzumab era. Oncologist 2006;11:878–86.

50. Bhargava R, Lal P, Chen B. Chromogenic in situ hybridisation for the detection of HER-2/neu gene amplification in breast cancer with an emphasis on tumors with borderline and low-level amplification: does it measure up to fluorescence in situ hybridisation? Am J Clin Pathol 2005;123:237–43.

51. Lin F, Shen T, Prichard JW. Detection of Her-2/neu oncogene in breast carcinoma by chromogenic in situ hybridisation in cytologic specimens. Diagn Cytopathol 2005;33:376–80.

52. Beatty BG, Bryant R, Wang W. HER-2/neu detection in fine-needle aspirates of breast cancer: fluorescent in situ hybridisation and immunocytochemical analysis. Am J Clin Pathol 2004;122:246–55.

53. Gu M, Ghafari S, Zhao M. Fluorescence in situ hybridisation for HER-2/neu amplification of breast carcinoma in archival fine needle aspiration biopsy specimens. Acta Cytol 2005;49:471–76.

54. Tomas AR, Praca MJ, Fonseca R, et al. Assessing HER-2 status in fresh frozen and archival cytological samples obtained by fine needle aspiration cytology. Cytopathology 2004;15:311–14.

55. Itoh H, Miyajima Y, Umemura S, et al. Lower HER-2/chromosome enumeration probe 17 ratio in cytologic HER-2 fluorescence in situ hybridisation for breast cancers: three-dimensional analysis of intranuclear localisation of centromere 17 and HER-2 signals. Cancer Cytopathol 2008;114:134–40.

56. Sauer T, Beraki K, Jebsen PW, et al. Ploidy analysis by in situ hybridisation of interphase cell nuclei in fine-needle aspirates from breast carcinomas: Correlation with cytologic grading. Diagn Cytopathol 1997;17:267–71.

57. Sauer T, Beraki K, Furu I, et al. Estimating loss of the wild-type p53 gene by in situ hybridisation of fine-needle aspirates from breast carcinomas. Diagn Cytopathol 1999;20:266–70.

58. Sauer T, Beraki K, Garred Ø, et al. EGFR gene copy number heterogeneity in FNAC from breast carcinomas determined by chromogenic in situ hybridisation. Diagn Cytopathol 2005;33:228–32.

59. Catania S, Boccato P, Bono A. Pneumothorax: a rare complication of the needle aspiration of the breast. Acta Cytol 1989;33:140.

60. Joshi A. FNA cytology in the management of male breast masses: nineteen years of experience. Acta Cytol 1999;43:334–38.

61. Bott S, Mohsen V, Wells C, et al. Needle tract metastases in breast cancer. Eur J Surg Oncol 1999;25:553.

62. Rytina ERC, Coady AT, Millis RR. Milk granuloma: an unusual appearance in lactational breast tissue. Histopathology 1991:466–67.

63. Khamapirad T, Hennan K, Leonard M, et al. Granulomatous lobular mastitis: two case reports with focus on radiologic and histopathologic features. Ann Diagn Pathol 2007;11:109–12.

64. Gupta D, Rajawanshi A, Gupta SK, et al. Fine needle aspiration cytology in the diagnosis of tuberculous mastitis. Acta Cytol 1999;43:191–94.

65. Veerysami M, Freeth M, Carmichael AR, et al. Wegener's granulomatosis of the breast. Breast J 2006;12:268–70.

66. Al-Khaffaf B, Knox F, Bundred NJ. Idiopathic granulomatous mastitis: a 25-year experience. J Am Coll Surg 2008;206:269–73.

67. Kaur AC, Dal H, Müezzinoglu B, et al. Idiopathic granulomatous mastitis. Report of a case diagnosed with fine needle aspiration cytology. Acta Cytol 1999;43:481–84.

68. Kobayashi TK, Sugihara H, Kato M, et al. Cytologic features of granulomatous mastitis. Report of a case with fine needle aspiration cytology and immunocytochemical findings. Acta Cytol 1998;42:716–20.

69. Kumarasinghe MP. Cytology of granulomatous mastitis. Acta Cytol 1997;41:727–30.

70. Martínez-Parra D, Nevado-Santos M, Meléndez-Guerrer B, et al. Utility of fine-needle aspiration in the diagnosis of granulomatous lesions of the breast. Diagn Cytopathol 1997;17:108–14.

71. Tse GM, Poon CS, Law BK, et al. Fine needle aspiration cytology of granulomatous mastitis. J Clin Pathol 2003;56:519–21.

72. Tse GM, Poon CS, Ramachandram K, et al. Granulomatous mastitis: a clinicopathological review of 26 cases. Pathology 2004;36:254–57.

73. Cakir B, Tuncbilek N, Karaka HM, et al. Granulomatous mastitis mimicking breast carcinoma. Breast J 2002;8:251–52.

74. Heer R, Shrimakar J, Griffith CD. Granulomatous mastitis can mimic breast cancer on clinical, radiological or cytological examination: a cautionary tale. Breast 2003;12:283–86.

75. Miralles TG, Gosalbez F, Menendez P. FNA of sclerosing lymphocytic lobulitis. Acta Cytol 1998;42:1447–50.

76. Sahoo S, Reeves W, DeMay RM. Amyloid tumor: a clinical and cytomorphologic study. Diagn Cytopathol 2003;28:325–28.

77. Dodd LG, Sneige N, Reece GP, et al. Fine-needle aspiration cytology of silicone granulomas in the augmented breast. Diagn Cytopathol 1993;9:498–502.

78. Vuong P. Fine needle aspiration cytology of subcutaneous cysticercosis of the breast. Acta Cytol 1989;33:659–62.

79. Kollur SM, El Hag IA. FNA of breast fibroadenoma: observer variability and review of cytomorphology with cytohistological correlation. Cytopathology 2006;17:239–44.

80. Shet TM, Reg JD. Aspiration cytology of tubular adenomas of the breast. An analysis of eight cases. Acta Cytol 1998;42:657–62.

81. Tavassoli FA, Soares J. Tumours of the breast. In: Tavassoli FA, Devilee P, editors Tumours of the breast and female genital organs. Lyon: IARC Press; 2003.

82. Doyle EM, Banville N, Quinn CM, et al. Radial scars/complex sclerosing lesions and malignancy in a screening programme: incidence and histological features revisited. Histopathology 2007;50:614.

83. Orell SR. Radial scar/complex sclerosing lesion – a problem in the diagnostic work-up of screen-detected breast lesions. Cytopathology 1999;10:250–58.

84. Chang A, Bassett L, Bose S. Adenomyoepithelioma of the breast: a cytologic dilemma. report of a case and review of the literature. Diagn Cytopathol 2002;26:196.

85. Iyengar P, Ali SZ, Brogi E. Fine-needle aspiration cytology of mammary adenomyoepithelioma: a study of 12 patients. Cancer Cytopathol 2006;108:250–56.

86. Kurashina M. Fine-needle aspiration cytology of benign and malignant adenomyoepithelioma: report of two cases. Diagn Cytopathol 2002;26:29–34.

87. Ng WK. Adenomyoepithelioma of the breast. A review of three cases with reappraisal of the fine needle aspiration biopsy findings. Acta Cytol 2002;46:324.

88. Gibbons D, Leitch M, Coscia J. FNA cytology and histologic findings of granular cell tumor of the breast: review of 19 cases with clinical/radiologic correlation. Breast J 2000;6:27–30.

89. Bunker JP, Houghton J, Baum M. Putting the risk of breast cancer in perspective. BMJ 1999;317:1307–9.

90. Dixon JM, Page DL. Ductal carcinoma in-situ of the breast. Breast 199; 7:242.

91. Jensen R, Page DL. Epithelial hyperplasia. In: Elston CW, Ellis IO, editors The Breast. 3rd edn Edinburgh: Churchill Livingstone; 1998. p. 65–90.

92. Feeley L, Quinn CM. Columnar cell lesions of the breast. Histopathology 2008;5:11–19.

93. Turasvili G, Hayes M, Gilks B, et al. Are columnar cell lesions the earliest histologically detectable non-obligate precursor of the breast?. Virchows Archiv 2008;452:589–98.

94. Cheng L, Lee WY, Chang TW. Benign mucocele-like lesion of the breast: how to differentiate from mucinous carcinoma before surgery. Cytopathology 2004;15:104–8.

95. Tan PH, Tse GM, Bay BH. Mucinous breast lesions: diagnostic challenges. J Clin Pathol 2008;61:11–19.

96. Wong NL, Wan SK. Comparative cytology of mucocele-like lesion and mucinous carcinoma of the breast in fine needle aspiration. Acta Cytol 2000;44:765–70.

97. Yeoh GP, Cheung PS, Chan KW. Fine-needle aspiration cytology of mucocele-like tumors of the breast. Am J Surg Pathol 1999;23:552–59.

98. Ustun M, Berner A, Davidson B, et al. Fine-needle aspiration cytology of lobular carcinoma in situ. Diagn Cytopathol 2002;27:22–26.

99. Karimzadeh M, Sauer T. Diagnostic accuracy of fine-needle aspiration cytology in histological grade 1 carcinomas: are we good enough? Cytopathology 2008;19:279–86.

100. Sauer T, Karimzadeh M. Characteristic cytological features of histological grade one (G1) breast carcinomas in fine needle aspirates. Cytopathology 2008;19:287–93.

101. Elston CW, Ellis IO, editors. Assessment of histological grade. In The Breast. 3rd edn Edinburgh: Churchill-Livingstone; 1998. p. 365–84.

102. Dey P, Luthra UK, Prasad A, et al. Cytologic grading and DNA image cytometry of breast carcinoma on fine needle aspiration cytology smears. Analyt Quant Cytol Histol 1999;21:17–20.

103. Dey P, Ghoshal S, Pattarai SK. Nuclear image morphometry and cytologic grade of breast carcinoma. Analyt Quant Cytol Histol 2000;22:483–85.

104. Fan F, Namiq A, Tawfik OW, et al. Proposed prognostic score for breast carcinoma on fine needle aspiration based on nuclear grade, cellular dyscohesion and bare atypical nuclei. Diagn Cytopathol 2006;34:542–46.

105. Jayaram G, Elsayed EM. Cytologic evaluation of prognostic markers in breast carcinoma. Acta Cytologica 2005;49:605–10.

106. Khan MZ, Haleem A, Al Hassani H, et al. Cytopathological grading as a predictor of histopathological grade in ductal carcinoma (NOS) of breast, on air-dried Diff-Quick smears. Diagn Cytopathol 2003;29:185–93.

107. Robinson IA, McKee G, Nicholsen A, et al. Prognostic value of cytologic grading of fine-needle aspirates from breast carcinomas. Lancet 1994;343:947–49.

108. Robles-Frias A, Gonzalez-Campora R, Martinez-Parra D, et al. Robinson cytologic grading of invasive ductal breast carcinoma: correlation with histologic grading and regional lymph node metastasis. Acta Cytologica 2005;49:149–53.

109. Skrbinc B, Babic A, Cufer T, et al. Cytological grading of breast cancer in Giemsa-stained fine needle aspiration smears. Cytopathology 2001;12:15–25.

110. Tahlan A, Nijhawan R, Joshi K. Grading of ductal breast carcinoma by cytomorphology and image morphometry with histologic correlation. Analyt Quant Cytol Histol 2000;22:193–98.

111. Taniguchi E, Yang Q, Tang W, et al. Cytologic grading of invasive breast carcinoma. Correlation with clinicopathologic variables and predictive value of nodal metastasis. Acta Cytologica 2000;44:587–91.

112. Robinson IA, McKee G, Nicholsen A, et al. Prognostic value of cytologic grading of fine-needle aspirates from breast carcinomas. Lancet 1994;343:947–49.

113. Silverstein MJ, Poller DN, Waisman J. Prognostic classification of breast ductal carcinoma-in situ. Lancet 1995;345:1154–57.

114. Bondeson L, Lindholm K. Prediction of invasiveness by aspiration cytology applied to nonpalpable breast carcinoma and tested in 300 cases. Diagn Cytopathol 1997;17:315–20.

115. Chhieng DC, Fernandez G, Cangiarella JF, et al. Invasive carcinoma in clinically suspicious breast masses diagnosed as adenocarcinoma by fine-needle aspiration. Cancer Cytopathol 2000;90:97–101.

116. Lee CH, Carter D, Philpotts LE, et al. Ductal carcinoma in situ diagnosed with stereotactic core needle biopsy: can invasion be predicted? Radiology 2000;217:466–70.

117. Verkooijen HM. Diagnostic accuracy of stereotactic large-core biopsy for nonpalpable breast disease: results of a multicenter prospective study with 95% surgical confirmation. Int J Cancer 2002;99:853–59.

118. Bofin AM, Lydersen S, Hagmar BM. Cytological criteria for the diagnosis of intraductal hyperplasia, ductal carcinoma in situ, and invasive carcinoma of the breast. Diagn Cytopathol 2004;31:207–15.

119. Bonzanini M, Gilioli E, Brancato B, et al. The cytopathology of ductal carcinoma in situ of the breast. A detailed analysis of fine needle aspiration cytology of 58 cases compared with 101 invasive ductal carcinomas. Cytopathology 2001;12:107–19.

120. Cangiarella J, Waisman J, Simsir A. Cytologic findings with histologic correlation in 43 cases of mammary intraductal adenocarcinoma diagnosed by aspiration biopsy. Acta Cytol 2003;47:965–72.

121. Cote JF, Klijanienko J, Meunier M, et al. Stereotactic fine-needle aspiration cytology of nonpalpable breast lesions. Curie's experience of 243 histologically correlated cases. Cancer Cytopathol 1998;84:77–83.

122. McKee GT, Tildsley G, Hammond S. Cytologic diagnosis and grading of ductal carcinoma in situ. Cancer Cytopathol 1999;87:203–9.

123. Shin HJ, Sneige N. Is a diagnosis of infiltrating versus in situ ductal carcinoma of the breast possible in fine-needle aspiration specimens?. Cancer Cytopathol 1998;84:186–91.

124. Sauer T, Garred Ø, Lømo J, et al. Assessing invasion criteria in fine needle aspirates from breast carcinoma diagnosed as DCIS or invasive carcinoma: can we identify an invasive component in addition to DCIS? Acta Cytol 2006;50:263–70.

125. Kumarasinghe MP, Poh WT. Differentiating non-high-grade duct carcinoma in situ from benign breast lesions. Diagn Cytopathol 2004;30:98–102.

126. Collins L, Carlo V, Hwang H, et al. Intracystic papillary carcinomas of the breast: a reevaluation using a panel of myoepithelial cell markers. Am J Surg Pathol 2006;30:1002–7.

127. Lui PC, Lau PP, Tse GM, et al. Fine needle aspiration cytology of invasive micropapillary carcinoma of the breast. Pathology 2007;39:401–5.

128. Madur B, Shet T, Chinoy R. Cytologic findings in infiltrating micropapillary carcinoma and mucinous carcinomas with micropapillary pattern. Acta Cytol 2007;51:25–32.

129. Gupta RK, Kenwright D, Naran S, et al. Fine needle aspiration cytodiagnosis of secretory carcinoma of the breast. Cytopathology 2000;11:496–502.

130. Das AK, Verma K, Aron M. Fine-needle aspiration cytology of glycogen-rich carcinoma of breast: Report of a case and review of literature. Diagn Cytopathol 2005;33:263–67.

131. Sauer T. Cytologic findings in malignant myoepithelioma: a case report and review of the literature. Cytojournal 2007;4:3.

132. Georgiannos SN, Aleong JC, Goode AW, et al. Secondary neoplasms of the breast. A survey of the 20th century. Cancer 2001;92:2259–66.

133. David MD, Gattuso P, Razan W, et al. Unusual cases of metastases to the breast: a report of 17 cases diagnosed by fine needle aspiration. Acta Cytol 2002;46:377–85.

134. Hejmadi RK, Day LJ, Young JA. Extramammary metastatic neoplasms in the breast: a cytomorphological study of 11 cases. Cytopathology 2003;14:191–94.

135. Kocjan G. Fine needle aspiration cytology: inadequate rates compromise success. Cytopathology 2003;14:307–8.

136. Levine T. Breast cytology – is there still a role? Cytopathology 2004;15:293–96.

137. Fessia L, Botta G, Arisio R, et al. Fine-needle aspiration of breast lesions: role and accuracy in a review of 7495 cases. Diagnostic Cytopathology 1987;3:121–25.

138. Kocjan G, Bourgain C, Fassina A, et al. The role of breast FNAC in diagnosis and clinical management: a survey of current practice. Cytopathology 2008;19(5):271–78.

139. Kocjan G, Chandra A, Cross P, et al. BSCC Code of Practice – fine needle aspiration cytology. Cytopathology 2009;20(5):283–96.

140. Perry N, Broeders M, de Wolf C, et al. European guidelines for quality assurance in breast cancer screening and diagnosis. Ann Oncol 2008;19:614–22.

141. N.I.H. The uniform approach to breast fine needle aspiration biopsy: a synopsis. The Breast 2007;2:357–63.

142. N.I.H. The uniform approach to breast fine needle aspiration biopsy. NIH Consensus Development Conference. Am J Surg 1997;174:371–85.

143. WHO histological classification of tumours of the breast. In: Tavassoli A, Devilee P (eds). Pathology and Genetics. Tumours of the breast and female genital organs. IARC Press, Lyon, 2003.

# Section 5

## Alimentary System

# Salivary glands

Gabrijela Kocjan and Ketan A. Shah

## Chapter contents

## Introduction

There is perhaps no tissue anywhere in the body that is subject to such a diverse and heterogeneous range of tumours and tumour-like conditions. While this results in fascinating cytopathology it also imposes limitations, which must be appreciated by both pathologists and clinicians if the extensive benefits of cytodiagnosis are to be fully and safely utilised in patient management. In recent years, advances in imaging techniques have contributed much to the assessment of salivary gland disease, but the findings are not uncommonly equivocal. Clinical management of salivary gland masses is increasingly relying on pre-treatment diagnosis derived from microscopic examination. Preoperative histological biopsy using a Vim-Silverman or Tru-Cut needle, or intraoperative frozen sections have their own hazards and organisational problems. In contrast, fine needle aspiration (FNA) is virtually risk free and offers enough information to plan appropriate patient management. This chapter discusses the cytological findings in commonly encountered salivary gland conditions along with diagnostic pitfalls and limitations. We hope that the algorithm provided at the end will be a useful guide in assessing salivary gland cytology.

## Aspiration technique

Standard fine needle aspiration (FNA) technique, using the capillary method without suction and direct spreading onto glass slides is the preference of the authors and is applicable to major and minor salivary glands.[1] The non-suction technique is advocated in order to avoid the post-FNA changes found in some lesions on histological examination after excision.[1] Alternatively, FNA samples may be rinsed in a solution and prepared either as cytospin preparations or as liquid based cytology (LBC). Immunosuppressed patients are prone to salivary gland disease and care should be taken to avoid needlestick injuries.[2] Cystic masses are best aspirated using a syringe attached to the needle, with or without a syringe holder. If possible, any residual mass should be re-aspirated in order to obtain representative cellular material. If microbiological culture or other ancillary investigations are required, repeat aspiration for this purpose is advised, as division of a single aspirate is seldom satisfactory. A combined approach of ultrasound-guided fine needle aspiration of head and neck masses, with immediate assessment of the material by a pathologist, can be more accurate than are specimens obtained in other ways.[3]

## Normal salivary gland components

### Acinar and ductal epithelium

Acinar cells are large, with abundant cytoplasm and small round uniform nuclei. The cytoplasm is finely granular in serous glands and clear or lightly vacuolated in mucous glands. Either type is fragile and easily disrupted by smearing, so that dispersed bare nuclei are found in the background. When complete acini are aspirated, the cells occur in compact lobulated groups (Fig. 5.1).

The larger ducts are lined by columnar and the smaller ones by cuboidal cells. The cells are usually arranged in flat sheets displaying good cohesion and uniform morphology. Small pointed nuclei arising from myoepithelial cells may occasionally be identified between the epithelium and the basement membrane.

### Intraparotid lymph nodes

Clinically, a frequently encountered problem is the distinction between enlarged lymph nodes and sialomegaly, particularly in the case of the parotid glands. Due to late encapsulation in foetal life, small lymph nodes are commonly enclosed within the parotid. It is not possible to distinguish between intraparotid lymphadenopathy and true salivary gland pathology reliably by palpation or imaging. FNA of a hyperplastic lymph node yields a mixed population of lymphocytes, follicle centre cells and 'tingible body' macrophages. When perinodal salivary tissue is also sampled, it becomes difficult to separate lymphadenopathy from salivary gland disease associated with lymphocytosis.

*The authors wish to acknowledge the privilege of having inherited from the previous edition a comprehensively written chapter by Drs J. Young and A. Warfield, both well known experts in this field.*

## Ectopic salivary glands

Ectopic (heterotopic) salivary gland tissue is commonly found in periparotid lymph nodes, middle ear and lower neck, but can also occur in more remote regions. Either normal acinar cells or material indicating benign or malignant disease can be encountered, as any of the salivary gland disorders found in normally placed salivary gland tissue can develop.[4,5]

## Non-neoplastic conditions

### Cysts

A systematic approach to the diagnosis of cystic salivary gland lesions by FNA can result in a correct diagnosis in >70% of cases.[6] Careful attention should be directed at identifying the extracellular fluid component (mucoid versus watery protein-aceous) as well as the predominant cellular component (e.g. lymphocytes, histiocytes, epithelial cells and oncocytes). Occasionally, epithelial cells may not be obtained on FNA of cystic salivary gland lesions.

#### Mucus cyst (mucocele)

Mucoceles result either from disruption of salivary ducts, often due to trauma, with salivary extravasation and reactive inflammation, or due to ductal obstruction and accumulation of saliva in dilated ducts. They commonly arise in minor salivary glands of the lip and oral cavity, and in the sublingual gland

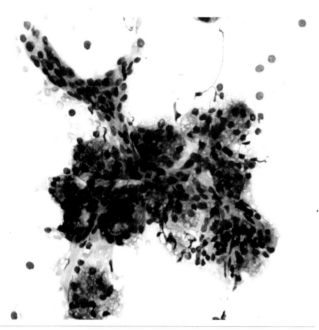

**Fig. 5.1** Acinar and ductal epithelium. Acinar cells are large, with abundant cytoplasm and small round uniform nuclei. The cytoplasm is finely granular in serous glands and clear or lightly vacuolated in mucous glands. Either type is fragile and easily disrupted by smearing, so that bare dispersed nuclei may be present in the background. When complete acini are aspirated the cells occur in lobulated groups. The larger ducts are lined by columnar epithelium and the smaller ones by cuboidal cells. Ductal epithelial cells are usually arranged in flat sheets displaying good cohesion and uniform morphology. Small pointed nuclei arising from myoepithelial cells may occasionally be identified between the epithelium and the basement membrane (MGG).

(ranula). When tense and deep seated, these may lead to clinical suspicion of neoplasia and are, therefore, not infrequently targets for FNA.

### Cytological findings: mucocele

- Watery or viscous fluid
- Scanty cellularity
- Leucocytes and macrophages in variable numbers
- Few epithelial cells
- Many leucocytes and epithelial atypia if secondarily infected.

The fluid is watery or viscous depending upon whether the epithelium is predominantly serous or mucinous (Fig. 5.2). It is relatively hypocellular, containing only a few leucocytes and macrophages and perhaps occasional sheets of columnar cells. Occasionally, leucocytosis is pronounced and the epithelial cells display reactive and inflammatory atypia. Collagenous spherulosis within a mucocele has been described.[7]

### Diagnostic pitfalls: mucocele

Cystic change occurs in both benign (Warthin's tumour, pleomorphic adenoma) and malignant (mucoepidermoid carcinoma, acinic cell carcinoma, high-grade carcinoma) salivary gland tumours.[8] Low-grade mucoepidermoid

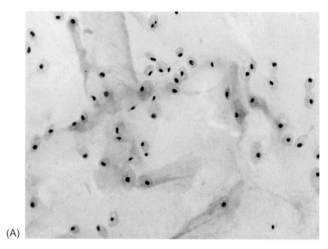

(A)

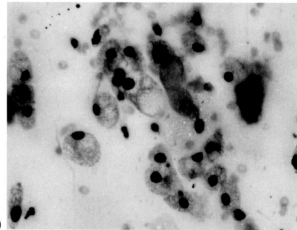

(B)

**Fig. 5.2** Mucocele. Fluid is relatively hypocellular, containing only a few leucocytes and macrophages (A) PAP, (B) MGG.

carcinoma cannot be excluded in aspirates diagnosed as mucinous cystic lesions.[6]

## Lymphoepithelial cyst

Bilateral and multiple lymphoepithelial cysts (LECs) of major salivary glands, in particular of parotid glands, are uncommon but are reported in human immunodeficiency virus (HIV) infected patients with an incidence of about 3–6% (Fig. 5.3). They represent an early manifestation of HIV infection and are rarely found in patients with advanced disease. They are the most common presentation (58.9%) of HIV infection in children.[9]

### Cytological findings: lymphoepithelial cyst

- Most aspirates are cystic
- Foamy macrophages and lymphocytes
- Squamous epithelial cells[2]
- Occasionally, multinucleated giant cells[10]
- Crystalloids.[11]

### Diagnostic pitfalls: lymphoepithelial cyst

Lymphoid hyperplasia may be florid and contain many centroblasts. It may therefore be mistaken for a non-Hodgkin lymphoma or other lymphoproliferative disorders.[12]

## Branchial cleft cyst

Branchial cysts are usually asymptomatic but one-third present acutely due to inflammation (Fig. 5.4). Aspirates yield abundant or scanty viscous fluid, which contains mature squamous cells and keratinous debris. Although lymphoid tissue is present in its wall, aspirates are usually taken from the centre of the lesion and therefore almost never contain lymphoid cells. Macrophages, cholesterol crystals and acute inflammatory cells are found in cysts where the epithelial lining has been disrupted. With associated inflammation, the squamous epithelial cells often exhibit mild nuclear atypia. In such cases, differentiation of a branchial cyst from cystic metastasis of a squamous cell carcinoma from upper aerodigestive tract and occasionally lungs becomes important. Examination of alcohol-fixed smears with better presentation of keratin and nuclear detail, and careful scrutiny for immature cells, dyskaryotic nuclei, pleomorphism and necrosis, should clarify the distinction in most cases. Well-differentiated squamous carcinoma metastasis with only mild nuclear abnormalities can be difficult to exclude and in such a case, radiological imaging and panendoscopy with biopsies should be recommended. Branchial cysts usually present before the age of 40 but so can some squamous carcinoma; age alone is not a reliable discriminator.

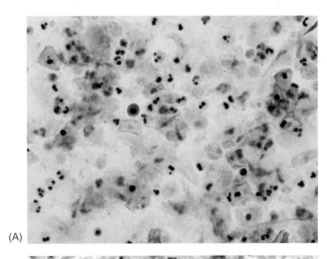

(A)

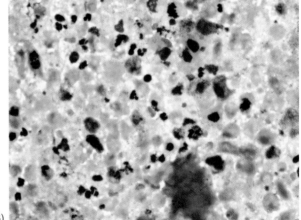

(B)

**Fig. 5.4** Branchial cleft cyst. (A) Cyst is usually lined by squamous and occasionally by columnar epithelium. It may contain variable numbers of inflammatory cells but usually does not contain necrotic background (PAP). (B) Aspirate from a squamous cell carcinoma shows marked degenerative changes, secondary inflammation and necrotic debris. The nuclei are irregular (PAP).

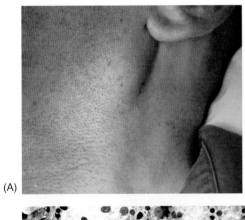

(A)

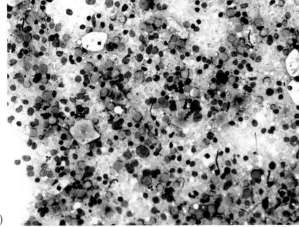

(B)

**Fig. 5.3** Lymphoepithelial cyst. (A) Bilateral and multiple lymphoepithelial cysts of major salivary glands, in particular of parotid glands, are quite rare and have been reported in HIV-infected patients. (B) The aspirates contain foamy macrophages, lymphoid cells, epithelial (squamous) cells and, occasionally, multinucleated giant cells (MGG).

# Sialadenitis

## Acute sialadenitis

Acute sialadenitis is due to specific bacterial or viral infection such as mumps parotitis. It is usually clinically obvious and FNA is not indicated. CMV sialadenitis should be considered in the differential diagnosis of painless salivary gland enlargement in patients with AIDS.[13] The presence of acute inflammatory cells in a salivary gland FNA does not always indicate acute sialadenitis; some salivary gland tumours may contain acute inflammation, either due to necrosis or as a result of a previous FNA. Such aspirates should be carefully assessed for other pathology that may be obscured by inflammation.

## Chronic sialadenitis

Calculi (sialoliths) form in the salivary ducts as the result of mineralisation of debris. The submandibular gland is the most common site. Clinically, calculi are associated with pain and swelling and retrograde infection results in acute or chronic sialadenitis. Changes in the duct wall include squamous, oncocytic and mucous cell metaplasia, and if obstruction is longstanding, atrophy and fibrosis of acinar tissue will ensue. Cystic change with a variety of crystalloids may occasionally be encountered.

Chronic sclerosing sialadenitis (CSS), also known as Kuttner tumour, is a cryptogenic tumour-like condition of the salivary glands. Immune-mediated processes are suspected in its pathogenesis and CSS is occasionally reported to be associated with sclerosing pancreatitis.[14]

### Cytological findings: chronic sialadenitis

- Scanty aspirate
- Ductal cells with possible metaplasia or atypia
- Paucity of acinar cells
- Inflammatory cells and background debris
- Possible cystic change and crystalloids.

Aspirates are generally hypocellular and epithelial cells, when present, are of ductal type. Acinar cells are unusual due to the atrophic changes (Fig. 5.5). Occasionally, large numbers of non-birefringent crystalloids (deep blue with May–Grünwald–Giemsa (MGG) or Diff-Quik and bright orange with Papanicolaou stain) of varying sizes and shapes are present. Lymphocytes, plasma cells, multinucleated histiocytes and neutrophils are also seen.[15,16]

### Diagnostic pitfalls: chronic sialadenitis

Severe inflammatory atypia of ductal cells with anisonucleosis and hyperchromasia may occur as does squamous metaplasia. With inflammatory cells and debris in the background, the appearance can be quite worrying and suggestive of a malignant neoplasm such as mucoepidermoid or squamous cell carcinoma.

## Granulomatous sialadenitis

Granulomatous involvement of salivary glands is present in about 6% of cases of sarcoidosis. Clusters of epithelioid cells, multinucleated histiocytes and lymphoid cells are seen in aspirates (Fig. 5.6). Duct obstruction with salivary leakage can incite a granulomatous reaction. Other causes include tuberculosis, fungal infection, cat scratch disease, brucellosis and toxoplasmosis. Granulomatous reaction to non-tyrosine crystalloids can be associated with both neoplastic and non-neoplastic

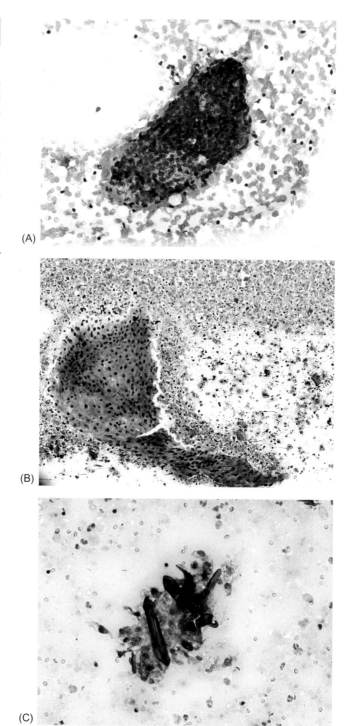

(A)

(B)

(C)

**Fig. 5.5** Chronic sialadenitis. (A) Aspirates are generally hypocellular and acinar cells are unusual due to the atrophic changes. Clusters of tightly cohesive ductal epithelium are seen (MGG). (B) Ductal cells may show squamous metaplasia with possible atypia (MGG). (C) Occasionally, aspirates from chronic sialadenitis contain large numbers of non-birefringent crystalloids of varying sizes and shapes (MGG).

salivary gland disease, and they may be a product of oncocytic cell secretion.[17]

## Myoepithelial sialadenitis

Myoepithelial sialadenitis (MESA) is commonest in middle-aged or elderly women and is usually bilateral and symmetrical,

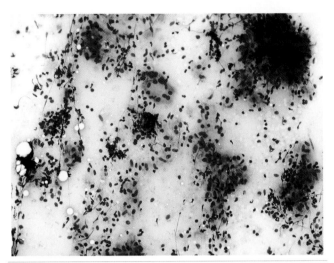

**Fig. 5.6** Sarcoidosis. Multinucleated giant cells and clusters of epithelioid cells against a background of lymphocytes are seen in aspirates (MGG).

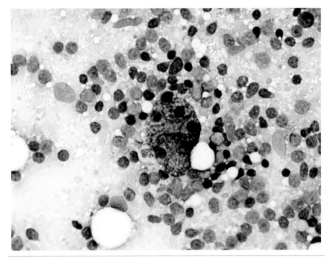

**Fig. 5.7** Myoepithelial sialadenitis (MESA). FNA preparations contain numerous lymphocytes mixed with follicle centre cells, plasma cells and histiocytes. Acinar cells are seen trapped in the infiltrate (MGG).

although sometimes initially unilateral. In cases of Sjögren's syndrome, other manifestations such as dryness of eyes and mouth, rheumatoid arthritis and hypergammaglobulinaemia are present.

Lymphoid lesions are uncommon and thus cytological experience on FNA is limited. A spectrum of diseases, ranging from benign lymphoepithelial lesion (localised myoepithelial sialadenitis or MESA) to systemic Sjögren's syndrome are included in this benign sialadenopathy, believed to be of autoimmune origin.

### Cytological findings: MESA

- Reactive lymphoid cells, plasma cells and histiocytes
- Clusters of myoepithelial cells are sometimes present.

FNA preparations contain numerous lymphocytes mixed with follicle centre cells, plasma cells and histiocytes (Fig. 5.7). Clusters of myoepithelial cells, if present, are a helpful pointer to the disease but are not always evident in aspirates. Florid lymphocytosis is seen in other conditions, including chronic sialadenitis, Warthin's tumour, mucoepidermoid carcinoma, acinic cell carcinoma and non-Hodgkin lymphoma.[18,19] Aspiration of perisalivary lymph nodes is another source of lymphoid tissue. Benign lymphoepithelial lesion can progress to malignant lymphoma; while high-grade lymphoma is easier to recognise, morphological differentiation from low-grade lymphoma can be difficult. Correlation with clinical findings and use of ancillary methods (flow cytometry, gene rearrangement studies) can help arrive at the diagnosis. FNA of lymphoid lesions with ancillary aids can make a definitive diagnosis.[20] The diagnosis of benign lymphoepithelial lesion is best established by correlating the clinical and cytopathological findings and using ancillary methods such as flow cytometry and gene rearrangement studies.[21,22]

## Miscellaneous conditions

### Sialadenosis

This is a non-inflammatory, often bilateral, swelling of the salivary glands, particularly of the parotid caused by hypertrophy of the acinar cells. It is associated with hormonal, nutritional or neurogenic disorders and with systemic diseases such as diabetes.[23]

Characteristically, numerous benign acinar cells are present and ductal cells are sparse. Care must be taken not to confuse this with well-differentiated acinic cell carcinoma.

### Sclerosing polycystic adenosis

Sclerosing polycystic adenosis is a recently described, rare lesion of the salivary gland. It can simulate a slow growing tumour. It is pseudoencapsulated and includes tubuloacinar adenosis with dilated ducts, apocrine metaplasia, epithelial hyperplasia and cystic changes associated with fibrosis, histologically resembling fibrocystic disease of the breast.[24] Recognition of this benign entity is important since the differential diagnosis includes other more common benign and malignant salivary gland neoplasms, particularly mucoepidermoid carcinoma and tumours with cystic and oncocytic features. The aspirates are characterised by flat cohesive sheets of epithelial cells with moderate amounts of finely granular oncocytic cytoplasm and enlarged round nuclei with indistinct nucleoli. Some epithelial groups form glandular structures with lumens, and the background contains small amounts of delicate mucoproteinaceous material. Occasional markedly vacuolated cells may be present, as well as many cells with apocrine change manifested by well-defined apical snouting.[25,26]

### Adenomatoid hyperplasia

Adenomatous ductal hyperplasia (ADH) of the salivary glands is rare, occurring almost exclusively in the palate. It is characterised histologically by the proliferating ducts which resemble intercalated duct epithelium. ADH is compared with adenomatoid acinar hyperplasia (AAH), a lesion found predominantly in intraoral salivary glands and histologically composed of hyperplastic acinar cells. The nature of these lesions is not clear. However, ADH may be a precursor lesion of salivary gland tumours (especially epithelial-myoepithelial carcinomas), whereas AAH may represent a reactive process of idiopathic nature. Clinically, it is generally misdiagnosed as a neoplasm.[27–29]

It is a potential source of a false positive diagnosis of mucoepidermoid carcinoma.

## Lipomatosis

The parotid and, to a lesser extent, the submandibular gland normally contain adipose tissue, which increases with advancing age. Lipomatosis is diffuse excess of interstitial fat, which may occur in obesity and diabetes and occasionally presents as a swelling. Fatty replacement of atrophic parenchyma, sialolipoma, periparotid lipomata and sialometaplasia in pleomorphic adenoma are other causes of fat cells in an aspirate.[30-35]

## Oncocytosis

Focal oncocytic change is common with increasing age. In diffuse hyperplastic oncocytosis of the parotid gland, extensive metaplasia of acinic and ductal cells leads to transformation of nearly all cells into oncocytes.[36] Cytologically, oncocytosis may be difficult to distinguish from oncocytoma or paucilymphocytic Warthin's tumour. Areas of oncocytic differentiation can occur in pleomorphic adenoma.

## Tumours of the salivary gland

Salivary gland tumours are uncommon. The annual incidence around the world is between 0.4 and 13.5 cases per 100 000 population, of which benign tumours represent between 54% and 79%. The majority of primary epithelial tumours occur in the parotid (up to 80%), followed by minor salivary glands, submandibular gland and sublingual gland. The relative incidence of malignancy is much higher in minor than in major salivary glands. The most recent WHO classification of salivary gland tumours is given in Box 5.1.[37]

## Benign salivary gland neoplasms

This is a diverse group of lesions where morphological variation occurs within each category and a degree of overlap exists between each tumour subtype. This makes the task of precise classification a challenge for histopathologists, and even more so for the cytopathologist.

### Pleomorphic adenoma

Pleomorphic adenoma (mixed tumour) is the commonest salivary gland neoplasm, accounting for 60% of all tumours. Most (80%) occur in the parotid and besides salivary glands, it is occasionally encountered in the nasal cavity, paranasal sinuses, upper respiratory tract and gastrointestinal tract.[37] The tumour occurs most often in patients aged 30–50 years and is slightly more common in females. Bilateral synchronous pleomorphic adenomas occur infrequently.[38] Histologically, the typical tumour consists of glandular structures composed of a double layer of epithelial and myoepithelial cells embedded in myxoid stroma. Cytology demonstrates most of the histological features of pleomorphic adenoma of salivary gland and is a useful tool in initial assessment of the tumour.[39] Squamous metaplasia, oncocytosis, mucus production, sebaceous or adipocytic differentiation[30-35] may occur and the mesenchymal component can undergo chondroid metaplasia or even ossification. Collagenous crystalloids may be a clue to the diagnosis of pleomorphic adenoma.[40]

---

**Box 5.1  WHO histological classification of tumours of the salivary glands**

Malignant epithelial tumours

- Acinic cell carcinoma
- Mucoepidermoid carcinoma
- Adenoid cystic carcinoma
- Polymorphous low-grade adenocarcinoma
- Epithelial-myoepithelial carcinoma
- Clear cell carcinoma, not otherwise specified
- Basal cell adenocarcinoma
- Sebaceous carcinoma
- Sebaceous lymphadenocarcinoma
- Cystadenocarcinoma
- Low-grade cribriform cystadenocarcinoma
- Mucinous adenocarcinoma
- Oncocytic carcinoma
- Salivary duct carcinoma
- Adenocarcinoma, not otherwise specified
- Myoepithelial carcinoma
- Carcinoma ex pleomorphic adenoma
- Carcinosarcoma
- Metastasising pleomorphic adenoma
- Squamous cell carcinoma
- Small cell carcinoma
- Large cell carcinoma
- Lymphoepithelial carcinoma
- Sialoblastoma

Benign epithelial tumours

- Pleomorphic adenoma
- Myoepithelioma
- Basal cell adenoma
- Warthin tumour
- Oncocytoma
- Canalicular adenoma
- Sebaceous adenoma
- Lymphadenoma
  - Sebaceous
  - Non-sebaceous
- Ductal papillomas
  - Inverted ductal papilloma
  - Intraductal papilloma
  - Sialadenoma papilliferum
- Cystadenoma

Soft tissue tumours

- Haemangioma

Haematolymphoid tumours

- Hodgkin lymphoma
- Diffuse large B-cell lymphoma
- Extranodal marginal zone B-cell lymphoma

Secondary tumours

(WHO 2005)

Cystic change in some tumours presents a diagnostic pitfall both in imaging and cytology.[41] Although a benign tumour, there are rare reports, in which these histologically benign tumours have inexplicably metastasised to distant sites.[42,43]

### Cytological findings: pleomorphic adenoma

- Cellular aspirates with large amount of myxoid background matrix
- Myoepithelial cells singly or in sheets
- Epithelial cells in form of tubules or as squamous or oncocytic cells
- Cell nuclei vary in size but have uniform chromatin
- Spindle-shaped mesenchymal cells
- Chondroid or other metaplastic changes are sometimes seen.

The cytological diagnosis of the great majority of pleomorphic adenomas is quite straightforward (Fig. 5.8). Aspirates contain plentiful myoepithelial cells, which are closely intermingled with fibrillary myxoid background substance. They lie singly or in sheets and have round to oval nuclei of uniform chromasia, although they may vary a little in size. A characteristic feature is the well-defined cytoplasmic membrane in the majority of these cells and bare nuclei are sparse. The background stromal substance is closely tangled with cells and stains

pinkish-grey with Papanicolaou and bright magenta with MGG due to metachromasia. Chondroid change is indicated by a blue reaction with the latter technique. The presence of abundant fibrillary matrix material with single myoepithelial cells in the background is highly diagnostic of pleomorphic adenoma. Published studies based on these criteria confirm a high level of accuracy for FNA diagnosis of pleomorphic adenoma.

### Diagnostic pitfalls: pleomorphic adenoma

- Dominance of one cell type
- Cytological atypia
- Globules of basement membrane material
- Cystic change
- Mucin production
- Squamous, mucinous, sebaceous metaplasia.

The histological heterogeneity of pleomorphic adenoma is reflected in its cytology. Problems in interpretation occur for two reasons: the predominance of one element over other components, or the presence of atypical cytomorphological features. If myoepithelial cells are numerous and mesenchymal material not readily apparent, the tumour may be classified as myoepithelioma. Clinically, this is of little significance. If the myxoid component is abundant, it may overwhelm the few

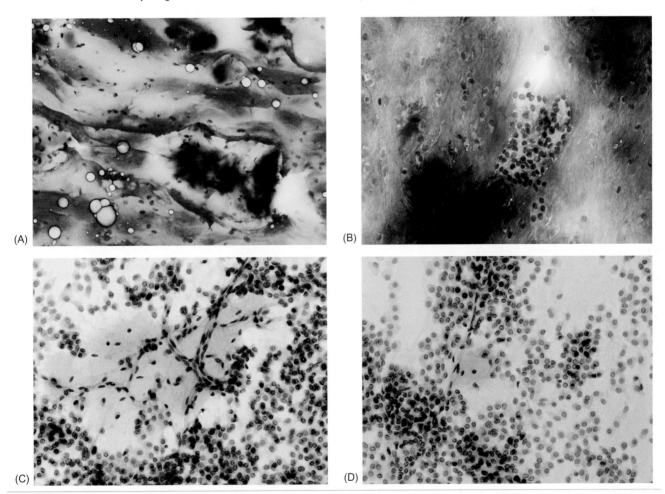

(A)  (B)  (C)  (D)

**Fig. 5.8** Pleomorphic adenoma. (A–D) Aspirates contain epithelial cells, which are closely intermingled with loose clusters of mesenchymal cells and fibrillary mucomyxomatous background substance. The epithelial cells lie singly or in sheets and have nuclei of uniform chromasia, although they may vary a little in size. The mesenchymal cells are rounded or spindly with elongated nuclei. The background substance is closely tangled with cells and stains pinkish-grey with Papanicolaou and bright magenta with MGG. (A) MGG. (B) MGG. (C) PAP, LP. (D) PAP.

epithelial cells present and the lesion may be mistaken for a retention cyst, nodular fasciitis,[44] schwannoma or intravenous pyogenic granuloma.[46] This is more likely to happen if only MGG-stained slides are examined, as strong metachromasia may mask other cellular components.

More serious is false suspicion of malignancy.[47] Some examples of pleomorphic adenoma are highly cellular and display marked cytological atypia. This is reflected in FNA specimens in which the myoepithelial cells can show loss of cohesion, nuclear enlargement and hyperchromasia to a worrying degree. It is important not to overdiagnose these changes. On histological examination, most such 'atypical' lesions are pleomorphic adenomas with mild cytological atypia within myoepithelial cells, which is acceptable in the spectrum of benign pleomorphic adenoma. If unequivocal cytological features of malignancy are present, the diagnosis of carcinoma ex-pleomorphic adenoma should be considered (see Carcinoma ex-pleomorphic adenoma, p. 245).

Some pleomorphic adenomas contain adenoid cystic-like areas.[48] Globules of basement membrane material may be seen in pleomorphic adenoma and basal cell adenoma, risking a misdiagnosis of adenoid cystic carcinoma, which could result in radical surgery.[49] Great caution must be exercised not to confuse the globules in pleomorphic adenoma with true adenoid cystic carcinoma. If the globules are few and other cellular features of pleomorphic adenoma are present, false suspicion of malignancy should not be raised. The seemingly naked nuclei of neoplastic cells in adenoid cystic carcinoma with their coarse nuclear chromatin and irregular nucleoli can reliably distinguish adenoid cystic carcinoma from cylindromatous adenomas[50] (see Adenoid cystic carcinoma, p. 243). Occasionally, pleomorphic adenoma may exhibit marked cystic change.[36,41,51]

Mucin production by pleomorphic adenomas is another difficulty and the differential diagnosis then includes Warthin's tumour and low-grade mucoepidermoid carcinoma. Pleomorphic adenoma occasionally reveals focal squamous metaplasia. When extensive, it may be misdiagnosed as metastatic well-differentiated squamous cell carcinoma or mucoepidermoid carcinoma in FNA.[52] Squamous cells can occur in other non-neoplastic and neoplastic lesions of the salivary such as chronic sialadenitis, lymphoepithelial cyst, Warthin's tumour, and squamous cell carcinoma.[53] The presence of squamous, mucinous, and/or sebaceous metaplasia, especially in the absence of chondromyxoid stroma, presents the potential for misinterpretation of the FNA as indicative of malignancy.[34,54]

Familiarity with the variable aspirate appearance of PA in addition to well-defined cytological and architectural criteria can help establish the proper diagnosis in the majority of cases.[55] There remain, however, few cases in which a definitive diagnosis is not possible.[56] Small tissue biopsies will not resolve these problems.[55]

## Myoepithelioma

Myoepithelioma (myoepithelial adenoma) is defined as a benign tumour composed almost exclusively of cells showing myoepithelial differentiation. They can be spindle celled, plasmacytoid, epithelioid or clear cell in morphology (Fig. 5.9).[37] Many authorities would accept a minor epithelial subpopulation, usually less than 5% tumour volume, within this definition.[57] The surrounding stroma can be collagenous or mucoid. About

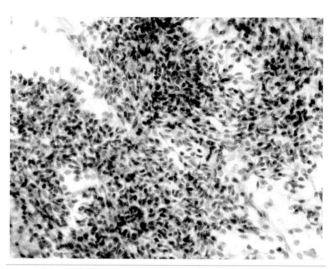

**Fig. 5.9** Myoepithelioma. Myoepithelioma (myoepithelial adenoma) in its pure form is a rare, benign tumour composed exclusively of myoepithelial cells, devoid of any stromal component (PAP).

40% occur in the parotid followed by the minor salivary glands, especially the palate.[37]

### Cytological findings: myoepithelioma

- Loosely cohesive fusiform or spindle cells
- Epithelioid, clear cell or hyaline (plasmacytoid) cells may be a component or predominate
- Ovoid nuclei with finely dispersed chromatin
- Little or no epithelial cell population
- Absent or scant stromal component.

Most myoepitheliomas are composed of a single cell type, though a combination of cell types may occur. Although a mild variation in nuclear size may occur with plasmacytoid cells, there is no coarseness of chromatin, prominence of nucleoli or pleomorphism. Stroma, if present, is scanty compared with pleomorphic adenoma. There is a convincing argument for regarding myoepithelioma and pleomorphic adenoma as different ends of a spectrum and discrimination between myoepithelial cell-rich pleomorphic adenoma and myoepithelioma is of little biological consequence.

### Diagnostic pitfalls: myoepithelioma

Myoepitheliomas are rarely diagnosed correctly on FNA. They are usually described as cellular pleomorphic adenomas, or benign spindle cell tumours depending on the predominant cell type. With experience the cytomorphological features of myoepithelioma are recognisable in FNA material.[57–63]

## Basal cell adenoma

Basal cell adenoma (BCA) is a rare benign epithelial tumour of the salivary gland. BCA is seen most frequently in the parotid gland and less commonly in the submandibular gland and minor glands of the upper lips, oral cavity and hard palate.[64]

### Cytological findings: basal cell adenoma

- Well-polarised basaloid cells, often with peripheral palisading
- Accompanying hyaline stroma (Fig. 5.10).

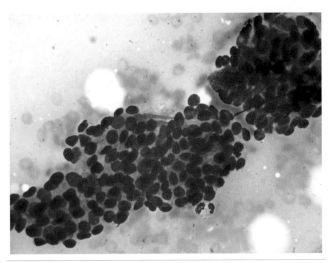

**Fig. 5.10** Basal cell adenoma. Aspirates contain well-polarised basaloid cells, often with peripheral palisading and accompanying hyaline stroma (MGG).

A variety of histological growth patterns such as solid, tubular, trabecular and membranous occurs and this diversity is recapitulated in FNA material. The membranous variant ('dermal analogue tumour') resembles an eccrine cylindroma of the skin and may occur either in isolation or in association with a variety of cutaneous adnexal neoplasms. The cells have uniform, round to oval nuclei with uniform chromasia. Scanty cytoplasm is often present as are bare nuclei in the background. Hyaline stroma is often in the form of small globules or finger-like fragments, to which cells adhere.

### Diagnostic pitfalls: basal cell adenoma

The potential of mistaking basal cell adenoma for adenoid cystic carcinoma is evident from the above description and must be kept in mind. Hyaline globules are smaller and fewer than those seen in adenoid cystic carcinoma and critical examination of the shape and intensity of staining of the stroma, the cytonuclear morphology and any background content of a smear may facilitate a correct diagnosis. The differences are at best subtle and, on occasion, definitive interpretation may not be feasible (see Adenoid cystic carcinoma, p. 243).[50,65,66]

The malignant counterpart of basal cell adenoma is basal cell adenocarcinoma.

## Warthin's tumour

The WHO recommends the use of this term over others (adenolymphoma, cystadenolymphoma, papillary cystadenoma lymphomatosum) in order to avoid confusion with a lymphoid malignancy and with lymphadenoma.[37] It occurs within the parotid and periparotid lymph nodes, with very rare examples at other sites.[37] The tumours are more common in males than in females; most occur in middle-aged or elderly individuals and have been associated with smoking.[67] They grow slowly, are often fluctuant and can be bilateral or unilaterally multicentric. Multiple tumours are detected in 20.5% of cases including the extraparotid sites.[68] Histologically, Warthin's tumour is composed of glandular, often cystic, papillary structures with a lymphoid stroma. The epithelium is double-layered and predominantly oncocytic but mucous or goblet cells and areas

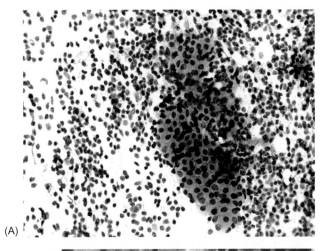

(A)

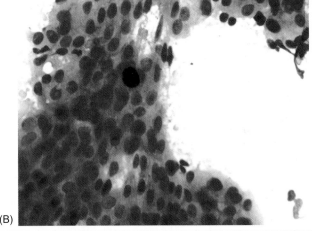

(B)

**Fig. 5.11** Warthin's tumour. (A) Aspirates are composed of glandular, often cystic, papillary structures with occasional lymphoid cells (MGG). (B) The epithelium is double-layered and predominantly oncocytic but mucous or goblet cells and areas of squamous metaplasia may be present (MGG).

of squamous metaplasia may be present (Fig. 5.11). Oncocytic cells are particularly susceptible to trauma and Warthin's tumours may show total or subtotal infarction and metaplastic transformation, either spontaneously or following FNA.[69–71] FNA without aspiration is a particularly valuable tool for the diagnosis of Warthin tumour.[1]

### Cytological findings: Warthin's tumour

- Watery or mucoid aspirate
- Sheets of oncocytic epithelial cells
- Admixture of lymphocytes
- Background debris.

The characteristic appearance comprises a background of proteinaceous and cell debris, with cellular elements represented by oncocytic, lymphoid and mast cells.[72] Oncocytic cells have abundant, pale grey (MGG) or green (PAP), granular cytoplasm. They occur in monolayered sheets, with a honeycombed pattern, frequently associated with mast cells with preserved granules in cytoplasm. Germinal centre structures and cholesterol crystals are often seen. Uncommon cellular findings include true squamous cells, atypical cells with vacuoles, osteoclastic giant cells, epithelioid cells and siderophages.[73] Uncommon findings in the background are corpora amylacea-like structures, homogeneous bright red droplets and tyrosine-rich crystals. The latter are associated with several oncocytic salivary gland neoplasms.[17,74,75]

## Diagnostic pitfalls: Warthin's tumour

Cystic lesions. Warthin's tumour represents one of the cystic parotid gland lesions in adults which also include benign lymphoepithelial lesions, mucus retention cyst, branchial cleft cyst, chronic sialadenitis, cystadenoma, cystic low-grade mucoepidermoid carcinoma, cystic pleomorphic adenoma, lymphangioma, cystadenocarcinoma, cystic acinic cell carcinoma, examples of polycystic disease of the parotid gland and lymphoma.[76–78] If the epithelial cells are few, Warthin's tumour can be mistaken for a non-neoplastic cyst. It may be associated with false positive diagnoses of malignancy on FNA.[79] The common location of Warthin's tumours within periparotid nodes may add to the clinical suspicion of metastasis.

When the lymphoid component, mucus and necrotic background are minimal or absent, the tumours can be confused with oncocytoma. In oncocytoma, the oncocytic epithelial cells are more often seen in papillary fragments, acini and singly in comparison to Warthin's tumour, where sheets of oncocytic cells are observed. Some degree of epithelial atypia can be seen in oncocyte-predominant benign lesions.[80]

Squamous metaplasia. Squamous metaplasia and cystic degeneration in Warthin's tumour are not uncommon. These features may be misinterpreted as mucoepidermoid or metastatic squamous carcinoma with cystic change.[81,82]

Mucin-containing lesions. The presence of extracellular or intracellular mucin in FNA specimens of salivary gland tumours may not be a reliable criterion for distinguishing Warthin's tumour from mucoepidermoid carcinoma.[83] The mixture of epithelial cell types that occurs in mucoepidermoid carcinoma is not seen (see Mucoepidermoid carcinoma, p. 242). However, a Warthin's tumour with squamous metaplasia may be difficult to differentiate cytologically from a mucoepidermoid carcinoma.

Other factors. Warthin's tumour may show I-131 increased uptake, despite a negative Tc-99m pertechnetate salivary gland scintigraphy, which may be misleading in patients investigated for thyroid carcinoma.[84] Clinicians and pathologists should consider an extraparotid Warthin's tumour in the differential diagnosis of multiple cervical masses.[79,85] Its laryngeal occurrence is rarely described.[86] Malignant transformation of Warthin's tumour is extremely rare, despite being the second most common benign tumour of the parotid gland.[87]

## Oncocytoma

Oncocytoma (oncocytic adenoma) is a rare, benign tumour composed of oncocytes (oxyphil cells). It differs from Warthin's tumour in that it is more usually unicentric, rarely cystic and contains no significant lymphocytic cell population. Its malignant counterpart is oncocytic carcinoma. The combination of oncocytomas and Warthin's tumour in the same patient has been described but is extremely rare.[88] FNA is fairly accurate in the preoperative diagnosis of Warthin's tumour. When the

lymphoid component, mucus and necrotic background are minimal or absent, the alternative diagnosis of an oncocytoma may be considered.

## Cytological findings: oncocytoma

- Oncocytic epithelial cells are more often seen in papillary fragments, acini and singly in comparison to Warthin's, where sheets of oncocytic cells are observed
- Some degree of epithelial atypia can be seen in oncocyte-predominant benign lesions.

## Diagnostic pitfalls: oncocytoma

Squamous metaplasia, especially if accompanied by atypia and necrosis, can prove challenging.[80] It is well recognised that benign oncocytic cells may exhibit a worrisome degree of nuclear atypia. Conversely, malignant oncocytes may appear deceptively monomorphic with bland nuclear features and, therefore, sometimes the best that can be attained is a diagnosis of 'oncocytic neoplasm', relaying the differential diagnosis with the caveat that malignancy cannot be excluded.

Other pitfalls include degenerate oncocytes (pyknocytes), which possess 'pseudokeratinised' orangeophilic cytoplasm masquerading as squamous cells and the problem of clear cell change. Metastatic renal, thyroid and apocrine mammary carcinoma should never be forgotten, particularly in the differential diagnosis of papillary cystic oncocytoma.[89]

Following the FNA, oncocytoma can histologically show a pseudomalignant change that mimics acinic cell carcinoma.[71]

Besides Warthin's tumour, oncocytic cells occur in mucoepidermoid carcinoma and acinic cell carcinoma.

## Sebaceous adenoma

Sebaceous adenoma and lymphadenoma are comparable with Warthin's tumour, albeit with sebaceous rather than oncocytic epithelium. Evidence of sebaceous differentiation may infrequently be seen in normal salivary parenchyma, pleomorphic adenoma, Warthin's tumour proper, myoepithelioma and mucoepidermoid carcinoma.[35] Voluminous, clear and microvacuolated cytoplasm with round, isomorphic nuclei are the hallmarks of benign sebaceous cells.

## Intraductal papilloma

Intraductal papillomas are rare, benign tumours most commonly encountered in minor salivary glands. They are cystic, solitary neoplasms that arise from ductal epithelium and produce painless swellings. They present as firm masses and are cytologically evocative of an adnexal tumour. Fluid may be aspirated.

## Cytological findings: intraductal papilloma

- Three-dimensional epithelial clusters, some with a papillary configuration
- Histiocytes
- The majority of cells show oncocytic differentiation; however, benign-appearing ductal cells in honeycomb sheets can also be present.

Awareness of the cytological features of intraductal papilloma of the salivary glands should prompt its inclusion in the differential diagnosis of papillary lesions of the head and neck.[90]

## Malignant salivary gland neoplasms

The global frequency of malignant salivary gland neoplasms ranges between 0.4 and 2.6/100 000 population.[37] In the UK, it was 0.7/100 000 population in 2004, with a mortality rate of 0.2/100 000 in 2005.[91] Between 21% and 46% of all salivary gland tumours are malignant, the incidence varying with site; 15–32% in parotid, 41–45% in submandibular, 70–90% in sublingual and 50% in minor salivary glands. Some 80–90% of intraoral salivary gland tumours are malignant.[37] Most are slow growing and present as a lump with no distinctive features. Pain, facial nerve involvement, rapid growth or associated lymphadenopathy, when present, are suggestive of malignancy. It is important to understand that cytological pleomorphism is not a feature of many malignant salivary gland tumours and that similar morphological patterns are shared by some benign and malignant tumours.

### Acinic cell carcinoma

Accounting for about 6.5% of all salivary gland tumours, 80% of acinic cell carcinomas arise in the parotid, 17% intraorally and 4% in the submandibular glands. They affect all age groups but commonly occur between the second and seventh decades. Histologically, they present varied architectural (solid/lobular, microcystic, papillary-cystic, follicular) and cellular (acinar, intercalated ductal, vacuolated, clear, non-specific glandular cell) patterns, the diagnostic feature being (at least focal) acinar cell differentiation.[37] This diversity is reflected cytologically and explains why tumours with prominent acinar differentiation are easiest to recognise.

---

**Cytological findings: acinic cell carcinoma**

- Cellular smears
- Clean background and many bare nuclei
- Loose aggregates of uniform epithelial cells.

The smear background lacks cell debris, inflammatory cells or extracellular mucin (Figs 5.12–5.14). Numerous bare nuclei are present, which are differentiated from lymphocytes by lack of a cytoplasmic rim. Fine granularity is seen in the background of tumours with prominent acinar cell differentiation. This and the bare nuclei are derived from fragile neoplastic cells. The tumour nuclei are 'bland,' round or oval and slightly larger than normal acinar nuclei but marked nuclear pleomorphism is not seen. Neoplastic cells occur in loose sheets of varying sizes that lack the well-defined, rounded outlines of normal acinar cell groups. Capillaries may be seen within cellular fragments. Moderate to abundant, finely granular/vacuolated cytoplasm is present. In tumours with prominent intercalated, ductal or non-specific glandular cells, the amount of cell cytoplasm and granularity vary, but on the whole, there is cellular uniformity. Non-specific glandular cells have scanty, finely granular cytoplasm and are arranged in multilayered cohesive clusters with indistinct cell borders.[92] Infrequent findings are lymphocytic infiltration, cystic change and oncocytic metaplasia.

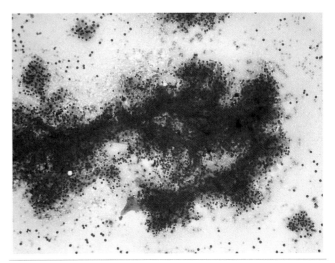

**Fig. 5.12** Acinic cell carcinoma. Loosely cohesive clusters of cells with vascular stroma in a clean background (MGG).

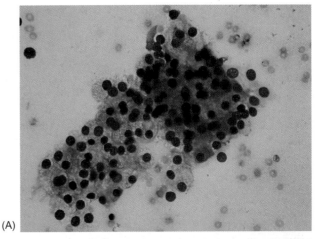

(A)

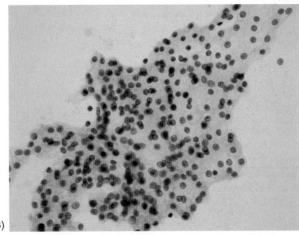

(B)

**Fig. 5.13** Acinic cell carcinoma. (A,B) Cells with acinar differentiation showing finely vacuolated cytoplasm and uniform nuclei. Note the finely granular background (MGG, PAP).

---

**Diagnostic pitfalls: acinic cell carcinoma**

Differentiation from normal salivary gland tissue: While they may be numerous, normal acinar cell groups are tightly cohesive with well-defined, rounded outlines unlike the

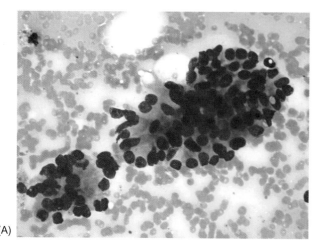

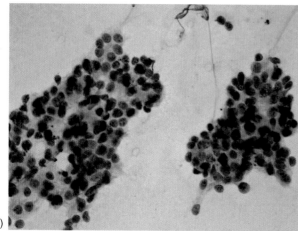

**Fig. 5.14** Acinic cell carcinoma. (A,B) Non-specific epithelia cells, where recognition as a carcinoma is easy but classification as acinic cell carcinoma difficult (MGG, PAP).

loosely structured sheets of acinic cell carcinoma. In addition, cohesive sheets of ductal cell are present, either isolated or attached to acini.

Aspirates from tumours composed predominantly of ductal or non-specific glandular cells are recognised as neoplastic and in most cases as carcinoma, but classification as acinic cell carcinoma may not be possible.[92]

Poorly differentiated or dedifferentiated variant: This is uncommon and occurs either as a primary lesion associated with differentiated acinic cell carcinoma, or as a recurrent tumour. It shows nuclear pleomorphism and is readily identified as a carcinoma; when present without classical acinic cell carcinoma, classification is difficult.

Papillary-cystic variant of acinic cell carcinoma: This variant is readily recognised histologically but its cytological diagnosis is often inaccurate.[93] The aspirates contain monolayered sheets or branching papillary clusters of uniform epithelial cells that generally lack acinar cell differentiation, set in a cystic background. They may be mistaken for a retention cyst, Warthin's tumour, mucoepidermoid carcinoma or cystadenocarcinoma.[93–95] Uniformity of epithelial cells is a useful feature but in an individual case, the diagnosis may not be apparent.

## Mucoepidermoid carcinoma

This most common salivary gland malignancy of childhood and adulthood accounts for 10–15% of all salivary gland tumours globally. Approximately half occur in major salivary glands (45% in the parotid).[37] Histologically, there is architectural and cellular heterogeneity; varying proportions of cystic and solid areas comprise mucous, intermediate and squamous cells that blend with each other. Clear and oncocytic cells occur and sometimes predominate. A commonly used three-tier grading system (low, intermediate or high grade) assesses cystic change, pleomorphism, mitoses, neural invasion and necrosis, but not the proportions of different cell types.[96]

### Cytological findings: mucoepidermoid carcinoma

- Variably cellular smears
- 'Dirty background'
- Mixture (mucous, squamous and intermediate) of epithelial cells.

Smear cellularity depends on proportion of solid or cystic areas aspirated (Figs 5.15, 5.16). The background, which variably contains mucin, evidence of cystic change (inflammatory cells, macrophages and cell debris) or necrosis, forms an important part of the diagnosis. Extracellular mucin appears pale grey on MGG and green or pink on Papanicolaou stain. The admixture of different epithelial cell types (mucous, intermediate, squamous) is a useful diagnostic feature, though their proportions vary. Mucous cells occur in cohesive sheets that show a honeycombed appearance. Their abundant cytoplasm is often finely vacuolated, with basally situated nuclei. They partially resemble endocervical cells on Papanicolaou stained smears. Squamous cells have abundant, 'plate-like' cytoplasm with variable intensity of keratin staining, best appreciated on Papanicolaou stains. They occur in small aggregates, or singly. However, prominent, widespread, single-cell keratinisation with intense cytoplasmic orangeophilia and nuclear atypia are not a feature of mucoepidermoid carcinoma (see below). Intermediate cells occur in cohesive sheets and have features in between mucous and squamous cells. They contain moderate amounts of cytoplasm and are usually the most numerous cells in an aspirate. They may show fine cytoplasmic vacuolation, which resembles that of macrophages, or contain a single mucin vacuole. Different cell types are easier to recognise in low-grade tumours. High-grade tumours with their nuclear pleomorphism can be diagnosed as a carcinoma, but classification as mucoepidermoid carcinoma may be difficult (see below). Tumour associated reactive lymphoid infiltrate may be present.

### Diagnostic pitfalls: mucoepidermoid carcinoma

Inflammatory cells and macrophages, if numerous, may mask neoplastic epithelial cells, resulting in an erroneous diagnosis of an inflammatory lesion. Intermediate cells with finely vacuolated cytoplasm may not be recognised as epithelial and be mistaken for macrophages. This difficulty arises in low-grade tumours with a large cystic component.[97]

Aspirates from high-grade tumours, recognised as a carcinoma, may be difficult to differentiate from other high-grade carcinomas such as salivary duct carcinoma and adenocarcinoma, not otherwise specified.[97] Epithelial heterogeneity, when seen, is a useful differentiating feature.

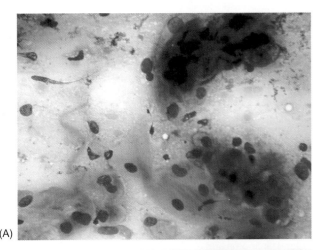

(A)

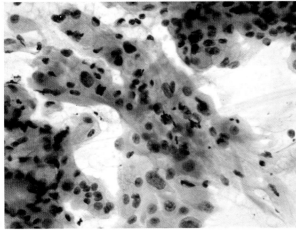

(B)

**Fig. 5.15** Mucoepidermoid carcinoma. On MGG, the squamous cells have plate-like, turquoise blue cytoplasm (A). The mucous cells contain faintly eosinophilic mucin vacuoles on Papanicolaou stain. The remaining cells represent intermediate cells and a few plate-like squamous cells are present at the periphery (B). This epithelial heterogeneity is characteristic of mucoepidermoid carcinoma (MGG, PAP).

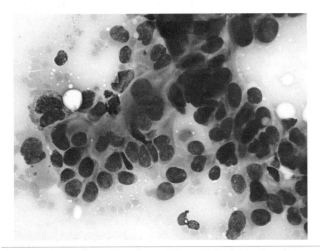

**Fig. 5.16** Mucoepidermoid carcinoma. This is a high-grade variant with nuclear atypia. There is a suggestion of squamous differentiation (MGG).

The background of mucin and cell debris along with groups of intermediate and squamous cells may be mistaken for Warthin's tumour.[98] In the latter, the oncocytic cells contain granular cytoplasm and generally show nuclear uniformity.

Apart from squamous metaplasia, other cell types are rare. A robust diagnosis of Warthin's tumour is possible when oncocytic cells, lymphocytes and cell debris are all present (see Warthin's tumour, p. 239).

Extensively keratinised malignant squamous cells are not a feature of mucoepidermoid carcinoma. When present, the possibility of squamous cell carcinoma, especially secondary involvement from an upper aerodigestive tract or lung tumour should be considered.

Rarely, aspirates from chronic sialadenitis may mimic a mucoepidermoid carcinoma. In sialadenitis, the ductal cell groups show straight edges with branching and contain scant cytoplasm with uniform nuclei. Squamous metaplasia may occur (see Chronic sialadenitis, p. 234) but epithelial heterogeneity is not seen.

## Adenoid cystic carcinoma

These comprise approximately 10% of all epithelial salivary gland tumours but 30% of epithelial minor salivary gland tumours.[37] Occurring in all age groups, they are commoner in the middle aged and elderly. Histologically, the tumours show three architectural patterns (cribriform, tubular and solid), which often coexist, and two cell types. Predominant are modified myoepithelial cells with hyperchromatic, angular nuclei and scanty, often clear cytoplasm. A smaller component of epithelial cells of columnar or cuboidal type is present. The myxoid and basement membrane-like stroma has characteristic cytological appearances, which form an important part of the diagnosis.

**Cytological findings: adenoid cystic carcinoma**

- Cellular smears
- Uniform basaloid cells
- Characteristic stroma.

The aspirates contain predominantly basaloid (myoepithelial) cells, which are present in tight clusters, rosette-like formations or adhering to globules (Figs 5.17, 5.18). Numerous dissociated tumour cells and bare nuclei are present in the background. Some cell clusters show peripheral nuclear palisading. The nuclei are usually uniform and round, oval or angular. Nuclear chromatin is dense or coarse and on Papanicolaou stained smears, small nucleoli may be seen but are never prominent. The epithelial cell component, being smaller, is difficult to identify. The stroma is characteristic and best appreciated on MGG stained smears, where it is magenta coloured (pale green or grey on Papanicolaou stain). Its commonest and widely recognised form is hyaline globules, which are often numerous and show variation in size, including large forms. They have firm, rounded edges and are surrounded by basaloid cells. Other forms of stroma comprise finger-like and membranous fragments with straight edges. A small amount of fibrillary material, similar to that seen in pleomorphic adenoma, is often present and the background (on MGG stain) contains granular, magenta coloured ground substance. Macrophages are seen with cystic degeneration. Necrosis is uncommon but may occur with the solid variant of the tumour.[99]

**Diagnostic pitfalls: adenoid cystic carcinoma**

Hyaline globules can be seen in other salivary gland tumours such as pleomorphic adenoma, basal cell neoplasms,

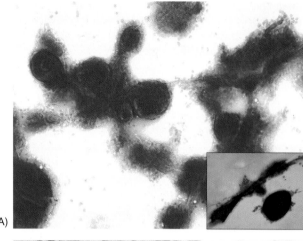

(A)

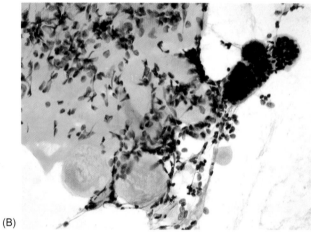

(B)

**Fig. 5.17** Adenoid cystic carcinoma. (A,B) This demonstrates the hyaline globules and finger/plate-like stromal material. Small basaloid cells are present adherent to the stroma (MGG, PAP).

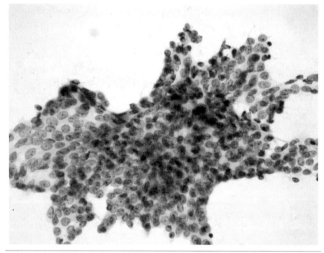

**Fig. 5.18** Adenoid cystic carcinoma. Note the uniform nuclei with granular chromatin and inconspicuous nucleoli (PAP).

epithelial-myoepithelial carcinoma and polymorphous low-grade adenocarcinoma.[99] In pleomorphic adenoma, they tend to be smaller, fewer in number and with less well-defined or 'hard' outlines. Pleomorphic adenoma contains myoepithelial cells with intact cytoplasm in the background, whereas most

of the dissociated 'cells' in adenoid cystic carcinoma are bare nuclei. In basal cell neoplasm, hyaline globules are small, less numerous and more uniform. The cells usually contain small amounts of cytoplasm and show uniform nuclear chromatin. Sometimes, a clear distinction from adenoid cystic carcinoma is not possible and in such instances, the possibility of a neoplasm with potential malignant behaviour should be raised. Hyaline globules in polymorphous low-grade adenocarcinoma (see Polymorphous low-grade adenocarcinoma, below) are small; smears are cellular and may contain papillary clusters of uniform basaloid cells and cells with moderate cytoplasm.[100] Solid variants of adenoid cystic carcinoma often lack hyaline globules and may show necrosis.

Prominent basaloid cells are a feature of cellular pleomorphic adenoma, basal cell neoplasms, polymorphous low-grade adenocarcinoma and epithelial-myoepithelial carcinoma. While differentiation from pleomorphic adenoma may be possible (fibrillary stroma and single myoepithelial cells), distinction from other entities may be difficult.

## Polymorphous low-grade adenocarcinoma

Polymorphous low-grade adenocarcinoma (PLGA) is the second most common intraoral malignant salivary gland tumour, accounting for 26% of all carcinomas. Approximately 60% involve the palate and 70% of patients are aged between 50 and 70 years.[37] Recently, cases have been reported in the parotid, either arising de-novo or as carcinoma ex-pleomorphic adenoma.[101,102] Histologically, tumours show a range of architectural patterns comprising sheets, cords, tubules, cribriform and papillary areas, composed of uniform, small- to medium-sized cells with bland appearing nuclei. Variable amounts of myxoid, hyaline or myxohyaline stroma are present.

### Cytological findings: polymorphous low-grade adenocarcinoma (Fig. 5.19)

- Cellular aspirates with branching papillary clusters and sheets of uniform cells
- Cells are basaloid or with moderate amount of cytoplasm
- The nuclei are regular, round to oval and with finely stippled chromatin
- Bare nuclei may be present
- Hyaline globules are often seen and fibrillary myxoid stromal material may be present in the background.[100]

### Diagnostic pitfalls: polymorphous low-grade adenocarcinoma

The cytological differential diagnoses of PLGA include cellular pleomorphic adenoma, basal cell neoplasms, adenoid cystic carcinoma (see Adenoid cystic carcinoma, p. 243), epithelial-myoepithelial carcinoma and papillary cystadenocarcinoma.[103] The possibility of PLGA should be considered in an intra-oral location but in an individual case, definitive diagnosis may not be possible.

## Salivary duct carcinoma

This highly aggressive adenocarcinoma is uncommon, representing 9% of salivary malignancies. Most patients present after the

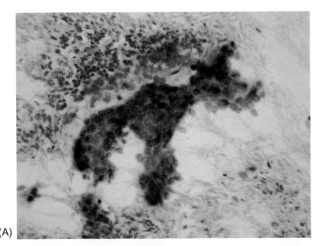

(A)

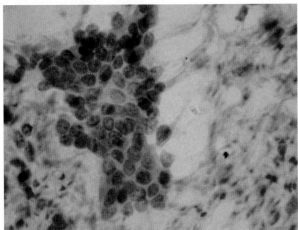

(B)

**Fig. 5.19** Polymorphous low-grade adenocarcinoma. (A,B) There are small hyaline globules that are surrounded by uniform cells with delicate cytoplasm. Bland nuclear features are seen on Papanicolaou stain (MGG, PAP). (This case was kindly provided by Dr Ivan Robinson.)

age of 50, parotid being the commonest site.[37] Histologically, it resembles high-grade intraductal and invasive breast carcinoma. Expanded duct-like structures with a cribriform proliferation of cells and central necrosis are present along with an infiltrative (tubular, papillary, solid or cribriform) component. Squamous differentiation may occur and the degree of cytological pleomorphism varies, both within and among different tumours.

- Cellular aspirates with loosely cohesive sheets of cytologically malignant epithelial cells
- Sieve-like pattern may be seen in cell sheets
- Necrosis often present in the background
- Most cells have uniform cytological features, though variation in nuclear size, coarse granular chromatin, giant nuclei and prominent nucleoli found
- Occasionally, squamous differentiation is seen.[104]

In a representative sample, the diagnosis of carcinoma is easily made. However, recognition as a salivary duct carcinoma

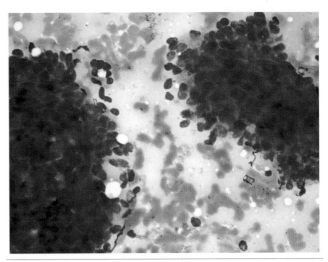

**Fig. 5.20** Salivary duct carcinoma. These cohesive cell clusters show cellular pleomorphism. This appearance is however, not specific for salivary duct carcinoma (MGG).

or differentiation from other high-grade carcinomas (mucoepidermoid carcinoma, adenocarcinoma not otherwise specified or metastatic carcinoma) may not be possible.[105]

## Carcinoma ex-pleomorphic adenoma

This refers to malignant transformation occurring within a longstanding pleomorphic adenoma. It is uncommon (approximately 3.6% of all salivary gland tumours; 12% of all salivary malignancies) and usually presents in the sixth or seventh decade.[37] Carcinoma is most frequently poorly differentiated adenocarcinoma, although any form of carcinoma may be found. Residual, benign pleomorphic adenoma must be identified in order to make this diagnosis.

- Smears are moderately to highly cellular
- Both benign (pleomorphic adenoma) and malignant (carcinomatous) elements are present, the former usually identified by its fibrillary, metachromatic stroma
- Malignant epithelial cells occur as discohesive sheets, adenoid or papilloid clusters, or as dissociated cells[106]
- Nuclear changes of malignancy are well established
- Occasionally, features of a mucoepidermoid carcinoma or other differentiated salivary gland carcinoma are seen.

This diagnosis is dependent on adequate sampling. The presence of carcinomatous elements alone, while not accurately classifying the tumour, would not affect clinical management, but diagnosis of the benign component alone would. In a pleomorphic adenoma with a long history or a sudden change in size, smears should be carefully assessed to identify malignant transformation. Benign pleomorphic adenoma can show atypia of myoepithelial cells, but this is never severe (see Pleomorphic adenoma, p. 236). The diagnosis of carcinoma ex-pleomorphic

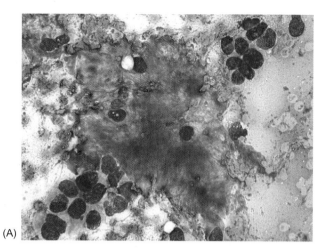

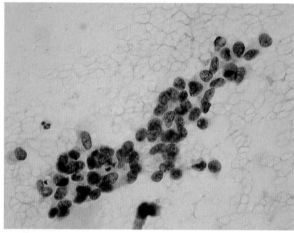

**Fig. 5.21** Carcinoma ex-pleomorphic adenoma. (A,B) The fibrillary matrix is best seen on MGG. Note the pleomorphic nuclei in the cells, which is more than would be acceptable for atypical myoepithelial cells in pleomorphic adenoma (MGG, PAP).

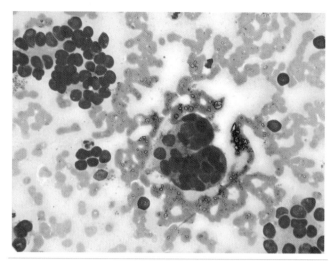

**Fig. 5.22** Epithelial-myoepithelial carcinoma. Single groups of epithelial cells surrounded by basaloid myoepithelial cells (MGG).

- Myoepithelial cells may appear as small, bland basaloid cells or as larger cells with pale, fragile cytoplasm. The latter can show variable nuclear atypia
- Single cells and bare nuclei are often a prominent feature
- A biphasic population may not always be present and myoepithelial cells may predominate
- Variable amounts of stroma, in the form of hyaline globules or chondromyxoid stroma, is present.[103,107]

### Diagnostic pitfalls: epithelial-myoepithelial carcinoma

While aspirates would be recognised as representing a salivary gland tumour, possibly malignant, differentiation from PLGA (see Polymorphous low-grade adenocarcinoma, p. 244), acinic cell carcinoma (see Acinic cell carcinoma, above) or metastatic renal cell carcinoma can be difficult. In addition, some cytological features are similar to those seen in cellular pleomorphic adenoma (see Pleomorphic adenoma, above).[103,107] In an aspirate that lacks characteristic cytological features of other common neoplasms, the possibility of epithelial-myoepithelial carcinoma may be considered.

## Lymphoid neoplasms

Lymphomas account for 1.7–7.7% of malignancies of major salivary glands.[108] Most non-Hodgkin lymphomas occurring in the salivary glands are B-cell lymphomas. Extranodal marginal zone B-cell lymphoma of MALT type is probably the most common type of primary salivary gland lymphoma; diffuse large B-cell lymphomas account for about 15% of salivary non-Hodgkin lymphoma. Anaplastic large cell lymphoma, peripheral T-cell lymphoma unspecified and extranodal NK/T cell lymphoma of nasal type can also affect the salivary glands. Involvement by Hodgkin lymphoma is very rare.[37]

Morphologically, high-grade lymphoma is easier to recognise while low-grade forms are difficult to differentiate from autoimmune lymphoepithelial sialadenitis (see Myoepithelial sialadenitis (MESA), p. 234). In this condition, there is an increased risk (44 times greater than the general population) of developing lymphoma.[108] Flow-cytometry, immunocytochemisty or tissue biopsy may be necessary to differentiate between

adenoma should only be made in the presence of unequivocal cytological features of malignancy.

## Epithelial-myoepithelial carcinoma

Representing 1% of salivary gland tumours, 60% occur in the parotid, with a peak incidence in the sixth and seventh decades. Histologically, this lobulated tumour contains characteristic, bi-layered duct-like structures with an inner layer of a single row of cuboidal cells surrounded by outer, single or multiple layers of polygonal cells with well-defined cytoplasm. The outer layer cells often show cytoplasmic clearing and stain with myoepithelial markers. Strands of eosinophilic, basement membrane-like stroma surround these structures. Some tumour lobules are composed of clear cells only and papillary-cystic foci may be present.[37]

### Cytological findings: epithelial-myoepithelial carcinoma (Fig. 5.22)

- The aspirates tend to be cellular
- Cells occur singly and in multilayered clusters
- The epithelial cells may form cohesive sheets or tubular structures and contain round, bland nuclei with scanty, well-defined cytoplasm

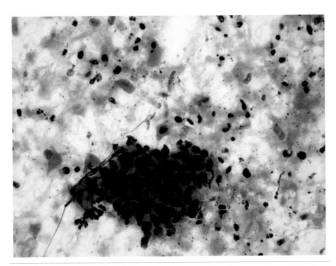

**Fig. 5.23** Metastatic squamous cell carcinoma. This degree of keratinisation is a feature of squamous cell carcinoma and not mucoepidermoid carcinoma (PAP).

reactive and neoplastic lymphoid infiltration. For a detailed description on cytomorphology of lymphoid neoplasms, please refer to Chapter 13.

## Other primary malignant tumours

### Squamous cell carcinoma (Fig. 5.23)

Primary squamous cell carcinoma of the salivary glands is rare (<1% of salivary gland tumours).[37] Numerous small, keratinised malignant cells and keratinous debris are often present and in a head and neck mass, cytological detection of squamous cell carcinoma warrants exclusion of metastatic disease from an upper aerodigestive tract or lung tumour.

### Basal cell adenocarcinoma

The differentiation of basal cell adenocarcinoma from a basal cell adenoma is histological and based on infiltration of surrounding tissue and nerves. The cytological findings in both entities are similar and as it is not possible to differentiate between the two, the term 'basal cell neoplasm' is used (see Basal cell adenoma, p. 238).

### Myoepithelial carcinoma

Most (75%) of these uncommon tumours occur in the parotid and are composed almost exclusively of cells with myoepithelial differentiation.[37] Cytologically, they may show a predominance of plasmacytoid, spindle or epithelioid cells, or a mixture of these cell types. Nuclear pleomorphism, coarse nuclear chromatin and prominent nucleoli are present in high-grade lesions, but may not be seen in all cases. In the latter instance, differentiation from a benign myoepithelioma may not be possible (see Myoepithelioma, p. 238).[109,110] Metastatic malignant melanoma remains an important differential diagnosis of cytologically malignant lesions.

### Other primary malignant tumours

These are uncommon and isolated case reports of their cytological features are present in the literature. It is beyond the scope of this chapter to cover all entities; however, recognition of a lesion as cytologically malignant is of clinical value (see Role of FNA in the management of salivary gland lesions, below). In cases of high-grade, poorly-differentiated or undifferentiated carcinoma, the possibility of metastatic disease should be considered.

## Secondary tumours

These comprise about 5% of all malignant tumours of salivary gland; the majority of cases are squamous cell carcinoma with melanoma second in frequency. Primary sites are frequently the upper and middle parts of the facial region (including skin, mucous membrane, deep soft tissues, eyes and ears). About 10% originate from distant sites such as lung (especially small cell carcinoma), kidney and breast. About 10% of tumours remain undefined as to their origin.[37]

## Role of FNA in the management of salivary gland lesions

The main goal of FNA of salivary gland lesions is to assist the clinician in the management of patients who present with a mass lesion. Cytological examination aims to determine if a process is of salivary or non-salivary origin, whether inflammatory and/or reactive, if neoplastic, whether benign or malignant, and if possible to render a specific diagnosis. The salivary glands are unique in their histological complexity and morphological variability of tumours, which is reflected in the cytological material. In addition to the overlapping morphological patterns of salivary gland tumours, they also represent relatively rare lesions, thus making it more difficult to acquire diagnostic expertise in FNA cytology. While almost all neoplastic salivary gland lesions will undergo surgical excision, knowing beforehand if a lesion is malignant or benign will aid in planning appropriate surgery and may prompt or postpone surgical intervention. A definitive diagnosis of a benign tumour would help determine mode of surgery (superficial parotidectomy for pleomorphic adenoma or enucleation for other tumours with lower potential for recurrence).[111]

In patients who are not undergoing surgery, FNA confirms both, benign and malignant disease, the latter in those unsuitable for attempted curative surgery or with recurrent disease prior to palliative treatment.[112] Overall, FNA can reduce the rate of salivary gland surgery by one-third to one-half.[113,114] In patients undergoing radical surgery, preoperative FNA determines the degree of urgency and helps plan the surgical approach, particularly in respect of the decision to preserve or sacrifice the facial nerve. Importantly, a preoperative diagnosis allows for counselling of the patient prior to surgery.

## Diagnostic accuracy

As will be appreciated by reading this text, FNA of the salivary glands presents many problems for the cytopathologist (Table 5.1) for differential diagnosis based on cellular morphology, but with experience and good team work, sensitivity and specificity are high. FNA series with good clinical and histological correlation indicate specificity as high as 94–100%

**Table 5.1** Common diagnoses based on type of salivary gland aspirate

| Type of aspirate | Non-neoplastic | | | Neoplastic | |
| --- | --- | --- | --- | --- | --- |
| | **Normal** | **Pathological** | **Benign** | **Malignant** | |
| Solid | Intraparotid lymph node | Sialadenosis | See Benign neoplasms | See Malignant neoplasms | |
| | Normal gland (lesion missed) | Sialadenitis | | | |
| Cystic | – | Retention cyst/mucocele | Warthin's tumour | Mucoepidermoid carcinoma | |
| Lymphoid | Intraparotid lymph node | Sialadenitis | Warthin's tumour | Reactive lymphoid infiltrate in primary salivary gland carcinoma | |
| | | | | Lymphoma | |
| Clean background | Normal gland | Sialadenosis | Basal cell neoplasms | Acinic cell carcinoma | |
| | | | | Adenoid cystic carcinoma | |
| Dirty background | – | Sialadenitis | Warthin's tumour | Mucoepidermoid carcinoma | |

and sensitivity of 81–100%.[1,3,6,9,18,48,49,55,77,78,82,98,111,112,115–139] When considered from the viewpoint of type-specific diagnostic accuracy of tumours the figure is approximately 80% and is better for benign than malignant neoplasms. Accuracy in diagnosis of pleomorphic adenoma is invariably high, which is important since this is by far the commonest FNA finding in routine practice. The diagnostic accuracy of ThinPrep LBC- (Cytyc Corporation, Marlborough, MA, USA) processed salivary gland FNA approaches that of the direct smears. However, there are several artifacts, such as diminished/distorted extracellular and stromal elements, cellular shrinkage and tissue fragmentation, that may lead to erroneous diagnoses.[116]

Causes of false negative and false positive errors and diagnostic problems have been reviewed in several papers. False negative results are generally due to unrepresentative sampling, especially from cystic tumours, and false positive reports from failure to appreciate the difficulties associated with pleomorphic adenoma and basal cell adenoma. Diagnostic problems in general are discussed by Young, and MacLeod and Frable.[140–142] They conclude that successful FNAC of the salivary glands depends on the recognition of the problem lesions.[141] Therefore, there are cases where a differential diagnosis is more appropriate than a definitive one and cytopathologists should use it remembering the dictum; 'Pathologists would be more accurate if they were less precise'. Despite this cautionary note, FNA of the salivary glands is an accurate, safe and clinically helpful technique.

## Approach to salivary gland cytology

Salivary gland cytology is useful in differentiating, first, salivary from non-salivary lesions, second, neoplastic from non-neoplastic lesions and, third, benign from malignant lesions. Specific diagnosis, while helpful, is not always essential.[134] Approached in a stepwise, logical manner, cytological assessment will ensure a satisfactory clinical outcome.[119,134]

When faced with interpreting a salivary gland FNA, we suggest the following approach:

- Is the aspirate from a salivary gland?
  - The commonest sites of salivary gland enlargement, parotid and submandibular regions, also contain lymph

nodes. An oncocytic neoplasm with lymphoid cells could represent a Warthin's tumour or a metastatic papillary thyroid carcinoma, to use one example. Masses related to skin (adnexal tumours) and soft tissue (nodular fasciitis, schwannoma) may mimic a salivary gland neoplasm, both clinically and cytologically.

- Is the aspirate diagnostic?
  - Sparsely cellular aspirates may contain enough diagnostic material, while cellular, but poorly spread smears may not be assessable or at worst, result in an incorrect diagnosis
  - Representative material may not be aspirated; small tumours could be missed on needling and only benign salivary gland tissue obtained. Clinical correlation is important in such cases
  - It is difficult to classify a cystic lesion when only cellular debris and macrophages are present. In such 'cystic lesions of uncertain pathogenesis,' absence of malignant cells does not exclude malignancy. Aspiration of a residual mass would help arrive at a specific diagnosis, as would correlation with clinical and imaging findings.

- Is it a non-neoplastic condition?
  - A well-defined mass could represent a reactive (intraparotid) lymph node, sialadenitis (chronic or granulomatous) or a specific cystic lesion
  - In diffuse salivary gland enlargement, cytology is of limited value but lymphoid infiltration or sialadenosis may be identified. Clinical correlation is important to establish a diagnosis in such cases.

- Does the aspirate contain cells from a neoplasm?
  - Basaloid cells: Consider cellular pleomorphic adenoma, basal cell neoplasm, adenoid cystic carcinoma, polymorphous low-grade adenocarcinoma and epithelial myoepithelial carcinoma
  - Squamous cells with little atypia: Consider chronic sialadenitis, pleomorphic adenoma, Warthin's tumour and mucoepidermoid carcinoma
  - Squamous cells with significant atypia: Consider mucoepidermoid and squamous cell carcinoma, primary or secondary
  - Oncocytic cells: Consider oncocytosis, Warthin's tumour, oncocytic neoplasm, mucoepidermoid carcinoma and acinic cell carcinoma

- Spindle cells: Consider pleomorphic adenoma, myoepithelioma, schwannoma, granulation tissue,[143] nodular fasciitis[44] and metastatic malignant melanoma.
- Is there cytological pleomorphism?
  - Consider high-grade mucoepidermoid carcinoma, salivary duct carcinoma, adenocarcinoma NOS, metastatic carcinoma, melanoma. Malignant salivary gland tumours such as acinic cell carcinoma, adenoid cystic carcinoma, low-grade mucoepidermoid carcinoma and polymorphous low-grade adenocarcinoma generally do not show cellular pleomorphism.
- What are the non-epithelial components?
  - Is stromal material present? Assess the type of stromal material (fibrillary, hyaline globules, etc.) and consider pleomorphic adenoma, adenoid cystic carcinoma, basal cell neoplasms, epithelial-myoepithelial carcinoma and polymorphous low-grade adenocarcinoma
  - What is the background like? Aspirates from acinic cell carcinoma have a clean background. Metachromatic, granular ground substance is present in pleomorphic adenoma, adenoid cystic carcinoma, epithelial myoepithelial carcinoma and basal cell neoplasms. Mucin is seen in mucoepidermoid carcinoma and some cases of Warthin's tumour have a mucoid background. Cystic change is present in Warthin's tumour and mucoepidermoid carcinoma. Less commonly, it occurs in pleomorphic adenoma, adenoid cystic carcinoma and acinic cell carcinoma
  - Is there a lymphoid infiltrate in the background? A reactive lymphoid infiltrate is an integral part of Warthin's tumour and sebaceous adenoma. Tumour associated lymphoid infiltration can occur in acinic cell carcinoma, mucoepidermoid carcinoma and non Hodgkin lymphoma.
- Can a specific diagnosis of a salivary gland neoplasm be made?
  - This is an important part of the examination, as not only does it influence management, it establishes the clinician's confidence in the test and the cytopathologist. However, given the morphological overlap between many salivary gland tumours, this confidence should not be put to the test unless characteristic cytological features are present and there is a high degree of clinical-radiological and pathological correlation. Otherwise, an indication that the cytological features are not characteristic of a single neoplasm is of greater clinical value.
- If a specific diagnosis is not possible, what differential diagnoses can be offered?
  - Pleomorphic adenoma is the commonest salivary gland tumour and its diagnosis is straightforward when characteristic features are present. However, it can show considerable morphological variation and may resemble other neoplasms cytologically. When so, this should be conveyed in the report and possible diagnoses listed
  - As malignant salivary gland tumours do not always show cellular pleomorphism, the cytology report could include differential diagnoses of both benign and malignant entities (e.g. basal cell neoplasm or adenoid cystic carcinoma). Such cases should be brought to the attention of a multidisciplinary team and discussed in the light of all available findings
  - Aspirates with malignant 'small round blue cells' can originate from lymphoma, small cell carcinoma, Merkel cell carcinoma, rhabdomyosarcoma, melanoma or other undifferentiated tumours. Morphologically, a diagnosis of malignancy is all that may be possible. Close correlation with clinical and radiological findings is necessary. When possible, immunocytochemistry should be carried out on additional material
  - In aspirates with 'small lymphoid cells,' differentiation of benign lymphoepithelial sialadenitis from a low-grade non-Hodgkin lymphoma requires additional investigations (flow cytometry, PCR, FISH, immunocytochemistry or a tissue biopsy).
- When making management decisions, should the clinicians rely on the FNA report alone?
  - While the experience of the cytopathologist is a critical factor, as in other spheres of medicine, cytologically complex and potentially malignant salivary gland lesions should be discussed at the multidisciplinary meetings along with the clinical and radiological findings. In this setting, the cytopathologist can alert the team of any potential pitfalls of morphological diagnosis.

## REFERENCES

1. Righi A, Foschini MP. Values and limits in fine needle aspiration in the diagnosis of Warthin tumour of the parotid gland. Pathologica 2006;98:635–39.

2. Chhieng DC, Argosino R, McKenna BJ, et al. Utility of fine-needle aspiration in the diagnosis of salivary gland lesions in patients infected with human immunodeficiency virus. Diagn Cytopathol 1999;21:260–64.

3. Robinson IA, Cozens NJ. Does a joint ultrasound guided cytology clinic optimize the cytological evaluation of head and neck masses? Clin Radiol 1999;54:312–16.

4. Gerber C, Zimmer G, Linder T, et al. Primary pleomorphic adenoma of the external auditory canal diagnosed by fine needle aspiration cytology. A case report. Acta Cytol 1999;43:489–91.

5. Ashraf MJ, Azarpira N, Khademi B. Diagnosis of pleomorphic adenoma in a heterotopic salivary gland: a case report. Acta Cytol 2007;51:197–99.

6. Edwards PC, Wasserman P. Evaluation of cystic salivary gland lesions by fine needle aspiration: an analysis of 21 cases. Acta Cytol 2005;49:489–94.

7. Henry CR, Nace M, Helm KF. Collagenous spherulosis in an oral mucous cyst. J Cutan Pathol 2008;35:428–30.

8. Closmann JJ, Torske KR. When a mucocele is not a mucocele: adenocarcinoma NOS. A case report and review of the literature. Gen Dent 2007;55:325–27.

9. Michelow P, Meyers T, Dubb M, Wright C. The utility of fine needle aspiration in HIV positive children. Cytopathology 2008;19:86–93.

10. Vicandi B, Jimenez-Heffernan JA, Lopez-Ferrer P, et al. HIV-1 (p24)-positive multinucleated giant cells in HIV-associated lymphoepithelial lesion of the parotid gland. A report of two cases. Acta Cytol 1999;43:247–51.

11. Lopez-Rios F, Ballestin C, Martinez-Gonzalez MA, et al. Lymphoepithelial cyst with

crystalloid formation. Cytologic features of two cases. Acta Cytol 1999;43:277–80.

12. Varnholt H, Thompson L, Pantanowitz L. Salivary gland lymphoepithelial cysts. Ear Nose Throat J 2007;86:265.

13. Wax TD, Layfield LJ, Zaleski S, et al. Cytomegalovirus sialadenitis in patients with the acquired immunodeficiency syndrome: a potential diagnostic pitfall with fine-needle aspiration cytology. Diagn Cytopathol 1994;10:169–72. discussion 72–74.

14. Kitagawa S, Zen Y, Harada K, et al. Abundant IgG4-positive plasma cell infiltration characterizes chronic sclerosing sialadenitis (Kuttner's tumor). Am J Surg Pathol 2005;29:783–91.

15. Saenz-Santamaria J, Catalina-Fernandez I, Fernandez-Mera JJ. Sialadenitis with crystalloid formation. Fine needle aspiration cytodiagnosis of 15 cases. Acta Cytol 2003;47:1–4.

16. Gupta RK, Green C, Fauck R, et al. Fine needle aspiration cytodiagnosis of sialadenitis with crystalloids. Acta Cytol 1999;43:390–92.

17. Nasuti JF, Gupta PK, Fleisher SR, et al. Nontyrosine crystalloids in salivary gland lesions: report of seven cases with fine-needle aspiration cytology and follow-up surgical pathology. Diagn Cytopathol 2000;22:167–71.

18. Stewart CJ, MacKenzie K, McGarry GW, et al. Fine-needle aspiration cytology of salivary gland: a review of 341 cases. Diagn Cytopathol 2000;22:139–46.

19. Chai C, Dodd LG, Glasgow BJ, et al. Salivary gland lesions with a prominent lymphoid component: cytologic findings and differential diagnosis by fine-needle aspiration biopsy. Diagn Cytopathol 1997;17:183–90.

20. Allen EA, Ali SZ, Mathew S. Lymphoid lesions of the parotid. Diagn Cytopathol 1999;21:170–73.

21. Cha I, Long SR, Ljung BM, et al. Low-grade lymphoma of mucosa-associated tissue in the parotid gland: a case report of fine-needle aspiration cytology diagnosis using flow cytometric immunophenotyping. Diagn Cytopathol 1997;16:345–49.

22. Kojima M, Nakamura S, Itoh H, et al. Kuttner's tumor of salivary glands resembling marginal zone B-cell lymphoma of the MALT type: a histopathologic and immunohistochemical study of 7 cases. Int J Surg Pathol 2004;12:389–93.

23. Ascoli V, Albedi FM, De Blasiis R, et al. Sialadenosis of the parotid gland: report of four cases diagnosed by fine needle aspiration cytology. Diagn Cytopathol 1993;9:151–55.

24. Bharadwaj G, Nawroz I, O'Regan B. Sclerosing polycystic adenosis of the parotid gland. Br J Oral Maxillofac Surg 2007;45:74–76.

25. Etit D, Pilch BZ, Osgood R, et al. Fine-needle aspiration biopsy findings in sclerosing polycystic adenosis of the parotid gland. Diagn Cytopathol 2007;35:444–47.

26. Imamura Y, Morishita T, Kawakami M, et al. Sclerosing polycystic adenosis of the left parotid gland: report of a case with fine needle aspiration cytology. Acta Cytol 2004;48:569–73.

27. Chen YK, Lin CC, Lin LM, et al. Adenomatoid hyperplasia in the mandibular retromolar area. Case report. Aust Dent J 1999;44:135–36.

28. Luna MA. Salivary gland hyperplasia. Adv Anat Pathol 2002;9:251–55.

29. Shimoyama T, Wakabayashi M, Kato T, et al. Adenomatoid hyperplasia of the palate mimicking clinically as a salivary gland tumor. J Oral Sci 2001;43:135–38.

30. Alos L, Cardesa A, Bombi JA, et al. Myoepithelial tumors of salivary glands: a

clinicopathologic, immunohistochemical, ultrastructural, and flow-cytometric study. Semin Diagn Pathol 1996;13:138–47.

31. Haskell HD, Butt KM, Woo SB. Pleomorphic adenoma with extensive lipometaplasia: report of three cases. Am J Surg Pathol 2005;29:1389–93.

32. Ide F, Kusama K. Myxolipomatous pleomorphic adenoma: an unusual oral presentation. J Oral Pathol Med 2004;33:53–55.

33. Kern MA, Kasper HU, Drebber U, et al. Report of a spindle cell myoepithelialioma of the minor salivary glands with extensive lipomatous component. Laryngorhinootologie 2005;84:432–35.

34. Seifert G, Donath K, Schafer R. Lipomatous pleomorphic adenoma of the parotid gland. Classification of lipomatous tissue in salivary glands. Pathol Res Pract 1999;195:247–52.

35. Skalova A, Starek I, Simpson RH, et al. Spindle cell myoepithelial tumours of the parotid gland with extensive lipomatous metaplasia. A report of four cases with immunohistochemical and ultrastructural findings. Virchows Arch 2001;439:762–67.

36. Behzatoglu K, Bahadir B, Huq GE, et al. Spontaneous infarction of a pleomorphic adenoma in parotid gland: diagnostic problems and review. Diagn Cytopathol 2005;32:367–69.

37. Barnes L, Eveson JW, Reichart P, et al. Pathology & Genetics: Head and Neck Tumours, WHO Blue Book Series. Geneva: WHO; 2005 9.

38. Keldahl ML, Zarif A, Gattuso P. Bilateral synchronous pleomorphic adenoma diagnosed by fine-needle aspiration. Diagn Cytopathol 2004;30:356–58.

39. Das DK, Anim JT. Pleomorphic adenoma of salivary gland: to what extent does fine needle aspiration cytology reflect histopathological features? Cytopathology 2005;16:65–70.

40. Sugihara K, Hirokawa M, Shimizu M, et al. Collagenous crystalloids in a fine needle aspirate of a pleomorphic adenoma of the minor salivary gland. A case report. Acta Cytol 1998;42:751–53.

41. Takeshita T, Tanaka H, Harasawa A, et al. Benign pleomorphic adenoma with extensive cystic degeneration: unusual MR findings in two cases. Radiat Med 2004;22:357–61.

42. Steele NP, Wenig BM, Sessions RB. A case of pleomorphic adenoma of the parotid gland metastasizing to a mediastinal lymph node. Am J Otolaryngol 2007;28:130–33.

43. Pitman MB, Thor AD, Goodman ML, et al. Benign metastasizing pleomorphic adenoma of salivary gland: diagnosis of bone lesions by fine-needle aspiration biopsy. Diagn Cytopathol 1992;8:384–87.

44. Saad RS, Takei H, Lipscomb J, et al. Nodular fasciitis of parotid region: a pitfall in the diagnosis of pleomorphic adenomas on fine-needle aspiration cytology. Diagn Cytopathol 2005;33:191–94.

45. Kapila K, Mathur S, Verma K. Schwannomas: a pitfall in the diagnosis of pleomorphic adenomas on fine-needle aspiration cytology. Diagn Cytopathol 2002;27:53–59.

46. Domanski HA. Intravenous pyogenic granuloma mimicking pleomorphic adenoma in a fine needle aspirate. A case report. Acta Cytol 1999;43:439–41.

47. Klijanienko J, Vielh P. Fine-needle sampling of salivary gland lesions. I. Cytology and histology correlation of 412 cases of pleomorphic adenoma. Diagn Cytopathol 1996;14:195–200.

48. Viguer JM, Vicandi B, Jimenez-Heffernan JA, et al. Fine needle aspiration cytology of pleomorphic adenoma. An analysis of 212 cases. Acta Cytol 1997;41:786–94.

49. Cerulli G, Renzi G, Perugini M, et al. Differential diagnosis between adenoid cystic carcinoma and pleomorphic adenoma of the minor salivary glands of palate. J Craniofac Surg 2004;15:1056–60.

50. Yang GC, Waisman J. Distinguishing adenoid cystic carcinoma from cylindromatous adenomas in salivary fine-needle aspirates: the cytologic clues and their ultrastructural basis. Diagn Cytopathol 2006;34:284–88.

51. Brachtel EF, Pilch BZ, Khettry U, et al. Fine-needle aspiration biopsy of a cystic pleomorphic adenoma with extensive adnexa-like differentiation: differential diagnostic pitfall with mucoepidermoid carcinoma. Diagn Cytopathol 2003;28:100–3.

52. Su CC, Chou CW, Yiu CY. Neck mass with marked squamous metaplasia: a diagnostic pitfall in aspiration cytology. J Oral Pathol Med 2008;37:56–58.

53. Mooney EE, Dodd LG, Layfield LJ. Squamous cells in fine-needle aspiration biopsies of salivary gland lesions: potential pitfalls in cytologic diagnosis. Diagn Cytopathol 1996;15:447–52.

54. Siddiqui NH, Wu SJ. Fine-needle aspiration biopsy of cystic pleomorphic adenoma with adnexa-like differentiation mimicking mucoepidermoid carcinoma: a case report. Diagn Cytopathol 2005;32:229–32.

55. Viguer JM, Jimenez-Heffernan JA, Vicandi B, et al. Cytologic diagnostic accuracy in pleomorphic adenoma of the salivary glands during 2 periods. A comparative analysis. Acta Cytol 2007;51:16–20.

56. Elsheikh TM, Bernacki EG. Fine needle aspiration cytology of cellular pleomorphic adenoma. Acta Cytol 1996;40:1165–75.

57. Ramdall RB, Cai G, Levine PH, et al. Fine-needle aspiration biopsy findings in epithelioid myoepithelioma of the parotid gland: a case report. Diagn Cytopathol 2006;34:776–79.

58. Bakshi J, Parida PK, Mahesha V, et al. Plasmacytoid myoepithelioma of palate: three rare cases and literature review. J Laryngol Otol 2007;121:e13.

59. Das DK, Haji BE, Ahmed MS, et al. Myoepithelioma of the parotid gland initially diagnosed by fine needle aspiration cytology and immunocytochemistry: a case report. Acta Cytol 2005;49:65–70.

60. De Las Casas LE, Hoerl HD, Oberley TD, et al. Myoepithelioma presenting as a midline cystic tongue lesion: cytology, histology, ancillary studies, and differential diagnosis. Diagn Cytopathol 2001;24:403–7.

61. DiPalma S, Alasio L, Pilotti S. Fine needle aspiration (FNA) appearances of malignant myoepithelioma of the parotid gland. Cytopathology 1996;7:357–65.

62. Dodd LG, Caraway NP, Luna MA, et al. Myoepithelioma of the parotid. Report of a case initially examined by fine needle aspiration biopsy. Acta Cytol 1994;38:417–21.

63. Kumar PV, Sobhani SA, Monabati A, et al. Myoepithelioma of the salivary glands. Fine needle aspiration biopsy findings. Acta Cytol 2004;48:302–8.

64. Ozcan C, Apa DD, Vayisoglu Y, et al. Unilateral parotid gland involvement with synchronous multiple basal cell adenomas. J Craniofac Surg 2007;18:1470–73.

65. Hara H, Oyama T, Saku T. Fine needle aspiration cytology of basal cell adenoma of the salivary gland. Acta Cytol 2007;51:685–91.

66. Stanley MW, Horwitz CA, Rollins SD, et al. Basal cell (monomorphic) and minimally pleomorphic adenomas of the salivary glands. Distinction from the solid (anaplastic) type

of adenoid cystic carcinoma in fine-needle aspiration. Am J Clin Pathol 1996;106:35–41.

67. Cennamo A, Falsetto A, Gallo G, et al. Warthin's tumour in the parotid gland (an inflammatory or a neoplastic disease?). Chir Ital 2000;52:361–67.

68. Maiorano E, Lo Muzio L, Favia G, et al. Warthin's tumour: a study of 78 cases with emphasis on bilaterality, multifocality and association with other malignancies. Oral Oncol 2002;38:35–40.

69. Bahar G, Dudkiewicz M, Feinmesser R, et al. Acute parotitis as a complication of fine-needle aspiration in Warthin's tumor. A unique finding of a 3-year experience with parotid tumor aspiration. Otolaryngol Head Neck Surg 2006;134:646–49.

70. Di Palma S, Simpson RH, Skalova A, et al. Metaplastic (infarcted) Warthin's tumour of the parotid gland: a possible consequence of fine needle aspiration biopsy. Histopathology 1999;35:432–38.

71. Skalova A, Starek I, Michal M, et al. Malignancy-simulating change in parotid gland oncocytoma following fine needle aspiration. Report of 3 cases. Pathol Res Pract 1999;195:399–405.

72. Klijanienko J, Vielh P. Fine-needle sampling of salivary gland lesions. II. Cytology and histology correlation of 71 cases of Warthin's tumor (adenolymphoma). Diagn Cytopathol 1997;16:221–25.

73. Jung SM, Hao SP. Warthin's tumor with multiple granulomas: a clinicopathologic study of six cases. Diagn Cytopathol 2006;34:564–67.

74. Flezar M, Pogacnik A. Warthin's tumour: unusual vs. common morphological findings in fine needle aspiration biopsies. Cytopathology 2002;13:232–41.

75. Gilcrease MZ, Nelson FS, Guzman-Paz M. Tyrosine-rich crystals associated with oncocytic salivary gland neoplasms. Arch Pathol Lab Med 1998;122:644–49.

76. Henke AC, Cooley ML, Hughes JH, et al. Fine-needle aspiration cytology of lymphangioma of the parotid gland in an adult. Diagn Cytopathol 2001;24:126–28.

77. Layfield LJ, Gopez EV. Cystic lesions of the salivary glands: cytologic features in fine-needle aspiration biopsies. Diagn Cytopathol 2002;27:197–204.

78. Raymond MR, Yoo JH, Heathcote JG, et al. Accuracy of fine-needle aspiration biopsy for Warthin's tumours. J Otolaryngol 2002;31:263–70.

79. Chae SW, Sohn JH, Shin HS, et al. Unilateral, multicentric Warthin's tumor mimicking a tumor metastatic to a lymph node. A case report. Acta Cytol 2004;48:229–33.

80. Verma K, Kapila K. Salivary gland tumors with a prominent oncocytic component. Cytologic findings and differential diagnosis of oncocytomas and Warthin's tumor on fine needle aspirates. Acta Cytol 2003;47:221–26.

81. Ballo MS, Shin HJ, Sneige N. Sources of diagnostic error in the fine-needle aspiration diagnosis of Warthin's tumor and clues to a correct diagnosis. Diagn Cytopathol 1997;17:230–34.

82. Parwani AV, Ali SZ. Diagnostic accuracy and pitfalls in fine-needle aspiration interpretation of Warthin tumor. Cancer 2003;99:166–71.

83. Goonewardene SA, Nasuti JF. Value of mucin detection in distinguishing mucoepidermoid carcinoma from Warthin's tumor on fine needle aspiration. Acta Cytol 2002;46:704–8.

84. Caglar M, Tuncel M, Usubutun A. Increased uptake on I-131 whole-body scintigraphy in Warthin tumor despite false-negative Tc-99m pertechnetate salivary gland scintigraphy. Clin Nucl Med 2003;28:945–46.

85. Wang MC, Tsai TL, Chen PC, et al. Extraparotid Warthin's tumor presented as a neck mass. J Chin Med Assoc 2003;66:752–54.

86. Jordan J, Babinski D, Sova J. Adenolymphoma (Warthin's tumor) of the larynx: coexistence with the bilateral laryngocele. Contribution to differential diagnosis with oncocytic papillary cystadenoma. Otolaryngol Pol 1999;53:213–16.

87. Yamada S, Matsuo T, Fujita S, et al. Mucoepidermoid carcinoma arising in Warthin's tumor of the parotid gland. Pathol Int 2002;52:653–56.

88. Araki Y, Sakaguchi R. Synchronous oncocytoma and Warthin's tumor in the ipsilateral parotid gland. Auris Nasus Larynx 2004;31:73–78.

89. Wackym PA, Gray GF Jr., Rosenfeld L, et al. Papillary cystic oncocytoma and Warthin's tumor of the parotid gland. J Laryngol Otol 1986;100:679–86.

90. Soofer SB, Tabbara S. Intraductal papilloma of the salivary gland. A report of two cases with diagnosis by fine needle aspiration biopsy. Acta Cytol 1999;43:1142–46.

91. Statistics CRUK. Incidence and Mortality 2004–2005.

92. Nagel H, Laskawi R, Buter JJ, et al. Cytologic diagnosis of acinic-cell carcinoma of salivary glands. Diagn Cytopathol 1997;16:402–12.

93. Ali SZ. Acinic-cell carcinoma, papillary-cystic variant: a diagnostic dilemma in salivary gland aspiration. Diagn Cytopathol 2002;27:244–50.

94. Shet T, Ghodke R, Kane S, et al. Cytomorphologic patterns in papillary cystic variant of acinic cell carcinoma of the salivary gland. Acta Cytol 2006;50:388–92.

95. Gonzalez-Peramato P, Jimenez-Heffernan JA, Lopez-Ferrer P, et al. Fine needle aspiration cytology of dedifferentiated acinic cell carcinoma of the parotid gland: a case report. Acta Cytol 2006;50:105–8.

96. Auclair PL, Goode RK, Ellis GL. Mucoepidermoid carcinoma of intraoral salivary glands. Evaluation and application of grading criteria in 143 cases. Cancer 1992;69:2021–30.

97. Klijanienko J, Vielh P. Fine-needle sampling of salivary gland lesions. IV. Review of 50 cases of mucoepidermoid carcinoma with histologic correlation. Diagn Cytopathol 1997;17:92–98.

98. Hughes JH, Volk EE, Wilbur DC. Pitfalls in salivary gland fine-needle aspiration cytology: lessons from the College of American Pathologists Interlaboratory Comparison Program in Nongynecologic Cytology. Arch Pathol Lab Med 2005;129:26–31.

99. Nagel H, Hotze HJ, Laskawi R, et al. Cytologic diagnosis of adenoid cystic carcinoma of salivary glands. Diagn Cytopathol 1999;20:358–66.

100. Gibbons D, Saboorian MH, Vuitch F, et al. Fine-needle aspiration findings in patients with polymorphous low-grade adenocarcinoma of the salivary glands. Cancer 1999;87:31–36.

101. Kemp BL, Batsakis JG, el-Naggar AK, et al. Terminal duct adenocarcinomas of the parotid gland. J Laryngol Otol 1995;109:466–68.

102. Ruiz-Godoy L, Suarez L, Mosqueda A, et al. Polymorphous low-grade adenocarcinoma of the parotid gland. Case report and review of the literature. Med Oral Patol Oral Cir Bucal 2007;12:E30–33.

103. Klijanienko J, Vielh P. Salivary carcinomas with papillae: cytology and histology analysis of polymorphous low-grade adenocarcinoma and papillary cystadenocarcinoma. Diagn Cytopathol 1998;19:244–49.

104. Moriki T, Ueta S, Takahashi T, et al. Salivary duct carcinoma: cytologic characteristics and application of androgen receptor immunostaining for diagnosis. Cancer 2001;93:344–50.

105. Khurana KK, Pitman MB, Powers CN, et al. Diagnostic pitfalls of aspiration cytology of salivary duct carcinoma. Cancer 1997;81:373–78.

106. Nigam S, Kumar N, Jain S. Cytomorphologic spectrum of carcinoma ex pleomorphic adenoma. Acta Cytol 2004;48:309–14.

107. Miliauskas JR, Orell SR. Fine-needle aspiration cytological findings in five cases of epithelial-myoepithelial carcinoma of salivary glands. Diagn Cytopathol 2003;28:163–67.

108. Ellis GL. Lymphoid lesions of salivary glands: malignant and benign. Med Oral Pathol Oral Cir Buccal 2007;12:E479–85.

109. Chhieng DC, Paulino AF. Cytology of myoepithelial carcinoma of the salivary gland. Cancer 2002;96:32–36.

110. Darvishian F, Lin O. Myoepithelial cell-rich neoplasms: cytologic features of benign and malignant lesions. Cancer 2004;102:355–61.

111. Gehrking E, Gehrking I, Moubayed P. Surgery of benign tumors of the parotid gland: the value of fine needle aspiration cytology. HNO 2007;55:195–201.

112. Elagoz S, Gulluoglu M, Yilmazbayhan D, et al. The value of fine-needle aspiration cytology in salivary gland lesions, 1994–2004. ORL J Otorhinolaryngol Relat Spec 2007;69:51–56.

113. Qizilbash AH, Elavathil LJ, Chen V, et al. Aspiration biopsy cytology of lymph nodes in malignant lymphoma. Diagn Cytopathol 1985;1:18–22.

114. Nettle WJ OS. Fine needle aspiration in the diagnosis of salivary gland lesions. Aust N Z J Surg 1989;59:47–51.

115. Aljafari AS, Khalil EA, Elsiddig KE, et al. Diagnosis of tuberculous lymphadenitis by FNAC, microbiological methods and PCR: a comparative study. Cytopathology 2004;15:44–48.

116. Al-Khafaji BM, Afify AM. Salivary gland fine needle aspiration using the ThinPrep technique: diagnostic accuracy, cytologic artifacts and pitfalls. Acta Cytol 2001;45:567–74.

117. Arabi Mianroodi AA, Sigston EA, Vallance NA. Frozen section for parotid surgery: should it become routine? ANZ J Surg 2006;76:736–39.

118. Bandyopadhyay A, Das TK, Raha K, et al. A study of fine needle aspiration cytology of salivary gland lesions with histopathological corroboration. J Indian Med Assoc 2005;103:312–14. 16.

119. Boccato P, Altavilla G, Blandamura S. Fine needle aspiration biopsy of salivary gland lesions. A reappraisal of pitfalls and problems. Acta Cytol 1998;42:888–98.

120. Cajulis RS, Gokaslan ST, Yu GH, et al. Fine needle aspiration biopsy of the salivary glands. A five-year experience with emphasis on diagnostic pitfalls. Acta Cytol 1997;41:1412–20.

121. Chhieng DC, Cangiarella JF, Cohen JM. Fine-needle aspiration cytology of lymphoproliferative lesions involving the major salivary glands. Am J Clin Pathol 2000;113:563–71.

122. Das DK, Petkar MA, Al-Mane NM, et al. Role of fine needle aspiration cytology in the diagnosis of swellings in the salivary gland regions: a study of 712 cases. Med Princ Pract 2004;13:95–106.

123. Daskalopoulou D, Rapidis AD, Maounis N, et al. Fine-needle aspiration cytology in tumors

and tumor-like conditions of the oral and maxillofacial region: diagnostic reliability and limitations. Cancer 1997;81:238–52.

124. David O, Blaney S, Hearp M. Parotid gland fine-needle aspiration cytology: an approach to differential diagnosis. Diagn Cytopathol 2007;35:47–56.

125. Ford L, Rasgon BM, Hilsinger RL Jr., et al. Comparison of ThinPrep versus conventional smear cytopreparatory techniques for fine-needle aspiration specimens of head and neck masses. Otolaryngol Head Neck Surg 2002;126:554–61.

126. Gupta RK, Naran S, Lallu S, et al. The diagnostic value of fine needle aspiration cytology (FNAC) in the assessment of palpable supraclavicular lymph nodes: a study of 218 cases. Cytopathology 2003;14:201–7.

127. Jayaram N, Ashim D, Rajwanshi A, et al. The value of fine-needle aspiration biopsy in the cytodiagnosis of salivary gland lesions. Diagn Cytopathol 1989;5:349–54.

128. Kraft M, Lang F, Mihaescu A, et al. Evaluation of clinician-operated sonography and fine-needle aspiration in the assessment of salivary gland tumours. Clin Otolaryngol 2008;33:18–24.

129. Layfield LJ. Fine-needle aspiration in the diagnosis of head and neck lesions: A review and discussion of problems in differential diagnosis. Diagn Cytopathol 2007;35:798–805.

130. Lioe TF, Elliott H, Allen DC, et al. The role of fine needle aspiration cytology (FNAC) in the investigation of superficial lymphadenopathy; uses and limitations of the technique. Cytopathology 1999;10:291–97.

131. Lu BJ, Zhu J, Gao L, et al. Diagnostic accuracy and pitfalls in fine needle aspiration cytology of salivary glands: a study of 113 cases. Zhonghua Bing Li Xue Za Zhi 2005;34:706–10.

132. Lukas J, Duskova J. Fine-needle aspiration biopsy in the diagnostic of the tumors and non-neoplastic lesions of salivary glands. Bratisl Lek Listy 2006;107:12–15.

133. Nasuti JF, Yu GH, Gupta PK. Fine-needle aspiration of cystic parotid glands lesions: an institutional review of 46 cases with histologic correlation. Cancer 2000;90:111–16.

134. Orell SR. Diagnostic difficulties in the interpretation of fine needle aspirates of salivary gland lesions: the problem revisited. Cytopathology 1995;6:285–300.

135. Owotade FJ, Fatusi OA, Adebiyi KE, et al. Clinical experience with parotid gland enlargement in HIV infection: a report of five cases in Nigeria. J Contemp Dent Pract 2005;6:136–45.

136. Postema RJ, van Velthuysen ML, van den Brekel MW, et al. Accuracy of fine-needle aspiration cytology of salivary gland lesions in the Netherlands cancer institute. Head Neck 2004;26:418–24.

137. Raghuveer CV, Leekha I, Pai MR, et al. Fine needle aspiration cytology versus fine needle sampling without aspiration. A prospective study of 200 cases. Indian J Med Sci 2002;56:431–39.

138. Rajwanshi A, Gupta K, Gupta N, et al. Fine-needle aspiration cytology of salivary glands: diagnostic pitfalls – revisited. Diagn Cytopathol 2006;34:580–84.

139. Seethala RR, LiVolsi VA, Baloch ZW. Relative accuracy of fine-needle aspiration and frozen section in the diagnosis of lesions of the parotid gland. Head Neck 2005;27:217–23.

140. Young J. Diagnostic problems in fine needle aspiration Cytopathology of the salivary glands. J Clin Pathol 1994;47:193–98.

141. MacLeod CB, Frable WJ. Fine needle aspiration biopsy of the salivary gland: problem cases. Diagn Cytopathol 1993;9:216–25.

142. Young J. Salivary glands. Fine Needle Aspiration. Oxford: Blackwell Scientific; 1993 48–67.

143. Maly B, Maly A, Doviner V, et al. Fine needle aspiration biopsy of intraparotid schwannoma. A case report. Acta Cytol 2003;47:1131–34.

# Oral cavity

Phillip Sloan and Alfred Böcking

## Introduction

Exfoliative cytology is increasingly being used for oral diagnosis and has been the subject of intense research over the last 5 years.[1] Significant advances have been made both in relation to screening for oral cancer and in the evaluation of oral precursor lesions. Mucosal biopsy is widely regarded as the gold standard for oral diagnosis but exfoliative cytology is also a valuable technique for the diagnosis of a range of pre-neoplastic, cancerous, infective and inflammatory mucosal disorders. Fine needle aspiration (FNA) also has an important role in the diagnosis of metastatic oral squamous carcinoma in the neck and can be used for cystic intraosseous jaw lesions and intraoral submucosal swellings.[2,3]

## Normal oral mucosa

Oral mucosa is heterogeneous and can be divided into masticatory, lining and specialised types.

### Masticatory mucosa

This covers the hard palate and gingivae and in places is bound directly to bone forming a mucoperiosteum. A fatty submucosa is present in the centre of the hard palate. The microanatomy of masticatory mucosa is related to its function of resisting compressive forces. Large connective tissue papillae are characteristic and the oral epithelium is cornified, most often showing parakeratosis. The keratin layer imparts a pale pink colour and if the keratin layer increases in thickness due to chronic irritation or trauma, the mucosa appears white and slightly spongy.

### Lining mucosa

This covers the ventral tongue, floor of mouth, soft palate and the buccal, labial and vestibular surfaces of the oral cavity. Again, the microanatomy of lining mucosa is related to its functions, shaping food for chewing and swallowing, and allowing movement for speech and other oral functions. Lining oral epithelium is non-keratinising in health and is almost transparent. Consequently, lining mucosa appears clinically red in colour due to blood in the vessels of the lamina propria. Lining oral epithelium is quite variable in thickness. Floor of mouth mucosa has poorly developed connective tissue papillae and the epithelium is thin. This contrasts with buccal mucosa where the connective tissue papillae are long, slender and curved, extending through a much thicker squamous epithelium. Most lining mucosa is located over a submucosa that contains minor mucus salivary glands.

### Specialised mucosa

This is found on the dorsum of the tongue. The mucosa is covered by filiform papillae and there are also larger fungiform, foliate and circumvallate papillae at specific locations. The dorsal lingual epithelium is keratinising and bacterial biofilm can be abundant on the surface of the filiform papillae.

### Sampling methods

Collection devices suitable to obtain cells from the superficial and intermediate layers may be conventional brushes, such as the CytoBrush, Orca-brush or others. Signs of dysplasia will be detected in the upper layers due to the principle of disturbed cell maturation that occurs in dysplasia in which a degree of nuclear abnormality (dyskaryosis) in the surface layers reflects the degree of disturbance of maturation of the whole thickness of the epithelium, i.e. dysplasia. It is the task of a cytopathologist to identify nuclear abnormalities in the cells collected in this way to predict the histological grade of dysplasia. The diagnostic criteria used are similar to cervical exfoliative cytology and are well known (Figs 6.1–6.3) (see Ch. 21).

Screening for oral cancer and precursor lesions can be performed by dentists and other healthcare professionals.

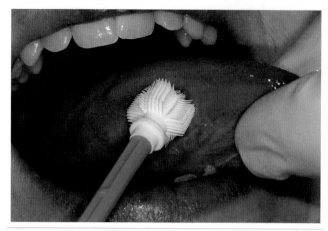

**Fig. 6.1** The Orcellex® device is placed firmly onto the oral mucosa and rotated 10 times to collect an adequate sample.

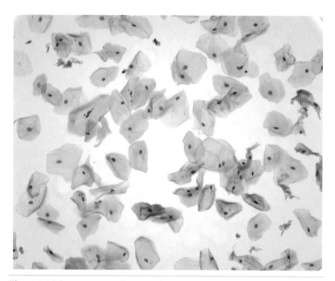

**Fig. 6.2** LBC preparation of normal floor of mouth mucosa showing superficial and intermediate squamous cells.

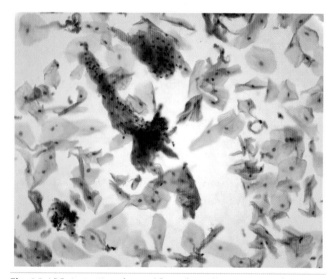

**Fig. 6.3** LBC preparation of normal floor of mouth mucosa using the Orcellex® brush showing intermediate and basal cells.

Tolonium chloride rinsing has been advocated in the past to distinguish between normal and abnormal oral mucosa and more recently tissue fluorescence has been employed effectively.[4] Exfoliative cytology is advocated for evaluation of suspicious lesions that are detected clinically by screening. This may be followed by a mucosal biopsy and transepithelial sampling. Exfoliative cytology of oral lesions may replace tissue biopsy in lesions that are clinically not obviously suspicious for malignancy but nevertheless need surveillance. As tissue biopsy is associated with low compliance (9%) and brush-biopsy not (100%),[5] this approach may lead to a higher rate of oral cancers identified in early stages.

## Oral precursor lesions

Oral carcinogenesis proceeds through a stepwise accumulation of genetic damage over time. Because the oral cavity is easy to examine and risk factors for oral cancer are known, there is great opportunity to improve patient outcomes through diagnosis and treatment of pre-malignant lesions before the development of invasive oral carcinoma.[6]

## Leukoplakia, erythroplakia and proliferative verrucous leukoplakia

An arbitrary distinction is often made between oral premalignant *conditions* and oral premalignant *lesions*. The former include a group of generalised mucosal disorders linked by epithelial atrophy and where there is an increased predisposition to oral cancer when mucosa is exposed to the known major risk factors such as sunlight exposure, smoking and alcohol consumption, areca or betel nut and also syphilis and sideropenic dysphagia.[7] Recently, strong evidence for an aetiological relationship between human papilloma virus and a subset of head and neck cancers has been noted.[8] Oral cancer risk is also associated with low socioeconomic status and related to lifestyle risk factors.[9] Where risk factors cannot be eliminated and lesions persist, then regular clinical follow-up should be considered. The need for follow-up and interval between visits will vary in individual cases. In contrast to the oral premalignant *conditions*, oral premalignant *lesions* are morphologically abnormal solitary or multiple areas of mucosa that are typically white, discoloured white, red, speckled or verrucous in appearance (Fig. 6.4). The WHO classification[10] combines leukoplakia and erythroplakia into 'precursor lesions', with the 6.8% estimated rate of transformation of oral leukoplakias to cancer.[11] It identifies proliferative verrucous leukoplakia (PVL) as a separate high-risk lesion with minimal cytological atypia.

## Assessment of dysplasia

There are several schemes for grading dysplasia in biopsies of oral precursor lesions. The WHO classification provides a five point system: hyperplasia, mild, moderate and severe dysplasia followed by carcinoma *in situ*.[10] The system can be mapped onto both the Ljubljana classification and the widely used three

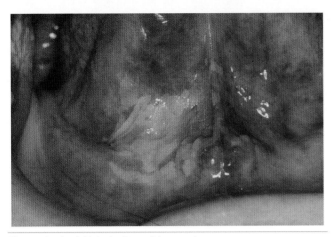

**Fig. 6.4** Leukoplakia in the floor of the mouth.

**Table 6.1** Current histological grading systems for oral dysplasia/squamous intraepithelial neoplasia (SIN)

| WHO | Ljubljana | SIN |
|---|---|---|
| Hyperplasia | Squamous hyperplasia | |
| Mild dysplasia | Basal/parabasal hyperplasia | 1 |
| Moderate dysplasia | Atypical (risky) hyperplasia | 2 |
| Severe dysplasia | Carcinoma *in situ* | 3 |
| Carcinoma *in situ* | Carcinoma *in situ* | 3 |

point squamous intraepithelial neoplasia (SIN) system (Table 6.1). For the first time the WHO set out criteria for diagnosis by defining both the architectural and cytological features of dysplasia.[10,11] However, there is good evidence in the literature favouring a binary system ('high-grade' and 'low-grade' categories) over multipoint scales for prediction of malignant transformation (Figs 6.5, 6.6).[12,13]

Squamous cell carcinoma will develop from antecedent dysplastic oral mucosal lesions if an early diagnosis has not been made and treatment given. Early diagnosis within stages I and II correspond to a vastly improved 5-year survival rate when compared with more advanced stage III and IV lesions.[14,15]

An accumulating body of evidence exists to show that oral cytology is a valuable technique for the assessment of oral premalignant lesions.[1,16,17] Exfoliative cytology has been shown to detect dysplasia in suspicious oral lesions with high sensitivity and specificity by several groups.[18–20] The use of auxiliary methods such as DNA image cytometry, AgNOR analysis, cytomorphometry[21] and cell cycle immunohistochemistry and semiautomated multimodal cell analysis using brush biopsies can increase accuracy even further.[17–19,22–24] Molecular genetics of each of the precursor lesions is being investigated for genetic alterations, which have been demonstrated in oral squamous cell carcinoma, to define their location on the continuum of changes, which lead to malignant transformation.[25]

Although the degree of dysplasia can be predicted on cytological samples, tissue biopsy is usually performed when dysplasia is detected, to confirm its grade and exclude the presence of invasion. The latter cannot be reliably assessed by exfoliative cytology alone. However, observer variability in the histological assessment of oral premalignant lesions is well described.[26]

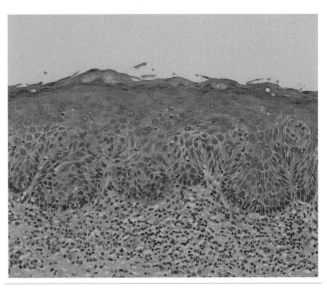

**Fig. 6.5** Low-grade epithelial dysplasia in the oral mucosa. Changes are restricted to the lower one-third of the oral epithelium. In an intra-observer study, there was variation between mild and moderate grades, but consensus that this lesion was low grade.

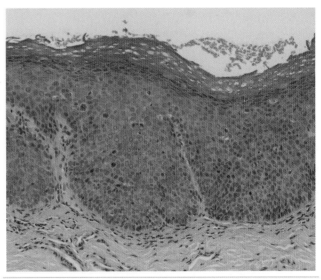

**Fig. 6.6** High-grade epithelial dysplasia in the oral mucosa. In an intra-observer study, there was variation between moderate, severe and severe amounting to CIS, but consensus that this lesion was high grade.

## Cytological findings: oral dysplasia

- Hyperchromasia of nuclei
- Increased nuclear to cytoplasmic ratio
- Anisonucleosis and nuclear pleomorphism
- Irregularities of nuclear membrane
- Nuclear crowding
- Nuclear moulding, clumping and irregular distribution of chromatin.

It is important to recognise regenerating oral epithelial cells which are typically found growing over the surface of clinically suspicious but benign oral ulcers and erosions. Regenerating cells form aggregates of immature keratinocytes often with increased nuclear to cytoplasmic ratios and sometimes prominent nucleoli, but with no other nuclear abnormalities.

Radiation and chemoradiation also induce cytological changes including micronucleation in both normal and malignant keratinocytes and care must be taken when cytology is performed in the immediate post-irradiation setting.[27]

## Auxiliary cytometry

Up to 5–14% of oral brush biopsies may yield equivocal cytological diagnoses.[18,28] Underlying diagnoses are mild, moderate or marked dysplasia, abnormal regenerating squamous epithelium or just scarcity of abnormal cells. In these cases, ancillary methods are desirable, that allow more definite, correct cytological diagnoses. Two such methods are: DNA image cytometry (DNA-ICM) and AgNOR analysis.

Diagnostic DNA-ICM is based on DNA measurements of several hundred atypical cells in routine cytological specimens. It aims to distinguish true prospectively malignant lesions from microscopically atypical or otherwise doubtful lesions. The biological basis of this ancillary method is chromosomal aneuploidy which is an accepted marker of malignant transformation of cells. Its cytometric equivalent, DNA aneuploidy, is

assumed if gains or losses of chromosomes or their parts result in a plus or minus of more than 10% of nuclear DNA mass in a growing cell population (stemline-aneuploidy) or if extremely high nuclear DNA values (single cell aneuploidy) occur. Measurements may be performed on previously stained slides after de-staining and Feulgen re-staining. Morphologically suspicious cells are interactively selected on a monitor and internal calibration is performed with normal (e.g. intermediate squamous) cells. The method has been internationally standardised and is applicable to many different epithelial dysplasias.[29] Papanicolaou, Feulgen and silver nitrate staining and respective measurements may sequentially be applied also on the same cells (multimodal cell analysis[19]) (Fig. 6.7).

Remmerbach et al.[28] reported a frequency of 13.9% of doubtful or suspicious oral cytological diagnoses due to different grades of squamous dysplasia or abnormal regenerating epithelium. Applying DNA aneuploidy as a marker for prospective malignancy on identical slides, they could improve diagnostic sensitivity for the detection of oral cancer from 91.3% to 97.8% and specificity from 95.1% to 100%. Thus 29.4% of oral cancers that clinically appeared as leukoplakias or erythroplakias were detected in stages Tis or T1. In a similar study,

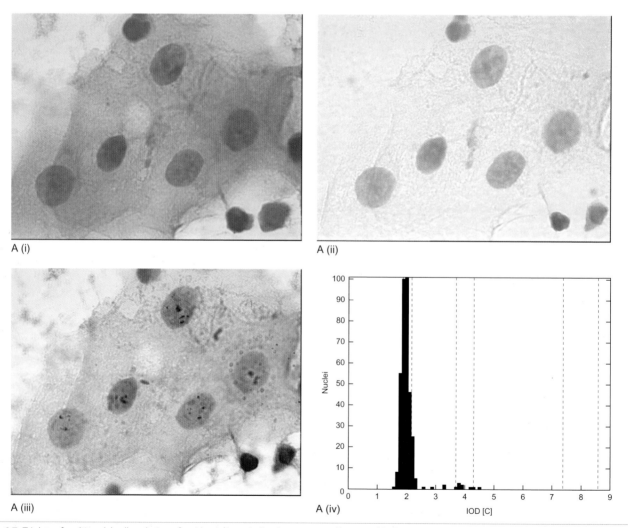

A (i)

A (ii)

A (iii)

A (iv)

**Fig. 6.7** Triplets of multimodal cell analysis on few identical atypical oral squamous cells, stained (A(i), B(i)) according to Papanicolaou for subjective inspection, (A(ii), B(ii)) according to Feulgen for DNA-ICM and (A(iii), B(iii)) with silver nitrate for AgNOR-analysis. Respective euploid (diploid) DNA-histogram in (A(iv)) and aneuploid with abnormal stemlines at 3.5c and 7.0c in (B(iv)). Mean AgNOR-counts per nucleus were 3.7 in (A) and 5.4 in (B). Final histological diagnoses were ulcer in (A) and in situ squamous cell carcinoma in (B). The displacements of images in (B) are due to computerised relocations of cells after repeated staining.

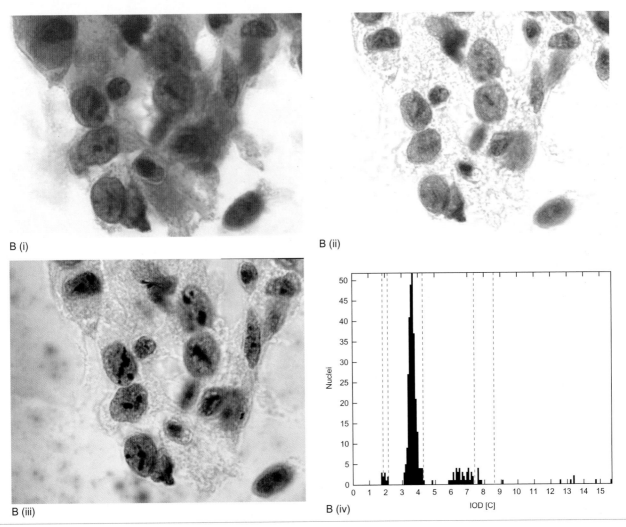

B (i)

B (ii)

B (iii)

B (iv)

**Fig. 6.7** (Continued)

Maraki et al.[17] described a sensitivity of 100% and specificity of 97.4% for the combined cytological and DNA cytometric evaluation of oral leukoplakias and erythroplakias. Some 8.1% of her cytological diagnoses had been equivocal. DNA-ICM was only applied, if one of the above mentioned diagnoses had occurred. Seven cases in which combined cytological/DNA cytometric diagnosis of early oral cancer was achieved up to 2.5 years before definitive biopsy diagnosis have been published.[17,23] Thus DNA-ICM may help to predict the prospective behaviour of cytological suspicious lesions, as the positive predictive values of DNA aneuploid findings was reported to be 100% and the negative value 98.1%.[18,23] DNA-ICM may be used for identification of tumour-free resection margins instead of histology.[30,31]

Another auxiliary method that allows assessment of potential malignancy of dysplastic or regenerating cells is AgNOR analysis. Remmerbach et al.[19,24] showed that counting the number of silver nitrate-stained nucleolar organiser regions (AgNORs) in about 100 atypical squamous cells allows 100% sensitivity and specificity of oral cancer detection on brush biopsies using a cut-off value to identify the precancerous from already cancerous cells among all dysplastic cells.[30] The AgNOR method can also be useful for grading dysplasia, for example a cut-off value of 2.3 separates mild and moderate dysplasia.[32]

Both methods, DNA-ICM and AgNOR analysis, may even be performed sequentially on identical cells. This type of multimodal cell analysis is especially useful, if only few atypical cells are available.[19] Thus, AgNOR analysis can be combined with DNA-ICM if the latter does not yield an unequivocal diagnosis (Fig. 6.7).

Immunohistochemical detection of cell cycle markers has also been proposed as a potential method of detecting cytological abnormality but no data on specificity and sensitivity in the routine clinical setting are available.[33,34] Molecular markers and techniques such as loss of heterozygosity in exfoliated cells can be used to detect clinically non-visible lesions in early dysplastic oral lesions.[35]

## Oral and oropharyngeal cancers

Oral cancer is an important health issue. The WHO predicts a continuing worldwide increase in the number of patients with oral cancer, extending this trend well into the next several decades. In the USA, the projected number of new cases of oral and oropharyngeal cancer will exceed 31 000 per year. Mortality due to cancers in this region exceeds the annual death rate in the USA caused by either cutaneous melanoma or cervical cancer. Significant agents involved in the aetiology of oral cancer in Western countries include sunlight exposure, smoking and alcohol consumption.[36]

Squamous cell carcinoma accounts for over 90% of oral and oropharyngeal malignancies. Diagnosis must always be confirmed by mucosal biopsy before treatment but both exfoliative and FNA cytology are particularly valuable for early detection, screening, surveillance and staging/mapping. Currently, histological grading is of little prognostic or predictive value, although there is now some evidence that HPV16 and related genome-driven carcinomas have a better prognosis than their non HPV counterparts, through increased radiosensitivity.[37] Detection of HPV by *in situ* hybridisation in biopsy tissue or in cytology preparations is likely to become routine practice in the future.[38] The limitation of HPV testing currently is that the genomic profile in HPV positive tumours is variable and is a more powerful determinant of response to therapy than the mere presence of HPV. Consequently, HPV positive and negative tumours have to be treated in an identical way. Cytometric analysis has the potential to provide a more objective method of predicting biological behaviour and more research is required in these areas.

Oral and oropharyngeal cancers often arise in a field of epithelial dysplasia that may be quite extensive (Figs 6.8, 6.9). Consequently, second primary cancers, often several centimetres from the originally treated area, are a major cause of overall treatment failure. The stepwise theory of carcinogenesis explains the existence of fields. Stem cells are thought to acquire a series of mutations that confer growth advantages, resulting in the lateral spread of precancerous epithelium with molecular lesions. Exfoliative cytology in combination with human tissue fluorescence provides one means to map the extent of the field at presentation with oral cancer, which in turn helps to determine surgical margins, radiotherapy fields and with post-treatment surveillance.[39]

## Cytological findings: invasive squamous carcinoma (Fig. 6.10)

- Hyperchromasia of nuclei
- Increased nuclear to cytoplasmic ratio
- Anisonucleosis and nuclear pleomorphism
- Irregularities of nuclear membranes
- Nuclear crowding
- Nuclear moulding, clumping and irregular distribution of chromatin
- Dyskeratosis
- Tadpole and strap cells.

As discussed above, auxiliary cytometry can be used to refine diagnosis and increase the sensitivity and specificity for recognising atypia. However, the distinction between invasive squamous carcinoma and dysplasia cannot be made reliably with current methods, particularly as oral squamous carcinomas can form a well-differentiated surface keratin layer while showing invasion on their deep aspect.

## Infections

### Fungal infections

Oral candidiasis is very common and presents in a variety of ways. *Candida albicans* is a dimorphic commensal organism and

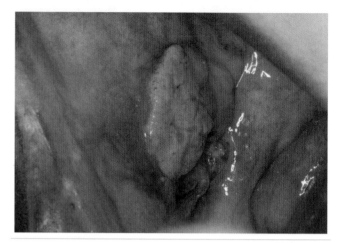
**Fig. 6.8** Squamous carcinoma of the left buccal mucosa arising in field change.

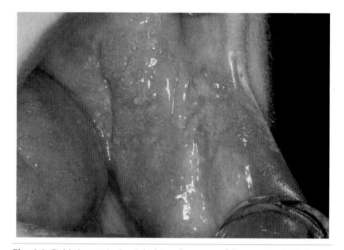
**Fig. 6.9** Field change in the right buccal mucosa of the same patient shown in Figure 6.8. Biopsy and cytology showed severe dysplasia.

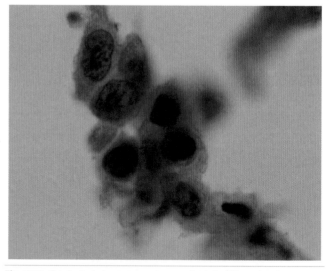
**Fig. 6.10** Cytological changes seen in a moderately differentiated squamous cell carcinoma of the tongue.

is found in healthy mouths in around 40% of the population. Consequently, occasional yeast forms may be found incidentally in any oral cytological preparation. The presence of pseudohyphae indicates that the yeast is actively proliferating and signals a disease state. Often the pseudohyphae are abundant and form tangles. Clinical reassessment of the oral mucosa is advised once the infection has been cleared, as *Candida* may secondarily colonise the keratin layer over dysplastic or inflammatory lesions.

There are reports in the literature of diagnosis of rarer oral fungal infections such as histoplasmosis, paracoccidioidomycosis, sporotrichosis and others by oral exfoliative cytology and these depend on morphological identification of the microorganism.[40]

## Viral exanthems

Herpes simplex (HHV-1) is the most frequent viral cause of acute oral eruption. In the initial infection the virus causes primary herpetic gingivostomatitis, characterised by grey blisters that break down to form small ulcers, crusted labial lesions, fever and tender cervical lymphadenopathy (Figs 6.11, 6.12) After the infection has cleared HHV-1 may remain in the trigeminal ganglion and on reactivation causes the familiar cold sores of herpes labialis.

### Cytological findings: herpes simplex

- Cell fusion with large multiple nuclei moulded together
- Margination of chromatin around generally 'empty' nuclei
- Large intranuclear inclusions in early lesions
- Older lesions show necrotic cells with degenerate nuclei
- Neutrophils are typically abundant in the background.

Herpetic infection can be identified using LBC or direct smears and either immunocytochemistry or *in situ* hybridisation can be used to identify the virus. Oral viral eruptions can less commonly be caused by Coxsackie viruses producing hand, foot and mouth disease or herpangina. Similar viral cytopathological features are seen.

## Hairy leukoplakia

This distinctive oral lesion was first identified in patients with HIV infection where it signalled transformation to AIDS. Subsequently it has been identified in a variety of immunosuppressive disorders, in patients receiving immunosuppressive therapy and as a transient infection. Clinically, white patches develop on the lateral borders of the tongue and these may be papillary or flat in form (Fig. 6.13). The Epstein-Barr virus (HHV-4) can be demonstrated by *in situ* hybridisation in routine biopsies and is restricted to the upper epithelial strata in characteristic koilocyte-like cells. *Candida* infection and parakeratosis is also frequently seen. Cytopathological diagnosis can be made in the clinical setting.[41]

### Cytological findings: hairy leukoplakia

- Cowdry type A inclusions
- Ground glass cytoplasm
- Nuclear chromatin margination
- *In situ* hybridisation can be used to confirm EBV (HHV-4) infection
- *Candida* pseudohyphae are commonly present.

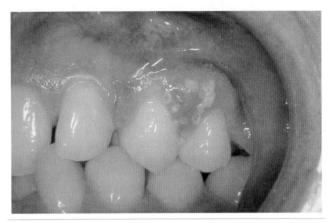

**Fig. 6.11** Herpes simplex vesicles on the gingival margin in primary herpetic stomatitis.

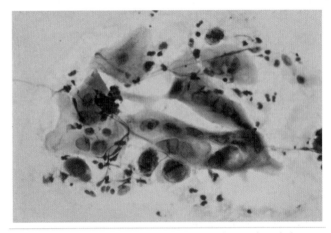

**Fig. 6.12** Viral cytopathic changes in a herpes simplex vesicle, including balloon nuclei and formation of multinucleated keratinocytes.

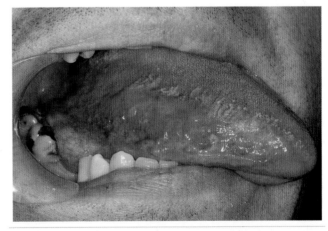

**Fig. 6.13** Oral hairy leukoplakia (courtesy of Dr Mike Pemberton, Manchester).

## Vesiculo-bullous disorders

Blisters in the oral cavity arise from a number of disease processes including trauma, viral infection, angina bullosa haemorrhagica, and autoimmune vesiculo-bullous disease. Close correlation with the clinical features is an essential part of the diagnostic process.

## Pemphigus vulgaris

Around 50% of cases with pemphigus vulgaris initially develop oral lesions. The oral phase of the disease may go unrecognised until increase in the titre and epitope spread of the autoantibodies results in a clinically severe cutaneous eruption. The oral lesions of pemphigus vulgaris are typically painful and bullae tend to occur in areas that are subject to trauma, such as the junction of the hard and soft palate and mucosa adjacent to single standing teeth or denture flanges. Intact bullae are not commonly seen because suprabasal splitting quickly leads to loss of the upper epithelial strata in the moist oral environment. Mucosal biopsy for direct immunofluorescence requires intact fresh tissue that can be difficult to obtain. Gentle brushing is normally sufficient to obtain adequate cytological samples for morphology and direct immunofluorescence (Figs 6.14, 6.15). The Tzanck cell characterises oral pemphigus and specificity can be increased if direct immunofluorescence is performed.[42]

### Cytopathological findings: pemphigus vulgaris

- Rounded shape due to acantholysis
- Cytoplasm basophilic and condensed at the cell periphery
- Increased nuclear size
- Hazy or absent nucleoli
- IgG circular cytoplasmic halo by direct IMF or immunoperoxidase
- Background of neutrophils and granular exudate
- Intercellular gaps and bridges.

## Mucous membrane pemphigoid

Cicatricial (mucosal) pemphigoid is a more frequently encountered oral vesiculo-bullous disorder than pemphigus and is main differential diagnosis when persistent oral blistering and erythema are encountered (Fig. 6.16). Cytological examination of the bulla fluid frequently shows numerous eosinophils with normal or regenerating keratinocytes from the bulla margins. However, neutrophils may predominate or cells may be scant in the preparation.

## Pigmented lesions

Cytology is generally not suitable for diagnosis of oral pigmented lesions. Mucosal biopsy is preferred for suspected melanocytic lesions but fine needle aspiration may be useful for distinguishing these from vascular malformations which are quite common in the oral cavity, particularly the tongue. However, mucosal nevi and malignant melanomas occur and may be confused clinically with squamous carcinoma. Cytology can detect oral naevus cell naevi and malignant melanomas. The latter diagnosis can be supported by immunocytochemistry. The cytological features of melanoma are similar to those described in cutaneous lesions (see Ch. 28).

## Jaw cysts

Many jaw cysts have characteristic clinical and radiographic features. Enucleation can usually be performed without prior

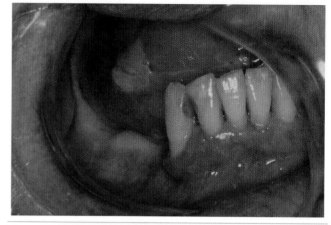

**Fig. 6.14** An oral lesion of pemphigus vulgaris on the lateral aspect of the tongue. Fluid filled blisters tend to break down quickly in the oral cavity and are rarely seen clinically.

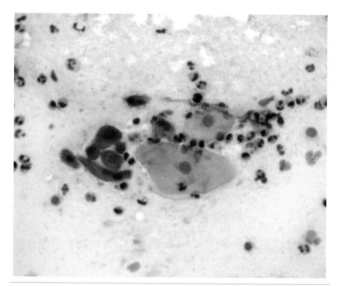

**Fig. 6.15** Tzanck cells are seen on the left of the field and can be compared with normal oral keratinocytes on the right.

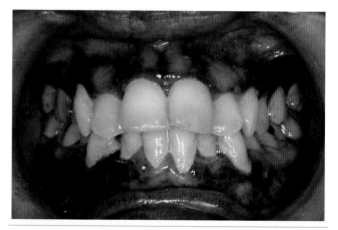

**Fig. 6.16** Mucous membrane pemphigoid presenting as red blistering lesions on the gingivae.

laboratory diagnosis and histological validation should then be undertaken. Aspiration of cystic lesions is useful for distinguishing between true intra-osseous lesions and the maxillary sinus, where air is obtained. Rarely odontogenic neoplasms simulate cysts and several including ameloblastoma can be predominantly cystic.

## Odontogenic keratocyst

Odontogenic keratocyst (cystic keratinising odontogenic tumour) can arise as a solitary sporadic lesion or as part of basal cell naevus syndrome. The cysts are often multilocular and tend to expand the buccal cortex of the jaw. FNA produces a creamy fluid.

### Cytological findings: odontogenic keratocyst (Fig. 6.17)

- Groups or isolated keratinocytes with normal or poorly defined nuclei
- Numerous anucleate squames
- Keratinocytes positive for pan-cytokeratin and CK19, negative for CK14.

## Inflammatory odontogenic cysts

The most common odontogenic cyst arises around the apex of a non-vital tooth and is known as the radicular cyst. Residual radicular cysts may be encountered from cyst remnants left behind in the jaw after tooth extraction. Dentigerous cysts are also common (Fig. 6.18), particularly around third molars, and non-odontogenic cysts may also arise from epithelium included in the jaws during embryonic development. All of these latter cysts share similar cytological features with the radicular cyst (Fig. 6.19) but the appearances are non-defining and close correlation with the radiographic and clinical features is essential for accurate diagnosis.

### Cytological findings: dentigerous cyst

- Brown glistening fluid with semisolid material
- Abundant cholesterol crystals are seen in polarised light
- Background of macrophages, neutrophils and granular debris
- Non-keratinising squames occasionally present.

## Odontogenic neoplasms

Ameloblastoma is the most common odontogenic neoplasm and it typically presents as a multilocular radiolucent lesion. Around two-thirds occur around the angle of the mandible, but they may arise in any part of the jaws.

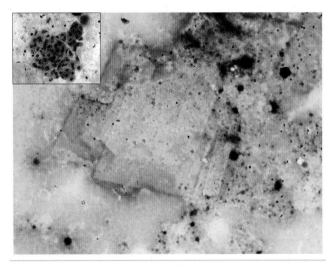

**Fig. 6.18** Dentigerous cyst. Male 32. Swelling of the cheek. Dentigerous cyst at the site of the unerupted tooth. Cytologically, a background of macrophages, neutrophils and granular debris with non-keratinising epithelium and debris are noted. Abundant cholesterol crystals are seen.

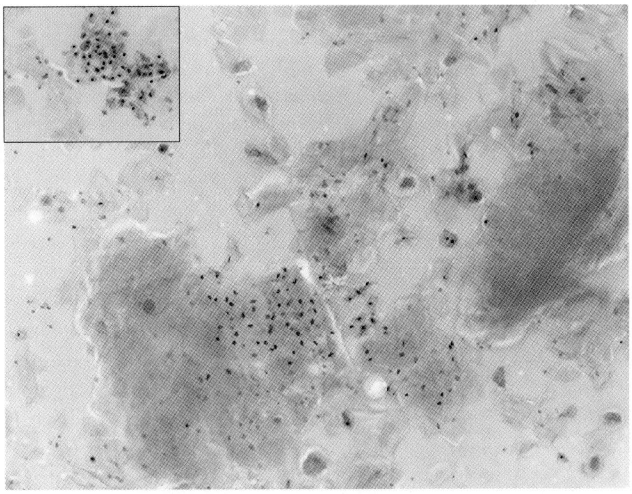

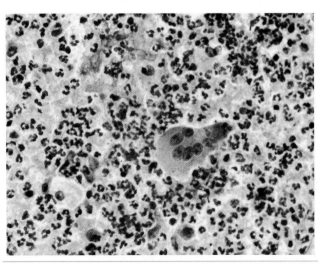

**Fig. 6.17** Odontogenic keratocyst. Male aged 24. On roentgenogram in the angle-third molar region. Pain and swelling. Cheese-like material aspirated. Cytologically anucleate squames and keratinased squamous cells are seen. Macrophages including giant cells are present. No inflammation.

**Fig. 6.19** Radicular cyst. Male 35. A well-circumscribed radiolucent area at the apex of tooth. Cytologically, neutrophils and macrophages including multinucleate giant cells are noted. No epithelium is seen.

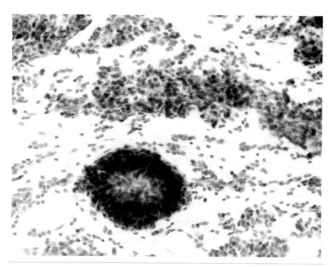

**Fig. 6.20** Ameloblastoma. Female 34. Multiple previous resections of ameloblastoma. Now as possible recurrence. Cytologically, hypercellular samples with granular background and occasionally tissue fragments of basaloid cells with peripheral palisading.

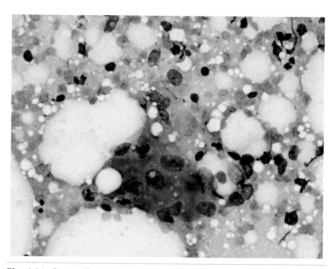

**Fig. 6.21** Giant cell granuloma. FNA of the swelling over the right ramus of mandible. Multinucleate giant cells suggesting a granulomatous process. Correlation with radiology is essential because many bone lesions contain osteoclast type giant cells.

## Cytological findings: ameloblastoma[3] (Fig. 6.20)

- Hypercellular samples with granular background
- Occasionally tissue fragments of basaloid cells with peripheral palisading
- A distinct, two-cell population consisting of small, hyperchromatic, basaloid-type cells and scattered larger cells with more open chromatin
- Occasional fragments of mesenchymal cells with more elongated nuclei and ample, clear cytoplasm may also be noted (Stellate reticulum-like cells)
- Islands of squamous cells
- Malignant cases that metastasise show prominent cytological pleomorphism, cellular crowding with moulding and a high mitotic index.

Single case reports or small series exist in the literature describing the diagnosis of rare variants of ameloblastoma,[43,44] including the unicystic type which behaves as cyst and also malignant ameloblastoma. In the right clinical setting and with proper radiological evidence, the cytological features of primary and metastatic ameloblastoma are unique. Diagnostic problems may arise when these lesions are pleomorphic and frankly malignant, especially at metastatic sites, such as the lung. A histological validation is essential to reach a definitive diagnosis.

## Bone lesions

Aspiration of suspected odontogenic cysts sometimes produces features of giant cell granuloma (Fig. 6.21), fibro-osseous lesion, solitary (unicameral) bone cyst, aneurysmal bone cyst, myeloma, metastasis and rarely primary bone neoplasms. The cytological diagnosis of bone lesions is discussed in Chapter 29.

## Oral submucosal swellings

In the oral cavity submucosal swellings can be caused by minor salivary gland lesions, including cysts and tumours, soft tissue lesions and bony prominences. The role of cytology for the diagnosis of salivary gland tumours is discussed in Chapter 5. The rate of salivary gland malignancy is relatively higher in the minor salivary glands than in the parotid and submandibular glands.

## Role of cytology in the management of oral cancer and precursor lesions

Given the natural history of oral cancer which, similar to that of the uterine cervix, is preceded by the preinvasive phase, this is an area potentially amenable to population screening. However, systematic reviews of screening for oral cancer have shown that there so far is insufficient evidence to justify implementation of population screening but benefits in mortality rates have been demonstrated in randomised controlled trials when high-risk subjects are targeted.[45,46] The known risk factors for oral and oropharyngeal cancer are tobacco use, alcohol, paan chewing, HPV and diet. Some countries do have national screening programmes and there are also invitational programmes as well as opportunistic screening when patients attend for routine dental check-ups.[45] However, there is considerable uncertainty in the parameters used in the evaluation of the cost-effectiveness of screening for oral cancer in primary care, particularly malignant transformation rate, disease progression, patterns of self-referral and costs. Evidence has been published to suggest that intervention has no greater benefit than 'watch and wait'.[47]

The concept of dysplasia/neoplasia surveillance has been applied to longstanding conditions associated with an increased risk of cancer. Although still controversial, periodic direct clinical examination as well as endoscopic techniques are currently performed in patients with inflammatory bowel diseases, Barrett's oesophagus, and melanocytic skin lesions in order to detect and treat dysplastic or early malignant changes and therefore improve the patients' prognosis. Unlike cervical screening, where the target tissue is anatomically discrete, screening of the wide area of oral and oropharyngeal mucosa for early microscopic change is problematic. Mignona et al.[14] have shown that dysplasia/neoplasia surveillance diagnosed most episodes (94.9%) of oral lichen planus malignant transformation in early intraepithelial and microinvasive phases, namely stage 0 and I oral cancers (T (is) N0M0 or T1N0M0). The 5-year survival rate, where applicable, has been 96.7%. Examination techniques that might improve the visualisation of suspicious lesions of the oral mucosa (ViziLite (R) system and VELscope (R) system) or that might facilitate the cytological identification of suspicious lesions (OralCDx (R) have been described.[48]

Currently, oral exfoliative cytology is a useful technique that can be used for detection and surveillance of oral precursor lesions, subject to the close collaboration between the clinicians and pathologists. Biopsy remains a gold standard on which management is based, although this suffers from interobserver variation.[26] Sensitivity and specificity of oral exfoliative cytology for the detection of dysplasia and oral cancer varies depending on the centre.[49] Currently, there are no evidence-based guidelines for the early detection, treatment or follow-up of oral precursor lesions.[50] The use of chemical adjuvants to diagnosis such as fluorescence and intraoral staining has been debated in the literature and there is a clear need for more research in the field. Large scale clinical trials to evaluate the role of oral cytology are needed to clarify its value and enable its potential to be exploited.[1]

## REFERENCES

1. Mehrotra R, Hullmann M, Smeets R, et al. Oral cytology revisited. J Oral Pathol Med 2009;38:161–66.

2. Goldenberg D, Sciubba J, Koch WM, et al. Cystic metastasis from head and neck squamous cell cancer: a distinct disease variant? Head & Neck 2006;28:633–38.

3. Tsamis I, Giatromanolaki A, Tamiolakis D, et al. Fine needle aspiration cytology in ameloblastoma of the mandible. Cytopathology 2002;13:375–78.

4. Poh CF, Ng SP, Williams PM, et al. Direct fluorescence visualisation of clinically occult high-risk oral premalignant disease using a simple hand-held device. Head & Neck 2007;29:71–76.

5. Velleuer E, Dietrich R, Böcking A, et al. A novel five step de-escalation procedure to enhance the compliance of FA patients for a regular oral cancer screening. 20th Annual Fanconi Anemia Research Fund Scientific Symposium, Eugene, Oregon, USA, 4–7 October, 2008. Book of abstracts.

6. Gillenwater A, Papadimitrakopoulou V, Richards-Kortum R. Oral premalignancy: new methods of detection and treatment. Curr Oncol Rep 2006;8:146–54.

7. Napier SS, Speight PM. Natural history of potentially malignant oral lesions and conditions: an overview of the literature. J Oral Pathol Med 2008;37:1–10.

8. Termine N, Panzarella V, Falaschini S, et al. HPV in oral squamous cell carcinoma vs head and neck squamous cell carcinoma biopsies: a meta-analysis (1988–2007). Ann Oncol 2008;19:1681–90.

9. Warnakulasuriya S. Significant oral cancer risk associated with low socioeconomic status. Evid Based Dent 2009;10:4–5.

10. Barnes L, Eveson JW, Reichart P, editors, et al. World Health Organization Classification of Tumours. Pathology and Genetics of Head and Neck Tumours. Lyon: IARC Press; 2005.

11. MacDonald G. Classification and histopathological diagnosis of epithelial dysplasia and minimally invasive cancer. In: Satellite symposium on epithelial dysplasia and borderline cancer of the head and neck: controversies and future directions. Joint BSOMP, BSOM, BAHNO Meeting 2003; Oxford.

12. Kujan O, Oliver RJ, Khattab A, et al. Evaluation of a new binary system of grading oral epithelial dysplasia for prediction of malignant transformation. Oral Oncol 2006;42:987–93.

13. Warnakulasuriya S, Reibel J, Bouquot J, et al. Oral epithelial dysplasia classification systems: predictive value, utility, weaknesses and scope for improvement. J Oral Pathol Med 2008;37:127–33.

14. Mignona MD, Fedele S, Russo LL. Dysplasia/neoplasia surveillance in oral lichen planus patients: A description of clinical criteria adopted at a single centre and their impact on prognosis. Oral Oncol 2006;42:819–24.

15. Huang CH, Chu ST, Ger LP, et al. Clinicopathologic evaluation of prognostic factors for squamous cell carcinoma of the buccal mucosa. J Chin Med Assoc 2007;70:164–70.

16. Navone R, Marsico A, Reale I, et al. Usefulness of oral exfoliative cytology for the diagnosis of oral squamous dysplasia and carcinoma. Minerva Stomatol 2004;53:77–86.

17. Maraki D, Becker J, Böcking A. Cytologic and DNA-cytometric very early diagnosis of oral cancer. J Oral Pathol Med 2004;33:398–404.

18. Remmerbach TW, Weidenbach H, Pomjanski N, et al. Cytologic and DNA-cytometric early diagnosis of oral cancer. Anal Cell Pathol 2001;22:211–21.

19. Remmerbach T, Meyer-Ebrecht D, Aach T, et al. Toward a multimodal cell analysis of brush biopsies for early detection of oral cancer. Cancer Cytopathol 2009;117:228–35.

20. Navone R, Burlo P, Pich A, et al. The impact of liquid-based oral cytology on the diagnosis of oral squamous dysplasia and carcinoma. Cytopathology 2007;18:356–60.

21. Ramaesh T, Mendis BR, Ratnatunga N, et al. Diagnosis of oral premalignant and malignant lesions using cytomorphometry. Odontostomatol Trop 1999;22:23–28.

22. Klanrit P, Sperandio M, Brown AL, et al. DNA ploidy in proliferative verrucous leukoplakia. Oral Oncol 2007;43:310–16.

23. Remmerbach T, Weidenbach H, Hemprich A, et al. Earliest detection of oral cancer using non-invasive brush-biopsy including DNA-image-cytometry: Report on four cases. Anal Cell Pathol 2003;25:159–66.

24. Remmerbach T, Weidenbach H, Müller C, et al. Diagnostic value of nucleolar organizer regions (AgNORs) in brush biopsies of suspicious lesions of the oral cavity. Anal Cell Pathol 2003;25:139–46.

25. Mithani SK, Mydlarz WK, Grumbine FL, et al. Molecular genetics of premalignant oral lesions. Oral Dis 2007;13:126–33.

26. Kujan O, Khattab A, Oliver RJ, et al. Why oral histopathology suffers inter-observer variability on grading oral epithelial dysplasia: an attempt to understand the sources of variation. Oral Oncol 2007;43:224–31.

27. Mehrotra R, Gupta A, Singh M, et al. Application of cytology and molecular biology in diagnosing premalignant or malignant oral lesions. Mol Cancer 2006;5:11–86.

28. Remmerbach T, Mathes SN, Weidenbach H, et al. Nichtinvasive Bürstenbiopsie als innovative Methode in der Früherkennung des Mundhöhlenkarzinoms. Mund-Kiefer-GesichtsChir 2004;8:229–36.

29. Böcking A, Giroud F, Reith A. Consensus Report of the ESACP task force on standardisation of diagnostic DNA image cytometry. Anal Cell Pathol 1995;8:67–74.

30. Depprich R, Handschel J, Wiesmann HP, et al. Use of bioreactors in maxillofacial tissue engineering. Br J Oral Maxillofac Surg 2008;46:349–54.

31. Handschel J, Öz D, Pomjanski N, et al. Additional use of DNA-image cytometry improves the assessment of resection margins. J Oral Pathol Med 2008;36:471–72.

32. Chattopadhyay A, Ray JG. AgNOR cut-point to distinguish mild and moderate epithelial dysplasia. J Oral Pathol Med 2008;37:78–82.

33. Scott IS, Odell E, Chatrath P, et al. A minimally invasive immunocytochemical approach to early detection of oral squamous cell carcinoma and dysplasia. Br J Cancer 2006;94:1170–75.

34. Thomson PJ, Hamadah O, Goodson ML, et al. Predicting recurrence after oral precancer treatment: use of cell cycle analysis. Br J Oral Maxillofac Surg 2008;46:370–75.

35. Bremmer JF, Braakhuis BJ, Brink A, et al. Comparative evaluation of genetic assays to identify oral pre-cancerous fields. J Oral Pathol Med 2008;37:599–606.

36. Sciubba JJ. Oral cancer. The importance of early diagnosis and treatment. Am J Clin Dermatol 2001;2:239–51.

37. Worden FP, Kumar B, Lee JS, et al. Chemoselection as a strategy for organ preservation in advanced oropharynx cancer: response and survival positively associated with HPV16 copy number. J Clin Oncol 2008;26:3138–46.

38. Zhang MQ, El-Mofty SK, Dávila RM. Detection of human papillomavirus-related squamous cell carcinoma cytologically and by in situ hybridisation in fine-needle aspiration biopsies

of cervical metastasis: a tool for identifying the site of an occult head and neck primary. Cancer 2008;114:118–23.

39. Poh CF, Zhang L, Anderson DW, et al. Fluorescence visualisation detection of field alterations in tumor margins of oral cancer patients. Clin Cancer Res 2006;12:6716–22.

40. Talhari C, de Souza JV, Parreira VJ, et al. Oral exfoliative cytology as a rapid diagnostic tool for paracoccidioidomycosis. Mycoses 2008;51:177–78.

41. Walling DM, Flaitz CM, Adler-Storthz K, et al. A non-invasive technique for studying oral epithelial Epstein-Barr virus infection and disease. Oral Oncol 2003;39:436–44.

42. Aithal V, Kini U, Jayaseelan E. Role of direct immunofluorescence on Tzanck smears in pemphigus vulgaris. Diagn Cytopathol 2007;35:403–7.

43. Walke VA, Munshi MM, Raut WK, et al. Cytological diagnosis of acanthomatous ameloblastoma. J Cytol 2008;25:62–64.

44. Mathew S, Rappaport K, Ali SZ, et al. Ameloblastoma. Cytologic findings and literature review. Acta Cytol 1997;41:955–60.

45. Kujan O, Glenny AM, Oliver RJ, et al. Screening programmes for the early detection and prevention of oral cancer. Cochrane Database Syst Rev 2006;3:CD004150.

46. Downer MC, Moles DR, Palmer S, et al. A systematic review of measures of effectiveness in screening for oral cancer and precancer. Oral Oncol 2006;42:551–60.

47. Speight PM, Palmer S, Moles DR, et al. The cost-effectiveness of screening for oral cancer in primary care. Health Technol Assess 2006;10. iii–iv, 1–144.

48. Trullenque-Eriksson A, Muñoz-Corcuera M, Campo-Trapero J, et al. Analysis of new diagnostic methods in suspicious lesions of the oral mucosa. Med Oral Pathol Oral Cir Bucal 2009;14:E210–16.

49. Hohlweg-Majert B, Deppe H, Metzger MC, et al. Sensitivity and specificity of oral brush biopsy. Cancer Invest 2009;27:293–97.

50. Epstein JB, Gorsky M, Fischer D, et al. A survey of the current approaches to diagnosis and management of oral premalignant lesions. J Am Dent Assoc 2007;138:1555–62.

# Oesophagus and gastrointestinal tract

Fernando Schmitt and Maria Helena Oliveira

## Chapter contents

## Introduction

Following the introduction of fibreoptic endoscopy, our knowledge of the gastrointestinal tract has changed, because we now have direct viewing and sampling of lesions. The pathological classification of gastrointestinal lesions is based on morphological criteria derived from surgical resection and biopsy specimens. Nevertheless, cytology can be very useful in the appropriate clinical context and, provided that the optimal sampling method for the particular clinical setting is chosen. Gastroenterologists may not be aware of the usefulness of cytology in this area so care must be taken that it is used in the appropriate clinical context with an understanding of the limitations of this approach (Box 7.1).

Nowadays, better sampling methods and cytological preparations can improve the sensitivity and specificity of the diagnosis of gastrointestinal lesions. Large lesions are more thoroughly sampled with a cytological brush passed through the endoscope, a less traumatic, easier and cheaper methodology. Lesions covered with normal mucosa or localised within the gut wall can be reached by fine needle aspiration (FNA) with or without endoscopic ultrasonographic (EUS) control.[1] Throughout the upper and lower gastrointestinal tract there are degenerative, inflammatory and neoplastic lesions that may be separately diagnosed by careful morphological study. Lesions such as lymphoma and gastrointestinal stromal tumours (GIST) can be reached by EUS-FNA needle.[2] The material obtained can be divided for direct preparations, cell blocks or liquid based cytology (LBC). Flow cytometry, molecular biology techniques and immunocytochemistry (ICC) can also be applied.

## Box 7.1  The advantages of cytology

- Survey of large mucosal areas
- Investigation of the cardiac region, not always accessible to endoscopic biopsy
- Exploration of large ulcers

## Normal anatomy and histology

### The oesophagus

The oesophagus begins at the cricoid cartilage (15 cm endoscopic length), passes within the posterior mediastinum and through the diaphragm where it extends for several centimetres, having a total length of about 40 cm from the incisors. Four layers characterise the gastrointestinal tract wall: mucosa, submucosa, muscularis propria and serosa. In the oesophagus, however, all four layers are only present in short abdominal and thoracic segments.[3] Each of these layers may have their own lesions but the mucosa is particularly exposed to external stimuli. Oesophageal mucosa consists of a non-keratinising stratified squamous epithelium, lamina propria and muscularis mucosae. The squamous epithelium is divided in three layers: basal cell, prickle cell (intermediate cells) and functional or superficial cell layer. There are normally also a few mononuclear cells, not classifiable by routine methods.

### The stomach

The stomach is a very distensible organ located in the left upper quadrant of the abdomen, between the oesophagus and the duodenum. Gastric mucosa consists of a superficial epithelium forming foveolae and a deeper layer of glands that empty into the base of the foveolae. The superficial cells are tall, columnar and mucus secreting with basally located nuclei. Glands differ in structure and function along the gross anatomical regions. Cardiac and pyloric (antral) glands are mucus secreting, with microvacuolated cytoplasm similar to Brunner's glands. Three types of cells are present in the fundic gland mucosa: zymogenic cells, which are cuboidal, basally located in the gland with a central nucleus and pale cytoplasm; parietal cells, triangular with centrally placed nuclei and dense cytoplasm; and mucous neck cells. Along with these are scattered endocrine cells, mostly located in the glands.[4]

### The duodenum

The duodenum is the most proximal segment of the small intestine and is, except proximally, a fixed retroperitoneal organ closely related to adjacent organs and structures. It surrounds the head of the pancreas and is divided in four portions: first or bulb, second or descending, third or horizontal and fourth or ascending. It ends at the angle of Treitz where the jejunum begins, at the level of the second lumbar vertebra. The common bile duct and the major and minor pancreatic ducts empty into the second portion through several anatomical variations, the ampulla of Vater being the major identifiable structure. Duodenal mucosa is poorly demarcated from gastric mucosa. In the first few millimetres it is antral in type, identical to gastric pyloric mucosa. Other areas are intestinal villous in type, covered by columnar absorptive cells with some goblet cells: and there are areas of transitional type where both are found. This transition extends for about 5 mm, beyond which the presence of pyloric type epithelium is referred to as gastric metaplasia. Submucosal Brunner's glands are lobular collections of tubulo-alveolar glands that sometimes extend to the deeper portions of the mucosa. These characterise the duodenal segment as they disappear towards the jejunum. The mucus secreting cells are cuboidal with pale cytoplasm and an oval nucleus located at the base. Also some scattered neuroendocrine cells can be seen.[5]

## The colon

The colon is the terminal segment of the gastrointestinal tract. The last portion is the rectum which enters the pelvis ending at the anal canal. Colonic superficial epithelial lining is composed of columnar cells covered by a layer of mucin, enzymes, lectins and glycans that form the glycocalyx. Crypts extend perpendicularly to the muscularis mucosae. Goblet cells, absorptive columnar cells, endocrine, Paneth and M cells line these structures. Also, lymphoid follicles are scattered along the colon with normal variations along it. Cellular turnover is highest in colonic mucosa, so apoptotic and mitotic cells can easily be found.[6]

## The anal canal

The anal canal has different lengths depending on whether it is defined anatomically or by histology (average 4.2 and 3 cm, respectively). Histologically four zones are described that can easily be seen on longitudinal sections and less easily macroscopically – the colorectal zone lined by intestinal type epithelium, the transitional zone lined by epithelial variants, the squamous zone lined by uninterrupted squamous epithelium, and the perianal skin and skin appendages. The macroscopic landmark is the dentate line, which is an important anatomical definition for common ground between clinicians and pathologists. It roughly corresponds to the transitional and squamous zone gathering point, varying in length around the circumference. Anal glands open in the transitional zone and can extend even to the external sphincter. The cells lining the different anatomical areas range from the intestinal type, already described, to the transitional type similar to urothelium, and squamous cells. Scattered Merkel and neuroendocrine cells, melanocytes and Langerhans cells are also found. Skin appendages include sebaceous, apocrine and sweat glands and hair.[7]

## Cytology sampling methods and preparation

Cells can be obtained through different sampling methods and a close dialogue with the endoscopists and knowledge of the clinical setting should influence the choice of method. Cytological sampling should be taken prior to any biopsy[8] and the main methods used include the following:

- Cytology balloons or sponges and sponge-mesh for screening for oesophageal squamous cell carcinomas have been extensively tested in Asia. These devices seem to be equally satisfactory for obtaining cellular yields, both squamous and glandular[9]
- Brushing under endoscopic view of the lesions is considered a good method to enhance detection of early lesions as it can represent more than the 1% of tissue obtained by biopsy alone.[10] The endoscopic brush should be employed like a needle rather than as a swab and jabbed through the surface mucosa or ulcer slough. Brush samples have advantages over the usual small biopsies since they include surface mucus or exudates from wider, sometimes unrelated mucosal surfaces and inevitably include exfoliated material. This is perhaps best explained by considering the identification of Helicobacter pylori in disposable brush wash preparations. The organisms are usually best seen in free wisps or trails of mucus rather than in close association with an epithelial surface as in histological sections. They are commonplace within oesophageal and duodenal brushes as a result of the wide inclusion of a sometimes cellular exudative gastric mucus sample within an otherwise directed brush sample. This of course considerably improves the yield from such samples on direct comparison with biopsy. Similarly, brush samples are superior to biopsy for the detection of the commoner types of epithelial malignancy in the oesophagus and stomach, and certainly for ulcerated epithelial malignancy. On the other hand, biopsy is superior for the detection of submucosal spread of signet-ring cell carcinoma of the stomach, for the rare submucosal glandular or endocrine tumours, primary lymphomas and for non-epithelial stromal tumours
- Imprint or crushing of biopsy fragments in addition to brushing, as previously mentioned, are well-documented techniques to detect H. pylori[11,12]
- Salvage cytology and washings are used much less often now. Salvage cytology is a procedure complementary to biopsies, intended to retrieve cells from the biopsy forceps and endoscopic tube
- Washings are generally badly tolerated by patients and clinicians do not feel comfortable with a morphological diagnosis that has no endoscopic correlation
- Endoscopic fine-needle aspiration biopsy with or without ultrasound-guidance (EUS-FNA) has gained relevance in the diagnosis of lesions not directly seen with the endoscope or in those where forceps biopsy failed to reach a diagnosis. It has clinical relevance because it changes diagnostic and therapeutic procedures, as for example, when staging oesophageal carcinoma. It is particularly important that cytopathologists assess the specimen adequacy and determine which ancillary studies will be needed at the time of the procedure.[2]

Cytological material can be prepared by direct smear with immediate fixation in alcohol or air-drying. Other authors prefer to rinse the brushes in a preservative liquid with the subsequent use of cytocentrifuge or liquid based cytology (LBC). Also cell blocks can be prepared either from the FNA needle or from other collecting devices. This methodology is particularly useful for immunocytochemistry and molecular biology studies.

Papanicolaou stain (PAP), May–Grünwald Giemsa (MGG) or similar stains and haematoxylin and eosin (H&E) are used according to local custom and which yield the best results. Ancillary techniques, including routine histochemistry for microorganisms, can also be applied, even on pre-stained slides. Immunocytochemistry, flow cytometry, molecular biology techniques and morphometry can be used in selected cases.

## General principles

One should always apply the principle of getting as much information as one can to establish a good rapport with clinicians and endoscopists. This is particularly important when dealing with EUS-FNA. Smears can be evaluated on site, which improves the cell yield and avoids repeating procedures later.[13]

At the microscope, both high- and low-power views are important. On low power we evaluate the background (mucous, inflammation, necrosis), overall architecture of the cell groups and how they are arranged on the smear. With high power we apply the classical cytological criteria for the nucleus, nucleoli and cytoplasm to categorise the cells as reactive, dysplastic, benign or malignant. Interpretation and diagnosis when possible should be based on surgical pathology terminology. Although we cannot always give a specific diagnosis, a clinically relevant comment should be given.

## Pitfalls

- One must bear in mind that heterotopias such as cardiac gastric glands, remnants of ciliated epithelium, sebaceous and pancreatic or endocrine cells in the oesophagus and stomach may occur and cause interpretive problems
- The cytological response to inflammation can be worrisome. Repair and malignancy can be very difficult to distinguish and criteria such as cell grouping, enlarged nuclei, prominent nucleoli and mitoses can be seen in both settings.[1] Tumour diathesis must be distinguished from ulceration slough. On the other hand, the presence of intact single cells, loss of polarity, irregular nuclear borders, irregular and multiple nucleoli and abnormal mitotic figures can be more reliable for the diagnosis of malignancy. Delicate chromatin is often seen in repair albeit with an enlarged nucleus and prominent nucleoli
- Granulation tissue from the base of an ulcer can pose a diagnostic problem with spindle cell tumours, particularly in HIV-positive patients where multiple infections and tumours occur together
- Radiation and chemotherapy can induce cytological atypia, most frequently described in the squamous epithelium of the oesophagus, as seen in the uterine cervix, but these changes can also occur in the glandular gastric lining[14]

- Contaminants rarely pose a diagnostic problem, unless they obscure and entrap the diagnostic cells. Vegetable cells and other food debris, tissue fragments and talc are among the commoner ones found.

## Oesophagus

### Normal cytological findings

The normal components of oesophageal cytology are the superficial and intermediate cells of the multilayered squamous epithelium. Oesophageal brush smears in the absence of disease are usually paucicellular. Superficial cells are eosinophilic while intermediate cells are more basophilic, both having voluminous delicate cytoplasm. The nucleus is pyknotic in the more mature cells while in the intermediate type it is slightly larger and the cytoplasm is finely granular. On vigorous sampling, parabasal cells can be present, having larger darker nuclei and basophilic cytoplasm. Sheets, clusters and pearl-like arrangements can be seen. Glandular cells from the gastric epithelium are often seen and should not raise the possibility of Barrett's oesophagus (Fig. 7.1). Oral bacteria, sometimes overlying superficial squamous cells from the oral mucosa, food contaminants and respiratory cells can also be seen (Box 7.2).

### Inflammatory conditions

Inflammation induces a cellular response that can be morphologically worrisome. Cells from the basal layer along with the more superficial layers can appear isolated or in small groups

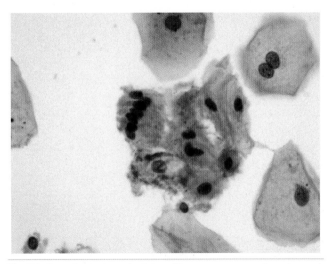

**Fig. 7.1** Normal oesophageal cytology. Observe squamous cells and normal glandular cells from gastric epithelium. Their presence does not imply a diagnosis of Barrett's epithelium (PAP).

---

**Box 7.2 Normal components of oesophageal brushings**

- Superficial and intermediate squamous cells
- Gastric epithelium
- Respiratory cells, macrophages
- Contaminants, food particles

---

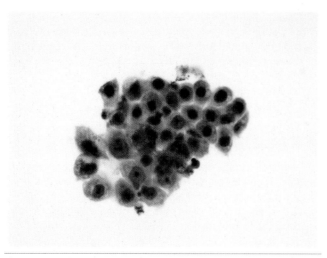

**Fig. 7.2** Oesophageal brush smear showing regenerative epithelium from basal layers. Observe the presence of nucleoli and cytoplasmic vacuolation (PAP).

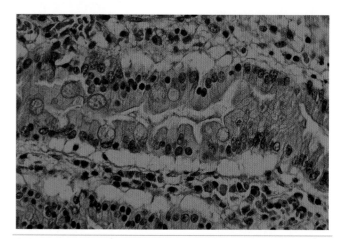

**Fig. 7.4** Intestinal type metaplasia in Barrett's oesophagus identified when goblet cells are present along with columnar cells, sometimes with an identifiable brush border (H&E). (Courtesy of Professor Paula Chaves, Instituto Português de Oncologia Francisco Gentil, Lisboa.)

## Cytological findings: reflux (peptic) oesophagitis

Typical brushing appearances in reflux oesophagitis will include some or all of the following features depending on a combination of the intensity or extent of the changes:

- Increased squamous cellularity and discohesiveness (squamous hyperplasia)
- Clumps of irregular parabasal type squamous cells with enlarged reactive hyperchromatic nuclei and multiple nucleoli
- Increased polymorphonuclear neutrophils and mucus admixed with the sheets of squamous cells, sometimes also associated with lymphocytes, plasma cells, macrophages and cell debris (Fig. 7.3)
- Eosinophils, which are associated with acid reflux and chemical inflammation
- Ulcer slough consisting of clumps of mixed inflammatory cells, macrophages, degenerate epithelial cells, fibroblasts, smooth muscle cells, red blood cells and small capillary or vein walls.

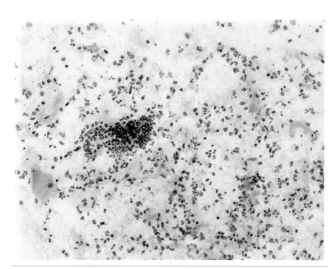

**Fig. 7.3** Oesophageal brush smear from a patient with reflux oesophagitis. Note the high proportion of polymorphonuclear neutrophils (PAP).

## Barrett's oesophagus

Barrett's oesophagus, a complication of chronic gastro-oesophageal reflux disease, is a pre-malignant condition for adenocarcinoma of the oesophagus and the oesophago-gastric junction. In the definition of the American College of Gastroenterology, Barrett's oesophagus is a change in the oesophageal epithelium of any length that can be recognised at endoscopy and is confirmed to have intestinal metaplasia by biopsy (Fig. 7.4). Three types of epithelium are recognised in Barrett's metaplasia: oxyntico-cardiac, cardiac and intestinal. Oxyntico-cardiac and cardiac types are identical to the corresponding gastric epithelial regions and one should be cautious in rendering a diagnosis of Barrett's metaplasia in lower oesophagus samples.

## Cytological findings: Barrett's oesophagus

- Intestinal type metaplasia is identified when goblet cells are present along with columnar or cuboidal cells. A considerable amount of epithelium folded or in sheets, is necessary for recognition of the 'portholes' which are mucus cells seen from above/below (Fig. 7.5). The villous border

reflecting regenerative epithelium (Fig. 7.2). Injury can be induced by infections, local action of chemicals and radiation.

## Reflux (peptic) oesophagitis

An incompetent sphincter mechanism, either transient or chronic, may lead to reflux of acid gastric contents into the lower oesophagus. A variety of conditions including sliding hiatus hernia, excessive alcohol consumption, pyloric stenosis, diabetic autonomic neuropathy, scleroderma and previous surgery, among others, may result in persistence of the reflux. The non-keratinised stratified squamous mucosa appears less resistant to acid or bile than the mucus and alkali-protected specialised columnar gastric glandular mucosa. This results in acute inflammation, regenerative squamous hyperplasia, keratosis and subsequent healing, gastric/intestinal type metaplasia or chronic ulceration.

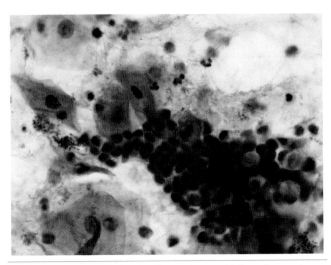

**Fig. 7.5** Oesophageal brush smear from a patient with Barrett's oesophagus. Observe glandular cells with goblet cells (PAP).

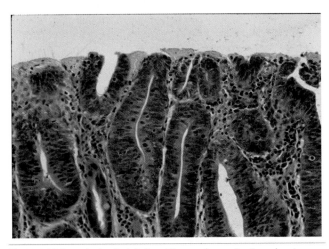

**Fig. 7.6** High-grade dysplasia in Barrett's oesophagus. Sections showing crypts lined by stratified columnar epithelium with mitoses readily distinguishable; loss of mucin production and nuclear enlargement with coarse chromatin can be appreciated (H&E). (Courtesy of Professor Paula Chaves, Instituto Português de Oncologia Francisco Gentil, Lisboa.)

is more difficult to see in cytology preparations than in sections

- Gastro-oesophageal reflux is the major cause for Barrett's metaplasia so one can expect to have some degree of inflammatory background
- There is debate about the feasibility of using cytology to diagnose glandular dysplasia in this setting.[15,16] While there is a good agreement concerning high-grade lesions and neoplasia, in low-grade lesions it is more difficult to reach good inter-observer concordance. Meanwhile, in most centres both cytology and histology are used to improve the sensitivity and specificity of the diagnosis (Fig. 7.6)
- The criteria used favouring dysplasia are, as described above, enlarged nuclei and apparent nucleoli with delicate chromatin (Fig. 7.7).

## Radiation changes

Oesophagitis coupled with typical radiation changes in squamous cells, or in any gastric cells present can be found in patients who receive chest irradiation for a variety of indications. Radiation changes may occasionally be present in the epithelial cells in conjunction with tumour cells if the tumour is being treated by irradiation or there may be accompanying ulcerative changes with or without additional infections such as *Candida*, cytomegalovirus (CMV) or Herpes simplex virus (HSV).

Radiation induced lesions are similar to those of the uterine cervix. Irradiation of the chest and mediastinum may be used in conjunction with chemotherapy. Lesions are dose related but some variation in individual susceptibility exists.[17] These lesions pose diagnostic problems with malignancy (Box 7.3). Enlarged cytoplasm and nucleus maintain a roughly normal N:C ratio. There are degenerative changes with cytoplasm and nuclear vacuolation, pyknosis or pale staining nucleus and regenerative changes with mitotic activity.

### Cytological findings: radiation changes

- Increased epithelial cellularity composed of ragged sheets and aggregates of superficial, intermediate and basal squamous cells, isolated and in trails of discohesive cells (hyperplasia)

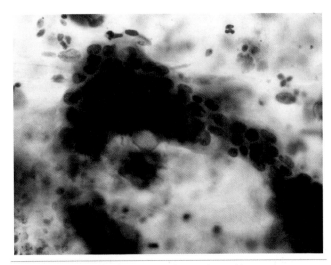

**Fig. 7.7** High-grade dysplasia in Barrett's oesophagus. Note on the cytological smears the presence of enlarged nuclei with delicate chromatin and some visible nucleoli (PAP).

---

**Box 7.3  Differential diagnosis of malignancy, radiation and chemotherapy**

- Malignancy
  - Hyperchromatic nuclei
  - Prominent and multiple nucleoli
  - High N:C ratio
- Radiation
  - Pale staining nuclei
  - Cytoplasmic and nuclear vesicular changes
  - Maintained N:C ratio
- Chemotherapy
  - Hyperchromatic nucleoli
  - Coarsely dense chromatin
  - Maintained N:C ratio

- Dense amphophilia or azurophilia (green) of squamous cells cytoplasm regardless of maturity reflecting a metachromatic stain response to cytoplasmic metabolic changes
- Multinucleation of epithelial cells and cellular gigantism of both mononuclear and multinucleated cells due to disruption of cell division
- Hydropic degeneration of nuclei and cytoplasm of the cells, with decreased uptake of stains and cytoplasmic vacuolation
- Hypo- or hyperchromatism of nuclei
- Dispersed prominent nucleoli (single or multiple)
- Normal nuclear/cytoplasmic (N:C) ratio despite increased nuclear and cytoplasmic diameters (unlike neoplasia)
- Variable or patchy occurrence of these changes within epithelial cells (heterogeneous cellular pleomorphism unlike the monotonous or homogeneous alterations in neoplasia)
- Degenerate dispersed-type mitoses
- Accompanying polymorphonuclear neutrophils with or without true ulcer slough
- Pump spindle or bizarre fibroblasts, macrophages and endothelial cells when ulceration is present.

## Infections

With the advent of transplantation and the acquired immuno-deficiency syndrome (AIDS), oesophageal infections are now a common medical problem. Cytology can be a very useful tool for diagnosing oesophageal infections with minimal trauma and high accuracy.

### *Candida* sp. and other fungi

*Candida* infection is the most frequent infection of the oesophagus. It has a typical endoscopic picture and on cytology variable amounts of yeast can readily be identified on H&E and Papanicolaou stains or with PAS and silver stains (Fig. 7.8). The epithelial cells are reactive with amphophilic squamous cells, parakeratotic whirls and increased granular layer squames. In HIV-positive patients, intense oesophageal candidiasis can occur and can be the first manifestation of the disease (Fig. 7.9).

### Cytological findings: *candida* sp. and other fungi

- 'Knotted' sheets of amphophilic squamous cells with admixed pseudohyphae and budding spores
- Increase in granular layer squames
- Parakeratotic rafts or whirls
- Increased diameter in superficial and intermediate cell nuclei
- Vesicular nuclei with multiple micronucleoli
- Entrapped neutrophil polymorphs and apoptotic debris within squames.

Rarely, other fungi such as *Mucor*, *Histoplasma* and *Actinomyces* spp. can produce oesophageal infections. Actinomycosis is an opportunistic infection, causing large ulcers. Sulphur granules characterise the morphology, as at other sites (Fig. 7.10).

### *Viral infections*

*Herpes simplex virus* infection can present with vesicles or well-demarcated ulcers, and lesions are seen in otherwise healthy individuals as well as immunosuppressed patients. Clinically, the plaque-like ulcerative slough is usually mistaken for *Candida*. Cytologically, the typical herpetic nuclear inclusions may be more difficult to identify unless immunocytochemistry or *in situ* hybridisation is used to highlight the cells. Otherwise they typically induce multinucleation with moulding, eosinophilic or basophilic intranuclear inclusions and ground glass nuclei (Fig. 7.11).

### Cytological findings: herpes simplex virus

- Separate mononuclear or bizarre syncytial-type giant, multinucleate squamous cells with moulded nuclei
- Eosinophilic or basophilic intranuclear inclusions or 'ground glass' nuclei

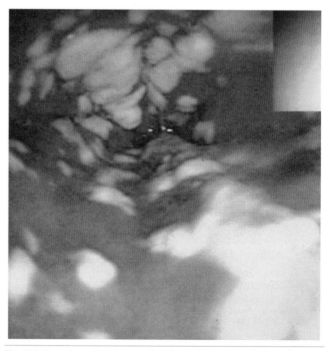

**Fig. 7.9** Oesophageal endoscopy showing yellow-white adherent plaque-like pseudomembranes that are characteristic of *Candida* infection. (Courtesy of Professor Paula Chaves, Instituto Português de Oncologia Francisco Gentil, Lisboa.)

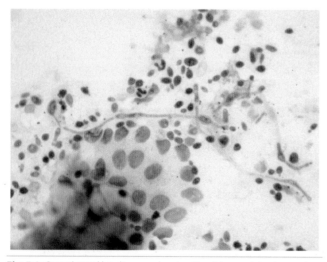

**Fig. 7.8** Oesophageal brush smear showing *Candida* pseudohyphae and spores. Note reactive epithelial cells (PAP).

- Beaded nuclear membranes with alternating marginated chromatin and nuclear chromatin holes or gaps.

*Cytomegalovirus* infection produces large ulcers frequently seen at the gastro-oesophageal junction and elsewhere within the gastrointestinal tract. The virus can infect epithelial squamous cells as well as stromal, endothelial and glandular cells, and, unlike HSV, ground-glass appearance and multinucleation are not seen. The hallmark is the nuclear inclusion.

### Cytological findings: cytomegalovirus

- Dissociated, amphophilic endothelial cells, often very degenerate or, rarely, changes in gastric epithelial cells
- Sometimes binucleate or trinucleate giant cells with inclusions

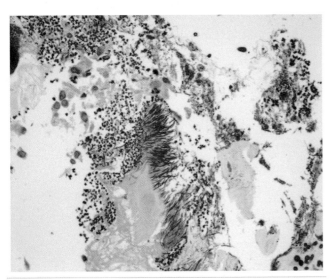

**Fig. 7.10** *Actinomyces* colonies form fungus-like branched networks of hyphae (PAS).

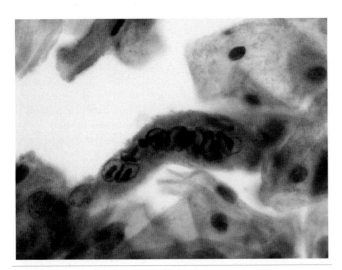

**Fig. 7.11** Oesophageal brush showing multinucleated cell with typical inclusion characteristic of *Herpes* virus (PAP). (Courtesy of Dr Evelina Mendonça, Instituto Português de Oncologia Francisco Gentil, Lisboa.)

- Large azurophilic 'owl's eye' nuclear inclusions, peri-inclusional clear nuclear halo, marginated nucleolus, intact nuclear envelope
- Cloud of smaller eosinophilic intracytoplasmic inclusions

*Human papillomavirus* (HPV) infection can be also detected in oesophageal brushes: the cellular changes include koilocytosis, parakeratosis, dyskeratosis and multinucleation. In some patients, especially HIV-positive or immunosuppressed patients following transplantation for example, as well as the HPV morphological changes, the virus can be identified antigenically or by demonstration of the viral DNA.

## Malignant neoplasms

### Squamous cell carcinoma

In spite of a decrease in incidence in the Western world, squamous cell carcinoma still represents 50% of all carcinomas of oesophagus. Most patients are male, in the seventh decade and present with dysphagia and weight loss. Alcohol, tobacco, chronic oesophagitis and possibly HPV-16 infections are associated risk factors. Most tumours occur in the middle and lower thirds of the oesophagus. The post-cricoid upper third carcinomas associated with the Plummer–Vinson syndrome are rare today. There is synchronous and asynchronous association with tumours in the oropharynx, larynx and respiratory tract, with similar aetiological risk factors. Macroscopically, the tumours have a variably ulcerating, exophytic or stricturing appearance.

The microscopic appearance of squamous tumours is similar to that in other sites. Papanicolaou stain is optimal cytologically to demonstrate the bright keratinised orangeophilic cytoplasm (Fig. 7.12). The chromatin can vary from coarse and hyperchromatic to pyknotic in appearance. Anucleated keratinised squamous cells may also be present. In less-differentiated tumours, scattered isolated cells with more cyanophilic cytoplasm, enlarged nuclei and more apparent nucleoli are commonly seen (Fig. 7.13).

### Cytological findings: squamous cell carcinoma

- Ragged solid microbiopsies and syncytial sheets
- Dissociated pleomorphic abnormal squamous cells

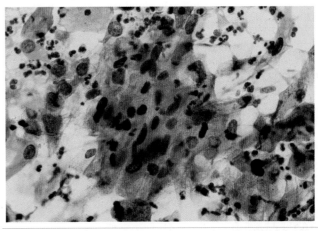

**Fig. 7.12** Oesophageal brush smear of well-differentiated squamous cell carcinoma. Note atypical squamous cells with inflammation on the background (PAP).

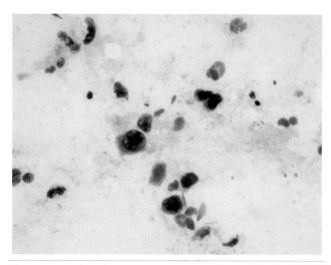

**Fig. 7.13** Oesophageal brush smear showing scattered isolated cells with enlarged nucleus in poorly differentiated squamous cell carcinoma (PAP).

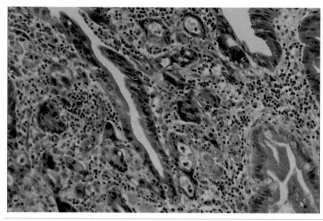

**Fig. 7.14** Histological sections from adenocarcinoma arising in Barrett's oesophagus. Presence of irregular glandular tubules growing in a back to back fashion; epithelium is severely atypical. Note the low-grade intestinal epithelial dysplasia on the right (H&E). (Courtesy of Professor Paula Chaves, Instituto Português de Oncologia Francisco Gentil, Lisboa.)

- Cell debris and/or slough
- Variable cytoplasmic differentiation or evidence of keratinisation.

Balloon cytology for the surveillance of squamous cell cancers has become accepted practice in high-incidence areas, especially in China. In addition, quantitative DNA fluorescence has been found to enhance detection of squamous cell cancers, including pre-invasive lesions, and can be applied to cytology taken in a high-risk population.

## Adenocarcinoma

There has been a striking increase in the incidence of this malignant neoplasm in Europe and USA in recent decades. Adenocarcinoma is most frequently localised at the gastro-oesophageal junction, generally being well-differentiated and only rarely having a signet-ring pattern. Apart from where there is a screening programme, staging at the time of diagnosis is high and the 5-year survival is low. The precursor lesion is dysplasia in Barrett's metaplasia, which is a risk factor along with reflux (Fig. 7.14). The changes of adenocarcinoma *in situ* in oesophageal brushings are similar to those described for endocervical adenocarcinoma *in situ* or colonic adenomatous *in situ* neoplastic changes. The histological descriptions are similar, although high-grade *in situ* changes are usually synchronous with adjacent invasive tumour at this site.

Cytological brushings show a background of necrosis within which there are dissociated columnar cells or small groups and more cuboidal or rounded cells, with enlarged hyperchromatic nucleus with one or more nucleoli (Fig. 7.15).

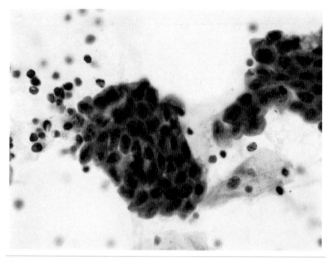

**Fig. 7.15** Cytological findings in oesophageal adenocarcinoma. Note cells with loss of polarity with increased N:C ratio and irregular nuclear contour; hyperchromatic nuclei with nucleoli (PAP).

## Other tumours

Rare histological variants of oesophageal cancer account for about 5% of cases. Other primary and secondary malignant tumours, epithelial and non-epithelial and certain inflammatory conditions that simulate cancer, occur in the oesophagus. These can be a diagnostic challenge but they are not common. Descriptions in the literature exist and one should keep these lesions in mind when dealing with particular clinical problems.[18-28]

## Stomach

### Normal cytological findings

Gastric brush samples are much more cellular than oesophageal brushings, even in the absence of disease. Normal components of gastric cytology comprise 'honeycomb' sheets of cells, columnar at the periphery with clear or dense cytoplasm, sometimes

---

### Cytological findings: adenocarcinoma

- Cellular aggregates with irregular outlines
- Loss of polarity
- Cuboidal/columnar cells
- Irregular nuclear contours
- Hyperchromatic nuclei with one or more large nucleoli
- Increased N:C ratio
- Tumour diathesis.

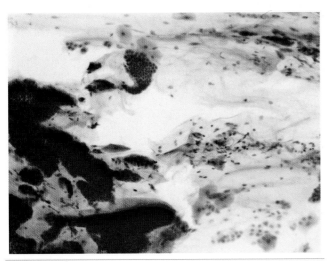

**Fig. 7.16** Normal components of gastric cytology comprising 'honeycomb' sheets of glandular cells (PAP).

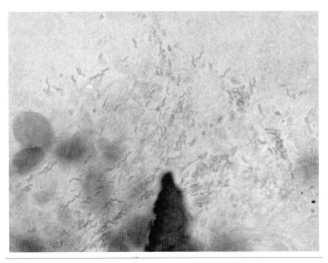

**Fig. 7.17** Spiral-like bacteria *(Hp)* are best seen entrapped in the mucus layer (PAP).

forming tubular structures (Fig. 7.16). Small nucleoli can be seen in the central located nucleus. Isolated naked nuclei may also be seen. Although not frequent, granular, eosinophilic, spherical acid-secreting parietal cells and more rarely recognisable pale cuboidal pepsinogen-secreting cells may be seen, depending on the site of the brushing and the depth of use of the brush. Inflammatory cells such as lymphocytes and neutrophils can also be present in variable amounts. As could be expected, food debris are often present and, not so frequently nowadays, fine or clumped refractile non-birefringent particles from the pre-endoscopy radiographic use of contrast medium (Box 7.4).

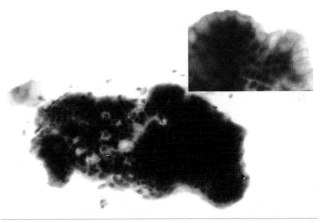

**Fig. 7.18** Gastric intestinal metaplasia characterised by a large sheet of epithelial cells with distinguishable 'portholes'. Inset shows a short brush border (PAP).

---

**Box 7.4  Normal components of gastric brushing**

- Sheets of cells with a honeycomb pattern
- Columnar cells of gastric superficial epithelium
- Macrophages and variable amounts of inflammatory cells
- Contaminants

---

## Inflammatory conditions

### Gastritis

The majority of cases of acute gastritis are self-limited, not requiring biopsy or cytological sampling for diagnosis.

Chronic gastritis is frequently sampled but an aetiological cause is not usually identified. The vast majority of cases are attributed to *Helicobacter pylori* infection. *Helicobacter pylori* plays a major role in upper gastrointestinal disorders, being a major cause of peptic ulcer disease and an important risk factor for gastric malignancy. It can be identified by several methods. While microbiological culture is the gold standard for the identification of the bacteria, biopsies are needed to classify the lesions according to the type of gastritis, inflammatory activity, lymphoid tissue and presence of tumour. The identification of the spiral bacteria by brush cytology, crush or imprint biopsies has been studied.[11] *Helicobacter pylori* spirals are best seen entrapped in the mucus layer, which is mostly removed by histological procedures. Cytology usually preserves this layer, so visualisation is easy with routine stains, such as

Papanicolaou or MGG methods and some reports show good results with Wright's stain (Fig. 7.17).[29]

Biopsies from *Helicobacter pylori* chronic gastritis show a diffuse plasma cell infiltrate, neutrophils permeating epithelial elements and lymphoid follicles. Cytology shows epithelial regenerative changes, sometimes with intestinal metaplasia in large cohesive groups of glandular cells. There may be some nuclear overlapping, slight nuclear enlargement and visible nucleoli. Cytoplasm can be dense and cells smaller. Brush smears may include some acute features, including increased mucous and fibrin meshes related to acute erosion and reactive (regenerative) epithelial sheets. This may raise the suspicion of dysplasia and neoplasia with a risk of false positive results. Favouring benign is the single layered cohesive group of cells and smooth nuclear membranes and only slightly variation in nuclear size.

Intestinal metaplasia may be recognised within sheets by the identification of an eosinophilic cuboidal or short columnar cell margin, a tenuous fused 'terminal bar' line and short brush border. Goblet cells are seen within the 'honeycomb', with the globule of mucus above or behind the nucleus (Fig. 7.18).

Other microorganisms can be identified, the majority being oral contaminants. If there is an ulcerated lesion, *Candida* sp.

and whorls of bacteria are often seen, raising the possibility of an underlying malignancy because of the frequent association. Descriptions of tuberculosis and syphilis, microfilaria and other parasites have been published.[1] CMV gastritis is associated with immunosuppression and the morphological aspects are as seen in other organs.

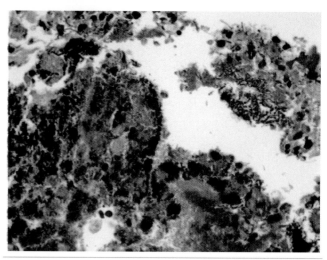

**Fig. 7.19** Ulcer slough composed of cell debris and haemorrhage where fungal spores and hyphae are readily seen (PAS).

---

### Cytological findings: gastritis

- Groups of epithelial cells with chronic inflammatory cell infiltration
- Discohesive epithelial cells
- Lymphocytes and plasma cells
- Variable acute inflammatory exudate
- Intestinal metaplasia may be seen.

## Peptic ulcer disease

This appears as compact fragments composed of mucus, histiocytes, epithelial cells and stromal material including small vessels, fibroblasts and lymphoid aggregates. The appearance of the deeper layers of the ulcer base is the critical element. In addition, there may be striated muscle from meat, vegetable matter or foreign crystalline debris from oral medications. Haemosiderin-laden macrophages may be seen, as evidence of old haemorrhage. *Candida* pseudohyphae may be present within the slough, representing secondary super infection as referred above (Fig. 7.19). Cells can show nuclear enlargement, visible nucleoli and mitosis reflecting regenerative epithelium.

This type of changes can be found in other gastric conditions like chronic atrophic gastritis and adenomas. They recapitulate what is seen in Barrett's epithelium and at the edge of ulcers, posing the same problems and challenges to reach a correct diagnosis.

Atrophic gastritis shows sheets of gastric epithelium, occasionally with intestinal metaplasia reflected by the presence of columnar and goblet cells intermingled with mixed inflammatory cells.

## Chemotherapy associated atypia

Acute gastric mucosal lesions can be caused by influx of anticancer agents into the regional blood stream, a type of therapy increasingly widely used. Systemic chemotherapy also induces gastric epithelial damage but lesions due to the more directed therapy are sampled more frequently.[1,14] Atypia can be severe and clinical information is crucial for the diagnosis.

# Neoplastic conditions

## Polyps

In general, isolated polyps are excised and only if multiple or large is there an attempt to screen the lesions using cytology. The majority are either hyperplastic or adenomatous and unless fragments are included it is not possible to diagnose these polyps on cytology alone. It is generally acknowledged that the natural course of hyperplastic polyps does not include transformation to carcinoma, although hyperplastic polyps are occasionally associated with gastric cancer.[30,31] Adenomas are indistinguishable from those of the lower gastrointestinal tract in that there are regenerative features with pseudostratification of elongated hyperchromatic epithelial cell nuclei and slough

---

### Box 7.5  Differential diagnosis of repair, dysplasia and neoplasia

- Repair
  - Monolayered groups of cells
  - Basophilic cytoplasm, often with no secretion
  - Intestinal metaplasia
  - Nucleus round and regular
  - (Evidence of *Helicobacter pylori*, ulcer slough)
- Dysplasia
  - Small clusters with piling up of cells
  - Obscured cytoplasmic boundaries
  - Larger, hyperchromatic nuclei
  - Atypia along with intestinal metaplasia
  - Presence of nucleoli (more evident in high grade)
  - Loss of polarity (more evident in high grade)
  - Anisonucleosis (more evident in high grade)
- Adenocarcinoma
  - Tumour diathesis
  - Isolated malignant cells or in small loose clusters
  - Severe anisonucleosis
  - Prominent nucleoli

---

from eventual ulceration. Occasionally, fragments of the fibrovascular core of the polyp is seen. The endoscopic features are essential to prevent the overdiagnosis of malignancy.

## Dysplasia

The difficulty of distinguishing cytologically between reparative changes, dysplasia and invasive neoplasia at any site cannot be overemphasised. There are few published data concerning this subject in gastric mucosa. In a review of 90 cases with cytology and histology available, the authors found that three degrees of cytological alteration would correspond to the three conditions.[32] Box 7.5 depicts these findings.

## Adenocarcinoma

Gastric adenocarcinoma is still one of the commonest forms of malignancy worldwide. The incidence and aetiological factors

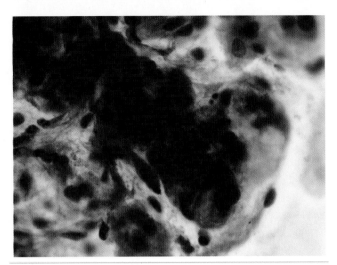

**Fig. 7.20** Gastric adenocarcinoma cytology showing three-dimensional groups of cells with loss of polarity, anisonucleosis and vacuolated cytoplasm (PAP).

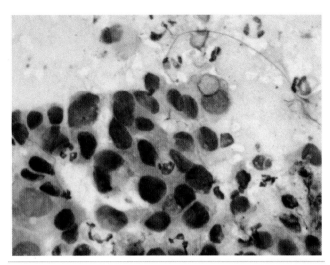

**Fig. 7.21** Gastric adenocarcinoma cytology showing group of atypical cells with a large vacuole in the cytoplasm (PAP).

differ in different parts of the world. *Helicobacter pylori* related tumours are declining while adenocarcinoma at the gastro-oesophageal junction, related to Barrett's metaplasia, is increasing in frequency.

The gross appearances of gastric cancer include polypoid, nodular, ulcerative and infiltrative plaque-like, or sclerosing forms. Combinations of these basic patterns may occur.

The best clue to the differential diagnosis of dysplasia and carcinoma is loss of cohesiveness. Single cells are easy to find and atypia is more readily appreciated. Desquamated cells with marked anisonucleosis, irregular nuclear contours, visible nucleoli and atypical mitotic figures can be seen. Three-dimensional groups of cells with loss of polarity and frayed contours will appear and the cells in groups will show moulding and overlapping. The N:C ratio is increased (Fig. 7.20). It is not always possible to assess with certainty the precise histological type of carcinoma, but the presence of large cells with an eccentric nucleus and a large vacuole implies a diffuse signet-ring cell type carcinoma (Fig. 7.21). However, care should be taken not to misinterpret macrophages with ingested mucus in the cytoplasm. Histiocytes have a bean-shaped nucleus with a normal N:C ratio. Transmucosal FNA has been used to sample those lesions that grow within the gastric wall.

### Cytological findings: adenocarcinoma

- Ulcer slough containing single malignant cells
- Presence of papillary or glandular formations
- Signet-ring cell carcinomas show a few dissociated cells, with a prominent mucous vacuole, open chromatin and large nucleoli
- Poorly differentiated tumours may have squamous features.

Knowledge of HER2 status is relevant to identify those patients who will benefit from specific therapies in gastric cancer.[33] Recently a score system, similar to the one used in breast cancer, is being validated using immunohistochemistry (IHC) and fluorescence *in situ* hybridisation (FISH).[34] For breast tumours, FISH has been applied to cytological samples to determine the over-expression of this receptor, so it is possible that in the near future directed cytological sampling of gastric

carcinoma will be used to assess HER2 because sampling is easier, faster and less expensive than biopsy.

### Neuroendocrine tumours

Carcinoid tumours of the stomach form a small percentage of this type of tumour in the gastrointestinal tract. In 2000, the WHO presented a classification scheme for all neuroendocrine tumours (NETs), which applied mainly to gastroentero-pancreatic tumours. The term carcinoid was replaced by (neuro) endocrine tumour, malignant carcinoid by well-differentiated (neuro) endocrine carcinoma, and the term 'small cell carcinoma' was changed to poorly differentiated NE carcinoma.

Small gastric NETs rarely give rise to symptoms and are diagnosed incidentally or in patients with pernicious anaemia. Larger carcinoids may bleed and occasionally, patients may complain of flushing, presenting with the 'atypical carcinoid syndrome'.[35] Histology is necessary for diagnosis. Cytology may be helpful, but should be confirmed by histology and ancillary tests. The cells are identical to those at other sites. The cytoplasm is finely granular, with a round nucleus and dispersed chromatin. There is little pleomorphism, necrosis or mitotic activity (Fig. 7.22). The differential diagnosis includes lymphoma and the diffuse type of adenocarcinoma. Histochemical and immunocytochemical stains can be used to distinguish these tumours.

### Gastrointestinal stromal tumours

Gastrointestinal stromal tumours (GIST) are the most common mesenchymal tumours of the gastrointestinal tract, with an annual incidence of 10–20 cases per million, being most commonly found in the stomach (40–70%). They occur with decreasing frequency in the small intestine (20–50%), in the colon and rectum (5–15%), and in the oesophagus (<2%). The tumour arises from the interstitial cells of Cajal, the pacemaker cells, forming the interface between the autonomic innervation of bowel and the smooth muscle itself.

Endoscopically they appear as a dome-shaped submucosal nodule, often with an ulcer at the centre (Fig. 7.23). Forceps biopsies frequently fail to sample diagnostic tissue because the mucosa slides over the underlying nodule. EUS-guided FNA is the best approach to reach the tumour.[36]

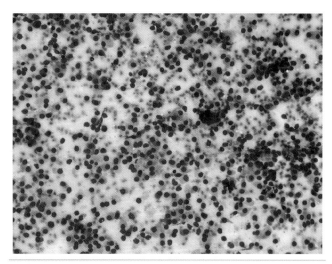

**Fig. 7.22** Well-differentiated neuroendocrine carcinoma, characterised by small discohesive cells and groups of cells with little pleomorphism, necrosis or mitotic activity (MGG).

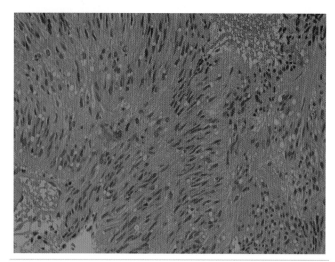

**Fig. 7.24** Cell block from GIST showing tissue fragments of a spindle cell neoplasm with dissecting fascicles. The tumour cells have ill-defined cytoplasmic borders, eosinophilic cytoplasm, uniform spindle nuclei with smooth nuclear membranes, and finely distributed even chromatin and inconspicuous nucleoli (H&E).

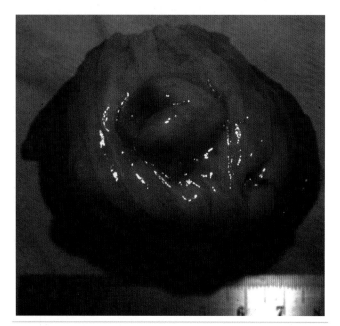

**Fig. 7.23** Typical gross aspect of a gastrointestinal stromal tumour forming a dome-shaped submucosal nodule with an ulcer at the centre.

Activating mutations of *c-kit* oncogene are the major genetic alterations in GISTs. The *c-kit* mutation is a proto-oncogene that codes for a transmembrane TK receptor: CD117. Once activated, *c-kit* propagates signalling events throughout the cell via multiple signal transduction pathways.

Until recently, the prognosis of patients with GISTs was poor due to their frequent recurrence and resistance to chemo- and radiotherapy regimens. The development and current treatment with specific RTK inhibitors is changing this scenario. Imatinib mesylate is a selective inhibitor of RTKs, by competing with adenosine triphosphate (ATP) for its binding site, preventing further phosphorylation of signalling molecules downstream of the receptor, responsible for the abnormal viability and proliferation signals in these cells. Several studies have linked different responses to the drug with *c-kit* alterations. In particular, tumours harboring exon 11 *c-kit* mutations are more likely to

respond to an Imatinib therapy than those with either exon 9 *c-kit* mutations or no detectable mutation. Currently, Imatinib is used for the treatment of Kit positive GIST patients with unresectable and/or metastatic malignant tumour. Besides Imatinib, another RTK inhibitor, Sunitinib (Sutent®, Pfizer), has recently been approved for the treatment of patients with GIST whose disease has progressed or who are unable to tolerate treatment with Imatinib.

It is a fact that obtaining an accurate diagnosis is of utmost importance for correct treatment, an earlier diagnosis being crucial for prompt therapy. EUS-FNA has been increasingly used for the assessment of diverse intra-abdominal and intra-thoracic tumours. The procedure not only allows meticulous representation of both extramural and intramural structures of the gastrointestinal tract but also permits tissue sampling from masses in these locations.

Recently, the authors analysed 85 patients with intramural gastrointestinal mesenchymal tumours and performed immunohistochemical and molecular analysis of both *c-kit* and *PDGFRA* genes in formalin-fixed paraffin embedded cell blocks obtained by EUS-FNA. Although cell blocks of the initial 85 cases were obtained, complete immunocytochemical and molecular analysis was only possible in 51 cases (Figs 7.24, 7.25). The mean age of patients was 62.4 (range, 26–92 years). Twenty (39.2%) patients were females and 31 (60.8%) were males. Topographically, 12 (23.5%) tumours were located in the oesophagus, 35 (68.6%) were gastric and four (7.8%) were located in the small intestine. The mean size of tumours documented by EUS was 33.9 mm (range 11–80 mm). Immunoreactivity for CD117 was detected in a majority of tumours pre-classified as GISTs. CD117 positivity in GIST cells was strongly present at the membrane and diffusely in the cytoplasm. CD117 was negative in 7/31 (22.6%) tumours pre-classified as GISTs. In two cases the immunostaining was not interpretable due the technical artefacts. PCR amplification and DNA sequencing revealed exon 11 mutations in 57.6% (19/33) GISTs, and exon 9 mutation in 3.0% (1/33). No *PDGFRA* activating mutations were detected in tumours bearing the *c-kit* wild type.

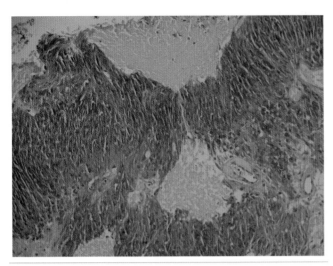

**Fig. 7.25** Cell block from GIST showing diffuse positivity for CD117 (immunohistochemistry).

In summary, our study demonstrated that 77.4% of GISTs strongly and diffusely express *c-kit*, irrespective of topography, age or gender. Although several studies indicate that 95–100% of GIST cases express kit, lower expression levels have been reported in Australian (78%) and Scandinavian studies (85%). Such differences in protein expression levels are probably due to different methodologies and population diversities. We identified *c-kit* mutations in 61% of GIST cases, in accordance with previously published ranges (30–90%). Nearly 95% (19/20) of *c-kit*-mutant tumours carried exon 11 mutations.[37]

EUS-FNA, a less costly, less risky and less invasive strategy than biopsy, is increasingly used for the diagnosis of gastrointestinal tumours, using cell block material for preoperative diagnosis, including immunocytochemistry and molecular analysis. With intraoperative cytology, it is possible to recognise the cellular characteristics of GIST and thereby narrow the differential diagnosis of a solid lesion in the gastrointestinal wall. This information can be useful for intraoperative management of the patient and establish the need for subsequent immunohistochemical and genetic studies.

Three histological types of GIST are described: spindle, epithelioid and mixed types, the first being the most frequent. The corresponding cytological aspects can equally be appreciated.

## Cytological findings: gastrointestinal stromal tumours

- Hypercellular smears
- Spindle-shaped cells in fascicles or whorls
- Scanty cytoplasm with cytoplasmic processes
- Elongated blunt-ended nuclei with granular chromatin
- Multiple nucleoli.

Hypercellularity with the majority of cells being spindle shaped while presenting in irregular outlined cell groups arranged in short fascicles or whorls is the commonest picture. The cells have elongated nuclei characterised by blunt ends. Their chromatin is finely to coarsely granular, with multiple small nucleoli (Figs 7.26, 7.27) The cytoplasm is scant with numerous wispy and fibrillary cytoplasmic processes.[38] The epithelioid type is characterised by loosely cohesive groups of intermediate-sized round to polygonal cells with nuclei

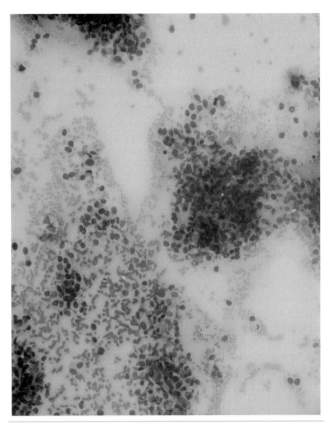

**Fig. 7.26** EUS-FNA from GIST showing highly cellular sample composed by tight aggregates and loosely cohesive cells, as well as isolated individual cells (PAP). (Courtesy of Dr Ricardo Fonseca, Instituto Português de Oncologia Francisco Gentil, Lisboa.)

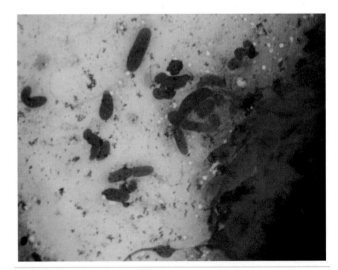

**Fig. 7.27** Cytological aspect of GIST characterised by uniform tumour cells with ill-defined cytoplasmic border. The nuclei are spindle and sometimes embedded in a fibrillary background. Necrosis is absent (MGG).

containing a coarsely granular chromatin. The nuclei generally have a solitary central nucleolus, irregular nuclear membranes, and variable degrees of nuclear pleomorphism.[39] The cells have abundant cytoplasm. Collagen bundles, as well as giant cells may also be noted. The mixed type contains spindle and epithelioid cells in separate areas.

### Diagnostic pitfalls: gastrointestinal stromal tumours

The differential diagnosis includes several mesenchymal and epithelial tumours and requires immunocytochemistry for confirmation. Smooth muscle, fibrous, vascular and neurogenic tumours are among the possibilities, as well as melanoma, lymphoma, neuroendocrine and metastatic tumours. From the point of view of ultrasonographics, who may be inclined to give a 'morphological' diagnosis, lipoma, duplication cyst and pancreatic rests are included in the differential diagnosis. The malignant potential of a GIST is difficult to establish on cytological sampling, especially if no positive markers of malignancy are present such as mitoses, necrosis, ulceration or infiltration of adjacent organs.

## Lymphoma

Cytology is not a first-line tool for diagnosis of gastric lymphoma. Most authors pay little attention to this diagnostic approach but despite this, some authors have published good results, with a definite diagnosis in half the patients (out of 27) where no low-grade lymphomas were included.[40] It is clinically relevant to differentiate MALT lymphoma from others that can have extra-nodal involvement such as large cell B cell lymphoma and, less frequently, Hodgkin's disease, because they will have different treatment approaches.

Primary gastric lymphomas usually present as single or multiple ulcerated nodular or polypoid masses in the gastric body or pyloric antrum. They may also take the form of incipiently ulcerating thickened rugae where the tumour is diffusely infiltrating.

The identification of lymphoma in brush smears requires the recognition of an unusual lymphoid population and whether that lymphoid population is reactive, derived from lymphocytic gastritis, or is neoplastic, that is, from a lymphoma of one of several particular cell types. Also, one must bear in mind that neuroendocrine carcinomas, poorly differentiated carcinomas and metastatic tumours to the gastric wall may be confused with lymphoma. In this setting, immunocytochemistry and flow cytometry are essential tools for a correct diagnosis. Unless lesions or lymph nodes are directly sampled this is not feasible in classical brush cytology. Morphology will show different types of lymphocytes, some reactive others suspicious of clonal proliferation; there may also be atypical changes in the epithelium due to the presence of ulcerated mucosa as seen clinically. The role of cytology is that of an ancillary technique.[8]

## Duodenum

### Normal cytological findings

Duodenal sampling is rare compared with other gastrointestinal sites. Normal components with brush sampling of the duodenum are similar to those obtained as contaminants with EUS-FNA.[41] They include sheets of epithelial cells with a honeycomb pattern, within which goblet cells can be seen. At the periphery, the cells are polarised and the cytoplasm is cyanophilic or eosinophilic with basal nuclei. A ciliated luminal surface may be seen. Goblet cells have finely vesicular cytoplasm and a basal nucleus (Fig. 7.28). Cells from pancreatic or bile ducts may be present and are indistinguishable from those from the duodenal surface (Box 7.6).

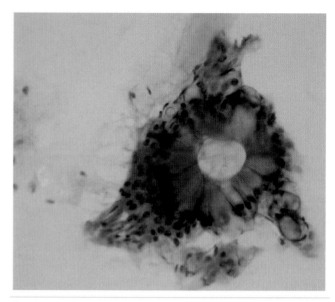

**Fig. 7.28** Normal components of duodenal cytology comprising goblet cells with finely vesicular cytoplasm and basally located nuclei (PAP).

### Box 7.6  Normal components of duodenal brushing

- Columnar epithelial cells isolated or in sheets with a honeycomb pattern
- Dissociated columnar cells with basally located round nucleus with delicate chromatin and small nucleoli
- Goblet cells
- Occasional Paneth cells
- Rare macrophages and other inflammatory cells

## Inflammatory conditions

### Duodenitis and peptic ulcer

In general duodenitis is non-specific. Usually there are inflammatory cells along with epithelial cells showing repair changes and increased cellularity with poorly preserved cells and stripped isolated nuclei.

In peptic disease ulcer slough appears along with degenerative and reparative epithelial changes as previously described in the stomach. Macrophages, leucocytes and red blood cells are present.

### Infectious diseases

Similar agents to those described in the oesophagus and stomach can be found at this site. Viral agents such as CMV produce the same cytological changes as already described in epithelial and stromal cells, affecting immunocompromised patients. The nuclei are enlarged with a halo surrounding the inclusion; sometimes cytoplasmic inclusions can also be seen.

*H. pylori* can colonise duodenal mucosa, either in the normal lining of the bulb or in gastric metaplastic epithelium in the distal duodenal segments.

Other agents may be seen especially in regions where prevalence of a particular microorganism is high and where cytological sampling greatly enhances a positive diagnosis. *Giardia lamblia* is seen as a pear-shaped microorganism with twin nuclei and a flagellum. Detection rate is even better than for *Hp*.[42]

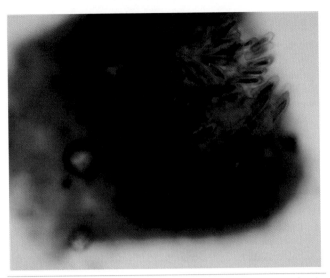

**Fig. 7.29** EUS-FNA from a duodenal mass showing the characteristics hooks of echinococcosis (Giemsa).

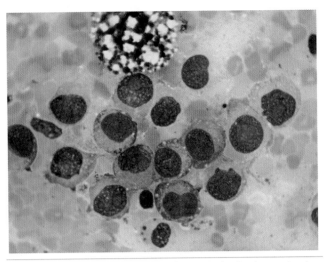

**Fig. 7.30** EUS-FNA from a metastatic melanoma in the duodenum showing malignant cells with abundant cytoplasm and prominent nucleoli (MGG).

*Cryptosporidium* sp. can infect an immunocompetent host but more often affects immunocompromised patients. The organisms are usually aligned over the mucosa so brush cytology can easily collect them.

Typical and atypical mycobacteria can infect the gastrointestinal tract and are a significant problem in many regions. Sampling is either obtained by endoscopic brushing or by EUS-FNA of masses and regional lymph nodes, allowing isolation of the microorganism in culture if enough material is obtained.[43] The smears either show the typical epithelioid granulomas with lymphocytes and a variable amount of necrosis or histiocytes with acid-fast bacilli of atypical mycobacterial infection, confirmed by acid-fast staining.

An unusual clinical presentation of *Taenia echinococcus* as an extra-mural mass in the gastrointestinal tract can be investigated by FNA cytology. The aspirate in general is clear and the tapeworms have characteristic hooks (Fig. 7.29).

## Neoplastic conditions

### Benign tumours

Adenomyomas and adenomas of the ampulla of Vater are the most frequent benign tumours of this region for which there are no confident criteria to make a cytological diagnosis, as with gastric polyps.

### Malignant tumours

Lymphoma and neuroendocrine tumours occur in the duodenum and their cytological features are similar to those seen at other sites.

Although a rare tumour in the small bowel, adenocarcinoma is more frequent in the duodenum where it involves the ampullary region. Their cytological features resemble those of the biliary tract (see Ch. 9). Three-dimensional groups of cells, with irregular outlines contrast with orderly benign epithelium, and there are numerous dissociated cells, more than expected in a benign lesion. The presence of normal epithelium is of enormous help. Atypia, anisokaryosis and anisocytosis are more pronounced the higher the grade. Low-grade adenocarcinomas pose the same problems as elsewhere, and at this site one should be aware of the reactive changes induced by the presence of 'stent' drainage or any diagnostic procedures.

There are few cytological reports concerning metastatic tumours to the small bowel but melanoma, breast, ovary and lung carcinomas are the most frequent primary sites.[1] These metastases can lie within the wall and in these cases, EUS-FNA is the best approach for diagnosis (Fig. 7.30).

## Colon

Large bowel cytology is not used for routine diagnosis or for prevention of colon cancer due to the extensive use of colonoscopy. Nevertheless, several authors report good results with direct brushing techniques especially for screening of the lesions of inflammatory bowel disease because these can be useful in the evaluation of extensive areas of damaged mucosa. Some tumoral strictures not amenable to forceps biopsy can be sampled with brush cytology and a diagnosis can be rendered. Liquid-based cytology from brush cytology can also be used with the advantage that molecular and immunohistochemical studies can be applied.[44] Lavage techniques described by some authors in the 1960s and 1970s no longer seem to have supporters.[8]

Percutaneous ultrasound-guided aspiration biopsy may be attempted for diagnosis of colonic lesions in situations where it may be the only means of obtaining a cytological diagnosis before surgery, for instance, in patients in whom colonoscopy is not possible or cannot be performed properly for various reasons.[45] Complications are rare but include haemorrhage, sepsis and needle tract seeding. EUS-FNA has also been used, especially for mural and extrinsic masses such as gastrointestinal stromal tumours, haemangioma, lymphoma, neuroendocrine carcinoma, lipoma, carcinoid tumour, recurrence of rectal carcinoma and recurrence of other distant malignancies, for example, gastric and ovarian carcinoma. EUS-FNA has been used to diagnose rectosigmoid endometriosis presenting as a subepithelial stricture or as a mass in the rectosigmoid region.

## Normal cytological findings

Normal components consist of columnar cells with a honey-comb pattern in flat sheets, tubular structures of intact crypts and as isolated cells. The nucleus is pale and centrally located. There may be Paneth cells, more often seen at the right colon. Goblet cells have barrel shaped vacuoles filling the cytoplasm and are more frequent than in the small bowel (Box 7.7).

---

**Box 7.7  Normal components of colonic brushings**

- Columnar cells with central pale nucleus
- Cells can be isolated, in flat sheets or in tubular profiles
- Mucous cells
- Macrophages, leucocytes and debris

---

## Inflammatory conditions

### Chronic inflammatory diseases

Both Crohn's disease (CD) and ulcerative colitis (UC), represent prototypical conditions whose most salient features are the presence of chronic inflammation involving various parts of the intestinal tract and an increased risk of cancer, which is a complication directly related to the duration and activity of gut inflammation. Clinically they are characterised by exacerbation and remission episodes. Diagnosis is based on clinical, serological, colonoscopic and morphological histology criteria but occasionally cytology can be used to rule out infections such as amoebiasis and tuberculosis.

Ulcerative colitis, and to a lesser extent CD, can be complicated by the development of adenocarcinoma, particularly in longstanding pancolitis. Cancers tend to be multiple, more anaplastic and extensively infiltrating, arising in a flat mucosa instead of the usual adenoma-carcinoma sequence.[46] Dysplasia in inflammatory bowel disease has an unpredictable course, which complicates efforts to develop molecular or histological markers of neoplastic progression or future cancer risk.[47]

Endoscopically, benign and malignant lesions can be indistinguishable in this setting. In order to have a more thoroughly sampled segment, particularly in stenotic lesions, cytology is incorporated in some centres to survey longstanding chronic inflammatory bowel disease,[48] but the categories of high-grade, low-grade and indefinite for dysplasia are defined for biopsy specimens.[1] Reparative, dysplasia and neoplasia pose the same problems discussed above in Barrett's oesophagus.

---

**Cytological findings: chronic inflammatory diseases**

Cytological samples from cases of CD and UC, when not complicated by dysplasia or carcinoma are nonspecific, with different findings depending on the stage of the disease. Ulcer slough and blood along with inflammatory cells and epithelial reactive changes may be seen. Enlarged cells with pale staining nuclei, thick nuclear membrane and visible nucleoli may be seen. Granulomas would aid the diagnosis of CD in the appropriate clinical and endoscopic setting.

---

**Diagnostic pitfalls: chronic inflammatory diseases**

The differential diagnosis between normal, dysplasia and neoplasia is based on several cytological features including cell grouping, presence or absence of mucin, normal cytoplasm, nuclei and nucleoli, as it is for the general cytological evaluation. In dysplasia, aggregates lose cell polarity and are slender with hyperchromatic nuclei and small to large nucleoli. Mucin and goblet cells are reduced. Isolated cells are more frequent in adenocarcinomas with obvious irregular cytoplasmic and nuclear contours and prominent nucleoli. The nucleus is hyperchromatic and there is variable amount of mucin. Cells aggregates are three-dimensional.

### Acute inflammatory diseases

Self-limited colitis is not usually sampled for cytological diagnosis. Some inflammatory conditions such as diverticulitis and amoebic colitis have been described; however, unless a specific agent is found, a descriptive diagnosis only should be rendered (Box 7.8).

Diverticulitis may present as a stenotic lesion, simulating neoplasia, and can be difficult to sample with forceps, making brush or FNA cytology alternative diagnostic approaches. *Entamoeba histolytica* colitis can be complicated by bowel perforation and endoscopic features can pose difficulties in the differential diagnosis with ulcerative colitis (Fig. 7.31). Also, CMV must be ruled out when ulcers are the major endoscopic feature. On the other hand, tuberculosis is one of the major differential diagnoses with CD (Fig. 7.32). In endemic areas, longstanding silent schistosomiasis has been associated with adenocarcinoma in the

---

**Box 7.8  Some causes of acute colitis reported cytologically**

- Diverticulitis
- *Entamoeba histolytica* colitis
- Schistosomiasis
- *Histoplasma capsulatum*
- CMV

---

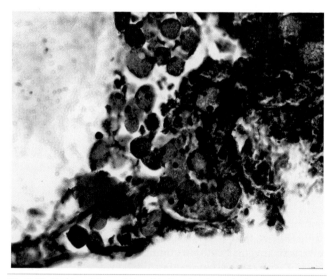

**Fig. 7.31** Cytology of amoebic colitis showing the typical parasite with its characteristic nucleus and phagocytised erythrocytes (PAS).

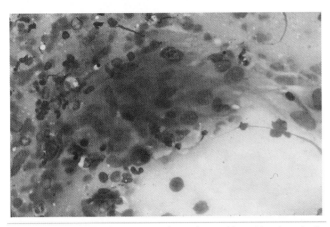

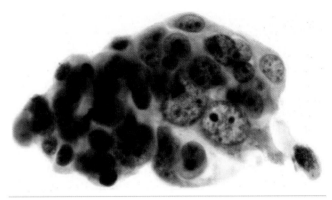

**Fig. 7.33** Colonic adenocarcinoma cytology showing group of atypical cells with prominent anisokaryosis (MGG).

**Fig. 7.32** Cytology illustrating a typical granuloma with multinucleated cells in a case of intestinal tuberculosis (MGG).

colon[49] and histoplasmosis has been found in an HIV patient presenting with a rectal mass. In this type of case, samples will yield inflammatory cells, debris, epithelial cells and sometimes the aetiological agent, normally entrapped in the mucous layer.

## Neoplastic conditions

Morphologically, normal colon mucosa in cancer patients is not metabolically normal. Based on these findings, some authors have suggested that analysis of the normal-looking mucosa by a rectal smear test or lavage, might be used as a simple, noninvasive screening test for colon cancer. Although a significantly higher or lower level of expression of a single gene might not be a very reliable indicator, multivariate analysis suggests that analysis of a group of genes might provide a much better indicator of increased risk. These genes are involved in several pathways related to cancer development, including the APC/β-catenin pathway, the nuclear factor-κB pathway, cell cycle, and inflammation.[50]

### Benign tumours

Although previous descriptions emphasise that in dysplasia, slender cell aggregates with loss of polarity and with hyperchromatic nuclei and small to large nucleoli are characteristics of benign colonic polyps, in our experience colonic polyps cannot be diagnosed by cytological sampling.

Although not a tumour, endometriosis is one of the greatest potential pitfalls in the diagnosis of recto-sigmoid wall masses. Reactive changes are worrisome and include nuclear enlargement and prominent nucleoli but the cell clusters are organised and there are variable amounts of haemorrhage. The clinical history is crucial for a correct diagnosis.

### Malignant tumours

Brush cytology is a sensitive technique in the diagnosis of colon cancer and combination with histology increases sensitivity and improves the overall accuracy.[51] Colonic carcinomas are mucus-producing adenocarcinomas with different levels of differentiation, ranging from well-defined glandular structures to solid growing anaplastic cancer cells (Fig. 7.33). Cells obtained by brushing or FNA correspond to this variation. Isolated cells

are more frequent in adenocarcinoma making it easier to identify irregular cytoplasmic and nuclear contours and prominent nucleoli. The nucleus is hyperchromatic and there is a variable amount of mucin. Cell aggregates are three-dimensional. The diagnosis is based mainly on nuclear abnormalities.

As previously described, other neoplasms such as neuroendocrine tumours, GISTs, lymphomas and metastatic tumours can be found in the colon and the cytological criteria are much the same as at other sites.

## Anal canal

Persistent infection with high-risk human papillomavirus is generally accepted as a necessary cause of cervical cancer. The natural history of anal intraepithelial neoplasia resembles that of cervical intraepithelial neoplasia.[52] Anal cytology has gained importance in recent years mainly because of the increased incidence of carcinoma in HIV patients, which parallels the incidence of carcinoma of the uterine cervix before screening programmes. Anal screening programmes for the 'at risk' population have been advocated but some issues still need to be clarified, including standardising of the collection of specimens, the criteria for adequacy of samples and how to classify lesions. Although several papers have been published on these matters, introducing such criteria, inter-observer and intra-observer reproducibility remain less than optimal. There seems to be no difference between liquid-based and conventional cytology. A range of opinions exists in the interpretation of anal cytology and biopsy specimens, but overall, there is only moderate agreement, even using the Bethesda System. In addition to standard Papanicolaou stained smears and directed biopsies, molecular markers such as p16 and aberrantly methylated tumour suppressor genes may help to improve reliability as well as accuracy.[53–55] Hybrid-capture II testing for high-risk human papillomavirus also seems to be a powerful tool, reducing the need for anoscopy in studies conducted in men with sexually transmitted disease.[56]

## Normal cytological findings

Normal components of anal cytology are nucleated and anucleated squamous cells and variable amounts of transitional and columnar cells from the rectum.

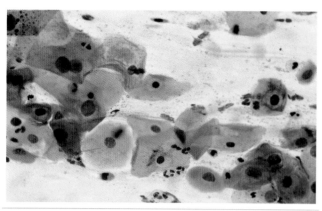

**Fig. 7.34** Smears from an anal lesion showing the presence of HPV-related changes in squamous cells (PAP).

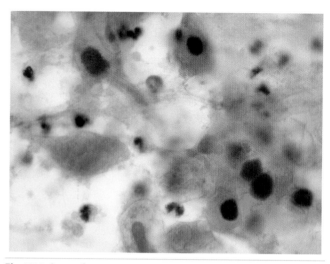

**Fig. 7.35** Smears from tumour mass in the anal canal showing atypical squamous cells, characterising a squamous cell carcinoma (PAP).

## Benign disorders

The vast majority of the clinical lesions of the anus are haemorrhoids, which are not a cytological problem.

Virus infections with herpes and human papillomavirus have been seen in men and women as sexual transmitted diseases with increasing incidence, particularly in HIV-positive patients. The most common is condylomata acuminata, which are similar to vulvar lesions and caused by HPV infection. Cytology samples show the same cells as described in other sites but with less obvious koilocytes and the presence of superficial anucleate squames is not helpful as they are to be expected in anal smears (Fig. 7.34).[57]

Pouchitis after ileal pouch-anal anastomosis for inflammatory bowel disease can be a serious problem. Several inflammatory and non-inflammatory conditions can mimic pouchitis, and endoscopy with biopsies is essential for distinguishing these various conditions.[58] Cytology may play a role in this setting. The risk of dysplasia is very low, but recent concerns regarding the malignant potential of the pouch require that surveillance be performed.[59]

## Malignant and pre-malignant lesions

The clinical appearance of anal/perianal dysplastic lesions is a poor predictor of the histological grade of disease. Anal intraepithelial neoplasia (AIN) is an HPV-related lesion. It has been shown that infection with high-risk human papillomavirus results in up-regulation of p16 and increased cellular proliferation. The presence of p16 immunoreactivity is a good predictor of dysplasia in anal specimens. However, the sensitivity and specificity of this marker are not high. Aberrant DNA methylation is a frequent event in anal high-grade squamous intraepithelial lesion (HSIL) and squamous cell carcinoma (SCC). Methylation of IGSF4 and DAPK1 is specific for HSIL and SCC, and may serve as a useful molecular biomarker.[60,61]

### Cytological findings: malignant and pre-malignant lesions

Anal canal cancers are composed predominantly of squamous cells or a mixture of squamous cells and transitional cells (cloacogenic carcinoma) (Fig. 7.35). Cloacogenic carcinomas arise in the transitional zone, where the cuboidal epithelium of rectum changes into stratified squamous epithelium of anal canal.[62]

Other lesions encountered in the perianal region include basal cell carcinoma, melanoma and extramammary Paget's disease of the perianal region.

## REFERENCES

1. Geisinger KR, Stanley MW, Raab SS, et al. Gastrointestinal system. In: Modern Cytopathology. Edinburgh: Churchill Livingstone; 2003. 1. , et al. .

2. Vander Noot MR 3rd, Eloubeidi MA, Chen VK, et al. Diagnosis of gastrointestinal tract lesions by endoscopic ultrasound-guided fine-needle aspiration biopsy. Cancer 2004;102:157–63.

3. DeNardi FG, Ridell RH. Esophagus. In: Mills SE, editor. Histology for Pathologists, 3rd ed. London: Lippincott Williams and Wilkins; 2007.

4. Owen DA. Stomach. In: Mills SE, editor. Histology for Pathologists. 3rd ed. London: Lippincott Williams and Wilkins; 2007.

5. Gramlich TL, Petras RE. Small intestine. In: Mills SE, editor. Histology for Pathologists. 3rd ed. London: Lippincott Williams and Wilkins; 2007.

6. Dahl J, Greenson JK. Colon. In: Mills SE, editor. Histology for Pathologists. 3rd ed. London: Lippincott Williams and Wilkins; 2007.

7. Fenger C. Anal canal. In: Mills SE, editor. Histology for Pathologists. 3rd ed. London: Lippincott Williams and Wilkins; 2007.

8. Melamed MR. The gastrointestinal tract. In: . Koss' Diagnostic Cytology and its Histopathologic Bases. 5th ed. Vol. 1. London: Lippincott Williams and Wilkins; 2005.

9. Sepehr A, Razavi P, Saidi F, et al. Esophageal exfoliative. Cytology Samplers – A comparison of three types. Acta Cytol 2000;44:797–804.

10. Wang KK, Wongkeesong M, Buttar N. American Gastroenterological Association Technical Review on the Role of the Gastroenterologist in the Management of Esophageal Carcinoma. Gastroenterology 2005;128:1471–505.

11. Misra SP, Misra V, Dwivedi M, et al. Diagnosing Helicobacter pylori by imprint cytology: can the same biopsy specimen be used for histology? Diagn Cytopathol 1998;18:330–32.

12. Cubukçu A, Günüllü NN, Erçin C, et al. Imprint cytology in the diagnosis of Helicobacter pylori. Does imprinting

damage the biopsy specimen? Acta Cytol 2000;44:124–27.

13. Klapman JB, Logrono R, Dye CE, et al. Clinical impact of on-site cytopathology interpretation on endoscopic ultrasound-guided fine needle aspiration. Am J Gastroenterol 2003;98:1289–94.

14. Brien TP, Farraye FA, Odze RD. Gastric dysplasia-like epithelial atypia associated with chemoradiotherapy for esophageal cancer: a clinicopathologic and immunohistochemical study of 15 cases. Mod Pathol 2001;14:389–96.

15. Hughes JH, Cohen MB. Is the cytologic diagnosis of esophageal glandular dysplasia feasible? Diagn Cytopathol 1998;18:312–16.

16. Kim R. Geisinger, Cytology in Barrett's esophagus. Diagn Cytopathol 1998;19:401–2.

17. Werner-Wasik M, Pequignot E, Leeper D, et al. Predictors of severe esophagitis include use of concurrent chemotherapy, but not the length of irradiated esophagus: a multivariate analysis of patients with lung cancer treated with nonoperative therapy. Int J Radiat Oncol Biol Phys 2000;48:689–96.

18. Leong QM, Kam JH. Primary malignant melanoma of the lower oesophagus presenting with dysphagia and upper gastrointestinal bleeding. Cases J 2008;11:1:28.

19. Johnson AD, Pambuccian SE, Andrade RS, et al. Ewing sarcoma and primitive neuroectodermal tumor of the esophagus: Report of a case and review of literature. Int J Surg Pathol 2008. May 21 [Epub ahead of print].

20. Narra SL, Tombazzi C, Datta V, et al. Granular cell tumor of the esophagus: report of five cases and review of the literature. Am J Med Sci 2008;335:338–41.

21. Ray S, Saluja SS, Gupta R, et al. Esophageal leiomyomatosis -an unusual cause of pseudoachalasia. Can J Gastroenterol 2008;22:187–89.

22. Mizuguchi S, Inoue K, Imagawa A, et al. Benign esophageal schwannoma compressing the trachea in pregnancy. Ann Thorac Surg 2008;85:660–62.

23. Pimenta AP, Preto JR, Gouveia AM, et al. Mediastinal tuberculous lymphadenitis presenting as an esophageal intramural tumor: a very rare but important cause for dysphagia. World J Gastroenterol 2007;13:6104–8.

24. Maezato K, Nishimaki T, Oshiro M, et al. Signet-ring cell carcinoma of the esophagus associated with Barrett's epithelium: report of a case. Surg Today 2007;37:1096–101.

25. Ku GY, Minsky BD, Rusch VW, et al. Small-cell carcinoma of the esophagus and gastroesophageal junction: review of the Memorial Sloan-Kettering experience. Ann Oncol 2008;19:533–37.

26. Hülagü S, Sentürk O, Aygün C, et al. Granular cell tumor of esophagus removed with endoscopic submucosal dissection. Turk J Gastroenterol 2007;18:188–91.

27. Kelly J, Leader M, Broe P. Primary malignant melanoma of the oesophagus: a case report. J Med Case Reports 2007;1:50.

28. Lee SS, Lee JL, Ryu MH, et al. Extra-pulmonary small cell carcinoma: single centre experience with 61 patients. Acta Oncol 2007;46:846–51.

29. Hashemi MR, Rahnavardi M, Bikdeli B, et al. Touch cytology in diagnosing Helicobacter

pylori: comparison of four staining methods. Cytopathology 2008;19:179–84.

30. Hirasaki S, Kanzaki H, Fujita K, et al. Papillary adenocarcinoma occurring in a gastric hyperplastic polyp observed by magnifying endoscopy and treated with endoscopic mucosal resection. Intern Med 2008;47:949–52.

31. Hirasaki S, Suzuki S, Kanzaki H, et al. Minute signet ring cell carcinoma occurring in gastric hyperplastic polyp. World J Gastroenterol 2007;13:5779–80.

32. Hustin J, Lagneaux G, Donnay M, et al. Cytologic patterns of reparative processes, true dysplasia and carcinoma of the gastric mucosa. Acta Cytol 1994;38:730–36.

33. Moutinho C, Mateus AR, Milanezi F, et al. Epidermal growth factor receptor structural alterations in gastric cancer. BMC Cancer 2008;8:10.

34. Hofmann M, Stoss O, Shi D, et al. Assessment of a HER2 scoring system for gastric cancer: results from a validation study. Histopathology 2008;52:797–805.

35. ENETS Guidelines Neuroendocrinology 2004; 80:394–424

36. Ando N, Goto H, Niwa Y, et al. The diagnosis of GI stromal tumors with EUS-guided fine needle aspiration with immunohistochemical analysis. Gastrointest Endosc 2002;55:37–43.

37. Gomes AL, Bardales RH, Milanezi F, et al. Molecular analysis of c-Kit and PDGFRA in GISTs diagnosed by EUS. Am J Clin Pathol 2007;127:1–8.

38. Wieczorek TJ, Faquin WC, Rubin BP, et al. Cytologic diagnosis of gastrointestinal stromal tumor with emphasis on the differential diagnosis with leiomyosarcoma. Cancer Cytopathol 2001;93:276–87.

39. Dong Q, McKee G, Pitman M, et al. Epithelioid variant of gastrointestinal stromal tumor: Diagnosis by fine-needle aspiration. Diagn Cytopathol 2003;29:55–60.

40. Sherman ME, Anderson C, Herman LM, et al. Utility of gastric brushing in the diagnosis of malignant lymphoma. Acta Cytol 1994;38:169–74.

41. Nagle JA, Wilbur DC, Pitman MB. Cytomorphology of gastric and duodenal epithelium and reactivity to B72.3: a baseline for comparison to pancreatic lesions aspirated by EUS-FNAB. Diagn Cytopathol 2005;33:381–86.

42. Patwari AK, Anand VK, Malhotra V, et al. Brush cytology: an adjunct to diagnostic upper GI endoscopy. Indian J Pediatr 2001;68:515–18.

43. Jain S, Kumar N, Jain SK. Gastric tuberculosis. Endoscopic cytology as a diagnostic tool. Acta Cytol 2000;44:987–92.

44. Kontzoglou K, Moulakakis KG, Alexiou D, et al. The role of liquid-based cytology in the investigation of colorectal lesions: a cytohistopathological correlation and evaluation of diagnostic accuracy. Arch Surg 2007;392:189–95.

45. Misra SP, Misra V, Dwivedi M, et al. Fine-needle aspiration biopsy of colonic masses. Diagn Cytopathol 1998;19:330–32.

46. Kornbluth A, Sachar DB. Practice Parameters Committee of the American College of Gastroenterology. Ulcerative colitis practice

guidelines in adults (update): American College of Gastroenterology, Practice Parameters Committee. Am J Gastroenterol 2004;99:1371–85.

47. Timothy LZ, David TR. Colorectal cancer and dysplasia in inflammatory bowel disease. World J Gastroenterol 2008;14:2662–69.

48. Itzkowitz SH, Present DH. Consensus conference: Colorectal cancer screening and surveillance in inflammatory bowel disease. Inflamm Bowel Dis 2005;11:314–21.

49. Li W-C, Pan Z-G, Sun Y-H. Sigmoid colonic carcinoma associated with deposited ova of Schistosoma japonicum: A case report. World J Gastroenterol 2006;12:6077–79.

50. Chen LC, Hao CY, Chiu YS, et al. Alteration of gene expression in normal-appearing colon mucosa of APC(min) mice and human cancer patients. Cancer Res 2004;64:3694–700.

51. Ehya H, O'Hara BJ. Brush cytology in the diagnosis of colonic neoplasms. Cancer 1990;66:1563–67.

52. Fox PA. Human papillomavirus and anal intraepithelial neoplasia. Curr Opin Infect Dis 2006;19:62–66.

53. Lytwyn A, Salit IE, Raboud J, et al. Interobserver Agreement in the Interpretation of Anal Intraepithelial Neoplasia. Cancer 2005;103:1447–56.

54. Colquhoun P, Nogueras JJ, Dipasquale B, et al. Interobserver and intraobserver bias exists in the interpretation of anal dysplasia. Dis Colon Rectum 2003;46:1332–38.

55. Walts AE, Thomas P, Bose S. Anal cytology: is there a role for reflex HPV DNA testing? Diagn Cytopathol 2005;33:152–56.

56. Goldstone SE, Kawalek AZ, Goldstone RN, et al. Hybrid Capture II detection of oncogenic human papillomavirus: a useful tool when evaluating men who have sex with men with atypical squamous cells of undetermined significance on anal cytology. Dis Colon Rectum 2008;51:1130–36.

57. Scholefield JH, Johnson J, Hitchcock A, et al. Guidelines for anal cytology – to make cytological diagnosis and follow up much more reliable. Cytopathology 1998;9:15–22.

58. Pardi DS, Shen B. Endoscopy in the management of patients after ileal pouch surgery for ulcerative colitis. Endoscopy 2008;40:529–33.

59. O'Riordain MG, Fazio VW, Lavery IC, et al. Incidence and natural history of dysplasia of the anal transitional zone after ileal pouch-anal anastomosis: results of a five-year to ten-year follow-up. Dis Colon Rectum 2000;43:1660–65.

60. Zhang J, Martins CR, Fansler ZB, et al. DNA methylation in anal intraepithelial lesions and anal squamous cell carcinoma. Clin Cancer Res 2005;11:6544–49.

61. Papaconstantinou HT, Lee AJ, Simmang CL, et al. Screening methods for high-grade dysplasia in patients with anal condyloma. J Surg Res 2005;127:8–13.

62. Herat A, Whitfeld M, Hillman R. Anal intraepithelial neoplasia and anal cancer in dermatological practice. Australas J Dermatol 2007;48:143–55.

# Section 6

## Hepatobiliary System and Pancreas

# Liver

Martha Bishop Pitman

## Chapter contents

## Introduction

Cytological analysis of the liver involves the aspiration of cells from focal mass lesions or from brushing the lining of strictured intrahepatic ducts primarily for the purpose of determining the presence or absence of malignancy. Fine needle aspiration (FNA) of focal mass lesions can be performed percutaneously or with endoscopic ultrasound guidance.[1,2] Intrahepatic ducts are brushed with the aid of endoscopic retrograde cholangiography.[3,4]

Needle aspiration of the liver was performed as long ago as 1833 when Roberts and Biett reported its use in the treatment of hepatic abscesses and echinococcal cysts.[5,6] Although the use of fine needles to obtain tissue for cytological diagnosis was first used by Lucatello in 1895 (cited in Lundquist 1971),[7] it was a technique refined in the 1920s by Martin and Ellis at the Memorial Hospital in New York.[8] Its utility in the liver was highlighted by Lundquist who published his experience using aspiration cytology in the evaluation of neoplastic and non-neoplastic disorders of the liver.[7,9,10] FNA biopsy is now the diagnostic procedure of choice for the diagnosis of focal mass lesions and is considered accurate and safe when performed and interpreted by experienced radiologists and pathologists.[1,11–13]

The diagnostic accuracy rate of FNA is reported at greater than 85% in most series.[14] False negative FNAs are most often due to sampling error. Proper specimen processing and staining optimises the preservation and presentation of the cells and is an important factor in reducing interpretation error. Routine supplementation of FNA with a cell block of tissue fragments or core biopsy is better than either method alone, especially for benign neoplasms and poorly differentiated neoplasms that require ancillary studies.[15–17]

## Contraindications

Contraindications for FNA of the liver are few but include a non-correctable bleeding diathesis, the lack of a safe access route, and an uncooperative patient[1,11] For EUS guided FNA, gastrointestinal obstruction is an absolute contraindication because of the risk of intestinal perforation.[18]

## Complications

With modern-day techniques, complications of FNA are uncommon. The most common complications include pain and haemorrhage.[14] The haemorrhage can be intraperitoneal, subcapsular, or intrahepatic and, if intrahepatic, can lead to haemobilia. There is a low risk of haematogenous dissemination of malignant cells after liver biopsy[19,20] as well as 'seeding' of the biopsy tract, complications that tend to be related to larger needle size.[14,21]

## Pre-biopsy assessment

Pre-biopsy assessment of patients undergoing FNA of the liver includes evaluation of the coagulation system to prevent excessive bleeding, generally complete blood count, prothrombin time and partial thromboblastin time.[1] Patients who are receiving intravenous sedation should not eat at least 6 hours before the biopsy.[1] Local anaesthetic is generally given down to the liver capsule. Discussing the procedure fully with the patient reduces patient anxiety, improves patient cooperation and increases the likelihood of a successful FNA procedure.

## Guidance systems

Percutaneous computed tomographic (CT) or ultrasound (US) guidance are the guidance systems used for most liver FNAs.[1,22–24] Endoscopic ultrasound guidance (EUS) is increasingly used for those lesions accessible through a transgastric approach, mostly in the left lobe.[2,25–28] Factors influencing the choice of the guidance system include the size, location and visibility of the mass, in addition to the experience and preference of the operator.[1,11] Ultrasound provides real-time needle visualisation, flexible patient positioning, variable imaging of the lesion, and is performed without ionising radiation.[1] CT facilitates biopsy of small, deep seated lesions not well demonstrated on ultrasound. CT more precisely demonstrates the anatomic relationships of a given lesion compared to US, improves the definition of tissue components and vascularity, and provides for accurate localisation of the needle tip immediately prior to sampling without the transmission of potential impediments such as drains, bone and gas.

*I dedicate this chapter to the loving memory of my father, George Benjamin Bishop, and to my family, Peter, Sarah, Katherine and Ben for their support.*

## Sampling techniques: percutaneous FNA, endoscopic ultrasound-guided FNA and bile duct brushing

Percutaneous FNA techniques generally vary depending on the location and size of the mass. Any mass lesion that is palpable can be directly aspirated without guidance in the usual manner for all palpable aspiration biopsies. The most common techniques using guidance include individual puncture, coaxial biopsy, and tandem needle biopsy.[1,11,29] The coaxial biopsy technique is most commonly used. This technique uses a coaxial introducer needle through which FNA and core needle biopsy are performed with only one puncture into the lesion and without the need for repeat imaging.

A concomitant core needle biopsy (CNB) following the FNA is recommended when at all possible. CNBs provide the necessary tissue architecture as well as readily available tissue for ancillary studies that aide in providing a more specific diagnosis in many cases. Combined with a preceding FNA, the accuracy in diagnosing focal mass lesions is significantly greater than that obtained with either method alone.[15–17,30]

Endoscopic ultrasound-guided FNA (EUS-FNA) of liver masses is confined to those lesions visible and accessible via the stomach or duodenum. Lesions in the right lobe of the liver and hilum are assessed via the duodenum and distal stomach while those in the left lobe are accessed via the proximal and mid-stomach.[31–34]

## Bile duct brushing

Biliary brushing cytology of suspicious biliary strictures is key to making an early diagnosis. Unfortunately, despite specificity of >95%, the technique has a low sensitivity ranging from 17–83%.[3] Low sensitivity can be attributed to difficult access, desmoplasia, associated inflammation (stents, primary sclerosing cholangitis ), scant specimen cellularity and poor cellular preservation and preparation.[4,35,36] If sufficient cells are present and the cells are properly preserved and prepared for cytological evaluation (direct smears, cytospins or liquid-based cytology (LBC)), the criteria for malignancy are universal: high N:C ratio, prominent nucleoli, nuclear membrane abnormalities and hyperchromasia yielding 100% specificity for malignancy.[37] LBC processing alone or in addition to direct smears has improved sensitivity and accuracy in some studies, but cytologists must be familiar with alterations to morphology and background elements that may make malignancy appear more subtle in some cases.[38–40]

Elevation in serum tumour markers CEA and CA19-9 have higher sensitivity for detecting carcinoma, but lower specificity (i.e. false positive tests).[37] Adding digital image analysis[35] and fluorescence in situ hybridisation (FISH)[41] show promise in improving the diagnostic value of biliary brush cytology.

## Specimen processing

As mentioned above, it is desirable to obtain both smears and cell block preparations in all FNAs of the liver. Smears are made from the aspiration part of the procedure using a small needle (<22 gauge) that provides a rapid means of evaluating the specimen, not only for cellular adequacy but frequently for diagnosis. Multiple FNAs can be performed with minimal morbidity. If well-fixed, adequately smeared slides are difficult to obtain, the aspirate can be expressed into a preservative and submitted to the laboratory as a liquid-based specimen for processing by either the ThinPrep® (Cytyc Corporation, Marlborough, MA) or Sure Path™ (TriPath Imaging, Burlington, NC) methods. Cell blocks are made from FNA rinsings, any tissue fragments that are obtained, and dedicated CNBs using a spring loaded 18–20 gauge CNB gun such as the ASAP Biopsy System (Meditech/Boston Scientific Corp, Watertown, MA) or the Coaxial Temno Biopsy System (Allegiance Healthcare Corp, McGaw Park, IL). This material provides a formalin fixed, paraffin embedded tissue sample from which special stains and immunohistochemical studies can be readily obtained. It also provides, in many cases, the architecture necessary for a specific diagnosis, particularly in benign liver lesions.

CNB specimens can also be used for rapid interpretation by touching the core to a glass slide in a touch prep fashion.[42] Despite the presence of thick, three-dimensional tissue fragments and the probability of some air-drying artifact due to the inherent time delay in preparing the slide, architectural clues may still be readily apparent for rapid diagnosis.

The cytopathologist is an important part of the overall team approach to FNA of the liver. The presence of a cytopathologist at the time of the FNA increases the overall accuracy of the procedure.[13,17,43] The time of the actual biopsy, when additional tissue is still readily available, is the time to evaluate the specimen for adequacy and to triage the tissue for special studies such as flow cytometry or electron microscopy studies. If a cytopathologist or cytotechnologist is not available to assist in the preparation of the specimen, it is imperative that the radiologist learn how to make proper smears. The most cellular specimen is useless if inadequately prepared for optimal interpretation.

## Tumour classification

The most recent WHO classification of tumours of the liver is presented in Table 8.1.[44] Correct diagnosis is imperative for proper patient management. Pyogenic abscesses are typically drained,[45,46] and smaller tumours are being treated with ablation techniques such as alcohol and thermal ablation.[47] Chemotherapy and radiation protocols require a tissue diagnosis and targeted gene therapy is under investigation.[48,49]

## Normal morphology

The liver is a complex organ with functional lobular units of hepatic parenchyma anchored by portal tracts containing branches of the hepatic artery, hepatic portal vein and bile duct. Sinusoids are lined by a discontinuous layer of endothelial cells that separate hepatic plates of 1–2 cells thick and that terminate in the central vein. Sinusoidal endothelial cells differ from vascular endothelial cells. Unlike the endothelial cells of true vessels, sinusoidal endothelial cells are not supported

**Table 8.1** WHO histological classification of tumours of the liver and intrahepatic bile ducts

| Epithelial tumours |
| --- |
| Benign |
| Hepatocellular adenoma (liver cell adenoma) |
| Focal nodular hyperplasia |
| Intrahepatic bile duct adenoma |
| Intrahepatic bile duct cystadenoma |
| Biliary papillomatosis |
| Malignant |
| Hepatocellular carcinoma (liver cell carcinoma) |
| Intrahepatic cholangiocarcinoma (peripheral bile duct carcinoma) |
| Bile duct cystadenocarcinoma |
| Combined hepatocellular and cholangiocarcinoma |
| Hepatoblastoma |
| Undifferentiated carcinoma |
| Non-epithelial tumours |
| Benign |
| Angiomyolipoma |
| Lymphangioma and lymphangiomatosis |
| Haemangioma |
| Infantile haemangioendothelioma |
| Malignant |
| Epithelioid haemangioendothelioma |
| Angiosarcoma |
| Embryonal sarcoma (undifferentiated sarcoma) |
| Rhabdomyosarcoma |
| Others |
| Miscellaneous tumours |
| Solitary fibrous tumour |
| Teratoma |
| Yolk sac tumour (endodermal sinus tumour) |
| Carcinosarcoma |
| Kaposi sarcoma |
| Rhabdoid tumour |
| Others |
| Haemopoietic and lymphoid tumours |
| Secondary tumours |
| Epithelial abnormalities |
| Liver cell dysplasia (liver cell change) |
| Large cell type (large cell change) |
| Small cell type (small cell change) |
| Dysplastic nodules (adenomatous hyperplasia) |
| Low grade |
| High grade (atypical adenomatous hyperplasia) |
| Bile duct abnormalities |
| Hyperplasia (bile duct epithelium and peribiliary glands) |
| Dysplasia (bile duct epithelium and peribiliary glands) |
| Intraepithelial carcinoma (carcinoma *in situ*) |
| Miscellaneous lesions |
| Mesenchymal hamartoma |
| Nodular transformation (nodular regenerative hyperplasia) |
| Inflammatory pseudotumour |

(From Hamilton SR, Aaltonen LA. Tumours of the liver and intrahepatic bile ducts. In: Hamilton SR, Aaltonen LA (eds) Pathology & Genetics Tumours of the Digestive System. Albany: WHO Publications Center; 2001: 158.)

by a basement membrane and do not express factor VIII, Ulex europaeus or CD 34.[50] Transformation of sinusoids with the acquisition of these properties leads to 'capillarisation' of the sinusoids, changes that are exploited in both histological and cytological evaluation for diagnosis (see below).

In order to appreciate an abnormality in liver FNA, it is imperative that the cytopathologist understands the components of the 'normal' liver.

## Cytological findings of 'normal liver'

The normal hepatocyte is a large polygonal cell with:

- Abundant granular cytoplasm
- One or two round to oval, centrally placed nuclei
- Even chromatin pattern and occasionally prominent nucleoli
- Generally appear as small clusters (Fig. 8.1) *or*
- Larger flat sheets with irregular jagged edges without endothelial cell wrapping (Fig. 8.2) *or*
- Single cells.

Benign bile duct epithelial cells present as:

- Varying sized flat monolayered sheets of epithelial cells (Fig. 8.3)
- On-edge or in small acinar structures or groups
- Smaller than benign hepatocytes
- With round regular nuclei
- Inconspicuous nucleoli
- Less abundant cytoplasm than hepatocytes (Fig. 8.4).

Endothelial cells of sinusoidal spaces and Kupffer cells are rarely appreciated in benign lesions.

## Pigments

Intracytoplasmic pigments in cytology preparations differ in appearance depending on the stain. Lipofuscin, which

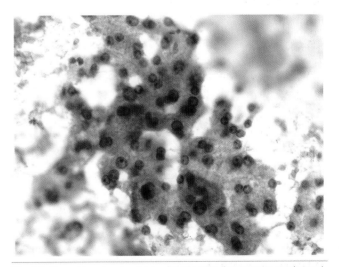

**Fig. 8.1** Normal hepatocytes. Benign hepatocytes demonstrate a polygonal shape, abundant granular cytoplasm, focal steatosis and 1–2 round to oval centrally placed nuclei, with an even chromatin pattern and small nucleoli (smear, PAP).

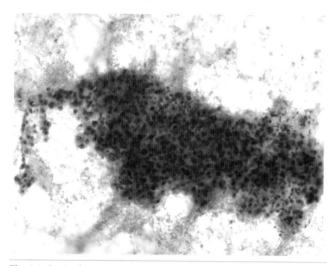

**Fig. 8.2** Benign hepatocytes. Smear pattern of benignity includes jagged, irregular shaped clusters of hepatocytes without peripherally wrapping endothelium (smear, PAP).

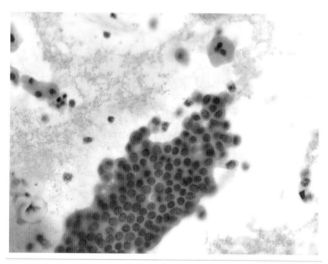

**Fig. 8.3** Benign bile duct epithelial cells. Flat, monolayered, honeycombed sheet with evenly spaced, round, regular nuclei typical of glandular cells of most sites (Cytospin, PAP).

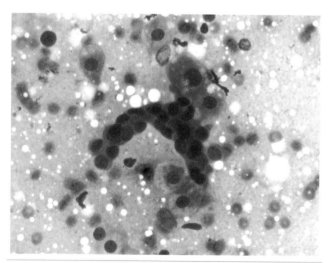

**Fig. 8.4** Benign bile duct epithelial cells. Bile duct epithelial cells are smaller than hepatocytes and display round regular nuclei with inconspicuous nucleoli and less abundant cytoplasm than in hepatocytes (smear, Diff-Quik).

constitutes the debris of intracellular lysosome breakdown, appears as a fine golden, granular, relatively non-refractile pigment in alcohol fixed, Papanicolaou (PAP) stained smears and is typically concentrated around the nucleus. This pigment is generally very common in the FNA of older adults and its absence should increase suspicion of a neoplasm on FNA of a mass lesion. Lipofuscin will stain darkly with a Fontana Mason stain creating a potential diagnostic pitfall with a metastatic melanoma.[51]

Bile pigment is produced by hepatocytes and is virtually pathognomonic of hepatocellular carcinoma when recognised within malignant cells. Bile appears as coarse, irregular, rather amorphous, non-refractile green to golden brown globular intracytoplasmic and extra-cytoplasmic deposits on Papanicolaou stain (Fig. 8.5). With Giemsa–Romanowsky stain, bile has a dark green to black hue. The distribution of the pigment is dependent on the degree of cholestasis, with pools of bile within canalicular spaces apparent in cases of extrahepatic obstruction (Fig. 8.6).

Iron or haemosiderin is a coarse, brown-black refractile pigment with Papanicolaou stain (Fig. 8.7A). While FNA can confirm the presence of heavy iron overload, it cannot replace CNB for histology and biochemical analysis to answer the clinical question of haemochromatosis. Malignant hepatocytes loose their ability to retain iron, and in the setting of haemachromatosis induced cirrhosis, where reactive hepatocyte atypia may be quite marked, it is helpful to use a special stain for iron like Prussian blue to highlight cells or clusters of cells without staining (Fig. 8.7B).[52]

## Non-neoplastic conditions

### Steatosis

Fatty change in hepatocytes is common in many conditions in the liver especially toxic/metabolic injury such as with alcohol abuse. Steatosis can result in the radiological appearance of a

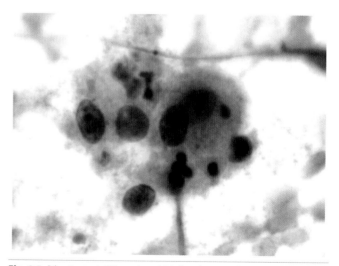

**Fig. 8.5** Bile pigment. Although variable in color, texture, size and density, bile is recognised by its globular, green-tinged non-refractile appearance (smear, PAP).

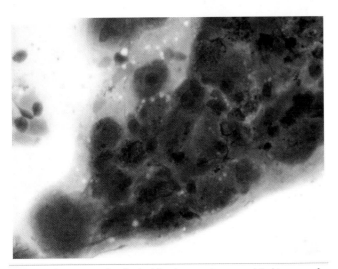

**Fig. 8.6** Bile pigment. Canalicular bile plugs can be appreciated in cases of extrahepatic obstruction (smear, Diff-Quik).

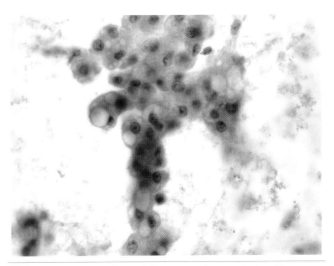

**Fig. 8.8** Steatosis. Fatty change in hepatocytes is recognised as either one or two large vacuoles (macrovesicular) or multiple small vacuoles (microvesicular) (smear, PAP).

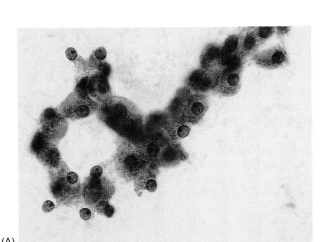

(A)

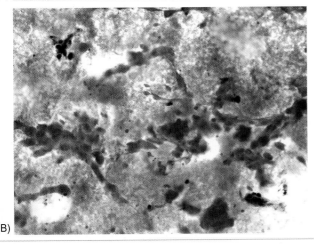

(B)

**Fig. 8.7** Haemosiderin pigment. (A) This pigment appears as coarse, brown-black refractile pigment on the standard Papanicolaou stain (smear, PAP). (B) Iron stain distinguishes the benign cells that stain blue and the malignant cells that do not (smear, Prussian blue).

**Fig. 8.9** Amyloid. Amyloid is recognised by its waxy or glassy green-tinged amorphous appearance (smear, PAP).

cytoplasm but do not indent the nucleus. A mixture of macro- and microvesicular steatosis is common (Fig. 8.8).

### Cytological findings: steatosis

- Benign appearing hepatocytes
- One-two large vacuoles (macrovesicular steatosis)
- Multiple small vacuoles (microvesicular steatosis).

## Amyloidosis

The deposition of amyloid in the liver can rarely cause the appearance of a mass lesion (amyloidoma) leading to FNA. Amyloid deposition in the liver is most often secondary to systemic diseases such as rheumatoid arthritis and plasma cell dyscrasias (multiple myeloma). Amyloid, regardless of type, is an extracellular amorphous hyaline material that has a pink or green waxy or glassy appearance on Papanicolaou stain (Fig. 8.9), and a magenta

mass lesion leading to FNA.[53] Fat may present in the form of macrovesicular steatosis, the most common form in which one or more large fat vacuoles fill the cytoplasm or microvesicular steatosis, in which multiple small lipid vacuoles expand the

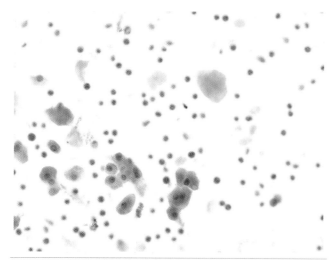

**Fig. 8.10** Amyloid. In liquid-based processing, amyloid may form hard rounded droplets that are easy to overlook (ThinPrep®, Papanicolaou).

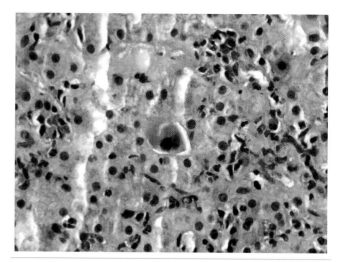

**Fig. 8.12** Extramedullary haemopoiesis. This cell block preparation demonstrates a megakaryocyte in the center surrounded by mixed haemopoietic cells infiltrating benign hepatic parenchyma (H&E).

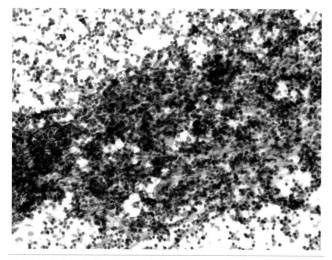

**Fig. 8.11** Splenosis. Smears are cellular and composed of well preserved mixed haemopoietic elements held together by a reticular network (smear, PAP).

colour on Giemsa–Romanowsky stain. Apple-green birefringence of Congo red stained smears will confirm the diagnosis. Amyloid can be recognised on LBC of FNAs, but like colloid, alteration of amyloid can occur causing it to appear as dense droplets (Fig. 8.10).[54]

## Cytological findings: amyloidosis

- Amorphous glassy or waxy extracellular material
- Rounded dense droplets on LBC
- Pink to green staining on Papanicolaou; magenta on Romanowsky
- Congo red stain is positive
- Apple-green birefringence with polarisation.

## Splenosis

Ruptured splenic tissue following trauma or splenectomy can result in implantation or auto-transplantation of splenic tissue

in the peritoneal cavity and even within parenchymal organs like the liver mimicking a neoplastic process, including hepatocellular carcinoma and especially metastatic malignancy given the typical multiple implants.[55,56] Although most patients are asymptomatic, these mass forming lesions are picked up incidentally and may be investigated by FNA. Smears that are cellular and well-preserved recapitulate the normal spleen demonstrating a mixture of normal haemopoietic cells in a bloody background supported by a reticular network[57] (Fig. 8.11). Lymphoid dominant FNAs, however, introduce small blue cell tumours into the differential diagnosis including small cell lymphoma and small cell carcinoma. An important clue to the diagnosis is a history of splenectomy and/or trauma.

## Cytological findings: hepatic splenosis

- Benign appearing haemopoietic cells: lymphocytes and neutrophils
- Lymphoid follicle
- Reticular network holding aggregates of cells together
- Bloody background.

## Extramedullary haemopoiesis

Extramedullary haemopoesis (EMH) is normal only within the first few weeks of life. After this point, EMH or myeloid metaplasia is an abnormal condition in which the liver attempts to produce the deficient blood cells that results when the normal bone marrow has been replaced by non-functioning tissue such as fibrosis in myeloproliferative diseases. EMH is also commonly associated with hepatoblastomas and hepatic angiosarcomas. EMH is often first considered with the recognition of megakaryocytes, large cells with abundant granular cytoplasm and lobulated nuclei. These cells are associated with normoblasts, red cell precursors, small cells with round, central pyknotic nuclei and dense eosinophilic cytoplasm, and myelocytes, slightly larger cells than normoblasts but smaller than megakaryocytes, a central round nucleus and granular cytoplasm (Fig. 8.12).[58]

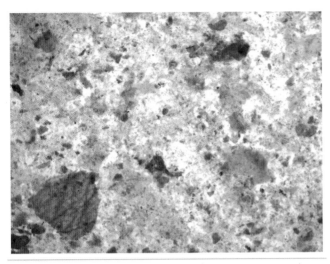

**Fig. 8.13** Echinococcal cyst. Aspirate smears of cyst contents can produce a thick and amorphous necrotic pattern often referred to as 'anchovy paste' (smear, PAP).

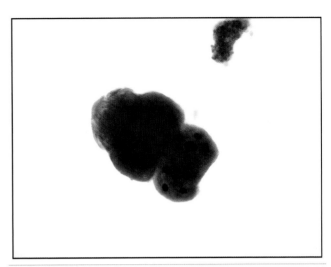

**Fig. 8.14** Echinococcal cyst. Protoscolices of the organism demonstrate a crown of characteristic 'shark tooth shaped' hooklets (ThinPrep®, PAP).

## Infection

Abscess formation in the liver is often suspected radiologically from the characteristic double target sign on computed tomography; however, organised abscesses can mimic hepatic tumours leading to FNA.[53] Pyogenic abscess is the most common and percutaneous biopsy is performed for tissue confirmation, culture and drainage.[45,59] FNA is an acceptable means of diagnosis for all abscess sizes, but for therapeutic drainage, FNA is recommended only for small abscesses <50 mm; larger abscesses require percutaneous catheter drainage for complete management.[45] Smears are dominated by nonspecific acute inflammatory cells and cellular debris. Cultures are helpful for identification of bacterial organisms.

Amoebic abscess is 10 times more common in men than in women and is rare in children.[60] The distinction between pyogenic and amoebic abscess is important for both therapy and prognosis. Pyogenic abscesses have a 20–60% morbidity due to an association with systemic infection, the tendency to produce multiple liver abscesses and an association with an older patient age.[61] Amoebic abscesses tend to occur as solitary liver masses in young patients, rarely require drainage and respond to metronidazole therapy.[60,61] Most patients with hepatic amoebiasis do not demonstrate intestinal symptoms, but hepatomegaly with point tenderness over the liver, below the ribs or in the intercostal spaces are typical presenting symptoms.[60] Identification of organisms in aspiration fluid of hepatic abscesses is uncommon and diagnosis rests on the constellation of presenting symptoms, high risk factors, typical radiological findings of a solitary right lobe mass and positive serum antibodies which are present in 70–80% of patients.[60] The single cell trophozoites of *E. histolytica* with round nucleus, condensed peripheral chromatin and central small nucleolus with foamy cytoplasm resemble histiocytes and can be easily overlooked.

Other infectious organisms may be recognised by unique characteristics such as the 'sulphur granules' of actinomyces and 'anchovy paste' smears (Fig. 8.13), echinococcal hooklets or scolices (Fig. 8.14) or laminated cyst wall (Fig. 8.15) in hydatid disease.[46]

Granulomatous inflammation may be related to infection such as with fungal or acid fast organisms, but the presence of

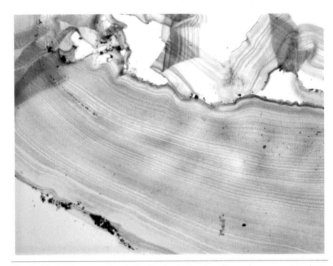

**Fig. 8.15** Echinococcal cyst. The laminated cyst wall may be appreciated on both smears and cell block (cell block, H&E).

granulomata in a liver FNA is in no way diagnostic of an infectious aetiology. The presence of granulomata may be related to many conditions including primary hepatobiliary disorders, sarcoidosis, and tumours such as lymphoma and metastatic carcinoma. Hepatic sarcoidosis is one of the most common causes of non-caseating granulomata of the liver.[62] Cytologically granulomata are composed of clusters of epithelioid histiocytes with oval to elongated, sometimes twisted nuclei and visible but indistinct, non-phagocytic, cytoplasm (Fig. 8.16). Special stains such as Grocott methenamine silver (GMS) and Ziehl Neelsen (ZN) for acid fast bacilli (AFB) can be performed on smears but are easier to perform on cell block preparations.

## Bile duct hamartoma

Bile duct hamartoma may present as a mass lesion mimicking a neoplasm, and as a result, may be encountered on FNA.[63]

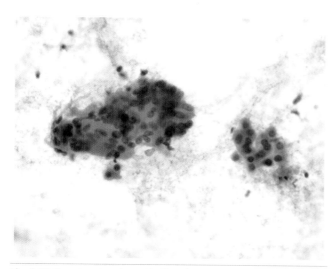

**Fig. 8.16** Granulomatous hepatitis. Granulomas are composed of cohesive clusters of epithelioid histiocytes with oval to elongated, often twisted nuclei and indistinct, but visible cytoplasm (smear PAP).

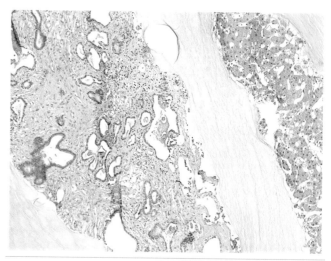

**Fig. 8.18** Bile duct hamartoma. Cell block preparations of core needle biopsies demonstrate the characteristic angulated proliferation of variably dilated bile ductules in a fibrotic background (H&E).

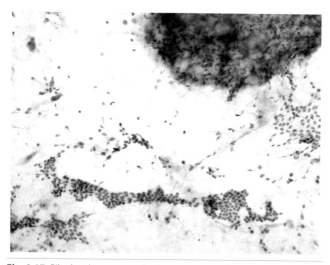

**Fig. 8.17** Bile duct hamartoma. Aspirate smears are dominated by benign-appearing bile duct epithelial cells with uncharacteristically scant numbers of associated hepatocytes (smear, PAP).

This lesion is often aspirated at the time of diagnostic EUS-FNA of pancreatic masses, so care must be taken to distinguish gastrointestinal contamination from bile duct epithelium as a means of ensuring the aspirate is representative of the lesion. Smears contain a predominant population of benign appearing bile duct epithelial cells often in the form of flat monolayered sheets of glandular cells with small uniformly spaced round nuclei (Fig. 8.17). Luminal edges with scant but visible non-mucinous cytoplasm are present. Benign hepatocytes are uncharacteristically few or absent as would be expected for a benign hepatic lesion such as focal nodular hyperplasia. Aspirates of bile duct adenoma have a similar appearance. Cell block preparations are helpful in rendering a diagnosis (Fig. 8.18).

### Cytological findings: bile duct hamartoma (adenoma)

- Benign appearing glandular epithelium, often in flat monolayered sheets

- Round, uniform, evenly spaced nuclei
- Scant but visible, non-mucinous cytoplasm
- Uncharacteristically few to no hepatocytes in the background.

## Mesenchymal hamartoma

Hepatic mesenchymal hamartoma is a benign mass forming lesion of malformed bile ducts and myxoid mesenchyme diagnosed in mostly male (70%) infants and children less than 5 years of age with rare cases reported in adults.[64,65] The aetiology is unclear with theories ranging from congenital plate abnormality to true neoplasm. These typically predominantly cystic masses are usually resected in childhood and complete resection is curative. Although serological tumour markers are usually normal, elevated AFP and atypical FNA cytology have been reported to lead to a preoperative diagnosis of hepatoblastoma, the primary tumour in the differential diagnosis.[12,66]

Reports of the cytological features are few[12,67,68] FNA produces scant smears composed of a loose myxoid mesenchymal stroma with benign-appearing spindle cells and sheets of benign glandular epithelium that reflects the histology of disorganised loose myxoid mesenchymal tissue surrounding variably sized benign bile ducts and occasionally hepatocytes (Fig. 8.19). Pseudocysts occur in the mesenchyme and are not lined by epithelial cells. Extramedullary haematopoesis may be noted. The patient's young age, male gender, cystic radiological appearance and benign-appearing myxoid spindled and glandular cell proliferation should lead to the correct diagnosis.

### Cytological findings: mesenchymal hamartoma

- Benign appearing glandular epithelium, often in flat monolayered sheets
- Myxoid stroma
- Benign appearing spindled cells
- Variable number of benign hepatocytes.

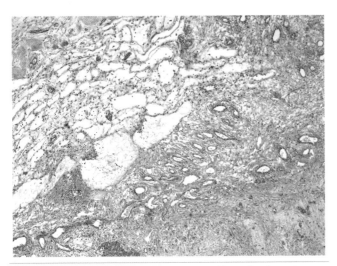

**Fig. 8.19** Mesenchymal hamartoma. Disorganised loose, focally cystic myxoid mesenchymal tissue surrounds variably sized benign bile ducts and occasionally hepatocytes (resection histology, H&E)

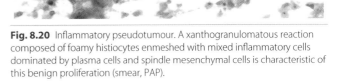

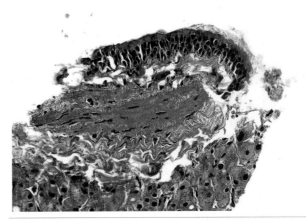

**Fig. 8.20** Inflammatory pseudotumour. A xanthogranulomatous reaction composed of foamy histiocytes enmeshed with mixed inflammatory cells dominated by plasma cells and spindle mesenchymal cells is characteristic of this benign proliferation (smear, PAP).

## Inflammatory pseudotumour

Inflammatory pseudotumour (IPT) of the liver is an uncommon, benign, mass-forming proliferation of mixed inflammatory cells and histiocytes dominated by polyclonal plasma cells infiltrating a stroma of fibroblasts, myofibroblasts and collagen. These lesions are reported in patients of both genders, but mostly males (70%), and all ages from infancy to the eighth decade.[69] The heterogeneity of these proliferations has led to many synonymous names, including plasma cell granuloma, inflammatory myofibrohistiocytic proliferation, fibroxanthoma and inflammatory myofibroblastic tumour. Although some reports of clonality and association with the Epstein–Barr virus have supported a neoplastic process in some cases,[70] the aetiology in most hepatic IPT is inflammatory or infectious.[71] More recently, pseudotumour is considered to be part of the IgG4 related sclerosing disease, often associated with autoimmune pancreatitis.[72–76]

These lesions are benign, but rare cases of biological aggressiveness and malignant transformation have been reported.[77]

Diagnosis by FNA is challenging due to the non-specific and variable nature of the mixed inflammatory sample.[78,79] Smears are often cellular composed of cohesive networks of spindle mesenchymal cells enmeshed with mixed inflammatory cells and foamy (xanthomatous) histiocytes that also populate the background. Plasma cells are usually prominent and neutrophils and eosinophils are minor components (Fig. 8.20). The spindle cell component may also be dominant and single spindle cells are noted. Atypia, especially in the mesenchymal cells and histiocytes, can be a pitfall.[78] The differential diagnosis includes spindle cell lesions of the liver including gastrointestinal stromal tumours and sarcomas. The typical high cellularity of the inflammatory component should preclude a false positive interpretation.

### Cytological findings: inflammatory pseudotumour

- Mixed inflammatory proliferation
- Numerous plasma cells and foamy histiocytes
- Benign appearing spindled cells in cohesive groups and singly

**Fig. 8.21** Ciliated hepatic foregut cyst. These unilocular subcapsular cysts are lined by stratified respiratory type epithelium (cell block, H&E). (From Sidawy MK, Syed ZA. Liver. In: Goldblum JR (ed.) Fine Needle Aspiration Cytology. Foundations in Diagnostic Pathology series. London: Elsevier; 2007.)

### Diagnostic pitfall: inflammatory pseudotumour

- Atypia, although usually focal and low grade, may suggest a spindle-cell neoplasm.

## Ciliated hepatic foregut cyst

This rare hepatic cyst is an embryological remnant of the foregut that differentiates along branchial lines to form a cyst lined by pseudostratified columnar epithelium. These cysts are predominantly unilocular, subcapsular and less than 4 cm.[80] Except for its hepatic location, the cytology is identical to a bronchogenic cyst (Fig. 8.21).[81]

### Cytological findings: ciliated hepatic foregut cyst

- Thin to mucoid cyst fluid
- Ciliated columnar cells
- Mucous cells
- Generally few to no hepatocytes

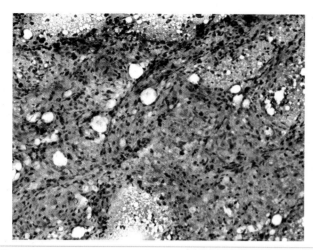

**Fig. 8.22** Angiomyolipoma. A combination of vessels, smooth muscle and adipocytes allows for a specific diagnosis on fine needle aspiration biopsy (smear, Diff-Quik). (From Odze RD, Goldblum JR. Surgical Pathology of the GI Tract, Liver, Biliary Tract and Pancreas, 1st edn. London: Elsevier; 2004.)

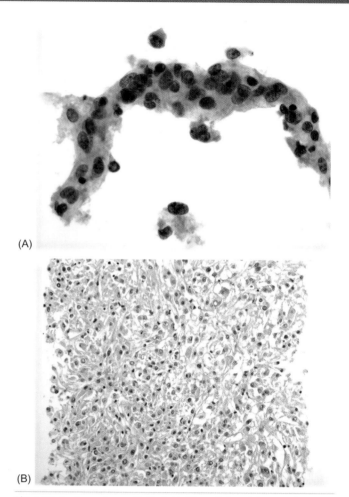

(A)

(B)

**Fig. 8.23** Angiomyolipoma. Epithelioid differentiation of the smooth muscle component can make diagnosis difficult on both (A) cytology and (B) histology. (A: ThinPrep, PAP; B: cell block, H&E.)

### Diagnostic pitfall: ciliated hepatic foregut cyst

- Mucoid contents and mucous cells could lead to diagnosis of hepatobiliary cystadenoma.

## Benign neoplasms

### Angiomyolipoma

This benign mesenchymal neoplasm is purported to arise from the perivascular epithelioid cell (PEC) and has been classified as a PEComa, one of several benign neoplasms of the tuberous sclerosis complex.[82] It is composed of varying combinations of fat, smooth muscle and vessels. When the fatty component is readily recognised radiologically, histologically and cytologically, the diagnosis is relatively straightforward (Fig. 8.22). In fact, it is usually the paucity of fat in the neoplasm that leads to a diagnostic dilemma and subsequent FNA.[83,84] The histological and cytological features of this tumour are similar in the liver and the kidney (see Ch. 11). Diagnostic difficulty on cytology arises when the fatty component is scant or focal and not sampled, and when solid epithelioid areas predominate (Fig. 8.23)[85,86] Cell block preparations provide not only architectural clues, but tissue for ancillary testing. Positive staining with HMB-45 confirms the diagnosis.[87] Other immunohistochemical markers that label this neoplasm include vimentin, desmin, actin and endothelial markers such as Factor VIII.[88]

### Cytological findings: angiomyolipoma

- Interlacing complex of smooth muscle, fat and blood vessels
- Immunocytochemical stain for confirmation: HMB-45.

### Diagnostic pitfalls: angiomyolipoma

- Smooth muscle may dominate smears and can demonstrate atypia
- Solid epithelioid areas may be dominant, can produce significant atypia and can lead to false positive interpretations.

### Haemangioma

Haemangiomas constitute the most common benign neoplasm of the liver. They occur in all ages and both genders. These mass lesions are generally small and asymptomatic, but can occasionally be large (>5 cm) and cause symptoms. Although radiological diagnosis has improved with enhanced imaging techniques, most are found incidentally during work-up for other conditions, including staging of malignancy, and can be difficult to distinguish from a metastasis radiologically.[89,90] Cytologically, FNA smears are frequently considered unsatisfactory or non-diagnostic due to either the aspiration of blood only, or the presence of nonspecific appearing connective tissue. It is this loose, rather than dense fibrous type connective tissue and smooth muscle fragments associated with blood and few to no background hepatocytes that should alert the pathologist to the diagnosis of haemangioma in the proper clinical setting. Cell block preparation of a core needle biopsy is crucial in making a specific diagnosis (Fig. 8.24).

### Cytological findings: haemangioma

- Bloody, scantily cellular smears
- Coils of loose connective tissue and smooth muscle

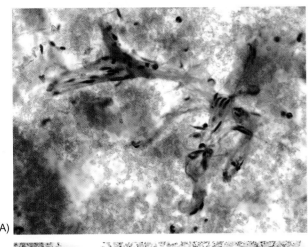

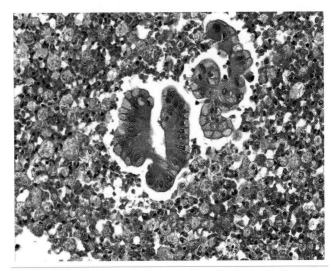

**Fig. 8.25** Hepatobiliary cystadenoma. Mucinous glandular epithelium and foamy histiocytes characterise the contents of this benign hepatic cyst (cell block, H&E) (From Sidawy MK, Syed ZA. Liver. In: Goldblum JR (ed.) Fine Needle Aspiration Cytology. Foundations in Diagnostic Pathology series. London: Elsevier; 2007.)

for diagnosis in the appropriate clinical setting (Fig. 8.25) Recognition of the malignant counterpart, hepatobiliary cystadenocarcinoma, is possible if the cytology is overtly malignant, but less than malignant cytology does not exclude malignancy and, as such, the treatment of choice is total resection.[92]

### Cytological findings: hepatobiliary cystadenoma

- Thin to mucoid cyst fluid
- Foamy histiocytes
- Benign appearing mucinous glandular cells
- Subepithelial ovarian type stroma is not aspirated
- Generally few to no hepatocytes

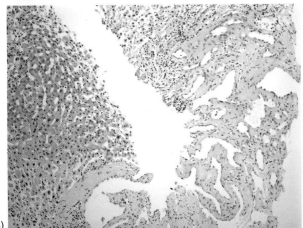

**Fig. 8.24** Haemangioma. (A) The presence of loose connective tissue and smooth muscle fragments associated with blood and few to no background hepatocytes, although considered non-diagnostic and often unsatisfactory for diagnosis, are typical findings in the aspiration of hepatic haemangioma. (B) A cell block preparation of a core needle biopsy is crucial in making a specific diagnosis.

- Generally few to no hepatocytes
- Smears commonly non-diagnostic; specific diagnosis dependent on cell block.

## Hepatobiliary cystadenoma

This benign cystic tumour is a solitary, multiloculated cystic neoplasm of the liver that is histologically similar to cysts found in the pancreas and ovary. Women are almost exclusively affected. These neoplasms can become very large and patients usually present with abdominal pain. The neoplasm does not communicate with the biliary system. The locules are filled with fluid that varies from thin and clear to bloody and turbid. The cyst lining is mucinous but the cells can become attenuated or denuded from fluid pressure. The characteristic subepithelial ovarian type stroma is not typically sampled on FNA which has been rarely reported.[91,92] The cytology is similar to mucinous cystic neoplasm of the pancreas, often scantily cellular and nondiagnostic on its own. Cyst fluid with foamy histiocytes and mucinous epithelium, even if very scant, are sufficient

## Benign hepatocytic nodules or masses

Benign hepatocytic mass-forming proliferations, including dysplastic nodule (DN), focal nodular hyperplasia (FNH) and hepatocellular adenoma (HCA), share in common many cytological features and distinction between them on smear cytology alone is difficult if not impossible.[93] As such, the cytological features of these lesions will be discussed together. In addition, all of these lesions share in common the same differential diagnosis, namely well-differentiated hepatocellular carcinoma. Taking into consideration the clinical and radiological presentation of the patient in conjunction with the cytohistology will typically lead to the correct interpretation (Table 8.2).

Dysplastic nodule is a diagnostic consideration in the clinical setting of a mass in a cirrhotic liver clinically suspicious for hepatocellular carcinoma. The nomenclature of dysplastic nodules has changed over the past decade and now is a term used for macroregenerative nodule, adenomatous hyperplasia and other terms used to describe nodules in the liver that are grossly and histologically larger than the surrounding cirrhotic nodules (usually ~1–3 cm).[94] Dysplastic nodules are sub-classified as low-grade dysplasia (macroregenerative nodule) and high-grade dysplasia (small cell dysplasia). High-grade dysplasia

**Table 8.2** Features typical of benign hepatic nodules versus well-differentiated hepatocellular carcinoma

| | | Benign hepatic nodules | | | |
| --- | --- | --- | --- | --- | --- |
| | | **DN, low grade** | **HCA** | **FNH** | **WDHCC** |
| Clinical | | | | | |
| | Gender | Males and females | Females≫males | Females≫males | Males > females |
| | Age | Adults | 15–45 years | All ages, mostly adult women | Adults |
| | Cirrhosis | Yes | No | No | Yes |
| | Other | | Oral contraceptive use; glycogen storage diseases | Hepatic haemangiomas | Alcohol abuse, viral hepatitis |
| Radiology | Nodule size | 0.8–3 cm nodules | 5–15 cm, solitary mass | <5 cm mass; stellate scar | >1 cm nodule |
| Serology | AFP | Not elevated | Not elevated | Not elevated | Elevated |
| Cytology | | | | | |
| | Hepatocytes | Irregular shaped clusters without peripheral or transgressing endothelial cells; single cells; bland appearing large hepatocytes ± cytoplasmic glycogen and/or fat; round regular nuclei without prominent nucleoli; scattered large dysplastic cells | | | Peripherally wrapping and transgressing vessels; monomorphic small hepatocytes; nucleoli, often macro; hyaline globules |
| | Bile ducts | Yes | No | Yes | No |
| Ancillary tests | | | | | |
| | Reticulin | Present, highlights normal 1–2 cell thick hepatic plates | | | Decreased to absent; highlights >3 cell thick plates when present |
| | AFP | Negative | Negative | Negative | Present (30–40%) |
| | Glypcian-3 | Negative | Negative (focal weak positive) | Negative | Positive |
| | CD34 | Negative | Positive, periportal/septal | Negative | Positive, diffuse |

WDHCC, well-differentiated hepatocellular carcinoma; DN, dysplastic nodule; HCA, hepatocellular adenoma; FNH, focal nodular hyperplasia; AFP, alpha-fetoprotein.

is thought to be the precursor to hepatocellular carcinoma. Low-grade dysplastic nodules contain anisonucleosis with large cell change with some portal tracts (Fig. 8.26) whereas high-grade dysplasia is a pure population of small hepatocytes without portal tracts (Fig. 8.27). Both types of dysplastic nodules retain the normal 1–2 cell thick hepatic plate architecture. A specific cytological diagnosis of a high-grade dysplastic nodule is rare given the overlapping cytological features with hepatocellular carcinoma.[93] The more typical cytological interpretation is 'negative', 'atypical hepatocytes' or 'suspicious for hepatocellular carcinoma' depending on the low-grade (polymorphous) or high-grade (monomorphous) proliferation of hepatocytes and the presence or absence of bile duct epithelium.

Focal nodular hyperplasia, a tumour most commonly found in adult women in a non-cirrhotic liver, is a well-circumscribed, non-encapsulated mass forming lesion composed of nodules of polyclonal, hyperplastic and normal appearing hepatocytes in one to two-cell thick hepatic plates supported by reticulin and separated by fibrous septa that often coalesce to form a stellate scar.[69] Thick-walled arteries and bile ductules proliferate within the fibrous tissue that provides the population of ductal epithelium so important in the cytological diagnosis and distinction from hepatocellular adenoma and carcinoma (Fig. 8.28).

Hepatocellular adenoma is a benign neoplasm of monoclonal hepatocytes arising in a non-cirrhotic liver that typically occurs in women 15–45 years old with a history of oral contraceptive use. When these neoplasms are multiple, a condition called liver adenomatosis applies.[69] These well-demarcated, non-encapsulated neoplasms of fatty and glycogenated hepatocytes are rarely associated with bile ductules and fibrous septa. Large arteries typical of the stellate scar of FNH are only found in the periphery, but the neoplasm is punctuated by medium- and small-sized arterioles, a clue to the diagnosis on cell block/CNB (Fig. 8.29). Haemorrhage and extramedullary haematopoesis are commonly encountered.

Cytologically, these benign reactive and neoplastic processes share in common features of reactivity. Smears are variably cellular with a smear pattern of benign appearing hepatocytes singly

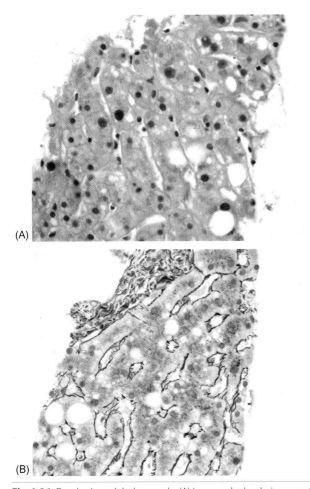

Fig. 8.26 Dysplastic nodule, low grade. (A) Low-grade dysplasia present in macroregenerative nodules is recognised by anisonucleosis with large cell change. (B) One to two cell layer hepatic plate architecture is maintained as illustrated by a reticulin stain (A: H&E; B: reticulin stain).

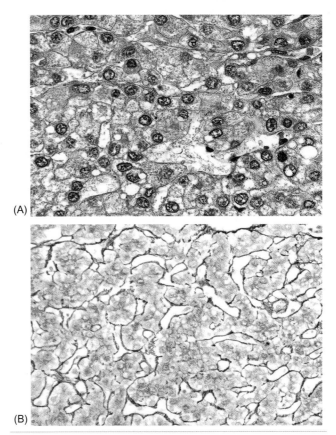

Fig. 8.27 Dysplastic nodule, high grade. Small cell dysplasia is recognised by a monomorphous population of small hepatocytes with an increased N:C ratio but maintained hepatic plate architecture (A: H&E; B: reticulin stain).

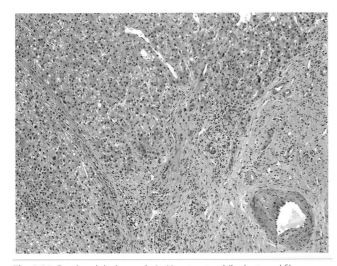

Fig. 8.28 Focal nodular hyperplasia. Hepatocytes, bile ducts and fibrous tissue in a disarray characterise this benign proliferation from other benign hepatocytic nodules (cell block, H&E).

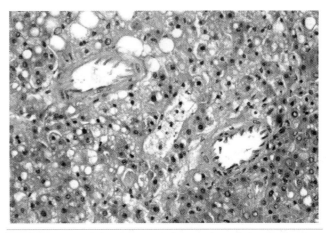

Fig. 8.29 Hepatocellular adenoma. Medium sized vessels punctuating hepatic parenchyma without bile duct epithelial cells characterises this benign neoplasm from other benign hepatocytic nodules (cell block, H&E).

or in irregularly shaped, jagged edged clusters without associated peripherally wrapping endothelial cells (Fig. 8.30). Proliferating or arborising vessels ('transgressing' endothelial cells) are focal at best[95–97] (see Fig. 8.38). Reactive and proliferative

bile duct epithelial cells may also be present in FNH or by contamination from the edges of other nodules, and their presence should greatly raise one's threshold for a malignant diagnosis (Fig. 8.31).

Cellular features of reactivity include an apparent hepatocytic pleomorphism rather than monomorphism (Fig. 8.32), an increased number of binucleated cells which tend to be decreased in hepatocellular carcinoma, a relatively low nuclear to cytoplasmic ratio, smooth nuclear membranes and prominent

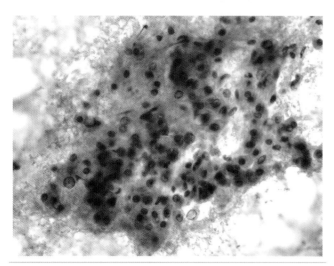

**Fig. 8.30** Hepatocellular adenoma. The benign hepatocytes form clusters with irregular contours without associated peripherally wrapping endothelial cells (smear, PAP).

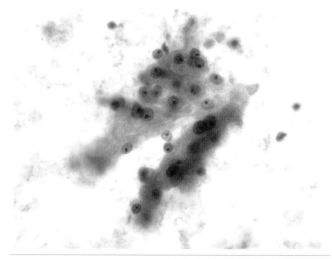

**Fig. 8.33** Reactive hepatocytes. Reactive hepatocytes demonstrate a low nuclear to cytoplasmic ratio and nuclei with smooth nuclear membranes and prominent but not macronucleoli (smear, PAP).

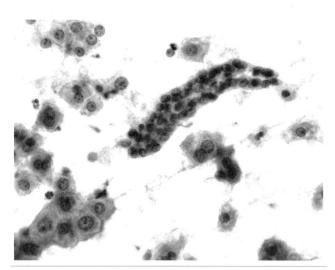

**Fig. 8.31** Focal nodular hyperplasia. Smears are composed of benign hepatocytes and bile duct epithelial cells (smear, PAP).

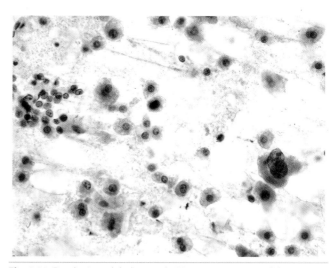

**Fig. 8.34** Dysplastic nodule, low grade. Macroregenerative nodules contain hepatocytes that demonstrate significant atypia or large cell change (low-grade dysplasia), cells that are recognised as benign by their sporadic placement among otherwise benign and reactive appearing hepatocytes. Note the bile duct cells in the upper left (smear, PAP).

but not large nucleoli (Fig. 8.33). Large cell change seen in low-grade dysplastic nodules are dysplastic hepatocytes recognised by their enlarged atypical nuclei and sporadic placement in a background of otherwise typically reactive appearing hepatocytes yielding a polymorphous and pleomorphic smear pattern (Fig. 8.34). Small cell dysplasia present in high-grade dysplastic nodules is extremely difficult to distinguish from the monomorphism of well-differentiated hepatocellular carcinoma but should be considered with small high N/C ratio hepatocytes without an abnormal vascular pattern of peripherally wrapping endothelial cells or transgressing endothelial cells.[93]

Due to the overlap in the components of these various benign entities on smear cytology, cell blocks as well as radiological and clinical correlation are crucial in making a specific diagnosis. The smallest fragment of tissue may be all that is necessary to render a specific diagnosis. This readily available tissue may be used for the few ancillary tests that can aid in the benign versus malignant differential diagnosis.

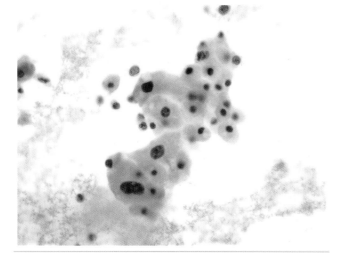

**Fig. 8.32** Reactive hepatocytes. Cellular and nuclear pleomorphism or anisonucleosis of benign, reactive hepatocytes is contrast to the monomorphism demonstrated by hepatocellular carcinoma (smear, PAP).

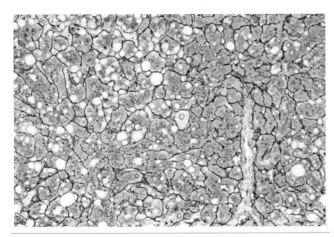

**Fig. 8.35** Hepatocellular adenoma. A reticulin stain highlights the maintained 1 to 2 cell layer thick hepatic plate architecture typical of benign hepatocytic processes. (cell block, reticulin stain).

## Ancillary tests

Cell block preparations of small tissue fragments or CNBs currently offer the best method of distinguishing between benign and malignant hepatocytic proliferations. Not only is the architecture available, but tissue is readily available for ancillary studies. The reticulin stain demonstrates a maintained 1–2 cell hepatic plate framework in all benign lesions even if in disarray and the sinusoids are not apparent[98] (Fig. 8.35; see also Figs 8.26B, 8.27B). Alpha-fetoprotein (AFP) staining is only focally and weakly positive at best in benign hepatocytic proliferations, but a negative stain does not exclude HCC. Serum levels of AFP >400 ng/mL are highly associated with the presence of HCC.[87] The immunostain hepatocyte paraffin 1 (HepPar 1)[99] does not distinguish between benign and malignant hepatocytes. Glypican-3, (GPC3), is an oncofetal protein shown to be overexpressed in HCC and can be detected in the serum and tissue of patients with HCC but not benign hepatic lesions, with the rare exception of weak focal staining in HCA.[100–104] Studies with immunohistochemistry staining with anti-GPC3 antibody, have indicated great promise in the distinction between benign and malignant hepatocytes on histological sections,[105,106] and on cytological material.[107] Immunostains that attempt to highlight capillarisation of the sinusoids such as CD34[108] Factor VIII[109], and laminin can also be helpful. CD34 can show significant sinusoidal positivity in HCA (Fig. 8.36), and this can present a pitfall in the interpretation of small tissue samples in cell block.

Molecular studies and image analysis studies have attempted to discriminate between benign and malignant hepatocytes. Flow cytometry has shown promise,[110] but there is still significant overlap in the ploidy patterns of benign and malignant processes. Proliferating cell nuclear antigen (PCNA) appears to have a better specificity in separating the two entities, however, there is still overlap in the PCNA positivity of small cell liver dysplasia and grades I and II hepatocellular carcinoma.[111,112] These methods, as well as polymerase chain reaction, FISH,[113] albumin messenger RNA,[114] and a combination of parameters[115] continue to be investigated.

### Cytological findings: benign hepatocytic nodules (DN, FNH, HCA)

- Hepatocytes in jagged irregular clusters and singly
- No peripherally wrapping endothelial cells

- Clusters may have focal transgressing endothelial cells
- Mild pleomorphism of cell and nuclear size; sporadically placed large, atypical cells (dysplastic hepatocytes/large cell change)
- Many binucleated hepatocytes
- Variably prominent nucleoli but no macroeosinophilic nucleoli
- Cytoplasm is generally abundant and granular but may show fatty change, lipofuscin pigment or iron deposition
- Reticulin stain will show retained 1–2 cell layer framework on cell block.

### Diagnostic pitfalls: benign hepatocytic nodules (DN, FNH, HCA)

- Marked steatosis may result in false negative reticulin stain
- AFP and glypican 3 are negative; weak focal staining may be noted
- CD34 generally does not stain sinusoids; focal strong staining in HCA.

## Malignant neoplasms – primary

## Hepatocellular carcinoma

Hepatocellular carcinoma (HCC) is the fifth most common cancer worldwide, and its incidence is increasing due to the widespread prevalence of hepatitis B and C virus infections, especially in Europe and the USA.[116,117] HCC almost always develops in the setting of cirrhosis, most often secondary to alcohol but with an incidence about 15% in patients with hepatitis C. The risk in patients with hepatitis C increases with concomitant metabolic injury from alcohol, obesity, diabetes and hepatitis B virus.[2] The prognosis of patients is poor for large symptomatic lesions, so early detection is key to long-term survival. Early detection of small, non-vascularly invasive tumours can improve survival from <10% to >50%.[118,119] In that regard, high-risk patients are routinely screened for suspicious nodules (≈1 cm) and FNA with CNB is typically used for diagnosis. Treatment options include liver transplantation for good surgical candidates, and percutaneous ablation for non-surgical candidates.[47,118,119] Percutaneous ablation techniques include ethanol injection and thermal ablation using radiofrequency, laser or microwave energy.[47]

The cytohistological diagnosis of hepatocellular carcinoma falls into two main categories: low-grade (well-differentiated) and high-grade (moderately and poorly differentiated) tumours.

### Well-differentiated hepatocellular carcinoma

Well-differentiated hepatocellular carcinoma is a tumour that looks hepatocytic but does not look obviously malignant. Given that the tumour cells of well-differentiated hepatocellular carcinoma are so similar to normal liver, the smear pattern proves to be a critical feature in evaluating these tumours.[95–97,120]

The three basic smear patterns are: (1) the cohesive, nested and trabecular pattern with peripherally wrapping endothelial cells, (2) loosely cohesive sheets with transgressing endothelial cells, or vessels and (3) the dispersed small cluster-single cell pattern without a recognisable vascular pattern.

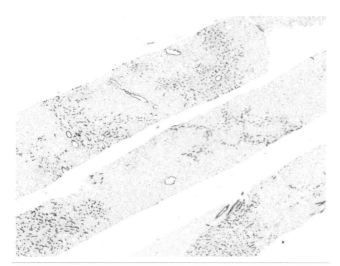

**Fig. 8.36** Hepatocellular adenoma. Capillarisation of sinusoids can occur in this benign neoplasm creating a pitfall on interpretation of immunoperoxidase stains for CD34 (cell block, antiperoxidase).

The most specific pattern is the peripherally wrapping endothelial pattern.[95,96] This pattern is one in which the endothelial cells of the sinusoids wrap around smooth edged, rounded nests and thickened hepatic trabeculae (Fig. 8.37). The endothelial cell nuclei may not be apparent in every plane of focus, but the presence of even one or two nuclei at the edge is sufficient. Although this pattern is only found in less than half of tumours,[95,96] when present, it has been found to be very specific for the diagnosis of hepatocellular carcinoma and proves to be one of the most important diagnostic clues in separating reactive non-neoplastic and benign neoplastic proliferations from well-differentiated hepatocellular carcinoma.[96,97]

The other pattern of endothelial proliferation has been termed transgressing,[96] arborising or central.[95] A complex network of small vessels is present in a loosely cohesive sheet of hepatocytes (Fig. 8.38). The appearance is similar to proliferating capillaries in other processes, such as granulation tissue, suggesting that the endothelial cells are associated with basement membranes, a feature of abnormal sinusoids as in hepatocellular carcinoma.[121] This pattern is not as specific for hepatocellular carcinoma as the peripherally wrapping endothelial pattern, but is highly associated with the presence of hepatocellular carcinoma. It is rarely seen in cases of cirrhosis and hepatitis.[96]

The dispersed small cluster-single cell pattern is completely non-specific and may be seen in all types of hepatocellular proliferations (Fig. 8.39). The smear pattern will not be helpful in all cases and other features need to be assessed.

Individual cellular features that support a malignant diagnosis include the presence of cellular monotony with a uniformly elevated nuclear to cytoplasmic ratio, e.g. all of the cells appear to have the same degree of atypia one to the other (Fig. 8.40). Macro-eosinophilic nucleoli and intracytoplasmic hyaline globules (Fig. 8.41).

Cell blocks of small tissue fragments and CNBs provide help in assessing the hepatic plate architecture and capillarisation of the sinusoids, either on routine H&E stain or with ancillary tests if necessary (see Fig. 8.37B and Ancillary tests, below).

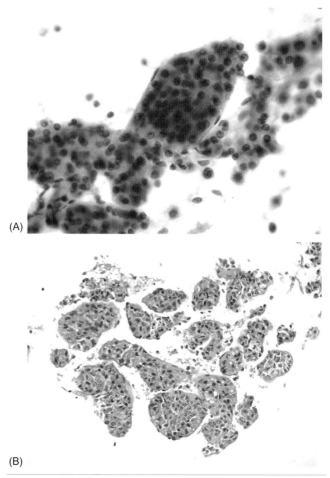

**Fig. 8.37** Well-differentiated hepatocellular carcinoma. (A) The peripherally wrapping endothelial cell pattern demonstrates the capillarised endothelial cells of sinusoids wrapping around smooth edged, rounded nests and thickened hepatic trabeculae of hepatocytes (smear, PAP). (B) This pathognomonic feature is also demonstrated in cell block preparations (H&E).

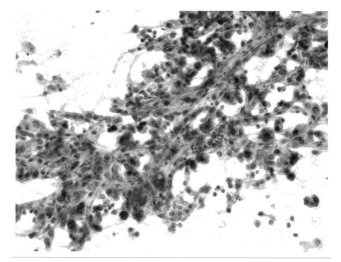

**Fig. 8.38** Well-differentiated hepatocellular carcinoma. The transgressing endothelial pattern demonstrates an arborising, proliferating or transgressing mesh work of capillaries in a loosely cohesive sheet of neoplastic hepatocytes (smear, PAP).

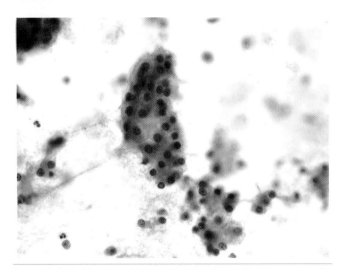

**Fig. 8.39** Well-differentiated hepatocellular carcinoma. The dispersed small cluster, single cell pattern shows malignant hepatocytes as predominantly large polygonal cells with preserved hepatocytic features that overall are deceptively bland (smear, PAP).

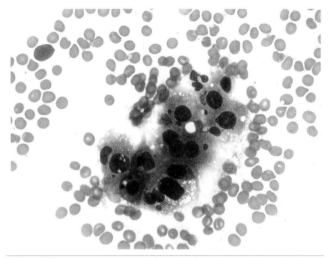

**Fig. 8.41** Well-differentiated hepatocellular carcinoma. Malignancy is supported by the presence of macronucleoli and increased intracytoplasmic hyaline globules (smear, Diff-Quik).

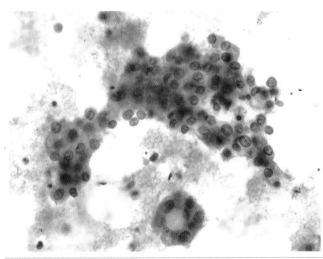

**Fig. 8.40** Well-differentiated hepatocellular carcinoma. Malignancy is supported by the presence of cellular monotony resulting from a relatively uniform population of cells with an elevated nuclear to cytoplasmic ratio. Note the acinar architecture in the bottom center of the image (smear, PAP).

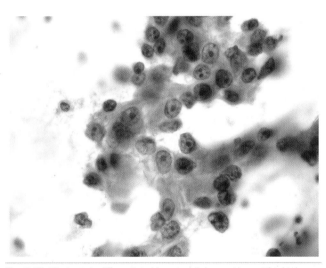

**Fig. 8.42** Moderately-differentiated hepatocellular carcinoma. This high-grade hepatocellular carcinoma maintains some hepatic preservation while displaying obvious malignant features (smear, PAP).

## Moderately to poorly differentiated hepatocellular carcinoma

High-grade hepatocellular carcinoma displays features of obvious malignancy, for example smears of high cellularity with cellular crowding and nuclear overlapping, nuclear membrane abnormalities, hyperchromasia and macronucleoli, which are many of the same features used to assess malignancy in a histological preparation. Moderately differentiated hepatocellular carcinoma is readily recognised as malignant by the nuclear atypia and there is some evidence of hepatic differentiation, such as abundant granular cytoplasm (Fig. 8.42). Poorly differentiated hepatocellular carcinoma is an obviously malignant tumour with little to no hepatic resemblance and as such difficult to distinguish from any other poorly differentiated tumour (Fig. 8.43).

Smear patterns are equally important in the diagnosis of high-grade HCC, especially the peripherally wrapping endothelial pattern. The presence of peripherally wrapping endothelial cells around the smooth edged nests and trabeculae of cells supports the diagnosis of HCC (Figs 8.43, 8.44). The peripheral pattern is not a feature of metastatic renal cell carcinoma, a morphological mimicker of hepatocellular carcinoma, but the transgressing pattern is the most common pattern of that tumour both in the kidney and in metastatic deposits[122] (see renal cell carcinoma, below).

Although present in less than half of cases, the presence of bile production by malignant tumour cells is a relatively pathognomonic finding for the diagnosis of HCC (Fig. 8.45).[95,123] A Hall's stain can be used to confirm the nature of the pigment as bile. The presence of intracytoplasmic mucin generally excludes hepatocellular carcinoma (except in the rare case of a combined hepatocellular-cholangiocarcinoma) and its presence should focus the differential diagnosis on adenocarcinoma.

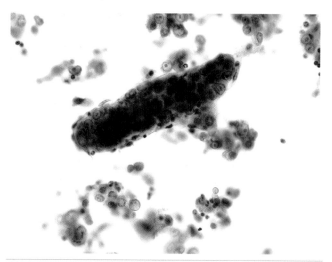

**Fig. 8.43** Poorly differentiated hepatocellular carcinoma. This high-grade hepatocellular carcinoma appears as an obviously malignant high-grade carcinoma, and there is little to no hepatic preservation. Note the peripherally wrapping endothelium, a feature that supports hepatic origin (ThinPrep, PAP).

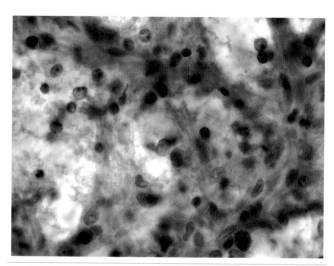

**Fig. 8.45** Poorly differentiated hepatocellular carcinoma. The recognition of malignant epithelial cells producing bile is essentially diagnostic of hepatocellular carcinoma (smear, PAP).

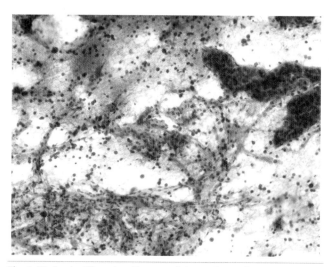

**Fig. 8.44** Poorly differentiated hepatocellular carcinoma. Smear pattern is important in the recognition of high-grade hepatocellular carcinomas and its recognition can preclude the need for ancillary studies. Note here the peripherally wrapping endothelium, the transgressing endothelium and the numerous naked nuclei in the background (smear, PAP).

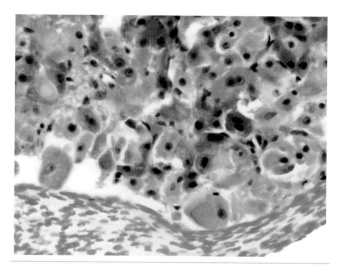

**Fig. 8.46** Fibrolamellar hepatocellular carcinoma. This variant is characterised by large polygonal hepatocytes with dense oxyphilic cytoplasm often containing intracytoplasmic pale bodies and a deceptively low nuclear to cytoplasmic ratio (cell block, H&E. Courtesy of Dr Edmond Cibas, Brigham & Women's Hospital).

## Hepatocellular carcinoma variants

Fibrolamellar variant is a variant of hepatocellular carcinoma that generally occurs in young patients as a solitary mass in a non-cirrhotic liver that lends itself more readily to excision, thereby improving the prognostic outlook.[124] It is a tumour associated with dense broad fibrous bands and large malignant hepatocytes with an abundance of dense oxyphilic cytoplasm. The presence of abundant dense oxyphilic type cytoplasm often with intracytoplasmic pale bodies, a deceptively low nuclear to cytoplasmic ratio and intranuclear inclusions are the key characteristic features on FNA cytology (Fig. 8.46). Due to the dense fibrous stromal component of this tumour, smears may be paucicellular and malignant hepatocytes may be individual, single, and widely scattered. Peripherally wrapping endothelium is not a feature of this tumour, but transgressing endothelium has been observed.[125]

The acinar cell variant is a morphological variant that presents a diagnostic challenge on cell block preparations. The frequently 'back to back' acini give the appearance of an adenocarcinoma (Fig. 8.47). There should be no mucin in the lumen of the acini or within the cytoplasm of the cells, and the acini should be separated by similarly malignant cells with no true cribriform architecture. Immunohistochemical stains will be helpful in establishing the correct diagnosis (see Ancillary studies, p. 305).

The clear cell variant is characterised by the abundance of intracytoplasmic fat and/or glycogen and introduces clear cell tumours metastatic from other sites into the differential diagnosis, especially from the kidney. Morphologically, the clear malignant hepatocytes are large polygonal cells with central nuclei, large nucleoli and abundant, clear, vacuolated cytoplasm. These neoplasms can be impossible to distinguish from

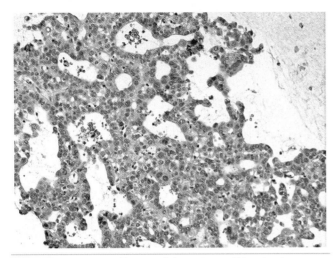

**Fig. 8.47** Acinar variant of hepatocellular carcinoma. This variant becomes apparent on cell block preparations with the demonstration of numerous variably sized back-to-back glandular spaces (H&E).

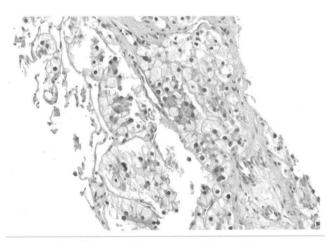

**Fig. 8.48** Clear cell hepatocellular carcinoma. This variant demonstrates polygonal cells with abundant vacuolated cytoplasm, mimicking other clear cell tumours, especially renal cell carcinoma. Compare with Fig. 8.61B (cell block, H&E).

clear cell renal cell carcinoma (Fig. 8.48). As mentioned above, the presence of the peripherally wrapping endothelial pattern is a finding that excludes renal cell carcinoma, but the transgressing pattern is not. Immunostains are usually required for diagnosis (see below).

### Ancillary studies

As mentioned above under 'Benign hepatocytic nodules', one of the most helpful ancillary tests in the diagnosis of well-differentiated hepatocellular carcinoma includes the use of the reticulin stain.[97,98,126] The reticulin stain can be used on either smears or cell block preparations. An abnormal reticulin staining pattern, usually in the form of an absence of reticulin staining (Fig. 8.49A, B), is highly associated with the presence of hepatocellular carcinoma.[97,98,126] Small, very early well-differentiated HCC may retain the reticulin staining pattern and cannot reliably be distinguished from small cell dysplasia.[127] Another pitfall in the interpretation of the reticulin stain is the presence of marked steatosis that can cause a false negative result.[98] Positive

staining with GPC3 also supports malignant over benign hepatocytes (see above). An iron stain such as the Prussian blue stain can highlight the normal, haemosiderin laden hepatocytes bright blue leaving malignant hepatocytes that have lost their ability to retain iron unstained (see Fig. 8.7B).

The basic immunocytochemical panel in the differential diagnosis of hepatocellular carcinoma and metastatic carcinoma, includes anti-hepatocyte antibody HepPar-1 that gives a strong diffuse chunky staining pattern (Fig. 8.49C),[128–130] MOC-31,[131–133] GPC3 (Fig. 8.49D),[105,106] AFP, low (CAM 5.2) and high (AE1) molecular weight (MW) cytokeratin (CK), polyclonal carcinoembryonic antigen (CEA) and neprilysin (CD10) staining, the latter two producing a canalicular staining pattern (Fig. 8.49E).[134–136] The hepatocytes markers Hep-Par 1 and GPC3 do not have 100% sensitivity or specificity for the diagnosis of malignancy of hepatic origin, so these markers should be used in a panel of markers to support a the diagnosis of HCC. The endothelial cell marker CD34 stains the sinusoids diffusely indicating capillarisation of the sinusoids and supporting the diagnosis of hepatocellular carcinoma (Fig. 8.49F). AFP staining is helpful if positive, but a negative stain does not rule out HCC as only about 40% of HCC are associated with a positive stain.[137] One must also keep in mind that AFP may occasionally be positive in reactive processes,[138] so a positive stain does not in itself diagnose malignancy. As mentioned earlier, serum levels of AFP >400 ng/mL are strongly associated with the presence of hepatocellular carcinoma, but not all tumours are associated with elevated levels, particularly the fibrolamellar variant.[124]

---

**Cytological findings: well-differentiated hepatocellular carcinoma**

- Low-power smear pattern with smooth-edged clusters and thickened trabeculae with peripherally wrapping endothelial cells (pathognomonic)
- Low-power smear pattern with more than focal loosely cohesive sheets of hepatocytes with transgressing vessels (highly suspicious finding)
- Monotonous, uniform hepatocytic cell population with subtle malignant features
- Acinar formation in cell clusters
- Increased nuclear to cytoplasmic ratio compared to normal hepatocytes
- Macroeosinophilic nucleoli
- Reduced number of binucleated cells
- Background free of bile duct epithelial cells
- Reticulin stain demonstrates a loss of the normal 1–2 cell thick hepatic plate architecture
- Iron stain fails to stain tumour in cases of haemachromatosis
- Positive glypican-3 immunostaining; AFP ± .

---

**Cytological findings: moderately to poorly differentiated hepatocellular carcinoma**

- Peripherally wrapping endothelial smear pattern is virtually pathognomonic
- Transgressing vessels are suggestive but cannot distinguish hepatocellular from renal cell carcinoma
- Presence of intracytoplasmic bile is pathognomonic

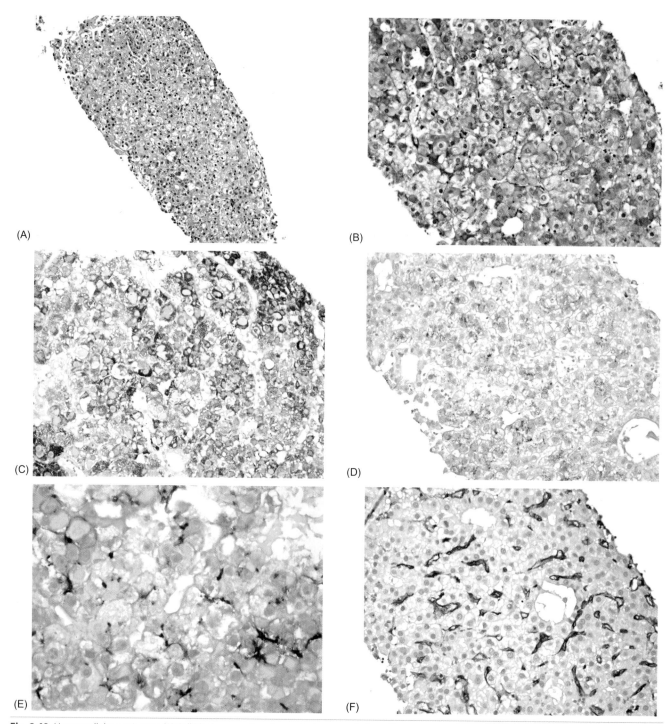

**Fig. 8.49** Hepatocellular carcinoma. (A) Cell block preparation demonstrates a population of hepatocytes with a solid, focally acinar growth pattern. (B) A reticulin stain demonstrates the loss of reticulin staining typical of hepatocellular carcinoma. (C) Immunoperoxidase staining shows coarse, granular diffuse staining with anti-hepatocyte antibody (Hep-Par-1). (D) Malignant hepatocytes also stain with antibodies to glypican-3. (E) Polyclonal CEA antibodies demonstrate a linear canalicular staining pattern as does CD10. (F) CD34 highlights the capillarisation of the sinusoids diffusely in hepatocellular carcinoma (A: H&E; B: reticulin; C–E peroxidase-antiperoxidase).

- Polygonal cells with central nuclei and prominent nucleoli with visible, granular to clear cytoplasm in moderately differentiated tumours; scant to no cytoplasm in poorly differentiated tumours
- Immunophenotype: low MW CK (Cam 5.2), polyclonal CEA, and CD10 (canalicular) HepPar-1 positive; AFP variable; high MW CK (AE1) negative.

## Cytological findings: variants

### Fibrolamellar hepatocellular carcinoma
- Population of large hepatocytes singly and in loose clusters
- Smears may be paucicellular due to fibrosis
- Transgressing vessels may be seen, but no peripherally wrapping endothelial cells

- Deceptively low nuclear to cytoplasmic ratio
- Large, variably atypical nuclei with prominent nucleoli and frequent intranuclear inclusions
- Cytoplasm is characteristically abundant and oncocytic appearing.

***Acinar variant***
- Back-to-back acini/rosettes of hepatocytes
- No mucin production.

***Clear cell variant***
- Cells with abundant vacuolated, clear cytoplasmic filled with glycogen and/or fat.

## Hepatoblastoma

Hepatoblastoma is the most common tumour of children with 75% occurring in males and 90% occurring before the age of 5 years.[69] There is a strong association with familial adenomatous polyposis syndrome and Beckwith-Wiedemann syndrome.[139] Patients generally present with an enlarging, often palpable mass that is usually single, lobulated and bulky. Serum AFP levels are almost always elevated and serve as a useful marker for recurrence and metastases.[69] Histologically, this tumour recapitulates the developing liver and may contain heterologous mesenchymal or epithelial elements.

Hepatoblastomas are classified as either epithelial or mixed epithelial-mesenchymal. The epithelial type consists of either immature embryonal and/or fetal hepatic epithelial cells; the mixed type typically contains both embryonal and foetal epithelial cells admixed with spindle cell mesenchyme.[94] Given this heterogeneity, the FNA smears of this tumour can have a varied appearance.[140,141] Smears of both types of hepatoblastoma are dominated by the epithelial cells. The fetal type cell resembles the normal hepatocyte but is generally smaller (Fig. 8.50A). The nuclei are central, round and bland appearing and the cytoplasm may contain fat and glycogen, unlike the embryonal cell type.[142] The embryonal cell is more primitive and undifferentiated with hyperchromatic nuclei and scant cytoplasm that may form rosettes and trabeculae[142] (Fig. 8.50B). Rarely the epithelial cells appear undifferentiated or anaplastic and resemble other small round blue cell tumours of childhood and are impossible to distinguish from neuroblastoma or Wilm's tumour on morphology alone.[143,144] The mesenchymal component, if present, presents as cellular spindle cell type mesenchyme, but heterologous elements may also be present including osteoid, cartilage, skeletal muscle and, particularly, extramedullary haematopoiesis.[142] A myxoid matrix has been described.[145]

The primary differential diagnosis rests most frequently between the fetal type hepatoblastoma and hepatocellular carcinoma, and embryonal or anaplastic hepatoblastoma and other paediatric small round blue cell tumours.[143]

### Ancillary tests

Ancillary studies and clinicopathological correlation are required. Hepatoblastomas will stain with high-molecular-weight cytokeratin,[146] whereas tumour cells of most hepatocellular carcinomas do not.[147] Both tumours stain with low-molecular-weight cytokeratin (CAM 5.2).[146] Polyclonal CEA stains hepatoblastomas

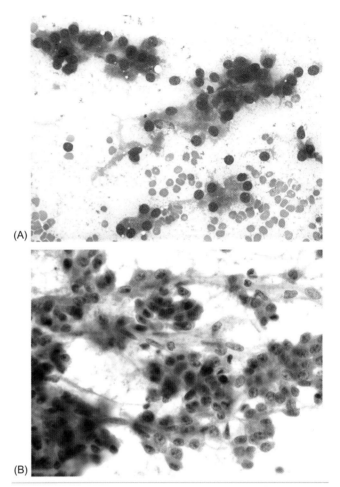

**Fig. 8.50** Hepatoblastoma. (A) The foetal type is composed of cells that resemble the normal hepatocyte but are generally smaller with central, round and bland nucleoli (smear, Diff-Quik). (B) The embryonal type is composed of more primitive cells with hyperchromatic nucleoli and scant cytoplasm (smear, PAP).

with a variable and inconsistent canalicular and/or cytoplasmic pattern depending on the type of hepatoblastoma.[148] This stain will not distinguish hepatoblastoma from hepatocellular carcinoma but can help in the distinction between a primary and metastatic tumours. HepPar-1 positivity supports a hepatic primary over other small round blue cell tumours of non-hepatic origin.[128–130,148]

### Cytological findings: hepatoblastoma

- Epithelial dominant smears
- Mesenchymal (spindle cell) component and/or heterologous elements, especially extramedullary haemopoesis and osteoid, relatively scant
- Epithelial cells are either small hepatocytic (fetal type), smaller immature, pleomorphic cells (embryonal type) or smaller still undifferentiated blue cells (anaplastic type)
- Epithelial cells form cohesive, crowded clusters, cords, ribbons or rosettes
- Immunophenotype: positive for low- and high-MW CK (CAM 5.2 and AE1), pCEA with variable canalicular/cytoplasmic staining, HepPar-1.

## Cholangiocarcinoma

Cholangiocarcinoma is an adenocarcinoma of the bile ducts that occurs predominantly in the noncirrhotic liver of the elderly population, most commonly of South-east Asia due to the high infestation with the liver fluke. Patients with primary sclerosing cholangitis (PSC) and cirrhosis due to hepatitis C are also at increased risk.[69,94] These neoplasms are classified by their location as peripheral (intrahepatic), hilar (Klatskin tumour), extra-hepatic and intraductal types. All but the intraductal type form a firm, white-tan mass that can become quite large when intrahepatic, but is usually small in the hilar or extra-hepatic locations due to obstruction causing early detection.[69] FNA is used to sample obvious masses while brush cytology is used to sample strictured or thickened ducts. EUS-FNA has been shown to add value to the diagnosis of hilar and extra-hepatic cholangiocarcinomas.[33] While the principal criteria for the diagnosis of adenocarcinoma on FNA smears are relatively standard regardless of location, the interpretation of bile duct brushings requires more stringent set of criteria and a higher threshold for the interpretation of malignancy. This is due to the difficulty in obtaining a specimen of quality and quantity sufficient for a confident malignant diagnosis. Sclerosis and inflammation inherent to the tumour or secondary to an underlying condition (PSC, stent placement, etc.) contribute to a paucicellular sample, and preparation artifact from obscuring blood, crush and air drying artifact limit optimal interpretation. Processing bile duct brushings in a liquid-based medium has shown improvement in diagnostic sensitivity and specificity (Fig. 8.51).[38–40]

The most common histological appearance of cholangiocarcinoma is a low-grade, well- to moderately differentiated adenocarcinoma forming tubules and cribriform glands infiltrating a sclerotic stroma. FNA smears generally produce a readily recognisable adenocarcinoma but with nonspecific features compared to those metastatic from the upper gastrointestinal tract and lung. Smears are variably cellular and demonstrate irregular, variably sized sheets of atypical to malignant appearing glandular cells that resemble bile duct epithelium (Fig. 8.52).

Clusters of tumour cells may show cytoplasmic vacuolisation and focal mucin production (Fig. 8.53). Cell block preparations are particularly helpful in this diagnosis because the characteristic common histological pattern described above may be recognised (Fig. 8.54).

### Ancillary tests

A simple mucin stain demonstrating the production of mucin will define the neoplasm as an adenocarcinoma and, with the rare exception of a mixed cholangiocarcinoma-hepatocellular carcinoma, exclude the diagnosis of hepatocellular carcinoma. The basic immunohistochemical panel discussed above under hepatocellular carcinoma will also help in this differential diagnosis. Distinguishing cholangiocarcinoma from metastatic adenocarcinomas relies primarily on clinical history, but a panel of immunohistochemical markers may be helpful for specific tumours (see Ch. 3).

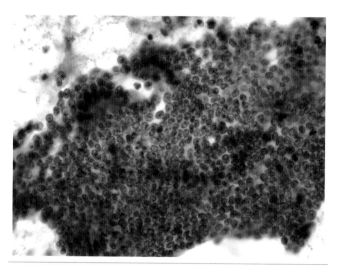

**Fig. 8.52** Cholangiocarcinoma. This adenocarcinoma demonstrates irregular, variably sized sheets of atypical to malignant appearing glandular cells that resemble bile duct epithelium (smear, PAP).

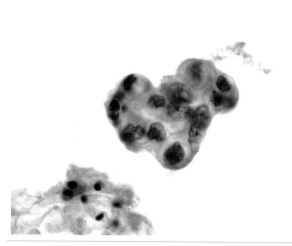

**Fig. 8.51** Cholangiocarcinoma. Intraductal and periductal tumours sampled by bile duct brushing often have better preservation with liquid-based processing (ThinPrep, PAP).

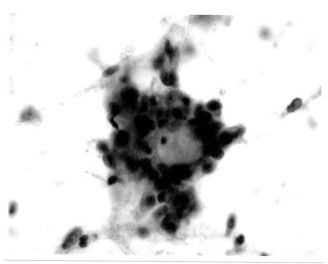

**Fig. 8.53** Cholangiocarcinoma. The recognition of three-dimensional cell clusters with mucin vacuoles confirms the diagnosis of adenocarcinoma and excludes hepatocellular carcinoma (smear, PAP).

## Cytological findings: cholangiocarcinoma

- Glandular cells in flat, angulated sheets
- Low-grade malignant nuclei with nuclear crowding, overlapping, slightly irregular nuclear membrane, parachromatin clearing
- A range of atypia may be seen from borderline malignant appearing to obviously malignant looking
- Exaggerated honeycombed pattern from uneven nuclear distribution in the sheet
- Cell blocks can help by demonstrating sclerotic stroma and cribriforming architecture
- Mucin stains positive at least focally in many cases
- Immunophenotype: keratin 7+,19+;20−; cytoplasmic pCEA, LeuM1, B72.3 +.

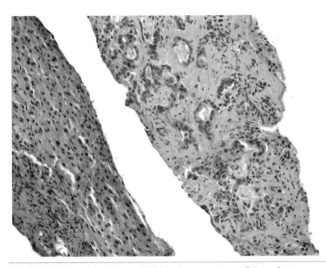

**Fig. 8.54** Cholangiocarcinoma. Cell block preparations of tissue fragments often demonstrate the characteristic angulated glands invading dense sclerosis (H&E).

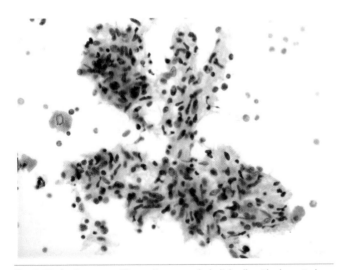

**Fig. 8.55** Angiosarcoma. The malignant endothelial cells with elongated spindle-shaped hyperchromatic nuclei are enmeshed with benign hepatocytes (smear, PAP).

## Angiosarcoma

Although extremely rare, angiosarcoma is the most common primary sarcoma of the liver occurring in older patients with a 3:1 ratio of men to women.[149] These neoplasms are believed to be secondary to exposure to hepatotoxic agents including vinyl chloride, Thorotrast, arsenic and anabolic steroids. The prognosis is poor. Histologically these neoplasms are single or multiple nodules of vascular channels lined by malignant endothelial cells. The malignant cells range from being widely spaced lining dilated sinusoidal channels to more solid growth filling the sinusoids and causing atrophy of the surrounding hepatocytes. An epithelioid appearance to the endothelial cells may also occur creating a pitfall and misdiagnosis of a carcinoma.[69] FNA smears are bloody and may be paucicellular.[150] Malignant endothelial cells can be seen interdigitating among reactive hepatocytes. They have elongated, spindled-shaped hyperchromatic nuclei that are easier to appreciate in small clusters (Fig. 8.55) than in large clusters where they tend to blend in with the hepatocytes. Tumour cells should stain positively for factor 8, CD31, CD34, or *Ulex europaeus lectin*.[151,152]

### Cytological findings: angiosarcoma

- Atypical to overtly malignant endothelial cells interspersed with hepatocyte clusters
- Spindle cell malignancy possibly with blood lakes
- Immunocytochemistry stains: Factor 8, CD31, CD34, ulex euroopaeus lectin.

## Embryonal sarcoma

Embryonal sarcoma is a rare malignancy of children typically between 6 and 10 years of age. Patients present with abdominal pain or with an abdominal mass. Histologically these neoplasms are composed of a myxoid stroma embedded with spindled to stellate cells which produces FNA smears composed of large, anaplastic cells (Fig. 8.56), multinucleated tumour giant cells and atypical spindle cells. Intracytoplasmic globules may be seen that are PAS positive but diastase resistant. Tumour cells also stain for vimentin, alpha-1-antitrypsin and alpha-1-antichymotrypsin.[153–156]

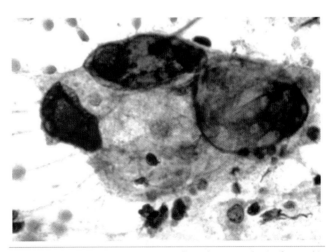

**Fig. 8.56** Embryonal sarcoma. Tumour cells are large, anaplastic often multinucleated tumour giant cells (smear, rapid H&E).

## Cytological findings: embryonal sarcoma

- Hypercellular smears
- Large, pleomorphic anaplastic cells with multinucleated giant cells and atypical spindle cells
- Intracytoplasmic globules that are PAS positive, diastase resistant
- Immunophenotype: vimentin, alpha-1-anti-trypsin and alpha-1-antichymotrypsin +.

## Malignant neoplasms – metastatic

The vast majority of malignancies in the liver are metastases,[157] and the distinction between a primary and metastatic malignancy is of both therapeutic and prognostic significance. Past medical history is of vital importance as most patients have a known history of a primary malignancy elsewhere. Metastatic tumours tend to recapitulate their appearance in the primary organ, and specific tumour types such as small cell carcinoma and lymphoma generally maintain a consistent cytological appearance. Adenocarcinoma, although frequently recognisable as an entity, presents the most difficulty in making a specific diagnosis as to site of origin. Adenocarcinoma from the colon is the most common metastasis to the liver.[157] The presence of an adenocarcinoma with a 'dirty necrosis' background is sufficient to diagnose adenocarcinoma consistent with colonic primary in a patient with a history of colonic cancer, and should direct the clinician to evaluate the colon first in a patient with an unknown primary. Other metastatic malignancies commonly encountered in the liver include those from the pancreas (adenocarcinoma and neuroendocrine tumours), stomach (adenocarcinoma and gastrointestinal stromal tumours), breast, lung (adenocarcinoma, small cell carcinoma and much less commonly squamous cell carcinoma), skin (melanoma) and bladder. Less common but diagnostically more challenging are metastases from the kidney and adrenal gland due to the morphological overlap with hepatocellular carcinoma. Sarcomas are the least encountered tumour type, the most common type being leiomyosarcoma, generally from the uterus, and it can be challenging but therapeutically important to distinguish metastatic GIST from leiomyosarcoma.[158,159] Lymphoma may also be seen in the liver, most commonly secondary to systemic disease, but can be a primary malignancy. If lymphoma is suspected on rapid interpretation, request should be made for a dedicated FNA for flow cytometry analysis, e.g. one that is not expressed onto a slide, rather one in which the aspirated tissue is rinsed into either buffered normal saline, cytolyte solution or RPMI. The combination of cytological evaluation and flow cytometry immunophenotyping is very often sufficient for diagnosis and subclassification of non-Hodgkin lymphoma.[160-164] The cytological features helpful in the diagnosis of a variety of metastatic tumours are presented below with accompanying supportive ancillary tests and illustrations.

## Cytological findings: adenocarcinoma (NOS)

- Polygonal to columnar glandular cells arranged in flat monolayered sheets, three-dimensional clusters or singly
- Lumens within clusters may be seen in some cases
- Nuclei are variably atypical ranging from quite bland in low-grade tumours to extremely atypical and obviously malignant in high-grade tumours

- Cytoplasm is delicate, frequently vacuolated, sometimes wispy
- Intracytoplasmic mucin may be seen; mucicarmine or other mucin stains can help identify focal mucin production.

## Cytological findings: colonic adenocarcinoma (Fig. 8.57)

- Cigar-shaped, often palisaded nuclei
- Variably prominent nucleoli but not macroeosinophilic nucleoli
- Dirty necrosis in the background (KEY)
- Immunocytochemistry: CK20+, CK7−, CEA+, CDX2.

## Cytological findings: breast carcinoma, ductal type

- Often low grade with a monomorphous cell population
- Flat angulated groups
- Single flame or cone-shaped cells
- Target cells (cells with intracytoplasmic lumen)
- Cell-in-cell arrangement
- Immunocytochemistry: oestrogen/progesterone ± and supportive if positive, but non-specific, gross cystic disease protein-15 is supportive if positive.

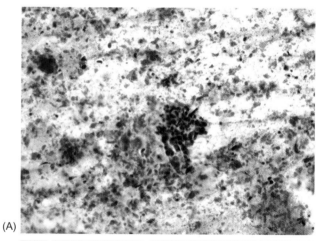
(A)

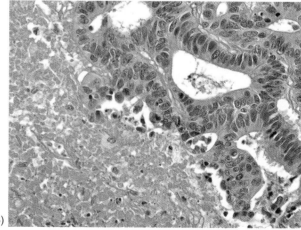
(B)

**Fig. 8.57** Metastatic colonic carcinoma. (A) This adenocarcinoma is recognised on smears by the background of dirty necrosis, a non-specific but characteristic feature. Viable aggregates of carcinoma may be few (smear, PAP). (B) Cell block shows malignant glands composed of tall, crowded columnar cells adjacent to cellular necrosis (H&E).

## Cytological findings: squamous cell carcinoma

- Relatively uncommon metastasis to the liver
- Large polygonal cells singly and in clusters
- Usually high grade with large, hyperchromatic nuclei with irregular nuclear membranes
- Cytoplasm is dense and non-vacuolated as opposed to that of adenocarcinoma
- Keratinising squamous cells stain orangophilic on Papanicolaou stain but this feature may not be present.

## Cytological findings: small cell undifferentiated carcinoma

- Small pleomorphic blue cells with little to no cytoplasm in clusters and singly
- Nuclei are hyperchromatic with coarse, stippled chromatin
- Nuclear moulding is common and characteristic
- Necrosis and apoptosis is common
- Smear or crush artifact is invariably present due to the fragile nature of the cells.

## Cytological findings: well-differentiated neuroendocrine carcinoma (e.g. metastatic pancreatic endocrine neoplasm (PEN) and carcinoid tumour) (Fig. 8.58)

- Small uniform blue cells with visible cytoplasm that tends to be scant and more evenly perinuclear in carcinoid tumours and more abundant and eccentric in PEN
- Nuclei with coarse stippled chromatin, more obvious in carcinoids than PEN
- Nucleoli generally not present in carcinoid tumours but visible in PEN
- No nuclear moulding, much less crush artifact, and no significant necrosis/apoptosis compared with small cell undifferentiated carcinoma
- Immunocytochemistry: keratin, synaptophysin and chromogranin positive.

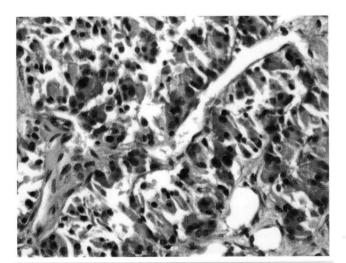

**Fig. 8.58** Metastatic well-differentiated neuroendocrine carcinoma. Neuroendocrine tumours can mimic hepatocellular carcinoma architecturally on cell block with 'endothelial wrapping' as well as cytologically with polygonal cell shape and relatively low-grade malignant nuclear features (cell block, H&E).

## Diagnostic pitfall: well-differentiated neuroendocrine carcinoma (e.g. metastatic pancreatic endocrine neoplasm (PEN) and carcinoid tumour)

- Cells can appear large and polygonal forming trabeculae with endothelial lining on cell block.

## Cytological findings: large cell lymphoma (Fig. 8.59)

- Mostly diffuse large B cell lymphoma, predominantly secondary but can be primary
- Discohesive, single cell population; may have pseudogroups, e.g. artifactual clustering
- Lymphoglandular bodies (clumps of stripped cytoplasm) in the background
- Coarse, frequently peripherally clumped chromatin
- Nucleoli may be present
- Cytoplasm is scant to invisible, but may be abundant in anaplastic large cell lymphoma
- Immunocytochemistry: leukocyte common antigen, CD20, CD19.

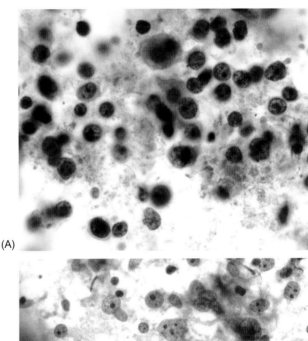

(A)

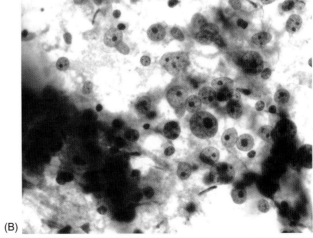

(B)

**Fig. 8.59** Large cell lymphoma. (A) Tumour cells disperse in a discohesive single cell pattern and display peripherally clumped chromatin, scant to no cytoplasm, occasionally prominent nucleoli and scattered lymphoglandular bodies (stripped cytoplasmic fragments) in the background (smear, PAP). (B) Numerous naked nuclei of high-grade hepatocellular carcinoma can look similar but are distinguished by the presence of large central macronucleoli (smear, PAP).

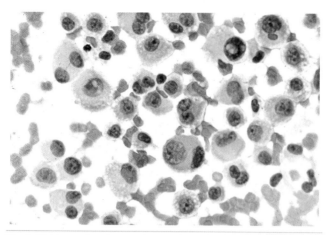

**Fig. 8.60** Metastatic melanoma. Large polygonal cells mimic hepatocellular carcinoma with polygonal cell shape, macronucleoli, intranuclear inclusions and abundant cytoplasm. Binucleated, 'mirror image' nuclei are distinctive for melanoma (cytospin, PAP).

## Cytological findings: melanoma (Fig. 8.60)

- Large polygonal cells singly and in clusters; may also be spindled or small blue cells with scant cytoplasm
- Central to eccentric nuclei with large nucleoli
- Intranuclear inclusions common
- Cytoplasm is commonly abundant, non-granular and frequently non-pigmented
- Immunocytochemistry: S100, HMB-45, Mart-1 and Melan-A positive; keratin negative.

## Diagnostic pitfall: melanoma

- Fontana–Masson stain will stain cytoplasmic melanin pigment black but will also stain lipofuscin pigment.

## Cytological findings: renal cell carcinoma (RCC) (Fig. 8.61)

- Large polygonal cells singly and in clusters
- Transgressing endothelial pattern the most common vascular pattern, but peripherally wrapping endothelial pattern is not a feature
- Round central nuclei with prominent macronucleoli ('owl's eye') in typical clear/granular cell type; papillary RCC type does not demonstrate prominent nucleoli
- Intranuclear inclusions can be seen and are frequent in chromophobe type
- Cytoplasm is commonly abundant and clear or granular; excessive and 'balloon- like' in chromophobe RCC and scant, often with haemosiderin in papillary RCC
- Immunocytochemistry: keratin, vimentin and EMA positive; CEA negative.

## Cytological findings: adrenal carcinoma (Fig. 8.62)

- Medium-sized polygonal cells singly and in clusters
- No transgressing endothelial pattern but peripherally wrapping endothelial pattern may be seen on cell block
- Nuclei are variably atypical with hyperchromasia and pleomorphism nucleoli do not tend to be macroeosinophilic as in hepatocellular carcinoma

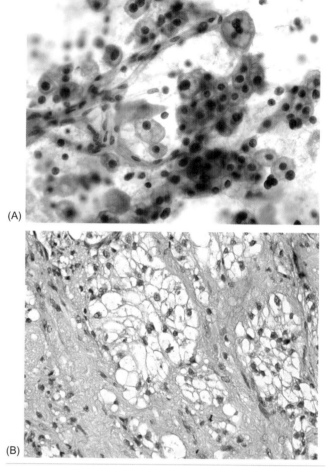

(A)

(B)

**Fig. 8.61** Metastatic renal cell carcinoma. (A) The classic appearance of renal cell carcinoma demonstrates large polygonal cells with clear to granular cytoplasm, central nuclei and large nucleoli. Note the transgressing endothelial pattern (smear, PAP). (B) Tissue fragments in cell blocks show aggregates of clear cell carcinoma. Compare with the clear cell hepatocellular carcinoma in Fig. 8.48 (H&E).

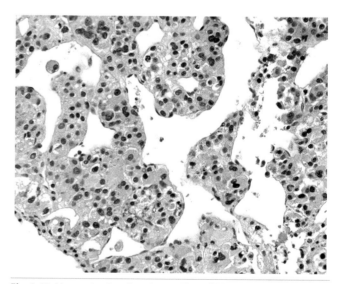

**Fig. 8.62** Metastatic adrenal carcinoma. This cell block preparation demonstrates the remarkable architectural similarity to hepatocellular carcinoma with large polygonal cells forming trabeculae with endothelial wrapping (H&E).

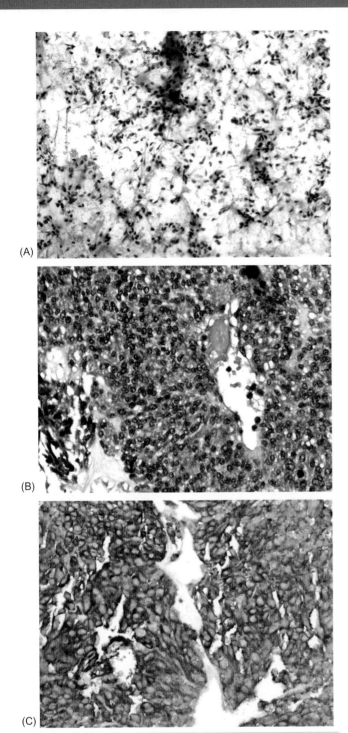

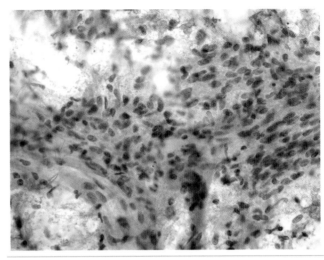

**Fig. 8.64** Metastatic leiomyosarcoma. Spindle cells in tightly cohesive groups or fascicles demonstrate elongated nuclei with blunted nuclear ends and more abundant cytoplasm than is typically seen in GIST (smear, PAP).

- Prominent vascular pattern
- Relatively bland nuclei without overt hyperchromasia or pleomorphism
- Delicate cytoplasmic processes
- Little to no crush artifact
- Immunophenotype: c-kit and CD34 positive; smooth muscle actin variably positive; desmin negative.

### Cytological findings: leiomyosarcoma (Fig. 8.64)

- Pleomorphic spindle cells in tightly cohesive three-dimensional groups and syncytia; occasional epithelioid features
- No prominent vascular pattern
- Hyperchromatic, pleomorphic nuclei with blunted nuclear ends
- Cytoplasm is more abundant than GIST
- Immunophenotype: desmin and smooth muscle actin positive; c-kit negative.

## Role of liver FNA in the management of liver lesions

Accurate diagnosis of focal mass lesions in the liver is essential for proper patient management. Assuming that a nodule in the liver in a patient with a known extrahepatic malignancy represents metastatic disease can lead to patient mismanagement and over-treatment. Even with classic clinical and radiological evidence of metastatic disease from a known primary malignancy, confirmation with tissue diagnosis is essential for patient enrollment in research protocols and for patients to qualify as candidates for new therapies such as ethanol ablation[47] and targeted gene therapy.[48,49] Infections and lymphomas are treated non-surgically and prompt diagnosis with FNA can expedite appropriate patient triage and treatment.

FNA is the diagnostic procedure of choice for focal liver lesions. When performed by experienced interventional radiologists and interpreted by experienced pathologists, the accuracy rivals that of frozen section. In institutions with considerable experience, the sensitivity of liver FNAB is as high as 90% with specificity approaching 100%.[1,11-13] Sampling error is the reason for most false negative results that are most often due to

**Fig. 8.63** Metastatic gastrointestinal stromal tumour. (A) Monomorphic spindle cells singly and in small groups with scant delicate cytoplasmic processes and oval to spindled nuclei (smear, PAP). (B) Cell block histology highlights the vascularity and perinuclear vacuoles typical of GIST (H&E). (C) Immunoperoxidase stain for ckit (CD117) confirms the diagnosis (peroxidase-antiperoxidase).

- Immunocytochemistry: keratin, EMA, CEA negative; vimetin, synaptophysin (±), inhibin and Melan-A positive.[165,166]

### Cytological findings: gastrointestinal stromal tumour (Fig. 8.63)

- Monomorphic spindle cells in loose groups and singly; occasional epithelioid features inexact needle localisation. As such, concomitant core biopsy improves accuracy, specificity and sensitivity, and both are better than either alone.[15,16,30,167–169]

The distinction between a primary and metastatic malignancy is also important for proper patient care. Access to the patient's past medical history is of vital importance as most patients have a known history of a primary malignancy elsewhere. Metastatic colon cancer should be high in the differential diagnosis with or without a known primary colon cancer as it is the most common malignancy in the liver. Recognition of the typical smear pattern of an adenocarcinoma with palisading columnar cells in a background of dirty necrosis (see Fig. 8.57) is usually sufficient to support the diagnosis in patients with a known history or to suggest clinical evaluation of the colon in patients without a known history. Familiarity of the typical appearance of extrahepatic malignancies is of benefit as most metastases recapitulate their appearance in the primary organ, and specific tumour types such as small cell carcinoma and lymphoma generally maintain a consistent cytological appearance.

A focal mass lesion in a cirrhotic liver places HCC at the top of the differential diagnosis and prepares the pathologist for the systematic smear evaluation. If not already a routine practice, procurement of tissue for cell block should be requested of the radiologist in anticipation of ancillary studies.

# REFERENCES

1. Gervais DA. Percutaneous image-guided biopsy: review of and emphasis on special approaches. In: Ray CE, Hicks ME, Patel N, editors Sir Syllabus Interventions in Oncology. Chicago: The Society of Interventional Radiology; 2003.

2. Thuluvath PJ. EUS-guided FNA could be another important tool for the early diagnosis of hepatocellular carcinoma. Gastroint Endosc 2007;66:274–76.

3. Baskin-Bey ES, Moreno LLE, Gores GJ. Diagnosis of cholangiocarcinoma in patients with PSC: A sight on cytology. J Hepatol 2006;45:476–79.

4. Siqueira E, Schoen RE, Silverman W, et al. Detecting cholangiocarcinoma in patients with primary sclerosing cholangitis. Gastrointest Endosc 2002;56:40–47.

5. Biett. Hydatides du foie avec developpement considerable, de cet organe; ponction explorative; incision; sortie d'une grande quantite d'acephalocystes; guerison. Gaz'd Hop 1833;7:383.

6. Roberts. Abscess of the liver, with hydatids. Operation. Lancet 1833;1:189–90.

7. Lundquist A. Fine-needle aspiration biopsy of the liver. Acta Med Scand 1971;520(Suppl):1–28.

8. Martin HE, Ellis EB. Biopsy by needle puncture and aspiration. Ann Surg 1930;92:169–81.

9. Lundquist A. Fine needle aspiration biopsy for cytodiagnosis of malignant tumour in the liver. Acta Med Scand 1970;188:465–70.

10. Lundquist A. Liver biopsy with a needle of 0.7 mm outer diameter: safety and quantitative yield. Acta Med Scand 1970;188:471–74.

11. Moulton JS, Leoni CJ, Quarfordt SD, et al. Percutaneous image-guided biopsy. In: Baum S, Pentecost MJ, editors Abrams' Angiography Interventional Radiology. Philadelphia: Lippincott Williams & Wilkins; 2006. p. 257–79.

12. Bakshi P, Srinivasan R, Rao KL, et al. Fine needle aspiration biopsy in pediatric space-occupying lesions of liver: a retrospective study evaluating its role and diagnostic efficacy. J Pediatr Surg 2006;41:1903–8.

13. Eloubeidi MA, Tamhane A, Jhala N, et al. Agreement between rapid onsite and final cytologic interpretations of EUS-guided FNA specimens: implications for the endosonographer and patient management. Am J Gastroenterol 2006;101:2841–47.

14. Wang P, Meng ZQ, Chen Z, et al. Diagnostic value and complications of fine needle aspiration for primary liver cancer and its influence on the treatment outcome – a study based on 3011 patients in China. Eur J Surg Oncol 2008;34:541–46.

15. Longchampt E, Patriarche C, Fabre M. Accuracy of cytology vs. microbiopsy for the diagnosis of well-differentiated hepatocellular carcinoma and macroregenerative nodule. Definition of standardized criteria from a study of 100 cases. Acta Cytol 2000;44:515–23.

16. Franca AV, Valerio HM, Trevisan M, et al. Fine needle aspiration biopsy for improving the diagnostic accuracy of cut needle biopsy of focal liver lesions. Acta Cytol 2003;47:332–36.

17. Ceyhan K, Kupana SA, Bektas M, et al. The diagnostic value of on-site cytopathological evaluation and cellblock preparation in fine-needle aspiration cytology of liver masses. Cytopathology 2006;17:267–74.

18. Quirk DW, Brugge WR. Endoscopic ultrasonography-directed fine needle aspiration. In: Centeno BA, Pitman MB, editors Fine Needle Aspiration Biopsy of the Pancreas. Boston: Butterworth-Heinemann; 1999. p. 13–16.

19. Yu SC, Lo DY, Ip CB, et al. Does percutaneous liver biopsy of hepatocellular carcinoma cause hematogenous dissemination? An in vivo study with quantitative assay of circulating tumor DNA using methylation-specific real-time polymerase chain reaction. AJR Am J Roentgenol 2004;183:383–85.

20. Rowe LR, Mulvihill SJ, Emerson L, et al. Subcutaneous tumor seeding following needle core biopsy of hepatocellular carcinoma. Diagn Cytopathol 2007;35:717–21.

21. Hamazaki K, Matsubara N, Mori M, et al. Needle track implantation of hepatocellular carcinoma after ultrasonically guided needle liver biopsy: A case report. Hepatogastroenterology 1995;42:601–6.

22. Crowe DR, Eloubeidi MA, Chhieng DC, et al. Fine-needle aspiration biopsy of hepatic lesions: computerized tomographic-guided versus endoscopic ultrasound-guided FNA. Cancer 2006;108:180–85.

23. Caletti G, Fusaroli P. Endoscopic ultrasonography. Endoscopy 2001;33:158–66.

24. Fritscher-Ravens A, Broering DC, Sriram PV, et al. EUS-guided fine-needle aspiration cytodiagnosis of hilar cholangiosarcoma: a case series. Gastrointest Endosc 2000;52:534–40.

25. Giovanni M, Seitz J, Monges Gea. Fine needle aspiration cytology guided by endoscopic ultrasonography: results in 141 patients. Endoscopy 1995;27:171–77.

26. Bentz JS, Kochman ML, Faigel DO, et al. Endoscopic ultrasound-guided real-time fine-needle aspiration: clinicopathologic features of 60 patients. Diagn Cytopathol 1998;18:98–109.

27. Wiersema MJ, Kochman ML, Cramer HM, et al. Endosonography-guided real-time fine-needle aspiration biopsy. Gastrointest Endosc 1994; 40:700–7.

28. Nguyen P, Feng JC, Chang KJ. Endoscopic ultrasound (EUS) and EUS-guided fine-needle aspiration (FNA) of liver lesions. Gastrointest Endosc 1999;50:357–61.

29. Strassburg CP, Manns MP. Approaches to liver biopsy techniques – revisited. Semin Liver Dis 2006;26:318–27.

30. Zainol H, Sumithran E. Combined cytological and histological diagnosis of hepatocellular carcinoma in ultrasonically guided fine needle biopsy specimens. Histopathology 1993;22:581–86.

31. Dewitt J, LeBlanc J, McHenry L, et al. Endoscopic ultrasound-guided fine needle aspiration cytology of solid liver lesions: a large single-center experience. Am J Gastroenterol 2003;98:1976–81.

32. Hollerbach S, Willert J, Topalidis T, et al. Endoscopic ultrasound-guided fine-needle aspiration biopsy of liver lesions: histological and cytological assessment. Endoscopy 2003;35:743–49.

33. Eloubeidi M, Chen V, Jhala N, et al. Endoscopic ultrasound-guided fine needle aspiration biopsy of suspected cholangiocarcinoma. Clin Gastroenterol Hepatol 2004;2:209–13.

34. Fritscher-Ravens A, Broering DC, Sriram PV, et al. EUS-guided fine-needle aspiration cytodiagnosis of hilar cholangiocarcinoma: a case series. Gastrointest Endosc 2000;52:534–40.

35. Rumalla A, Baron TH, Leontovich O, et al. Improved diagnostic yield of endoscopic biliary brush cytology by digital image analysis. Mayo Clin Proc 2001;76:29–33.

36. Boberg KM, Jebsen P, Clausen OP, et al. Diagnostic benefit of biliary brush cytology in cholangiocarcinoma in primary sclerosing cholangitis. J Hepatol 2006;45:568–74.

37. Furmanczyk PS, Grieco VS, Agoff SN. Biliary brush cytology and the detection of cholangiocarcinoma in primary sclerosing cholangitis: evaluation of specific cytomorphologic features and CA19–CA19 levels. Am J Clin Pathol 2005;124:355–60.

38. Volmar KE, Vollmer RT, Routbort MJ, et al. Pancreatic and bile duct brushing cytology

in 1000 cases: review of findings and comparison of preparation methods. Cancer 2006;108:231–38.

39. Siddiqui MT, Gokaslan ST, Saboorian MH, et al. Comparison of ThinPrep and conventional smears in detecting carcinoma in bile duct brushings. Cancer 2003;99:205–10.

40. Ylagan LR, Liu LH, Maluf HM. Endoscopic bile duct brushing of malignant pancreatic biliary strictures: retrospective study with comparison of conventional smear and ThinPrep techniques. Diagn Cytopathol 2003;28:196–204.

41. Kipp BR, Stadheim LM, Halling SA, et al. A comparison of routine cytology and fluorescence in situ hybridisation for the detection of malignant bile duct strictures. Am J Gastroenterol 2004;99:1675–81.

42. Hahn PF, Eisenberg PJ, Pitman MB, et al. Cytopathologic touch preparations (imprints) from core needle biopsies: accuracy compared with that of fine-needle aspirates. AJR Am J Roentgenol 1995;165:1277–79.

43. Pupulim LF, Felce-Dachez M, Paradis V, et al. Algorithm for immediate cytologic diagnosis of hepatic tumors. AJR Am J Roentgenol 2008;190:W208–12.

44. Hamilton SR, Aaltonen LA. Tumours of the liver and intrahepatic bile ducts. In: Hamilton SR, Aaltonen LA, editors Pathology & Genetics Tumours of the Digestive System. Albany: WHO Publications Center; 2001:158.

45. Zerem E, Hadzic A. Sonographically guided percutaneous catheter drainage versus needle aspiration in the management of pyogenic liver abscess. AJR Am J Roentgenol 2007;189:W138–42.

46. Babu KS, Goel D, Prayaga A, et al. Intraabdominal hydatid cyst: a case report. Acta Cytol 2008;52:464–66.

47. Lencioni R, Crocetti L, Bozzi E, et al. Thermal (heat) ablation of hepatocellular cancer. In: Mauro MA, editor. Image-guided interventions. Philadelphia: Elsevier; 2008.

48. Roh V, Laemmle A, Von Holzen U, et al. Dual induction of PKR with E2F-1 and IFN-alpha to enhance gene therapy against hepatocellular carcinoma. Cancer Gene Ther 2008.

49. Calvisi DF, Pascale RM, Feo F. Dissection of signal transduction pathways as a tool for the development of targeted therapies of hepatocellular carcinoma. Rev Recent Clin Trials 2007;2:217–36.

50. Roskams T, Desmet VJ, Verslype C. Development, structure and function of the liver. In: Burt A, Portmann BC, Ferrell LD, editors MacSween's Pathology of the Liver. Philadelphia: Elsevier; 2007:12.

51. Brennick JB, O'Connell JX, Dickersin GR, et al. Lipofuscin pigmentation (so-called) 'melanosis') of the prostate. Am J Surg Pathol 1994;18:446–54.

52. Terada T, Nakanuma Y. Iron-negative foci in siderotic macroregenerative nodules in human cirrhotic liver. A marker of incipient neoplastic lesions. Arch Pathol Lab Med 1989;113:916–20.

53. Kim KW, Kim MJ, Lee SS, et al. Sparing of fatty infiltration around focal hepatic lesions in patients with hepatic steatosis: sonographic appearance with CT and MRI correlation. AJR Am J Roentgenol 2008;190:1018–27.

54. Michael CW, Hunter B. Interpretation of fine-needle aspirates processed by the ThinPrep technique: cytologic artifacts and diagnostic pitfalls. Diagn Cytopathol 2000;23:6–13.

55. Imbriaco M, Camera L, Manciuria A, et al. A case of multiple intra-abdominal splenosis with computed tomography and magnetic resonance imaging correlative findings. World J Gastroenterol 2008;14:1453–55.

56. Choi GH, Ju MK, Kim JY, et al. Hepatic splenosis preoperatively diagnosed as hepatocellular carcinoma in a patient with chronic hepatitis B: a case report. J Korean Med Sci 2008;23:336–41.

57. Galloro P, Marsilia GM, Nappi O. Hepatic splenosis diagnosed by fine-needle cytology. Pathologica 2003;95:57–59.

58. Lemos LB, Baliga M, Benghuzzi HA, et al. Nodular hematopoiesis of the liver diagnosed by fine-needle aspiration cytology. Diagn Cytopathol 1997;16:51–54.

59. Giorgio A, de Stefano G, Di Sarno A, et al. Percutaneous needle aspiration of multiple pyogenic abscesses of the liver: 13-year single-center experience. AJR Am J Roentgenol 2006;187:1585–90.

60. Haque R, Huston CD, Hughes M, et al. Amebiasis. N Engl J Med 2003;348:1565–73.

61. Lodhi S, Sarwari AR, Muzammil M, et al. Features distinguishing amoebic from pyogenic liver abscess: a review of 577 adult cases. Trop Med Int Health 2004;9:718–23.

62. Ishak KG. Granulomas of the liver. In: Toacham HL, editor. Pathology of Granulomas. New York: Raven Press; 1983. p. 307–69.

63. Iha H, Nakashima Y, Fukukura Y, et al. Biliary hamartomas simulating multiple hepatic metastasis on imaging findings. Kurume Med J 1996;43:231–35.

64. Siddiqui MA, McKenna BJ. Hepatic mesenchymal hamartoma: a short review. Arch Pathol Lab Med 2006;130:1567–69.

65. Yesim G, Gupse T, Zafer U, et al. Mesenchymal hamartoma of the liver in adulthood: immunohistochemical profiles, clinical and histopathological features in two patients. J Hepatobiliary Pancreat Surg 2005;12:502–7.

66. Boman F, Bossard C, Fabre M, et al. Mesenchymal hamartomas of the liver may be associated with increased serum alpha foetoprotein concentrations and mimic hepatoblastomas. Eur J Pediatr Surg 2004;14:63–66.

67. Jimenez-Heffernan JA, Vicandi B, Lopez-Ferrer P, et al. Fine-needle aspiration cytology of mesenchymal hamartoma of the liver. Diagn Cytopathol 2000;22:250–53.

68. al-Rikabi AC, Buckai A, al-Sumayer S, et al. Fine needle aspiration cytology of mesenchymal hamartoma of the liver. A case report. Acta Cytol 2000;44:449–53.

69. Goodman ZD, Terracciano LM. Tumours and tumour-like lesions of the liver. In: Burt A, Portmann BC, Ferrell LD, editors MacSween's Pathology of the liver. Philadelphia: Elsevier; 2007: p. 762–800.

70. Dehner LP. Inflammatory myofibroblastic tumor: the continued definition of one type of so-called inflammatory pseudotumor. Am J Surg Pathol 2004;28:1652–54.

71. Chan J. Inflammatory pseudotumor: A family of lesions of diverse nature and etiologies. Adv Anat Pathol 1996;3:156–71.

72. Kanno A, Satoh K, Kimura K, et al. Autoimmune pancreatitis with hepatic inflammatory pseudotumor. Pancreas 2005;31:420–23.

73. Uchida K, Satoi S, Miyoshi H, et al. Inflammatory pseudotumors of the pancreas and liver with infiltration of IgG4-positive plasma cells. Intern Med 2007;46:1409–12.

74. Neild GH, Rodriguez-Justo M, Wall C, et al. Hyper-IgG4 disease: report and characterisation of a new disease. BMC Med 2006;4:23.

75. Kamisawa T, Okamoto A. IgG4-related sclerosing disease. World J Gastroenterol 2008;14:3948–55.

76. Zen Y, Harada K, Sasaki M, et al. IgG4-related sclerosing cholangitis with and without hepatic inflammatory pseudotumor, and sclerosing pancreatitis-associated sclerosing cholangitis: do they belong to a spectrum of sclerosing pancreatitis? Am J Surg Pathol 2004;28:1193–203.

77. Coffin CM, Humphrey PA, Dehner LP. Extrapulmonary inflammatory myofibroblastic tumor: a clinical and pathological survey. Semin Diagn Pathol 1998;15:85–101.

78. Hosler GA, Steinberg DM, Sheth S, et al. Inflammatory pseudotumor: a diagnostic dilemma in cytopathology. Diagn Cytopathol 2004;31:267–70.

79. Malhotra V, Gondal R, Tatke M, et al. Fine needle aspiration cytologic appearance of inflammatory pseudotumor of the liver. A case report. Acta Cytol 1997;41(Suppl):1325–28.

80. Vick DJ, Goodman ZD, Deavers MT, et al. Ciliated hepatic foregut cyst: a study of six cases and review of the literature. Am J Surg Pathol 1999;23:671–77.

81. Lubrano J, Rouquette A, Huet E, et al. Ciliated hepatic foregut cyst discovered after kidney transplantation in a hepatitis C virus-infected patient: a report of one case and review of the literature. Eur J Gastroenterol Hepatol 2008;20:359–61.

82. Bonetti F, Pea M, Martignoni G, et al. The perivascular epithelioid cell and related lesions. Adv Anat Pathol 1997;4:343–58.

83. Sawai H, Manabe T, Yamanaka Y, et al. Angiomyolipoma of the liver: case report and collective review of cases diagnosed from fine needle aspiration biopsy specimens. J Hepatobiliary Pancreat Surg 1998;5:333–38.

84. Cha I, Cartwright D, Guis M, et al. Angiomyolipoma of the liver in fine-needle aspiration biopsies: its distinction from hepatocellular carcinoma. Cancer 1999;87:25–30.

85. Mai KT, Yazdi HM, Perkins DG, et al. Fine needle aspiration biopsy of epithelioid angiomyolipoma. A case report. Acta Cytol 2001;45:233–36.

86. Tsui WM, Colombari R, Portmann BC, et al. Hepatic angiomyolipoma: a clinicopathologic study of 30 cases and delineation of unusual morphologic variants. Am J Surg Pathol 1999;23:34–48.

87. Sturtz CL, Dabbs DJ. Angiomyolipomas: the nature and expression of the HMB45 antigen. Mod Pathol 1994;7:842–45.

88. Ma TK, Tse MK, Tsui WM, et al. Fine needle aspiration diagnosis of angiomyolipoma of the liver using a cellblock with immunohistochemical study. A case report. Acta Cytol 1994;38:257–60.

89. Guy CD, Yuan S, Ballo MS. Spindle-cell lesions of the liver: Diagnosis by fine-needle aspiration biopsy. Diagn Cytopathol 2001;25:94–100.

90. Layfield LJ, Mooney EE, Dodd LG. Not by blood alone: diagnosis of hemangiomas by fine-needle aspiration. Diagn Cytopathol 1998;19:250–54.

91. Pinto MM, Kaye AD. Fine needle aspiration of cystic liver lesions. Cytologic examination and carcinoembryonic antigen assay of cyst contents. Acta Cytol 1989;33:852–56.

92. Del Poggio P, Buonocore M. Cystic tumors of the liver: A practical approach. World J Gastroenterol 2008;14:3616–20.

93. Lin CC, Lin CJ, Hsu CW, et al. Fine-needle aspiration cytology to distinguish dysplasia

from hepatocellular carcinoma with different grades. J Gastroenterol Hepatol 2008;23(7 Pt 2):e146–52.

94. Ferrell LD. Benign and malignant tumors of the liver. In: Odze RD, Goldblum JR, Crawford JM, editors Surgical Pathology of the GI Tract, Liver, Biliary Tract, and Pancreas. Philadelphia: Saunders; 2004.

95. Kung ITM, Chan SK, Fung KH. Fine-needle aspiration in hepatocellular carcinoma: combined cytologic and histologic approach. Cancer 1991;67:673–80.

96. Pitman MB, Szyfelbein WM. The significance of endothelium in the FNA diagnosis of hepatocellular carcinoma. Diagn Cytopathol 1995;12:208–14.

97. deBoer WB. Cytodiagnosis of well-differentiated hepatocellular carcinoma: can indeterminate diagnoses be reduced? Cancer Cytopathol 1999;87:270–77.

98. Bergman S, Graeme-Cook F, Pitman MB. The usefulness of the reticulin stain in the differential diagnosis of liver nodules on fine-needle aspiration biopsy cellblock preparations. Mod Pathol 1997;10:1–7.

99. Lamps LW, Folpe AL. The diagnostic value of hepatocyte paraffin antibody 1 in differentiating hepatocellular neoplasms from nonhepatic tumors: A review. Adv Anat Pathol 2003;10:39–43.

100. Zhu Z, Friess H, Wang L, et al. Enhanced glypican-3 expression differentiates the majority of hepatocellular carcinomas from benign hepatic disorders. Gut 2001;48:558–64.

101. Nakatsura T, Yoshitake Y, Senju S, et al. Glypican-3 overexpressed specifically in human hepatocellular carcinoma, is a novel tumor marker. Biochem Biophys Res Commun 2003;20:16–25.

102. Capurro M, Wanless I, Sherman M, et al. Glypican-3 a novel serum and histochemical marker for hepatocellular carcinoma. Gastroenterology 2003;125:89–97.

103. Hippo Y, Watanabe K, Watanabe A, et al. Identification of soluble NH2-terminal fragment of glypican-3 as a serological marker for early-stage hepatocellular carcinoma. Cancer Res 2004;64:2418–23.

104. Ligato S, Mandich D, Cartun RW. Utility of glypican-3 in differentiating hepatocellular carcinoma from other primary and metastatic lesions in FNA of the liver: an immunocytochemical study. Mod Pathol 2008;21:626–31.

105. Libbrecht L, Severi T, Cassiman D, et al. Glypican-3 expression distinguishes small hepatocellular carcinomas from cirrhosis, dysplastic nodules, and focal nodular hyperplasia-like nodules. Am J Surg Pathol 2006;30:1405–11.

106. Wang XY, Degos F, Dubois S, et al. Glypican-3 expression in hepatocellular tumors: diagnostic value for preneoplastic lesions and hepatocellular carcinomas. Hum Pathol 2006;37:1435–41.

107. Kandil D, Leiman G, Allegretta M, et al. Glypican-3 immunocytochemistry in liver fine-needle aspirates: a novel stain to assist in the differentiation of benign and malignant liver lesions. Cancer 2007;111:316–22.

108. de Boer WB, Segal A, Frost FA, et al. Can CD34 discriminate between benign and malignant hepatocytic lesions in fine-needle aspirates and thin core biopsies? Cancer 2000;90:273–78.

109. Gottschalk-Sabag S, Ron N, Glick T. Use of CD34 and factor VIII to diagnose hepatocellular carcinoma on fine needle aspirates. Acta Cytol 1998;42:691–96.

110. Ng IOL, Lai ECS, Ho JCW, et al. Flow cytometric analysis of DNA ploidy in hepatocellular carcinoma. Am J Clin Pathol 1994;102:80–86.

111. Adachi E, Hashimoto H, Tsuneyoshi M. Proliferating cell nuclear antigen in hepatocellular carcinoma and small cell liver dysplasia. Cancer 1993;72:2902–9.

112. Ojanguren I, Ariza A, Llatjós M, et al. Proliferating cell nuclear antigen expression in normal, regenerative, and neoplastic liver: A fine needle aspiration cytology and biopsy study. Hum Pathol 1993;24:905–8.

113. Cajulis RS, Frias-Hidvegi D, Yu GH, et al. Detection of numerical chromosomal abnormalities by fluorescence in situ hybridisation of interphase cell nuclei with chromosome-specific probes on archival cytologic samples. Diagn Cytopathol 1996;14:178–81.

114. Krishna M, Lloyd RV, Batts KP. Detection of albumin messenger RNA in hepatic and extrahepatic neoplasms. A marker of hepatocellular differentiation. Am J Surg Pathol 1997;21:147–52.

115. Deprez C, Vangansbeke D, Fastrez R, et al. Nuclear DNA content, proliferation index, and nuclear size determination in normal and cirrhotic liver, and in benign and malignant primary and metastatic hepatic tumors. Am J Clin Pathol 1993;99:558–65.

116. Sherman M. Hepatocellular carcinoma: epidemiology, risk factors, and screening. Semin Liver Dis 2005;25:143–54.

117. Anthony PP. Hepatocellular carcinoma: an overview. Histopathol 2001;39:109–18.

118. Mazzaferro V, Regalia E, Doci R, et al. Liver transplantation for the treatment of small hepatocellular carcinomas in patients with cirrhosis. N Engl J Med 1996;334:693–99.

119. Yoo HY, Patt CH, Geschwind JF, et al. The outcome of liver transplantation in patients with hepatocellular carcinoma in the United States between 1988 and 2001: 5-year survival has improved significantly with time. J Clin Oncol 2003;21:4329–35.

120. Sóle M, Calvet X, Cuberes T, et al. Value and limitations of cytologic criteria for the diagnosis of hepatocellular carcinoma by fine needle aspiration biopsy. Acta Cytol 1993;37:309–16.

121. Haratake J, Hisaoka M, Yamamoto O, et al. An ultrastructural comparison of sinusoids in hepatocellular carcinoma, adenomatous hyperplasia, and fetal liver. Arch Pathol Lab Med 1992;116:67–70.

122. Weir P, Pitman MB. The vascular architecture of renal cell carcinoma in fine-needle aspiration biopsies. An aid in its distinction from hepatocellular carcinoma. Cancer 1997;81:45–50.

123. Bottles K, Cohen MB, Holly EA, et al. A step-wise logistic regression analysis of hepatocellular carcinoma. Cancer 1988;62:558–63.

124. Craig JR, Peters RL, Edmondson HA, et al. Fibrolamellar carcinoma of the liver: A tumor of adolescents and young adults with distinctive clinico-pathologic features. Cancer 1980;46:372–79.

125. Perez-Guillermo M, Masgrau NA, Garcia-Solano J, et al. Cytologic aspect of fibrolamellar hepatocellular carcinoma in fine-needle aspirates. Diagn Cytopathol 1999;21:180–87.

126. Ljung BM, Ferrell LD. Fine-needle aspiration biopsy of the liver: diagnostic problems. In: Pathology: State of the Art Reviews. Philadelphia: Hanley & Belfus Inc; 1996. p. 365–88.

127. Kondo F, Kondo Y, Nagato Y, et al. Interstitial tumour cell invasion in small hepatocellular carcinoma. Evaluation in microscopic and low magnification views. J Gastroenterol Hepatol 1994;9:604–12.

128. Minervini MI, Demetris AJ, Lee RG, et al. Utilisation of hepatocyte-specific antibody in the immunocytochemical evaluation of liver tumors. Mod Pathol 1997;10:686–92.

129. Leong AS, Sormunen RT, Tsui WM, et al. Hep Par 1 and selected antibodies in the immunohistological distinction of hepatocellular carcinoma from cholangiocarcinoma, combined tumours and metastatic carcinoma. Histopathology 1998;33:318–24.

130. Zimmerman RL, Burke MA, Young NA, et al. Diagnostic value of hepatocyte paraffin 1 antibody to discriminate hepatocellular carcinoma from metastatic carcinoma in fine-needle aspiration biopsies of the liver. Cancer (Cancer Cytopathol) 2001;93:288–91.

131. Niemann TH, Hughes JH, DeYoung BR. MOC-31 aids in the differentiation of metastatic adenocarcinoma from hepatocellular carcinoma. Cancer 1999;87:295–98.

132. Porcell AI, DeYoung BR, Proca DM, et al. Immunohistochemical analysis of hepatocellular and adenocarcinoma in the liver: MOC31 compares favorably with other putative markers. Mod Pathol 2000;13:773–78.

133. Kakar S, Gown AM, Goodman ZD, et al. Best practices in diagnostic immunohistochemistry: hepatocellular carcinoma versus metastatic neoplasms. Arch Pathol Lab Med 2007;131:1648–54.

134. Borscheri N, Roessner A, Rocken C. Canalicular immunostaining of neprilysin (CD10) as a diagnostic marker for hepatocellular carcinomas. Am J Surg Pathol 2001;25:1297–303.

135. Ahuja A, Gupta N, Kalra N, et al. Role of CD10 immunochemistry in differentiating hepatocellular carcinoma from metastatic carcinoma of the liver. Cytopathology 2008;19:229–35.

136. Wang L, Vuolo M, Suhrland MJ, et al. HepPar1, MOC-31, pCEA, mCEA and CD10 for distinguishing hepatocellular carcinoma vs. metastatic adenocarcinoma in liver fine needle aspirates. Acta Cytol 2006;50:257–62.

137. Imoto M, Nishimura D, Fukuda Y, et al. Immunohistochemical detection of alpha-fetoprotein, carcinoembryonic antigen and ferritin in formalin-paraffin sections from hepatocellular carcinoma. Am J Gastroenterol 1985;80:902–6.

138. Roncalli M, Borzio M, DeBiagi G, et al. Liver cell dysplasia and hepatocellular carcinoma: a histological and immunohistochemical study. Histopathol 1985;9:209–21.

139. Fletcher JA, Kozakewich HP, Pavelka K, et al. Consistent cytogenetic aberrations in hepatoblastoma: a common pathway of genetic alterations in embryonal liver and skeletal muscle malignancies? Genes Chromosomes Cancer 1991;3:37–43.

140. Ersoz C, Zorludemir U, Tanyeli A, Gumurdulu D, Celiktas M. Fine needle aspiration cytology of hepatoblastoma. A report of two cases. Acta Cytol 1998;42:799–802.

141. Parikh B, Jojo A, Shah B, et al. Fine needle aspiration cytology of hepatoblastoma: a study of 20 cases. Indian J Pathol Microbiol 2005;48:331–36.

142. Us-Krasovec M, Pohar-Marinsek Z, Golouh R, et al. Hepatoblastoma in fine needle aspirates. Acta Cytol 1996;40:450–56.

143. Kaw YT, Hansen K. Fine needle aspiration cytology of undifferentiated small cell ('anaplastic') hepatoblastoma. A case report. Acta Cytol 1993;37:216–20.

144. Philipose TR, Naik R, Rai S. Cytologic diagnosis of small cell anaplastic hepatoblastoma: a case report. Acta Cytol 2006;50:205–7.

145. Cangiarella J, Greco MA, Waisman J. Hepatoblastoma. Report of a case with cytologic, histologic and ultrastructural findings. Acta Cytol 1994;38:455–58.

146. Van Eyken P, Sciot R, Callea F, et al. A cytokeratin-immunohistochemical study of hepatoplastoma. Hum Pathol 1990;21:302–8.

147. Johnson DE, Herndier BG, Medeiros LJ, et al. The diagnostic utility of the keratin profiles of hepatocellular carcinoma and cholangiocarcinoma. Am J Surg Pathol 1988;12:187–97.

148. Fasano M, Theise ND, Nalesnik M, et al. Immunohistochemical evaluation of hepatoblastomas with use of the hepatocyte-specific marker, hepatocyte paraffin 1, and the polyclonal anti-carcinoembryonic antigen. Mod Pathol 1998;11:934–38.

149. Ishak KG, Goodman ZD, Stocker JT. Tumors of the liver and intrahepatic bile ducts. Atlas of tumor pathology 2001; 3rd series: Fascicle 31.

150. Liu K, Layfield LJ. Cytomorphologic features of angiosarcoma on fine needle aspiration biopsy. Acta Cytol 1999;43:407–15.

151. Saleh HA, Tao LC. Hepatic angiosarcoma: aspiration biopsy cytology and immunocytochemical contribution. Diagn Cytopathol 1998;18:208–11.

152. Boucher LD, Swanson PE, Stanley MW, et al. Cytology of angiosarcoma. Findings in fourteen fine-needle aspiration biopsy specimens and one pleural fluid specimen. Am J Clin Pathol 2000;114:210–19.

153. Sharifah NA, Muhaizan WM, Rahman J, et al. Fine needle aspiration cytology of undifferentiated embryonal sarcoma of the liver: a case report. Malays J Pathol 1999;21:105–9.

154. Pollono DG, Drut R. Undifferentiated (embryonal) sarcoma of the liver: fine-needle aspiration cytology and preoperative chemotherapy as an approach to diagnosis and initial treatment. A case report. Diagn Cytopathol 1998;19:102–6.

155. Garcia-Bonafe M, Allende H, Fantova MJ, et al. Fine needle aspiration cytology of undifferentiated (embryonal) sarcoma of the liver. A case report. Acta Cytol 1997;41:1273–78.

156. Lack EE, Schloo BL, Azumi N, et al. Undifferentiated (embryonal) sarcoma of the liver. Clinical and pathologic study of 16 cases with emphasis on immunohistochemical features. Am J Surg Pathol 1991;15:1–16.

157. Edmondson HA, Craig JR. Neoplasms of the liver. In: Schiff L, Schiff ER, editors Diseases of the Liver. Philadelphia: JB Lippincott; 1987: p. 1109–16.

158. Rader AE, Avery A, Wait CL, et al. Fine-needle aspiration biopsy diagnosis of gastrointestinal stromal tumors using morphology, immunocytochemistry, and mutational analysis of c-kit. Cancer 2001;93:269–75.

159. Wieczorek TJ, Faquin WC, Rubin BP, et al. Cytologic diagnosis of gastrointestinal stromal tumor with emphasis on the differential diagnosis with leiomyosarcoma. Cancer 2001;93:276–87.

160. Dong HY, Harris NL, Preffer FI, et al. Fine-needle aspiration biopsy in the diagnosis and classification of primary and recurrent lymphoma: a retrospective analysis of the utility of cytomorphology and flow cytometry. Mod Pathol 2001;14:472–81.

161. Young NA, Al-Saleem TI, Ehya H, et al. Utilisation of fine-needle aspiration cytology and flow cytometry in the diagnosis and subclassification of primary and recurrent lymphoma. Cancer 1998;84:252–61.

162. Moriarty AT, Wiersema L, Synder W, et al. Immunophenotyping of cytologic specimens by flow cytometry. Diagn Cytopathol 1993;9:252–58.

163. Lui K, Mann KP, Vitellas KM, et al. Fine-needle aspiration with flow cytometry immunophenotyping for primary diagnosis of intra-abdominal lymphomas. Diagn Cytopathol 1999;21:98–104.

164. Robins DB, Katz RL, Swan F, et al. Immunotyping of lymphoma by fine-needle aspiration. A comparative study of cytospin preparations and flow cytometry (comments). Am J Clin Pathol 1994;101:569–76.

165. Busam KJ, Iversen K, Coplan KA, et al. Immunoreactivity for A103, an antibody to melan-A (Mart-1), adrenocortical and other steroid tumors. Am J Surg Pathol 1998;22:57–63.

166. Iezzoni JC, Mills SE, Pelkey TJ, et al. Inhibin is not an immunohistochemical marker for hepatocellular carcinoma. Anat Pathol 1999;111:229–34.

167. Isler RJ, Ferucci JT, Wittenberg J, et al. Tissue core biopsy of abdominal tumors with a 22 gauge cutting needle. Am J Roentgenol AJR 1981;136:725–28.

168. Bell DA, Carr CP, Szyfelbein WM. Fine needle aspiration cytology of focal liver lesions. Results obtained with examination of both cytologic and histologic preparations. Acta Cytol 1986;30:397–402.

169. Guo Z, Kurtycz DFI, Salem R, et al. Radiologically guided percutaneous fine-needle aspiration biopsy of the liver: retrospective study of 119 cases evaluating diagnostic effectiveness and clinical complications. Diagn Cytopathol 2002;26:283–89.

# Gall bladder and extrahepatic bile ducts

Gabrijela Kocjan

## Chapter contents

## Introduction

Gall bladder cancer is the fifth most common cancer involving the gastrointestinal tract, but it is the most common malignant tumour of the biliary tract worldwide. The percentage of patients diagnosed as having gall bladder cancer after simple cholecystectomy for presumed gall bladder stone disease is 0.5–1.5%. This tumour is traditionally regarded as a highly lethal disease with an overall 5-year survival of less than 5%. The marked improvement in the outcome of patients with gall bladder cancer in the last decade is because of the aggressive radical surgical approach that has been adopted, and due to improvements in surgical techniques and perioperative care.[1]

Carcinoma of the hepatobiliary ducts is associated with cholelithiasis and chronic cholecystitis, hepatitis B and C, cirrhosis and alcohol, primary sclerosing cholangitis (PSC), which carries an increased risk of 10–20%, and biliary papillomatosis.[2,3] It develops through a multistep histopathological sequence. Historically, premalignant or non-invasive neoplastic lesions of bile ducts have been called biliary dysplasia or atypical biliary epithelium. In 2005, a conceptual framework and diagnostic criteria for biliary intraepithelial neoplasia (BilIN) were proposed using the livers of patients with hepatolithiasis. In 2007, consensus was reached for the terminology of BilIN and a three-grade classification system (BilIN-1, BilIN-2 and BilIN-3) based on the degree of atypia was proposed.[4]

Cholangiocarcinomas (CC) are broadly classified into intrahepatic tumours, (extrahepatic) hilar tumours and (extrahepatic) distal bile duct tumours. There has been recent progress in identifying potential risk factors for the tumour, and in the use of emerging technologies for diagnosis and palliative treatment. Diagnosis may be improved by new approaches to enhance the diagnostic yield and utility of biliary cytology. The role of new imaging approaches such as positron emission tomography scanning, endoscopic ultrasound and optical coherence tomography for diagnosis are being examined and defined. Long-term results for transplantation protocols for curative intent in non-resectable localised disease have been described. Photodynamic therapy looks extremely promising for adjunct therapy of intrahepatic mass lesions.[5]

Intrahepatic cholangiocarcinoma (ICC), also known as cholangiocellular carcinoma or peripheral bile duct carcinoma, is an intrahepatic malignant tumour that consists of cells resembling the biliary epithelium (see Ch. 8, p. 308). The proportion of ICC among primary hepatic malignancies is approximately 10% worldwide. Some ICCs arising from the large biliary duct are likely to exhibit an aggressive course even in cases of small tumour size.[6] ICC is reportedly a late complication of primary sclerosing cholangitis. Most of the preceding pathological conditions are forms of chronic cholangitis, and longstanding inflammation, chronic injury, and regenerative hyperplasia of the biliary epithelium. Biliary epithelial dysplasia is encountered in the intrahepatic bile ducts both near and remote from ICC foci in the liver and near and remote from the chronically inflamed biliary tree.[7]

Carcinoma of the extrahepatic bile ducts constitutes one-third of biliary tract cancers.[8] In contrast to gall bladder cancer, gallstones are present in only 20% of cases.[8] There is, however, an association between carcinoma and sclerosing cholangitis or chronic suppurative cholangitis, biliary parasites such as liver flukes, ulcerative colitis and choledochal cysts.[8] A proportion of carcinomas may arise in pre-existing benign papillary neoplastic lesions, which may be localised or multifocal; papillary tumours have a better prognosis.[8]

A range of other neoplastic and tumour-like processes occurs in the region (Box 9.1).[8,9]

## Endoscopic techniques

Malignancies of the bile duct are often suspected in patients with abnormal serum hepatic enzyme levels and obstruction of the biliary system. Although cross-sectional imaging can provide evidence for biliary obstruction and a malignancy arising from the bile duct, a definitive diagnosis is often obtained through the use of endoscopic procedures.[10] Endoscopic retrograde cholangiopancreatography (ERCP), the most commonly performed procedure for cholangiocarcinoma, can provide a

*I wish to acknowledge the privilege of having inherited from the previous edition a comprehensively written chapter by Drs G. Sterrett, D. Whitaker and K. Shilkin.*

## Box 9.1   Primary tumours of the gall bladder and extrahepatic bile ducts[8,9]

Epithelial neoplasms
Benign

- Adenoma
- Papillomatosis
- Cystadenoma

Epithelial dysplasia and carcinoma *in situ*
Malignant

- Adenocarcinoma
  - Papillary, intestinal, gastric foveolar
  - Clear cell, mucinous, signet ring
  - Cystadenocarcinoma
- Adenosquamous carcinoma
- Squamous cell carcinoma
- Small cell carcinoma (neuroendocrine, undifferentiated)
- Large cell neuroendocrine carcinoma
- Large cell undifferentiated carcinoma
  - Spindle and giant cell/sarcomatoid
  - With osteoclast-like giant cells

Neuroendocrine neoplasms

- Carcinoid
- Adenocarcinoid (goblet-cell carcinoid)
- Carcinoid-adenocarcinoma (mixed)
- Paraganglioma, gangliocytic paraganglioma

Non-epithelial neoplasms
Benign

- Leiomyoma
- Lipoma
- Haemangioma
- Lymphangioma
- Osteoma
- Granular cell tumour
- Neurofibroma
- Ganglioneuroma

Malignant

- Rhabdomyosarcoma
- Malignant fibrous histiocytoma
- Angiosarcoma
- Leiomyosarcoma
- Kaposi's sarcoma

Miscellaneous
Carcinosarcoma
Malignant melanoma
Malignant lymphoma
Germ cell tumours
Tumour-like lesions
Regenerative epithelial atypia
Papillary hyperplasia
Squamous metaplasia
Adenomyomatous hyperplasia
Mucocoele
Heterotopias
Cholesterol polyp
Inflammatory polyp
Fibrous polyp
Myofibroblastic proliferations
Xanthogranulomatous cholecystitis
Cholecystitis with lymphoid hyperplasia

## Box 9.1   (Continued)

Malakoplakia
Congenital cyst
Amputation neuroma
Primary sclerosing cholangitis
Aspiration of gastric/duodenal contents

diagnosis through brush cytology of the bile duct. Duct brushing cytology is an important tool in evaluation of the extrahepatic biliary tract and large pancreatic ducts. The emergence of neoadjuvant therapies underscores the importance of accurate preoperative diagnosis by noninvasive means.[11]

Procedures for collecting cytological material from the biliary tree are the following:

- *Bile sampling*: three bile samples should be obtained on successive days from any patient undergoing percutaneous drainage; as large a volume as can be aspirated should be collected and sent promptly to the laboratory. Bile obtained from drainage bags shows bacterial overgrowth and loss of cell detail and is usually not suitable for cytological assessment. In patients with external biliary drains, bile for cytology should be aspirated directly from the drainage catheter, or collected over a short period

- *Brush or catheter samples*: This material is obtained during ERCP. Any stricture is first negotiated with a guide wire, and a brush passed over the wire and drawn back and forth along the stricture. Multiple samples improve sensitivity. Washing the brushes in saline and cytocentrifuging the elutant may increase the yield from ductal brush samples as may 'salvage' cytology of endoscopic brush sheaths. Liquid-based cytology (LBC) either alone or in combination with direct smears is promising to reduce technical artefact and increase accuracy of biliary brushings cytology[11,12]

- *FNA samples*: Material is obtained by EUS-FNA. Multiple samplings may be necessary and multiple imaging procedures are of value in combination. The presence of the pathologist at the procedure for rapid reporting can reduce the number of needle passes. The practice of on-site cytology interpretation varies across endoscopic ultrasound (EUS) programmes in the USA and Europe but is generally considered beneficial to the level of diagnostic accuracy.[13,81]

Transcatheter brush sampling is preferred for hilar lesions of the liver and biliary strictures, whereas FNA samples are more sensitive for pancreatic head masses. Intraoperative FNA is useful when less invasive procedures have proved negative, to provide a diagnosis before major surgery.

Preparation of samples from this region requires some flexibility on the part of the cytology laboratory. Bile samples and duodenal contents containing gastroduodenal and pancreatic secretions provide a hostile cell medium, and necessitate rapid transport to the laboratory to reduce degeneration. Transport to the laboratory within an hour gives quite satisfactory cell preservation. Where delay is unavoidable, alcohol prefixation may aid in cell preservation, although this renders membrane filter preparations unsatisfactory.

Relief from biliary obstruction can be provided with temporary plastic stenting or permanent metal stenting. Photodynamic therapy guided by ERCP may provide improved palliation from biliary obstruction in the future. Endoscopic ultrasonography (EUS) complements the role of ERCP and may provide a tissue diagnosis through EUS-FNA and staging through ultrasound imaging. High-resolution ultrasound images can provide detailed information regarding the relationship between a mass and the bile duct wall. Despite these advances in endoscopic techniques and imaging of the bile duct, a tissue diagnosis often remains elusive in many patients.

## Complications and contraindications

The overall complication rate of ERCP in non-selected patients in one series was 12.6%, consisting of post-ERCP pancreatitis (5.1%), bleeding (3.7%), cholangitis (1.9%), cardiopulmonary complications (0.9%), and perforation (0.5%); procedure-related mortality was 0.1%.[14] The postprocedural complications of EUS-FNA, include abdominal pain, nausea, vomiting and gastrointestinal bleeding. They are considered to be rare but require further evaluation with prospective studies.[13,15–18]

Gall bladder FNA can result in bile leaks, particularly in association with common bile duct obstruction. This technique is thus not usually advised except in the immediate preoperative period or unless special precautions are taken. However, ultrasound or laparoscopically guided FNA of gall bladder for collection of bile, apparently without significant complications, has been described.

## Normal cytology

### Duodenal aspirates

- Biliary epithelium in monolayered sheets
- Duodenal cells with brush borders or goblet cell forms
- 'Matchstick' cells of gall bladder origin
- Cuboidal pancreatic acinar cells
- Degenerate cells of indeterminate origin.

The normal cell components of this sample site include cells from the stomach, duodenum and those shed from bile ducts and the pancreas. Most often, specific identification of the epithelium of origin will not be possible. Ductal cells from all sites are shed as small monolayered sheets with moderately dense cytoplasm. Duodenal cells have a more prominent brush border and are taller columnar cells with a goblet cell component; gall bladder cells are described as 'matchstick' cells with a columnar morphology and bulging terminal nuclei. Pancreatic acinar cells are cuboidal and lie in small clusters. Cells showing round densely hyperchromatic nuclear fragments within rounded-up cell bodies are considered to be degenerate epithelial cells.

### Bile

- Scanty cellular material
- Background of bile pigment and crystals
- Cholesterol crystals in some conditions
- Sheets of gall bladder epithelium, especially after saline irrigation.

Normal bile contains little cellular material, though bile and pancreatic secretion stimulated by secretin, pancreozymin, cholecystokinin or magnesium sulphate result in increased cell shedding. Bile pigment and crystals are observed in the background.

Cholesterol crystals are present in patients with a variety of disorders of the biliary tree including cholelithiasis or cholecystitis; they are said to be absent from patients with diseases of the liver or pancreas. Gall bladder epithelium presents in sheets or aggregates with dense cytoplasm; saline irrigated samples are more cellular and contain better preserved abraded sheets.

### Bile duct brushings

Normal bile duct or pancreatic ductal epithelium has the following features in bile duct brushings: (Figs 9.1–9.4).

- Regular arrangement in flat sheets
- Sheets architecturally complex
- Cells tall columnar
- Nuclei oval, round, basal
- Fine chromatin pattern
- Nucleoli inconspicuous.

### FNA samples

As with percutaneous FNA of other intra-abdominal sites, epithelium of multiple types may be encountered as the needle traverses tissues such as bowel mucosa, liver or pancreatic acinar and ductal tissue.

## Benign conditions

### Inflammatory and reactive processes

- Slight overlapping of epithelial cells in sheets
- Small nucleoli
- Low N:C ratio
- Variable inflammatory cell component
- Degenerative and regenerative changes in epithelial cells
- Extreme reactive changes may simulate malignancy.

Inflammatory changes and organisms have been demonstrated in bile by gall bladder FNA preoperatively in cholecystitis. Intraoperative FNA has been used to diagnose abscess and

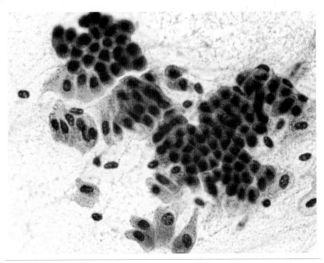

**Fig. 9.1** Normal bile duct epithelium shows regular arrangement in flat sheets. Cells are tall columnar, nuclei oval, round, basal with fine chromatin pattern and inconspicuous nucleoli (PAP).

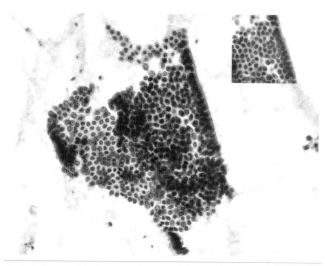

**Fig. 9.2** Biliary epithelium showing smooth luminal border (PAP).

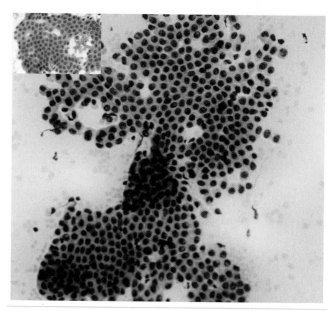

**Fig. 9.4** Monolayered sheet with enlarged nuclei and prominent nucleoli, but retained honeycomb structure and low nuclear/cytoplasmic ratio. Sheets may be architecturally complex and show 'holes'. Bile duct brushings (MGG and PAP).

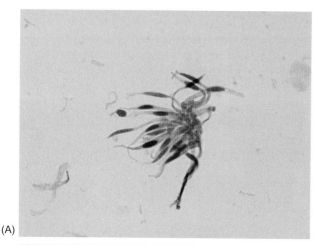

(A)

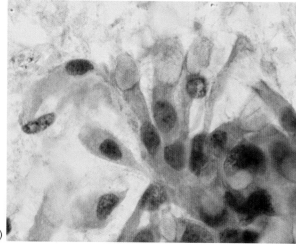

(B)

**Fig. 9.3** Biliary epithelium. (A) Slender columnar cells (matchstick cells) are often seen as single and in small clusters (PAP). (B) Duodenal epithelium show tall columnar cells with goblet type cytoplasm.

xanthogranulomatous cholecystitis by finding a mixed inflammatory cell component in company with large numbers of foamy histiocytes and surrounding capillary blood vessels.[19] Chronic pancreatitis is discussed later in Chapter 10.

Changes due to primary sclerosing cholangitis (PSC), stent placement and postoperative effect are similar in all types of cytological samples and include a range of regenerative and degenerative alterations in bile duct epithelium, with cells reminiscent of squamous metaplasia, nuclear enlargement, nuclear size variation, prominent nucleoli and cellular disorganisation (Fig. 9.5A–C).

More extreme changes have been reported in parasitic infestation. Reactive papillary clusters may be seen; the lack of nuclear irregularity, nuclear hyperchromasia, or high nuclear/cytoplasmic ratio will generally allow a distinction from neoplastic change.

## Parasitic infestation

### Cytological findings: parasitic infestation

- Parasitic ova
- Inflammatory and necrotic debris
- Worms, fragmented or entire
- Epithelial hyperplasia, metaplasia
- Late risk of cholangiocarcinoma.

In the samples of bile submitted for cytological examination, ova of liver flukes (e.g. *Clonorchis sinensis* and *Opisthorchis viverrini*) may be identified against a background of granular necrotic debris, neutrophils and eosinophils.[20] *Fasciola hepatica* infestation may also be identified. Criteria for recognition of *Clonorchis* ova include small size, laminated walls, opercula with prominent shoulders and spinous processes (Fig. 9.6). Whole worms, or parts thereof, may also be seen.[21] Biliary infestation with *Clonorchis* is also associated with epithelial hyperplasia, goblet cell metaplasia, squamous metaplasia and adenomatous hyperplasia.[21] The high mucin content of the bile is associated with bacterial superinfection, stone formation and, later, cholangiocarcinoma may supervene. All these conditions may coexist.

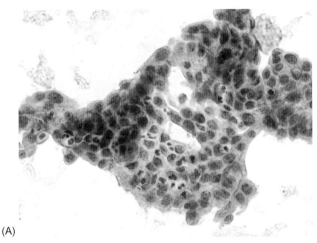

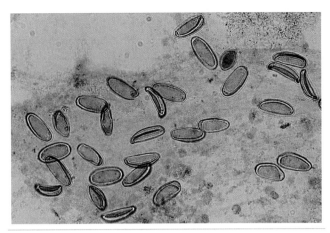

**Fig. 9.6** Ova of *Clonorchis sinensis* in bile (PAP).

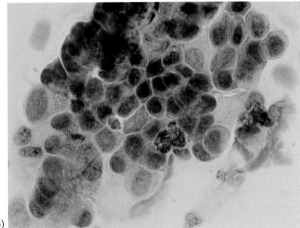

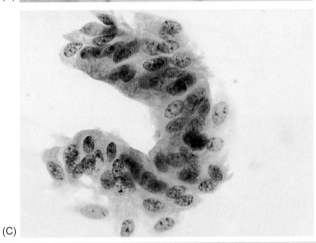

**Fig. 9.5** (A) Biliary brushings. Inflammatory exudate and biliary epithelium showing mild cytological and architectural atypia (PAP). (B,C) Primary sclerosing cholangitis, stent placement and postoperative effect produce similar changes in all types of cytological samples and include a range of regenerative and degenerative alterations in bile duct epithelium, with cells reminiscent of squamous metaplasia, nuclear enlargement, nuclear size variation, prominent nucleoli and cellular disorganisation (PAP).

## Dysplasia

Premalignant changes in bile ductal or gall bladder epithelium, dysplasia and carcinoma *in situ* are now recognised in the gall bladder and extrahepatic bile ducts. These lesions are considered

to be the precursors of the corresponding invasive carcinomas.[9] Layfield et al. have shown that premalignant lesions, that is dysplasia and carcinoma *in situ*, can be diagnosed on bile duct brushings. Dysplasia has been graded as high and low. Since biopsy of small mucosal lesions may be technically difficult, brushings are often the only way to diagnose premalignant lesions.[22]

The main cytological criteria for detection of premalignant and malignant conditions of bile ducts are the following:

- Nuclear overlapping and crowding
- Small but distinct nucleoli
- Moderate N:C ratio.

### Cytological findings: low-grade dysplasia (Fig. 9.7)

- Sheets and clusters with nuclear crowding and overlapping
- Smooth nuclear outline, moderate N:C ratio
- Granular chromatin with mild clumping
- 1–2 small distinct nucleoli.

### Cytological findings: high-grade dysplasia (Fig. 9.8)

- Clusters and groups with prominent nuclear crowding and overlapping
- Irregular nuclear membranes, high N:C ratio
- Coarse chromatin
- Distinct prominent nucleoli.

Gall bladder FNA or bile may show premalignant cellular changes of biliary duct epithelium. There is a high correlation between the cytological and histological diagnosis of carcinoma *in situ* and invasive carcinoma but lower correlation for a cytological diagnosis of hyperplasia and dysplasia. Most authors do not consider it possible to diagnose precursors of carcinoma accurately or to distinguish between intraepithelial and invasive tumours in brush samples.[23,24]

## Biliary papillomatosis/intraductal papillary neoplasm

Intraductal papillary neoplasm is a rare neoplasm of the intrahepatic and extrahepatic biliary tree, and its findings have been reported by Tsui et al.[25]

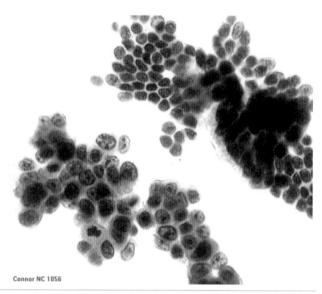

Connor NC 1056

**Fig. 9.7** Low-grade dysplasia. The lower sheet of epithelium showing nuclear crowding and overlapping, granular chromatin with mild clumping and clearing and 1–2 small distinct nucleoli. However, they have a smooth nuclear outline and a moderate N:C ratio. Differential diagnosis includes reactive conditions and low-grade dysplasia (PAP).

### Cytological findings: intraductal papillary neoplasm:

- Hypercellular smear
- Very broad and often double-cell layered sheets of ductal cells
- Papillary configuration
- Preserved honeycomb pattern with even nuclear spacing
- Some nuclear overlapping but no frankly malignant nuclear features.

The constellation of these features is highly characteristic of intraductal papillary mucinous neoplasia (IPMN) (Fig. 9.9) and helpful in distinguishing it from cholangiocarcinoma and other differential diagnoses. A firm preoperative diagnosis can thus be achieved, allowing better planning in management of this borderline malignant tumour. Because of its distinct clinicopathological features and a favourable prognosis that can be expected after complete surgical resection, it has been suggested that intraductal papillary neoplasia should be distinguished from other types of peripheral cholangiocarcinoma, as a distinct entity, like its counterparts in the pancreas (see Ch. 10).[26] Similarly, other authors stress that mucin-hypersecreting bile duct tumour is characterised by a striking homology with an IPMN of the pancreas (see Ch. 10).[27,28] A diagnosis of IPMN (biliary) is usually made in patients with biliary dilatation by radiological study. The prognosis, especially of the benign category, is excellent. Aggressive surgical resection is the treatment of choice for IPMN.[29]

## Adenocarcinoma

Primary carcinoma of the gall bladder is a rare neoplasm that is frequently difficult to diagnose preoperatively. The obstacles to diagnosis include vague symptoms and the relative inaccessibility of the gall bladder and cystic duct to biopsy. Cytological

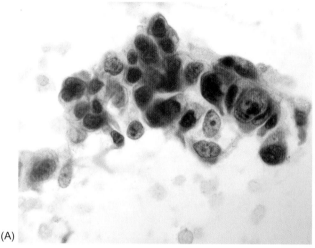

(A)

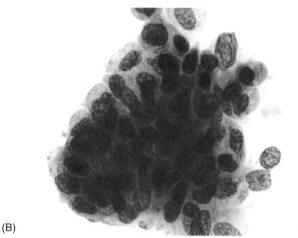

(B)

**Fig. 9.8** High-grade dysplasia. (A) The epithelium shows loss of honeycomb structure in the cluster on the left as opposed to a relatively normal looking bile duct epithelium on the right. Dysplastic epithelium shows prominent overlapping, crowding, irregular nuclear membrane, coarse chromatin and distinct or prominent nucleoli. Features are suspicious of malignancy (PAP). (B) MGG stained smear shows crowding and overlapping.

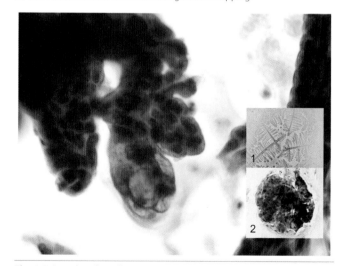

**Fig. 9.9** Intraductal papillary mucinous neoplasm. Hypercellular smear with very broad and often double-cell layered sheets of ductal columnar epithelium in papillary configuration and with preserved honeycomb pattern with even nuclear spacing showing dysplastic but not frankly malignant nuclear features (PAP). Ferning effect of mucus (inset 1), PASd positivity in the cytoplasm (inset 2).

descriptions of gall bladder carcinoma are sparse and are largely confined to malignant cells identified in aspirated bile. Examination of bile is a fairly insensitive technique for diagnosing carcinoma, partly due to the effect of biliary salts on cellular morphology.[30] However, with the widespread use of more sophisticated imaging techniques, the gall bladder is becoming more readily accessible to visualisation. In view of this, FNA holds promise as a non-invasive technique in the diagnosis of gall bladder neoplasms.[31]

## Diagnosis of adenocarcinoma from bile

Adenocarcinoma of gall bladder, bile duct or pancreatic origin presents as single cells and small three-dimensional clusters showing moulding, cell-in-cell arrangements, nuclei with irregular nuclear outlines and pleomorphism, prominent nucleoli and increased nuclear/cytoplasmic ratio. Poorly differentiated tumours show more cell dispersal and, occasionally, a purely single cell pattern, or marked pleomorphism including giant cell forms. In contrast, benign reactive cells present as larger more cohesive sheets. The background may show variable numbers of inflammatory cells and histiocytes, necrotic material and degenerating cells.

## Biliary brush samples

### Cytological findings: adenocarcinoma

- Clusters of cells, disorganised sheets, loose aggregates, small acinar groups and single pleomorphic cells
- Marked overlapping and crowding
- Nuclear enlargement, moulding and irregular nuclear outlines
- Prominent nucleoli
- High N:C ratio
- Coarse chromatin
- Background of necrotic debris.

Architectural features of malignancy include disorganisation within clusters, loss of cohesion, small acinar groups and single cells (Figs 9.10–9.12).[23] Marked nuclear enlargement within sheets, nuclear crowding, moulding, irregularity of nuclear outline and nuclear pleomorphism permit a definitive diagnosis of malignancy when there is adequate well-preserved material.[23] A background of necrotic debris may be helpful in some cases. Very well-differentiated tumours present as cohesive monolayered sheets which are much more difficult to evaluate and unequivocal nuclear criteria of malignancy may not be present. Cell block assessment of architecture may allow a diagnosis of malignancy in well-differentiated tumours. Cohen et al. consider nuclear moulding, chromatin clumping and increased N:C ratio to be the most important criteria in diagnosing malignancy.[32] In Renshaw's study, both an 'overall assessment of malignancy' and features of chromatin clumping, increased N:C ratio, nuclear moulding and loss of honeycombing had equally high predictive values and reproducibility between pathologists; an 'overall assessment' had the highest sensitivity.[33]

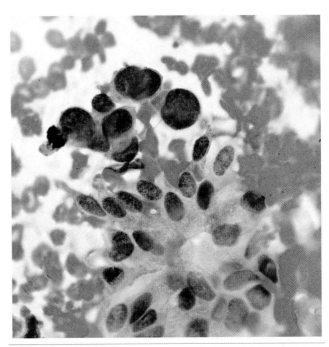

**Fig. 9.10** Adenocarcinoma. A contrast between the benign bile duct epithelium (below) and malignant (above). Malignant cells are arranged as single atypical cells and clusters with marked overlapping and crowding, coarse chromatin, distinct prominent nucleoli, high N:C ratio, occasionally abundant cytoplasm (PAP).

## Special tumour types

### Adenosquamous and squamous cell carcinoma

The region of the gall bladder, extrahepatic bile ducts and pancreas is well known for mixed tumours and, more rarely, pure squamous cell carcinoma (Fig. 9.13).

### Villous adenoma and well-differentiated papillary carcinoma

Villous adenoma and well-differentiated papillary carcinoma with a predominantly exophytic growth are rare, albeit well described.

### Cytological findings: villous adenoma

- Numerous clusters of hypercrowded columnar cells
- Irregular feathered edges
- Coarser chromatin than the surrounding normal bile duct epithelium.

Brush samples of villous adenoma are described as yielding cellular specimens with pavement-like sheets and some three-dimensional papillary clusters with elongated columnar cells.[34] Bardales et al. observed that some cases showed features indistinguishable from invasive adenocarcinoma.[34] Stewart et al. reported on brush findings in three patients with adenomas of bile duct or ampulla with sufficient cytological atypia for a 'positive' diagnosis.[23] The features of intraductal papillary neoplasm were described earlier (see p. 323). Cytological features may be indistinguishable from villous adenoma or normal duodenal mucosa. The findings may be reported as suspicious of adenocarcinoma.

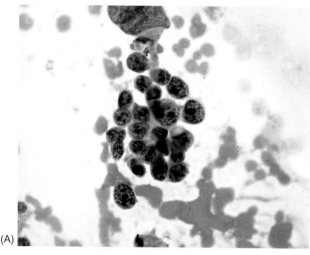

(A)

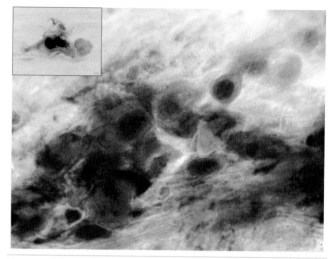

**Fig. 9.13** Keratinous debris and malignant cells from an adenosquamous carcinoma of the bile duct. Inset: keratinised malignant cells (PAP).

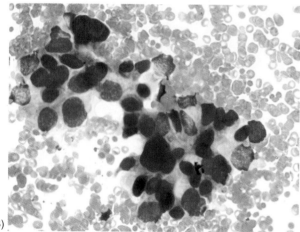

(B)

**Fig. 9.11** Adenocarcinoma. (A,B) Malignant epithelial cells showing marked nuclear pleomorphism, irregularity of nuclear outlines and multinucleation. Sheet of ductal epithelial cells with slight disorganisation and loss of honeycomb structure, some nuclear pleomorphism and enlargement, and hyperchromasia; suspicious of malignancy (PAP, MGG).

## Cystadenoma and cystadenocarcinoma

### Cytological and clinical findings: cystadenoma and cystadenocarcinoma

- Biliary cystadenoma
  - Tends to occur in women
  - Has a well-known tendency for malignant transformation
  - Columnar or cuboidal mucin-secreting epithelium
  - Mostly uniform
- Mucinous cystadenocarcinoma
  - Cells differ in size
  - Nuclei show a coarse chromatin pattern
  - Haphazard arrangement.

Cystic mucinous neoplasms of extrahepatic bile duct origin are morphologically identical to those described in the pancreas and intrahepatic ducts (see Chs 8, 10).[35]

## Other neoplasms

Metastatic carcinomas from the upper and lower gastrointestinal tract and liver are diagnosed by all the methods described above,[36] although brush and bile samples have a lower reported sensitivity than percutaneous or direct intraoperative FNA.

### Diagnostic pitfalls

The most commonly encountered pitfalls in cytological diagnosis of the hepatobiliary tree are the following:[22]

- Benign versus well-differentiated carcinoma
  - Sclerosing cholangitis
  - Dysplasia
  - Carcinoma *in situ*
- Special tumour types
  - e.g. Mucinous cystadenocarcinoma
  - Papillary adenocarcinoma versus adenoma of the ampulla.

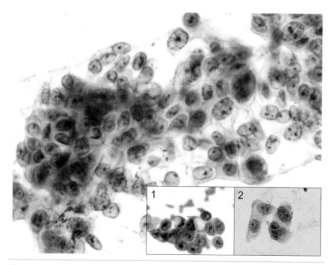

**Fig. 9.12** Adenocarcinoma. Markedly enlarged nuclei of malignant cells, with dense cytoplasm showing focal mucin vacuolation (inset 1). Poorly differentiated bile duct adenocarcinoma has large pleomorphic cells (inset 2).

## False positive findings

Bile duct brushing cytology is the primary screening technique for cholangiocarcinoma. It is associated with a relatively low sensitivity but high specificity. Few false positive bile duct brushings have been reported in the literature, with the majority of these having occurred in a background of primary sclerosing cholangitis.[37]

Non-traumatic inflammatory hilar strictures are uncommon, but are known to mimic malignancy. Some of the examples are: lymphoplasmacytic sclerosing pancreatitis and cholangitis, primary sclerosing cholangitis, granulomatous disease, non-specific fibrosis/inflammation and stone disease.[38]

## False negative findings

Review of 'false negative cases' reveals four main reasons for the relatively modest sensitivity of biliary brush cytology in diagnosis of malignancy: poor sampling, lack of diagnostic criteria for dysplasia-carcinoma *in situ*, difficulties in recognition of special tumour types, and underestimating the significance of the smear background.[39]

Special types of cholangiocarcinoma with bland nuclear features pose a diagnostic challenge on cytological evaluation, particularly the well-differentiated cholangiocarcinoma with tubular architecture and the gastric foveolar type cholangiocarcinoma with mucin-producing tumour cells.[40]

The difficulty of distinguishing reactive bile duct epithelium from well-differentiated adenocarcinoma has been examined by Stewart et al., who, in reviewing previous series of duct brushings, quote misinterpretation of low-grade dysplasia, reactive papillary changes with epithelial atypia, intestinal metaplasia of biliary epithelium and the effects of previous bile duct stenting as causes of false positive reports.[23] These authors describe in detail three cases leading to presumed false positive diagnoses, in patients with sclerosing cholangitis, bile duct stones and pancreatitis. In one case there were crowded three-dimensional clusters, nuclear moulding, a coarse chromatin pattern and distinct nucleoli. Pronounced degenerative changes were seen in some of the atypical epithelium and in associated normal epithelium. In a second case, small numbers of highly atypical but somewhat degenerate cell groups were reported as consistent with adenocarcinoma, and in the third, there were small numbers of highly atypical cells with some degenerative changes. The degenerative changes present and the small amounts of material in two of the specimens were features that might have led to an equivocal rather than definite malignant diagnosis.[23]

The presence of a stent in the bile duct can result in highly atypical epithelial cells in brushings from this site. There is usually marked cellular and nuclear enlargement but the lack of nuclear hyperchromasia, nuclear membrane irregularity or high nuclear/cytoplasmic ratio are features against a diagnosis of malignancy. Parasitic infestation of ducts may be a source of similar difficulty as may papillitis or inflammatory changes in the region of ampulla of Vater.[20] Primary sclerosing cholangitis often gives rise to worrying regenerative change and inflammatory changes associated with other benign lesions such as bile duct cysts may also afford diagnostic difficulty. Bardales reports 'false positive' diagnoses of malignancy from cytology of adenoma of the duodenal papilla.[24] Stewart argues

that such diagnoses are not 'false positive' because the lesions need to be identified as neoplastic and to proceed to operative resection.[23]

Underdiagnosis of malignancy may result from inexperience, particularly in duct brushings, whereby an overcautious approach in an area of known diagnostic difficulty leads to 'suspicious' reports on material with nuclear criteria of malignancy. Concentration of experience will reduce this problem, although for many centres, the number of cases seen may not be enough to acquire expertise. In FNA samples, well-differentiated carcinomas presenting in monolayered sheets with a retained honeycomb structure may be underdiagnosed. Tumours of unusual type such as mucinous and papillary intraductal lesions may have a particularly bland appearance.[39]

## The role of cytology in management of diseases of hepatobiliary ducts

Management of patients with *malignant hilar biliary obstruction* is challenging for all specialists involved in their care.[41] Evaluation should focus on potential surgical resection, which offers the principal chance of cure; liver transplantation is offered as an experimental treatment at a few centres. Attempt at curative surgical resection is appropriate for selected tumours and often requires partial hepatectomy. Diagnosis and staging is now facilitated by the use of magnetic resonance cholangiopancreatography, spiral computed tomography and endoscopic ultrasonography, which should largely supplant invasive cholangiography. Use of endoscopic retrograde cholangiopancreatography and percutaneous transhepatic cholangiography should be limited primarily to palliation of jaundice in patients with unresectable tumours and to establish a tissue diagnosis in ambiguous cases.

The increased risk of malignancy in *primary sclerosing cholangitis* also applies to *polypoid lesions of the gall bladder*. Cholecystectomy and intensified screening for *dysplasia of the bile ducts and colon* may be advisable in primary sclerosing cholangitis patients with neoplasia of the gall bladder.[42] Brush cytology from bile duct strictures in primary sclerosing cholangitis patients can detect *cholangiocarcinoma in situ*. Patients with cytological low-grade and high-grade dysplasia/adenocarcinoma are currently referred for liver transplantation in some institutions.[43,44] Lal et al. have found bile duct brushing is a sensitive method of detecting neoplasia in the setting of primary sclerosing cholangitis.[45] Furmanczyk et al. found that combining biliary brush cytology findings and CA19-9 serum levels helped improve sensitivity.[46] In suspected cases, the diagnosis can be established with non-invasive imaging studies. Biliary invasion should be reserved for patients with obstruction. In high-risk patients, advanced cytological tests of aneuploidy (digital image analysis and fluorescent *in situ* hybridisation) aid early diagnosis.[47] Patients with unresectable cholangiocarcinoma or pre-existing primary sclerosing cholangitis should be considered for liver transplantation with neoadjuvant chemoirradiation.[48] For gall bladder lesions, preoperative US-guided FNAC is safe, rapid, reliable, cost-effective and accurate in diagnosing *xanthogranulomatous cholecystitis*.[49]

The role of cytology in this area is therefore mainly to provide a definitive diagnosis of malignancy to support a clinical or endoscopic diagnosis. This will allow palliative therapy, particularly for bile duct obstruction by tumour, and it will ensure the avoidance of more extensive investigations. Cytodiagnosis by a single technique or on a single sample has a lower sensitivity in the detection of malignancy here than in some other sites and the area is one of acknowledged difficulty in diagnosis. Cellular degeneration in bile or duodenal contents and the well-differentiated and fibrosing growth pattern of many cancers render obtaining sufficient material for unequivocal diagnosis difficult.

Definitive diagnosis of *benign processes* is limited, although FNA diagnosis of *xanthogranulomatous cholecystitis*,[49] *cholesterol polyps*,[50] *abscess*, and even *Pneumocystis infection*[51] are reported. *Liver fluke infestation* may be recognised in bile. This is an important clinical problem in some geographic areas or in areas with high South-east Asian immigration.[20]

## Diagnostic accuracy

*Biliary tract brush specimens* are fast becoming the method of choice in the evaluation of patients who present with biliary tract strictures.[52] Although the specificity is high, sensitivity rates for the detection of malignancy are generally low on cytological sampling.[53] The combination of both brush cytology and forceps biopsy results in only a minor increase in diagnostic sensitivity.[54] Improvement in diagnostic sensitivity for carcinoma of pancreaticobiliary tract in biliary duct brushings was achieved by identifying the key malignant cytomorphological features: three-dimensional micropapillae, anisonucleosis, nuclear contour irregularity, prominent nucleoli, and high N/C ratio.[55] Sensitivity and specificity of CA19-9 at a cut off of 186 IU/mL are 100% and 94%, respectively. Serum trypsinogen-2 is also a useful marker for diagnosing patients with cholangiocarcinoma, and is superior to serum CA19-9 and CEA.[56] In a review of 1000 cases of pancreatic and bile duct brushing cytology Volmar et al. found 52.6% sensitivity, 99.4% specificity, 98.9% positive predictive value, 67.1% negative predictive value, and 75.7% accuracy.[11] New liquid-based preparations and ancillary tests have emerged with the intent of addressing the relatively low sensitivity. The combination of direct smear and the liquid-based cytology method (ThinPrep, Hologic, Bedford, Massachusetts, USA) showed superior sensitivity and accuracy.[11] The use of the additional diagnostic category 'suspicious' increased the sensitivity to 90.4%, at the expense of a fall of the specificity to 66.7%.[57] The combination of a positive brush cytology and an abnormal CA19-9 had a sensitivity and specificity of, respectively, 87.5% and 97.3% in detecting carcinoma in patients with primary sclerosing cholangistis.[58]

Among the factors that influence the accuracy of biliary cytology are interpathologist variation for the biliary cytology interpretation and the knowledge of the patient's clinical information, which appears to clarify cytology interpretation resulting in fewer equivocal results.[59] Neither stricture dilation nor increasing brush size and bristle stiffness seem to improve the sensitivity of brush cytology for the detection of cancer. On the contrary, repeat brushing increases the diagnostic yield and should be performed when sampling biliary strictures with a cytology brush at ERCP.[60,61] Predictors of positive yield include older age, mass size >1 cm, and stricture length of >1 cm.[62] Dumonceau et al. showed that biliary sampling at ERCP using a dedicated basket provided a significantly higher sensitivity

for cancer detection than brushing.[63] Logrono et al. analysed the causes of false negative cytology of biliary brushings and found that sampling error was a major cause of false negative diagnoses (67%), followed by interpretive (17%) and technical errors (17%).[64] They conclude that improvements in sensitivity and diagnostic accuracy for cancer of the pancreatobiliary tract can be achieved by optimising slide preparatory techniques. Also, enhancement of the cytologist's diagnostic skills enables the identification of the morphological features of premalignant lesions. Repeat brushings are indicated for suspicious or negative results not consistent with the clinical or radiological findings.[64]

*EUS-FNA* has added to the diagnostic power of EUS for other gastrointestinal tumours. It is highly specific (100%) with sensitivity rates of 87% and 80% from clinically suspected malignancies of biliary tract and gall bladder, respectively. Sampling error and associated acute inflammation may results in false negative diagnoses.[65] EUS-FNA is a sensitive method for the diagnosis of primary biliary stenosis following negative results or unsuccessful ERCP brush cytology. The low negative predictive value does not permit reliable exclusion of malignancy following a negative biopsy.[66,67] The overall diagnostic accuracy of preoperative US-guided FNA of gall bladder carcinoma and xanthogranulomatous cholecystitis (XGC) is reported as 96.77%.[49] The overall possibility of missing XGC was 3.33% and that of carcinoma, 12.01%. Both of the endoscopic EUS-guided tissue sampling techniques, FNA and Tru-Cut biopsy, have advantages and limitations. A sequential sampling strategy, in which EUS-guided Tru-Cut biopsy is attempted first, and FNA performed only when Tru-Cut biopsy fails to obtain a macroscopically adequate sample, achieves a diagnostic accuracy of 92%, with 11% of patients requiring both sampling procedures.[68]

False positive diagnoses of malignancy are infrequent, but occasionally occur even for very experienced workers.[23] The difficulty in diagnosis in this region and the frequency of reactive changes, which may resemble malignancy, also lead to a proportion of 'atypical' or inconclusive reports. Stewart et al. report 10.1% such reports in their series, with no reduction over the course of the study. Two-thirds of patients with these reports were shown later to have carcinoma.[23]

A combination of techniques in a given case allows a higher sensitivity for a malignant diagnosis, and the selection of which to apply first depends on the individual case. Single bile samples are of inherently lower sensitivity than brush or FNA specimens; the latter can be accurately directed to the site of abnormality.[69] For example, *intraoperative FNA*, even of small tumours at the confluence of the biliary tree, has a high sensitivity.

The reasons for false negative results for bile samples include enzymatic digestion and degeneration of tumour cells, and obstruction of ducts by external compression, which prevents cell shedding. Where there is concentrated experience, bile aspirates from patients with percutaneous bile drainage give sensitivities of the order of 60% for diagnosing malignancy.[70]

*Brush cytology during ERCP* is the most useful method of cytological diagnosis in pancreato-biliary strictures. Stewart et al. in a study of 406 patients found an overall sensitivity of 60% in the diagnosis of neoplasm, and a 70% sensitivity in the last-third of their experience.[23] Layfield achieved diagnostic sensitivity of 44% and specificity 98%.[22] Our own results show 75% sensitivity and 96% specificity for diagnosis of malignancy in the hepatobiliary tract.

Other recent smaller studies found somewhat lower sensitivities ranging from 35% to 48%.[39,64,71,72] Stewart et al. found similar sensitivities for pancreatic carcinoma (59.6%) and cholangiocarcinoma (62.5%).[23] Satisfactory samples can be obtained in up to 94.7% of brushings.[23] Failure to cannulate the desired duct is now less often a usual cause of unsatisfactory specimens due to improvements in guidewire bypass instruments. The absence of a luminal component may be the cause in some cases.[23] As mentioned earlier, poor sampling, lack of criteria for the distinction between dysplasia/carcinoma *in situ* and invasive carcinoma, difficulties in recognising special tumour types and underestimating the significance of the smear background were described as other reasons for the 'modest' sensitivity of bile duct brushings in diagnosing malignancy.[39,64] Stewart et al. improved their sensitivity of diagnosis of malignancy from 44.3% in the initial third of the study to 70.7% in the final third.[23] In the author's view, this area of diagnosis perhaps more than any other, requires concentration of experience for optimal results.

*Cell block preparations* of aspirated material or material expressed from obstructed stent tubes may yield a diagnosis in several of our cases when previous procedures were unhelpful. Material adherent to stent removers may also be diagnostic.[70]

*Larger needle biopsy techniques* are generally contraindicated in this anatomical region, mainly due to the higher rate of complications. Some authors consider them complementary to cytology whereas others found no increase in sensitivity over cytology alone.[54]

## The future

Other modalities have been used to increase the sensitivity of cytological diagnosis. *DNA ploidy analysis* may increase sensitivity but with increased false positives.[73] *Mutations in p53 and ras oncogenes* are a common finding in biliary carcinomas,[74] however the diagnostic value of their detection in cytological preparations either by PCR or immunocytochemistry is debated. Some workers found no increase in sensitivity over cytology for p53 immunocytochemistry.[75,76] Others were able to increase the sensitivity over cytological diagnosis alone, but with a relatively low overall sensitivity.[77] Assessing K-ras mutations by PCR of brushings may be limited by the presence of such changes in hyperplasias, by intratumoral heterogeneity and by their low frequency in bile duct compared to pancreatic carcinoma.[71] *Telomerase activity* has also been associated with bile duct carcinoma and can be measured in cytological samples.[78] Diagnostic sensitivities for brushing cytology have ranged from 18% to 90%. Positive diagnoses of malignancy are of great clinical value but a negative result is of relatively little clinical aid when the radiographic or clinical findings are suspicious for a malignancy. A variety of techniques have been used in an attempt to improve diagnostic sensitivity for brushing cytology. These have included *immunohistochemistry and various molecular diagnostic techniques*. Using the *high resolution melting curve technique*, Willmore-Payne et al. performed mutational analysis on bile duct brushing specimens for *mutations in p53, K-ras, BRAF, and EGFR genes*. No mutations were detected in benign lesions or dysplasia. Only 8% of specimens from adenocarcinomas had p53 mutations and only 33% of cases had K-ras mutations. Mutational analysis did not appear to improve the cytological detection of adenocarcinoma by bile duct brushings.[79] Ayaru et al. demonstrate that *minichromosome maintenance (MCM) replication proteins* (MCM5) in bile detected by a simple automated test is a more sensitive indicator of pancreaticobiliary malignancy than routine brush cytology.[80]

## REFERENCES

1. Lai CH, Lau WY. Gall bladder cancer – a comprehensive review. Surgeon 2008;6:101–10.

2. Cox H, Ma M, Bridges R, et al. Well-differentiated intrahepatic cholangiocarcinoma in the setting of biliary papillomatosis: a case report and review of the literature. Can J Gastroenterol 2005;19:731–33.

3. Gupta SC, Misra V, Singh PA, et al. Gall stones and carcinoma gall bladder. Indian J Pathol Microbiol 2000;43:147–54.

4. Zen Y, Adsay NV, Bardadin K, et al. Biliary intraepithelial neoplasia: an international interobserver agreement study and proposal for diagnostic criteria. Mod Pathol 2007;20:701–9.

5. Singh P, Patel T. Advances in the diagnosis, evaluation and management of cholangiocarcinoma. Curr Opin Gastroenterol 2006;22:294–99.

6. Aishima S, Kuroda Y, Nishihara Y, et al. Proposal of progression model for intrahepatic cholangiocarcinoma: clinicopathologic differences between hilar type and peripheral type. Am J Surg Pathol 2007;31:1059–67.

7. Shimonishi T, Sasaki M, Nakanuma Y. Precancerous lesions of intrahepatic cholangiocarcinoma. J Hepatobiliary Pancreat Surg 2000;7:542–50.

8. Albores-Saavedra J, Henson DE, Klimstra DS. Tumours of the gall bladder, extrahepatic bile ducts and ampulla of VaterFascicle 27. In: Atlas of Tumour Pathology, 3rd Series. Washington DC: Armed Forces Institute of Pathology; 2000. Fascicle 27.

9. Albores-Saavedra J, Henson DE, Sobin LH. The WHO histological classification of tumors of the gall bladder and extrahepatic bile ducts. A commentary on the 2nd edn. Cancer 1992;70:410–14.

10. Brugge WR. Endoscopic techniques to diagnose and manage biliary tumors. J Clin Oncol 2005;23:4561–65.

11. Volmar KE, Vollmer RT, Routbort MJ, et al. Pancreatic and bile duct brushing cytology in 1000 cases: review of findings and comparison of preparation methods. Cancer 2006;108:231–38.

12. Sheehan MM, Fraser A, Ravindran R, et al. Bile duct brushings cytology – improving sensitivity of diagnosis using the ThinPrep technique: a review of 113 cases. Cytopathology 2007;18:225–33.

13. Eloubeidi MA, Tamhane A, Varadarajulu S, et al. Frequency of major complications after EUS-guided FNA of solid pancreatic masses: a prospective evaluation. Gastrointest Endosc 2006;63:622–29.

14. Kapral C, Duller C, Wewalka F, et al. Case volume and outcome of endoscopic retrograde cholangiopancreatography: results of a nationwide Austrian benchmarking project. Endoscopy 2008;40:625–30.

15. Al-Haddad M, Wallace MB, Woodward TA, et al. The safety of fine-needle aspiration guided by endoscopic ultrasound: a prospective study. Endoscopy 2008;40:204–8.

16. Fernandez-Esparrach G, Gines A, Garcia P, et al. Incidence and clinical significance of hyperamylasemia after endoscopic ultrasound-guided fine-needle aspiration (EUS-FNA) of pancreatic lesions: a prospective and controlled study. Endoscopy 2007;39:720–24.

17. Mortensen MB, Fristrup C, Holm FS, et al. Prospective evaluation of patient tolerability, satisfaction with patient information, and complications in endoscopic ultrasonography. Endoscopy 2005;37:146–53.

18. Storch I, Shah M, Thurer R, et al. Endoscopic ultrasound-guided fine-needle aspiration and Trucut biopsy in thoracic lesions: when tissue is the issue. Surg Endosc 2008;22:86–90.

19. Krishnani N, Shukla S, Jain M, et al. Fine needle aspiration cytology in xanthogranulomatous cholecystitis, gall bladder adenocarcinoma and coexistent lesions. Acta Cytol 2000;44:508–14.

20. Papillo JL, Leslie KO, Dean RA. Cytologic diagnosis of liver fluke infestation in a

patient with subsequently documented cholangiocarcinoma. Acta Cytol 1989;33:865–69.

21. Lim MK, Ju YH, Franceschi S, et al. Clonorchis sinensis infection and increasing risk of cholangiocarcinoma in the Republic of Korea. Am J Trop Med Hyg 2006;75:93–96.

22. Layfield LJ, Wax TD, Lee JG, et al. Accuracy and morphologic aspects of pancreatic and biliary duct brushings. Acta Cytol 1995;39:11–18.

23. Stewart CJ, Mills PR, Carter R, et al. Brush cytology in the assessment of pancreatico-biliary strictures: a review of 406 cases. J Clin Pathol 2001;54:449–55.

24. Bardales RH, Stanley MW, Simpson DD, et al. Diagnostic value of brush cytology in the diagnosis of duodenal, biliary, and ampullary neoplasms. Am J Clin Pathol 1998;109: 540–48.

25. Tsui WM, Lam PW, Mak CK, et al. Fine-needle aspiration cytologic diagnosis of intrahepatic biliary papillomatosis (intraductal papillary tumor): report of three cases and comparative study with cholangiocarcinoma. Diagn Cytopathol 2000;22:293–98.

26. Ji Y, Fan J, Zhou J, et al. Intraductal papillary neoplasms of bile duct. A distinct entity like its counterpart in pancreas. Histol Histopathol 2008;23:41–50.

27. Zen Y, Fujii T, Itatsu K, et al. Biliary papillary tumors share pathological features with intraductal papillary mucinous neoplasm of the pancreas. Hepatology 2006;44:1333–43.

28. Shibahara H, Tamada S, Goto M, et al. Pathologic features of mucin-producing bile duct tumors: two histopathologic categories as counterparts of pancreatic intraductal papillary-mucinous neoplasms. Am J Surg Pathol 2004;28:327–38.

29. Paik KY, Heo JS, Choi SH, et al. Intraductal papillary neoplasm of the bile ducts: the clinical features and surgical outcome of 25 cases. J Surg Oncol 2008;97:508–12.

30. Dodd LG, Moffatt EJ, Hudson ER, et al. Fine-needle aspiration of primary gall bladder carcinoma. Diagn Cytopathol 1996;15: 151–56.

31. Gupta RK, Naran S, Lallu S, et al. Fine needle aspiration cytodiagnosis of primary squamous cell carcinoma of the gall bladder. Report of two cases. Acta Cytol 2000;44:467–71.

32. Cohen MB, Wittchow RJ, Johlin FC, et al. Brush cytology of the extrahepatic biliary tract: comparison of cytologic features of adenocarcinoma and benign biliary strictures. Mod Pathol 1995;8:498–502.

33. Renshaw K. Malignant Neoplasms of the Extrahepatic Biliary Ducts. Ann Surg 1922;76:205–21.

34. Bardales RH. Fine needle aspiration cytology of papillary neoplasms. Clin Lab Med 1998;18:373–99. v.

35. Hruban RH, Takaori K, Klimstra DS, et al. An illustrated consensus on the classification of pancreatic intraepithelial neoplasia and intraductal papillary mucinous neoplasms. Am J Surg Pathol 2004;28:977–87.

36. Dusenbery D. Combined hepatocellular-cholangiocarcinoma. Cytologic findings in four cases. Acta Cytol 1997;41:903–9.

37. Layfield LJ, Cramer H. Primary sclerosing cholangitis as a cause of false positive bile duct brushing cytology: report of two cases. Diagn Cytopathol 2005;32:119–24.

38. Corvera CU, Blumgart LH, Darvishian F, et al. Clinical and pathologic features of proximal biliary strictures masquerading as hilar cholangiocarcinoma. J Am Coll Surg 2005;201:862–69.

39. Kocjan G, Smith AN. Bile duct brushings cytology: potential pitfalls in diagnosis. Diagn Cytopathol 1997;16:358–63.

40. Chaudhary HB, Bhanot P, Logrono R. Phenotypic diversity of intrahepatic and extrahepatic cholangiocarcinoma on aspiration cytology and core needle biopsy: case series and review of the literature. Cancer 2005;105:220–28.

41. Freeman ML, Sielaff TD. A modern approach to malignant hilar biliary obstruction. Rev Gastroenterol Dis 2003;3:187–201.

42. Karlsen TH, Schrumpf E, Boberg KM. Gall bladder polyps in primary sclerosing cholangitis: not so benign. Curr Opin Gastroenterol 2008;24:395–99.

43. Boberg KM, Jebsen P, Clausen OP, et al. Diagnostic benefit of biliary brush cytology in cholangiocarcinoma in primary sclerosing cholangitis. J Hepatol 2006;45:568–74.

44. Baskin-Bey ES, Moreno Luna LE, Gores GJ. Diagnosis of cholangiocarcinoma in patients with PSC: a sight on cytology. J Hepatol 2006;45:476–79.

45. Lal A, Okonkwo A, Schindler S, et al. Role of biliary brush cytology in primary sclerosing cholangitis. Acta Cytol 2004;48:9–12.

46. Furmanczyk PS, Grieco VS, Agoff SN. Biliary brush cytology and the detection of cholangiocarcinoma in primary sclerosing cholangitis: evaluation of specific cytomorphologic features and CA19–CA19 levels. Am J Clin Pathol 2005;124:355–60.

47. Kipp BR, Stadheim LM, Halling SA, et al. A comparison of routine cytology and fluorescence in situ hybridisation for the detection of malignant bile duct strictures. Am J Gastroenterol 2004;99:1675–81.

48. Malhi H, Gores GJ. Review article: the modern diagnosis and therapy of cholangiocarcinoma. Aliment Pharmacol Ther 2006;23:1287–96.

49. Krishnani N, Dhingra S, Kapoor S, et al. Cytopathologic diagnosis of xanthogranulomatous cholecystitis and coexistent lesions. A prospective study of 31 cases. Acta Cytol 2007;51:37–41.

50. Wu SSLK, Soon MS, Yeh KT. Ultrasound guided percutaneous transhepatic fine needle aspiration cytology study of gall bladder polypoid lesions. Am J Gastroenterol 1996;91:1591–94.

51. Yang G. Pneumocystis carinii infection presents as common bile duct mass biopsied by fine needle aspiration. Diagn Cytopathol 2000;22:25–26.

52. Selvaggi SM. Biliary brushing cytology. Cytopathology 2004;15:74–79.

53. Macken E, Drijkoningen M, Van Aken E, et al. Brush cytology of ductal strictures during ERCP. Acta Gastroenterol Belg 2000;63:254–59.

54. Weber A, von Weyhern C, Fend F, et al. Endoscopic transpapillary brush cytology and forceps biopsy in patients with hilar cholangiocarcinoma. World J Gastroenterol 2008;14:1097–101.

55. Ylagan LR, Liu LH, Maluf HM. Endoscopic bile duct brushing of malignant pancreatic biliary strictures: retrospective study with comparison of conventional smear and ThinPrep techniques. Diagn Cytopathol 2003;28:196–204.

56. Lempinen M, Isoniemi H, Makisalo H, et al. Enhanced detection of cholangiocarcinoma with serum trypsinogen-2 in patients with severe bile duct strictures. J Hepatol 2007;47:677–83.

57. Wight CO, Zaitoun AM, Boulton-Jones JR, et al. Improving diagnostic yield of biliary brushings cytology for pancreatic cancer

and cholangiocarcinoma. Cytopathology 2004;15:87–92.

58. Siqueira E, Schoen RE, Silverman W, et al. Detecting cholangiocarcinoma in patients with primary sclerosing cholangitis. Gastrointest Endosc 2002;56:40–47.

59. Harewood GC, Baron TH, Stadheim LM, et al. Prospective, blinded assessment of factors influencing the accuracy of biliary cytology interpretation. Am J Gastroenterol 2004;99:1464–69.

60. de Bellis M, Fogel EL, Sherman S, et al. Influence of stricture dilation and repeat brushing on the cancer detection rate of brush cytology in the evaluation of malignant biliary obstruction. Gastrointest Endosc 2003;58:176–82.

61. Fogel EL, deBellis M, McHenry L, et al. Effectiveness of a new long cytology brush in the evaluation of malignant biliary obstruction: a prospective study. Gastrointest Endosc 2006;63:71–77.

62. Mahmoudi N, Enns R, Amar J, et al. Biliary brush cytology: factors associated with positive yields on biliary brush cytology. World J Gastroenterol 2008;14:569–73.

63. Dumonceau JM, Macias Gomez C, Casco C, et al. Grasp or brush for biliary sampling at endoscopic retrograde cholangiography? A blinded randomized controlled trial. Am J Gastroenterol 2008;103:333–40.

64. Logrono R, Kurtycz DF, Molina CP, et al. Analysis of false-negative diagnoses on endoscopic brush cytology of biliary and pancreatic duct strictures: the experience at 2 university hospitals. Arch Pathol Lab Med 2000;124:387–92.

65. Meara RS, Jhala D, Eloubeidi MA, et al. Endoscopic ultrasound-guided FNA biopsy of bile duct and gall bladder: analysis of 53 cases. Cytopathology 2006;17:42–49.

66. DeWitt J, Misra VL, Leblanc JK, et al. EUS-guided FNA of proximal biliary strictures after negative ERCP brush cytology results. Gastrointest Endosc 2006;64:325–33.

67. Byrne MF, Gerke H, Mitchell RM, et al. Yield of endoscopic ultrasound-guided fine-needle aspiration of bile duct lesions. Endoscopy 2004;36:715–19.

68. Aithal GP, Anagnostopoulos GK, Tam W, et al. EUS-guided tissue sampling: comparison of 'dual sampling' (Tru-Cut biopsy plus FNA) with 'sequential sampling' (Tru-Cut biopsy and then FNA as required). Endoscopy 2007;39: 725–30.

69. Kurzawinski TR, Deery A, Dooley JS, et al. A prospective study of biliary cytology in 100 patients with bile duct strictures. Hepatology 1993;18:1399–403.

70. Mansfield JC, Griffin SM, Wadehra V, et al. A prospective evaluation of cytology from biliary strictures. Gut 1997;40:671–77.

71. Sturm PD, Hruban RH, Ramsoekh TB, et al. The potential diagnostic use of K-ras codon 12 and p53 alterations in brush cytology from the pancreatic head region. J Pathol 1998;186:247–53.

72. Ponchon T, Gagnon P, Berger F, et al. Value of endobiliary brush cytology and biopsies for the diagnosis of malignant bile duct stenosis: results of a prospective study. Gastrointest Endosc 1995;42:565–72.

73. Ryan ME, Baldauf MC. Comparison of flow cytometry for DNA content and brush cytology for detection of malignancy in pancreaticobiliary strictures. Gastrointest Endosc 1994;40(2 Pt 1):133–39.

74. Itoi T, Takei K, Shinohara Y, et al. K-ras codon 12 and p53 mutations in biopsy specimens

and bile from biliary tract cancers. Pathol Int 1999;49:30–37.

75. Stewart CJ, Burke GM. Value of p53 immunostaining in pancreatico-biliary brush cytology specimens. Diagn Cytopathol 2000;23:308–13.

76. Ponsioen CY, Vrouenraets SM, van Milligen de Wit AW, et al. Value of brush cytology for dominant strictures in primary sclerosing cholangitis. Endoscopy 1999;31:305–9.

77. Tascilar M, Sturm PD, Caspers E, et al. Diagnostic p53 immunostaining of endobiliary brush cytology: preoperative cytology compared with the surgical specimen. Cancer 1999;87:306–11.

78. Niiyama H, Mizumoto K, Kusumoto M, et al. Activation of telomerase and its diagnostic application in biopsy specimens from biliary tract neoplasms. Cancer 1999;85: 2138–43.

79. Willmore-Payne C, Volmar KE, Huening MA, et al. Molecular diagnostic testing as an adjunct to morphologic evaluation of pancreatic ductal system brushings: potential augmentation for diagnostic sensitivity. Diagn Cytopathol 2007;35:218–24.

80. Ayaru L, Stoeber K, Webster GJ, et al. Diagnosis of pancreaticobiliary malignancy by detection of minichromosome maintenance protein 5 in bile aspirates. Br J Cancer 2008;98:1548–54.

81. Kocjan G, Chandra A, Cross P, et al. BSCC Code of Practice: fine needle aspiration cytology. Cytopathology 2009;20(5):283–96.

# Pancreas

Martha Bishop Pitman

## Chapter contents

## Introduction: technical aspects

Pancreatic cancer causes over 200 000 deaths per year and is the eighth leading cause of cancer deaths worldwide.[1] The incidence of pancreatic cancer is relatively uniform among different countries and has a peak incidence in the seventh to eighth decades of life.[2] Age, male gender, obesity, cigarette smoking and genetic conditions such as familial pancreatitis, Peutz–Jegher's syndrome and familial adenomatous multiple mole melanoma syndrome are associated with an increased risk of pancreatic cancer.[3] Although the vast majority (80–90%) of tumours in the pancreas are conventional ductal adenocarcinomas, there is a wide variety of non-neoplastic, benign neoplastic and malignant solid and cystic lesions in the pancreas that are analysed preoperatively for diagnosis. Modern imaging techniques such as high-resolution spiral computed tomography (CT), magnetic resonance imaging and endoscopic ultrasound (EUS) have improved our ability to recognise and delineate pancreatic masses and to detect them earlier as smaller mass lesions.

## Indications for fine needle aspiration (FNA)

FNA is a well-established technique to procure tissue for diagnosis in patients with unresectable disease and in those patients who may be eligible for therapeutic protocols.[4] Preoperative biopsy of mass lesions in resectable patients, however, is more controversial.[5] The potential delay in diagnosis, low negative predictive value and purported increased costs are cited as arguments for resection without confirmation if the clinical diagnosis in straightforward.[5] Accuracy of the clinical and radiological diagnosis is not 100%,[6–9] however, and the morbidity of pancreatic surgery, although improved over the past 25 years, is still fairly significant especially in the elderly population.[10] In addition, not all malignancies are surgically managed – lymphoma for example – and non-surgical management of patients with pre-malignant disease is increasingly common.[11–14] The accuracy and utility of preoperative FNA is dependent on the quality of the sample as well as the quality of the interpretation. Cytology interpretation requires training in cytological principles and criteria, and most importantly requires experience in pancreatic cytology using a multimodal approach that incorporates the clinical, radiological and ancillary laboratory tests into the overall interpretation of the specimen.[15,16]

## Biopsy techniques

Unlike other abdominal organs such as the liver and kidney, a core biopsy (CB) of the pancreas is associated with a significant risk of complications. As such, FNA remains the primary means of establishing a tissue diagnosis preoperatively. Before the development of interventional EUS, pancreatic biopsies were performed using either CT or transabdominal US guidance. With the advent of EUS, transgastric or transduodenal FNA of pancreatic masses has provided an alternative procedure for acquiring tissue to confirm the presence of pancreatic cancer and, in many centres, has entirely replaced CT-guided biopsies. It should be recognised, however, that CT is perhaps the most widely used and most important single test used in preoperative staging of pancreatic cancer and in assessment of tumour resectability, and has been shown to be superior to most other imaging modalities in accurately predicting resectability and staging of pancreatic adenocarcinoma.[17,18] Although a recent randomised, prospective crossover trial of EUS-guided FNA versus CT- or US-guided FNA for diagnosing cancer showed no statistically significant difference in the sensitivity or accuracy of CT/US-FNA and EUS-FNA,[19] there are several advantages of an EUS-FNA over percutaneous FNA. Perhaps the greatest advantage is that it allows biopsy of small (0.5 cm) lesions that are not evident by conventional imaging studies.[20] The enhanced resolution is, in part, from the proximity of the transducer to the organ examined. The short needle path decreases potential complications as well. The tissue around the needle path is resected at the time of surgery in the typical adenocarcinoma of the pancreatic head, and this reduces the possibility of tumour dissemination. EUS also simultaneously allows for accurate staging of pancreatic malignancy by sampling suspicious peripancreatic nodes and liver lesions. However, both techniques are robust and the eventual choice is dependent on several factors including availability of EUS and local expertise both in procuring and interpreting the FNA sample.

*The author wishes to thank Dr V. Deshpande, the author of this chapter in the previous edition, for his help with tables and images. I dedicate this chapter to the faculty and staff of the Massachusetts General Hospital for their support.*

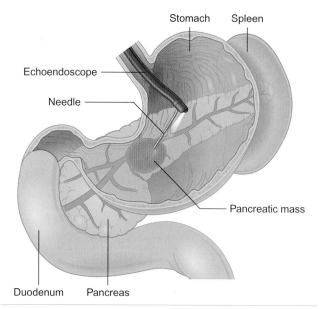

Stomach    Spleen

Echoendoscope

Needle

Pancreatic mass

Duodenum    Pancreas

**Fig. 10.1** The FNA needle is guided by the echoendoscope. Aspirates of masses in the pancreatic head are performed through the duodenum, and those in the body and tail of the gland via the stomach.

The EUS equipment consists of an image guidance system and the echoendoscope that is placed into the stomach or duodenum (Fig. 10.1). Using the guidance of the high-frequency ultrasound transducer on the tip of the echoendoscope, a small 19–25 gauge needle is passed through the wall of the gastrointestinal tract and into the pancreatic mass or cyst. Masses in the pancreatic head use a transduodenal approach and those in the pancreatic body and tail use a transgastric approach. The biopsy channel is oriented so that the biopsy needle is advanced into the imaging plane allowing for real-time imaging of the biopsy. Once in the lesion, the stylet is removed, suction is applied using a syringe, and the needle is moved back and forth within the lesion to dislodge cells and pull them into the needle. If cystic, the cyst fluid is drained as much as possible. Depending on volume, cyst fluid can be submitted for routine cytology, biochemical and molecular analysis (see Pancreatic cysts, p. 350). Any visible mural nodule or solid component should be separately sampled. Obtaining formalin fixed paraffin embedded tissue from needle rinses or CB provides not only additional morphological information about the lesion, but readily available tissue for ancillary studies.[21]

In addition to CT and EUS-guided FNA, there are several other techniques that can provide tissue for interpretation. These techniques are no longer the procedures of choice, although they can be of value in selected clinical situations. For example, intraoperative FNA is a highly effective method of establishing a diagnosis of pancreatic malignancy.[22] It, however, requires a surgeon to perform a laparotomy. Endoscopic retrograde cholangiopancreatography (ERCP) allows for sampling of the pancreatic juice. Although cytological examination of pancreatic juice can provide a tissue diagnosis, this is seldom the procedure of choice in the post-EUS era.[23] EUS-guided pancreatic duct aspiration is safe and can provide diagnostic material in a patient with pancreatic duct dilation.[24] Brushing cytology of the pancreatic duct has been reported to show high specificity for carcinoma, however, the sensitivity is lower than EUS-guided FNA.[25]

## Rapid on-site interpretation

Rapid on-site cytopathology interpretation has been shown to improve the diagnostic yield of EUS-guided FNA.[22,26,27] Interpretation of selected smears is routinely performed at our institution by a cytopathologist for all solid lesions that provide a sample from which adequate smears can be made. On-site assessment allows for appropriate triage of the specimen for ancillary studies, most importantly flow cytometry analysis of unfixed tissue and rarely for electron microscopy.[22] Cyst fluids can produce direct smears if the fluid is thick, but thin watery or bloody fluids are sent to the laboratory fresh and undiluted, from which cytospins are made for routine stains and special stains for mucin (see Pancreatic cysts, p. 350). Triage of cyst fluid for biochemical analysis or molecular analysis can be performed either by the gastroenterologist or the pathology laboratory.

## Complications

The overall risk of complications from EUS-FNA is relatively low at approximately 2%, with no severe or fatal incidents reported, and the risk appears only slightly higher than that for standard EUS alone.[28,29] The most common complications arising from FNA of the pancreas are haemorrhage and pancreatitis.[29–31] With percutaneous FNA, tumour seeding along the cutaneous needle track is an extremely rare event. Transperitoneal rather than needle track spread may be of greater concern.[32] Subsequent to the work of Warshaw et al.,[32] prospective studies of peritoneal washings, an indicator of transperitoneal seeding, in patients undergoing pancreatic surgery with or without prior FNA have concluded that CT-guided FNA does not appear to increase the risk for positive peritoneal washings.[33]

## Accuracy and limitations of a pancreatic FNA

EUS guided FNA of the pancreas is a technically difficult procedure and yields aspirates that are diagnostically challenging. Thus, the sensitivity of this procedure is variable, averaging 80% but ranging from 60% to 100%.[34–49] Sensitivity of the procedure can increase over time, reflecting increasing experience with this technique.[50] The specificity of diagnosis in the setting of a solid pancreatic mass is greater than 90%. The adequacy and sensitivity rates are generally higher when rapid onsite assessment is performed.[51]

It is difficult to compare the sensitivity of FNA among studies because of the wide variability in factors such as needle size, operator experience and improvement in radiological equipment. Additionally, the atypical and suspicious categories have been variably interpreted as negative or positive for the purposes of statistical analysis. The inaccuracies of pancreatic FNA appear to be almost entirely due to false negative reports. The sensitivity for cystic neoplasms is lower than that for solid neoplasms primarily due to the low cellularity of most of these cystic lesions.[52]

Brush cytology has close to 100% specificity; it has about a 50% sensitivity rate due to false negative sampling and interpretation.[25] Definitive malignant interpretations are hindered by preparation artifact leading to indeterminate interpretations, as well as strict criteria and a high threshold for malignancy given the well-known atypia that generally occurs in inflamed, often stented ducts.[53,54]

## Normal histology and cytology

The bulk of the pancreas is composed of an exocrine component comprised of acini arranged in lobules. Acinar cells secrete digestive enzymes into an excretory ductal system lined by epithelium that varies from cuboidal to tall columnar cells depending on the calibre of the duct. A dense zone of connective tissue surrounds the islets that probably accounts for the absence of endocrine cells in most FNA smears. Acinar epithelium dominates smears of normal pancreas and early pancreatitis. In late chronic pancreatitis, the acinar tissue is largely destroyed, leaving behind scar tissue, ductal epithelium and endocrine cells (see Ductal epithelium, below).

### Acinar epithelium

FNA samples from normal pancreas are of moderate cellularity and are composed mainly of acinar cells arranged in tight grape-like clusters or balls often attached to tissue fragments with ill-defined fibrovascular stroma (Fig. 10.2A), but also as individual acinar units, single cells and bare nuclei. Appreciation of this typical, organised, low-power architecture is important for distinguishing benign from malignant acinar proliferations, as well as acinar from endocrine proliferations. Cellular aspirates in which acinar cells present a solid cellular smear pattern of monomorphic cells can be mistaken for a neoplasm (Fig. 10.2B). Acinar cells are polygonal cells with ample cytoplasm which is dense and blue green with the standard Papanicolaou stain and purple and more obviously granular with a Wright–Giemsa stain (Fig. 10.2C). Nuclei are round with finely stippled chromatin. Small and eccentric nucleoli are often easily identified. The presence of these nucleoli helps in the identification of stripped acinar cells as epithelial and not lymphoid in nature.

### Ductal epithelium

Ductal cells tend to be sparse in FNA smears from normal pancreas, but are more noticeable in the presence of duct obstruction secondary to tumour or chronic pancreatitis. They are readily identified in pancreatic duct brushings. These cuboidal to columnar cells are larger than acinar cells and are often arranged as monolayer sheets or strips of cells with a luminal edge of non-mucinous cytoplasm. Viewed en face the sheets have a honeycomb appearance with a uniform, geometric distribution of round, regular nuclei without crowding and well-defined cell borders (Fig. 10.3). The nuclei display evenly distributed finely granular chromatin and inconspicuous nucleoli that may become enlarged and prominent when reactive. The cytoplasm varies in amount from scanty to moderate and is dense and non-mucinous to the eye.

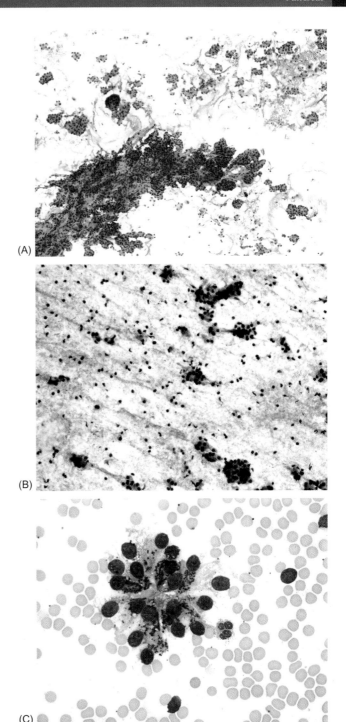

(A)

(B)

(C)

**Fig. 10.2** Pancreatic acinar cells. (A) Cohesive grape-like clusters of benign acinar cells are attached to a fibrovascular stroma and dispersed in the background (PAP). (B) When dispersed in small clusters and numerous single cells, cellular aspirates of benign acinar cells can be mistaken for a solid cellular neoplasm such as a pancreatic endocrine neoplasm (PAP). (C) Acinar cells are recognised by the typical acinar arrangement of polygonal cells with eccentric small round uniform nuclei, small nucleoli and abundant granular cytoplasm (Wright–Giemsa stain).

### Islet cells

Islet cells are not usually recognised on FNA with routine stains, requiring special stains to highlight the neurosecretory granules for identification.

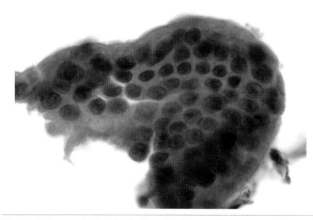

**Fig. 10.3** Pancreatic ductal cells. Ductal cells most often appear as flat monolayered sheets of non-mucinous glandular cells with evenly distributed round uniform nuclei (PAP).

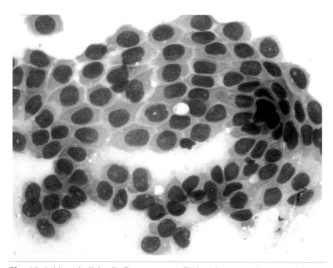

**Fig. 10.4** Mesothelial cells. Percutaneous FNA with an anterior approach may retrieve mesothelial cells as a contaminant that resembles ductal cells. Mesothelial cells are recognised by the presence of intercellular spaces or 'windows' (Wright–Giemsa).

## Contaminants

The principal contaminant of percutaneous FNA is mesothelium. Mesothelial cells may contaminate the FNA specimen when the lesion is approached anteriorly as peritoneum envelopes the anterior aspect of the pancreas. Mesothelial cells resemble benign ductal cells presenting in FNA smears with a similar flat, monolayered sheet-like arrangement. They are distinguished by their characteristic intercellular spaces or 'windows' (Fig. 10.4). Mesothelial cells can create a diagnostic pitfall especially when reactive and atypical leading to a false positive interpretation of carcinoma.

EUS-FNAs are invariably contaminated by epithelium and mucus from the gastrointestinal (GI) tract. Being able to recognise duodenal and gastric epithelium is essential for accurate interpretation of these specimens.[55,56] GI contamination from the duodenum and the stomach typically presents as flat monolayer sheets with a honeycomb pattern. Duodenal epithelium usually presents in large sheets studded with goblet cells, which have the appearance of a fried egg on alcohol-fixed

preparations where the round central nucleus is surrounded by a clear halo (Fig. 10.5A). Gastric epithelium is more often present in small groups of glandular epithelium in which surface foveolar cells display mucinous cytoplasm that makes distinction from low-grade mucinous cyst lining epithelium virtually impossible (see below). One clue that may help is to appreciate the location of the cytoplasmic mucin, which tends to be limited to the upper third of the cytoplasmic compartment in gastric epithelium as opposed to more unevenly distributed mucin often filling the cytoplasmic compartment of cyst lining epithelium (Fig. 10.5B).

GI contamination can lead to under or over-interpretation of pancreatic FNAs. Mistaking benign GI groups as benign ductal cells can lead to interpreting an inadequate sample as adequate, contributing to a false negative interpretation. Conversely, reactive atypical GI groups can be mistaken for well-differentiated adenocarcinoma leading to a false positive interpretation. Both contaminating epithelia may appear complex and atypical from folding and discohesion or, in the case of duodenum, presenting as intact villi creating a diagnostic pitfall for over-interpretation as carcinoma (Fig. 10.5C). These groups of cells are generally distinguishable from ductal adenocarcinomas as they lack the characteristic nuclear features of malignancy, and contain goblet cells and lymphocytes within the epithelium.

---

### Cytological findings: gastrointestinal cells in EUS-FNA of the pancreas

*Duodenum*

- Flat and cohesive monolayered sheet with a honeycomb pattern; occasionally papillary groups (intact villi, smaller groups and single cells)
- Sporadically placed goblet cells
- Non-mucinous glandular cells with brush border
- Lymphocytes ('sesame seeds') in the epithelium (variable).

*Stomach*

- Small sheets, strips and occasionally single cells and gastric pits
- Apical mucin cups in foveolar cells.

---

### Diagnostic pitfalls: GI cells in FNA of the pancreas

- Pancreatic ductal cells leading to adequate interpretation of an inadequate sample
- Well-differentiated adenocarcinoma
- Mucinous cysts.

---

## Reactive and inflammatory processes

## Acute pancreatitis

Acute pancreatitis is a disease of sudden onset, which may follow episodes of alcohol abuse, trauma or obstruction of the pancreatic duct by stones or tumour. Release of destructive digestive enzymes causes extensive necrosis and inflammation of the parenchyma and surrounding tissue. Acute pancreatitis commonly involves the parenchyma diffusely and is a relative contraindication for FNA as there is a slight risk of exacerbation of the pancreatitis. However, the sequelae of acute pancreatitis,

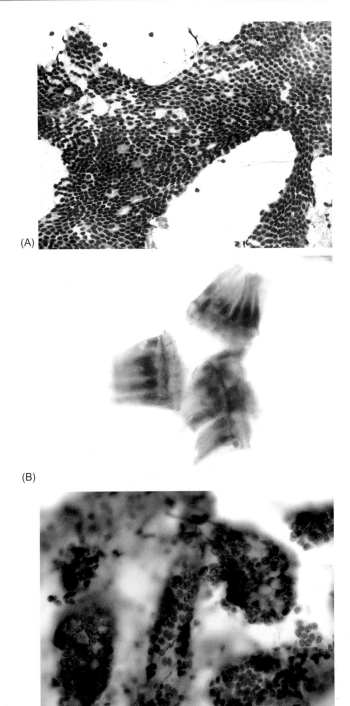

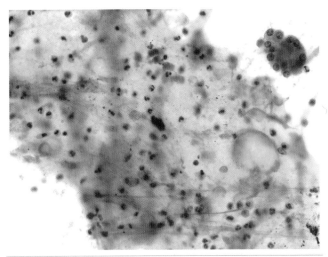

**Fig. 10.6** Acute pancreatitis. Inflammatory debris, fat necrosis and benign pancreatic tissue support this interpretation. Note the single group of acinar cells (upper right) (PAP).

prominent inflammatory component on the slide admixed with benign pancreatic tissue should prevent potential pitfalls in diagnosis (Fig. 10.6).

### Cytological findings: acute pancreatitis

- Acute inflammatory cells predominate
- Cellular debris
- Macrophages and fat necrosis
- Degenerated epithelial cells
- Granulation tissue including capillaries and reactive fibroblasts are seen in the healing phase.

### Diagnostic pitfalls: acute pancreatitis

- Regenerative epithelial atypia
- Reactive mesothelial cells.

## Chronic pancreatitis

Chronic pancreatitis is the result of repeated bouts of acute pancreatitis that lead to destruction of the acinar component and irreversible scarring of the parenchyma. A relative prominence of the endocrine component is seen on histology due to destruction of the acinar component, collapse of the remaining parenchyma and subsequent islet cell aggregation. The most common cause is alcohol abuse, but chronic pancreatitis is also commonly caused by chronic duct obstruction (e.g. from stones, thick secretions in cystic fibrosis, pancreatic divisum).[3] The most important disease to be distinguished from chronic pancreatitis is pancreatic adenocarcinoma, which it can mimic clinically, on imaging, intraoperatively and on FNA. Aspiration of normal or injured acinar tissue may simulate a pancreatic endocrine neoplasm by yielding a solid cellular smear pattern (see Fig. 10.2B). Such a pattern may also be noted from FNA of a focus of islet cell aggregation. Replacement fibrosis may also hinder adequate sampling with a fine needle. When the FNA smear shows a predominantly inflammatory background with fibrosis and mixed acinar and ductal cells or only scant benign appearing ductal epithelium, the diagnosis is relatively straightforward

**Fig. 10.5** (A) Duodenal epithelium. Flat monolayered sheets of non-mucinous epithelium studded with goblet cells distinguish duodenal epithelium from pancreatic ductal cells or cyst lining epithelium (PAP). (B) Gastric epithelium. Gastric foveolar cells may appear mucinous and often demonstrate mucin in the upper third of the cytoplasmic compartment forming an apical cup of mucin (PAP). (C) Duodenal epithelium. Duodenal villi may be misinterpreted as carcinoma or papillae of IPMN. Appreciation of goblet cells and intraepithelial lymphocytes will help identify the cells as duodenal in origin (PAP).

such as pseudocyst and abscess formation, and the hard nodular gland of chronic pancreatitis, may simulate cancer. Active chronic pancreatitis with a focal mass lesion is more likely to have an FNA performed to rule out tumour. Attention to the

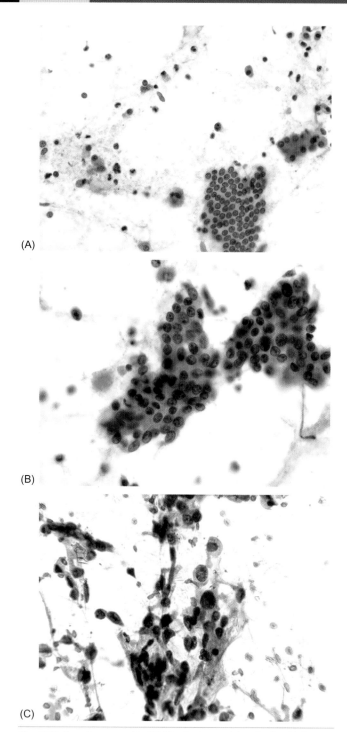

(A)

(B)

(C)

**Fig. 10.7** Chronic pancreatitis. (A) Mixed acinar and ductal cells with few inflammatory cells and histocytes in the background (PAP). (B) Ductal cells with reactive atypia illustrated by slightly irregular nuclei, uneven spacing and nucleoli (PAP). (C) Glandular cells with marked atypia in chronic pancreatitis is a pitfall for false positive diagnosis (PAP).

(Fig. 10.7(A). However, a largely pure population of ductal cells with even mild atypia as defined by slight nuclear irregularity, uneven spacing and nucleoli (Fig. 10.7B) raises the possibility of well-differentiated adenocarcinoma. Prominent epithelial regeneration and reactive atypia of ducts and acini may cause difficulty in excluding carcinoma, and many of these

cases are interpreted as indeterminate (atypical or suspicious) for malignancy.[57,58] Such atypia can be quite marked (Fig. 10.7C).

### Cytological findings: chronic pancreatitis

- Scant cellularity
- Fragments of tissue composed of collagen and fibroblasts
- Scant chronic inflammatory cell component in the fibrotic tissue fragments
- Admixture with other pancreatic cells including acinar epithelium
- Ductal groups may be predominate cells on the smears
- Uniform distribution of cells in the group
- Minimal anisonucleosis
- Relatively even chromatin without parachromatin clearing
- Non-mucinous cytoplasm mostly
- Variable nuclear atypia.

Key cytological features to help distinguish benign reactive ducts from well-differentiated adenocarcinoma centre on cell group architecture, e.g. the arrangement of the cells within the groups and the nuclear features of the cells. GI contamination, which may be indistinguishable from ductal epithelium, can further confound this issue by indicating adequate sampling of the mass lesion when, in fact, the sampling is inadequate and thus contributing to a false negative interpretation.

### Diagnostic pitfalls: chronic pancreatitis

- Regenerative epithelial atypia simulating adenocarcinoma
- Islet cell aggregation and benign acinar cells versus islet cell tumour
- GI epithelium.

## Autoimmune pancreatitis (AIP)

AIP is a sclerosing inflammatory, pancreatocentric autoimmune disease of the pancreas that frequently presents as a mass forming lesion.[59] The majority of individuals present with obstructive jaundice, and thus this lesion frequently mimics pancreatic adenocarcinoma both clinically and radiologically. A tissue diagnosis of autoimmune pancreatitis is essential as this is a steroid responsive disease, and pancreatectomy is rarely justified. Histology is characterised by a periductal collar of lymphoplasmacytic inflammation, diffuse interlobular and/or lobular chronic inflammation, dense fibrosis and obliterative phlebitis (lymphoplasmacytic sclerosing pancreatitis).[59,60] Cell block preparations of small tissue fragments obtained at FNA or core biopsy are important for the recognition of these features (Fig. 10.8A). The cytological features sufficient to diagnose the condition on FNA are present in less than one-third of cases, and thus an FNA only occasionally provides a diagnosis of AIP.[57] The key cytological feature that should alert the pathologist to this diagnosis is the presence of cellular stromal fragments, the cellularity being due predominantly to embedded lymphocytes and plasma cells (Fig. 10.8B). Ductal cells with atypia in this setting should be interpreted with caution as such ductal atypia aspirated from the pancreas of an individual with AIP presenting with obstructive jaundice and a

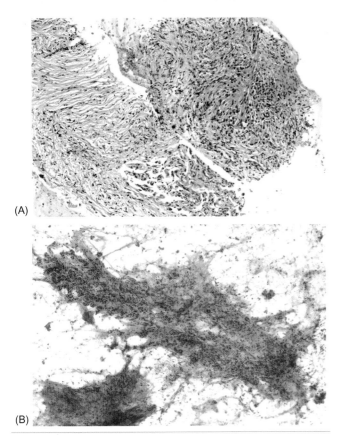

(A)

(B)

**Fig. 10.8** Autoimmune pancreatitis. (A) Core biopsy or tissue fragments in cell block are very helpful in recognising the cellular stroma with embedded lymphocytes and plasma cells characteristic of this disease (H&E). (B) A clue to the diagnosis on FNA smears is recognising the characteristic cellular stroma with embedded lymphocytes and plasma cells (PAP). (From Hruban RH, Pitman MB, Klimstra DS. Tumors of the Pancreas. Atlas of Tumor Pathology, 4th series, Fascicle 6. Washington, DC: American Registry of Pathology; Armed Forces Institutes of Pathology; 2007.)

pancreatic 'mass' could be misdiagnosed as adenocarcinoma. Additionally, injured acinar epithelial cells may produce a solid cellular smear pattern resembling the parenchyma rich-stroma poor tumours of the pancreas such as pancreatic endocrine neoplasm. Serum IgG4 levels are usually elevated in AIP. A review of the imaging by an experienced radiologist and correlation with serum IgG4 levels should help avoid this pitfall. Additionally, FNA from AIP show none of the cardinal features of a well-differentiated ductal adenocarcinoma, namely nuclear anisonucleosis and nuclear membrane irregularities.

### Cytological findings: autoimmune pancreatitis

- Cellular stromal fragments of tissue containing reactive fibroblasts and embedded lymphocytes and plasma cells
- Background lymphocytes and plasma cells are scant
- Reactive ductal epithelium
- Acinar groups.

### Diagnostic pitfalls: autoimmune pancreatitis

- Reactive ductal cells mistaken for adenocarcinoma
- Injured acinar cells resulting in a solid cellular smear pattern of a neoplasm.

## Bacterial infections

Abscess formation may result from infected necrotic pancreatic tissue or superinfection of a pseudocyst secondary to acute pancreatitis. A CT scan cannot distinguish sterile inflammation from an infectious process. FNA of the fluid collection under aseptic conditions has become the procedure of choice for verification of bacterial infection.[61] Immediate cytological examination may support the clinical diagnosis of an abscess if the smears consist of a marked acute inflammatory exudate and necrotic cellular debris. Drainage of a pancreatic abscess is a surgical emergency. Identification of bacteria with a rapid Gram stain is sufficient evidence for prompt surgical intervention and drainage.

Isolated forms of tuberculosis may rarely mimic a pancreatic malignancy.[62] Such a diagnosis is prompted by the recognition of necrotising granulomas and confirmed with the identification of acid fast organisms, either on smears with an acid fast stain or by culture.

## Solid malignant neoplasms

Classification of tumours of the pancreas is listed in Table 10.1.[63] The differential diagnosis of solid malignancies of the pancreas includes ductal adenocarcinoma and pancreatic endocrine tumours most commonly, and less commonly, acinar cell carcinoma, pancreatoblastoma and metastatic neoplasms. The vast majority (90%) of solid malignancies in the pancreas represent ductal adenocarcinoma or one its variants. Patient presentation and the radiographic appearance of the mass should be considered at the time of diagnosis. An ill-defined irregular hypoechoic mass in the pancreatic head of a 65-year-old male engenders a different differential diagnosis from that of a well-defined, round mass in the pancreatic tail of a 35-year-old female.

## Ductal adenocarcinoma

Adenocarcinoma arising from the exocrine pancreas constitutes ~90% of all pancreatic malignancies, with more than 60% located in the head region. They are highly aggressive tumours occurring mainly in the fifth to seventh decades of life. Radiologically most adenocarcinomas appear as poorly defined, hypodense (CT) or hypoechoic (EUS) masses that distort the normal lobular architecture of the pancreas.[64] When located in the pancreatic head, they may be associated with pancreatic and bile duct stricture and downstream dual dilatation of both ducts ('double-duct' sign).[64] Rarely, a *de-novo* adenocarcinoma may appear cystic.

### High-grade ductal adenocarcinoma

The majority of high-grade adenocarcinomas – that is, moderately and poorly differentiated adenocarcinomas – are easily diagnosed as malignant due to the characteristic high-grade features of carcinoma: crowded groups, cells with high nuclear to cytoplasmic ratio, irregular nuclear membranes, coarse irregular chromatin, single malignant cells, mitotic activity

**Table 10.1** Histological classification of tumours of the pancreas

I.   Epithelial neoplasms
    *A.  Exocrine neoplasms*
      1.   Serous cystic neoplasms
      2.   Mucinous cystic neoplasms
        a)   mucinous cystadenoma
        b)   mucinous cystadenoma with moderate dysplasia
        c)   mucinous cystic neoplasm with carcinoma *in situ*
        d)   mucinous cystadenocarcinoma
      3.   Intraductal papillary mucinous neoplasms
        e)   IPMN-adenoma
        f)   IPMN with moderate dysplasia
        g)   IPMN with carcinoma *in situ*
        h)   IPMN with an associated invasive carcinoma
        i)    Intraductal oncocytic papillary neoplasm
      4.   Invasive ductal adenocarcinoma and variants
      5.   Acinar cell neoplasms

    *B.  Endocrine neoplasms*
      1.   Adenoma (<0.5 cm)
      2.   Well-differentiated pancreatic endocrine neoplasm of uncertain malignant potential
      3.   Malignant well-differentiated pancreatic endocrine neoplasm
      4.   Small cell carcinoma

    *C.  Epithelial neoplasms (of uncertain differentiation)*
      1.   Solid pseudopapillary neoplasm
      2.   Pancreatoblastoma

    *D.  Miscellaneous*
      1.   Teratoma
      2.   Lymphoepithelial cyst

II.  Non-epithelial neoplasms
    a.   Haemangioma
    b.   Lymphangioma
    c.   Leiomyosarcoma
    d.   Malignant fibrous histiocytoma
    e.   Lymphoma
    f.   Paraganglioma
    g.   Other

III. Secondary neoplasms (metastases to the pancreas)

(Modified from Hruban RH, Pitman MB, Klimstra DS. Tumors of the Pancreas. Atlas of Tumor Pathology, 4th Series, Fascicle 6. Washington, DC: American Registry of Pathology; Armed Forces Institutes of Pathology; 2007.)

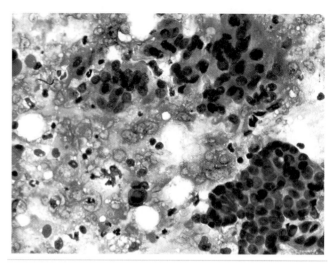

**Fig. 10.9** High-grade adenocarcinoma. Epithelial cells with overtly malignant features including cellular clusters, large cells with high nuclear to cytoplasmic ratio, large irregular nuclei, single malignant cells and necrosis (Wright–Giemsa).

and background necrosis (Fig. 10.9). Rarely poorly differentiated adenocarcinomas may present with a prominent dispersed cell population that mimics acinar cell carcinoma, neuroendocrine tumour and lymphoma. Immunohistochemical stains such as cytokeratin and chromogranin as well as flow cytometry may be necessary to differentiate carcinoma from these tumours.

## Well-differentiated ductal adenocarcinoma

Well-differentiated adenocarcinomas are more problematic as these lesions often show a deceptively bland appearance. The under diagnosis of well-differentiated adenocarcinoma as reactive epithelial changes is probably the greatest contributing factor for the relative low sensitivity of FNA. Several studies performed over the last two decades have addressed this issue.[65–67] Robins et al.[65] confirmed the diagnostic criteria for pancreatic adenocarcinoma, described by Mitchell and Carney:[68] three major criteria (nuclear crowding and overlap, irregular chromatin distribution and nuclear contour irregularity) and four minor criteria (nuclear enlargement, single malignant cells, necrosis and mitosis) to assist in making a diagnosis of adenocarcinoma. The presence of two or more major criteria or one major and three minor criteria were diagnostic of malignancy. Lin and Staerkel[66] identified four criteria that were consistently present in well-differentiated adenocarcinoma: (1) nuclear volume variation in cells within the same group, (2) nuclear membrane abnormalities, (3) nuclear crowding/overlap/three-dimensional fragments and (4) nuclear enlargement ($>1.5 \times$ RBC). On low magnification, sheets of tumour may initially resemble gastrointestinal contaminating epithelium. However, at the same low magnification, recognition of the uneven distribution of cells in the sheet or 'drunken honeycomb' appearance (Fig. 10.10), in contrast to the nuclei within the monolayers of gastrointestinal contaminating epithelium or benign pancreatic ductal epithelium that are evenly and geometrically spaced with the sheet (Fig. 10.11). Well-differentiated adenocarcinoma may also demonstrate crowded, overlapped, irregularly shaped nuclei with anisonucleosis of 4:1 in a single sheet of cells (Fig. 10.12). The cells of reactive ductal epithelium, however, generally lack the other nuclear features of carcinoma such a variable enlargement in one sheet, parachromatin clearing and irregular nuclear membranes required for the diagnosis of adenocarcinoma (see Fig. 10.7B). Additionally, FNA smears from chronic pancreatitis tend to be less cellular, are associated with an inflammatory component, and show admixed acinar cells. Thus, aspirates with a significant number of non-ductal cells should be viewed with caution.

GI contamination can result in cellular smears, also producing a diagnostic challenge. Reactive changes in GI epithelium may result in slight nuclear irregularity, nuclear grooves and nuclear enlargement ($>2 \times$ RBC) (Fig. 10.13). The two most

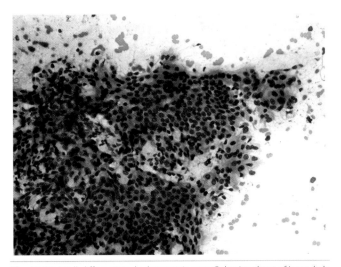

**Fig. 10.10** Well-differentiated adenocarcinoma. Cohesive sheet of irregularly spaced nuclei in a 'drunken honeycomb' pattern (Wright–Giemsa).

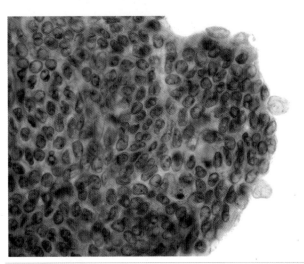

**Fig. 10.12** Well-differentiated adenocarcinoma. Nuclear crowding and overlap, anisonucleosis of 4:1 in the same group and irregular nuclear membranes supports a malignant interpretation (PAP).

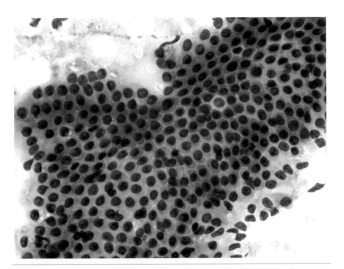

**Fig. 10.11** Benign glandular epithelium. GI contamination and benign ductal cells appear as flat monolayered sheets of evenly spaced non-mucinous epithelium in contrast to the 'drunken honeycomb' pattern of adenocarcinoma illustrated in 10.10 (Wright–Giemsa).

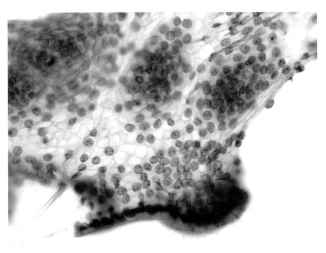

**Fig. 10.13** Gastric epithelium. Uneven spacing can be seen due to normal gastric mucosal architecture. Note the islands of cells denoting gastric crypts (PAP).

reliable features of a well-differentiated adenocarcinoma have been shown to be nuclear membrane irregularities and anisonucleosis, as defined by at least a 4:1 variation in nuclear size within a tissue fragment.[67]

A *foamy gland pattern* of adenocarcinoma is an exceptionally deceptively bland pattern of pancreatic adenocarcinoma characterised by abundant microvesicular ('foamy') cytoplasm (Fig. 10.14A).[69,70] The clue to recognising these cells as abnormal initially rests with the cytoplasm which is abundant and mucinous to the eye, an abnormal finding as normal pancreatic ductal epithelium is non-mucinous to the eye (see Fig. 10.2C). Subsequent close attention to the nuclear features should show sufficient irregularities to support a malignant interpretation (Fig. 10.14B).

## Cytological findings: ductal adenocarcinoma

*High-grade ductal adenocarcinoma*

- Three-dimensional groups with nuclear crowding and overlap
- Easily identified intact malignant single cells
- Obvious nuclear membrane irregularities, hyperchromasia and coarse chromatin
- Mitosis and necrosis.

*Well-differentiated ductal adenocarcinoma*

- Nuclear contour irregularities
- Nuclear variation (>4:1) within a single group of cells

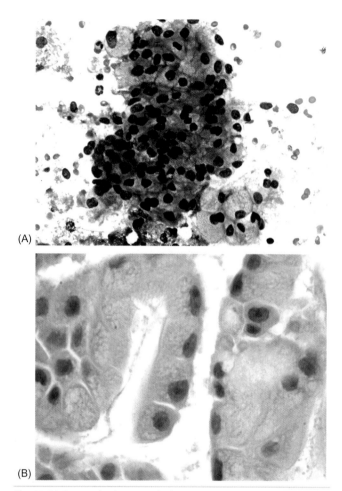

**Fig. 10.14** Foamy gland pattern of adenocarcinoma. (A) These deceptively malignant glandular cells demonstrate bland round nuclei but abnormally voluminous and visibly mucinous (foamy) cytoplasm (Wright–Giemsa). (B) Despite the low nuclear to cytoplasmic ratio, nuclear abnormalities are apparent as is abundant microvesicular mucinous cytoplasm on this cell block preparation (H&E).

- Chromatin clearing and/or clumping
- 'Washed-out' nuclear chromatin (parachromatin clearing)
- Monolayer sheets with nuclear overlapping
- 'Drunken honeycomb' appearance
- Mitosis, necrosis and discohesion with single cells are useful but rarely present.

Surgery remains the mainstay of treatment of pancreatic ductal adenocarcinomas and remains the only therapy that offers long-term survival.[71] Unfortunately, a significant number of patients are inoperable, and the radiation and/or chemotherapy that is offered to these individuals is rarely curative. The encouraging improvement in survival of patients undergoing neoadjuvant therapy has spurred a renewed interest in preoperative chemoradiation protocols.[72]

### Diagnostic pitfalls: ductal adenocarcinoma

- GI contaminating epithelium
- Reactive ductal groups in chronic pancreatitis
- Autoimmune pancreatitis.

### Ancillary studies: ductal adenocarcinoma

Because of advances in our understanding of the molecular underpinnings of pancreatic carcinoma, numerous genes and proteins have been examined as diagnostic markers for pancreatic carcinoma. Currently, however, these tests have not been integrated into routine clinical practice.

- Oncogenes. K-ras mutations are detected in more than 90% of pancreatic adenocarcinomas, and thus could serve as a sensitive marker of pancreatic ductal adenocarcinoma.[73] Unfortunately, K-ras mutations are also detected in pre-neoplastic diseases of the pancreas, such as pancreatic intraepithelial neoplasia (PanIN) and chronic pancreatitis

- Tumour suppressor genes frequently inactivated in pancreatic cancer include p53, SMAD4 and p16. Loss of p53 and SMAD4, as documented by immunohistochemistry, can supplement traditional cytological diagnosis of pancreatic FNA.[74,75] In addition, loss of nuclear expression of SMAD4 can distinguish pancreatic adenocarcinomas from other adenocarcinomas, as SMAD4, while lost in >80% of pancreatic ductal adenocarcinomas, is only infrequently lost in adenocarcinomas of the ovary, colon, endometrium and lung[76]

- Mucin markers: While normal pancreatic ductal epithelium generally lacks expression of apomucins, pancreatic ductal adenocarcinomas frequently overexpress these mucins, particularly MUC1 and MUC4.[77] In one study, the combination of MUC1 + /MUC2 − /MUC5AC+ was identified in 70% of pancreatic ductal adenocarcinomas, and was not observed in reactive samples[78]

- Global expression profiling studies have lead to the identification of a number of biomarkers. Among these, mesothelin, S100P and prostate stem cell antigen show promise; these protein are either absent or under-expressed in non-neoplastic pancreas, while over-expressed in pancreatic adenocarcinomas.[79–81]

## Variants of ductal adenocarcinoma

While numerous morphological variants have been recognised, the identification of these variants, albeit immensely gratifying to the cytopathologist, are seldom of clinical relevance with few exceptions. Clinically these variants behave at least as aggressively as, if not more so, than conventional tubular ductal adenocarcinoma, and surgery remains the mainstay of treatment.

### Undifferentiated carcinoma (pleomorphic carcinoma, pleomorphic giant cell carcinoma)

Undifferentiated carcinoma is a large and aggressive malignant neoplasm, that although may appear to show little evidence of epithelial differentiation, is both genetically and biologically a variant of pancreatic adenocarcinoma.[3] The tumour is composed of large, pleomorphic cells, giant cells with malignant nuclei and/or ovoid to spindle shaped cells that form poorly cohesive groups supported by scant fibrous stroma (Fig. 10.15).[82] The undifferentiated nature of the tumour raises a wide differential diagnosis, and while the majority of these lesions stain for cytokeratin, this reactivity may be focal and may not be identified on the FNA or in scant cell block preparations.

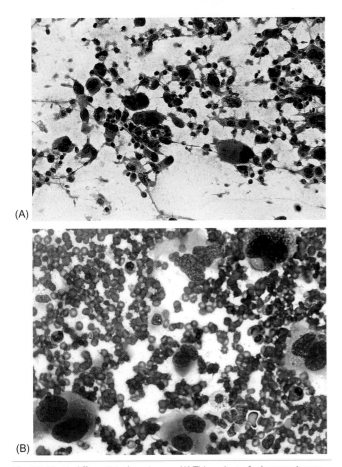

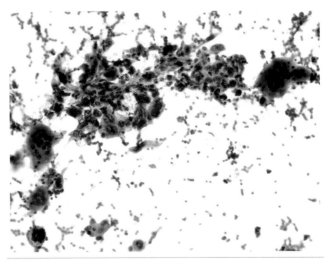

**Fig. 10.16** Undifferentiated carcinoma with osteoclast-like giant cells. Malignant mononuclear cells are associated with usually readily apparent osteoclast-type giant cells (PAP).

**Fig. 10.15** Undifferentiated carcinoma. (A) This variant of adenocarcinoma is composed of large bizarre discohesive epithelioid to spindled giant malignant cells. A rare osteoclast-type giant cell may be noted (PAP). (B) The large bizarre malignant cells may be few and widely scattered (Wright–Giemsa).

Immunohistochemical stains for cytokeratin may be required to confirm the epithelial nature of the specimen and differentiate this neoplasm from metastatic melanoma (S100 and HMB-45 positive), haemopoietic (leucocyte common antigen positive, among other more specific markers), mesenchymal (vimentin and other more specific markers such as desmin for smooth muscle and CD31 for vascular tumours), and germ cell tumours (alpha-fetoprotein, beta-HCG, placental alkaline phosphatase, among others).

**Cytological findings: undifferentiated carcinoma**

- Marked cellularity with prominent tumour diathesis
- Predominantly isolated and poorly cohesive cells with few cell clusters
- Bizarre pleomorphic single cells
- Scattered multinucleated giant cells with malignant nuclei
- Osteoclast-type giant cells are few
- Spindled cells
- Bizarre mitotic figures.

## Undifferentiated carcinoma with osteoclast-like giant cells

Undifferentiated carcinoma with osteoclast-like giant cells (UCOGC) is the currently accepted nomenclature that reflects the understanding that these tumours are fundamentally malignant epithelial neoplasms associated with benign appearing multinucleated giant cells that resemble the giant cells of a giant cell tumour of the bone.[3] The presence of K-ras point mutations, and the association of many of these neoplasms with either conventional ductal adenocarcinoma or mucinous cystic neoplasms, is indicative of their epithelial differentiation.[3,83] On histology and cytology, the tumour is composed of osteoclast-like giant cells and atypical to overtly malignant polygonal to spindle-shaped epithelioid mononuclear cells (Fig. 10.16).[84] The malignant mononuclear cells are positive for cytokeratin, while the osteoclast-like giant cells are not. However, the cytokeratin reactivity is variable and some tumour cells may demonstrate either limited reactivity or complete lack of keratin expression. Thus, the absence of cytokeratin expression does not exclude this diagnosis.

**Cytological findings: undifferentiated carcinoma with osteoclast-like giant cells (UCOGC)**

- Dual cell population
- Spindle to polygonal epithelioid atypical mononuclear cells
- Bland multinucleated osteoclast-like giant cells
- Osteoid may be present.

Benign and malignant processes in which multinucleated giant cells are a prominent feature should be distinguished from this tumour. The primary differential diagnosis is with undifferentiated (pleomorphic) carcinoma of the pancreas. Although undifferentiated carcinoma of the pancreas may show overlapping features with UCOGCs, undifferentiated carcinomas contain giant cells predominantly with malignant nuclei and only rare benign appearing osteoclast-like giant cells in contrast to the benign appearing osteoclast-like giant cells predominating in UCOGC tumours. Other malignant tumours that may yield bizarre multinucleated malignant cells include metastatic anaplastic carcinoma of the thyroid, malignant melanoma, hepatocellular carcinoma, high-grade sarcomas and trophoblastic tumours. Tuberculosis, fat necrosis, pseudocysts, fungal infections and foreign body giant cell reactions are among the benign lesions in which multinucleated giant cells may be seen.[82] However, these benign entities are extremely rare in the pancreas and are not associated with the usually overtly malignant stromal mononuclear cells of UCOGC.

### Diagnostic pitfalls: undifferentiated carcinoma with osteoclast-like giant cells

- Undifferentiated (pleomorphic) carcinoma of the pancreas
- Other high-grade primary and metastatic malignant neoplasms with tumour giant cells
- Benign conditions with reactive stroma and giant cells.

## Adenosquamous carcinoma

This rare neoplasm is characterised by the presence of a variable proportion of mucin-producing glandular and squamous epithelial cells.[85,86] The squamous component should accounts for at least 30% of the tumour.[63] A few reports have described the FNA findings of adenosquamous carcinoma.[86,87] As in histology, the proportions of squamous and glandular cells vary. The squamous element may dominate or may be the only cell type seen, and single cells with cytoplasmic mucin vacuoles may be the only evidence of glandular differentiation (Fig. 10.17). Pure squamous cell carcinomas of the pancreas are virtually non-existent. Hence, if glandular differentiation cannot be identified, a metastatic squamous cell carcinoma should be considered in the differential diagnosis.

### Cytological findings: adenosquamous carcinoma

- Malignant glandular cells
- Malignant squamous cells; may not be keratinising.

### Diagnostic pitfalls: adenosquamous carcinoma

- Metastatic squamous cell carcinoma.

## Signet ring carcinoma

This is an extremely rare carcinoma composed almost exclusively of mucin filled signet ring cells. Metastasis from a gastric primary should be excluded before making this diagnosis.[3]

## Mucinous non-cystic carcinoma

Mucinous non-cystic carcinoma or colloid carcinoma is an uncommon carcinoma dominated by a background of abundant mucin with foci of conventional adenocarcinoma constituting less than 20% of the tumour.[3] When carefully examined, almost all colloid carcinomas can be shown to arise from an intraductal papillary mucinous neoplasm (IPMN).[88] The aspirates resemble those from colloid carcinoma of the breast with aggregates of well-differentiated tumour cells floating in pools of mucin. When strictly defined (>80% mucinous component), the prognosis of colloid carcinoma is significantly better than conventional ductal adenocarcinoma.[3,88]

## Acinar cell carcinoma

Acinar cell carcinoma is a rare aggressive tumour that occurs predominantly in adults with a mean age of 62 years, but also represents about 15% of pancreatic neoplasms in children (Table 10.2).[3] A few patients develop a syndrome characterised by subcutaneous fat necrosis and polyarthralgia caused by excessive lipase in the serum secreted by this type of tumour. Because of their large size and relatively sharply circumscribed round to ovoid shape, acinar cell carcinomas can usually be distinguished from ductal carcinomas radiologically. Grossly cystic lesions are termed acinar cell cystadenocarcinoma. Median survival is 18 months.[3] On histology, the most common patterns are acinar (composed of small glandular acinar units) and solid.[89]

Malignant acinar cells are deceptively bland and can resemble benign acinar cells. Conversely, normal acinar cells may be mistaken for acinar cell carcinoma. Unlike the malignant counterpart, normal acinar cells are organised into cohesive grape-like clusters on FNA and do not display the high nuclear to cytoplasmic ratio or macronucleoli that are often noted in acinar cell carcinoma (see Fig. 10.2A). In acinar cell carcinoma the relatively cohesive, organoid arrangement of benign acinar cells is replaced by cellular sheets and/or numerous single cells and stripped tumour nuclei (Fig. 10.18A). Tumour cells of acinar cell carcinoma are polygonal cells with round nuclei, coarse chromatin, prominent nucleoli and granular cytoplasm that may spill into the background (Fig. 10.18B). The absence of striking cytoplasmic granularity and large, prominent nucleoli are not, however, a situation that typically leads to diagnostic difficulty with other solid cellular neoplasms, particularly endocrine tumours.[90,91]

### Cytological findings: acinar cell carcinoma

- Cellular smears, solid cellular smear pattern
- Loosely cohesive clusters and vague acini
- Single cells, including stripped naked nuclei
- Granular background of zymogen granules from stripped cytoplasm
- Monomorphic cells with round nuclei and prominent nucleoli
- Scant to moderate cytoplasm with granularity (best seen on air-dried smears).

The primary neoplasms in the differential diagnosis of acinar cell carcinoma include the other parenchymal rich, stromal poor tumours of the pancreas- endocrine neoplasms, pancreatoblastoma and solid pseudopapillary neoplasm (Table 10.2). All of these tumours can produce a very similar solid cellular, discohesive smear pattern of monomorphic polygonal cells. Pancreatoblastoma may be impossible to distinguish from acinar cell carcinoma based on cytology alone as acinar

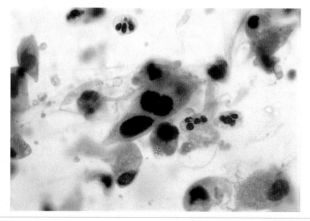

**Fig. 10.17** Adenosquamous carcinoma. Cluster of malignant squamous cells and neoplastic mucin-containing glandular cells (PAP).

**Table 10.2** Solid cellular neoplasms

| | Pancreatic endocrine neoplasm | Acinar cell carcinoma | Solid pseudopapillary neoplasm | Pancreatoblastoma |
|---|---|---|---|---|
| Clinical features | | | | |
| | 40–60 years old M = F; 50% functional | Adults in their 60s ≫ children; M:F = 4:1; lipase hypersecretion syndrome in some | 20–30 years old F≫M | 2–3 years old ≫ 40 years old M = F; 50% Asian |
| CT/EUS features | | | | |
| | Round, generally small (1–2 cm) well-defined and circumscribed solid, occasionally cystic masses | Well-defined and circumscribed, often lobulated homogeneous solid, occasionally cystic masses, avg. 10 cm | Well-defined and circumscribed solid and cystic masses, avg. 10 cm; often in the tail | Well-defined and circumscribed masses, avg. 10 cm |
| Cytological features | | | | |
| Smear background | Generally clean | Clean or granular from stripped cytoplasm | Clean or filled with hemorrhagic debris, foamy histiocytes and giant cells | Generally clean |
| Smear pattern | Dyshesive, single cell pattern; few small clusters | Solid sheets and groups, acinar structures, single cells; loss of organoid grape-like clustering | Highly cellular with papillary fragments, loose clusters and single cells; fibrovascular cores with myxoid stroma | Cellular with clusters and single cells; ± stroma with vessels; recognising squamoid corpuscles require cell block |
| Nuclei | Round to oval and eccentrically placed in the cell | Round and uniform with mild anisonucleosis | Uniform, oval with nuclear grooves and indentations | Tri-lineage epithelial differentiation with most cells demonstrating acinar features |
| Nuclear chromatin | Coarse, stippled, 'salt-n-pepper' | Coarse | Even and finely granular | Variable |
| Nucleoli | None or small but can be prominent | Usually prominent but may be absent | Absent to inconspicuous | Usually prominent |
| Mitoses | Variable but usually none or rare | None to rare | Absent | Variable |
| Cytoplasm | Dense to finely granular, rarely clear or oncocytic | Relatively abundant and granular | Scant to moderate with occasional perinuclear vacuole or hyaline globule | Generally granular |
| Immunohistochemical stains | Pan-keratin, chromogranin, synaptophysin, CD56, Leu7, NSE, variable hormonal markers | Trypsin, chymotrypsin, lipase and elastase, pan-keratin | Vimentin, alpha-1-antitrypsin, CD10, NSE, CD56; beta-catenin | Dependent on differentiation; squamoid corpuscles are usually not immunoreactive |

(From Pitman MB, Deshpande V. Endoscopic ultrasound-guided fine needle aspiration cytology of the pancreas: a morphological and multimodal approach to the diagnosis of solid and cystic mass lesions. Cytopathology 2007; 18:331–347, Wiley.)

cell differentiation is the dominate line of differentiation in this trilineage tumour and squamous corpuscles are impossible to appreciate on smears.[92] Their distinction relies on individual cellular features and immunohistochemical stains (Table 10.2). The primary ancillary tests include those that highlight the exocrine nature of the cells: PAS/dPAS histochemical stains and trypsin, chymotrypsin and lipase immunohistochemical stains.[3]

### Diagnostic pitfalls: acinar cell carcinoma

- Pancreatic endocrine neoplasm
- Solid pseudopapillary tumour
- Pancreatoblastoma
- Normal acinar cells.

## Pancreatoblastoma

Pancreatoblastoma is a rare malignant epithelial tumour generally affecting young children and occasionally adults.[93] It is the most common malignant pancreatic neoplasm of childhood.[3] On histology, the tumour is composed of solid nests of polygonal cells with acinar and to a lesser extent endocrine and ductal differentiation with intervening cellular fibrous stromal bands. The diagnostic feature is the squamoid corpuscle that is an aggregate of cells with squamous differentiation. This key diagnostic finding has not been described on FNA smears and requires a cell block preparation of tissue fragments for identification (Fig. 10.19). Immunohistochemistry for exocrine differentiation (trypsin is

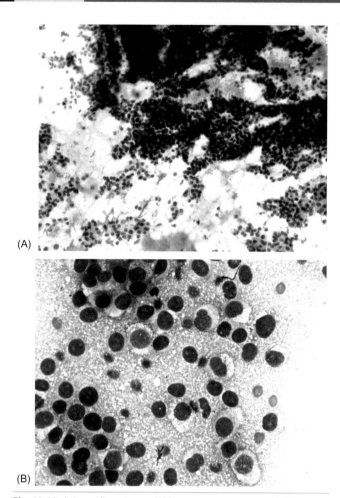

(A)

(B)

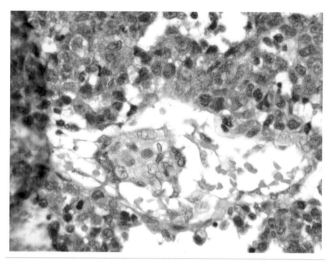

**Fig. 10.19** Pancreatoblastoma. The squamoid corpuscle in the centre of the solid nests of acinar appearing cells is the diagnostic findings and is best recognised on cell block (H&E).

**Fig. 10.18** Acinar cell carcinoma. (A) Low-power smear pattern helps to distinguish malignant from benign acinar cells. Compare this cellular crowded sheet pattern to the organoid, grape-like pattern in Fig. 10.2A (PAP) (B) The characteristic granular cytoplasm of acinar cells may be dispersed in the background from stripped cells and is best noted on air-dried smears (Wright–Giemsa).

usually sufficient) and/or electron microscopy is required to either demonstrate or confirm acinar cell differentiation (Table 10.2). Foci of endocrine cell differentiation may also be present as noted by endocrine immunohistochemical markers such as chromogranin and synaptophysin. The stromal component is immunoreactive with vimentin. The squamoid corpuscles are typically not immunoreactive but may show focal staining with cytokeratin, endocrine and CEA antibodies.[3]

### Cytological findings: pancreatoblastoma

- Cellular and biphasic tumour
- Epithelial component
- Syncytial groups and dissociated cells
- Monomorphic cell with moderate amount of cytoplasm
- Squamoid corpuscle
- Stromal component
- Primitive spindle-shaped cells
- Occasionally heterologous elements such as cartilage.

Pancreatoblastoma shows significant overlap with acinar cell carcinoma, and also enters the differential diagnosis of the other solid cellular neoplasms of the pancreas – pancreatic endocrine neoplasm (PEN) and solid pseudopapillary neoplasm (see Acinar cell carcinoma, p. 344). Identification of squamous corpuscles and primitive stroma are key differentiating features. In the absence of these elements, it may be virtually impossible to distinguish a pancreatoblastoma from an acinar cell carcinoma. In children, the clinical importance of distinguishing these two entities is minimal, as their genetic and biological behaviour are remarkably similar. Additionally, morphologically similar tumours of the adjacent kidney such as Wilms tumour and neuroblastoma warrant clinical consideration.

### Diagnostic pitfalls: pancreatoblastoma

- Acinar cell carcinoma
- Pancreatic endocrine neoplasm
- Solid pseudopapillary neoplasm
- Wilm's tumour
- Neuroblastoma.

## Pancreatic endocrine neoplasm (PEN)

Except for benign microadenomas (<5 mm nonfunctioning islet cell tumourlets unlikely to be sampled by FNA), PENs are well-differentiated low-grade neoplasms of the endocrine cells with malignant potential. The WHO recognises a three-tier classification – well-differentiated endocrine neoplasms, well-differentiated endocrine carcinoma and poorly differentiated endocrine carcinoma.[63,94] The most reliable feature of malignant behaviour in PENs is metastasis to regional lymph nodes or liver. Other recognised adverse prognostic parameters include angioinvasion, perineural invasion, mitoses (>2/50HPF), Ki67 labelling index (>2%), and tumour necrosis. Cytological features on FNA do not correlate with biological behaviour and, as such, FNA samples are interpreted as 'pancreatic endocrine neoplasms' rather than carcinoma in most cases. With modern imaging techniques detecting an increasing number of asymptomatic patients with PENs, many of which measure less than 1 cm, there is now a significant need to identify prognostic parameters on FNA.[95] It has been shown that microsatellite loss analysis on EUS-FNA material may have value in the preoperative assessment and risk stratification of patients with PEN.[96]

PENs can occur at any age, but peak around 50 years of age and are uncommon in children. While in the past the majority of PENs were functional, today non-functional tumours predominate, and smaller, non-functioning neoplasms are increasingly incidental findings.[3,95] Among the functional tumours, insulinomas are the most common, followed by gastrinomas, VIPomas, glucagonomas and somatostatinomas.[95] The cytological features of functional and non-functional PENs are the same.

Radiologically, PENs are well-circumscribed and homogenous lesions. They are typically solitary, and when multiple, invariably occur in individuals with MEN-1 syndrome. Rarely, they may present as a cystic mass.[97] On histology, the most common patterns are trabecular or gyriform, glandular and solid.

The characteristic cytological features of PENs on FNA include discohesive solid cellular smears (Fig. 10.20A) with some loose clusters, single cells and stripped naked nuclei (Fig. 10.20B). Monomorphic plasmacytoid cells with coarse, stippled 'salt and pepper' chromatin are the key features (Fig. 10.21) and association with prominent vasculature may be seen (Fig. 10.22) as can rosette formation. Vacuolated (clear cell and lipid-rich) and oncocytic variants have been described (Fig. 10.23).[98–101] Clear cell variants of PEN are typically associated with patients with von Hippel–Lindau disease, but the similar appearing lipid rich variant of PEN may have a different pathogenesis.[101] Nucleoli can also be noted, especially if the specimen is processed as liquid-based cytology (Fig. 10.24).[102–106]

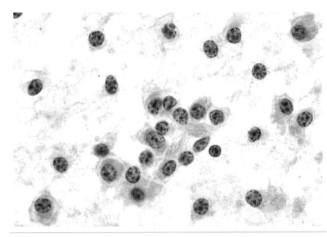

**Fig. 10.21** Pancreatic endocrine tumour. A predominantly dispersed pattern of plasmacytoid tumour cells with eccentric nuclei, minor variation in nuclear size, stippled nuclear chromatin and dense and granular cytoplasm is typical of PEN (PAP).

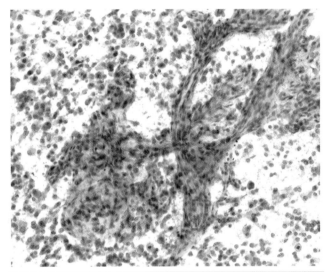

**Fig. 10.22** Pancreatic endocrine neoplasm. Prominent vascularity may be noted but papillary formation as seen in solid pseudopapillary neoplasms (Fig. 10.26B) should not be present. (From Sidawy MK, Syed ZA. Liver. In: Goldblum JR (ed.) Fine Needle Aspiration Cytology. Foundations in Diagnostic Pathology Series. Elsevier, 2007.)

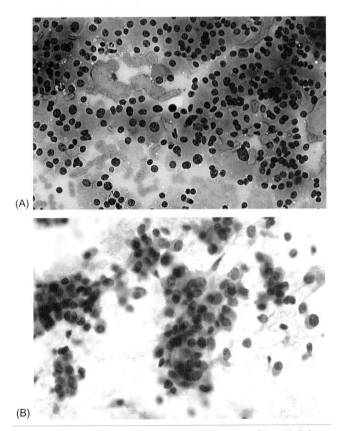

**Fig. 10.20** Pancreatic endocrine neoplasm. (A) Monomorphic epithelial cells in a discohesive single cell smear pattern shared by the solid cellular neoplasms of the pancreas (Wright–Giemsa). (B) Monomorphic epithelial cells in loose clusters and singly (PAP).

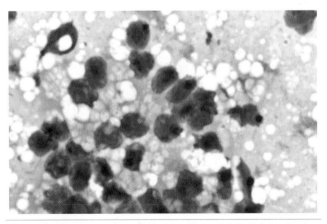

**Fig. 10.23** Pancreatic endocrine neoplasm. Clear cell or lipid rich variant of PEN must be distinguished from metastatic renal cell carcinoma (Wright-Giemsa).

The presence of prominent nucleoli and pleomorphism introduces adenocarcinoma into the differential diagnosis and support of endocrine differentiation with immunohistochemical stains (chromogranin and/or synaptophysin) may be necessary to confirm the neuroendocrine nature of the tumour.[107]

## Cytological findings: well-differentiated PEN

- Cellular smears, solid cellular smear pattern
- Predominantly single cells, some with stripped nuclei
- Loose or more rarely tightly cohesive clusters
- Blood vessels
- Rosette-like structures
- Monomorphic plasmacytoid population of small to medium-sized cells with occasional larger cells
- Round nuclei with finely stippled chromatin and smooth nuclear membranes, some binucleation
- Nucleoli small and inconspicuous, occasionally prominent
- Scant to moderate amounts of delicate cytoplasm (rarely vacuolated or oncocytic)
- Metachromatic cytoplasmic granules (on air-dried material)
- Mitoses, marked nuclear pleomorphism and necrosis absent or rare.

FNAs from benign pancreatic parenchyma composed predominantly of disrupted acinar cells with prominent nucleoli and stripped cytoplasm yielding a monomorphic smear pattern may resemble a PEN (see Fig. 10.2B).[108] To prevent a false positive interpretation, correlation with the radiological findings and immunohistochemical confirmation of endocrine differentiation is warranted.

As outlined in Table 10.2, acinar cell carcinomas, solid pseudopapillary tumours and PENs constitute the primary differential diagnosis of solid cellular smear patterns as seen in aspirates of PENs. Individual cellular features may be sufficient to distinguish these tumours in many cases, but, in others, immunohistochemistry is required (Table 10.2). For PEN, positivity with endocrine markers such as chromogranin

and synaptophysin are the standard antibodies used in most practices. Clear cell or lipid rich variants of PEN need to be distinguished from metastatic renal cell carcinoma, a neoplasm that may present as a round solitary metastatic deposit decades following nephrectomy, mimicking a primary tumour.[100]

## Diagnostic pitfalls: well-differentiated PEN

- Cystic degeneration
- Acinar cell carcinoma
- Solid pseudopapillary tumour
- Benign acinar cells
- Metastatic renal cell carcinoma.

## Poorly differentiated endocrine carcinoma (small cell carcinoma)

Primary undifferentiated small cell carcinoma of the pancreas is extremely rare and is readily distinguishable from well-differentiated endocrine neoplasm/carcinoma.[109] The histological features are indistinguishable from small cell carcinomas of the lung.[109,110] Consequently, the cytological features are identical to small cell carcinomas of the lung. Nuclear moulding, finely granular chromatin, inconspicuous nucleoli and scant cytoplasm are characteristic features (Fig. 10.25). Tumour necrosis, an uncommon finding in well-differentiated endocrine tumours, is commonly noted on smears. The differential diagnosis includes metastatic small cell carcinomas, especially from the lung. It is important to distinguish these poorly differentiated endocrine carcinomas from well-differentiated endocrine tumours as the survival in these individuals is measured in months, unlike patients with even metastatic well-differentiated PENs, whose prognosis is considerably better.

## Solid pseudopapillary neoplasm (SPN)

This tumour, also referred to as Frantz's tumour, occurs predominantly in adolescent girls and young women with a mean

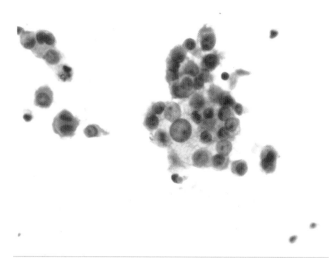

**Fig. 10.24** Pancreatic endocrine neoplasm. Nucleoli may be prominent and the cells may lack the characteristic chromatin pattern, especially if processed by liquid based cytology (PAP).

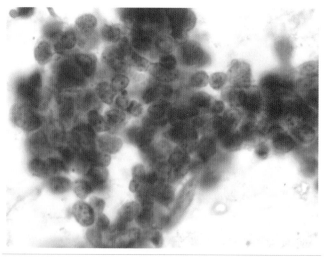

**Fig. 10.25** High-grade pancreatic endocrine carcinoma (small cell carcinoma). Markedly irregular hyperchromatic cells with nuclear moulding are noted in this high-grade neuroendocrine carcinoma (PAP).

age of 28 years, but a range of 7–79 years. Radiologically SPNs are well-circumscribed, generally large tumours with variably solid and cystic components located throughout the pancreas, but often in the body and tail. This tumour is an indolent tumour of low-grade malignancy with metastases present in 10–15% of cases.[111] Long-term survival has been reported even in patients with metastases to the liver and peritoneum.[112] Complete resection of node negative patients is considered curative. Despite the cystic nature of this neoplasm it is included here under solid malignancies due to its primary solid nature and the similar appearance of this neoplasm on FNA to other solid cellular neoplasms. Because the cystic component can be dominant, SPN must also be considered in the differential diagnosis of primary cystic pancreatic lesions.

As the name suggests, the predominant histological patterns are solid and pseudopapillary, with the papillary areas resulting from degenerative change occurring in a fundamentally solid tumour with rich vasculature. The tumour is composed of small uniform cells that frequently loosely surround fibrovascular cores composed of variably myxoid stroma (Fig. 10.26A). The presence of such papillary fragments on FNA smears makes the diagnosis straightforward (Fig. 10.26B). The smear background may be clean or filled with cyst debris. The vascular papillary cores may not be prominent or even present on FNA, however, yielding a solid cellular smear pattern very similar to PEN, acinar cell carcinoma and pancreatoblastoma. Diagnosis in such cases rests with evaluation of the cellular features and in some cases immunohistochemistry (Table 10.2).[113–116] The cells of SPN are oval to round with uniform euchromatic nuclei without prominent nuclei. Nuclear grooves and indentations are a characteristic finding. The cytoplasm is scant to moderate and may contain a perinuclear vacuole or a hyaline globule (Fig. 10.27). SPNs are variably positive with cytokeratin and show nuclear reactivity with beta-catenin, but not for E-cadherin, while PENs show a membranous pattern of reactivity with both beta-catenin and E-cadherin.[117] In conjunction with a chromogranin stain, this pattern of immunoreactivity can distinguish SPN from PEN.

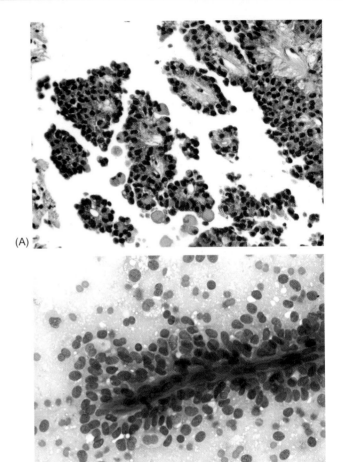

(A)

(B)

**Fig. 10.26** Solid pseudopapillary neoplasm. (A) Papillary fragments with myxoid stromal cores are characteristic of this tumour (H&E). (B) Papillary fragments in an otherwise solid cellular smear pattern of monomorphic cells distinguishes SPN from its mimickers (Wright–Giemsa).

### Cytological findings: solid pseudopapillary neoplasm

- Solid cellular smear pattern
- Papillary clusters with slender central fibrovascular cores with myxoid or collagenous stroma and loosely cohesive tumour cells
- Balls or globules of myxoid (metachromatic with Wright–Giemsa stain) stroma with or without a surrounding thick layer of neoplastic cells
- Monomorphically round to oval nuclei with nuclear grooves and indentations
- Finely granular chromatin and small to no nucleoli
- Cytoplasm is scanty and may contain perinuclear vacuoles and hyaline globules
- Foamy macrophages and necrosis (evidence of cystic change).

### Diagnostic pitfalls: solid pseudopapillary neoplasm

- PENs
- Acinar cell carcinoma
- Pancreatoblastoma.

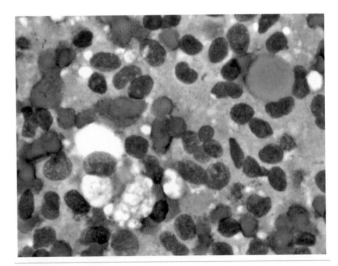

**Fig. 10.27** Solid pseudopapillary neoplasm. Characteristic features of individual tumour cells include bland round to oval nuclei with nuclear grooves and indentations and occasional cytoplasmic perinuclear vacuoles and hyaline globules (Wright–Giemsa).

## Metastatic tumours

Secondary neoplasms involving the pancreas are rare, and pancreatic involvement as the sole site of metastasis is even more uncommon. In autopsy sees the common primary neoplasms that metastasise to the pancreas include melanoma, and carcinomas from the lung, colorectum and breast.[3] Direct extension from cancer of the stomach, duodenum, gall bladder, liver and retroperitoneum may also occur.

## Renal cell carcinoma

Renal cell carcinoma is notorious for giving rise to a late solitary metastasis, even decades later, and is the primary site most likely to metastasise to the pancreas and mimic a primary neoplasm.[100,118] The cytological findings of metastatic renal cell carcinoma are similar to those seen in the kidney with bland polygonal cells, round slightly eccentric nuclei, prominent nucleoli and vacuolated cytoplasm (Fig. 10.28). Distinction from clear cell or lipid-rich PEN is warranted as the morphology of these two neoplasms may be indistinguishable (see Figs 10.23, 10.28).[100]

## Haemopoietic malignancies

Most haemopoietic malignancies involve the pancreas secondarily but can be primary, although extremely rarely.[119] Pancreatic lymphomas are most commonly non-Hodgkin lymphoma that can clinically mimic pancreatic adenocarcinoma as does metastatic renal cell carcinoma. It is essential to recognise pancreatic lymphomas, as the mainstay of therapy is not surgery, but chemotherapy. Primary pancreatic lymphomas are most commonly diffuse large B-cell lymphomas.[119] While the cytomorphological features may suggest lymphoid differentiation, there may be overlapping features with other neoplasms that produce a solid cellular smear pattern (Fig. 10.29). Ancillary tests such as flow cytometry and immunohistochemistry are typically necessary for diagnosis and especially for subclassification (see Chs 13 and 14).

## Pancreatic cysts

Cysts of the pancreas constitute a broad spectrum of entities from benign to pre-malignant to malignant cysts (Table 10.3). Until recently, cysts of the pancreas were thought to be relatively rare, but with the routine use of cross-sectional imaging, there has been a dramatic increase in the detection of often asymptomatic cysts.[6,120–125] Historically it has been advocated that all pancreatic cysts be resected due to the uncertainty in preoperative diagnosis and the fear of malignant degeneration of a mucinous cyst.[123] Management algorithms are evolving, however. As we gain in knowledge about the biological behaviour of these neoplasms and improve our ability to diagnose these cysts accurately, alternative treatment options to surgery become available.[13,14,126–128]

## Multimodal approach to cytological diagnosis of cystic lesion of the pancreas

Although cyst cytology alone is often non-diagnostic, when evaluated in the context of the clinical history, radiological features and gross cyst fluid observations and ancillary tests such as special stains for mucin, biochemical testing for CEA and amylase and increasingly molecular analysis, accuracy can be greatly improved.[129–136] An educated and experienced cytopathologist is critical for accurate interpretation.[14,123,135,137–143] The purpose of these preoperative investigations is primarily to distinguish mucinous neoplasms from pseudocysts and serous cystadenomas, distinctions that directly affect patient management decisions.[13,14,128,144,145] Table 10.3 outlines the multimodal parameters of the most commonly encountered pancreatic cysts.

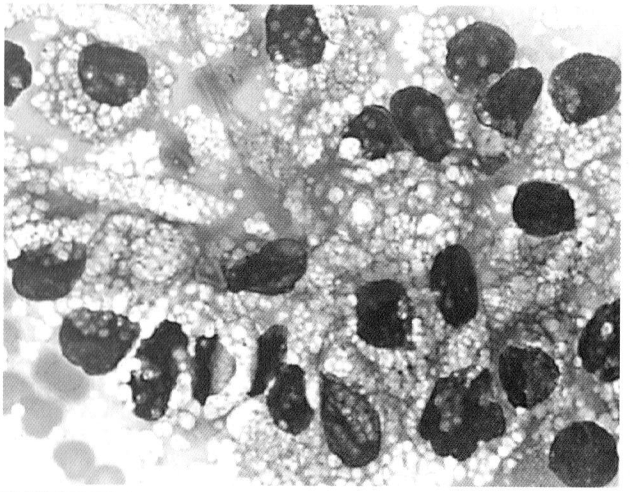

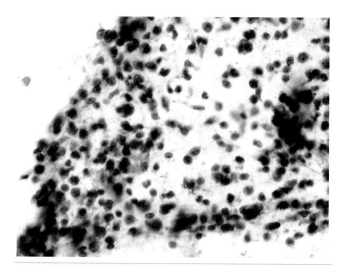

**Fig. 10.28** Metastatic renal cell carcinoma. Monomorphic cells with bland nuclei and cytoplasm with defined small vacuoles are characteristic of this tumour but must be distinguished from clear cell variant of PEN, which can look identical (Wright–Giemsa).

**Fig. 10.29** Primary pancreatic peripheral T-cell lymphoma. The discohesive single cell pattern places lymphoma in the differential diagnosis of solid cellular neoplasms and the pleomorphism of the cells mimics adenocarcinoma (PAP).

**Table 10.3** Cystic mass lesions

| | Pseudocyst | Serous cystadenoma | Mucinous cystic neoplasm | Intraductal papillary mucinous neoplasm |
|---|---|---|---|---|
| Clinical features | | | | |
| | Associated with pancreatitis and trauma; most pancreatitis related to alcohol | 65 years old F >>M | 40–50 years old female | 65 years old M > F |
| CT/EUS features | | | | |
| | Most are single, unilocular, thin-walled cysts without septations | Large, mostly microcystic; some with central stellate scar with star-burst calcifications; some with few and large cysts | Thick-walled, often calcified solitary, multiloculated, well-circumscribed cysts in the body or tail; no communication with the pancreatic duct | Main duct, branch duct and combined types. Cysts are single or multiple and connect to the main pancreatic duct; 70% in the head; thick wall, multiple septations and mural nodule correlate with high grade |
| Cytological features | | | | |
| Smear background | Amorphous cyst debris | Clean to bloody | Variably thick mucin; mucin may be thin and clear | Variably thick mucin; mucin may be thin and clear |
| Smear pattern | Variably cellular without epithelial cell component | Hypocellular; frequently acellular | Acellular to hypocellular in low-grade neoplasms bland mucinous cells; variably atypical glandular cells in higher grade neoplasms | Acellular to hypocellular in low-grade neoplasms bland mucinous cells; variably atypical glandular cells in higher grade neoplasms; may see papillary structures |
| Nuclei | NA | Round and regular; bland | Bland to variably atypical | Bland to variably atypical |
| Nuclear chromatin | A | Smooth and even | Variable | Variable |
| Nucleoli | NA | None | Absent to conspicuous | Absent to conspicuous |
| Mitoses | none | None | Generally absent | Generally absent |
| Cytoplasm | Histiocytes may have dense cytoplasm and mimic epithelial cells | Scant but visible and finely vacuolated | Mucinous, more obvious in low-grade neoplasms | Mucinous, more obvious in low-grade neoplasms; |
| Cyst fluid analysis | High amylase in thousands U/L; low CEA < 200 ng/mL | Low amylase and low CEA <200 ng/mL | Variable amylase, typically low; CEA usually >200 ng/mL | Amylase generally high; CEA usually >200 ng/mL |

(From Pitman MB, Deshpande V. Endoscopic ultrasound-guided fine needle aspiration cytology of the pancreas: a morphological and multimodal approach to the diagnosis of solid and cystic mass lesions. Cytopathology 2007; 18:331–347, Wiley).

## Biochemical analysis of cyst fluid

The biochemical analysis of usually at least 1 mL of fresh, unfixed and undiluted fluid aspirated from cystic lesions of the pancreas is very helpful in distinguishing cystic neoplasms from pseudocysts, serous cysts from mucinous cysts, and benign from malignant mucinous cystic neoplasms.[138,141,146,147] Observation of the gross characteristics of the cyst is also very informative. Pseudocysts are typically thin and watery, brown to green and occasionally turbid.[148] This translates into a relatively low viscosity compared with serum and the fluid of mucinous cysts. Conversely, as the name implies, mucinous cysts very frequently produce a thick viscous fluid that can be clear or white in colour, that is difficult to aspirate and express onto the slide due to the high viscosity.[148] From the early studies of

various tumour markers, CEA has yielded the best results in discriminating between a mucinous and non-mucinous cyst.[141] Pseudocysts and serous cystadenomas have low levels of CEA (<25 ng/mL at MGH). In contrast, neoplastic mucinous cysts usually have CEA values above 200 ng/mL (at MGH).[141] The results of biochemical analysis of CEA as well as the resulting threshold levels may be laboratory dependent. In a meta-analysis evaluating CEA levels in mucinous cysts, a level of 800 ng/mL was found to have a 79% accuracy rate separating mucinous and non-mucinous cysts.[138] Raising the cut-off value for CEA for this distinction decreases the sensitivity of detection albeit increasing the specificity. Amylase is the second test that is very helpful in the preoperative interpretation of pancreatic cysts. Pseudocysts invariably have an elevated amylase level, usually in the thousands.[141,146] As such, an amylase level of <250 U/L virtually excludes the diagnosis of a pseudocyst. The use of amylase to distinguish MCN from IPMN is surprisingly inaccurate, although there is a trend towards IPMN having higher values compared with MCN.[141]

## Molecular analysis of cyst fluid

Our understanding of the diagnostic value of the genetic mutations in pancreatic cyst fluid is evolving. Commercial molecular tests are available but controversial as there have been few published reports.[130,136,149,150]

As currently reported[130,149] malignant cysts require either *KRAS* gene point mutation, two or more LOH or high quantity/quality of DNA with *KRAS* or LOH mutation present at a high amplitude (>75%) suggesting a significant clonal expansion. Mucinous cysts show either *KRAS* gene point mutation, two or more LOH or high quantity/quality of DNA, and non-mucinous cysts do not show any of these molecular changes and little, poor-quality DNA. Validation studies on cysts diagnosed histologically to confirm the value of these findings are needed before wide use of these methods are utilised for diagnosis. A recent study comparing the molecular classification of cysts into general categories of non-mucinous, benign mucinous and malignant mucinous cysts with the current practice using clinical, radiological and cyst fluid parameters shows good concordance, however.[136]

## Non-neoplastic cysts

### Pseudocyst

A pancreatic pseudocyst by definition has no epithelial lining, hence the prefix 'pseudo'. These fluid collections of pancreatic secretions, necrotic debris and blood occur from damage to the pancreatic parenchyma secondary to the release and activation of pancreatic enzymes. The incidence of pseudocysts is highest in patients with a well-established history of acute and chronic pancreatitis. Approximately 10% of patients with pancreatitis will develop a pseudocyst.[3,151] The most common aetiology of pancreatitis is alcohol abuse and alcohol-related pseudocysts are more common in middle-aged men. Although some pseudocysts may be medically managed, most are drained or resected, given the potential risk of complications such as rupture and haemorrhage due to erosion into a vessel, obstruction of surrounding structures and infection.[152]

Radiologically, pseudocysts usually appear as solitary, small to very large (up to 20 cm) well-demarcated, thick to thin walled, unilocular cysts. They can occur anywhere in the pancreas, however most (~65%) occur in the pancreatic tail.[3,153] The cyst fluid aspirated from an uncomplicated pseudocyst is generally thin, brown to green and non-mucinous. A complicated pseudocyst, however, may produce thick mucoid appearing fluid due to the presence of inflammation and fibrin.[148]

Cytologically, the characteristic features include degenerative cyst debris without thick extracellular mucin, but with acute and chronic inflammatory cells, histiocytes, and haemosiderin-laden macrophages. No cyst lining epithelial cells should be present; however, contaminating gastric or duodenal epithelium and even extracellular mucin may be present presenting a diagnostic pitfall for the misinterpretation of a mucinous cyst. It should be remembered that, except for the goblet

cells in duodenal epithelium, the enterocytes of the duodenum are non-mucinous to the eye. Epithelial cells with apical mucin cups in the upper third of the cytoplasmic compartment should be regarded as gastric contamination (see Fig. 10.5B).[154] Complicated pseudocysts may appear mucoid due to inflammatory debris and it can be quite challenging to distinguish fibrinous mucoid debris from neoplastic mucin. Additionally, histiocytes may appear quite epithelioid mimicking serous cells when finely vacuolated and mucinous cells when large vacuoles are present (Fig. 10.30). Amylase is consistently elevated (usually in thousands of U/L) in pseudocysts with an undetectable or very low CEA level.[15,148,155]

### Lymphoepithelial cyst

Lymphoepithelial cyst is a rare benign squamous-lined cyst with subepithelial non-neoplastic lymphoid tissue. This cyst

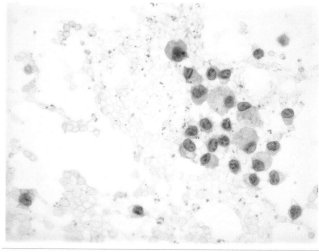

**Fig. 10.30** Pseudocyst. The characteristic contents of a pseudocyst include proteinaceous debris and a variable number of inflammatory cells, which may be dominated by epithelioid histiocytes that must be distinguished from epithelial cells (PAP).

is much more common in middle-aged men with a 4:1 male to female ratio.[3,156,157] Radiologically lymphoepithelial cyst may present anywhere in the pancreas as a unilocular or multilocular cyst, generally with a thick appearing wall and internal debris that corresponds to the keratinous debris. These cysts have a wide size range of little over 1 cm to 17 cm, averaging 5 cm.[3,156,157]

The cytological appearance is similar to that of an epidermal inclusion cyst with nucleated and anucleate squamous cells, keratinous and cholesterol debris. Histiocytes and lymphocytes may be noted in the background (Fig. 10.31A). An intact cyst wall with subepithelial lymphoid tissue may also be seen (Fig. 10.31B).[3,15,148,158,159]

### Cytological findings: lymphoepithelial cyst

- Anucleate squames and abundant keratinous debris
- Mature superficial squamous cells
- Lymphocytes are usually present but amount is variable and may be quite scant
- $\pm$ Cholesterol clefts.

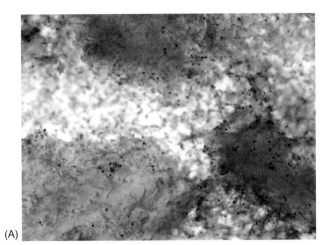

(A)

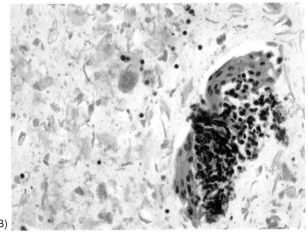

(B)

**Fig. 10.31** Lymphoepithelial cyst. (A) A background of anucleated squamous cells and keratinous debris are typical of the contents of a lymphoepithelial cyst. Note the sprinkling of lymphocytes in the background (PAP). (B) The presence of an intact cyst wall with squamous cell lining and subepithelial lymphoid tissue may occasionally be seen, as shown here in this cell block preparation (H&E).

The differential diagnosis is with other squamous-lined cysts such as a dermoid cyst of the pancreas and splenic epidermoid cyst, both benign cysts more rare than lymphoepithelial cyst.[156,160] The distinction between these entities may frequently not be possible, and are not clinically relevant. A pseudocyst is also in the differential diagnosis due to the necrotic appearance of the keratinous debris. Conservative resection is curative.

### Diagnostic pitfalls: lymphoepithelial cyst

- Complicated pseudocyst
- Other squamous lined cysts in the region of the pancreas such as dermoid cysts and epidermoid cysts.

## Retention cysts

Retention cysts are small cysts that form from cystically dilated segments of pancreatic ducts as a consequence of focal duct obstruction. They are typically unilocular, small (<1 cm), and are lined by ductal epithelium which is often denuded.[3,153] The cytological features are non-diagnostic, showing few ductal epithelial cells and inflammatory cells. They are unlikely to be confused with a mucinous neoplasm either clinically or on imaging studies. It is, however, conceivable that aspirates of these lesions, when focally lined by metaplastic mucinous epithelium, may show a few mucinous epithelial cells and muciphages.[161]

## Cystic neoplasms

### Serous cystadenoma

Serous cystadenoma (microcystic or glycogen-rich cystadenoma) is a benign, typically microcystic, neoplasm that produces serous fluid. This neoplastic cyst is estimated to account for about 25% of all cystic neoplasms and occurs more frequently in elderly females with a mean age of 65 years, but in a wide age range of 18–91 years.[3] There is an association with von Hippel–Lindau syndrome.[162] These neoplasms are benign with very rare reports of malignant transformation.[163,164] Variants of this neoplasm include unilocular and oligocystic subtypes, depending on the number and size of the cysts. Solid variants are also rarely encountered.[165] Complete surgical resection is curative and is recommended for any symptomatic neoplasm or neoplasm greater than 4 cm due to the faster growth rate of larger neoplasms and the risk of rupture or erosion into a large vessel that can cause death. Asymptomatic neoplasms less than 4 cm can be followed without resection making cytological confirmation of the diagnosis very important.[166,167]

Microcystic serous cystadenoma may demonstrate very characteristic radiological findings.[123,168] Cross-sectional imaging demonstrates a 'soap bubble' pattern due to the numerous microcysts that average less than 2 cm each. Many neoplasms will contain a central stellate scar, and about 30% of these will demonstrate a 'star burst pattern' of microcalcifications within the scar.[169] Not all microcystic neoplasms present so characteristically, however, and they can be confused radiologically with carcinoma.[170] Oligocystic and unilocular variants of serous cystadenomas also cannot be distinguished from other cysts in the pancreas radiologically.[171] Reports of an accurate diagnosis of serous cystadenoma based on imaging studies vary from approximately 27% to 87%.[168,172–174] It is these radiologically uncharacteristic serous cystadenomas that are often the ones that are evaluated by FNA, increasing the diagnostic difficulty for the pathologist.

The fluid aspirated from a serous cystadenoma is clear and thin and may be quite bloody, but is not mucoid as in most mucinous cysts. Smears are frequently very paucicellular and it is not uncommon for smears to be acellular.[174,175] Identification of even a couple of small clusters of cells with bland cuboidal morphology can be very helpful in the appropriate clinical setting, even if not technically considered 'diagnostic'. Tumour cells are uniform cuboidal cells in small clusters and flat sheets with round central to slightly eccentric nuclei and scant but visible cytoplasm that is homogenous to clear (Fig. 10.32A). The nuclei have smooth nuclear membranes, an even chromatin pattern, and inconspicuous to no nucleoli. Importantly, mucin is not present within these cells. Haemosiderin-laden macrophages may be a prominent component of the aspirate, and when identified in an aspirate without

the typical proteinaceous debris expected of a pseudocyst, may serve as a surrogate marker and clue to the diagnosis of this neoplasm.[174] If sufficient cells are procured for cell block preparation, PAS stain with and without diastase will confirm the presence of cytoplasmic glycogen and exclude the presence of mucin (Fig. 10.32B).

### Cytological findings: serous cystadenoma

- Hypocellular
- Cuboidal non-mucinous epithelial cells
- Flat sheets with a honeycomb pattern, small flat clusters or single cells
- Bland, round or oval euchromatic nuclei without prominent nucleoli
- Clear, finely vacuolated cytoplasm
- Cytoplasmic glycogen demonstrated by PAS with and without diastase
- No intracellular or extracellular mucin
- Association with haemosiderin-laden macrophages in some cases.

A cyst fluid CEA of <5 ng/mL and a low amylase level provide strong evidence for a serous cystadenoma. Conversely, a CEA of >200 ng/mL would for all practical purposes exclude a serous cystadenoma.[155] Molecular analysis of the cyst fluid should fail to demonstrate *KRAS* or significant LOH mutations, although 3p deletions tend to confirm the diagnosis and signify an association with VHL disease.[130]

### Diagnostic pitfalls: serous cystadenoma

- Acellular and hypocellular samples
- Epithelioid histiocytes
- Gastrointestinal contaminating epithelium.

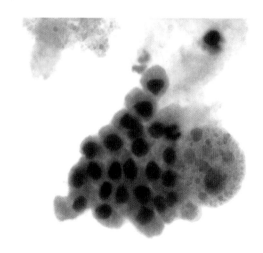

(A)

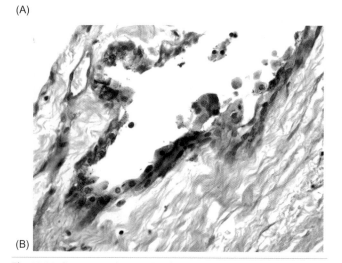

(B)

**Fig. 10.32** Serous cystadenoma. (A) The tumour cells are uniform cuboidal cells with bland central nuclei, smooth nuclear membranes and even chromatin. The cytoplasm is delicate and may appear clear and finely vacuolated but is non-mucinous. Haemosiderin-laden macrophages are not uncommonly associated with this neoplasm and offer a clue to the diagnosis (PAP). (B) Uniform cuboidal cells may be very few, but are typical of serous cystadenoma and when in a cell block provide cells to confirm the intracytoplasmic glycogen (PAS + /PAS with diastase negative) and absence of mucin (mucicarmine or Alcian blue ph 2.5 negative) (H&E).

## Intraductal papillary mucinous neoplasm (IPMN)

IPMN is a mucin-producing neoplastic cyst that arises from and is directly connected with the pancreatic ductal system, either the main duct and/or side branch duct, and is lined by typically papillary and variably atypical mucinous epithelium. These neoplasms are not associated with subepithelial ovarian-type stroma as is required for the diagnosis of MCN.[14] Most IPMN occur in elderly men and women with a peak age of close to 65 years and a slight male predominance. Complete surgical resection is currently the treatment of choice, although treatment options are evolving for branch duct IPMN due to the more often low-grade nature of these neoplasms.[126] Prognosis is directly related to the presence or absence of an invasive carcinoma.[3] As such, complete and thorough histological sampling is essential to rule out an invasive component given that these neoplasms tend to be very heterogeneous in their lining, and that an invasive component may not be apparent grossly. Non-invasive IPMN have a greater than 90% 5-year survival rate, but this rate drops to 40% with invasive carcinoma, a rate that is still significantly better than conventional ductal adenocarcinoma.[3]

Radiological and EUS features can be diagnostic when a markedly distended main pancreatic duct is noted to have filling defects or when there are multiple branch duct cysts.[176,177] The visualisation of copious amounts of mucin from a patulous ampulla is pathognomonic of IPMN.[178] The appearance of an isolated branch duct IPMN, however, is almost impossible to distinguish from other cysts in the pancreas.[6,142,144] Unlike MCN that are rare in the pancreatic head and uncinate process, branch duct IPMN cysts are non-septated, unilocular cysts often less than 5 cm that occur more commonly in the pancreatic head, especially the uncinate process.[14,142,179,180] The recognition of an associated mural nodule is an independent predictor of malignancy.[177,181]

The epithelial lining of IPMN includes gastric-foveolar type, intestinal type, pancreatobiliary type and oncocytic type. Most main duct IPMN are lined by cells with intestinal differentiation, but branch duct IPMN are most commonly associated with gastric-foveolar type epithelium, the epithelial subtype least associated with carcinoma, hence the better prognosis of branch duct IPMN compared with the main duct type.[182] Distinguishing these varying types of lining epithelium in cytological preparations is not necessary. Distinguishing cyst lining epithelium from GI contamination is important. Consideration of cyst location, organ traversed and other clinical and radiological features makes the distinction possible in many cases (Table 10.3).

FNA of IPMN produce variable amounts of mucin and cyst lining epithelium, and, as such, may not accurately reflect the histological grade of the cyst.[135,181,183–187] A specific diagnosis of IPMN, therefore, is a less common cytological interpretation than a more general diagnosis of a neoplastic mucinous cyst that includes MCN. This is primarily due to hypocellularity of the mucinous contents aspirated and/or a lack of architectural specificity of the glandular epithelium, for example, absence of papillary fragments. In addition, the lining of the cysts is often heterogeneous, so it is important to emphasise that regardless of the cytological diagnosis, a higher-grade neoplasm cannot be excluded.[135,181]

Thick and viscous, typically white cyst fluid grossly indicates mucin in most cases and, when reflected on the slide as a thick sheet of 'colloid-like' mucin (Fig. 10.33), is diagnostic of a mucinous cyst regardless of the presence of an epithelial component. Gastrointestinal mucin may appear focally thick but not 'colloid-like'. Degenerate inflammatory cells and histiocytes within the mucin also help to distinguish cyst mucin from contaminating mucin.[188] Wisps of thick mucin containing entrapped epithelial fragments with columnar cells displaying apical mucin cups should be interpreted as gastric contamination when aspirated from a cyst in the body or tail of the pancreas (see Fig. 10.5B): but given that the gastric-foveolar type of lining is the most common type of lining in branch duct IPMN that most often occur in the pancreatic head, the typical transduodenal approach is not likely to produce foveolar appearing contamination.[154,181] Air-dried smears of thin mucin may produce 'ferning', an indication of its mucinous nature (Fig. 10.34). Thin, clear fluid may not be recognised at all if the fluid is processed by liquid-based methods. When processed as cytospin preparations, mucin stains (mucicarmine and/or Alcian blue pH 2.5) can help to identify and distinguish proteinaceous fluid from mucin (Fig. 10.35). Negative mucin stains, however, do not exclude the diagnosis of IPMN.

*IPMN with low-grade dysplasia (adenoma)* typically produces scantily cellular aspirates composed of bland columnar

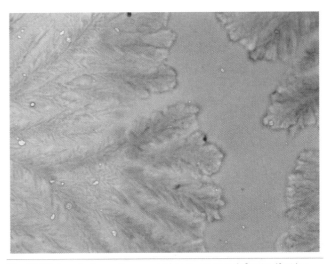

**Fig. 10.34** Neoplastic mucinous cyst. Thin mucin may define itself with a 'ferning' pattern, which distinguishes it from a proteinaceous background (Wright–Giemsa).

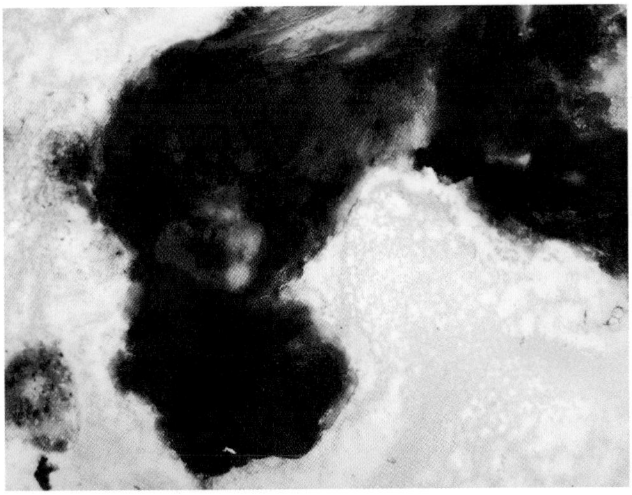

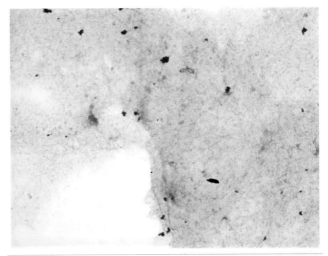

**Fig. 10.35** Neoplastic mucinous cyst. Background mucin that mimics proteinaceous debris may be confirmed with special stains for mucin (Mucicarmine stain).

**Fig. 10.33** Neoplastic mucinous cyst. Colloid-like mucin is typical of a neoplastic mucinous cyst, both MCN and IPMN. This quality and quantity of mucin is not seen from GI contamination (Wright–Giemsa).

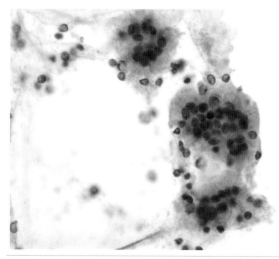

**Fig. 10.36** Intraductal papillary mucinous neoplasm – with low-grade dysplasia. Bland mucinous epithelium have round, regular nuclei, abundant mucinous cytoplasm and a low nuclear to cytoplasmic ratio (PAP).

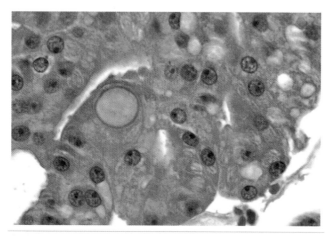

**Fig. 10.37** Intraductal papillary mucinous neoplasm – oncocytic variant. Oncocytic epithelium demonstrates round, regular nuclei, prominent nucleoli and abundant granular cytoplasm (H&E).

mucinous glandular cells arranged in small clusters and flat to folded sheets with a honeycombed pattern. Clusters of columnar cells with round basal nuclei and mucinous cytoplasm are most often noted (Fig. 10.36). Single cells may also be seen. Papillary epithelial fragments must be distinguished from villi of duodenal contamination for transduodenal EUS-guided aspirates. Recognition of intraepithelial lymphocytes and sporadically placed goblet cells supports duodenal epithelium (see Fig. 10.5C), whereas the recognition of a mucinous (to the eye) luminal edge supports lesional epithelium. Single cells with visible mucinous cytoplasm also support lesional cells. Dense, oncocytic cytoplasm is consistent with intraductal oncocytic papillary neoplasm (Fig. 10.37).

### Cytological findings: intraductal papillary mucinous neoplasm with low-grade dysplasia (adenoma)

- Variable amounts of mucin
- Thick, colloid-like mucin with or without mucinous epithelium

- Thin, watery mucin
- Low cellularity
- ± Papillary fragments
- Mucinous glandular epithelium with mucin occupying more than one-third of the columnar cytoplasmic compartment
- Absence of nuclear atypia
- No background necrosis.

*IPMN-moderate dysplasia and IPMN-carcinoma* (in situ and invasive) are lined by atypical to malignant appearing glandular epithelium with variable amounts of cytoplasmic mucin. Although malignant IPMN typically have increased overall cellularity with respect to low-grade neoplasms, not all carcinomas produce cellular aspirates. In fact, the typical heterogeneity of these neoplasms may produce aspirate specimens with a range of cellular atypia from adenoma to carcinoma making accurate cytological diagnosis a challenge.[135] Atypical cells display nuclear crowding, loss of polarity, nuclear elongation and hyperchromasia. Hyperchromatic cells with irregular nuclear membranes and high nuclear to cytoplasmic ratios may be arranged in elongated to papillary clusters where the length is usually twice the width of the group (Fig. 10.38), small relatively bland epithelial cell clusters (Fig. 10.39) or singly. Even if very scant in amount, recognition of just one small group of such atypical epithelial cells is important for classifying the cyst as at least moderate dysplasia.[15,135,181] Open chromatin, irregular nuclear membranes and nucleoli, significant background inflammation and necrosis supports the interpretation of an *in situ* or invasive carcinoma (Fig. 10.40). Only necrosis appears to correlate with the presence of invasion, but this distinction cannot be made on aspirates of cyst contents alone.[135] A mural nodule is indicative of an invasive carcinoma and, currently, aspiration of this nodule is necessary to document an invasive carcinoma cytologically.

### Cytological findings: intraductal papillary mucinous neoplasm with moderate dysplasia and higher

In addition to the above findings for lesions with low-grade dysplasia:

- ± Increased cellularity relative to adenoma
- Recognisable cytological atypia with increased cellularity and atypia correlating with increased grade: single intact cells, doublets and small cell clusters, cellular papillary groups, nuclear irregularity, increased nuclear: cytoplasmic ratio, decreased cytoplasmic mucin, irregular nuclear membranes and nucleoli
- Abundant background inflammation and necrosis support malignancy.

Cyst fluid analysis for CEA and amylase levels should be performed on all cyst fluids, and is especially important in the interpretation of cyst fluids that are thin and not grossly mucoid and likely to have few cells. CEA levels above 200 ng/mL are reported to distinguish non-mucinous from mucinous cysts with very high levels of CEA correlating with malignancy.[123,147] Increasing the cut-off value for CEA increases the specificity but decreases the sensitivity of the test.[138] Amylase levels tend to be high in IPMN due to the connectivity of IPMN with the pancreatic duct, but amylase levels may also be high in MCN and pseudocysts so other factors need to be taken into consideration when making an overall interpretation. Molecular

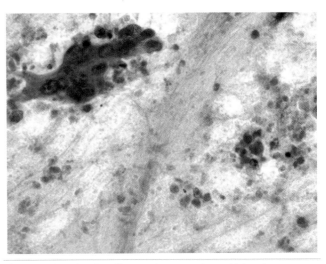

**Fig. 10.40** Intraductal papillary mucinous neoplasm with invasive carcinoma. Clusters of markedly atypical epithelial cells are present in a background of extracellular mucin and coagulative cellular necrosis (PAP).

**Fig. 10.38** Intraductal papillary mucinous neoplasm with moderate dysplasia. Even if very few and relatively bland appearing, recognising these tiny clusters and single epithelial cells with nuclear atypia and vacuolated cytoplasm signify a neoplastic mucinous cyst of at least moderate dysplasia (PAP).

- Obscuring inflammation, necrosis and debris
- GI contamination in EUS-guided aspirates
- Low CEA levels
- Peripancreatic cysts such as duplication cysts
- Secondarily cystic solid neoplasms.

## Mucinous cystic neoplasm (MCN)

MCN is a neoplastic mucin producing cyst that, in almost all cases, occurs in a female, does not communicate with the pancreatic ductal system, is lined by mucinous epithelial cells with varying degrees of atypia, and by definition contains subepithelial ovarian type stroma.[14] Most MCN occur in middle age (50 years old) and most are low grade.[127] All MCN are believed to eventually progress to malignancy if not resected, so complete surgical resection is the treatment of choice. Regardless of the atypia of the lining epithelium, like IPMN, the prognosis is directly related to the presence or absence of an invasive carcinoma.[3] Complete and thorough histological sampling is essential to rule out an invasive component given that these neoplasms tend to be very heterogeneous in their lining, and that an invasive component may not be apparent from gross inspection of the resected cyst. Complete resection of thoroughly evaluated, non-invasive cysts is considered curative.[3]

Radiologically the vast majority of MCN occur in the tail or body of the pancreas as solitary, isolated macrocystic masses (5–10 cm).[127,190] Multiloculation with visible septations and no connection to the pancreatic ductal system also support MCN. Larger macrocysts (>5 cm) with the radiological identification of peripheral eggshell calcifications in the cyst wall is considered specific for MCN and highly predictive of malignancy.[142]

On a pure cytological level, FNA of MCNs for all practical purposes are identical to those described above for IPMN. The subepithelial ovarian-type stroma typically is not appreciated on cytology smears. Unlike IPMN that can have different types of epithelium lining the cyst, the mucinous lining epithelium

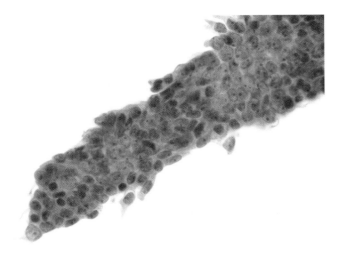

**Fig. 10.39** Intraductal papillary mucinous neoplasm with carcinoma *in situ*. This elongated group of epithelium twice as long as wide shows nuclear enlargement and crowding, open chromatin and nucleoli consistent with carcinoma. The background is free of inflammation and necrosis (PAP).

analysis of the cyst fluid demonstrating *KRAS* and LOH mutations also supports an interpretation of a mucinous cyst with malignancy correlating with elevated quantity DNA, *KRAS* 2-gene mutation and/or with numerous LOH mutations.[130,136] Further validation of the diagnostic utility of molecular testing of pancreatic cyst fluid is needed.

IPMN involving the main duct solely, or in combination with one or more branch duct cysts is relatively specific for radiological diagnosis. Branch duct IPMN most often need to be distinguished from pseudocysts, gastrointestinal duplication cysts, macrocystic serous cysts and secondarily cystic solid neoplasms, especially cystic endocrine neoplasms.[189]

### Diagnostic pitfalls: IPMN

- Scant and under-representative sample
- Thin or non-detectable mucin

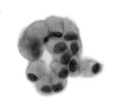

**Fig. 10.41** Mucinous cystic neoplasm with low-grade dysplasia. Low-grade epithelium displays small, round basal nuclei and cytoplasmic mucin that fills the cytoplasmic compartment in contrast to the apical mucin cup noted in foveolar cells that may contaminate the specimen as shown in Fig. 10.5B (PAP).

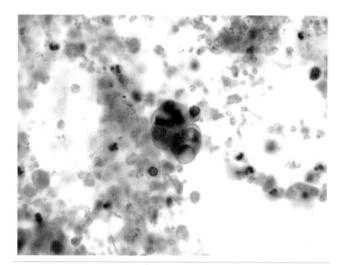

**Fig. 10.42** Mucinous cystic neoplasm with invasive carcinoma (mucinous cystadenocarcinoma). Cluster of malignant cells with irregular nuclear membranes residual mucin vacuoles in a background with coagulative necrosis supports the interpretation of malignancy (PAP).

of MCN is generally a single layer of uniform appearing columnar mucinous epithelium that increases in nuclear atypia with increasing grade of the neoplasm (Figs 10.41, 10.42). The cyst lining cells may become attenuated from pressure decreasing the mucinous appearance of the cells. Additionally, the lining of some MCN can become denuded yielding only cyst debris and foamy histiocytes and, as such, aspirates may be devoid of identifiable mucin and epithelial cells causing misdiagnosis as a pseudocyst or serous cyst. Transgastric FNA makes distinction of bland-appearing mucinous cyst lining epithelium and foveolar gastric epithelium difficult, if not impossible. Cyst fluid analysis is particularly important in this circumstance. Consideration of patient sex, cyst location and EUS features (the multimodal) can help to make the diagnosis more specific.

## Cytological findings: MCN

- Thick, colloid-like mucin with or without mucinous epithelium
- Thin, watery mucin
- Often low cellularity due to typically low-grade neoplasms
- Mucinous epithelium with mucin filling cytoplasmic space (low-grade neoplasms)
- Variable nuclear atypia, background inflammation and necrosis.

Biochemical analysis of the cyst fluid showing CEA levels above 200 ng/mL support the interpretation of a mucinous cyst and very high levels of CEA correlate with (but are not diagnostic of) malignancy.[147,155] Amylase levels may or may not be elevated in MCN.[155] Similar to IPMN, molecular analysis of the cyst fluid demonstrating *KRAS* 2-gene mutation and LOH mutations also supports an interpretation of a mucinous cyst with malignancy correlating with elevated quantity DNA and numerous mutations.[130,136]

## Diagnostic pitfalls: MCN

- Thin or undetectable mucin
- GI contamination in EUS-guided aspirates
- Low CEA levels
- Peripancreatic cysts such as duplication cysts
- Secondarily cystic solid neoplasms.

# The role of FNA in the management of pancreatic lesions

As pointed out in this chapter, the cytopathologist plays a critical role in the management of patients with pancreatic lesions. There is significant overlap in the clinical and radiological features of solid and cystic mass lesions of the pancreas precluding definitive management decisions based on clinical and radiological features alone in many cases.[19] Management options for patients are broad and dependent on many factors including patient age, symptoms, malignant potential of the lesion and co-morbid conditions of the patient that affect surgical risk.[12] These factors combined with our evolving knowledge of the biological behaviour and growth patterns of the many varied diseases of the pancreas have increasingly called for a pathological diagnosis prior to therapy.[14] Clinical management of patients with neoplastic cysts is based on the preoperative distinction of non-mucinous and mucinous cysts in general, and benign and malignant cysts in particular. Histological diagnosis often requires surgical intervention. A cytological diagnosis can be obtained with minimally invasive techniques that utilise CT, US or EUS. EUS-guided FNA is evolving as the diagnostic method of choice due to the higher resolution, shorter biopsy trajectory, decreased risk of tumour seeding and ability to more accurately stage the patient during a single procedure using EUS. Diagnostic accuracy with sufficiently high sensitivity and specificity depends on a multimodal team approach that combines the clinical and radiological patient information with the cytological impression and the results of ancillary studies.[15] A general diagnostic algorithm for the cytopathologist is outlined in Figure 10.43.

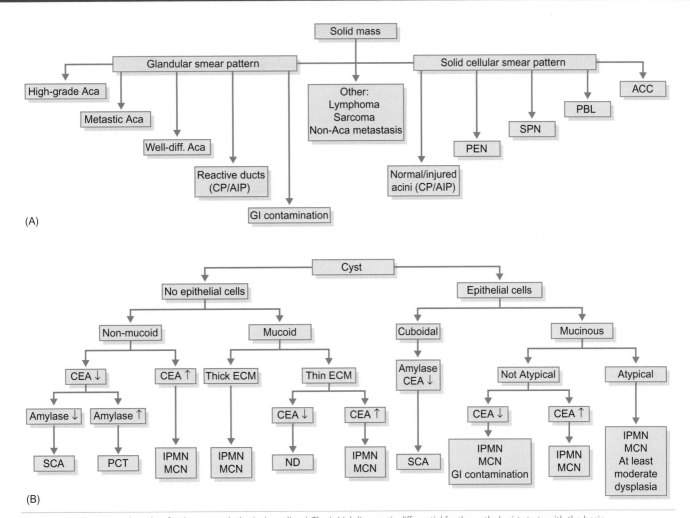

**Fig. 10.43** A diagnostic algorithm for the cytopathologist is outlined. The initial diagnostic differential for the pathologist starts with the basic information from the radiological image: Is the lesion (A) solid or (B) cystic? (A) Aca, adenocarcinoma; CP, chronic pancreatitis; AIP, autoimmune pancreatitis; GI, gastrointestinal; PEN, pancreatic endocrine neoplasm; SPN, solid pseudopapillary neoplasm; PBL, pancreatoblastoma; ACC, acinar cell carcinoma. (B) CEA, carcinoembryonic antigen; ECM, extracellular mucin; SCA, serous cystadenoma; PCT, pseudocyst; IPMN, intraductal papillary mucinous neoplasm; MCN, mucinous cystic neoplasm; ND, non-diagnostic; SCA, serous cystadenoma.

## REFERENCES

1. Parkin DM, Bray F, Ferlay J, et al. Estimating the world cancer burden: Globocan 2000. Int J Cancer 2001;94:153–56.

2. Ahlgren JD. Epidemiology and risk factors in pancreatic cancer. Semin Oncol 1996;23:241–50.

3. Hruban RH, Pitman MB, Klimstra DS. Tumors of the pancreas. In: Armed Forces Institutes of Pathology (eds.), Atlas of Tumor Pathology. Washington, DC: American Registry of Pathology 2007; 4th series: Fascicle 6.

4. Hartwig W, Schneider L, Diener MK, et al. Preoperative tissue diagnosis for tumours of the pancreas. Br J Surg 2009;96:5–20.

5. Goldin SB, Bradner MW, Zervos EE, et al. Assessment of pancreatic neoplasms: review of biopsy techniques. J Gastrointest Surg 2007;11:783–90.

6. Brugge WR. Cystic pancreatic lesions: can we diagnose them accurately what to look for? FNA marker molecular analysis resection, surveillance, or endoscopic treatment? Endoscopy 2006;38(Suppl 1):S40–7.

7. Fisher WE, Hodges SE, Yagnik V, et al. Accuracy of CT in predicting malignant potential of cystic pancreatic neoplasms. HPB (Oxford) 2008;10:483–90.

8. Peddu P, Quaglia A, Kane PA, et al. Role of imaging in the management of pancreatic mass. Crit Rev Oncol Hematol 2009;70:12–23.

9. Sachs T, Pratt WB, Callery MP, et al. The incidental asymptomatic pancreatic lesion: nuisance or threat? J Gastrointest Surg 2009;13:405–15.

10. Ouaissi M, Sielezneff I, Pirro N, et al. Pancreatic cancer and pancreaticoduodenectomy in elderly patient: morbidity and mortality are increased.

Is it the real life? Hepatogastroenterology 2008;55:2242–46.

11. Brugge WR, Lauwers GY, Sahani D, et al. Cystic Neoplasms of the Pancreas. N Engl J Med 2004;351:1218–26.

12. Spinelli KS, Fromwiller TE, Daniel RA, et al. Cystic pancreatic neoplasms: observe or operate. Ann Surg 2004;239:651–57. discussion 7–9.

13. Scheiman JM. Management of cystic lesions of the pancreas. J Gastrointest Surg 2008;12:405–7.

14. Tanaka M, Chari S, Adsay V, et al. International consensus guidelines for management of intraductal papillary mucinous neoplasms and mucinous cystic neoplasms of the pancreas. Pancreatology 2006;6:17–32.

15. Pitman MB, Deshpande V. Endoscopic ultrasound-guided fine needle aspiration

cytology of the pancreas: a morphological and multimodal approach to the diagnosis of solid and cystic mass lesions. Cytopathology 2007;18:331–47.

16. Sahani DV, Lin DJ, Venkatesan AM, et al. Multidisciplinary approach to diagnosis and management of intraductal papillary mucinous neoplasms of the pancreas. Clin Gastroenterol Hepatol 2009;7:259–69.

17. Horton KM, Fishman EK. Adenocarcinoma of the pancreas: CT imaging. Radiol Clin North Am 2002;40:1263–72.

18. Pappas S, Federle MP, Lokshin AE, et al. Early detection and staging of adenocarcinoma of the pancreas. Gastroenterol Clin North Am 2007;36:413–29.

19. Horwhat JD, Paulson EK, McGrath K, et al. A randomised comparison of EUS-guided FNA versus CT or US-guided FNA for the evaluation of pancreatic mass lesions. Gastrointest Endosc 2006;63:966–75.

20. Volmar KE, Vollmer RT, Jowell PS, et al. Pancreatic FNA in 1000 cases: a comparison of imaging modalities. Gastrointest Endosc 2005;61:854–61.

21. Wittmann J, Kocjan G, Sgouros SN, et al. Endoscopic ultrasound-guided tissue sampling by combined fine needle aspiration and Tru-Cut needle biopsy: a prospective study. Cytopathology 2006;17:27–33.

22. Leiman G. My approach to pancreatic fine needle aspiration. J Clin Pathol 2007;60:43–49.

23. Goodale RL, Gajl-Peczalska K, Dressel T, et al. Cytologic studies for the diagnosis of pancreatic cancer. Cancer 1981;47(Suppl):1652–55.

24. Lai R, Stanley MW, Bardales R, et al. Endoscopic ultrasound-guided pancreatic duct aspiration: diagnostic yield and safety. Endoscopy 2002;34:715–20.

25. Volmar KE, Vollmer RT, Routbort MJ, et al. Pancreatic and bile duct brushing cytology in 1000 cases: review of findings and comparison of preparation methods. Cancer 2006;108:231–38.

26. Klapman JB, Logrono R, Dye CE, et al. Clinical impact of on-site cytopathology interpretation on endoscopic ultrasound-guided fine needle aspiration. Am J Gastroenterol 2003;98:1289–94.

27. Jhala NC, Eltoum IA, Eloubeidi MA, et al. Providing on-site diagnosis of malignancy on endoscopic-ultrasound-guided fine-needle aspirates: should it be done? Ann Diagn Pathol 2007;11:176–81.

28. O'Toole D, Palazzo L, Arotcarena R, et al. Assessment of complications of EUS-guided fine-needle aspiration. Gastrointest Endosc 2001;53:470–74.

29. Eloubeidi M, Varadarajulu S, Desai S, et al. The negative predictive value of EUS-Guided FNA in patients with suspected pancreatic cancer. Gastrointest Endosc 2006;63:AB279.

30. Eloubeidi M, Chen V, Jhala N, et al. Endoscopic ultrasound-guided fine needle aspiration biopsy of suspected cholangiocarcinoma. Clin Gastroenterol Hepatol 2004;2:209–13.

31. Varadarajulu S, Eloubeidi MA. Frequency and significance of acute intracystic hemorrhage during EUS-FNA of cystic lesions of the pancreas. Gastrointest Endosc 2004;60:631–35.

32. Warshaw AL. Implications of peritoneal cytology for staging of early pancreatic cancer. Am J Surg 1991;161:26–29. discussion 9–30.

33. Leach SD, Rose JA, Lowy AM, et al. Significance of peritoneal cytology in patients with potentially resectable adenocarcinoma of the pancreatic head. Surgery 1995;118:472–78.

34. Mallery JS, Centeno BA, Hahn PF, et al. Pancreatic tissue sampling guided by EUS,

CT/US, and surgery: a comparison of sensitivity and specificity. Gastrointest Endosc 2002;56:218–24.

35. Chang KJ. Endoscopic ultrasound-guided fine needle aspiration in the diagnosis and staging of pancreatic tumors. Gastrointest Endosc Clin North Am 1995;5:723–34.

36. Erickson RA, Sayage-Rabie L, Avots-Avotins A. Clinical utility of endoscopic ultrasound-guided fine needle aspiration. Acta Cytol 1997;41:1647–53.

37. Faigel DO, Ginsberg GG, Bentz JS, et al. Endoscopic ultrasound-guided real-time fine-needle aspiration biopsy of the pancreas in cancer patients with pancreatic lesions. J Clin Oncol 1997;15:1439–43.

38. Bhutani MS, Hawes RH, Baron PL, et al. Endoscopic ultrasound guided fine needle aspiration of malignant pancreatic. Endoscopy 1997;29:854–58.

39. Bentz JS, Kochman ML, Faigel DO, et al. Endoscopic ultrasound-guided real-time fine-needle aspiration: clinicopathologic features of 60 patients. Diagn Cytopathol 1998;18:98–109.

40. Suits J, Frazee R, Erickson RA. Endoscopic ultrasound and fine needle aspiration for the evaluation of pancreatic masses. Arch Surg 1999;134:639–42. discussion 42–43.

41. Williams DB, Sahai AV, Aabakken L, et al. Endoscopic ultrasound guided fine needle aspiration biopsy: a large single centre experience. Gut 1999;44:720–26.

42. Sahai AV, Schembre D, Stevens PD, et al. A multicenter U.S. experience with EUS-guided fine-needle aspiration using the Olympus GF-UM30P echoendoscope: safety and effectiveness. Gastrointest Endosc 1999;50:792–96.

43. Erickson RA, Sayage-Rabie L, Beissner RS. Factors predicting the number of EUS-guided fine-needle passes for diagnosis of pancreatic malignancies. Gastrointest Endosc 2000;51:184–90.

44. Ylagan LR, Edmundowicz S, Kasal K, et al. Endoscopic ultrasound guided fine-needle aspiration cytology of pancreatic carcinoma: a 3-year experience and review of the literature. Cancer 2002;96:362–69.

45. Shin HJ, Lahoti S, Sneige N. Endoscopic ultrasound-guided fine-needle aspiration in 179 cases: the M. D. Anderson Cancer Center experience. Cancer 2002;96:174–80.

46. Eloubeidi MA, Jhala D, Chhieng DC, et al. Yield of endoscopic ultrasound-guided fine-needle aspiration biopsy in patients with suspected pancreatic carcinoma. Cancer 2003;99:285–92.

47. Frossard JL, Amouyal P, Amouyal G, et al. Performance of endosonography-guided fine needle aspiration and biopsy in the diagnosis of pancreatic cystic lesions. Am J Gastroenterol 2003;98:1516–24.

48. Eloubeidi MA, Tamhane A. EUS-guided FNA of solid pancreatic masses: a learning curve with 300 consecutive procedures. Gastrointest Endosc 2005;61:700–8.

49. Eloubeidi MA, Varadarajulu S, Desai S, et al. A prospective evaluation of an algorithm incorporating routine preoperative endoscopic ultrasound-guided fine needle aspiration in suspected pancreatic cancer. J Gastrointest Surg 2007;11:813–19.

50. Agrawal D, Moparty B, Brugge WR. EUS-FNA Cytology of Pancreatic Masses: Performance Characteristics Improve with Time (Nine Years) and Experience (712 Patients). Gastrointest Endosc 2007;65:AB306.

51. Jhala NC, Jhala D, Eltoum I, et al. Endoscopic ultrasound-guided fine-needle aspiration biopsy: a powerful tool to obtain samples from small lesions. Cancer 2004;102:239–46.

52. Brandwein SL, Farrell JJ, Centeno BA, et al. Detection and tumor staging of malignancy in cystic, intraductal, and solid tumors of the pancreas by EUS. Gastrointest Endosc 2001;53:722–27.

53. Logrono R, Kurtycz DF, Molina CP, et al. Analysis of false-negative diagnoses on endoscopic brush cytology of biliary and pancreatic duct strictures: the experience at 2 university hospitals. Arch Pathol Lab Med 2000;124:387–92.

54. Logrono R, Wong JY. Reporting the presence of significant epithelial atypia in pancreaticobiliary brush cytology specimens lacking evidence of obvious carcinoma: impact on performance measures. Acta Cytol 2004;48:613–21.

55. Nagle JA, Wilbur DC, Pitman MB. Cytomorphology of gastric and duodenal epithelium and reactivity to B72.3: a baseline for comparison to pancreatic lesions aspirated by EUS-FNAB. Diagn Cytopathol 2005;33:381–86.

56. Nawgiri RS, Nagle JA, Wilbur DC, et al. Cytomorphology and B72.3 labeling of benign and malignant ductal epithelium in pancreatic lesions compared to gastrointestinal epithelium. Diagn Cytopathol 2007;35:300–5.

57. Deshpande V, Mino-Kenudson M, Brugge WR, et al. Endoscopic ultrasound guided fine needle aspiration biopsy of autoimmune pancreatitis: diagnostic criteria and pitfalls. Am J Surg Pathol 2005;29:1464–71.

58. Stelow EB, Bardales RH, Lai R, et al. The cytological spectrum of chronic pancreatitis. Diagn Cytopathol 2005;32:65–69.

59. Finkelberg DL, Sahani D, Deshpande V, et al. Autoimmune pancreatitis. N Engl J Med 2006;355:2670–76.

60. Chari ST, Smyrk TC, Levy MJ, et al. Diagnosis of autoimmune pancreatitis: the Mayo Clinic experience. Clin Gastroenterol Hepatol 2006;4:1010–16. quiz 934..

61. Mithofer K, Mueller PR, Warshaw AL. Interventional and surgical treatment of pancreatic abscess. World J Surg 1997;21:162–68.

62. Loya AC, Prayaga AK, Sundaram C, et al. Cytologic diagnosis of pancreatic tuberculosis in immunocompetent and immunocompromised patients: a report of 2 cases. Acta Cytol 2005;49:97–100.

63. Aaltonen LA, Hamilton SR. International Agency for Research on Cancer. Pathology and Genetics of Tumours of the Digestive System. World Health Organization. Oxford: Oxford University Press; 2000.

64. Gangi S, Fletcher J, Nathan M. Time interval between abnormalities seen on CT and the Clinical diagnosis of pancreatic cancer: Retrospective review of CT scans obtained before diagnosis. AJR Am J Roentgenol 2004;182:897–903.

65. Robins DB, Katz RL, Evans DB, et al. Fine needle aspiration of the pancreas. In quest of accuracy. Acta Cytol 1995;39:1–10.

66. Lin F, Staerkel G. Cytologic criteria for well-differentiated adenocarcinoma of the pancreas in fine-needle aspiration biopsy specimens. Cancer 2003;99:44–50.

67. Hysell C, Belsley NVD. EUS guided fine needle aspiration biopsies of solid ductal adenocarcinomas of the pancreas: a critical look at the atypical and suspicious categories. Cancer 2007;111:351.

68. Mitchell ML, Carney CN. Cytologic criteria for the diagnosis of pancreatic carcinoma. Am J Clin Pathol 1985;83:171–76.

69. Adsay V, Logani S, Sarkar F, et al. Foamy gland pattern of pancreatic ductal adenocarcinoma:

a deceptively benign-appearing variant. Am J Surg Pathol 2000;24:493–504.

70. Stelow EB, Pambuccian SE, Bardales RH, et al. The cytology of pancreatic foamy gland adenocarcinoma. Am J Clin Pathol 2004;121:893–97.

71. Merchant N, Berlin J. Past and future of pancreas cancer: are we ready to move forward together? J Clin Oncol 2008;26:3478–80.

72. Evans DB, Varadhachary GR, Crane CH, et al. Preoperative gemcitabine-based chemoradiation for patients with resectable adenocarcinoma of the pancreatic head. J Clin Oncol 2008;26:3496–502.

73. Maluf-Filho F, Kumar A, Gerhardt R, et al. K-ras mutation analysis of fine needle aspirate under EUS guidance facilitates risk stratification of patients with pancreatic mass. J Clin Gastroenterol 2007;41:906–10.

74. van Heek T, Rader AE, Offerhaus GJ, et al. K-ras, p53, and DPC4 (MAD4) alterations in fine-needle aspirates of the pancreas: a molecular panel correlates with and supplements cytologic diagnosis. Am J Clin Pathol 2002;117:755–65.

75. Shen J, Cibas ES, Qian X. The immunohistochemical expression pattern of SMAD4, p53, and CDX2 is helpful in diagnosing pancreatic ductal adenocarcinoma in endoscopic ultrasound-guided fine needle aspirations (EUS-FNA). Mod Pathol 2007;20(Suppl. 2):83A.

76. Ali S, Cohen C, Little JV, et al. The utility of SMAD4 as a diagnostic immunohistochemical marker for pancreatic adenocarcinoma, and its expression in other solid tumors. Diagn Cytopathol 2007;35:644–48.

77. Chhieng DC, Benson E, Eltoum I, et al. MUC1 and MUC2 expression in pancreatic ductal carcinoma obtained by fine-needle aspiration. Cancer 2003;99:365–71.

78. Giorgadze TA, Peterman H, Baloch ZW, et al. Diagnostic utility of mucin profile in fine-needle aspiration specimens of the pancreas: an immunohistochemical study with surgical pathology correlation. Cancer 2006;108:186–97.

79. McCarthy DM, Maitra A, Argani P, et al. Novel markers of pancreatic adenocarcinoma in fine-needle aspiration: mesothelin and prostate stem cell antigen labeling increases accuracy in cytologically borderline cases. Appl Immunohistochem Mol Morphol 2003;11:238–43.

80. Baruch AC, Wang H, Staerkel GA, et al. Immunocytochemical study of the expression of mesothelin in fine-needle aspiration biopsy specimens of pancreatic adenocarcinoma. Diagn Cytopathol 2007;35:143–47.

81. Deng H, Shi J, Wilkerson M, et al. Usefulness of S100P in diagnosis of adenocarcinoma of pancreas on fine-needle aspiration biopsy specimens. Am J Clin Pathol 2008;129:81–88.

82. Layfield LJ, Bentz J. Giant-cell containing neoplasms of the pancreas: an aspiration cytology study. Diagn Cytopathol 2008;36:238–44.

83. Sakai Y, Kupelioglu AA, Yanagisawa A, et al. Origin of giant cells in osteoclast-like giant cell tumors of the pancreas. Hum Pathol 2000;31:1223–29.

84. Molberg KH, Heffess C, Delgado R, et al. Undifferentiated carcinoma with osteoclast-like giant cells of the pancreas and periampullary region. Cancer 1998;82:1279–87.

85. Kardon DE, Thompson LD, Przygodzki RM, et al. Adenosquamous carcinoma of the pancreas: a clinicopathologic series of 25 cases. Mod Pathol 2001;14:443–51.

86. Rahemtullah A, Misdraji J, Pitman MB. Adenosquamous carcinoma of the pancreas:

cytologic features in 14 cases. Cancer 2003;99:372–78.

87. Layfield LJ, Bentz JS, Gopez EV. Immediate on-site interpretation of fine-needle aspiration smears. A cost and compensation analysis. Cancer (Cancer Cytopathol) 2001;93:319–22.

88. Seidel G, Zahurak M, Iacobuzio-Donahue C, et al. Almost all infiltrating colloid carcinomas of the pancreas and periampullary region arise from *in situ* papillary neoplasms: a study of 39 cases. Am J Surg Pathol 2002;26:56–63.

89. Klimstra DS, Heffess CS, Oertel JE, et al. Acinar cell carcinoma of the pancreas. A clinicopathologic study of 28 cases. Am J Surg Pathol 1992;16:815–37.

90. Labate AM, Klimstra DL, Zakowski MF. Comparative cytologic features of pancreatic acinar cell and islet cell tumor. Diagn Cytopathol 1997;16:112–16.

91. Stelow EB, Bardales RH, Shami VM, et al. Cytology of pancreatic acinar cell carcinoma. Diagn Cytopathol 2006;34:367–72.

92. Pitman MB, Faquin WC. The fine-needle aspiration biopsy cytology of pancreatoblastoma. Diagn Cytopathol 2004;31:402–6.

93. Klimstra DS, Wenig BM, Adair CF, et al. Pancreatoblastoma. A clinicopathologic study and review of the literature. Am J Surg Pathol 1995;19:1371–89.

94. Capella C, Oberg K, Papotti M, et al. Pancreatic endocrine tumours: mixed exocrine-endocrine carcinomas. In: DeLellis RA, Lloyd RV, Heitz PU, Eng C, editors World Health Organization Classification of Tumours Pathology and genetics of tumours of endocrine organs. Lyon: IARC Press; 2004. p. 205–6.

95. Vagefi PA, Razo O, Deshpande V, et al. Evolving patterns in the detection and outcomes of pancreatic neuroendocrine neoplasms: the Massachusetts General Hospital experience from 1977 to 2005. Arch Surg 2007;142:347–54.

96. Nodit L, McGrath KM, Zahid M, et al. Endoscopic ultrasound-guided fine needle aspirate microsatellite loss analysis and pancreatic endocrine tumor outcome. Clin Gastroenterol Hepatol 2006;4:1474–78.

97. Ligneau B, Lombard-Bohas C, Partensky C. Cystic endocrine tumors of the pancreas: clinical, radiologic and histopathological features in 13 cases. Am J Surg Pathol 2001;25:752–60.

98. Ordonez NG, Silva EG. Islet cell tumour with vacuolated lipid-rich cytoplasm: a new histological variant of islet cell tumour. Histopathology 1997;31:157–60.

99. Pacchioni D, Papotti M, Macri L, et al. Pancreatic oncocytic endocrine tumors. Cytologic features of two cases. Acta Cytol 1996;40:742–46.

100. Hoang MP, Hruban RH, Albores-Saavedra J. Clear cell endocrine pancreatic tumor mimicking renal cell carcinoma: a distinctive neoplasm of von Hippel–Lindau disease. Am J Surg Pathol 2001;25:602–9.

101. Singh R, Basturk O, Klimstra DS, et al. Lipid-rich variant of pancreatic endocrine neoplasms. Am J Surg Pathol 2006;30:194–200.

102. Bell DA. Cytologic features of islet-cell tumors. Acta Cytol 1987;31:485–92.

103. Collins BT, Cramer HM. Fine-needle aspiration cytology of islet cell tumors. Diagn Cytopathol 1996;15:37–45.

104. Jimenez-Heffernan JA, Vicandi B, Lopez-Ferrer P, et al. Fine needle aspiration cytology of endocrine neoplasms of the pancreas. Morphologic and immunocytochemical findings in 20 cases. Acta Cytol 2004;48:295–301.

105. Gu M, Ghafari S, Lin F, et al. Cytological diagnosis of endocrine tumors of the pancreas by endoscopic ultrasound-guided fine-needle aspiration biopsy. Diagn Cytopathol 2005;32:204–10.

106. Chang F, Vu C, Chandra A, et al. Endoscopic ultrasound-guided fine needle aspiration cytology of pancreatic neuroendocrine tumours: cytomorphological and immunocytochemical evaluation. Cytopathology 2006;17:10–17.

107. Zee SY, Hochwald SN, Conlon KC, et al. Pleomorphic pancreatic endocrine neoplasms: a variant commonly confused with adenocarcinoma. Am J Surg Pathol 2005;29:1194–200.

108. Young NA, Mody DR, Davey DD. Misinterpretation of normal cellular elements in fine-needle aspiration biopsy specimens: observations from the College of American Pathologists Interlaboratory Comparison Program in Non-Gynecologic Cytopathology. Arch Pathol Lab Med 2002;126:670–75.

109. Berkel S, Hummel F, Gaa J, et al. Poorly-differentiated small cell carcinoma of the pancreas. A case report and review of the literature. Pancreatology 2004;4:521–26.

110. Reyes CV, Wang T. Undifferentiated small cell carcinoma of the pancreas: a report of five cases. Cancer 1981;47:2500–2.

111. Martin RC, Klimstra DS, Brennan MF, et al. Solid pseudopapillary tumor of the pancreas: a surgical enigma? Ann Surg Oncol 2002;9:35–40.

112. Tang LH, Aydin H, Brennan MF, et al. Clinically aggressive solid pseudopapillary tumors of the pancreas: a report of two cases with components of undifferentiated carcinoma and a comparative clinicopathologic analysis of 34 conventional cases. Am J Surg Pathol 2005;29:512–19.

113. Naresh KN, Borges AM, Chinoy RF, et al. Solid and papillary epithelial neoplasm of the pancreas. Diagnosis by fine needle aspiration cytology in four cases. Acta Cytol 1995;39:489–93.

114. Pelosi G, Iannucci A, Zamboni G, et al. Solid and cystic papillary neoplasm of the pancreas: a clinico-cytopathologic and immunocytochemical study of five new cases diagnosed by fine-needle aspiration cytology and a review of the literature. Diagn Cytopathol 1995;13:233–46.

115. Bardales RH, Centeno B, Mallery JS, et al. Endoscopic ultrasound-guided fine-needle aspiration cytology diagnosis of solid pseudopapillary tumor of the pancreas: a rare neoplasm of elusive origin but characteristic cytomorphologic features. Am J Clin Pathol 2004;121:654–62.

116. Pettinato G, Di Vizio D, Manivel JC, et al. Solid pseudopapillary tumor of the pancreas: a neoplasm with distinct and highly characteristic cytological features. Diagn Cytopathol 2002;27:325–34.

117. Kim MJ, Jang SJ, Yu E. Loss of E-cadherin and cytoplasmic-nuclear expression of beta-catenin are the most useful immunoprofiles in the diagnosis of solid pseudopapillary neoplasm of the pancreas. Hum Pathol 2008;39:251–58.

118. Thompson LD, Heffess CS. Renal cell carcinoma to the pancreas in surgical pathology material. Cancer 2000;89:1076–88.

119. Volmar KE, Routbort MJ, Jones CK, et al. Primary pancreatic lymphoma evaluated by fine-needle aspiration: findings in 14 cases. Am J Clin Pathol 2004;121:898–903.

120. Mallery JS, Centeno BA, Hahn P, et al. Pancreatic tissue sampling guided by EUS, CT/US, and surgery: a comparison of

sensitivity and specificity. Gastrointest Endosc 2002;56:218–24.

121. Eloubeidi M, Chen V, Eltoum I, et al. Endoscopic ultrasound-guided fine needle aspiration biopsy of patients with suspected pancreatic cancer: diagnostic accuracy and acute and 30-day complications. Am J Gastroenterol 2003;98:2663–68.

122. Brugge WR. Role of endoscopic ultrasound in the diagnosis of cystic lesions of the pancreas. Pancreatology 2001;1:637–40.

123. Brugge WR, Lauwers GY, Sahani D, et al. Cystic neoplasms of the pancreas. N Engl J Med 2004;351:1218–26.

124. Lee LS, Saltzman JR, Bounds BC, et al. EUS-guided fine needle aspiration of pancreatic cysts: a retrospective analysis of complications and their predictors. Clin Gastroenterol Hepatol 2005;3:231–36.

125. Adsay NV. Cystic neoplasia of the pancreas: pathology and biology. J Gastrointest Surg 2008;12:401–4.

126. Gan SI, Thompson CC, Lauwers GY, et al. Ethanol lavage of pancreatic cystic lesions: initial pilot study. Gastrointest Endosc 2005;61:746–52.

127. Crippa S, Salvia R, Warshaw AL, et al. Mucinous cystic neoplasm of the pancreas is not an aggressive entity: lessons from 163 resected patients. Ann Surg 2008;247:571–79.

128. Liao T, Velanovich V. Asymptomatic pancreatic cysts: a decision analysis approach to observation versus resection. Pancreas 2007;35:243–48.

129. Van Heek T, Rader A, Offerhaus G. K-ras, p53, and DPC4 (MAD4) alterations in fine-needle aspirates of the pancreas: a molecular panel correlates with and supplements cytologic diagnosis. Am J Surg Oncol 2002;117:755–65.

130. Khalid A, McGrath KM, Zahid M, et al. The role of pancreatic cyst fluid molecular analysis in predicting cyst pathology. Clin Gastroenterol Hepatol 2005;3:967–73.

131. Buchholz M, Kestler HA, Bauer A, et al. Specialised DNA arrays for the differentiation of pancreatic tumors. Clin Cancer Res 2005;11:8048–54.

132. Fukushima N, Walter KM, Uek T, et al. Diagnosing pancreatic cancer using methylation specific PCR analysis of pancreatic juice. Cancer Biol Ther 2003;2:78–83.

133. Pearson AS, Chiao P, Zhang L, et al. The detection of telomerase activity in patients with adenocarcinoma of the pancreas by fine needle aspiration. Int J Oncol 2000;17:381–85.

134. Tada M, Komatsu Y, Kawabe T, et al. Quantitative analysis of K-ras gene mutation in pancreatic tissue obtained by endoscopic ultrasonography-guided fine needle aspiration: clinical utility for diagnosis of pancreatic tumor. Am J Gastroenterol 2002;97:2263–70.

135. Michaels PJ, Brachtel EF, Bounds BC, et al. Intraductal papillary mucinous neoplasm of the pancreas: cytologic features predict histologic grade. Cancer 2006;108:163–73.

136. Shen J, Brugge WR, Dimaio CJ, et al. Molecular analysis of pancreatic cyst fluid: a comparative analysis with current practice of diagnosis. Cancer Cytopathol 2009;117:217–27.

137. Alsibai KD, Denis B, Bottlaender J, et al. Impact of cytopathologist expert on diagnosis and treatment of pancreatic lesions in current clinical practice. A series of 106 endoscopic ultrasound-guided fine needle aspirations. Cytopathology 2006;17:18–26.

138. van der Waaij LA, van Dullemen HM, Porte RJ. Cyst fluid analysis in the differential diagnosis of pancreatic cystic lesions: a pooled analysis. Gastrointest Endosc 2005;62:383–89.

139. Jacobson BC, Baron TH, Adler DG, et al. ASGE guideline: The role of endoscopy in the diagnosis and the management of cystic lesions and inflammatory fluid collections of the pancreas. Gastrointest Endosc 2005;61:363–70.

140. Brugge WR. Should all pancreatic cystic lesions be resected? Cyst-fluid analysis in the differential diagnosis of pancreatic cystic lesions: a meta-analysis. Gastrointest Endosc 2005;62:390–91.

141. Brugge WR, Lewandrowski K, Lee-Lewandrowski E, et al. Diagnosis of pancreatic cystic neoplasms: a report of the cooperative pancreatic cyst study. Gastroenterology 2004;126:1330–36.

142. Sahani DV, Kadavigere R, Saokar A, et al. Cystic pancreatic lesions: a simple imaging-based classification system for guiding management. Radiographics 2005;25:1471–84.

143. Sarr MG, Murr M, Smyrk TC, et al. Primary cystic neoplasms of the pancreas. Neoplastic disorders of emerging importance-current state-of-the-art and unanswered questions. J Gastrointest Surg 2003;7:417–28.

144. Volmar KE, Creager AJ. Fine needle aspiration of pancreatic cysts: Use of ancillary studies and difficulty in identifying surgical candidates. Acta Cytol 2006;50:647–55.

145. Fernandez-del Castillo C, Targarona J, Thayer SP, et al. Incidental pancreatic cysts: clinicopathologic characteristics and comparison with symptomatic patients. Arch Surg 2003;138:423–27. discussion 33–34.

146. Ryu JK, Woo SM, Hwang JH, et al. Cyst fluid analysis for the differential diagnosis of pancreatic cysts. Diagn Cytopathol 2004;31:100–5.

147. Linder JD, Geenen JE, Catalano MF. Cyst fluid analysis obtained by EUS-guided FNA in the evaluation of discrete cystic neoplasms of the pancreas: a prospective single-center experience. Gastrointest Endosc 2006;64:697–702.

148. Pitman MB. The pancreas. In: Sidawy M, Ali S, editors Fine Needle Aspiration Cytology. Philadelphia: Churchill Livingstone; 2007.

149. Khalid A, Finkelstein S, McGrath K. Molecular diagnosis of solid and cystic lesions of the pancreas. Gastroenterol Clin North Am 2004;33:891–906.

150. Schoedel KE, Finkelstein SD, Ohori NP. K-Ras and microsatellite marker analysis of fine-needle aspirates from intraductal papillary mucinous neoplasms of the pancreas. Diagn Cytopathol 2006;34:605–8.

151. Aghdassi A, Mayerle J, Kraft M, et al. Diagnosis and treatment of pancreatic pseudocysts in chronic pancreatitis. Pancreas 2008;36:105–12.

152. Barthet M, Lamblin G, Gasmi M, et al. Clinical usefulness of a treatment algorithm for pancreatic pseudocysts. Gastrointest Endosc 2008;67:245–52.

153. Kloppel G. Pseudocysts and other non-neoplastic cysts of the pancreas. Semin Diagnost Pathol 2000;17:7–15.

154. Nagle J, Wilbur DC, Pitman MD. The cytomorphology of gastric and duodenal epithelium and reactivity to B72.3: A baseline for comparison to pancreatic neoplasms aspirated by EUS-FNAB. Diagn Cytopathol 2005;33:381–86.

155. Brugge WR. Evaluation of pancreatic cystic lesions with EUS. Gastrointest Endosc 2004;59:698–707.

156. Adsay NV, Hasteh F, Cheng JD, et al. Lymphoepithelial cysts of the pancreas: a report of 12 cases and a review of the literature. Mod Pathol 2002;15:492–501.

157. Nasr J, Sanders M, Fasanella K, et al. Lymphoepithelial cysts of the pancreas:

an EUS case series. Gastrointest Endosc 2008;68:170–73.

158. Centeno BA, Stockwell JW, Lewandrowski KB. Cyst fluid cytology and chemical features in a case of lymphoepithelial cyst of the pancreas: a rare and difficult preoperative diagnosis. Diagn Cytopathol 1999;21:328–30.

159. Liu J, Shin HJ, Rubenchik I, et al. Cytologic features of lymphoepithelial cyst of the pancreas: two preoperatively diagnosed cases based on fine-needle aspiration. Diagn Cytopathol 1999;21:346–50.

160. Servais EL, Sarkaria IS, Solomon GJ, et al. Giant epidermoid cyst within an intrapancreatic accessory spleen mimicking a cystic neoplasm of the pancreas: case report and review of the literature. Pancreas 2008;36:98–100.

161. Centeno BA, Pitman MB. Fine Needle Aspiration Biopsy of the Pancreas. Boston: Butterworth-Heinemann; 1999.

162. Mohr VH, Vortmeyer AO, Zhuang Z, et al. Histopathology and molecular genetics of multiple cysts and microcystic (serous) adenomas of the pancreas in von Hippel-Lindau patients. Am J Pathol 2000;157:1615–21.

163. Strobel O, Z'Graggen K, Schmitz-Winnenthal FH, et al. Risk of malignancy in serous cystic neoplasms of the pancreas. Digestion 2003;68:24–33.

164. Compton CC. Serous cystic tumors of the pancreas. Semin Diagn Pathol 2000;17:43–55.

165. Reese SA, Traverso LW, Jacobs TW, et al. Solid serous adenoma of the pancreas: a rare variant within the family of pancreatic serous cystic neoplasms. Pancreas 2006;33:96–99.

166. Tseng JF, Warshaw AL, Sahani DV, et al. Serous cystadenoma of the pancreas: tumor growth rates and recommendations for treatment. Annals of Surgery 2005;242:413–19. discussion 9–21.

167. Galanis C, Zamani A, Cameron JL, et al. Resected serous cystic neoplasms of the pancreas: a review of 158 patients with recommendations for treatment. J Gastrointest Surg 2007;11:820–26.

168. Lee SE, Kwon Y, Jang JY, et al. The morphological classification of a serous cystic tumor (SCT) of the pancreas and evaluation of the preoperative diagnostic accuracy of computed tomography. Ann Surg Oncol 2008;15:2089–95.

169. Bassi C, Salvia R, Molinari E, et al. Management of 100 consecutive cases of pancreatic serous cystadenoma: wait for symptoms and see at imaging or vice versa? World J Surg 2003;27:319–23.

170. Colonna J, Plaza JA, Frankel WL, et al. Serous cystadenoma of the pancreas: clinical and pathological features in 33 patients. Pancreatology 2008;8:135–41.

171. O'Toole D, Palazzo L, Hammel P, et al. Macrocystic pancreatic cystadenoma: the role of EUS and cyst fluid analysis in distinguishing mucinous and serous lesions. Gastrointest Endosc 2004;59:823–29.

172. Curry CA, Eng J, Horton KM, et al. CT of primary cystic pancreatic neoplasms: can CT be used for patient triage and treatment? AJR Am J Roentgenol 2000;175:99–103.

173. Ahmad NA, Kochman ML, Brensinger C, et al. Interobserver agreement among endosonographers for the diagnosis of neoplastic versus non-neoplastic pancreatic cystic lesions. Gastrointest Endosc 2003;58:59–64.

174. Belsley NA, Pitman MB, Lauwers GY, et al. Serous cystadenoma of the pancreas: limitations and pitfalls of endoscopic

ultrasound-guided fine-needle aspiration biopsy. Cancer 2008;114:102–10.

175. Huang P, Staerkel G, Sneige N, et al. Fine-needle aspiration of pancreatic serous cystadenoma: cytologic features and diagnostic pitfalls. Cancer 2006;108:239–49.

176. Silas AM, Morrin MM, Raptopoulos V, et al. Intraductal papillary mucinous tumors of the pancreas. AJR Am J Roentgenol 2001;176:179–85.

177. Kawamoto S, Lawler LP, Horton KM, et al. MDCT of intraductal papillary mucinous neoplasm of the pancreas: evaluation of features predictive of invasive carcinoma. AJR Am J Roentgenol 2006;186:687–95.

178. Yamaguchi K, Tanaka M. Mucin-hypersecreting tumor of the pancreas with mucin extrusion through an enlarged papilla. Am J Gastroenterol 1991;86:835–39.

179. Kobari M, Egawa S, Shibuya K, et al. Intraductal papillary mucinous tumors of the pancreas comprise 2 clinical subtypes: differences in clinical characteristics and surgical management. Arch Surg 1999;134:1131–36.

180. Sohn TA, Yeo CJ, Cameron JL, et al. Intraductal papillary mucinous neoplasms of the pancreas: an updated experience. Ann Surg 2004;239:788–97. discussion 97–99.

181. Pitman MB, Michaels PJ, Deshpande V, et al. Cytological and cyst fluid analysis of small (< or =3 cm) branch duct intraductal papillary mucinous neoplasms adds value to patient management decisions. Pancreatology 2008;8:277–84.

182. Adsay NV, Merati K, Basturk O, et al. Pathologically and biologically distinct types of epithelium in intraductal papillary mucinous neoplasms: delineation of an 'intestinal' pathway of carcinogenesis in the pancreas. Am J Surg Pathol 2004;28:839–48.

183. Layfield LJ, Cramer H. Fine-needle aspiration cytology of intraductal papillary-mucinous tumors: a retrospective analysis. Diagn Cytopathol 2005;32:16–20.

184. Dodd LG, Farrell TA, Layfield LJ. Mucinous cystic tumor of the pancreas: an analysis of FNA characteristics with an emphasis on the spectrum of malignancy associated features. Diagn Cytopathol 1995;12:113–19.

185. Recine M, Kaw M, Evans DB, et al. Fine-needle aspiration cytology of mucinous tumors of the pancreas. Cancer 2004;102:92–99.

186. Sole M, Iglesias C, Fernandez-Esparrach G, et al. Fine-needle aspiration cytology of intraductal papillary mucinous tumors of the pancreas. Cancer 2005;105:298–303.

187. Emerson RE, Randolph ML, Cramer HM. Endoscopic ultrasound-guided fine-needle aspiration cytology diagnosis of intraductal papillary mucinous neoplasm of the pancreas is highly predictive of pancreatic neoplasia. Diagn Cytopathol 2006;34:457–62.

188. Lau SK, Lewandrowski KB, Brugge WR, et al. Diagnostic significance of mucin in fine needle aspiration samples of pancreatic cysts. Mod Pathol 2000;13:48A.

189. Bordeianou L, Vagefi PA, Sahani D, et al. Cystic pancreatic endocrine neoplasms: a distinct tumor type? J Am Coll Surg 2008;206:1154–58.

190. Sarr MG, Carpenter HA, Prabhakar LP, et al. Clinical and pathologic correlation of 84 mucinous cystic neoplasms of the pancreas: can one reliably differentiate benign from malignant (or premalignant) neoplasms? Ann Surg 2000;231:205–12.

# Section 7

## Kidney and Urinary Tract

# Kidney and retroperitoneal tissues

Beatrix Cochand-Priollet

## Chapter contents

## Introduction

As is apparent throughout this third edition of *Diagnostic Cytopathology*, fine needle aspiration (FNA) cytology of deep-seated organs is an extremely useful technique, widely used especially preoperatively to ensure that the patient is given the most appropriate treatment. However, long-term results over a number of years show that FNA has been less successful for the kidney than for other organs.

About 20 years ago, renal FNA was rarely considered worthwhile because tumours were very large when discovered, requiring total nephrectomy whatever the final diagnosis. Preoperative diagnoses are more frequently required now, as many renal tumours are incidental, discovered on ultrasound or CT scan (Fig. 11.1) and usually detected as small masses in asymptomatic patients.[1,2] Even so, microbiopsies are often preferred to FNA, as highlighted by a number of recently published series,[3–11] sometimes associated with cytological analysis, but more often not.

However, renal FNA is a safe method, providing accurate results with high levels of sensitivity and specificity when performed by well-trained, skilled cytopathologists.[12–14] The diagnostic accuracy of FNA has been shown to range from 70% to 100%,[12,13] whereas its specificity ranges from 91.9% to 99% and its sensitivity from 80% to 94%.[12,14] Only a few series of renal FNA analyses have been published over the last 10 years, the largest of which include 180 and 108 cases,[13,14] with most consisting of less than 20 cases or even of reports of single cases.

We have chosen to follow the 2004 World Health Organization classification for the cytological description of the different tumours (see Box 11.1). This classification is based on the correlation between results for morphological analysis, immunohistochemistry, electron microscopy, cytogenetics and molecular genetics.[15] Some of the tumours are quite rare and have not yet been described cytologically, although illustrated in histological textbooks. These tumours will not be discussed in this chapter.

## Indications and contraindications for FNA of kidney

For solid renal masses, the indications include:

- To establish the diagnosis, and especially the malignant potential, of a renal tumour that cannot be resected due to its size or the patient's inability to tolerate surgery, or because there are already metastases at the time of diagnosis
- To make a diagnosis of a metastasis or diagnose a second primary renal tumour in the presence of an already known cancer
- To decide on the surgical strategy in cases of small tumours located at the upper or lower poles of the kidney (whether partial or total nephrectomy or non-surgical treatment)[2]
- To select small benign renal neoplasms in order to facilitate optimal patient management.[16]

For cystic lesions of the kidney, FNA is virtually always indicated in order to eliminate or confirm malignancy.[17]

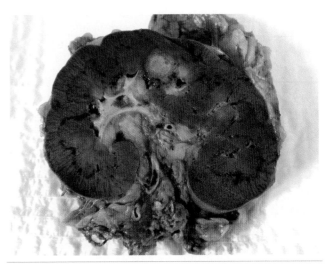

**Fig. 11.1** Tumour 1.4 cm in diameter discovered incidentally on CT scan.

Contraindications are in general the same as those for FNA of other deep-seated organs. In addition though, FNA is contraindicated in patients with only one kidney.

## FNA technique

In the past, radiological investigations included intravenous pyelography, angiography, ultrasonography, computed tomography and magnetic resonance imaging. Nowadays, contrast enhanced sonography and PET/computed tomography are likely to be used as they are more efficient techniques.[18–20] Renal arteriography is no longer the procedure of choice for the evaluation of renal masses. These investigations are very useful for detecting renal masses, to appreciate their solid or cystic/partially cystic appearance, to detect an extension into the surrounding adipose tissue or renal pelvis as well as extension into the renal vein. However, there are very few cases where radiological techniques can specify the histological type of the tumour, apart from angiomyolipoma if this mixed tumour includes a substantial component of adipose tissue. In order to determine the histological type of a renal tumour, cytological or histological material has to be available.

Renal FNAs are usually performed with a 23–25-gauge needle attached to a 20 mL syringe. When aspiration is completed the cytological material is usually expelled directly onto slides in order to obtain air-dried smears for staining with Diff-Quik or May–Grünwald Giemsa (MGG) and some alcohol-fixed smears to be stained by the Papanicolaou (PAP) method. Liquid-based preparation is also widely used, rinsing the needle directly into an appropriate preservative (Hologic® or Tripath Imaging®). For cystic lesions, centrifugation is recommended with cytospin slides then prepared for both Diff-Quik and PAP staining.

Cell block preparation is a valuable technique for FNA of deep-seated organs. It offers the opportunity to obtain some embedded cytological material previously fixed with formalin and recovered after centrifugation or to include some very small hardly discernible fragments of tissue. Tissue sections obtained from these cell blocks may be stained by haematoxylin and eosin or may be used for histochemistry as well as immunohistochemistry. These ancillary techniques are useful in selected cases and may replace core biopsy material.

Complications that may occur include transient haematuria, haemorrhage with pain, pneumothorax or infection. Some cases of cutaneous seeding have been reported in the past but none have been published recently, probably due to improvements in FNA technique. Very rare cases of massive tumour infarction have also been reported.[21]

## The unsatisfactory specimen

This category has rarely been described in detail and even though most articles give a percentage of unsatisfactory specimens, ranging from 5% to 21%, yet the criteria used are not adequately reported. A few authors have tried to validate some criteria considered as helpful guidelines.[13] These are summarised as follows:

- An adequate sample from a solid mass has to contain 'representative material,' that is a large number of

**Table 11.1** Cytological features of normal renal cells

|  | Cellular arrangement | Nuclear pattern | Cytoplasmic features |
|---|---|---|---|
| Tubular cells | Usually small flat of cells | Round, regular nuclei, | Well-defined cell borders |
|  | Rarely isolated cells | Small nucleoli, |  |
|  |  | Anisokaryosis may be observed |  |
| Glomerules | Three-dimensional groups of cells | Small regular nuclei | Scant cytoplasm |
|  | Sometimes tiny blood vessels |  |  |

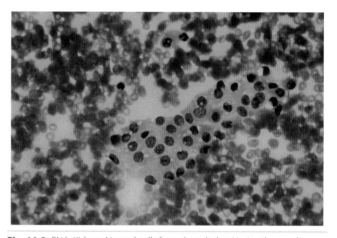

**Fig. 11.2** FNA: Kidney. Normal cells from the tubules. Notice the regular round nuclei (MGG).

well-preserved cells, but they should not be normal cells and must present the characteristics and features of a diagnostic category
- A cyst fluid aspirate, even if devoid of cells, is not necessarily unsatisfactory
- Normal cells are quite often observed in kidney FNAs and these must be identified in order to avoid any confusion with abnormal or tumour cells. These normal cells are described in Table 11.1 (Fig. 11.2).

## Malignant tumours of kidney

Renal cell carcinomas (RCC) represent over 90% of all malignancies in the kidney that occur in adults of both sexes, but are two to three times more frequent in men than in women.[15] These carcinomas account for 3% of adult malignancies overall (Box 11.1).[22] Tobacco smoking is one of the major aetiological factors. Workers in the rubber industry also have a higher incidence of RCC. Nephroblastoma, the most frequent malignant tumour in infancy, affects about one child in every 8000.[15]

## Box 11.1 2004 WHO classification of the renal tumours of adulthood[15]

1 Malignant renal cell tumours
  1.1 Clear cell RCC
  1.2 Multilocular cystic renal cell carcinoma (MCRCC)
  1.3 Papillary renal cell carcinoma (PRCC)
  1.4 Chromophobe renal cell carcinoma (CRCC)
  1.5 Carcinoma of the collecting ducts of Bellini
  1.6 Renal medullary carcinoma
  1.7 Renal carcinoma associated with Xp11.2 translocations/ TFE3 gene fusions
  1.8 Renal cell carcinoma associated with neuroblastoma
  1.9 Mucinous, tubular and spindle cell carcinoma
  1.10 Renal cell carcinoma, unclassified
2 Benign tumours
  2.1 Papillary adenoma
  2.2 Oncocytoma
3 Metanephric neoplasms
4 Mixed epithelial and mesenchymal tumours
5 Other adult tumours

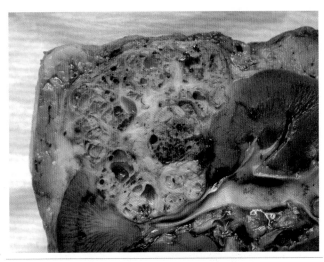

**Fig. 11.3** Large tumour with necrosis and haemorrhagic areas, very suggestive of a clear cell renal cell carcinoma (CCRCC).

## Clear cell renal cell carcinoma (CCRCC)

As the commonest histological type, this tumour is found in about 70% of all adult renal carcinomas.[22] CCRCCs are very rare in infancy.[23] The tumour is randomly distributed in the cortex and occurs with equal frequency in either kidney, usually as a solitary tumour but sometimes multiple.[15] CCRCCs may occur in patients with von Hippel–Lindau disease, which is inherited through an autosomal dominant trait and caused by germine mutations of the VHL tumour suppressor gene, located on chromosome 3p25-26. Recently, 3p deletions have also been described for the sporadic CCRCCs (3p25.1-25.3, 3p21.3-22.3; 3p14.1-14.2). They underline the role of chromosome 3 in renal cancer development, and are frequently associated with a trisomy 5q.[24] The mean age for sporadic CCRCCs is 61 years versus 37 years for CCRCCs in von Hippel–Lindau disease.

Macroscopically, these tumours are typically golden yellow with haemorrhagic and necrotic areas as well as patchy calcification (Fig. 11.3). Histologically, CCRCCs are composed of cells with clear cytoplasm filled with lipid and glycogen which are dissolved during routine histological processing. The cells show solid or acinar or more rarely papillary patterns with a thin network of small blood vessels between the cells groups.

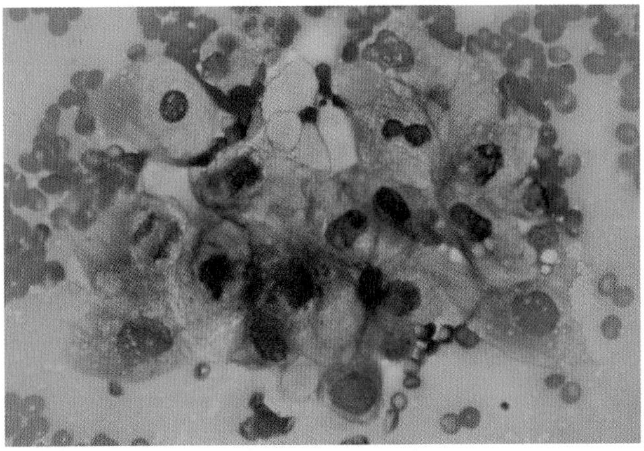

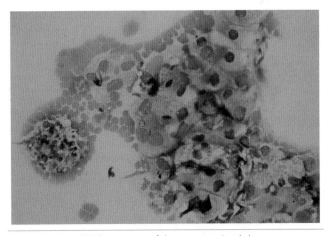

**Fig. 11.4** FNA: CCRCC; clusters of cells with microvacuolated cytoplasm and both regular and irregular nuclei (MGG).

**Fig. 11.5** FNA: CCRCC; same type of clusters as previously but note a macrophage with cellular debris from necrosis (MGG).

### Cytological findings: CCRCC (Figs 11.4, 11.5)

- Isolated cells in association with some clusters of cells, rarely with papillary clusters
- Cells with irregular borders
- Nuclear atypia ranging from small to large nuclei with regular or irregular borders
- Abundant cytoplasm, either vacuolated or granular
- Many naked nuclei, but usually without necrosis.

### Diagnostic pitfalls: CCRCC

Problems may occur in cases of chromophobe renal cell carcinoma with a clear component when the perinuclear clear rim of the chromophobe cells is enlarged. CCRCCs may also be misdiagnosed for xanthogranulomatous pyelonephritis but xanthoma cells are more foamy than clear;[25] however, when xanthogranulomatous pyelonephritis is associated with keratinising squamous metaplasia, the risk of misdiagnosing malignancy is higher.[26] Adrenocortical carcinomas may also be hard to differentiate from CCRCCs but the radiological findings should be helpful.

## Chromophobe renal cell carcinoma (CRCC)

This carcinoma represents approximately 5% of all renal carcinomas.[15] The mean age of incidence is in the sixth decade. Only a few cases of metastases have been described. Extensive chromosomal losses have been shown, especially -1,-2,-6,-10, -13,-17,-21.[27] In addition, mutations in BHD and TP53 genes have been described.[28]

Macroscopically, these tumours are typically light brown when fresh and light grey after formalin fixation, with no or few haemorrhagic areas (Fig. 11.6). Histologically, CRCCs are composed of cells with polygonal, transparent usually microvacuolated cytoplasm. A perinuclear clear rim is often observed. The cytoplasmic borders are clearly defined, making the cells appear to be framed. The nuclei are often irregular and wrinkled; bi- or multinucleated cells are common. These cells show an essentially solid pattern with a network of thick-walled blood vessels between the cells groups. In fact, there are two types of chromophobe cell carcinoma: one composed of relatively clear cells, the other of large eosinophilic cells mimicking oncocytomas. Mixed types have been described.

### Cytological findings: CRCC (Figs 11.7, 11.8)[13,29,30]

- Isolated cells in association with some small clusters of cells
- Variable-sized tumour cells
- Cells with well-defined borders or even thickened cell membranes
- Nuclei often have irregular borders, sometimes with cytoplasmic nuclear inclusions or grooves
- Binucleation
- Abundant cytoplasm, either clear but microvacuolated or eosinophilic and granular
- Perinuclear clearing of the cytoplasm.

### Diagnostic pitfalls: CRCC

Problems may occur in cases of CRCC-eosinophilic variant when the cytoplasm is granular and eosinophilic, resembling that of oncocytic cells. It is then necessary to be cautious and to look for the nuclear irregularities not usually seen in oncocytoma. Difficulties may also arise between CCRCCs and chromophobe cell carcinomas in cases of chromophobe cell carcinoma-clear variant (Fig. 11.9). Cytochemistry and/or immunocytochemistry can then be helpful.

## Papillary renal cell carcinoma (PRCC)

This carcinoma represents approximately 10% of all renal carcinomas.[15] As with the chromophobe renal cell carcinoma, the mean age of incidence is in the sixth decade. Five-year survival

for all stages ranges from 49% to 84%. Two types of PRCC have been described. *Type 1* is usually a low-grade tumour with a favourable clinical outcome and *type 2* a high-grade tumour with a poor prognosis. Trisomy or tetrasomy 7, trisomy 17

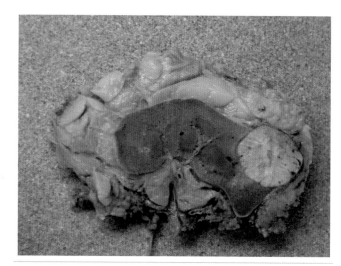

**Fig. 11.6** Light grey tumour suggestive for a chromophobe renal cell carcinoma (CRCC).

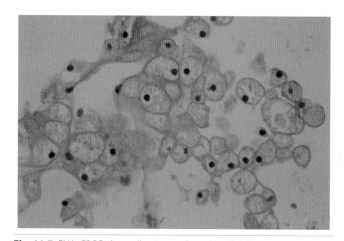

**Fig. 11.7** FNA: CRCC-clear cell variant; cells with well-defined borders and microvacuolated cytoplasm (cell block, H&E).

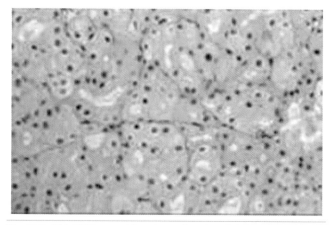

**Fig. 11.8** FNA: CRCC-oncocytic variant; cells with well-defined borders but granular eosinophilic cytoplasm and irregular nuclei. Note a nuclear cytoplasmic inclusion (cell block, H&E).

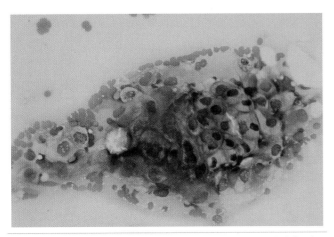

**Fig. 11.9** FNA: CRCC–CCRCC variant. Note the few cells with well-defined borders and binucleation (MGG).

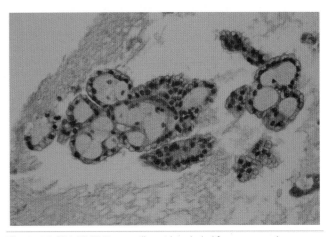

**Fig. 11.10** FNA: PRCC. Few papillae with included foamy macrophages (cell block; H&E).

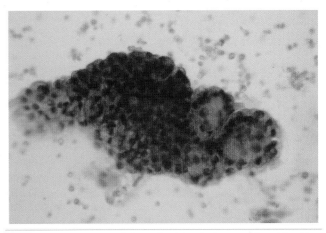

**Fig. 11.11** FNA: PRCC. Small clear cuboidal and columnar cells arranged in clusters with some tubular arrangements (PAP).

and loss of chromosome Y are the usual karyotypic changes in *type 1* PRCC. Additional trisomies may be observed, most frequently trisomies 16, 12 and 20.[31] These abnormalities are not observed in *type 2*, which seems to be more heterogeneous. Recently, MYC activation has been revealed in these high-grade papillary carcinomas.[32]

Macroscopically the *type 1* PRCC tumours are well-circumscribed, partially cystic with some haemorrhagic and necrotic areas. Bilaterality and multifocality are more often encountered than with the other primitive renal tumours. Histologically, the *type 1* PRCC are characterised by a papillary and tubular architecture. Foamy macrophages are often observed within the fibrovascular core of the papillae, as well as some microcalcifications. The haemorraghic and necrotic areas include some cholesterol crystals. In *type 1* tumours the papillae are covered by small, regular, sometimes clear or eosinophilic cells (Fig. 11.10) whereas in *type 2* PRCCs the papillary architecture is often not obvious and the cells are tall with eosinophilic cytoplasm and enlarged nuclei including prominent nucleoli. Hyperexpression of Topo II has been described.

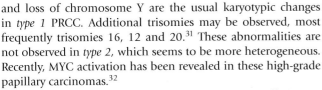

### Cytological findings: PRCC (Figs 11.11, 11.12)[13,33]

- Clusters of cells with papillary and/or tubular arrangement in *type 1* PRCC
- Numerous foamy macrophages sometimes included in the clusters
- Cells with scant cytoplasm in *type 1* and deeply basophilic cytoplasm in *type 2* PRCCs
- Variable numbers of enlarged nuclei, sometimes grooved
- Psammoma bodies.

### Diagnostic pitfalls: PRCC

Problems arise mostly with clear cell carcinomas in PRCCs with clear cytoplasm.[25] Transitional cell carcinoma may also cause difficulty when the cytoplasm is more basophilic and the nuclei enlarged. FNA is especially useful in patients with multiple renal tumours in order to eliminate metastases whether or not the presence of a primary cancer has been established.

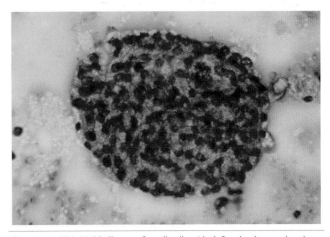

**Fig. 11.12** FNA: PRCC. Cluster of small cells with defined columnar border typical of a papillary arrangement (MGG).

## Collecting duct carcinoma

This carcinoma is rare (<1% of all renal carcinomas) and its prognosis is poor.[15] The mean age of incidence is about 55 years. Molecular events are variable and not well known as few cases have been studied. LOH have been identified on many chromosomes such as 1q, 6p, 8p, 13q, 21q. These tumours are usually located in the central area of the kidney. Histologically, they show a papillary and tubulopapillary architecture. The cells have a high nuclear/cytoplasmic ratio and are characterised by a hobnail pattern. Sarcomatoid features are commonly observed.[15] Recently, some controversies have appeared concerning this entity.[34]

### Cytological findings: collecting duct carcinoma[35–37]

- Three-dimensional sheets of cells with numerous tubules
- Atypical nuclei
- Low nuclear/cytoplasmic ratio
- Elongated sarcomatoid cells
- Prominent nucleoli and chromatin clearing
- Desmoplastic component.

### Diagnostic pitfalls: collecting duct carcinoma

These occur mainly with transitional cell renal carcinoma when the tubular structures are absent and also with metastatic poorly differentiated carcinomas. The lack of distinctive cytological features is a diagnostic challenge for the cytopathologist. But the previously described cytological criteria may be helpful in suggesting the diagnosis when correlated with radiological criteria and immunocytochemistry.

## Wilms tumour (nephroblastoma)

This is a malignant embryonal tumour composed of blastemal cells, usually occurring between the ages of 1 and 3 years and rarely in adults. The tumour may be unilateral or bilateral. The development of nephroblastoma is strongly linked with genetic abnormalities located on 11p13 and designated as WT1 alterations in syndromic cases; their role in sporadic cases of nephroblastoma is less obvious, suggesting other genetic abnormalities. Histologically, this tumour reveals a combination of three types of cells: blastemal, epithelial and stromal cells. The proportion and the degree of differentiation of these cells vary from specimen to specimen.[22]

### Cytological findings: Wilms tumour (Figs 11.13, 11.14)[38]

- Sheets of cells with nuclear overlapping and crowding
- Three-dimensional clusters with some tubular features
- Pleomorphic nuclei with irregular membranes
- Clumped chromatin
- Enlarged nucleoli
- Numerous mitoses.

### Diagnostic pitfalls: Wilms tumour

The problems that arise in diagnosis of these tumours are discussed in the chapter on the cytology of childhood tumours (see Ch. 33, Figs 33.12–33.14).

## Miscellaneous malignant primitive renal tumours

Over recent years, various authors have published the cytopathological findings of some of the rare malignant primitive renal tumours. These include, three cases of childhood

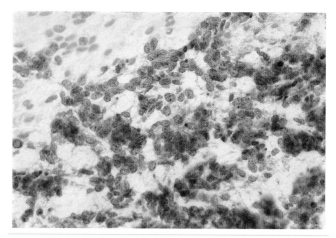

**Fig. 11.13** FNA: Wilms tumour. Small undifferentiated cells are seen here, some in small clusters. Very little cytoplasm is seen (PAP).

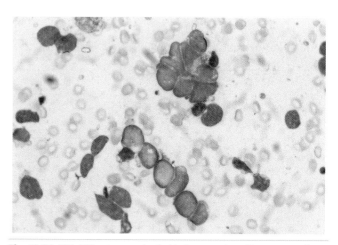

**Fig. 11.14** FNA: Wilms tumour. In air-dried smears the cells appear small with no visible cytoplasm and may be mistaken for lymphoid cells, except that they are in small clusters (MGG).

rhabdoid tumour[39] and nine cases of clear cell sarcoma.[40–42] In adults there have been reports of two cases of mucinous tubular and spindle cell carcinoma[43,44] and one case of Xp11.2 translocation/TFE3 fusion renal cell carcinoma (Fig. 11.15).[45] Haemangiopericytoma has been diagnosed by FNA in five cases,[46] and there have been single case reports on FNA of renal medullary carcinoma[47] and angiosarcoma.[48] Four cases of PNET have also been described.[49–51] These case reports underline the accuracy of renal FNA for cancer typing.[12]

Transitional renal cell carcinoma (TCC) is not part of the WHO kidney tumour classification, but it may be encountered in renal FNA. These tumours are characterised by three-dimensional clusters of large cells with anisokaryosis and strongly basophilic cytoplasm (Figs 11.16, 11.17) (see Ch. 12).[13]

Several cases of lymphoma have also been described,[4,13] constituting 3% of a series of 407 renal lesions. They were predominantly of B cell type (see Chs 13, 14).

## Renal metastases

Metastases into the kidney are not infrequent. In cases of extrarenal primary cancer metastatic deposits occur in about 7% of cases. The primary tumour is usually known but occasionally renal metastases are the first manifestation. The commonest primary sites are: lung, breast, skin, contralateral kidney, gastrointestinal tract, liver, ovary and testis.[22,52] FNA is essential in cases presenting as a single renal mass and it is important to recognise metastases on FNA cytology because chemotherapy is usually preferred over the surgical option.

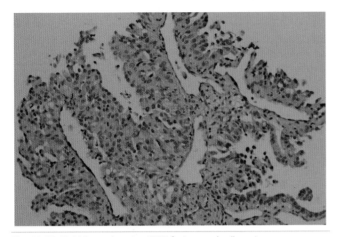

**Fig. 11.15** Xp11.2 translocation/TFE3 fusion renal cell carcinoma (microbiopsy, H&E).

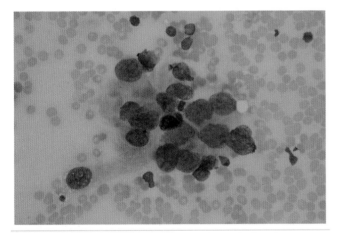

**Fig. 11.16** FNA: transitional cell carcinoma. A cluster of cells with anisocytosis and anisokaryosis (MGG).

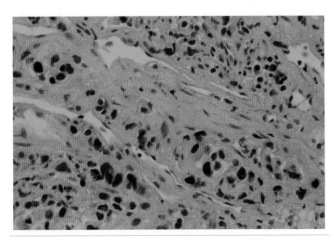

**Fig. 11.17** FNA: transitional cell carcinoma (microbiopsy, H&E).

### Cytological findings: renal metastases[52,53]

- Lack of the usual features observed in primary renal tumours
- Three-dimensional clusters of cells, resembling those of the primary tumour if known
- Few isolated cells
- Necrosis.

## Benign primitive renal tumours

The commonest tumours in this group are angiomyolipoma and oncocytoma. The importance of recognising these entities on FNA cannot be underestimated as it is critical for the subsequent management of patients.

## Angiomyolipoma

Angiomyolipoma is the most common benign mesenchymal tumour of the kidney. It is typically a neoplasm composed of an admixture in variable amounts of mature adipocytes, smooth muscle cells and thick-walled vessels. This neoplasm occurs in patients between 45 and 55 years, younger if associated with tuberous sclerosis. There is a 4:1 female predominance. The diagnosis is usually achieved by ultrasonography or computed tomography, hence these lesions represent only 1% of resected tumours because their treatment is often conservative, especially if they are small tumours.

### Cytological findings: angiomyolipoma (Figs 11.18, 11.19)[54–58]

- Oval to spindle-shaped cells, singly or in groups
- Mature adipocytes
- Stromal component
- Branching blood vessels
- Sometimes foamy macrophages and giant cells
- Nuclear cytoplasmic inclusions and nuclear pleomorphism.

This diagnosis may be a cytological challenge in the absence of adipocytes and when the smooth muscle cells are enlarged mimicking epithelial cells and malignancy (Fig. 11.20).

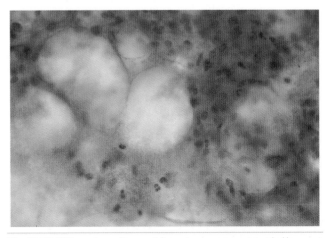

**Fig. 11.18** FNA: angiomyolipoma. Adipocytes are seen surrounded by smooth muscle cells in this fragment of aspirated tissue (PAP).

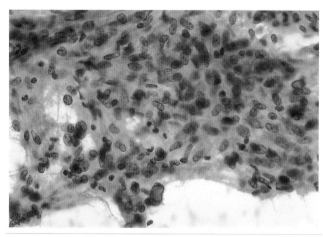

**Fig. 11.19** FNA: angiomyolipoma. Thick clusters of smooth muscle cells are seen in this field (PAP).

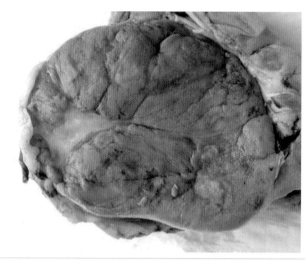

**Fig. 11.21** Oncocytoma. Brown pale tumour with a central fibrous scar.

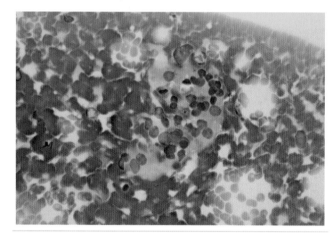

**Fig. 11.20** FNA: angiomyolipoma. Atypical smooth muscle cells mimicking epithelial cells (MGG).

## Oncocytoma

Oncocytoma is a benign renal epithelial neoplasm and represents about 5% of all renal neoplasms. About 50% of these tumours have no cytogenetic abnormalities. When cytogenetic abnormalities exist, two categories of gene alterations can be found: either 1p deletion with Y loss in male, or specific translocations: t(5;11)(q35;q13); (t(6;11)(p21;q13).[59] Macroscopically, it is typically a tan mahogany-brown tumour, usually well delimited without necrosis and haemorrhagic areas and sometimes with a central scar (Fig. 11.21). It may be partially cystic. Histologically, it is composed of large uniform cells with abundant eosinophilic and granular cytoplasm. There are round, enlarged eccentric nuclei, usually with prominent nucleoli and sometimes areas with bizarre, hyperchromatic nuclei. In spite of the very atypical nuclei the tumour remains benign. The granularity of the cytoplasm is due to the presence of numerous mitochondria.

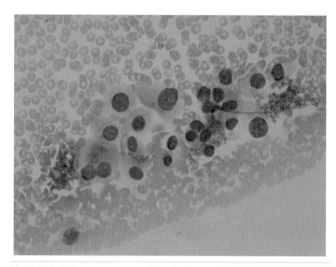

**Fig. 11.22** FNA: oncocytoma with single large cells, basophilic cytoplasm with blue granulations and round nuclei with prominent nucleoli (MGG).

### Cytological findings: oncocytoma (Figs 11.22, 11.23)[60,61]

- Numerous large single cells
- Pale basophilic and granular cytoplasm with sometimes dark blue granulations

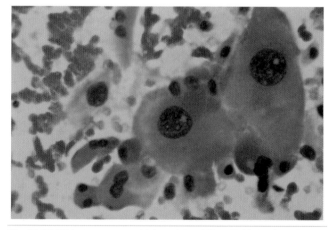

**Fig. 11.23** FNA: oncocytoma with large basophilic cells. Notice binucleation and anisokaryosis (MGG).

- Round regular nuclei
- Bi- and multinucleation
- Prominent nucleoli
- Sometimes nuclear atypia.

The most challenging differential diagnosis is to distinguish oncocytoma from CCRCC and CRCC.

## Metanephric adenoma

A few cases of metanephric adenoma diagnosed by FNA have been described recently.[62,63] This tumour is more frequent in children than in young adults. It is a solid grey-white tumour, varying in size. It shares some cytogenetic data with papillary tumours, for instance chromosome Y loss and trisomies 7 or 17, as well as some histological features such as papillary or microcystic architecture and psammoma bodies. More typically it is characterised by the association of tubules and glomeruloid structures (Fig. 11.24). As the cells have small uniform nuclei and scant cytoplasm, it may resemble nephroblastoma.[22]

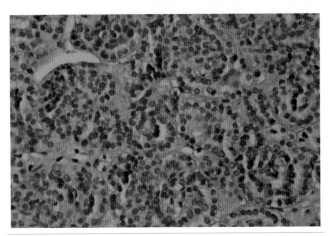

**Fig. 11.24** Metanephric adenoma with glomeruloid features (microbiopsy, H&E).

### Cytological findings: metanephric adenoma (Fig. 11.25)[64]

- Tightly packed cells with tubular structures and sometimes rosettes
- Scant cytoplasm
- Round uniform nuclei with finely dispersed chromatin
- Nuclear grooves and pseudo-inclusions may be observed
- Psammoma bodies
- No or infrequent mitoses.

The cytological findings in aspirates from metanephric adenoma may be hard to distinguish from those of Wilms tumour. Usually the diagnosis can be suggested, allowing a conservative surgical excision.

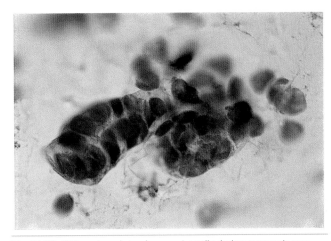

**Fig. 11.25** FNA: metanephric adenoma. A small tubular structure is seen, composed of cells with little cytoplasm (H&E).

## Cystic neoplasms

RCCs and benign renal cysts are the two commonest causes of renal masses, about 15% of RCCs being cystic. Renal FNA has a useful part to play in distinguishing benign renal cysts from multilocular cystic RCCs. The cystic neoplasms consist predominantly of multilocular CCRCC (Fig. 11.26) and cystic nephroma in adults, while in children they are either a cystic partially differentiated nephroblastoma or a cystic Wilms tumour.

The multilocular CCRCC is called 'carcinoma' but so far there has never been a report of recurrence or metastasis.[15] The cells are identical to those seen in CCRCC of low grade and have to be distinguished from histiocytes. Only one case of cystic nephroma and one case of cystic partially-differentiated nephroblastoma[65,66] have been described. In both cases it is essential to recognise the blastemal cell component. However, the lack of blastemal cells does not prove a tumour to be a cystic nephroma, while their presence excludes a diagnosis of cystic nephroma.

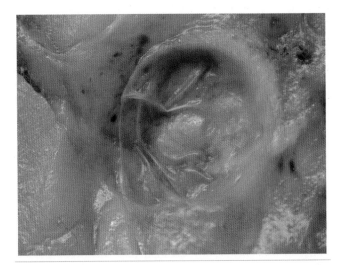

**Fig. 11.26** Renal cyst of benign appearance, but lined by a few clusters of clear cells on histology (cystic CCRCC).

## Ancillary techniques

### Cytochemistry

Routine cytochemistry such as stains for mucin or melanin can be useful particularly for identifying metastatic deposits when the primary tumour type is already known. With primary renal tumours too, cytochemical stains can contribute, for instance, using Hale's colloidal iron stain in order to distinguish oncocytoma from CRCC. Both tumours are positive with this stain but there is a cytoplasmic microvesicular positivity with oncocytoma and an apical or perinuclear positivity with CRCC.[60]

### Immunocytochemistry

With the above-listed categories of renal tumours described cytologically, we have underlined how much a specific diagnosis is essential for therapeutic purposes. Recently, some very rare or quite difficult diagnoses have been achieved by FNA. This increase in renal tumour typing on FNA is strongly linked to the use of immunocytochemistry. Most of the antibodies available for histological diagnosis can be used for cytological samples too, either with the cell block technique, which is similar to the routine histological technique, or using liquid-based cytological material. The latter technique presents two advantages: optimal cellular preservation and the use of higher antibody dilutions.[67]

Some antibodies are especially useful for the diagnosis of renal tumours: CD10 (for CCRCCs); cytokeratin 7 (Fig. 11.27); AMACR (PRCC); CD117 (CRCC); HMB45 (angiomyolipoma); EMA, low-molecular-weight cytokeratin, UEA (collecting duct carcinoma), CD57 (metanephric adenoma); vimentin (CCRCCs, PRCC, clear cell sarcoma); CD99 (PNET); TFE3 (Xp11.2 translocation/TFE3 fusion renal cell carcinoma), CD45, CD20, CD30, CD5 (lymphomas), CD68 (xanthogranulomatous pyelonephritis; some benign cysts). To distinguish one tumour from another, the association of three or four of these antibodies, taking account of the positive as well as the negative results, is usually recognised as the most helpful method.[68,69] A summarising list of the most useful antibodies is given in Table 11.2.

The monoclonal antibody against RCC produced in 1985, known as renal cell carcinoma marker (RCC Ma), is described by some authors as highly specific and helpful on FNA. Its sensitivity is variable, ranging from 33% to 85%. It is used to detect primary as well as metastatic renal malignant tumours.[70–72] In addition, Pax-2 has been tested in cytological material as an immunohistochemical marker for renal cell carcinoma. Its sensitivity and specificity for RCC are reported as 61% and 97%, respectively.[73]

### Cytogenetics

Most of the renal malignant tumours offer some specific genetic changes, as obviously listed in the relevant previous paragraphs. Therefore, the question that arises consequently concerns the role one should give to molecular studies for typing renal tumours routinely. Apart from the additional cost of these techniques, cytogenetic studies are not useful systematically for several reasons: (1) most of the renal tumours are easily recognised by their histological characteristics; (2) when some 'morphological overlapping' occurs suggesting a different diagnostic possibility, cytochemistry and immunocytohistochemistry are very useful and usually sufficient for a conclusive diagnosis; (3) many cytogenetical characteristics are not specific for only one tumour type: trisomies 7 and 17 are found in both PRCC and metanephric adenoma; oncocytomas often do not offer any specific cytogenetical change; PRCC type 2 have not yet been characterised by any specific cytogenetic profile. Nevertheless cytogenetic studies may be useful to detect a von Hippel–Lindau disease in young people or in cases of renal cell carcinoma, unclassified.

## The retroperitoneum

Retroperitoneal and pelvic masses include a wide range of benign and malignant lesions most of which are not specific to the retroperitoneum. Their importance in the present

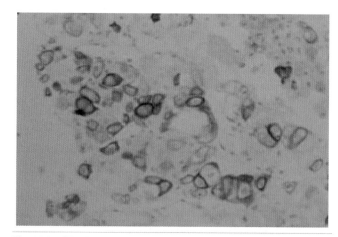

**Fig. 11.27** FNA: CRCC. Membranous and cytoplasmic positivity of cytokeratin 7 (cell block).

**Table 11.2** Immunocytochemical markers for renal tumours

| Antibodies | Tumours |
| --- | --- |
| CD10 | CCRCC |
| CD20 | Lymphoma |
| CD30 | Lymphoma |
| CD45 | Lymphoma |
| CD68 | Histiocytes |
| CD99 | PNET |
| CD117 | CRCC |
| Cytokeratin 7 | PRCC |
| AMARC | PRCC |
| HMB45 | Angiomyolipoma; melanoma (metastases) |
| EMA | Carcinoma of the collecting ducts; metastases |
| UEA | Carcinoma of the collecting ducts |
| TFE3 | RCC with Xp11.2 translocations/TFE3 gene fusions |

chapter lies in awareness on the part of the cytopathologist of all the possibilities when presented with an FNA from this region.

Benign masses most frequently arise from an abscess or tuberculosis (Fig. 11.28); malignant masses include many different tumours, such as primitive and metastatic carcinomas; neuroendocrine carcinomas, lymphomas (Fig. 11.29), sarcomas (Fig. 11.30) and melanoma. All these tumours are covered fully with detailed descriptions of their cytology in other appropriate chapters. In this section, the discussion will only cover idiopathic retroperitoneal fibrosis. It is noticeable that very few studies have been published about retroperitoneal FNA cytology, suggesting that it is under-used in comparison with FNA of deep-seated organs.[74]

## Idiopathic retroperitoneal fibrosis

Idiopathic retroperitoneal fibrosis is a rare disease affecting males more often than females, and occurring in the fourth and fifth decades of life. The disease commonly presents with a feeling of weakness, abdominal and/or flank pain, weight loss and urinary disturbances. Radiographic imaging features may suggest the diagnosis but the findings are non-specific. Therefore, FNA or biopsy is required to exclude other diagnoses (see Ch. 29).

### Cytological findings: idiopathic retroperitoneal fibrosis[75]

- Moderately cellular smears
- Cohesive aggregates of spindle cells
- Numerous small lymphocytes
- Scattered plasma cells and histiocytes
- Absence of necrosis and mitoses.

### Diagnostic pitfalls: idiopathic retroperitoneal fibrosis

Problems may occur with the nodular sclerosing variant of Hodgkin's disease. The lack of Reed–Sternberg cells and the use of immunocytochemistry with CD15 and CD30 antibodies to search for hidden Hodgkin cells are helpful. If many lymphocytes are present non-Hodgkin lymphoma should also be considered. In cases with atypical spindle cells, a diagnosis of sarcoma could be suggested, but with idiopathic retroperitoneal fibrosis there are no mitoses or other worrying features (Fig. 11.31). In these cases the non-committal term 'fibrous lesion' could be used.

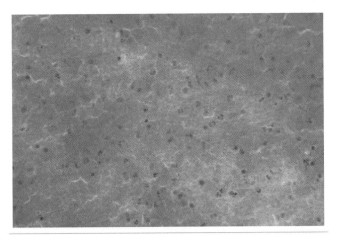

**Fig. 11.28** FNA: retroperitoneal paravertebral mass. Eosinophilic granular necrosis including few leucocytes suggestive of tuberculosis (PAP).

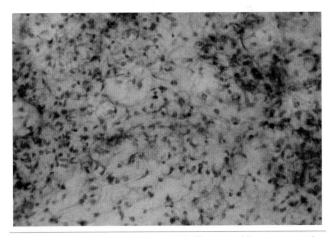

**Fig. 11.30** FNA: retroperitoneal mass. Well-differentiated liposarcoma with numerous lipoblasts (PAP).

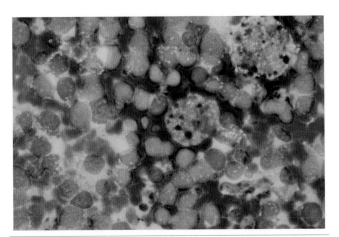

**Fig. 11.29** FNA: retroperitoneal paravertebral mass. Burkitt lymphoma: note the microvacuolated lymphoblasts and the macrophages (MGG).

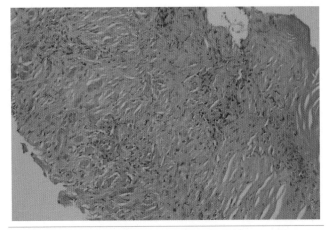

**Fig. 11.31** FNA: retroperitoneal mass. Spindle cells proliferation with collagen and some inflammatory cells suggestive for an idiopathic retroperitoneal fibrosis (H&E).

## The role of the cytopathologist in clinical management

Renal and retroperitoneal FNAs are less often performed compared with the large series of FNAs from other deep organs. This might be linked to the perception of a high morbidity risk of the technique, coupled with a low specificity for FNA of kidney masses, as well as with a higher risk of an unsatisfactory or inconclusive specimen in cases of fibrosis or sarcomas of the retroperitoneum. Therefore, cytology has until now been largely replaced by surgical excision or core biopsies.

However, with recent technical improvements, including liquid-based cytology, immunocytochemistry and the use of cell blocks, cytological diagnoses should be more widely accepted since the technique offers many diagnostic opportunities and new developments.

Furthermore, changes in surgical practice such as minimal excision or partial nephrectomy for low-grade small tumours require a reliable diagnosis preoperatively, offering a new role for FNA in patient management.

Histological as well as cytological diagnoses are enhanced by knowledge of the clinical and biological data and correlation with the radiological features. The cytopathologist has to be informed about all the available data at the time the FNA is performed and should take part in clinical decision-making for patients with an FNA from this region. Kidney and retroperitoneal FNAs in particular require this approach due to the variety of lesions that may be discovered. This reinforces the need for regular multidisciplinary team meetings, attended by clinicians, radiologists and pathologists, so that clinicians understand what the pathologist is reporting and the pathologist sees the full clinical picture as well as having feedback on the interpretation of the findings.

## REFERENCES

1. Volpe A, Jewett MA. The natural history of small renal masses. Nat Clin Pract Urol 2005;2:384–90.

2. Silverman SG, Israel GM, Herts BR, et al. Management of the incidental renal mass. Radiology 2008;249:16–31.

3. Caoili EM, Bude RO, Higgins EJ, et al. Evaluation of sonographically guided percutaneous core biopsy of renal masses. AJR Am J Roentgenol 2002;179:373–78.

4. Hunter S, Samir A, Eisner B, et al. Diagnosis of renal lymphoma by percutaneous image guided biopsy: experience with eleven cases. J Urol 2006;176:1952–56.

5. Jaff A, Molinié V, Mellot F, et al. Evaluation of imaging-guided fine-needle percutaneous biopsy of renal masses. Eur Radiol 2006;15:1721–26.

6. Johnson PT, Nazarian LN, Needleman L, et al. Sonographically guided renal mass biopsy: indications and efficacy. Ultrasound Med 2001;20:749–53.

7. Neuzillet Y, Lechevallier E, Andre M, et al. Accuracy and clinical role of fine needle percutaneous biopsy with computerized tomography guidance of small (less than 4.0 cm) renal masses. J Urol 2004;171:1802–5.

8. Reichelt O, Gajda M, Chyhrai A, et al. Ultrasound-guided biopsy of homogenous solid renal masses. Eur Urol 2007;52:1421–26.

9. Schmidbauer J, Remzi M, Memarsadeghi M, et al. Diagnostic accuracy of computed tomography-guided percutaneous biopsy of renal masses. Eur Urol 2008;53:1003–11.

10. Volpe A, Kachura JR, Geddie WR, et al. Techniques, safety and accuracy of sampling of renal tumors by fine needle aspiration and core biopsy. J Urol 2007;178:379–86.

11. Wunderlich H, Hindermann W, Al Mustafa AM, et al. The accuracy of 250 fine needle biopsies of renal tumors. J Urol 2005;174:44–46.

12. Garcia-Solano J, Acosta-Ortega J, Perz-Guillermo M, et al. Solid renal masses in adults: image-guided fine-needle aspiration cytology and imaging techniques. '

Two heads better than one?' Diagn Cytopathol 2008;36:8–12.

13. Truong LD, Todd TD, Dhurandar B, et al. Fine-needle aspiration of renal masses in adults: Analysis of results and diagnostic problems in 108 cases. Diagn Cytopathol 1999;20:339–49.

14. Zardawi IM. Renal fine needle aspiration cytology. Acta Cytol 1999;43:184–90.

15. Eble JN, Sauter G, Epstein JI, et al. Pathology and genetics of tumours of the urinary system and male genital organs. In: World Health Organization classification of tumours. Lyon, France: IARC Press; 2004. 15.

16. Prasad SR, Surabhi VR, Menias VO, et al. Benign renal neoplasms in adults: cross-sectional imaging findings. AJR Am J Roentgenol 2008;190:158–64.

17. Wolf JS. Evaluation and management of solid and cystic renal masses. J Urol 1998;159:1120–33.

18. Quaia E, Bertolotto M, Cioffi V, et al. Comparison of contrast-enhanced sonography with unenhanced sonography and contrast-enhanced CT in the diagnosis of malignancy in complex cystic renal masses. AJR Am J Roentgenol 2008;191:1239–49.

19. Lebret T, Poulain JO, Molinié V, et al. Percutaneous core biopsy for renal masses: indications, accuracy and results. J Urol 2007;178:1184–88.

20. Bouchelouche K, Oehr P. Positron emission tomography and positron emission tomography/computerized tomography of urological malignancies: an update review. J Urol 2008;179:34–45.

21. Fulcinetti F, Mascolo M, Insabato L, et al. Massive infarction of papillary carcinoma of the kidney after fine needle aspiration biopsy: report of a case with cytohistologic correlation. Acta Cytol 2006;50:563–66.

22. Murphy WM, Grignon DJ, Perlman EJ. Tumors of the Kidney, Bladder and Related Urinary Structures. Washington, DC: Armed Forced Institute of Pathology; 2004.

23. Barroca H, Farinha N, Carvalho JL. Renal cell carcinoma: Cytologic diagnosis in a child. Diagn Cytopathol 1999;21:362.

24. Banks BR, Tirukonda P, Taylor C, et al. Genetic and epigenetic analysis of von Hippel Lindau gene alterations and relationship with clinical variables in sporadic renal cancer. Cancer Res 2006;66:2000–11.

25. Masoom S, Venkataraman G, Jensen J, et al. Renal FNA-based typing of renal masses remain a useful adjunctive modality: evaluation of 31 renal masses with correlative cytology. Cytopathology 2009;1:50–55.

26. Dhingra KK, Singal S, Jain S. Rare coexistence of keratinising squamous metaplasia with xanthogranulomatous pyelonephritis. Report of a case with the role of immunocytochemistry in the differential diagnosis. Acta Cytol 2007;51:92–94.

27. Gunawan B, Bergmann F, Braun S, et al. Polyploidisation and losses of chromosomes 1, 2, 6, 13, and 17 in three cases of chromophobe renal cell carcinomas. Cancer Genet Cytogenet 1999;110:57–61.

28. Gad S, Lefevre SH, Khoo SK, et al. Mutations in BHD and TP53 genes, but not in HNF1 beta gene in a large series of sporadic chromophobes renal cell carcinoma. Clin Cancer Res 2006;96:336–40.

29. Salamanca J, Alberti N, Lopez-Rios F, et al. Fine needle aspiration of chromophobe renal cell carcinoma. Acta Cytol 2007;51:9–15.

30. Sharma SG, Mathur SR, Aron M, et al. Chromophobe renal cell carcinoma with calcification: report of a case with rare finding on aspiration smears. Diagn Cytopathol 2008;36:647–50.

31. Yang XJ, Tan MH, Kim HL, et al. A molecular classification of papillary renal cell carcinoma. Cancer Res 2005;65:5628–37.

32. Furge KA, Chen J, Koeman J, et al. Detection of DNA copy number changes and oncogenic signalling abnormalities from gene expression data reveals MYC activation in high-grade papillary carcinoma. Cancer Res 2007;67:3171–76.

33. Lim JC, Wojcik EM. Fine-needle aspiration cytology of papillary renal cell carcinoma: the association with concomitant secondary malignancy. Diagn Cytopathol 2006;34:797–800.

34. Kafe H, Verbavatz JM, Cochand-Priollet B, et al. Collecting duct carcinoma: an entity to be redefined? Virchows Arch 2004;445:637–40.

35. Sarode VR, Islam S, Wooten D, et al. Fine needle aspiration cytology of collecting duct carcinoma of the kidney: report of a case with distinctive features and differential diagnosis. Acta Cytol 2004;48:843–48.

36. Sironi M, Delpiano C, Claren R, et al. New cytologic findings on fine-needle aspiration of renal collecting duct carcinoma. Diagn Cytopathol 2003;29:239–40.

37. Ono K, Nishino E, Nakamine H. Renal collecting duct carcinoma. Report of a case with cytologic findings on fine needle aspiration. Acta Cytol 2000;44:380–84.

38. Goregaonkar R, Shet T, Ramadwar M, et al. Critical role of fine needle aspiration cytology and immunocytochemistry in preoperative diagnoses of pediatric renal tumors. Acta Cytol 2007;51:721–29.

39. Barrocca HM, Costa MJ, Carvalho JL. Cytologic profile of rhabdoid tumor of the kidney. A report of 3 cases. Acta Cytol 2003;47:1055–58.

40. Iyer VK, Agarwala S, Verma K. Fine needle aspiration cytology of clear cell sarcoma of the kidney: study of eight cases. Diagn Cytopathol 2005;33:83–89.

41. Iyer VK, Kapila K, Verma K. Fine needle aspiration cytology of clear cell sarcoma of the kidney with spindle cell pattern. Cytopathology 2003;14:160–64.

42. Portugal R, Barroca H. Clear cell sarcoma, cellular mesoblastic nephroma, metanephric adenoma: cytological features and differential diagnosis with Wilms tumour. Cytopathology 2008;19:80–85.

43. Ortega JA, Solano JG, Perez-Guillermo M. Cytologic aspects of mucinous tubular and spindle-cell renal carcinoma in fine needle aspirates. Diagn Cytopathol 2006;34:660–62.

44. Owens CL, Argani P, Ali SZ. Mucinous tubular and spindle-cell renal carcinoma of the kidney: cytopathologic findings. Diagn Cytopathol 2007;35:593–96.

45. Schintsine M, Fillie AC, Torres-Cabala C, et al. Fine needle aspiration of a Xp11.2 translocation/TFE3 fusion renal cell carcinoma metastatic to the lung: report of a case and review of the literature. Diagn Cytopathol 2006;34:751–56.

46. Chhieng D, Cohen JM, Waisman J, et al. Fine needle aspiration cytology of hemangiopericytoma. A report of five cases. Cancer 1999;87:190–95.

47. Qi J, Shen PU, Rezuke WN, et al. Fine needle aspiration cytology diagnosis of renal medullary carcinoma: a case report. Acta Cytol 2001;45:735–39.

48. Johnson VV, Gaertner EM, Crothers BA. Fine-needle aspiration of angiosarcoma. Arch Pathol Lab Med 2002;126:478–80.

49. Kang SH, Perle MA, Nonaka D, et al. Primary Ewing sarcoma/PNET of the kidney: fine needle aspiration, histology and dual color break apart FISH assay. Diagn Cytopathol 2007;35:353–57.

50. Premalata CS, Gayathri Devi M, Biswas S, et al. Primitive neuroectodermal tumor of the kidney. A report of two cases diagnosed fine needle aspiration cytology. Acta Cytol 2003;47:457–59.

51. Maly B, Maly A, Reinhartz T, et al. Primitive neuroectodermal tumor of the kidney. Report of a case diagnosed by fine needle aspiration cytology. Acta Cytol 2004;48:264–68.

52. Giashuddin S, Cangiarella J, Elgert P, et al. Metastases to the kidney: eleven cases diagnosed by aspiration biopsy with histological correlation. Diagn Cytopathol 2005;32:325–29.

53. Gattuso P, Ramzy I, Truong LD, et al. Utilisation of fine needle aspiration in the diagnosis of metastatic tumours to the kidney. Diagn Cytopathol 1999;21:35–38.

54. Singh D, Kashyap S, Kaur S. Renal angiomyolipoma, a diagnostic dilemma: a case report. Indian J Pathol Microbiol 2007;50:622–23.

55. Handa U, Nanda A, Mohan H. Fine-needle aspiration of renal angiomyolipoma: a report of four cases. Cytopathology 2007;18:250–54.

56. Pancholi V, Munjal K, Jain M, et al. Preoperative diagnosis of renal angiomyolipoma with fine needle aspiration cytology: a report of 3 cases. Acta Cytol 2006;50:466–68.

57. Crapanzano JP. Fine needle aspiration of renal angiomyolipoma: cytological findings and diagnostic pitfalls in a series of five cases. Diagn Cytopathol 2005;32:53–57.

58. Kulkarni B, Desai SB, Dave B, et al. Renal angiomyolipomas-a study of 18 cases. Indian J Pathol Microbiol 2005;48:459–63.

59. Jhang JS, Narayan G, Murty VV, et al. Renal oncocytomas with 11q13 rearrangements: cytogenetic, molecular and immunohistochemical analysis of cyclin D1. Cancer Genet Cytogenet 2004;149:114–19.

60. Liu J, Fanning CV. Can renal oncocytomas be distinguished from renal cell carcinoma on fine needle aspiration specimens? A study of conventional smears in conjunction with ancillary studies. Cancer 2001;93:390–97.

61. Deshpande A, Munshi M. Renal oncocytoma with hyaline globules: cytologic diagnosis by guided fine needle aspiration, a case report. Indian J Pathol Microbiol 2005;48:230–35.

62. Bosco M, Galliano D, La Saponara F, et al. Cytologic features of metanephric adenoma of the kidney during pregnancy: a case report. Acta Cytol 2007;51:468–72.

63. Khayyata S, Grignon DJ, Aulicino MR, et al. Metanephric adenoma vs. Wilms' tumor: a report of 2 cases by fine needle aspiration and cytologic comparisons. Acta Cytol 2007;51:464–67.

64. Xu X, Acs G, Yu GH, et al. Aspiration cytology of metanephric adenoma of the kidney. Diagn Cytopathol 2000;22:330–31.

65. Nayak A, Iyer VK, Agarwala S, et al. Fine needle aspiration cytology of cystic partially-differentiated nephroblastoma of the kidney. Cytopathology 2006;17:145–48.

66. Gupta R, Dhingra K, Singh S, et al. Multicystic nephroma: a case report. Acta Cytol 2007;51:651–53.

67. Fadda G, Rossi ED, Mule A, et al. Diagnostic efficacy of immunocytochemistry on, fine needle aspiration biopsies processed by thin-layer cytology. Acta Cytol 2006;17:145–48.

68. Allory Y, Bazille C, Vieillefond A, et al. Profiling and classification tree applied to renal epithelial tumours. Histopathology 2008;2:158–66.

69. Zhou M, Roma A, Magi-Galluzzi C. The usefulness of immunohistochemical markers in the differential diagnosis of renal neoplasms. Clin Lab Med 2005;25:247–57.

70. Gokden N, Mukunyadzi P, James JD, et al. Diagnostic utility of renal cell carcinoma marker in cytopathology. Appl Immunohistochem Mol Morphol 2003;11:116–19.

71. Yang B, Ali SZ, Rosenthal SD. CD10 facilitates the diagnosis of metastatic renal cell carcinoma from primary adrenal cortical neoplasm in adrenal fine needle aspiration. Diagn Cytopathol 2002;27:149–52.

72. Simsir A, Chhieng D, Wei XJ, et al. Utility of CD10 and RCCma in the diagnosis of metastatic conventional renal-cell adenocarcinoma by fine needle aspiration biopsy. Diagn Cytopathol 2005;33:3–7.

73. Gokden N, Kemp SA, Gokden M. The utility of Pax-2 as an immunohistochemical marker for renal cell carcinoma. Diagn Cytopathol 2008;36:473–77.

74. Guo Z, Kurtycz DF, De Las Casas LE, et al. Radiologically guided percutaneous fine-needle aspiration biopsy of pelvic and retroperitoneal masses: a retrospective study of 68 cases. Diagn Cytopathol 2001;25:43–49.

75. Dash RC, Liu K, Sheafor DH, et al. Fine needle aspiration findings in idiopathic retroperitoneal fibrosis. Diagn Cytopathol 1999;21:22–26.

# Urine cytology

Stephen S. Raab

## Chapter contents

## Introduction

For practical purposes, clinicians obtain urinary tract cytology specimens for evaluation for the presence or absence of cancer. Urine specimens provide a critical role in the evaluation of patients who have signs such as haematuria and/or symptoms such as painful urination suggestive of pathology within the urinary tract. In some regions with high industrial exposure to known bladder carcinogens, urine cytology is used as the initial test for screening for early detection of bladder cancer.[1,2] Urine cytology is also currently a mainstay in the surveillance of patients who have a history of urinary tract malignancy.

The organisation of this chapter follows the clinical practice of diagnosing or excluding cancer. Following a discussion of the preparation and the cytological findings in routine urine specimens, the criteria for diagnosis of the various types of neoplasms encountered in urinary tract specimens and the pitfalls that lead to false positive and false negative diagnoses are discussed. Recent technological developments are reviewed and finally, an approach to laboratory quality control in this branch of cytology is included.

## Specimen types

Urinary tract cytology specimens are classified as either voided or instrumented and the proportion of each type for a given cytology practice depends on the patient population and clinician subspecialty. This separation is important as the cytological appearance of cancers and the diagnostic pitfalls are often unique for different specimen types. The majority of urine specimens are voided. However, cytology practices that receive specimens from urologists who perform cystoscopic examinations generally receive more instrumented specimens, as the patient population either has signs or symptoms highly suspicious for cancer or has been previously treated for cancer. An important point to remember is that some clinicians obtain a post-cystoscopy urine that may inadvertently be classified as a 'voided urine'. The cytological findings in post-cystoscopic voided urines are essentially the same as in instrumented urines.

The separation of urine specimens into the categories of voided and instrumented follows the classic cytological separation into those specimens obtained through a normal cellular shedding mechanism and those collected by scraping, the first being of low cellularity, unless the patient has disease and the second being more cellular.

A final type of urine specimen is the 'conduit' specimen, procured in a patient who had a cystectomy with a conduit constructed from other body tissues, such as the ileum. The conduit connects the upper urinary tract to a body outlet. As clinicians obtain conduit specimens to track disease in the upper tract (renal pelves, calyces or ureters), the cells of interest are urothelial cells (not the intestinal cells), which tend to be few in number, similar to the findings in classical voided specimens.

## Voided urine samples

Voided specimens are also known as clean catch specimens and are obtained in patients who have a variety of clinical histories. A random specimen (and not an early morning specimen) is recommended to limit cellular degeneration.[3] As mentioned above, voided urine specimens tend to be of low cellularity, unless the patient has:

- A high-grade urothelial cell carcinoma of the bladder but only in some cases, as high-grade cancers often do not shed many cells
- An irritative lesion, such as lithiasis
- An infectious process, or
- Contaminated urine, most frequently procured from a woman, in which the predominant component is non-urinary tract cells.

Highly cellular specimens require thorough evaluation, and the cytomorphology of these four conditions will be discussed below. Voided urines are superior to instrumented urines in detecting malignancies of the urethra.

## Instrumented urine samples

Instrumented urine specimens are further divided into different types, which are procured through a catheter or after an instrument (such as a cystoscope) is introduced into the urinary tract. Instrumented specimens include catheterised urines, bladder washings, brushings and upper urinary tract urines obtained by ureteric catheterisation. As noted above, a post-cystoscopy urine specimen may be considered a type of instrumented specimen and is similar to a washing specimen in terms of cellular findings. Instrumented urines are superior to voided urines in detecting malignancies of the bladder and upper tract.

### Catheterised specimens

Catheterised specimens are collected for a variety of reasons, such as the work-up of patients who may have a urinary tract infection, determining the cause of haematuria, or for cancer screening in patients who have in-dwelling catheters.

### Washing specimens

A washing may be performed of any part of the urinary tract, although the most common washing specimen is of the bladder. Washing specimens may be directed or undirected and in a washing procedure, a solution (e.g. electrolyte or saline) is injected into the cavity of interest and then withdrawn. Washing specimens are often performed as a method for examining a large area for cancer. Washings are the most sensitive cytological method for cancer detection. *Upper tract specimens* are a type of washing specimen, but often are discussed separately because the cytological findings of the upper tract differ from those of the bladder, the upper tract consisting of the renal collecting ducts, pelves and ureters.

### Brushing specimens

A brushing is performed under cystoscopic guidance of a specific area of concern. Brushing sampling may be performed on any portion of the urinary tract and are often collected in conjunction with a washing. The brushing specimen is either placed directly on a slide or placed into a fixative.

## Specimen processing

Laboratories process urine specimens in a variety of ways, depending on available technology and preference. In the USA, laboratories predominantly use centrifugation and monolayer methods. Other methods include the use of filters or the preparation of a cell block. The different findings using monolayer and centrifugation methods are discussed when appropriate throughout this chapter.

As close inspection of nuclear detail is critical for the diagnosis of urothelial cancer, most laboratories use the Papanicolaou stain as the sole stain for evaluation. Some laboratories use other stains, such as a modified Wright–Giemsa stain to evaluate for entities other than urothelial cell nuclei.

## Diagnostic categories

As in all cytology, an adequate sample is critical to making a proper interpretation.[4] Although cytopathologists and cytotechnologists intuitively assess the adequacy of urine specimens, well-established criteria for specimen adequacy are lacking for different specimen types and preparation methods. The greatest difficulty arises in the adequacy assessment of voided urine specimens, as they are of lower cellularity compared to other specimen types. Optimally, the cellularity of voided samples should be described, e.g. reporting no cells, a less than optimal number of cells and numerous cells, in addition to rendering a diagnosis. Adequacy is currently assessed informally, based on a number of factors including experience. If no urothelial cells are seen, specimen re-preparation should be considered. Generally speaking, most voided urines contain at least a few urothelial and inflammatory cells or acellular components such as crystals or debris.

Clinicians use urinary tract cytology diagnostic categories (Box 12.1) to triage patients for additional follow-up and treatment.[5] At present, there is neither general agreement on the use of these categories by cytopathologists nor coherent clinical recommendations on how patients with different clinical histories, signs, and/or symptoms should be managed, based on specific diagnoses. Currently used diagnostic categories confer specific risks of malignancy, and these risks depend on cytopathologist experience and other factors. In the ideal practice setting, clinicians behave in a Bayesian fashion and use their pre-urine test probability of malignancy with the specific diagnostic category risk of malignancy to calculate the post-urine test probability of malignancy.[6,7] As expected, the categories of benign, atypical, suspicious, and malignant confer an increasing probability of malignancy, although the actual patient risk of malignancy depends on far more than the cytopathologist's interpretation. Published articles on the use of diagnostic categories and clinical decision-making describe the complexity of this process.[6–8]

One of the most understudied areas in urine cytology is in the cytopathologist's use and meaning of indeterminate diagnoses, especially the diagnosis of atypical. Providing cytomorphological criteria for atypia is extremely difficult, and to state the obvious, atypical cells do not have definitive features of benignity or malignancy.[9,10] Compared with cervical smear test cytology in which the risk of pre-neoplasia is relatively well established for an 'atypical squamous cells – undetermined

---

**Box 12.1  Urinary tract diagnostic categories**

Benign

Atypical

Suspicious

Malignant

- Urothelial carcinoma
  - High-grade urothelial carcinoma
  - Low-grade urothelial carcinoma
- Squamous cell carcinoma
- Adenocarcinoma
- Other malignancies

significance' (ASC-US) interpretation, the risk of neoplasia/malignancy associated with an atypical urine is not. Throughout this chapter, the concept of atypia is discussed.

## Cytomorphological criteria of benign and neoplastic urinary tract specimens

### Non-neoplastic or 'normal' urine specimens

The cytological features of 'normal' urine specimens serve as a basis for comparison to neoplastic conditions. Features of reactive/reparative/infection-associated urines will be discussed in the differential diagnosis of neoplastic conditions. Completely 'normal' urines are obtained in some patients who undergo screening and in some patients who undergo cystoscopic examination and do not have disease, for example, in the routine cystoscopic follow-up in some patients who have a history of bladder cancer. Below, the similarities and differences in the benign cytomorphological findings are discussed by specimen type.

#### Voided urine specimens

Voided urine specimens sample the entire urinary tract, including the kidneys, renal pelves, ureters, bladder and urethra. As these urinary tract regions may be lined by different cell types, voided urine specimens from a non-diseased tract may exhibit a variety of appearances, reflecting the fact that different portions of the urinary tract are lined by urothelial cells, squamous cells, and glandular cells.

*Urothelial cells.* Like squamous epithelium, urothelium is divided into three cell layers: superficial, intermediate and basal/parabasal. Urothelium varies in thickness from two to three cells in the renal pelvis to five to six in the bladder (Fig. 12.1). The superficial urothelial cell layer is a single cell in thickness and superficial cells are large, sometimes multinucleated, and also known as umbrella cells because of their contours. Superficial urothelial cells may be larger than 100 μm in diameter, although their nuclear to cytoplasmic ratio is low, except in reactive conditions or in degenerate specimens. Most

superficial cells contain from one to three nuclei, although it is not unusual to see more nuclei, as these cells respond to a variety of insults. Overall, a superficial urothelial cell is approximately the size of an intermediate squamous cell. The cytoplasm of superficial cells is variable, but tends to be finely granular (Fig. 12.2); cytoplasmic vacuolation is fairly common, especially in reparative processes. The cytoplasmic borders are well defined and the cells have a rounded appearance. Superficial cells are the most common urothelial cell type seen in voided urine specimens from non-diseased individuals. Seeing cells from other urothelial layers is a sign of disease in a voided urine specimen.

The intermediate cell layer is variable in thickness and the cells are cuboidal and much smaller than intact superficial cells. The basal/parabasal cell layer also is a single layer in thickness and the cells are a similar shape but slightly smaller compared to intermediate urothelial cells (Fig. 12.3).

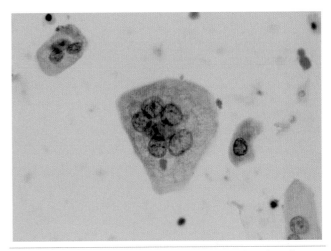

**Fig. 12.2** Urine, voided: superficial cells. Several large multinucleated superficial cells with abundant cytoplasm are admixed with inflammatory cells and debris. The superficial cell nuclei are enlarged and lack significant hyperchromasia. A few of these nuclei contain a prominent nucleolus (PAP).

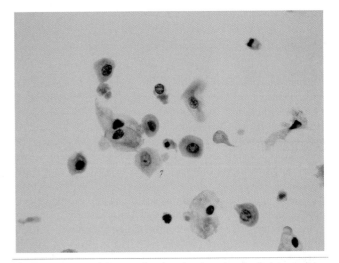

**Fig. 12.3** Urine, wash: intermediate, basal, and parabasal cells. Intermediate, basal and parabasal urothelial cells are considerably smaller than superficial cells and contain a small to moderate amount of cyanophilic cytoplasm that is finely vacuolated. Their nuclei are round to oval and may also contain a prominent nucleolus in reactive processes. The nuclei shown here are about twice the size of red blood cells (PAP).

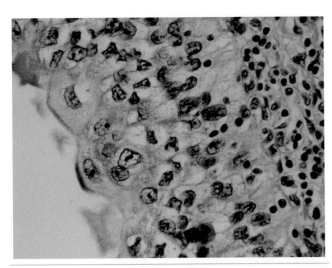

**Fig. 12.1** Histology: section of bladder. A full-thickness section of reactive urothelium is shown. The superficial urothelial cells show abundant cytoplasm, large nuclei and prominent nucleoli. Several of the superficial cells show multinucleation (H&E).

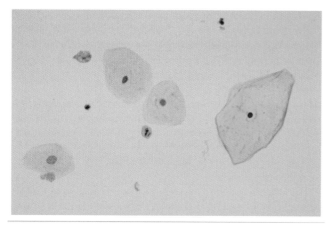

**Fig. 12.4** Urine, voided: benign squamous cells. Three superficial squamous cells with small nuclei and abundant cytoplasm are admixed with a few inflammatory cells. This voided urine is from a man who has a history of lithiasis (PAP).

| Box 12.2  Sources of glandular cells in urine specimens |
| --- |
| Normal lining |
| Cystitis glandularis |
| Periurethral glands |
| Prostate |
| Kidney |
| Seminal vesicle |
| Epididymis |
| Vas deferens |
| Female genital tract |
| Nephrogenic adenoma |
| Adenocarcinoma |
| Urothelial carcinoma with adenocarcinomatous differentiation |

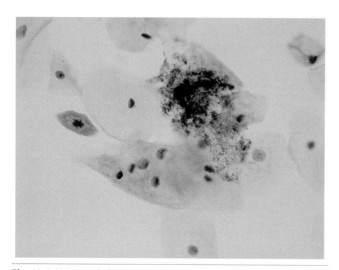

**Fig. 12.5** Urine, voided: squamous cell contaminant. In this voided urine from a 45-year-old woman with haematuria, squamous cells are admixed with abundant bacteria. There is an absence of acute inflammation. Note the single, slightly degenerate, reactive urothelial cell with densely granular nuclear chromatin (PAP).

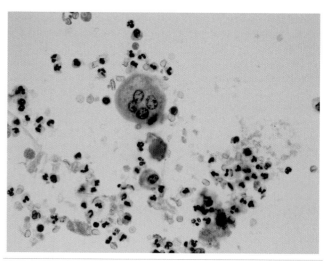

**Fig. 12.6** Urine, voided: inflammatory cells and red cells. Acute inflammatory cells are admixed with red cells and several reactive urothelial cells. The nuclei in the superficial urothelial cell show degenerative features with foci of nuclear membrane thickening and breaks (PAP).

*Squamous cells.* The female urethra is entirely lined by stratified squamous epithelium, and the male urethra is lined by stratified squamous epithelium at the orifice of the penile (spongy) portion. The remainder of the penile portion and the membranous portion are lined partially by stratified squamous epithelium and partially by urothelium. Squamous epithelium also may be found in the bladder, and is normally seen in the trigone in 10% of men and 50% of women.[11] In voided urine specimens, superficial squamous cells from the urothelial tract may be present (Fig. 12.4). In women, the urinary tract squamous cells are often confused with benign squamous cell contaminant from the gynecological tract. The presence of bacteria associated with squames, in the absence of reactive changes and inflammation, is usually a sign that the squamous cells are not of urinary tract origin (Fig. 12.5).

*Glandular cells.* Glandular cells are more frequently seen in instrumented urine specimens and have a number of sources (Box 12.2).[12,13] Most glandular cells arise from the urothelial lining itself, as the urothelium is capable of differentiating along several pathways. Glandular epithelium also may arise as a response to chronic irritation. Mucous-secreting glands are normally found in the spongy portion of the male urethra and in the female urethra, hence these cells may be shed in voided urine specimens. Glandular cells exhibit oval, basal nuclei with finely granular blue to green cytoplasm. Cytoplasmic vacuolation and even cilia may be seen. Renal tubular cells are observed in casts or small sheets and reflect kidney disease such as infarct or tubular necrosis.

A variety of cells other than urothelial, squamous and glandular cells and other structures may be seen in voided urine specimens. These cells include inflammatory cells, red blood cells (Fig. 12.6) and sperm. Other structures include crystals (Fig. 12.7), casts (Fig. 12.8) and corpora amylacea.

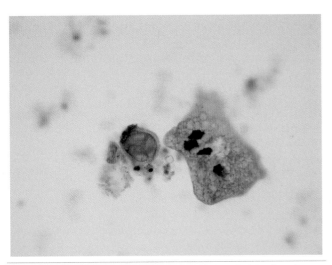

**Fig. 12.7** Urine, voided: crystals. A large superficial urothelial cell is adjacent to a large crystal. Red blood cells and debris are present in the background (PAP).

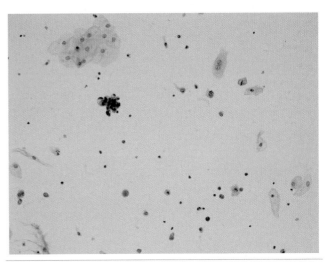

**Fig. 12.9** Urine, washing: high cellularity. At a low power, this bladder washing specimen in a patient with a history of lithiasis shows a variety of urothelial cell types. Superficial and intermediate urothelial cells are admixed with inflammatory cells and squamous cells (PAP).

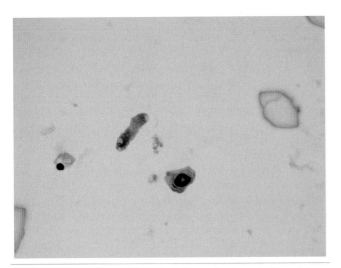

**Fig. 12.8** Urine, voided: cast. A renal tubular cast is admixed with crystals and a reactive intermediate urothelial cell (PAP).

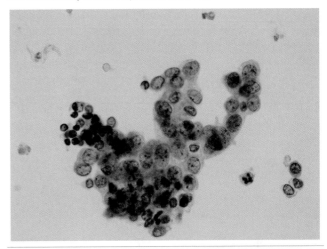

**Fig. 12.10** Urine, washing: three-dimensional cell group. A large staghorn cluster of urothelial cells is infiltrated by a few acute and chronic inflammatory cells. The urothelial cell nuclei are round to oval and contain thickened nuclear rims, although the chromatin pattern is hypochromatic. A small red nucleolus is present in most of the nuclei. The urothelial cell cytoplasm is finely granular and not homogeneous (PAP).

## Instrumented urine specimens

Instrumented specimens are characterised by high cellularity, as the method of cellular procurement forcibly removes epithelium (Fig. 12.9). These specimens show large groups of cells, small cell clusters and single cells from all urothelial cell layers. The large groups of urothelial cells often demonstrate all cell layers, with superficial cells overlying intermediate and basal/parabasal cells (Fig. 12.10). These groups are termed 'instrumentation artefact' and may be confused with low-grade urothelial carcinomas.[14] At high power, the smaller groups of urothelial cells lack significant atypia (Fig. 12.11).

Catheterised urines tend to show more inflammation than other instrumented urine types, as indwelling catheters cause irritation and inflammation (Fig. 12.12).

## Ileal conduit specimens

Ileal conduit specimens are predominantly composed of numerous intestinal glandular cells and inflammatory cells that often have a degenerate appearance (Fig. 12.13).[15,16] The

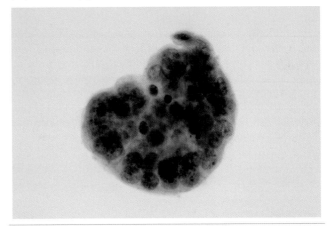

**Fig. 12.11** Urine, washing: benign urothelial cells. A three-dimensional group of urothelial cells shows round nuclei with evenly distributed granular nuclear chromatin. Although the nuclei show overlapping, other characteristics of neoplasia are lacking (PAP).

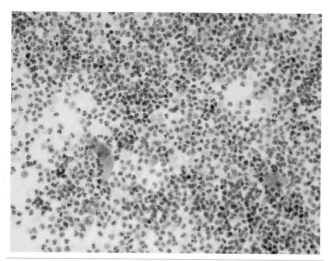

**Fig. 12.12** Urine, catheterised: acute inflammation. This patient has an indwelling catheter and a secondary infection, characterised by marked acute inflammation. A reactive superficial cell with a moderate amount of cytoplasm showing bichromasia is present (PAP).

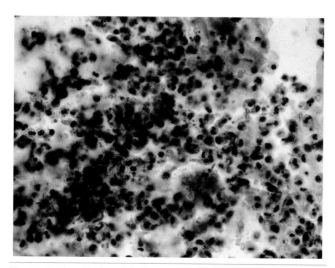

**Fig. 12.13** Urine, ileal conduit: degenerate cells. Most ileal conduit urines are cellular and contain few urothelial cells, abundant degenerate glandular cells, and debris. The degenerate ileal cells contain small, hyperchromatic nuclei and a moderate amount of cytoplasm (PAP).

high cellularity arises from the natural sloughing of the intestinal epithelium, as glandular cells lack the hardiness to withstand the toxicity of urine. The glandular cells may form flat sheets, similar to the findings in colonic brushing specimens. The degenerate glandular cells contain a pyknotic and eccentrically placed nucleus. The nuclear to cytoplasmic ratios are not increased, but the smudged hyperchromasia may be alarming. Occasional upper tract superficial urothelial cells are seen.

## Malignancy and its pitfalls

### Urothelial cancer

Urothelial carcinoma is the most common cancer detected by urine cytology and the most common site of origin is the bladder. Worldwide, over 390 000 bladder cancers are detected

---

> **Box 12.3  Surgical pathological diagnostic categories for urothelial lesions**
>
> Normal
>
> Hyperplasia
>
> Flat lesions with atypia
>
> - Reactive atypia
> - Atypia of unknown significance
> - Dysplasia (low grade)
> - Carcinoma *in situ*
>
> Papillary lesions
>
> - Papilloma
> - Papillary neoplasm of low malignant potential (PNLMP)
> - Low-grade urothelial carcinoma
> - High-grade urothelial carcinoma
>
> Invasive neoplasms
>
> - Lamina propria invasion
> - Muscularis propria invasion

annually.[17] In most parts of the world, 90% of bladder cancers are urothelial in origin, 5% squamous and 5% mixed urothelial and squamous. Primary adenocarcinoma of the bladder is rare. Bladder cancer often presents insidiously, with more than 75% of patients having haematuria, which is often painless.[18] Symptoms include urinary frequency, dysuria and urgency.

Most cytological diagnostic systems classify urothelial carcinomas into the categories of high grade and low grade. This system is far less complex than the currently used histopathological diagnostic grading systems (Box 12.3).[19–21] Although the low-grade/high-grade cytological grading system does not precisely map to the histopathological grading systems, there generally is correlation between the better-differentiated tumours on histopathology with cytologically low-grade carcinomas and the more poorly differentiated tumours on histopathology with cytologically high-grade carcinomas.

As Oosterhuis et al. wrote, tumour progression may occur in all patients with all tumour types, except for those with papillomas, which often are not diagnosed on urine specimens.[19] The key to the cytological diagnostic system is in flagging this risk, as clinicians use triage protocols based on clinical findings and the cytological diagnosis of low or high-grade urothelial carcinoma. For example, on a voided urine specimen, the diagnosis of a high-grade urothelial carcinoma generally results in additional follow-up, such as cystoscopic examination. On a bladder wash specimen, the diagnosis of low- or high-grade urothelial carcinoma is used in conjunction with the cystoscopic impression.

### Diagnostic accuracy

Koss et al. reported that the sensitivity of voided urine for the diagnosis of high-grade urothelial carcinoma was 94.2%.[22] The sensitivity increased as the number of voided urine specimens increased, with 79% of cancers detected on the first specimen, 14% on the second specimen and 7% on the third specimen. Other authors have confirmed this high level of sensitivity.[2,23–25]

Monolayer preparation methods detect high-grade lesions at a similar percentage,[26] although indeterminate rates may initially rise after implementation.[27]

The calculation of the specificity of voided urine cytology for high-grade urothelial carcinoma depends on how indeterminate diagnoses are assessed, although the false positive rate of an outright diagnosis of high-grade urothelial carcinoma is extremely low. In some patients, lesions are not visualised on cystoscopic examination even following a positive urine cytology, indicating the limits of cystoscopy and biopsy as a gold standard.[4]

In a study using histological follow-up as the gold standard, 40% (55 of 136) patients had an indeterminate voided urine diagnosis (atypical or suspicious) and follow-up of a high-grade urothelial carcinoma; only 26% of patients had a benign lesion.[4] Although this study involved a number of high-risk patients who had a history of cancer, the data indicate that indeterminate diagnoses harbour a relatively high risk of cancer.

The sensitivity of bladder wash specimens for the diagnosis of high-grade urothelial carcinoma is higher than that seen in voided urine specimens.[4,28,29]

The sensitivity and specificity of the diagnosis of low-grade urothelial carcinoma in instrumented urine specimens is controversial. The reported sensitivity (based on making a definitively malignant diagnosis) in the literature ranges from 0% to 73%, although in experienced hands, the sensitivity is over 50%.[23,30–32] Based on the same follow-up study listed above, 67% (14 of 21) patients had a diagnosis of atypical, suspicious or malignant and a low-grade urothelial carcinoma on follow-up.[4]

The literature is virtually unanimous that the outright diagnosis of a low-grade urothelial carcinoma is exceedingly difficult to make on a voided urine specimen. However, one study showed that 48% of biopsy proven low-grade urothelial carcinomas had a voided urine diagnosis of atypical or suspicious.[4] In this study, 11% of all institutional voided urine cases had an indeterminate diagnosis, as the vast majority of patients did not have histology follow-up. These data indicate that indeterminate diagnoses raise the post-test probability of low-grade cancer, even in voided urine specimens.

## High-grade urothelial carcinoma

### Cytological findings: high-grade urothelial carcinoma

- Increased cellularity usually present
- Single pleomorphic malignant cells, a few groups
- Raised nuclear:cytoplasmic ratio
- Coarse dense nuclear chromatin
- Nuclear membrane irregularities.

The diagnosis of high-grade urothelial carcinoma corresponds to either an *in situ* or an invasive lesion. As a rule, the cytological features are not definitive in making this separation, although the more anaplastic the tumour, the more likely it is that the tumour is invasive.[24,25] Invasive high-grade urothelial carcinomas have a tendency to be clinically aggressive and most cancer deaths from papillary urothelial carcinomas are from the high-grade types.[33]

### Voided urine specimens

The malignant cells of a high-grade urothelial carcinoma are generally observed singly, although loose clusters also may

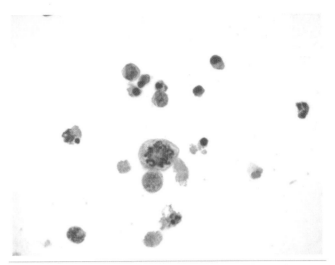

**Fig. 12.14** Urine, voided: high-grade urothelial carcinoma. The malignant urothelial cells vary in size and shape and exhibit variable degrees of degeneration. A large atypical mitotic figure is seen in the centre of the field (PAP).

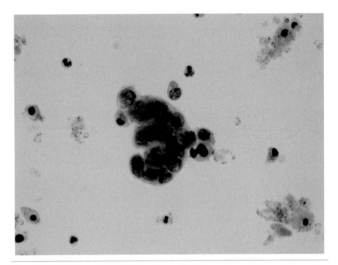

**Fig. 12.15** Urine, voided: high-grade urothelial carcinoma. The malignant urothelial cells contain a thin rim of homogeneous cytoplasm. There is an absence of cytoplasmic vacuoles (PAP).

be present.[24,34] In voided urines, only rare cells may be seen, indicating that careful screening, as for cervical smear tests, is necessary.

The malignant cells vary in size and shape, and in some cases, huge malignant cells may be seen (Fig. 12.14). The nuclear:cytoplasmic ratio is increased, and most malignant cells have only a thin rim of dense, homogeneous or non-vacuolated cytoplasm (Fig. 12.15).[32] Cytoplasmic vacuolation is not a typical feature, but may be observed in cases with abundant acute inflammation. The cytoplasmic membranes are easily distinguished in high-grade urothelial carcinomas.

The appearance of the nucleus is the defining feature of high-grade urothelial carcinoma. The nucleus is large and exhibits marked nuclear membrane irregularities (Fig. 12.16). The nuclear chromatin is extremely coarse and some cells have a West Virginia 'coal black' appearance, indicating that the chromatin is uniformly dark and impenetrable in appearance due to degenerative changes (Fig. 12.17).[32,35] When present,

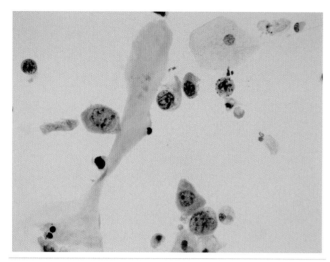

**Fig. 12.16** Urine, voided: high-grade urothelial carcinoma. The malignant cell nuclei are large and the nuclear membranes are irregular. The nuclear membranes show focal thickening. Several of the nuclei show multiple prominent nucleoli (PAP).

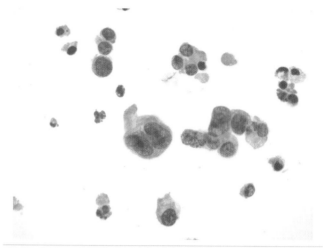

**Fig. 12.18** Urine, voided: high-grade urothelial carcinoma. The malignant urothelial cell nuclei are large and prominent nucleoli are seen (PAP).

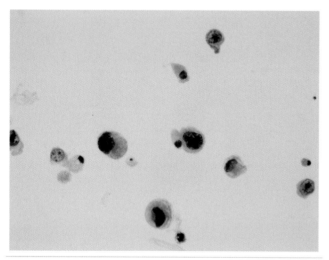

**Fig. 12.17** Urine, voided: high-grade urothelial carcinoma. Occasional malignant urothelial cell nuclei have a 'coal black' appearance with densely hyperchromatic chromatin patterns (PAP).

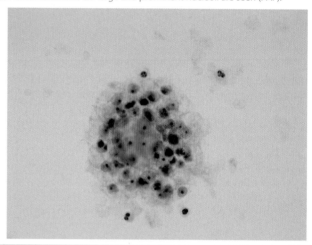

**Fig. 12.19** Urine, voided: high-grade urothelial carcinoma. The malignant cells show glandular differentiation with finely vacuolated cytoplasm, similar to the cytoplasmic presentation seen in clear cell carcinoma of the kidney. A multinucleated malignant urothelial cell with densely homogeneous cytoplasm is present in the center of the group of malignant cells showing glandular differentiation (PAP).

nucleoli are large and prominent and cytophagocytosis may be present (Fig. 12.18).[36] Nassar et al. reported that greater smudging of cancer cells was observed in monolayer preparations, although monolayer preparations also showed more even disbursement of malignant cells.[37]

High-grade urothelial carcinomas occasionally exhibit squamous or glandular differentiation, squamous being the more frequent (Fig. 12.19).[23] Squamous differentiation is characterised by keratinisation, sometimes manifested by parakeratosis or keratin pearls (Fig. 12.20). Malignant glandular differentiation is difficult to recognise but is discernible by cytoplasmic vacuolation. Although invasive high-grade urothelial carcinomas may exhibit sarcomatoid differentiation, the malignant cells are not typically observed in voided urine specimens but may be seen in washing specimens (Fig. 12.21).

## Ileal conduit urine specimens

High-grade urothelial carcinoma cells tend to be few and are admixed with the numerous degenerate glandular cells, as

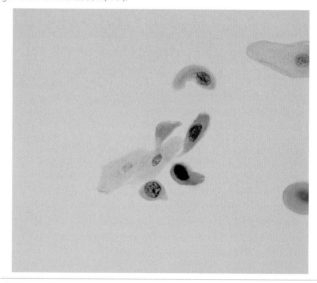

**Fig. 12.20** Urine, voided: high-grade urothelial carcinoma. Several of the malignant cells show squamous differentiation. Note the presence of a malignant urothelial cell showing dense cytoplasm without keratinisation (PAP).

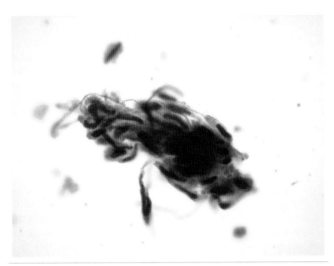

**Fig. 12.21** Urine, washing: high-grade urothelial carcinoma. The malignant cells show a spindled appearance consistent with low-grade sarcomatous differentiation. The malignant spindle cells have densely hyperchromatic nuclei that vary in size and shape. The degree of mesenchymal differentiation may vary considerably. There is an absence of inflammation in the background (PAP).

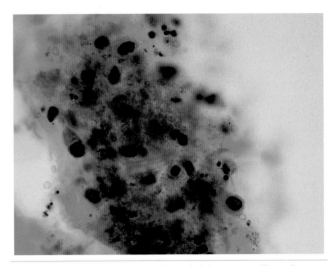

**Fig. 12.23** Urine, washing: high-grade urothelial carcinoma. The malignant cells are numerous and pleomorphic. Tumour diathesis and debris are admixed with malignant cell nuclei showing a coal black appearance (PAP).

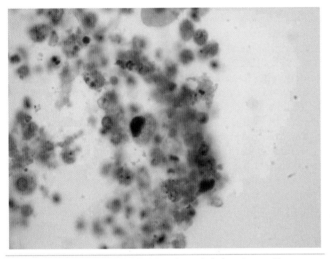

**Fig. 12.22** Urine, ileal conduit: high-grade urothelial carcinoma. The malignant cells show non-degenerate features in a background of degenerate ileal cells. The size of the malignant urothelial cell nuclei is considerably larger than the degenerate glandular cell nuclei (PAP).

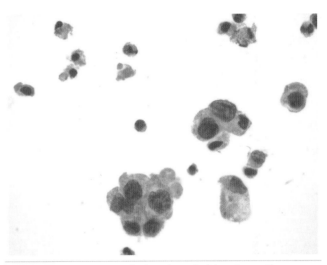

**Fig. 12.24** Urine, upper tract: high-grade urothelial carcinoma. The malignant cells show marked nuclear atypia in a background of slightly atypical urothelial cells (PAP).

described above. The malignant cells often are better preserved, are larger, and maintain crisper nuclear membranes, compared to the degenerate cells (Fig. 12.22).[15,16]

### Instrumented urine specimens

In instrumented urine specimens, numerous malignant cells usually are seen (Fig. 12.23) and the malignant cells have the same cytological features as described for voided urine specimens. Small- to moderate-sized clusters of malignant cells may be seen, but large groups of malignant cells are unusual, as high-grade urothelial carcinomas typically show extensive cellular dissociation.

### Upper tract specimens

Benign urothelial cells of the upper tract, compared with their lower tract counterparts, show higher nuclear:cytoplasmic ratios, more prominent nuclear membrane irregularities and larger nuclei (Fig. 12.24). Instrumentation produces large groups of cells. Nonetheless, the diagnosis of high-grade urothelial carcinoma tends to be straightforward, as the nuclear size, hyperchromasia and membrane irregularities exceed the changes of benign urothelium.[38–40] Potts et al reported that the criteria of high nuclear:cytoplasmic ratios, anisonucleosis and nuclear overlapping were among the most important criteria in diagnosing high-grade urothelial carcinoma of the upper tract (Fig. 12.25).[41]

---

**Diagnostic pitfalls: high-grade urothelial carcinoma**

- Degenerative changes
- Chemotherapy and radiation therapy changes
- Lithiasis
- Human polyoma virus effects
- Reactive changes from other causes.

## Urothelial cellular degeneration

Urothelial cells may undergo degeneration with nuclear pyknosis and hyperchromasia that may mimic a high-grade urothelial cancer. Degeneration is most problematic in voided urinary tract specimens (Fig. 12.26).[35] The degree of urothelial cell degeneration is related to urine acidity and accompanying inflammatory conditions.[23] The most degenerate specimens tend to be first morning voids and those obtained from collection bags.

High-grade urothelial carcinomas may display considerable degenerative features, but one should always be able to find a handful of malignant cells that have intact nuclear membranes. Renshaw et al. reported that coal block nuclei with intact nuclear membranes are seen almost exclusively in malignancy.[10] Degenerate cells are the main cause of the use of non-definitive diagnoses, such as atypical.

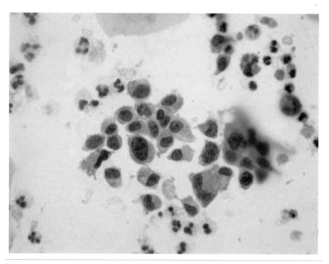

**Fig. 12.25** Urine, upper tract: high-grade urothelial carcinoma. The malignant cells show high nuclear:cytoplasmic ratios and variation in nuclear size. Tumour necrosis is present in the background (PAP).

## Chemotherapy and radiation therapy effect

Chemotherapy and radiation therapy may induce a variety of cellular changes that mimic those seen in a high-grade urothelial carcinoma. Chemotherapeutic effect results from agents administered systemically, such as cyclophosphamide and busulfan, or intravesically. The changes may therefore be seen in patients being treated specifically for urothelial cancer or in patients being treated for other malignancies. Radiation therapy may be targeted in those patients who have unresectable urothelial cancers or in patients with tumours adjacent to the urinary tract, such as those arising in the uterine cervix or prostate.

The cytomorphology of urinary tract specimens is similar for both chemotherapy and radiation therapy, regardless of the specimen type. In the first stages of treatment, the cells are sloughed and are accompanied by blood and copious acute inflammatory cells. Specimens obtained after this early phase are more problematic, especially in patients who have had radiation therapy, as the cellular atypia may occur years after the last treatment.

The cytomorphological features of chemotherapy and radiation therapy include increased cellularity, cellular degeneration, frayed cytoplasmic borders, increased nuclear:cytoplasmic ratios, nuclear hyperchromasia, nuclear multilobation, nuclear pseudoinclusions, karyorrhexis and karyolysis.[42–47] Nuclear hyperchromasia and nuclear membrane irregularities are the most worrisome features that may be confused with malignancy (Fig. 12.27). Cytomorphological features most helpful in identifying treatment effect are overall cellular enlargement with abundant cytoplasm (Fig. 12.28). In treatment effect, the cellular nuclei often have a homogeneously dark nucleus, whereas in high-grade urothelial carcinoma, the nuclear chromatin is more textured (Fig. 12.29). If only rare, large, bizarre appearing cells are present, high-grade urothelial carcinoma is less likely (Fig. 12.30).

Bacillus Calmette–Guérin (BCG) vaccine is the main chemotherapeutic agent for treating many bladder cancers, particularly carcinoma *in situ*. BCG is derived from *Mycobacterium*

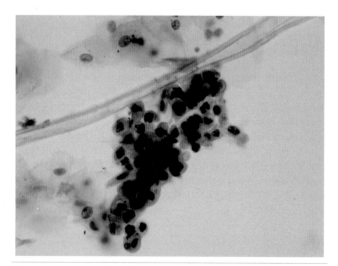

**Fig. 12.26** Urine, voided: degeneration. A large cluster of degenerate urothelial cells contain hyperchromatic nuclei with irregular nuclear membranes. These cells contain a moderate amount of cytoplasm and lack the high nuclear:cytoplasmic ratio of high-grade urothelial carcinoma cells. Background squamous cells are hardier and show fewer degenerative features (PAP).

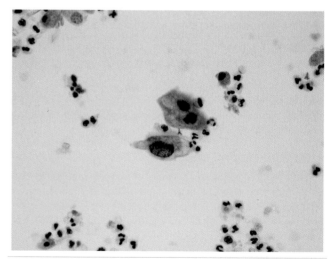

**Fig. 12.27** Urine, voided: chemotherapy effect. The urothelial cell shows nuclear enlargement, slight hyperchromasia and nuclear membrane irregularities. The nuclear membrane is not markedly thickened and the nuclear hyperchromasia is less than that seen in a high-grade urothelial carcinoma. This patient was receiving systemic chemotherapy for leukaemia (PAP).

*bovis* and causes a granulomatous response with extensive epithelial sloughing and degeneration. The cytological response to BCG has been well documented and consists of an initial acute inflammatory response followed by an increase in the number of chronic inflammatory cells in urinary tract specimens. In the later phases, histiocytes and true granulomas may be seen, sometimes noticeable in instrumented urine specimens (Fig. 12.31).[48,49]

The cellular atypia in non-neoplastic urothelial cells associated with BCG treatment is less pronounced than that associated with other chemotherapeutic agents. The challenge in interpreting urine specimens in patients who have or are being treated with BCG is in separating rare tumour cells from degenerate benign cells (Fig. 12.32), as the presence of malignant cells is indicative that the tumour has not been completely eradicated or has recurred. Definitively malignant cells with intact, crisp nuclear chromatin should be present before making a diagnosis of high-grade urothelial carcinoma.

## Lithiasis

Lithiasis is the most common non-neoplastic process that may yield a urine specimen mimicking a high-grade urothelial carcinoma. Up to 85% of urinary tract stones are composed of calcium phosphate or calcium oxalate. Less frequently, calculi are composed of cystine, struvite or uric acid. Individuals of all ages may have lithiasis and urine specimens should be interpreted cautiously when patients have clinical histories suggestive of lithiasis such as pain, previous history of stones or pyuria. Marked cellular atypia in urine specimens from younger patients, especially if under 40 years of age, should also raise the suspicion of lithiasis.

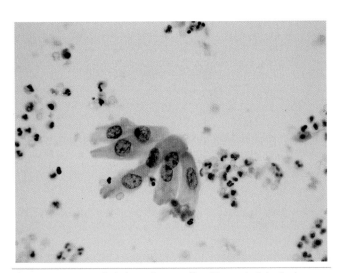

**Fig. 12.28** Urine, washing: radiation therapy effect. The urothelial cell shows cellular enlargement, binucleation and abundant cytoplasm. One nucleus contains a prominent nuclear groove and the other nucleus is slightly degenerated with gaps in the nuclear membrane. This patient was receiving radiation therapy for prostate cancer and the washing specimen shows abundant acute inflammation and red blood cells (PAP).

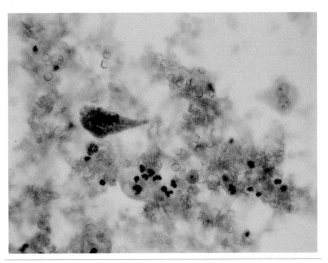

**Fig. 12.30** Urine, voided: chemotherapy effect. A urothelial cell shows an enlarged, bizarre, degenerate nucleus with abundant cytoplasm. Large cytoplasmic fragments are admixed with blood and acute inflammation. This patient had systemic chemotherapy for a germ cell neoplasm (PAP).

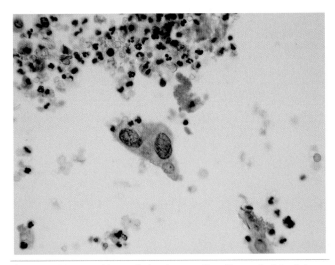

**Fig. 12.29** Urine, voided: chemotherapy effect. The urothelial cells show degenerate nuclei with irregular, thickened nuclear membranes. The cytoplasm is densely homogeneous, although the nuclear:cytoplasmic ratios are low. The cells have an elongated shape, similar to the shape of glandular cells. One of the reactive cells shows binucleation (PAP).

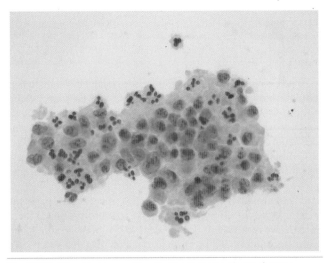

**Fig. 12.31** Urine, bladder washing: Bacillus Calmette–Guérin therapy effect. Histiocytes and granulomas in latter stage therapy may be seen in instrumented urine specimens. Numerous histiocytes are admixed with neutrophils in this loosely formed granuloma. In later stages of BCG therapy effect, the granulomas have more of an epithelioid appearance (PAP).

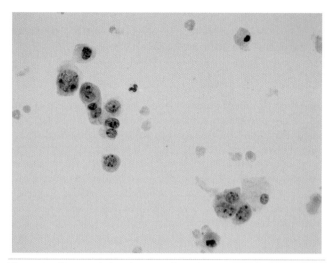

**Fig. 12.32** Urine, voided: malignant cells in a background of Bacillus Calmette–Guérin therapy effect. The malignant urothelial cells show marked nuclear hyperchromasia in a background of degenerated cells and chronic inflammatory cells. In this patient, numerous malignant cells are seen; in more diagnostically challenging cases, only rare degenerated malignant cells are appreciated (PAP).

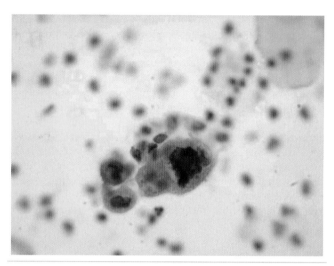

**Fig. 12.34** Urine, voided: lithiasis. The urothelial cells show enlarged bizarre nuclei with abundant cytoplasm. The acute inflammatory response is brisk. The large urothelial cell nucleus has a degenerate appearance, similar to findings seen in chemotherapy or radiation effect. This patient was 29 years old (PAP).

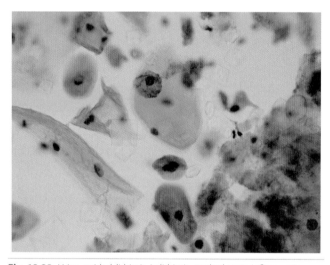

**Fig. 12.33** Urine, voided: lithiasis. In lithiasis, marked acute inflammation, squamous metaplasia, and reactive squamous cells may be seen. The urothelial cells often have slightly hyperchromatic nuclei (PAP).

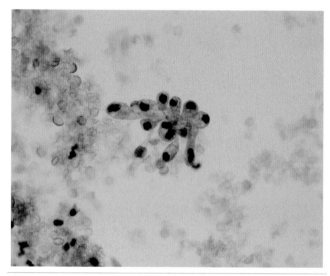

**Fig. 12.35** Urine, voided: lithiasis. The urothelial cells show vacuolated cytoplasm and degenerative features. The nuclei are hyperchromatic, but small and not larger than the accompanying red cells. The cytoplasm of these reactive cells is often known as 'bubbly' (PAP).

In voided urine specimens, lithiasis is characterised by hypercellularity, pseudopapillary groups, acute and chronic inflammation, squamous metaplasia, blood, and acellular fragments possibly representing stone fragments (Fig. 12.33).[50,51] Stone fragments may be calcified and laminated.

Urothelial cells in patients with lithiasis may exhibit significant cellular atypia consisting of nuclear enlargement and nuclear hyperchromasia. The urothelial cell nuclei in lithiasis tend to have smooth and thin nuclear membranes, lack the extreme hyperchromasia seen in high-grade urothelial cell carcinoma, have moderate to low nuclear to cytoplasmic ratios, and more frequently have prominent nucleoli (Fig. 12.34).[50,51] In lithiasis, there is generally an absence of single markedly hyperchromatic cells as the atypical cells tend to remain in groups or small clusters and inflammation and/or blood is much more abundant. The presence of cytoplasmic bichromasia, vacuolated cytoplasm, and cellular debris also is more supportive

of lithiasis than high-grade urothelial carcinoma (Fig. 12.35). High-grade urothelial carcinomas exhibit a dual population of malignant cells and benign urothelial cells, whereas in lithiasis, a spectrum of atypical cellular changes is seen (Fig. 12.36).

## Human polyoma (BK) virus

Human polyomavirus is a DNA virus and a member of the Papovirus family. Human polyomavirus may be detected in all urinary specimen types. The virus is first acquired in childhood but may be reactivated and cause infection in immunocompromised patients or even in those who have no underlying disorder. Human polyomavirus infects urothelial cells and/or renal tubular cells, especially in renal transplant patients.

Urothelial cells infected with human polyomavirus are always seen singly and are generally small (Fig. 12.37), although larger

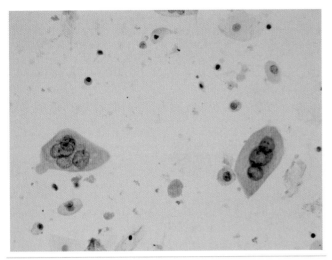

**Fig. 12.36** Urine, voided: lithiasis. The superficial urothelial cells show enlarged nuclei with slight nuclear membrane irregularities, but lack the marked hyperchromasia seen in high-grade urothelial carcinoma. The background has a 'dirty' appearance with debris and chronic inflammatory cells (PAP).

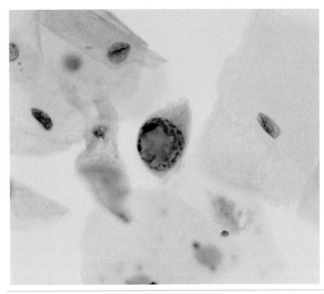

**Fig. 12.38** Urine, voided: human polyomavirus. A nuclear inclusion in a human polyomavirus infected urothelial cell is seen. In this infected cell, the inclusion occupies only a portion of the nucleus and the surrounding chromatin is granular (PAP).

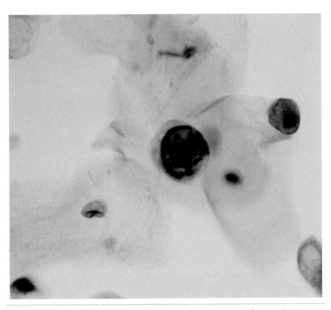

**Fig. 12.37** Urine, voided: human polyomavirus. Human polyomavirus infected urothelial cells are seen singly and are generally small (PAP).

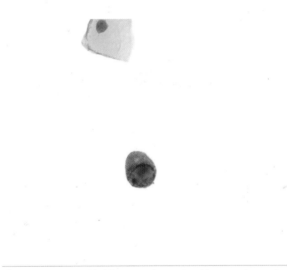

**Fig. 12.39** Urine, voided: human polyomavirus. Human polyomavirus infected urothelial cells contain smoothly contoured nuclear membranes. The nuclear membrane appears thickened, as the residual chromatin is compressed at the nuclear edge (PAP).

infected cells may be similar in size to high-grade urothelial carcinoma cells.[52] The nuclei are hyperchromatic, which is the reason why infected urothelial cells may be mistaken for high-grade urothelial carcinoma, especially when the nuclei are somewhat degenerate. Thus, the term 'decoy' cell is used to describe infected urothelial cells.[53,54]

The nuclear hyperchromasia arises from the presence of a nuclear inclusion that is homogeneous in texture and stains blue to black (Fig. 12.38).[52–54] The inclusion occupies almost the entire nucleus and compresses the residual nuclear chromatin against the nuclear rim to produce the appearance of a thickened nuclear membrane. Notably, the nuclear membrane of an infected cell is not irregular in contour in contrast to the membrane of a high-grade urothelial carcinoma cell (Fig. 12.39).

Human polyomavirus infected cells have a high nuclear to cytoplasmic ratio and the blue to green cytoplasm is often

eccentrically visible along one side of the cell to give the appearance of a comet (Fig. 12.40). The inclusions may be so degenerate that the infected cell nuclei have a cleared or empty appearance. The inclusions may be seen without associated cytoplasm, imitating a stripped nucleus (Fig. 12.41), which is unusual for a high-grade urothelial carcinoma.

The most challenging specimen is a voided urine from a patient recently treated for high-grade urothelial carcinoma, which shows rare cells with degenerate hyperchromatic nuclei suspicious for either high-grade urothelial carcinoma or human polyomavirus infection. In the latter case, the degenerate cells tend to be small; for the definitive diagnosis of carcinoma, well-preserved, intact cells with discernible nuclear chromatin should be appreciated.

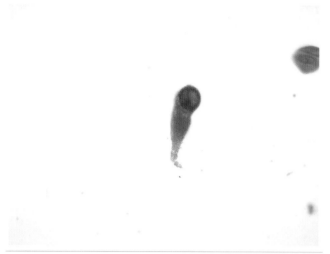

**Fig. 12.40** Urine, voided: human polyomavirus. The human polyomavirus infected urothelial cell shows an eccentrically placed nucleus. The cell has the appearance of a comet with a long tail (PAP).

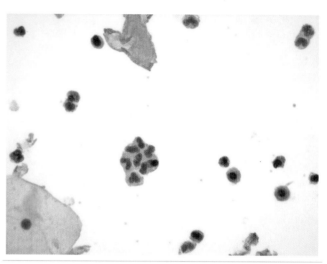

**Fig. 12.42** Urine, voided: bacterial infection. Degenerate urothelial and inflammatory cells are seen in a background of bacterial cystitis. Numerous neutrophils are present (PAP).

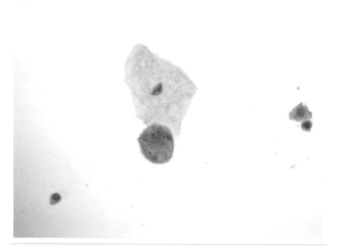

**Fig. 12.41** Urine, voided: human polyomavirus. A stripped nuclear inclusion in human polyomavirus infection is seen. The nucleus appears intact and the cytoplasm is completed absent. In some specimens, the stripped nuclear inclusions appear degenerate and hyperchromatic, raising the suspicion of a high-grade urothelial carcinoma (PAP).

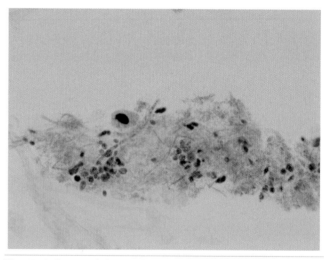

**Fig. 12.43** Urine, voided: *Candida* sp. infection. *Candida sp.* yeast and pseudohyphal forms with degenerate acute inflammatory cells and urothelial cells are seen. It may be difficult to separate a true bladder infection from contaminant if only a few yeast forms are present (PAP).

## Reactive changes from other causes

Reactive changes may be seen in a variety of conditions in addition to lithiasis, radiation therapy, chemotherapy and viral effect. The atypia in reactive conditions is commonly secondary to inflammation and/or cellular degeneration. Several of these causes are listed below.

*Bacterial infection.* Bacterial cystitis is usually caused by faecal flora, Gram-negative organisms such as *Escherichia coli* (80% of infections), *Proteus, Klebsiella* and *Pseudomonas aeruginosa*. Bacterial infections occur mostly in adult females but also may occur in patients with urinary tract obstruction,[55] such as stones, or men with prostatic hypertrophy, and patients with nerve damage.

In most cases, voided urine specimens show abundant bacteria and acute inflammation. Urothelial cells typically are few and are poorly preserved, showing a hyperchromatic, small nucleus and frayed cytoplasm. The absence of nuclear detail is the key to not making a diagnosis of high-grade urothelial carcinoma (Fig. 12.42). The observation of rare tumour cells and marked inflammation is unusual for high-grade urothelial carcinoma. Occasionally, large groups of reactive urothelial cells are detached, which also is an unusual feature of high-grade tumours.

*Fungal infection.* Voided urine specimens in patients who have a urinary tract fungal infection are similar in appearance to the findings in bacterial cystitis, with pronounced acute inflammation and rare degenerate urothelial cells. The most common fungal form seen in a voided urine specimen is *Candida*, which in women is most often secondary to vaginal contamination; these preparations show squamous cells and bacteria, in addition to *Candida*, and the urothelial cells are greater in number and non-reactive in appearance. Patients may present with *Candida* cystitis (Fig. 12.43), although other fungi, including *Histoplasma, Aspergillus, Cryptococcus* and *Blastomyces* have been reported.[56]

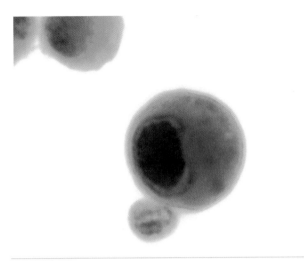

**Fig. 12.44** Urine, voided: cytomegalovirus infection. A cytomegalic infected cell shows a very large nuclear inclusion (PAP).

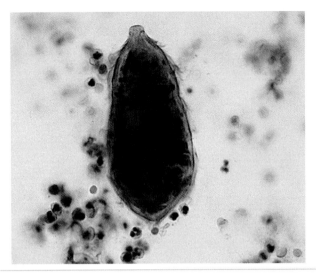

**Fig. 12.45** Urine, voided: *Schistosoma haematobium* ovum. The schistosome ovum is not well preserved and the typical spine is not clearly visible. The background contains inflammatory cells (PAP). (Courtesy of Dr G McKee).

*Mycobacterial infection.* The principal site of *Mycobacterium tuberculosis* infection of the urinary tract is the kidney, although the bladder may be involved secondarily. Bladder wash and voided urine specimens show a chronic inflammatory response, similar to that seen in BCG therapy. The urothelial cells display enlarged, hyperchromatic nuclei, although they are usually also degenerate.[57,58]

*Viral infection.* In addition to human polyomavirus and human papillomavirus (discussed later), other viruses that may be identified in urinary tract specimens include cytomegalovirus (CMV) and herpes simplex virus (HSV). CMV infects renal convoluted tubular cells in immunosuppressed patients and very young patients and the cytomorphological appearance is described elsewhere in this text (see Chs 18, 23). Very few virally infected cells are seen in urinary tract specimens and these cells often have a degenerate appearance (Fig. 12.44).[59,60] When CMV-infected cells degenerate, they may mimic a high-grade urothelial carcinoma.

HSV infects urothelial cells but more often is seen in genital infections as a contaminant in urinary tract specimens. HSV infections are characterised by abundant acute inflammation and degenerated cellular debris.[61,62] Other viruses that have been identified in urinary tract specimens include measles virus and adenovirus.

*Parasitic infections.* Parasitic infections of the urinary tract include *Trichomonas* and *Schistosoma*. *Trichomonas vaginalis* usually is a contaminant in women and the organisms are seen in association with intermediate squamous cells and acute inflammation. In men, *Trichomonas* most likely is seen in the urethra and is a cause of non-gonococcal urethritis;[63] voided urines in these patients show abundant acute inflammation and sloughed urothelial cells that exhibit marked reactive changes.

Schistosomiasis of the bladder is most common in the Middle East and is mainly caused by *Schistosoma haematobium*. The eggs of *Schistosoma* may be observed in urinary tract specimens (Fig. 12.45).[64] Schistosomal infections are characterised by exuberant acute inflammation, blood, squamous metaplasia, and marked reactive urothelial and squamous cell changes. Schistosomal infections are a risk factor for squamous cell carcinoma of the bladder. Other parasites infecting the urinary tract are also accompanied by a marked inflammatory response.

*Malakoplakia.* Malakoplakia is a chronic granulomatous disease caused by a defect in the phagolysosomal processing of bacteria and predominantly occurs in middle-aged women. On cystoscopic examination, the bladder surface is lined by confluent yellow nodules or plaques,[65] which represent granulomas composed of histiocytes and multinucleated giant cells known as von Hansemann histiocytes. These giant cells contain abundant granular cytoplasm that stains positively with periodic acid Schiff (PAS). This staining is caused by the presence of phagolysosomes containing partially digested bacteria. The diagnosis of malakoplakia depends on the observation of Michaelis–Gutmann bodies, which are round, laminated cytoplasmic inclusions ranging from 4–10 μm in diameter (Fig. 12.45).[66] The Michaelis–Gutmann body is PAS positive and may calcify and become encrusted with iron. Voided urine specimens show abundant inflammation including neutrophils and histiocytes.

## Low-grade urothelial carcinoma

The majority of low-grade urothelial carcinomas do not behave aggressively. Jordan et al. estimated that approximately 5% of patients who have a low-grade urothelial carcinoma die of their disease.[33] However, 50–75% of patients with low-grade urothelial carcinoma have recurrence within 2 years of the initial diagnosis.[67] Low-grade cancers progress to high-grade cancers in up to 20% of cases, necessitating close clinical follow-up.[33] In most patients, low-grade urothelial carcinomas have a frond-like papillary appearance and are easily identified on cystoscopic examination. Clinicians may wash and/or biopsy these lesions when seen on cystoscopic examination. In some instances, the papillary fronds cannot be seen, as they lie behind folds.

### Cytological findings: low-grade urothelial carcinoma (instrumented specimens)

- Metaplastic cytoplasm
- Slightly increased nuclear to cytoplasmic ratio
- Nuclear membrane irregularities
- Eccentrically placed nodule

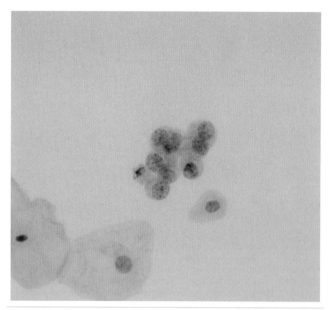

**Fig. 12.46** Urine, voided: atypical urothelial cells. The urothelial cells are small, but have finely granular chromatin with slightly thickened nuclear membranes. In several of the cells, the nucleus is eccentrically placed and the cytoplasm ranges from finely granular to slightly dense. On cystoscopic and histological follow-up, the patient had a low-grade urothelial carcinoma (PAP).

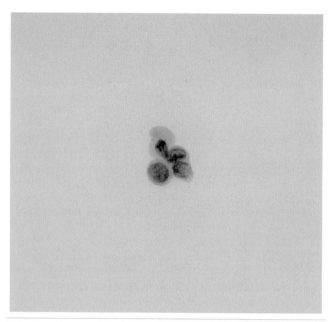

**Fig. 12.47** Urine, voided: urothelial cell cluster. A small cluster of atypical urothelial cells with homogeneous cytoplasm is seen. The relative paucity of these atypical cells often precludes the ability to make a definitively neoplastic diagnosis. On cystoscopic and histological follow-up, the patient had a low-grade urothelial carcinoma (PAP).

## Voided urine specimens

The published criteria for the diagnosis of low-grade urothelial carcinoma are based on studies of instrumented urine specimens and not on voided urine specimens.[30] A definitive diagnosis of a low-grade urothelial carcinoma is therefore problematic on voided urine specimens.

Several research groups found that over 50% of atypical voided urine specimens show low-grade urothelial carcinoma on follow-up.[4,35] Deshpande and McKee noted that cytological criteria more indicative of low-grade urothelial carcinoma included increased specimen cellularity, cell clusters, and nuclear membrane irregularities.[35] The presence of moderate to large cell clusters with relatively bland nuclei was concerning for low-grade urothelial carcinoma; however, these cell clusters were seen in reactive and reparative conditions as well. Thus, most cytopathologists choose to classify these groups as atypical (Fig. 12.46).

Nasuti et al. reported that monolayer preparations artificially cause both clustering of cells and disruption of true tissue fragments.[68] Deshpande and McKee reported that pseudoclusters are difficult to distinguish from true cell clusters on monolayer preparations, limiting interpretation (Fig. 12.47).[35] These findings indicate that definitive criteria for low-grade urothelial carcinoma are elusive on voided urine specimens, although features suggestive of neoplasm can be identified.

## Instrumented urine specimens

In histological sections, low-grade urothelial carcinoma is a well-differentiated neoplasm and the tumour cells are arranged on papillary fronds (Fig. 12.48). The cells exhibit an increased number of layers, have slightly increased nuclear to cytoplasmic ratios and display mild nuclear changes.

Published criteria for the diagnosis of low-grade urothelial carcinoma on instrumented urine specimens are shown in Box 12.4.[30–32] With bladder wash specimens, the search for tumour

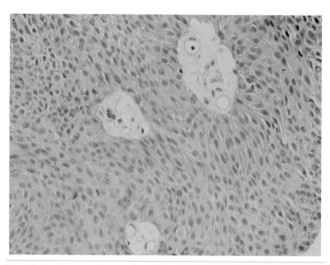

**Fig. 12.48** Histology: low-grade urothelial carcinoma. Several fibrovascular cores are surrounded by well-differentiated neoplastic cells. The malignant cells have abundant cytoplasm with monotonous round to oval nuclei (H&E).

should begin with single cells or cells in small clusters and not in the larger groups.[69] The reason for this is that criteria for malignancy, both cytoplasmic and nuclear, are subtle and large groups with cellular overlap limit definitive assessment. In addition, low-grade urothelial cell carcinomas are more likely to dissociate than non-neoplastic conditions.[70]

For low-grade urothelial carcinoma, the use of the combined criteria of increased nuclear to cytoplasmic ratios (Fig. 12.49), cytoplasmic homogeneity (Fig. 12.50), and irregular nuclear membranes (Fig. 12.51) have been shown to result in considerable accuracy in bladder washing specimens.[30] Murphy argued that the criterion of an eccentrically placed nucleus (Fig. 12.52) is also a very helpful feature.[32] Some cytopathologists look for distinct populations of cells, with the low-grade tumour cells

## Box 12.4 Cytomorphological criteria for the diagnosis of low-grade urothelial carcinoma

Hypercellularity

Papillary clusters and single cells

Uniformity of cell size

Absence of cytoplasmic vacuolation (homogeneous cytoplasm)

Increased nuclear to cytoplasmic ratio (slight)

Enlarged nuclei (slight)

Irregular nuclear membranes

Finely granular chromatin

Eccentric nucleus

Absent to small nucleolus

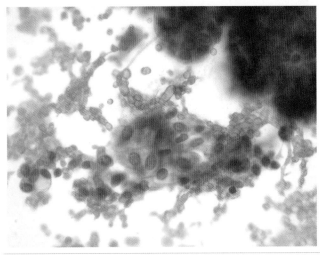

**Fig. 12.50** Urine, bladder washing: low-grade urothelial carcinoma. A cluster of cells of low-grade urothelial carcinoma shows densely homogeneous cytoplasm. The nuclear:cytoplasmic ratio is only slightly enlarged and the nuclear membranes are irregular in contour (PAP).

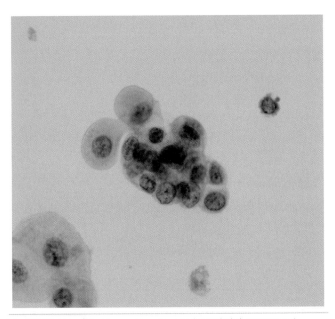

**Fig. 12.49** Urine, bladder washing: low-grade urothelial carcinoma. A cluster of low-grade carcinoma cells lies inferior to two benign intermediate urothelial cells. The low-grade carcinoma cells have high nuclear to cytoplasmic ratios, slightly thickened nuclear membranes and finely granular chromatin. The cytoplasm is difficult to see, but is metaplastic and non-vacuolated. Note that the size of the malignant cell nuclei is about the same as the benign intermediate cell nuclei, but the cytoplasm is considerably scantier (PAP).

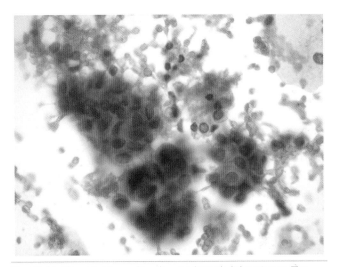

**Fig. 12.51** Urine, bladder washing: low-grade urothelial carcinoma. The urothelial cell nuclear membranes show irregularities and slight thickening. The malignant cells are seen in moderate-sized groups and singly. The criteria for malignancy are easier to identify in the single cells (PAP).

showing more uniformity compared with reactive or benign urothelial cells. Xin et al. reported that low-grade urothelial carcinomas in monolayer preparations exhibit similar findings to those in centrifugation specimens.[71]

The exclusion of low-grade urothelial carcinoma is based on other criteria. The presence of a marked inflammatory background limits interpretation in bladder wash specimens, as the urothelial cells, whether neoplastic or not, exhibit too much reactivity to classify definitively. Low-grade urothelial carcinoma should not be diagnosed in cells that show noticeable cytoplasmic vacuolation (Fig. 12.53) nor if the nuclei exhibit too much hyperchromasia (Fig. 12.54). The nuclear membranes may be

thick, but coarse chromatin is not seen. The outright diagnosis of low-grade urothelial carcinoma should be avoided in poorly preserved specimens.

### Diagnostic pitfalls: low-grade urothelial carcinoma

- Instrumentation artifact
- Reactive conditions.

### Instrumentation artifact

Instrumentation produces large groups of urothelial cells that may mimic papillary or pseudopapillary fragments (Box 12.5) (Fig. 12.55). As the primary diagnosis of low-grade urothelial carcinoma depends on the careful observation of nuclear and cytoplasmic features, the definitive diagnosis of a low-grade urothelial carcinoma should not rest solely on the presence of large groups in which individual cell characteristics are difficult to see.[14]

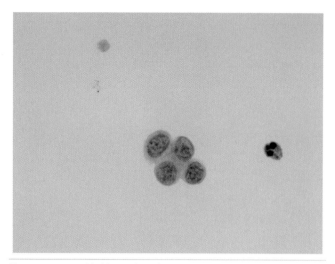

**Fig. 12.52** Urine, bladder washing: low-grade urothelial carcinoma. The urothelial cell nuclei of low-grade urothelial carcinoma are eccentrically placed. These low-grade urothelial cancer cells contain only a small rim of cytoplasm (PAP).

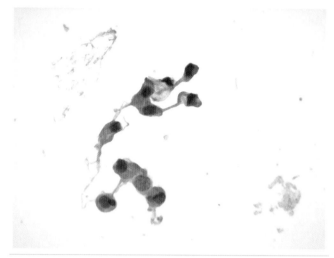

**Fig. 12.54** Urine, bladder washing: reactive urothelial cells. The urothelial cells show hyperchromatic and eccentrically placed nuclei. However, the degree of nuclear hyperchromasia is too pronounced for a low-grade urothelial carcinoma and the nuclear:cytoplasmic ratios are too low for a high-grade urothelial carcinoma (PAP).

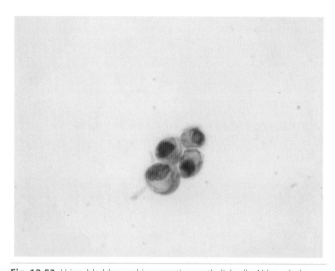

**Fig. 12.53** Urine, bladder washing: reactive urothelial cells. Although these urothelial cells show nuclear hyperchromasia, increased nuclear:cytoplasmic ratios, and nuclear membrane irregularities, the presence of cytoplasmic vacuolisation indicates a reactive process (PAP).

| **Box 12.5  Cytomorphological features of instrumentation artifact** |
|---|
| Large pseudopapillary groups |
| Three-dimensional balls |
| Cytoplasmic collars |
| Nuclear overlap |
| Distinct cytoplasmic membranes |
| Groups lined by superficial cells |
| Cells with low nuclear:cytoplasmic ratios |
| Finely granular nuclear chromatin |

## Reactive conditions

A variety of reactive conditions, such as lithiasis, infections, or chemotherapy effect, may produce slight cytoplasmic or nuclear atypia that raise suspicion for a low-grade urothelial carcinoma. Instrumented urines of these conditions produce large groups of cells, slight nuclear hyperchromasia and nuclear membrane irregularities. The presence of inflammation and the lack of single cells that exhibit the classic features of homogeneous cytoplasm with slight nuclear enlargement and nuclear membrane irregularity are signs that the atypia is secondary to reactive change rather than a low-grade urothelial carcinoma (Fig. 12.56). Most reactive conditions are associated with cytoplasmic vacuolation and prominent nucleoli, which are not features of a low-grade lesion.

Other reactive conditions include inverted papilloma, non-specific cystitis, interstitial cystitis, eosinophilic cystitis, urethral caruncle and inflammatory pseudotumour. These conditions are diagnosed on histological biopsy, as the inflammatory and/or proliferative changes are seen beneath the urothelial surface. On cystoscopic examination, some of these lesions may appear as mass lesions, for instance, inverted papilloma or inflammatory pseudotumour; others may be seen as patches of erythema. Both of these findings are worrisome for urothelial carcinoma. Certain lesions such as eosinophilic cystitis or caruncle may ulcerate producing inflammation and reactive urothelial changes. Instrumented urine specimens from the patients who have non-ulcerated mass lesions typically show benign urothelial cells and knowledge of the clinical history can lead to over-diagnosis of low-grade lesions, especially if slight atypia is seen.

## Squamous cell carcinoma

Urothelial carcinoma with squamous cell differentiation is far more common than a primary squamous cell carcinoma of the urinary tract. A squamous cell carcinoma arising in an

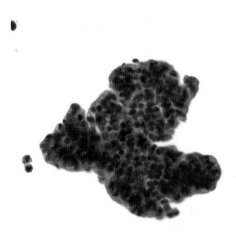

**Fig. 12.55** Urine, bladder washing: instrumentation artifact. Large groups of benign urothelial cells often are dislodged with instrumentation. In this group, superficial urothelial cells overly numerous intermediate urothelial cells. The urothelial cells are crowded but do not exhibit significant atypia (PAP).

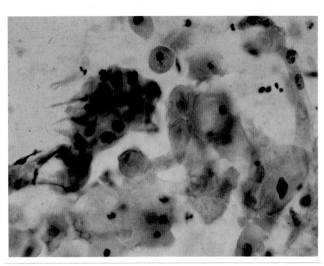

**Fig. 12.57** Urine, voided: squamous cell carcinoma. The malignant cells show keratinising and non-keratinising features. The malignant keratinised cells show either small, hyperchromatic nuclei or enlarged nuclei with irregular cytoplasmic shapes (PAP).

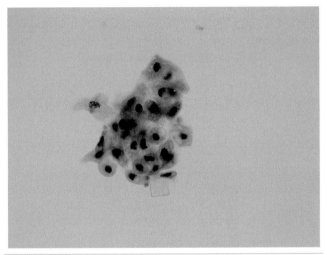

**Fig. 12.56** Urine, bladder washing: reactive findings. The urothelial cells show vacuolated cytoplasm and low nuclear:cytoplasmic ratios, although nuclear hyperchromasia and nuclear membrane irregularities are present. The patient has a history of lithiasis (PAP).

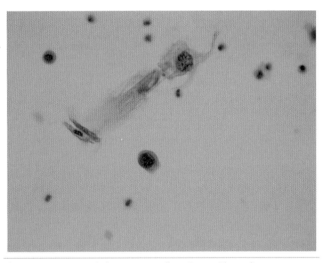

**Fig. 12.58** Urine, voided: squamous cell carcinoma. The malignant squamous cells show bizarre shapes with cytoplasmic protrusions. Parakeratosis and hyperkeratosis also are seen (PAP).

adjacent organ (e.g. uterine cervix) also must be excluded from a primary cancer. Most squamous cell carcinomas arise in the anterior wall and are well differentiated.

### Cytological findings: squamous cell carcinoma

- Cellular sample
- Mature squamous cells, slight atypia or anucleate if well-differentiated
- Obvious malignant features if moderately/poorly differentiated.

## Voided urine specimens

Well-differentiated squamous cell carcinomas are difficult to diagnose because they show little cytological atypia. The majority of squamous cell carcinomas arising in the bladder are keratinising.[72] On voided urine specimens, anucleated squamous cells, normal parakeratosis and atypical parakeratosis are seen (Fig. 12.57). The presence of squamous cells showing definitively malignant features, such as nuclear hyperchromasia, nuclear enlargement and nuclear membrane irregularity, may be rare.

In contrast, moderately and poorly differentiated squamous cell carcinomas are more easily diagnosed and the malignant cells appear similar to those observed in sputum specimens. In keratinising squamous cell carcinoma, highly atypical parakeratotic cells are more prevalent and bizarre squamous forms and keratin pearls are seen (Fig. 12.58). Cells similar in appearance to high-grade dysplastic cells seen in cervical smears may also be present. In non-keratinising squamous cell carcinoma, clusters of cells with high nuclear:cytoplasmic ratios and enlarged nuclei are seen. The cytoplasm has a metaplastic appearance and prominent nucleoli are common (Fig. 12.59).

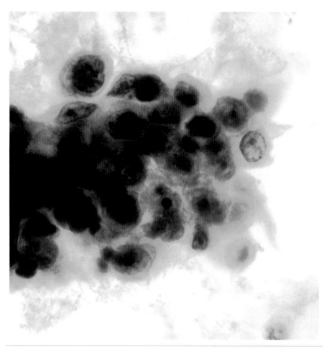

**Fig. 12.59** Urine, bladder washing: squamous cell carcinoma. Prominent nucleoli are seen in the malignant cells of this non-keratinising squamous cell carcinoma of the bladder (PAP).

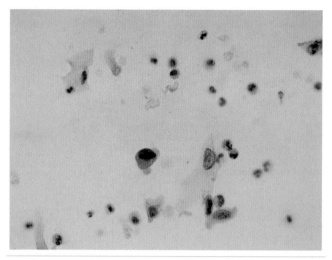

**Fig. 12.60** Urine, voided: squamous cell carcinoma. The non-keratinised cells of squamous cell carcinoma have a densely metaplastic appearance. The malignant cell nuclei are irregular in shape and a background of acute inflammation is present (PAP).

## Instrumented urine specimens

In well-differentiated squamous cell carcinomas, the specimens are highly cellular and show large numbers of anucleated squamous cells. Definitively malignant squamous cells also tend to be present in larger numbers in both well-differentiated and poorly differentiated tumours (Fig. 12.60).

| Diagnostic pitfalls: squamous cell carcinoma |
| --- |

- Atypical squamous metaplasia
- Contaminant squamous cells
- Human papillomavirus
- Other carcinomas with squamous features.

## Atypical squamous metaplasia

Squamous metaplasia may occur in a number of settings including lithiasis, indwelling catheters, chronic inflammatory conditions and inflammatory conditions admixed with metaplasia may result in cellular atypia within squamous cells (Fig. 12.61). Although poorly differentiated squamous cell carcinomas are sometimes associated with marked inflammation secondary to ulceration and invasion, well-differentiated squamous cell carcinomas generally are not associated with an acute inflammatory component. Thus, atypical parakeratotic squamous cells associated with inflammation are more likely to be reactive than neoplastic (Fig. 12.62). Again, the clinical history is paramount in separating reactive atypia from possible neoplasia.

## Contaminant

In women, a pitfall for over diagnosing squamous cell carcinoma is when vaginal contaminant squamous cells have an atypical appearance, especially when abundant inflammation is present.

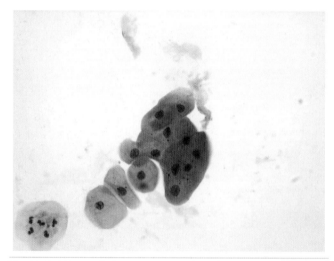

**Fig. 12.61** Urine, voided: squamous metaplasia. These metaplastic squamous cells have abundant cytoplasm with keratohyaline granules. The metaplastic nuclei are round or only slightly irregular in appearance (PAP).

## Human papillomavirus (HPV) infection

Bladder HPV infections typically involve areas of squamous metaplasia and the cytological appearance is identical to that seen in cervicovaginal PAP tests (Fig. 12.63). HPV infection is usually manifested by low-grade atypia/dysplasia due to the presence of a condyloma. In voided urine specimens, high-grade dysplastic cells associated with atypical parakeratosis may mimic a squamous cell carcinoma. In either scenario, the cytological diagnosis should be sufficient to result in cystoscopy. The more difficult problem is in separating cervico vaginal dysplasia introduced through gynaecological tract contamination from urinary tract squamous dysplasia.

## Urothelial carcinoma and other carcinomas

As mentioned previously, high-grade urothelial carcinomas may exhibit areas of squamous differentiation making separation difficult. If only a few malignant cells are seen in voided

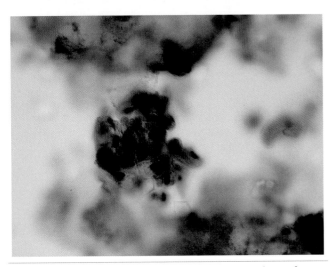

**Fig. 12.62** Urine, bladder washing: atypical parakeratosis. A cluster of squamous cells showing slightly enlarged, hyperchromatic nuclei is seen. The large, eosinophilic structure at the top of the microscopic field is a stone fragment. The parakeratotic cell group is representative of reactive change. The patient is 35 years old (PAP).

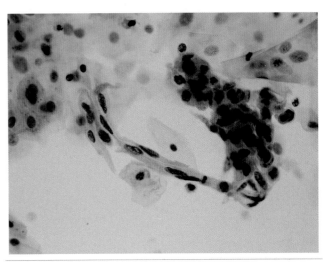

**Fig. 12.64** Urine, washing: poorly differentiated carcinoma. The malignant cells have a spindled appearance with hyperchromatic, enlarged, elongated nuclei. Although the cells show a lack of keratinisation, a non-keratinising squamous cell carcinoma cannot be excluded. The malignant cells appear adjacent to groups of urothelial cells. Histologic follow-up showed that the patient had a non-keratinising squamous cell carcinoma (PAP).

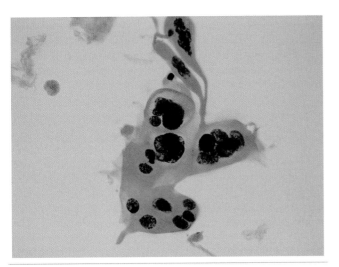

**Fig. 12.63** Urine, voided: human papillomavirus infection. Human papillomavirus findings in the bladder are similar to those seen in the cervix or vagina. In this specimen, the infected cells show multinucleation, nuclear hyperchromasia, and peri-nuclear cytoplasmic halos (PAP).

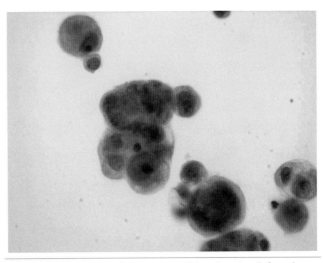

**Fig. 12.65** Urine, voided: adenocarcinoma. The malignant cells form three-dimensional clusters with cytoplasmic vacuolisation. Many of the malignant cells display a prominent nucleolus (PAP).

urine samples or if many non-keratinised malignant cells are seen on instrumented specimens a diagnostic comment should indicate that specific classification of the tumour type is not possible (Fig. 12.64). Metastatic malignancies and malignancies growing from adjacent tissues also should be considered in this differential diagnosis.

## Adenocarcinoma

Adenocarcinomas comprise less than 1% of all primary bladder cancers and the presence of malignant glandular differentiation is most likely to indicate glandular differentiation in a high-grade urothelial carcinoma.[73] Primary adenocarcinomas are subdivided into carcinomas that resemble colonic carcinomas, which make up 85% of primary adenocarcinomas, signet-ring

cell carcinomas and clear cell carcinomas.[73,74] Approximately 25% of signet-ring cell carcinomas are of urachal origin.[73]

### Cytological findings: adenocarcinoma

The findings are similar in voided and instrumented specimens and vary with the type of adenocarcinoma present. For the colonic carcinoma variant, groups and single cells show cuboidal or columnar shapes, hyperchromatic nuclei, nuclear membrane irregularities and cytoplasmic vacuolisation (Fig. 12.65).[74,75] Picket fence type nuclei may be observed. The signet-ring and clear cell variants are extremely rare.

### Diagnostic pitfalls: adenocarcinoma

Cells from metastases, contamination from the female genital tract and non-malignant glandular process are in the

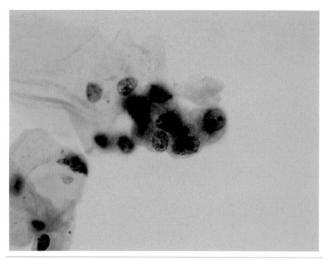

**Fig. 12.66** Urine, voided: reactive endocervical cells. The reactive endocervical cells contain a moderate amount of granular cytoplasm. The nuclear membranes of these endocervical cells are smooth and regular (PAP).

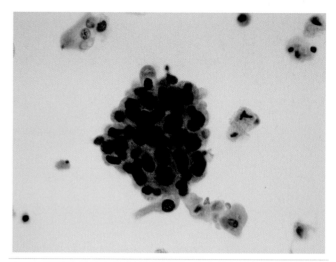

**Fig. 12.68** Urine, voided: prostatic adenocarcinoma. In this prostatic adenocarcinoma, the nuclei contain prominent nucleoli (PAP).

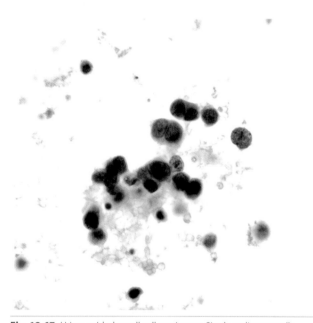

**Fig. 12.67** Urine, voided: small cell carcinoma. Single malignant cells and small clusters of malignant cells are present. The malignant cells have granular chromatin and high nuclear:cytoplasmic ratios (PAP).

differential diagnosis of the finding of malignant glandular cells in urinary tract specimens.[74] Markedly atypical glandular cells may be seen in endometriosis of the bladder wall[13] and in reactive endocervical cells contaminating voided urine specimens (Fig. 12.66). These conditions are usually associated with marked acute inflammation, which is unusual in many primary bladder adenocarcinomas.

## Other malignancies

Other malignancies that can be recognised in urine samples include small cell carcinoma (Fig. 12.67), haematolymphoid lesions and malignancies secondarily involving the urinary

tract. These malignancies include prostatic adenocarcinoma (Fig. 12.68), renal, colonic and gynaecological tumours by direct spread and also metastases.[73,74] The commonest primary sites metastasising to the urinary tract are melanoma and tumours of ovarian, testicular, and breast origin. It is difficult to separate metastatic tumours from high-grade urothelial carcinomas if the metastases are poorly differentiated.

## Urinary biomarkers

In cases of bladder cancer, life-long surveillance is required to detect subsequent tumour recurrence. Current surveillance protocols consist of cystoscopic evaluation and urine cytology every 3–4 months for the first 2 years and at longer intervals in subsequent years.[76] As discussed earlier, voided urine cytology has excellent sensitivity for high-grade bladder cancers and lower sensitivity for low-grade cancers. Cystoscopic examination has a sensitivity as low as 70%, is expensive and causes considerable patient discomfort.[77] For these reasons, researchers and clinicians have advocated the need for non-invasive and accurate biomarkers for the surveillance of patients who have a history of bladder cancer and also for primary screening.[76]

In the last decade, the United States Federal Drug Administration approved biomarker assays specific for the detection of bladder cancer.[78,79] These assays include: (1) assays for urine proteins (proteomic) such as NMP22®, BTA stat®, and BTA TRAK®; (2) immunocytochemical assays such as ImmunoCyt®; and (3) fluorescence *in situ* hybridisation (FISH).[78–84] The development of these assays has reflected the remarkable advances in proteomics and genomics. Lam and Nabi wrote that the ideal biomarker should be able to replace cystoscopic examination and be cost effective: in the current environment, existing protein or molecular biomarkers have not fully met this challenge.[77]

The sensitivity and specificity of currently available biomarkers is shown in Table 12.1.[76,78–84] The utility of biomarkers generally is assessed by comparing the sensitivity and specificity with urine cytology. For example, the UroVysion® test relies on chromosomal alterations associated with bladder cancer by the

**Table 12.1** Sensitivity and specificity of urinary markers[76,78–84]

| Test | Marker | Sensitivity (%) | Specificity (%) |
|------|--------|-----------------|-----------------|
| Fibrin degradation product (FDP) | Fibrin degradation product | 78–91 | 75–90 |
| ImmunoCyt® | High-molecular-weight carcinoembryonic antigen and mucins | 70–95 | 70–85 |
| UroVysion® | Chromosomal probes | 69–75 | 82–85 |
| Bladder tumour antigen (BTA) stat® | Human complement factor H-related protein | 60–70 | 50–75 |
| Bladder tumour antigen (BTA) TRAK® | Human complement factor H-related protein | 60–70 | 50–75 |
| Nuclear matrix proteins (NMP) 22® | Nuclear matrix apparatus proteins | 60–75 | 70–85 |

use of fluorescent probes to centromeres on chromosomes 3, 7, 17, and 9p21.[78] The protocol for test performance is both labour-intensive and operator dependent, requiring expertise of the person who counts and examines the slides. In a meta-analysis of diagnostic accuracy, Hajdinjak reported that excluding Ta tumours, the sensitivity for UroVysion and cytology was 86% and 61%, respectively.[83] Differences in test performance disappeared when superficial cases were excluded from the analysis. Hajdinjak concluded that cytology results were highly specific, although a negative cytology result did not meaningfully change the post-test probability of urothelial cancer. UroVysion results did not provide conclusive evidence of the presence or absence of cancer, but both positive and negative results altered the post-test probability of malignancy.[83]

A number of genetic markers have been studied to determine their role in bladder cancer development and progression.[76] These markers include tumour-suppressor genes (e.g. p53), cell cycle regulators (e.g. Ki-67), protooncogenes and oncogenes (e.g. c-myc or EGFR), and cell adhesion molecules (E-cadherin). Some of these markers have potential prognostic value for cancer recurrence, progression and survival.

Epigenetics is the study of inherited reversible changes in gene function or other cell phenotypes that occur without any change in DNA sequence. An epigenetic mechanism for long-term silencing of gene expression is DNA methylation. Molecular diagnosis may allow for the detection of some epigenetic events that occur early in the disease process.[76] Methylation analysis in urine is being studied for cancer detection and prognosis. Promotor hypermethylation occurs in bladder cancer and methylation-specific polymerase chain reaction is being used to detect specific methylation markers in the urine. Lastly, gene-expression analysis using microarray technology is currently being studied as an approach to determine the biological behaviour of bladder cancer, including tumour growth, progression and metastatic potential.[76] In the future, these research efforts may alter ancillary testing in urine cytology specimens.

## Quality assurance and improvement

Pathology laboratories play a critical role in the quality assurance and quality improvement of the total testing process (TTP)[85–88] for the diagnosis of neoplasms and other diseases of the urinary tract. The TTP is complex and involves numerous clinical decisions involving the ordering of several tests (in addition to urine cytology) and procedures.

For any particular test, the TTP is divided into the phases of:

- Pre-pre-analytical (deciding which test should be performed)
- Pre-analytical (performing the test)
- Analytical (laboratory processing and interpretation)
- Post-analytical (result reporting)
- Post-post-analytical (acting on the test result).

Failures in any step in the process result in testing errors that may have a number of consequences.[85]

Many of the steps in the TTP, including the pre- and post-analytical steps, are not standardised.[9] Some analytical laboratory steps also are not standardised, such as diagnostic category use, preparation methods, and the involvement of cytotechnologists in screening. The lack of standardisation is indicative of practice variability, which in turn means that optimal processes are not uniformly practiced.[89,90] This is a source of error and inefficiency.[91,92]

Based on cytohistological correlation[93] data of urine and follow-up bladder biopsy specimens ($n = 208$), 60% of non-correlating cases were caused by a sampling failure, although interpretive defects were not insignificant, generally signifying differential use of diagnostic criteria.[4] Over 12% of testing failures were secondary to sampling or interpretation defects in cystoscopic examination and or biopsy interpretation following an appropriately interpreted urine specimen.[4]

Some 49% of urine/biopsy testing failures led to some degree of patient harm, generally consisting of additional diagnostic testing (either repeat urines or biopsies) to establish the diagnosis, delays in treatment or unnecessary cystoscopic examination.[4,9]

Laboratories are performing quality improvement initiatives to improve and standardise practice (Box 12.6). Initiatives for the preparation, screening and interpretation processes of the laboratory are shown. These initiatives target different specific or groups of steps in the TTP. As laboratories move forward with the implementation of new technologies, such as biomarkers, they are also advancing in the study of process characteristics and the implementation of process change.

## The role of the cytopathologist in patient management

As is clear from the above, it is essential that the interpretation and reporting of urinary tract cytology take full account of the clinical details and the results of all other investigations. Optimal patient management depends upon close working relationships between clinicians and pathologists to ensure full appreciation of the advantages and limitations of cytology and to provide feedback on patient outcome. This is best achieved by attendance at regular multidisciplinary-team meetings for discussing individual patients, such as are now widely held in all fields of clinical and laboratory medicine.

## Box 12.6  Quality improvement initiatives

Specimen processing

- Performing multiple methods of specimen preparation
- Re-preparing less than optimal specimens
- Re-preparing specimens diagnosed as the cytotechnologist as atypical
- Requiring complete patient history prior to accessioning
- Using different methods to prepare less than optimal specimens (e.g. bloody)
- Grading specimen preparation quality
- Proficiency testing for preparation

Screening/interpretation

- Devising assessments of specimen adequacy
- Rapid screening by multiple cytotechnologists
- Standardising diagnostic category use
- Creating feedback loops to clinicians who procure less than optimal specimens

- Using tools (e.g. photomicrographs) for uniform approaches to diagnosis
- Attending special conferences to address specific diagnostic categories
- Screening and interpreting unknown test cases
- Creation of educational modules
- Proficiency testing
- Rapid double review for second cytotechnologist
- Blinded double review for pathologists
- Forced second opinion for all non-negative diagnoses
- Forced second opinion for all negative cases with a history of urinary tract cancer
- Formal root cause analysis of all non-correlating cases
- Immediate assessments at time of procedure (centrifugation and rapid PAP test)
- Creation of clinician/pathologist/cytotechnologist scorecards of failures

# REFERENCES

1. Brown FM. Urine cytology. Is it still the gold standard for screening? Urol Clin North Am 2000;27:25–37.

2. Bastacky S, Ibrahim S, Wilczynski SP, et al. The accuracy of urine cytology in daily practice. Cancer (Cancer Cytopathol) 1999;87:118–28.

3. Murphy WM. Urinary cytology in diagnostic pathology. Diagn Cytopathol 1985;1:173–75.

4. Raab SS, Grzybicki DM, Vrbin CM, et al. Urine cytology discrepancies. Frequency, causes, and outcomes. Am J Clin Pathol 2007;127:946–53.

5. Ooms EC, Veldhuizen RW. Cytological criteria and diagnostic terminology in urinary cytology. Cytopathology 1993;4:51–54.

6. Winkler RL, Smith JE. Uncertainty in medical testing. Med Decis Making 2004;24:654–58.

7. Bianchi MT, Alexander BM, Cash SS. Incorporating uncertainty into medical decision making: an approach to unexpected test results. Med Decis Making 2009;29:116–24. [Epub ahead of print].

8. Ashby D. Bayesian statistics in medicine: a 25 year review. Stat Med 2006;25:3589–631.

9. Raab SS, Grzybicki DM, Janosky JE, et al. Clinical impact and frequency of anatomic pathology errors in cancer diagnoses. Cancer 2005;104:2205–13.

10. Renshaw AA. Subclassifying atypical urinary cytology specimens. Cancer (Cancer Cytopathol) 2000;90:222–29.

11. Wiener DP, Koss LG, Sablay B, et al. The prevalence and significance of Brunn's nests, cystitis cystica and squamous metaplasia in normal bladders. J Urol 1979;122: 317–21.

12. Schumann GB, Johnston WL, Weiss MA. Renal epithelial fragments in urine sediment. Acta Cytol 1981;25:147–52.

13. Schneider V, Smith MJ, Frable WJ. Urinary cytology in endometriosis of the bladder. Acta Cytol 1980;24:30–33.

14. Kannan V, Bose S. Low-grade transitional carcinoma and instrumentation artifact. A challenge in urinary cytology. Acta Cytol 1993;37:899–902.

15. Anagnostopoulou I, Rammou-Kinia R, Likourinas M. Urine cytology evaluation in cases of uretero-ileal cutaneous diversion. Cytopathology 1995;6:268–72.

16. Wolinska WH, Melamed MR. Urinary conduit cytology. Cancer 1973;32:1000–6.

17. World Health Organization. Global cancer rates could increase by 50% to 15 million by 2020. Online. Available at: http://www.who. int/mediacentre/news/releases/2003/pr27/en/ print.html (accessed: 17 October, 2008).

18. Hall D. Bladder cancer: VIII Urinary tract disorders. Philadelphia: WB Saunders; 1998 563–565.

19. Oosterhuis JWA, Schapers RFM, Janssen-Heijnen MLG, et al. Histologic grading of papillary urothelial carcinoma of the bladder: prognostic value of the 1998 WHO/ISUP classification system and comparison with conventional grading systems. J Clin Pathol 2002;55:900–5.

20. Epstein JI, Amin MB, Reuter VR, et al. The bladder consensus conference committee: the world health organization/international society of urological pathology consensus classification of urothelial (transitional cell) neoplasms of the urinary bladder. Am J Surg Pathol 1998;22:1435–48.

21. Busch C, Algaba F. The WHO/ISUP 1998 and WHO 1999 systems for malignancy grading of bladder cancer. Scientific foundation and translation to one another and previous systems. Virchows Arch 2002;441:105–8.

22. Koss LG, Deitch D, Ramanathan R, et al. Diagnostic value of cytology of voided urine. Acta Cytol 1985;29:810–16.

23. Murphy WM. Current status of urinary cytology in the evaluation of bladder neoplasms. Hum Pathol 1990;21:886–95.

24. Shenoy UA, Colby TV, Schumann GB. Reliability of urinary cytodiagnosis in urothelial neoplasms. Cancer 1985;56:2041–45.

25. Highman WJ. Flat in situ carcinoma of the bladder: cytological examination of urine in diagnosis, follow-up and assessment of response to chemotherapy. J Clin Pathol 1988;41:540–46.

26. Wright RG, Halford JA. Evaluation of thin-layer methods in urine cytology. Cytopathology 2001;12:306–13.

27. Voss JS, Kipp BR, Kreuger AK, et al. Changes in specimen preparation method may impact urine cytologic evaluation. Am J Clin Pathol 2008;130:428–33.

28. Trott PA, Edwards L. Comparisons of bladder washings and urine cytology in the diagnosis of bladder cancer. J Urol 1973;110:664–66.

29. Matzkin H, Moinuddin S, Soloway M. Value of urine cytology versus bladder washings in bladder cancer. Urology 1992;39:201–3.

30. Raab SS, Lenel JC, Cohen MB. Low-grade transitional cell carcinoma of the bladder. Cytologic diagnosis by key features as identified by regression analysis. Cancer 1994;74:1621–26.

31. Raab SS, Slagel DD, Jensen CS, et al. Low-grade transitional cell carcinoma of the urinary bladder: application of select cytologic criteria to improve diagnostic accuracy. Mod Pathol 1996;9:225–32.

32. Murphy WM, Soloway MS, Jukkola AF, et al. Urinary cytology and bladder cancer. The cellular features of transitional cell neoplasms. Cancer 1984;53:1555–65.

33. Jordan A, Weingarten J, Murphy W. Transitional cell neoplasms of the urinary bladder: can biologic potential be predicted from histologic grading? Cancer 1987;60:2766–74.

34. Rosa B, Cazin M, Dalian G. Urinary cytology for carcinoma in-situ of the urinary bladder. Acta Cytol 1985;29:117–24.

35. Deshpande V, McKee GT. Analysis of atypical urine cytology in a tertiary care center. Cancer (Cancer Cytopathol) 2005;105:268–75.

36. Kojima S, Sekine H, Fukui I, et al. Clinical significance of 'cannibalism' in urinary cytology of bladder cancer. Acta Cytol 1998;42:1365–69.

37. Nassar H, Ali-Fehmi R, Madan S. Use of ThinPrep® monolayer technique and cytospin preparation in urine cytology: a comparative analysis. Diagn Cytopathol 2003;28:115–18.

38. Highman W. Transitional carcinoma of the upper urinary tract: a histological and cytopathological study. J Clin Pathol 1986;39:297–305.

39. Kannan V. Papillary transitional-cell carcinoma of the upper urinary tract: a cytological review. Diagn Cytopathol 1990;6:204–9.

40. Bian Y, Ehya H, Bagley D. Cytologic diagnosis of upper urinary tract neoplasms by ureteroscopic sampling. Acta Cytol 1995;39:733–40.

41. Potts SA, Thomas PA, Cohen MB, et al. Diagnostic accuracy and key cytologic features of high-grade transitional cell carcinoma in the upper urinary tract. Mod Pathol 1997;10:657–62.

42. Stella R, Battistelli S, Marcheggiani F, et al. Urothelial cell changes due to busulfan and cyclophosphamide treatment in bone marrow transplantation. Acta Cytol 1990;34:885–90.

43. Koss L, Melamed M. The effect of Busulfan on human epithelia. Am J Clin Pathol 1965;44:385–97.

44. Murphy W, Soloway M, Lin C. Morphologic effects of thiotepa on mammalian urothelium: changes in abnormal cells. Acta Cytol 1978;22:550–54.

45. Pagano F, Bassi P, Milani C, et al. Pathologic and structural changes in the bladder after BCG intravesical therapy in men. Prog Clin Biol Res 1989;310:81–91.

46. Loveless K. The effects of radiation upon the cytology of benign and malignant bladder epithelia. Acta Cytol 1973;17:355–60.

47. O'Morchoe P, Riad W, Cowles L, et al. Urinary cytological changes after radiotherapy of renal transplant. Acta Cytol 1976;20:132–36.

48. Betz SA, See WA, Cohen MB. Granulomatous inflammation in bladder wash specimen after intravesical bacillus Calmette-Guerin therapy for transitional cell carcinoma of the bladder. Am J Clin Pathol 1993;99:244–48.

49. Bhan R, Pisharodi LR, Gudlaugsson E, et al. Cytological, histological, and clinical correlations in intravesical Bacillus Calmette-Guerin immunotherapy. Ann Diagn Pathol 1998;2:55–60.

50. Highman W, Wilson E. Urine cytology in patients with calculi. J Clin Pathol 1982;35:35–356.

51. Kannan V, Gupta D. Calculus artifact. A challenge in urinary cytology. Acta Cytol 1999;43:794–800.

52. Coleman DV. The cytodiagnosis of human polyoma virus infection. Acta Cytol 1975;19:93–96.

53. Crabbe JG. 'Comet' or decoy' cells found in urinary sediment smears. Acta Cytol 1971;15:303–5.

54. Minassian H, Schinella R, Reilly JC. Polyomavirus in the urine: follow-up study. Diagn Cytopathol 1994;10:209–11.

55. Swedlund S. Acute urinary tract infection in adults. Urinary Tract Dis 1998;VIII:544–46.

56. Orr WA, Mulholland SG, Walzak MP Jr.. Genitourinary tract involvement with systemic mycosis. J Urol 1972;107:1047–50.

57. Piscioli F, Pusiol T, Polla E, et al. Urinary cytology of tuberculosis of the bladder. Acta Cytol 1985;29:125–31.

58. Kapila K, Verma K. Cytologic detection of tuberculosis of the urinary bladder. Acta Cytol 1984;28:90–91.

59. Chang SC. Urinary cytologic diagnosis of cytomegalic inclusion disease in childhood leukemia. Acta Cytol 1970;14:338–43.

60. Bancroft J, Seyboldt JF, Windhager HA. Cytologic diagnosis of cytomegalic inclusion disease: a case report. Acta Cytol 1961;5:182–86.

61. Murphy WM. Herpesvirus in bladder cancer. Acta Cytol 1976;20:207–10.

62. Gomousa-Michael M, Rammou-Kinia R. Herpesvirus infection of the male urethra identified by cytology. Acta Cytol 1992;36:270–71.

63. Krieger JN. Urologic aspects of trichomoniasis. Invest Urol 1981;18:411–17.

64. Dimmette RM, Sproat HF, Klimt CR. Examination of smears of urinary sediment for detection of neoplasms of bladder: survey of an Egyptian village infested with Schistosoma hematobium. Am J Clin Pathol 1955;25:1032–42.

65. Curran FT. Malakoplakia of the bladder. Br J Urol 1987;59:559–63.

66. Ashton PR, Lambird PA. Cytodiagnosis of malakoplakia. Report of a case. Acta Cytol 1970;14:92–94.

67. Lee R, Droller MJ. The natural history of bladder cancer. Implications for therapy. Urol Clin North Am 200; 27:1–13.

68. Nasuti JF, Fleisher SR, Gupta PK. Significance of tissue fragments in voided urine specimens. Acta Cytol 2001;45:147–52.

69. Sack M, Artymyshyn RL, Tomaszewski JE, et al. Diagnostic value of bladder washing cytology, with special reference to low-grade urothelial neoplasms. Acta Cytol 1995;39:187–94.

70. Hughes JH, Raab SS, Cohen MB. The cytologic diagnosis of low-grade transitional cell carcinoma. Am J Clin Pathol 2000;114(Suppl):S59–67.

71. Xin W, Raab SS, Muchael CW. Low-grade urothelial carcinoma: reappraisal of the cytologic criteria on ThinPrep®. Diagn Cytopathol 2006;29:125–29.

72. Lagwinski N, Thomas A, Stephenson AJ, et al. Squamous cell carcinoma of the bladder: a clinicopathologic analysis of 45 cases. Am J Surg Pathol 2007;31:1777–87.

73. Murphy WM, Beckwith JB, Farrow GM. Tumors of the urinary bladder: adenocarcinoma. In: Rosai J, editor. Tumors of the Kidney, Bladder, and Related Structures. Washington, DC: Armed Forces Institute of Pathology; 1994. p. 255–59.

74. Bardales RH, Pitman MB, Stanley MW, et al. Urine cytology of primary and secondary urinary bladder adenocarcinoma. Cancer 1998;84:335–43.

75. Shinagawa T, Tadokoro M, Abe M, et al. Papillary urothelial adenocarcinoma of the bladder demonstrating prominent signet ring cells in a smear. A case report. Acta Cytol 1998;42:407–12.

76. Kim W-J, Bae S-C. Molecular biomarkers in urothelial bladder cancer. Cancer Sci 2008;99:646–52.

77. Lam T, Nabi G. Potential of urinary biomarkers in early bladder cancer diagnosis. Expert Rev Anticancer Ther 2007;7:1105–15.

78. Halling KC, Kipp BR. Bladder cancer detection using FISH (UroVysion assay). Adv Anat Pathol 2008;15:279–86.

79. Black PC, Brown GA, Dinney CP. Molecular markers of urothelial cancer and their use in monitoring of superficial urothelial cancer. J Clin Oncol 206; 24:5528–5535.

80. Sozen S, Biri H, Sinik Z, et al. Comparison of the nuclear matrix protein 22 with voided urine cytology and BTA stat test in the diagnosis of transitional cell carcinoma of the bladder. Eur Urol 1999;36:225–29.

81. Ramakumar S, Bhuiyan J, Besse JA, et al. Comparison of screening methods in the detection of bladder cancer. J Urol 1999;161:388–94.

82. Lokeshwar VB, Habuchi T, Grossman HB, et al. Bladder tumor markers beyond cytology: international consensus panel on bladder tumor markers. Urology 2005;66:215–21.

83. Hajdinjak T. UroVysion FISH test for detecting urothelial cancers: meta-analysis diagnostic accuracy and comparison with urinary cytology testing. Urol Oncol 2008;26:646–51.

84. Heicappell R, Müller M, Fimmers R, et al. Qualitative determination of urinary complement factor H-related (hcfHrp) in patients with bladder cancer, healthy controls, and patients with benign urologic disease. Urol Int 2000;65:181–84.

85. Stroobants AK, Goldschmidt AM, Plebani M. Error budget calculations in laboratory medicine: linking the concepts of biological variation and allowable medical errors. Clin Chim Acta 2003;333:169–76.

86. Howanitz PJ. Errors in laboratory medicine: practical lessons to improve patient safety. Arch Pathol Lab Med 2005;129:1252–61.

87. Lundberg GD. Acting on significant laboratory results. JAMA 1981;245:1762–63.

88. Zarbo RJ, Jones BA, Friedberg RC, et al. Q-tracks: a College of American Pathologists program of continuous laboratory monitoring and longitudinal tracking. Arch Pathol Lab Med 2003;126:1036–44.

89. Kohn LT, Corrigan JM, Donaldson MS. To err is human: building a safer health system. Washington, DC: National Academy Press; 1999.

90. Raab SS, Grzybicki DM. Measuring quality in anatomic pathology. Clin Lab Med 2008;28:245–59.

91. Zarbo RJ, D'Angelo R. The Henry Ford production system: effective reduction of process defects and waste in surgical pathology. Am J Clin Pathol 2007;128:1015–22.

92. Raab SS, Grzybicki DM, Condel JL, et al. Effect of lean method implementation in the histopathology section of an anatomic pathology laboratory. J Clin Pathol 2008;61:1193–99.

93. Department of Health and Human Services, Health Care Financing Administration. Clinical laboratory improvement amendments of 1988: final rule 57, Federal Register 7146; 1992 (codified at 42 CFR S.493).

# Section 8

## Lymphoreticular System

# Lymph nodes

Lambert Skoog and Edneia Tani

## Chapter contents

## Introduction

Enlarged lymph nodes were the first organs to be sampled by fine needle aspiration (FNA); today, they are one of the most frequently sampled tissues. In 1904 Greig and Gray reported that trypanosomes could be demonstrated in smears from lymph node aspirates,[1] and for some years afterwards, the technique was used to identify various organisms in infected lymph nodes. The earliest report of a wider application of needle aspiration came from the USA in 1921 when Guthrie described using aspirated material to diagnose a variety of diseases causing lymphadenopathy.[2] Over the next 30 years the technique was slowly adopted by clinicians and pathologists, resulting in a number of reports on its usefulness. The first study of FNA to show a convincingly high sensitivity was presented by Morrison and co-workers in 1952.[3]

We now have a large body of evidence supporting the use of FNA as a primary method of diagnosis in reactive, infective and metastatic lymphadenopathy, but the diagnosis of malignant lymphoma by FNA has been much more controversial. However, several recent studies have shown conclusively that a combined cytological and immunological evaluation of aspirated lymphoid cells results in distinctly improved diagnostic accuracy in cases of lymphoma.[4-26] This had inevitably lead to acceptance of FNA cytology as a method which is comparable to histopathology in diagnostic accuracy.

## The role of cytology in lymph node diagnosis

Lymph nodes react to a variety of microorganisms and non-specific stimuli by expansion of the follicle centres and/or interfollicular tissue. This results in enlargement of nodes, which may be considerable. The clinical management of patients with enlarged lymph nodes varies with factors such as age, the presence of known infection and the previous medical history. For example, children can present with massive local lymphadenopathy even after mild infections. Accordingly, medical treatment and a period of observation should precede the request for FNA in a child with persistent lymph nodes after a recent history of infection.

In contrast, adult or elderly patients often react to infections with only slight to modest lymph node enlargement: therefore distinct lymphadenopathy in an elderly patient will arouse suspicion of malignancy and justify immediate needle biopsy. For patients between these two extreme clinical settings it is more difficult to decide which patient is more likely to have a reactive or neoplastic lymphadenopathy.

FNA was introduced in most medical centres with a view to reducing the number of excisional biopsies of lymph nodes. Although a routine procedure, surgical excision is considerably more expensive and time consuming, and is afflicted with a distinctly higher morbidity than FNA. Using cytomorphology alone it is often possible to decide if the lymphadenopathy has resulted from reactive lymphadenitis, metastatic malignancy or lymphoma. Patients with reactive lymph node enlargement or metastasis from a known malignancy can thus be spared lymph node excision. In cases with indeterminate cytology or diagnosis of lymphoma, surgical excision has usually been regarded as mandatory.

Today, this still seems to be the prevailing application of FNA cytology in patients with lymphadenopathy. There has, however, been a trend towards accepting cytomorphology alone as sufficient for diagnosis in patients with abdominal or mediastinal lymphomas. Obviously, this is not because lymphomas at these sites are easier to diagnose than those found in superficial sites, but results rather from clinical considerations. The laparotomy and mediastinotomy or mediastinoscopy otherwise required have a distinct morbidity and can also lead to delay in therapy.

Aspirated cells perform excellently in immunocytochemistry, flow cytometry and gene rearrangement analysis, as has been demonstrated by a number of authors.[4-30] This has increased the accuracy of lymphoma diagnosis on FNA material to the same level as histopathology in some series.[23-25] However, it should be pointed out that the correct subclassification of lymphomas on cytological material requires experience and optimal material, both of which may be difficult to obtain at centres with relatively few lymphoma patients. In principle this variation in reliability of cytological diagnosis means that FNA cytology can be exercised in the management of patients with lymphadenopathy either at a basic or an advanced level.

At a basic level, aspirated cells are evaluated on routine smears alone. This will allow a conclusive diagnosis in the majority of patients with metastatic tumours and in many cases of reactive lymphadenopathy. Most high-grade lymphomas should also

*The authors gratefully acknowledge their debt to the late T. Löwhagen, whose contribution to the first edition of this chapter provided a substantial basis for the revised editions.*

be recognisable, while many of the low-grade lymphomas and some cases of reactive lymphadenopathy will not be identified reliably. From this it is clear that conventional FNA cytology should be used to select patients for open biopsy where tissue is needed for histology and immunological evaluation.

At an advanced level, aspirated cells are evaluated on smears and the diagnosis is then substantiated by immunocytochemistry, flow cytometry and/or gene rearrangement analysis (see Algorithm below). This approach allows a conclusive diagnosis in the vast majority of metastatic tumours, reactive processes and lymphomas. Confirmation by histology is then only necessary in a minority of lymphomas, namely follicular lymphoma Grade III in which choice of treatment is currently based on whether growth pattern, is nodular or diffuse. Even at this advanced diagnostic level some cases of lymphadenopathy cannot be diagnosed conclusively. In such cases our experience is that lymph node excision with subsequent histology will rarely be of additional diagnostic value. It is accordingly advisable to perform a repeat FNA biopsy after 2–3 weeks. This time is obviously not fixed but will be determined by various factors including any active infection, the condition of the patient and patient anxiety.

In the opinion of the authors, all laboratories involved in the diagnosis of patients with lymphadenopathy should use FNA cytology in conjunction with immunological characterisation. This diagnostic approach will have a substantial impact on the diagnostic accuracy and consequently the clinical management of such patients.

## Technical aspects

### Smear making

Aspiration biopsies of lymph nodes should preferably be performed with a 23 gauge (0.6 mm) needle. In most cases this will provide enough cells for smears as well as cytospin preparations. The use of larger needles usually results in admixture of peripheral blood which may preclude cytological and immunological evaluation of the lymphoid cells.

Lymph node aspirates are usually cellular, making it difficult to prepare smears of good quality. The smear should be thin to ensure instant fixation, which will allow an optimal evaluation of cytological details. However, care must be exercised not to use too much pressure in preparing such thin smears. Lymphoid cells are fragile and readily lose their cytoplasm. Fragmented cytoplasm will appear as small pale grey structures with Romanowsky stains, and these are often called 'lymphoglandular bodies'. Sometimes identical structures can also be seen in smears from other fragile cells; they are thus not pathognomonic for cells of lymphoid origin.

Whenever possible, both air-dried and alcohol-fixed smears should be prepared for May–Grünwald–Giemsa (MGG) and Papanicolaou (PAP) staining, respectively. These stains complement each other and allow an optimal evaluation of cytological details. If mycobacterial or fungal infections are suspected, extra material should be sent for PCR and/bacteriology.

### Cytospin preparations

After using parts of the aspirates for smear making, the remainder should be suspended in a buffered balanced salt (BBS) solution at pH 7.4 for cytospin preparations. An ordinary aspirate from an enlarged lymph node will yield several millions of cells. The number of suspended cells should therefore be calculated and the concentration adjusted to $1$–$2 \times 10^6$ cells/ml. Cell-rich suspensions can be diluted to optimal concentration by adding BBS solution. Vigorous mixing should be avoided since it can destroy lymphoid cells, particularly the large immature cells seen in high-grade lymphomas. If the cell concentration is low the cells can be concentrated by centrifugation at 700 rpm for 3–5 min. The resulting pellet is then gently resuspended in a reduced volume of BBS solution. To prepare the cytospin slides the cell suspension is spun in a cytocentrifuge at 700 rpm for 3 min. Each cytospin should contain $1$–$2 \times 10^5$ nucleated cells.

One of the cytospins should always be stained with MGG and compared with the smears to monitor recovery of all cell components. If the suspension contains a rich admixture of red blood cells, it is possible to purify the lymphoid cells by

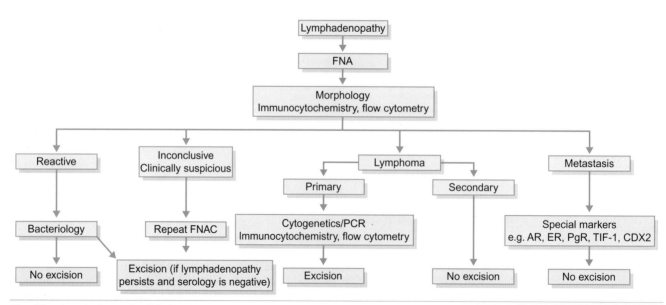

**Algorithm**  Lymphadenopathy clinical management.

density gradient centrifugation. Normally this procedure does not result in any significant cell loss except in some cases of large cell lymphomas which may be fragile and therefore lost in density gradient centrifugation.

Air dried cytospin preparations can be stored at room temperature for up to 1 week without detrimental effect on the immunological staining. Alternatively the cytospin can be stored at −20°C either in a plastic box or wrapped in aluminium foil. Under these conditions lymphoid cells retain their immunological and morphological characteristics for at least 1–2 years. It is important that the slides are kept wrapped until fully thawed when brought out for use otherwise the cells are prone to disintegration. Both immunoalkaline phosphatase and immunoperoxidase methods are suitable for cytospin preparations.

## Flow cytometry

Aspirated cells can also be immunologically characterised by flow cytometry (FC).[14,15,18–20,23,26] As in the case of immunocytochemistry on cytospin preparations one part of the aspirate should be used for smear making. The second part should be suspended in BBS solution at pH 7.4. A cell concentration of approximately 1 million cells per ml buffer will be sufficient for a complete characterisation of reactive lesions as well as most B- and T-cell lymphomas. At the moment four colour FC is standard in immunophenotyping of lymphomas. Evaluation of scattering light allows elimination of dead cells and granulocytes. Several studies have shown a good agreement between FC on FNA material and surgical biopsy specimen.[21,25]

FC is a rapid and sensitive technique which can detect small abnormal cell populations in a reactive background. Since FC does not allow an evaluation of cytomorphology it is of importance that the results are correlated to cytomorphology on routinely stained smears. Lymphomas with large cells are often fragile and such cells are destroyed during FC analysis. A close cooperation between the FC laboratory and the cytopathologist is therefore strongly recommended.

## Molecular biology

Aspirated cells also perform well in PCR rearrangement analysis.[27,28,30] After the aspirated cells have been suspended in BBS at pH 7.4 they should be pelleted immediately, snap frozen and stored at −70°C until used for rearrangement analysis. Cytospin preparations can also be used for FISH analysis of specific translocations to aid subtyping of lymphomas.

## Normal lymph node histology and cytology

Knowledge of the structural, histological and cytological features of normal lymph nodes is essential in the evaluation of FNA smears from enlarged nodes, whether the pathology is reactive, infective or due to a lymphoproliferative disorder. A brief outline of the structure of a normal lymph node is therefore included, followed by a more detailed description of the normal cell population.

## Normal histology

The lymph node parenchyma is surrounded and divided by a fibrous capsule with attached septa. The parenchyma is composed of the cortex, medulla and paracortex. B cells predominate in the cortex and medulla whereas T cells are mainly found in the paracortical tissues.

The cortex contains primary and secondary follicles, the proportions varying with the state of activity of the node. Primary follicles, composed of aggregates of small resting B cells, are found in the unstimulated node. Secondary follicles develop after antigen stimulation and are composed of a narrow mantle zone of small B lymphocytes surrounding a germinal centre. Several types of cells are found in the germinal centre, the vast majority being B cells in the form of centroblasts and centrocytes. Macrophages containing phagocytosed cellular debris are also present.

Mature immunoglobulin secreting B cells, familiar as plasma cells, are the principal cell type found in the medulla. The paracortex contains many small lymphoid cells which are of T phenotype. In addition activated T cells and immunoblasts are present.

## Normal cytology (Fig. 13.1)

As could be predicted from the description of the normal histology, aspirates from normal lymph nodes and from some reactive nodes are dominated by different types of lymphocytes, but plasma cells, macrophages and granulocytes are also found.

- Mature lymphocytes of either B or T phenotype measure around 8 μm in air-dried smears. They have a dense nucleus with coarse chromatin and a pale-blue rim of cytoplasm
- Plasma cells are characterised by their eccentrically placed nucleus with its chromatin arranged in a cartwheel-like pattern. The abundant cytoplasm often shows a less intense basophilic staining in the paranuclear area
- Centrocytes are B cells which measure around 10 μm and have sparse, weakly stained basophilic cytoplasm. The nucleus has a fine chromatin pattern, is usually irregular in shape and may be cleaved
- Centroblasts are larger than centrocytes and have a characteristic round nucleus usually with several marginal nucleoli. The cytoplasm is sparse and may contain some vacuoles
- Immunoblasts of either B or T phenotype are the largest of the lymphoid cells and measure 20–30 μm. They have a round nucleus, often eccentrically placed, with 1–3 large strongly basophilic nucleoli. The cytoplasm is usually also intensely basophilic but may be lacking
- Macrophages have a round to oval nucleus with evenly distributed chromatin and an inconspicuous nucleolus. The poorly defined cytoplasm varies markedly in size but may measure up to 45 μm. In stimulated lymph nodes the macrophages contain phagocytosed cellular debris consisting of darkly stained particles, often referred to as tingible bodies.

## Reactive lymphadenopathy

Lymph nodes respond to many different agents by enlarging and becoming more active. Depending on the type of stimulus, a node may react with one of three basic histological and cytological patterns: reactive hyperplasia, suppurative lymphadenitis or granulomatous lymphadenitis. In some cases it is possible

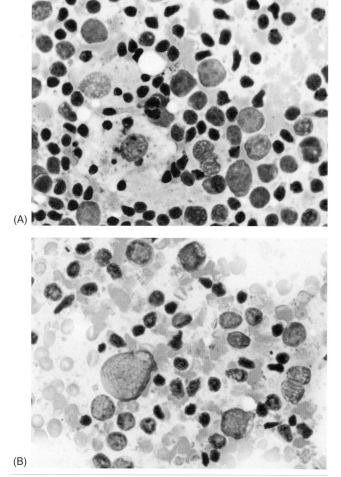

(A)

(B)

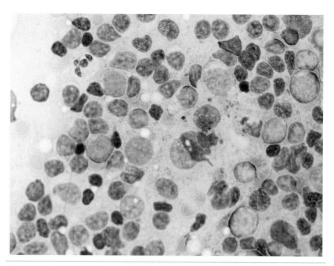

**Fig. 13.2** Reactive lymphadenitis. Mixed lymphoid cells, granulocytes, plasma cells and tingible body macrophages (MGG).

**Fig. 13.1** Lymph node aspirates with normal lymphoid cells (A). A macrophage with plentiful clear cytoplasm containing 'tingible bodies' is surrounded by large round centroblasts with sparse cytoplasm. Medium-sized centrocytes with irregular nuclei and smooth chromatin and small mature lymphocytes with condensed chromatin are also present (MGG). (B). One large immunoblast with an eccentrically placed nucleus and well developed basophilic cytoplasm is surrounded by smaller centroblasts and mature plasma cells (MGG).

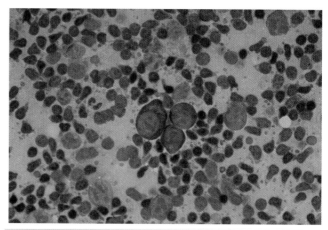

**Fig. 13.3** Infectious mononucleosis. Several atypical immunoblasts are present in a background of small lymphocytes (MGG).

to identify the causative agent, either in routine preparations or by special stains such as those for mycobacteria, leishmania, histoplasma and trypanosomes, but the majority of reactive nodes show non-specific changes.

## Reactive hyperplasia

Histologically, this response may take the form of enlargement of the lymphoid follicles which develop active germinal centres. These are characterised by numerous centroblasts and centrocytes, a rich admixture of macrophages with a poorly defined pale cytoplasm containing tingible bodies, and a surrounding cuff of small lymphocytes. Alternatively, there may be expansion of the interfollicular tissue by numerous mature lymphocytes, lymphoplasmacytoid cells, plasma cells and varying numbers of immunoblasts. A mixture of both patterns is present in some cases. Nodes draining tumours or other sources of tissue breakdown may be further expanded by the presence of numerous histiocytes in the sinusoids, a picture referred to as sinus histiocytosis.

## Cytological findings: reactive hyperplasia (Figs 13.2, 13.3)

### Non-specific hyperplasia

Non-specific hyperplasia yields a cytological pattern on FNA which depends on the proportions of follicular and interfollicular tissue in the aspirate, and this in turn usually correlates with the histological findings described above. Thus, smears from a node composed predominantly of large follicles with active germinal centres contain many centroblasts and centrocytes, while the interfollicular tissue is comparatively sparse and represented by mature lymphocytes, plasma cells and immunoblasts (Fig. 13.2).

In extreme cases, the pattern may mimic a mixed lymphoma of centroblastic/centrocytic type. The presence or absence of tingible body macrophages is of little diagnostic value. Immunocytochemical evaluation of the lymphoid population may be the only way to resolve this diagnostic problem.

In contrast, when interfollicular tissue predominates, the smears are rich in lymphocytes, plasma cells, lymphoplasmacytoid cells and some immunoblasts. Such smears are difficult to differentiate from those of a low-grade

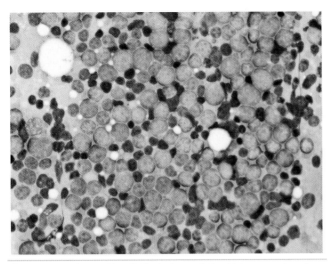

**Fig. 13.4** HIV infection. Florid follicular hyperplasia with large number of immature follicle centre cells mixed with mature lymphocytes and one macrophage with tingible bodies (MGG).

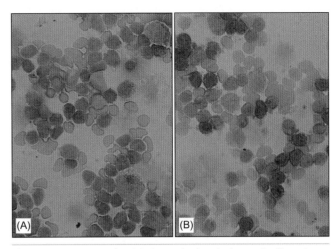

**Fig. 13.5** Immunocytochemistry in reactive lymphadenopathy. Cytospin material from the aspirate shown in Figure 13.2. B- and T-cell markers identify a mixed population of lymphoid cells (A). B cells of varying sizes (B). Small mature T cells (alkaline phosphatase).

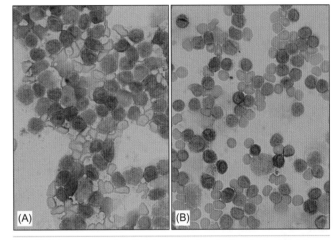

**Fig. 13.6** Immunocytochemistry in reactive lymphadenopathy showing polyclonal light chain expression with no predominance of either kappa or lambda to suggest lymphoma. (A) Kappa; (B) Lambda (alkaline phosphatase).

lymphoma. Analysis of light chain immunoglobulin restriction is usually required to arrive at a conclusive diagnosis.

Some conditions lead to a cytological pattern which clearly deviates from the general types described above. A description of the best recognised of these follows. It is important to remember that definitive diagnosis is dependent on good clinical correlation.

### Viral and post-vaccinial lymphadenitis

These conditions cause intense reactivity in the interfollicular tissue which presents with a prominent immunoblastic proliferation in addition to lymphoplasmacytoid cells and plasma cells.

### HIV infection

Generalised lymphadenopathy is common in patients with acquired immunodeficiency syndrome (AIDS).[31] There is a florid follicular hyperplasia with immature follicle centre cells in a background of mature lymphocytes, plasma cells and macrophages (Fig. 13.4). Immunoblasts are always present. The pattern is non-specific and thus not diagnostic for AIDS.

The lymphoid cells are mostly polyclonal B cells but some mature T cells are also present.

### Infectious mononucleosis

Infectious mononucleosis can also cause lymphadenitis, which is mainly confined to the interfollicular tissue (Fig. 13.3). Cytologically, it is characterised by numerous immunoblasts, some of which are atypical with large irregular nuclei.[32] In rare cases the pattern may even be suggestive of Hodgkin's disease.[32] Serological tests can be helpful, but phenotyping of the atypical cell population may be the only way to rule out a lymphoma.

### Rheumatoid arthritis, systemic lupus erythematosus and secondary syphilis

All of these conditions can cause massive lymphadenopathy. Cytologically, there is a reactive pattern with numerous plasma cells, some containing Russell bodies, which may lead to a suspicion of a low-grade lymphoma with plasmacytic

differentiation. In such cases, it may be impossible to arrive at a conclusive diagnosis without resorting to immunocytochemistry.

### Dermatopathic lymphadenopathy

This is a special variant of reactive lymphadenitis which is observed in patients with chronic skin disorders such as psoriasis or dermatitis. The germinal centres are hyperplastic and the interfollicular tissue is expanded by cells of histiocytic appearance.[33] Smears from such lymph nodes show numerous small lymphocytes, plasma cells, eosinophils and occasional blast cells. There are numerous histiocyte-like cells, also known as interdigitating reticulum cells, with pale indistinct cytoplasm. Macrophages containing brown melanin pigment from the damaged skin are always present.

## Immunocytochemistry (Figs 13.5–13.7)

In reactive lymphadenitis the small lymphocytes are mostly T cells of which the helper type predominate. The B cells are of various sizes and are polyclonal, expressing both kappa and lambda light chains. Atypical immunoblasts are either of T or B phenotype, some of which may also express CD30 (Ki-1). They do not

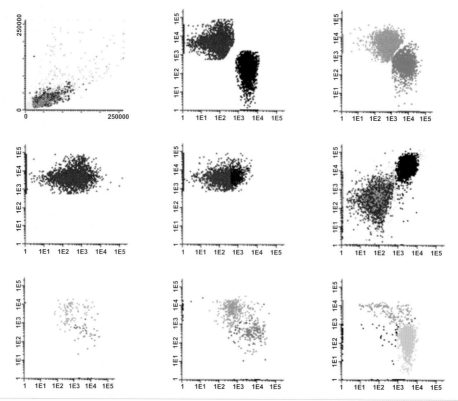

**Fig. 13.7** 8-colour flow cytometry analysis of fine needle aspirate from a lymph node with reactive follicular hyperplasia. The following antibody panel was used: Lambda FITC/ Kappa PE/CD19 PerCP-Cy5/ CD10 APC/ CD5 PE-Cy7/ CD4 APC-Cy7/ CD8 AM-Cyan/ CD3 Pacific Blue. Data were acquired using FACS-Canto and DIVA software (Becton Dickinson). Data analysis was done using Infinicyt (Cytognos, Salamanca, Spain) software. Upper row: Left: forward scatter/side scatter plot shows that most cells were in the lymphocyte area. Dead cells (yellow) are excluded from analysis. Middle: CD19 vs CD3 plot shows 47% B cells (red) and 43% T cells (blue). Right: Kappa (orange)/ Lambda (green) analysis in CD19/SSC gated B cells shows normal kappa/lambda ratio 1.3. Middle row: Left: CD19 vs CD5 plot within CD19/SSC gate shows a small population of CD5+ B cells that correspond to mantle zone B cells (5% of B cells). Middle: CD19 vs CD10 plot within CD19/SSC gate shows a somewhat larger population of CD10+ B cells that correspond to germinal center cells (20% of B cells). Right: CD3 vs CD5 plot shows that most T cells were positive for both markers (blue). Lower row: Left: Kappa/lambda analysis of CD5+ B cells shows normal kappa/lambda ratio (1.2). Middle: Kappa/lambda analysis of CD10+ B cells shows normal kappa/lambda ratio (1.5). Right: CD4 and CD8 expression in CD3-gated T-cell population. CD4/CD8 ratio was increased to 8.5 (Courtesy Professor A. Porwit, Hematopathology Division, Dept Pathology and Cytology, Karolinska University Hospital Solna, Stockholm, Sweden).

express CD15 (Leu M1). This phenotype is inconsistent with that of the neoplastic cells in Hodgkin lymphoma, where the mixed cellular infiltrate might be mistaken for a reactive picture.

The flow cytometry pattern of reactive lymphadenitis is seen in Figure. 13.7.

## Sinus histiocytosis

This is a very common finding in reactive lymph nodes and often associated with follicular hyperplasia but may also be seen in its absence. Characteristic is dilatation of subcapsular and trabecular sinuses, which are partially or completely filled with histiocytes/macrophages. This type of hyperplasia is observed in lymph nodes which drain areas with cancer as well as inflammatory lesions but in many cases the cause is unknown.

### Cytological findings: sinus histiocytosis

The sinus histiocytosis is characterised by mixture dominated by small lymphocytes, some blasts and numerous, sometime multinucleated, macrophages with abundant foamy cytoplasm and round, oval or kidney-shaped nuclei.

## Sinus histiocytosis with massive lymphadenopathy

This is a rare, extreme form of sinus histiocytosis that was first described by Rosai and Dorfman in 1969.[34] The disorder is seen most often in black children and adolescents. Most patients are in good health and develop massive bilateral non-tender enlargement of the cervical lymph nodes followed by fever. Extra nodal involvement has also been described. The cause is unknown but the disorder has a prolonged course and spontaneous regression of the nodes usually takes place.

### Cytological findings: sinus histiocytosis with massive lymphadenopathy (Fig. 13.8)

There are numerous lymphocytes and large pale histiocytes which have vesicular nuclei with small nucleoli and an abundant vacuolated cytoplasm. The histiocytes often have well-preserved lymphocytes in the cytoplasm which is referred to as lymphocytophagocytosis or emperipolesis.[35–38]

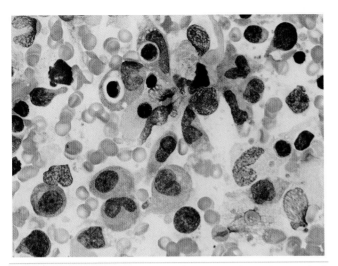

**Fig. 13.8** Rosai–Dorfman's disease. Large histiocyte with prominent nucleoli and lymphophagocytosis (MGG).

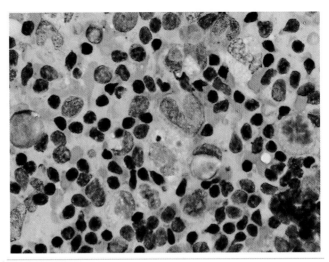

**Fig. 13.9** Kikuchi's lymphadenitis. Lymphocytes mixed with phagocytic histiocytes with vacuolated cytoplasm and irregular punched-out nuclei (MGG).

## Immunocytochemistry

Some mature T cells are present. The B cells and plasma cells are polyclonal. A strong S-100 positivity and lack of lysozyme reactivity is characteristic for the large histiocytes.

## Kikuchi's disease

Histiocytic necrotising lymphadenitis is a rare well-defined clinical entity which was first described by Kikuchi and Fujimoto et al. in 1972.[39,40] It affects mainly young women presenting with fever and enlargement of one or more cervical nodes. It is a benign, self-limiting disease and its aetiology is still unknown.

### Cytological findings: Kikuchi's disease (Fig. 13.9)

Numerous foamy macrophages as well as 'tingible body' macrophages containing karyorrhectic debris in a background of necrotic material. Small lymphocytes, as well as activated lymphocytes are found. Neutrophils, epithelioid cells and plasma cells, when present, are few in number.[41]

## Acute infective lymphadenopathy

A more definitive morphological categorisation of lymph node disease is sometimes possible in certain infections directly involving nodes and in the group of inflammatory or infective disorders associated with granuloma formation. It is of the utmost importance in these conditions, however, that microbiological culture is undertaken for confirmation of the infectious agent.

## Acute suppurative lymphadenitis

Lymph nodes draining or adjacent to a focus of bacterial infection, may be directly invaded by the organisms, causing acute lymphadenitis followed in some cases by suppuration. Initially a light infiltrate of neutrophil polymorphs is present but as the tissues undergo necrosis the node becomes a suppurative mass. Appropriate treatment may result in resolution or scarring.

### Cytological findings: acute suppurative lymphadenitis

- In the initial phase slightly turbid fluid is aspirated
- Smears show a proteinaceous background with cell debris, mixed lymphocytes and sparse granulocytes
- Later the aspirate becomes purulent with many degenerate neutrophils in a thick background of cell debris.

## Suppurative non-tuberculous mycobacteriosis

This variant of infectious lymphadenitis occurs often in otherwise healthy children without clinical signs of infection. They present with a firm, often non-tender enlarged lymph node in the neck. The most common pathogen in non-tuberculous mycobacteriosis is *Mycobacterium avium*.[42]

Aspirated material is often purulent and it is important to recognise the need for mycobacterial culture.

### Cytological findings: suppurative non-tuberculous mycobacteriosis (Fig. 13.10)

- Thick smear with cellular debris and granulocytes
- Variable amount of lymphocytes
- Few macrophages and epithelioid histiocytes
- Multinucleated giant cells are rarely seen.

## Granulomatous lymphadenopathy

### Aetiology and pathogenesis

The most common cause of granulomatous lymphadenitis in developed countries is sarcoidosis, but in many tropical areas, and in patients with immunodeficiency, other aetiologies are more

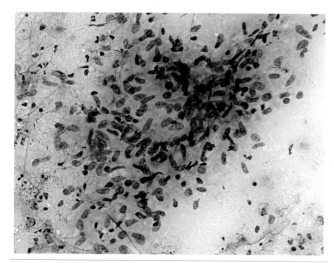

**Fig. 13.10** Suppurative non-tuberculous mycobacterial lymphadenitis. Cellular debris, neutrophil granulocytes, mature lymphocytes and epithelioid histiocytes in irregular clusters (MGG).

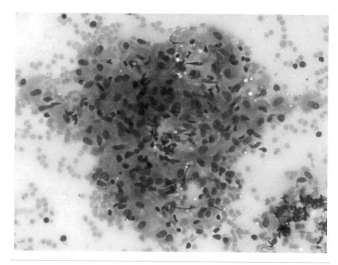

**Fig. 13.11** Sarcoidosis. Cluster of epithelioid cells forming a granuloma (MGG).

common. Infections are a particularly important group and tuberculosis is the commonest of these, although many other organisms can present with granulomatous lymphadenopathy, including leprosy, cat scratch disease, paracoccidioidomycosis, histoplasmosis, leishmaniasis, lymphogranuloma venereum, brucellosis and tularemia. Granulomatous lymphadenitis can also be caused by foreign bodies such as talc or silica. Furthermore, granulomas may form part of a reactive background in the presence of malignant lymphoma or may occur in nodes draining a carcinoma.

### General cytological findings

The general cytological picture of granulomatous lymphadenitis is characterised by clusters of epithelioid cells which have elongated nuclei, picturesquely described as banana, footprint or carrot shaped, arranged in a syncytial fashion with abundant ill-defined cytoplasm. A variable number of multinucleated Langhans giant cells may be present, their nuclei polarised in an arc at one part of the cell border. The presence or absence of pale amorphous necrosis is of diagnostic significance in establishing the aetiology of the granulomatous reaction.

## Sarcoidosis

This systemic disorder of young adults is characterised histologically by the presence of non-caseating giant cell granulomata and tends to affect lungs and lymph nodes mainly but most organs can be involved. A similar reaction is sometimes seen in nodes draining a primary carcinoma whether or not metastases to the node have occurred. This finding is referred to as a sarcoidal reaction.

### Cytological findings: sarcoidosis (Fig. 13.11)

- The aspirate contains cohesive clusters of epithelioid cells and numerous small mature lymphocytes
- In most cases multinucleated giant cells are present
- The background is free from necrosis, a finding strongly suggestive of sarcoidosis.

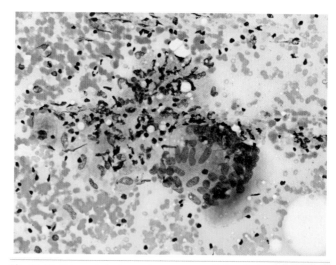

**Fig. 13.12** Tuberculosis. A granuloma composed of epithelioid cells is present in a background of necrosis with numerous granulocytes (MGG).

### Diagnostic pitfalls: sarcoidosis

If Langhans giant cells are absent the differential diagnosis should include Hodgkin's disease and low-grade T-cell lymphoma. Techniques such as PCR and special stains for organisms such as mycobacteria and fungi, as well as immunocytochemistry to characterise the lymphoid cells are of value in reducing the number of diagnostic alternatives. In sarcoidosis, the lymphoid population is dominated by T cells, with a normal ratio of helper to suppressor cells, while the B cells are polyclonal.

## Tuberculous lymphadenitis

Infection of lymph nodes by *Mycobacterium tuberculosis* is usually the result of spread from primary lung infection and can present clinically with massive generalised lymphadenopathy, especially of the cervical nodes, even to the extent of simulating lymphoma. The hallmark of tuberculosis histologically is the presence of caseating necrosis associated with epithelioid giant

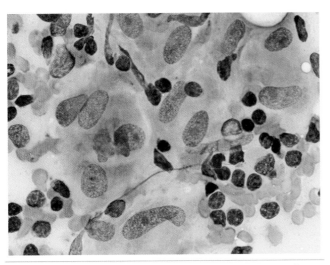

**Fig. 13.13** Tuberculosis. This field contains a mixture of epithelioid cells, plasma cells, lymphocytes and macrophages (MGG).

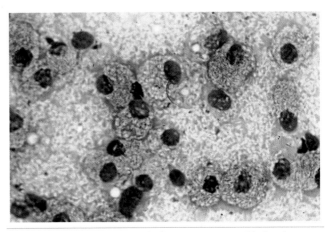

**Fig. 13.14** Atypical mycobacterial infection. Histiocytes with abundant 'foamy' cytoplasm are seen. In an immunocompromised patient this picture should arouse suspicion of an atypical mycobacterial organism (MGG).

cell granulomata. Early diagnosis is particularly important since the condition is treatable.

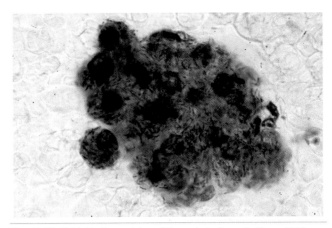

**Fig. 13.15** Ziehl–Neelsen staining of the aspirate shown in Figure 13.15, revealing numerous acid fast bacilli distending the histiocytic cells.

### Cytological findings: tuberculous lymphadenitis (Figs 13.12, 13.13)

Aspiration smears from tuberculous lymphadenitis show three major cell patterns:

- Epithelioid granulomas without necrosis, in which there are small clusters of epithelioid histiocytes and single forms, mixed with reactive lymphocytes, but Langhans giant cells are not often seen
- Epithelioid granulomas with necrosis, showing similar features, but in addition there is a variable amount of pale stained amorphous material in the background
- Necrosis without epithelioid granuloma. This type shows thin necrotic debris containing large numbers of polymorphonuclear cells and scattered histiocytes.

For definitive diagnosis, acid fast bacilli can be identified using the Ziehl–Neelsen (ZN) stain or other stains for acid fast bacilli.[43–45] These stains have a relatively low sensitivity and are nowadays mostly replaced by PCR techniques to identify the mycobacteria.

## Atypical mycobacterial infection

Immunodeficient patients, including those with AIDS, suffer from many of the infectious causes of lymphadenitis and are especially predisposed to tuberculosis, but may also be infected by less common organisms which are rarely encountered in the general population. Infection due to *Mycobacterium avium intracellulare* is an example of this type of lymphadenitis and is recognised with increasing frequency in this group of patients.

Histologically, the lymphoid tissue is replaced by large histiocytes with voluminous finely vacuolated, ill-defined cytoplasm containing numerous bacilli.

### Cytological findings: atypical mycobacterial infection (Figs 13.14, 13.15)

- Smears show histiocytic cells with abundant pale cytoplasm

- In MGG-stained preparations the mycobacteria present as cylindrical non-stained 'negative images' of bacilli that are diagnostic of mycobacterial infection[46]
- The presence of bacilli can sometimes be demonstrated using the ZN stain. Characteristically, they are arranged randomly within the cytoplasm.

## Leprosy

Leprosy is a chronic destructive systemic infection due to *Mycobacterium leprae* and is now mainly seen in third world countries. As in the histology of this disease, two different types of reaction are seen cytologically in affected lymph nodes, referred to as lepromatous and tuberculoid.[47]

In the lepromatous or Virchow's form of leprosy, the enlarged lymph nodes yield syncytial histiocytes with abundant clear cytoplasm containing numerous acid fast bacilli. In leprosy, the bacilli are present in parallel disposition in the form of globi in the cytoplasm of the histiocytes which are sometimes referred to as Virchow's or globus cells. The arrangement of organisms is important in distinguishing leprosy from atypical mycobacterial infection.[47,48]

In the tuberculoid form of leprosy, the predominant cytological picture is a granulomatous process, containing

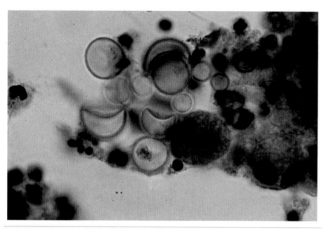

**Fig. 13.16** Paracoccidioidomycosis. Multinucleated giant cell and histiocytes in a necrotic background with granulocytes. The spores are seen as rounded structures with birefringent capsules (MGG). (Courtesy of Dr RM Viero, Dept Pathology, Faculdade de Medicina de Botucatu UNESP, Brazil.)

epithelioid histiocytes in a background of lymphocytes. Organisms are present in low numbers, and are more difficult to identify than in the lepromatous form.

## Paracoccidioidomycosis (Figs 13.16, 13.17)

Paracoccidioidomycosis is a fungal infection endemic in South America. *P. brasiliensis* often causes massive lymphadenopathy which results from a granulomatous reaction. Epithelioid cells, multinucleated giant cells, neutrophils and eosinophils are found in varying numbers. The diagnosis is established by identification of multiple budding spores, 5–15 μm in diameter, with birefringent cell membranes.[49] A Gomori–Grocott silver stain will readily identify the spores.

## Histoplasmosis (Fig. 13.18)

*Histoplasma capsulatum* is another fungal infection that can give rise to a granulomatous reaction. The yeast form is oval and 2–3 μm in diameter and resides in the cytoplasm of macrophages.

## Cryptococcosis

*Cryptococcus neoformans* is also one of the fungal infections that may lead to a granulomatous reaction in lymph nodes. However, most cases present with an inflammatory infiltrate dominated by neutrophils and histiocytes.

## Actinomycosis

Actinomycosis, the condition caused by filamentous bacterial organisms of the *Actinomyces* species, is a further source of granulomatous inflammation to be considered in the differential diagnosis.[50] The organisms are best shown by Gram-stain.

## Foreign body granulomas

Talc, silicone or beryllium can induce massive lymphadenopathy which is impossible to differentiate clinically from metastatic lymph node disease. The aspirated material consists

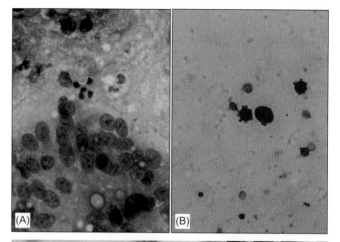

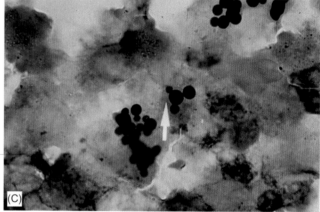

**Fig. 13.17** Paracoccidioidomycosis. (A) Multinucleated giant cell with spores visible in the cytoplasm (MGG). (B) Spores with pathognomonic multiple budding (Gomori). (Courtesy of Dr RM Viero, Dept Pathology, Faculdade de Medicina de Botucatu UNESP, Brazil.)

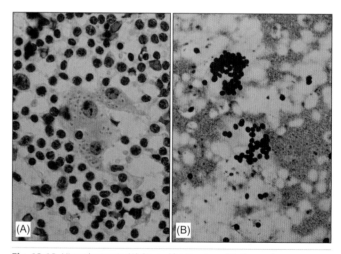

**Fig. 13.18** Histoplasmosis. (A) Several histiocytes with tiny oval spores characteristically within the cell cytoplasm (Shorr). (B) Multiple spores identified by Gomori. (Courtesy of Dr RM Viero, Dept Pathology, Faculdade de Medicina de Botucatu UNESP, Brazil.)

mainly of giant cells containing foreign body particles, together with lymphocytes of mature type and mononuclear histiocytes.[51,52] Antibodies to vimentin, and epithelial, lymphoid, melanocytic and myogenic differentiation markers should be used to corroborate the diagnosis.

## Malignant lymphomas

### Introduction

Malignant lymphomas are divided into two major categories: Hodgkin lymphoma and non-Hodgkin lymphomas. They can be further divided into several subgroups, which are important to identify because of their different clinical behaviour. Hodgkin lymphoma is most commonly subclassified according to the Rye scheme which was proposed in 1966,[53] which is also followed in the recent WHO classification.[54]

The classification of non-Hodgkin lymphomas has been more controversial. The Kiel classification propounded in 1975 and the 1982 Working Formulation have been the two most commonly used schemes for this group of tumours.[55,56] Histological assessment of architectural and cytological features has traditionally formed the basis for all of the classifications. The updated Kiel classification, published in 1988, also incorporated data from immunophenotypic analysis.[57] In the REAL (Revised European-American classification of Lymphoid neoplasms) an attempt was made to define clinical relevant subgroups of lymphomas that could be recognised with available morphological, immunological and genetic techniques.[58] The 'WHO classification of tumours of haematopoetic and lymphoid tissues' is based on the same parameters as the REAL classification and is today generally accepted.[54]

### The role of cytology in lymphoma diagnosis

Much effort has been spent on the diagnosis of malignant lymphomas by FNA, attempts which have until recently been only partially successful. One major reason for this is that most neoplastic lymphoid cells lack the traditional cytological features of malignancy. Such cells are close replicas of their benign counterparts. In many instances the cytological diagnosis therefore rests on evaluation of whether or not the smears show a spectrum of cells in proportions typical of benign conditions.

If the FNA sample is composed of only one cell type a confident diagnosis of non-Hodgkin lymphoma can usually be made. However, some lymphomas are composed of several types of neoplastic cells, while others contain a confusing admixture of benign lymphoid cells with neoplastic elements, which obviously obscures the picture. The complexity of such samples may be an overwhelming task even for the most experienced cytopathologist. In the case of Hodgkin lymphoma the finding of cells with large atypical nuclei and multilobated nuclei has been considered diagnostic.

At present no system of classification has been constructed for FNA cytology material. From published data, it seems clear that a histological diagnosis based on the Kiel classification correlates very well with FNA findings.[59] This partly results from the fact that the Kiel classification has only two subgroups in which growth pattern is of importance for diagnosis and choice of therapy. In both the REAL and WHO classification systems there is a much greater emphasis on cytomorphology, immunophenotyping and molecular studies than on architecture growth pattern. Growth pattern, whether nodular or diffuse, contributes to diagnosis in only one subtype. Thus this system will allow a conclusive diagnosis and subtyping of most lymphomas on cytological material if the morphological evaluation is combined with immunophenotypic studies and sometimes cytogenetics.[60-62]

Diagnosis and subclassification of Hodgkin lymphoma have been attempted on FNA material.[63-65] Again, the classification schemes in current use are based on both architectural and cytological features in excised tissue, making their application to FNA material somewhat difficult.

The reported accuracy of cytological diagnosis and classification of lymphomas on FNA samples varies between 10% and 90%.[66] Not surprisingly, this degree of variation has impeded the acceptance of FNA cytology as the sole diagnostic modality in patients with suspected lymphoma. However, as previously pointed out, FNA cytology is more readily accepted for evaluation of patients with suspected recurrent lymphoma, or deep-seated primary lymphomas. This attitude is somewhat puzzling since the diagnostic difficulties encountered in these special circumstances are identical irrespective of the fact that the lymphoma is primary or recurrent, superficial or deep-seated.

The use of ancillary techniques including immunocytochemistry, cytogenetics and DNA hybridisation has greatly increased the utility of cytological material for conclusive diagnosis of lymphoma. In fact, cytology specimens seem ideal for immunological evaluation; recent studies show a high diagnostic accuracy if the cytological findings are combined with results from immunophenotyping and clonal restriction analysis.

## Hodgkin lymphoma

### Clinical background

Hodgkin lymphoma accounts for approximately 1% of all malignancies in the Western world. It shows a bimodal age incidence curve with the first peak between 15 and 30 years of age, followed by a second peak in elderly people. This bimodal pattern, together with differences in histological subtype, has led to the suggestion that Hodgkin lymphoma is, in fact, two separate malignancies. Speculations about the aetiology have included environmental agents, Epstein–Barr virus infection and genetic factors such as impaired immunocompetence.

Most patients present with localised lymphadenopathy which affects cervical or mediastinal nodes in approximately 70% of cases. Axillary or inguinal nodes are less often the primary site, accounting for 15% of cases each. Primary extranodal manifestation is very rare. Systemic symptoms such as weight loss, fever, itching and night sweats are relatively frequent.

The histological diagnosis of Hodgkin lymphoma rests on the identification of mononuclear Hodgkin cells and giant cells with lobated nuclei, the so called Reed–Sternberg cells. These two cell types can occur in different background settings, which form the basis for subtyping. The following subtypes are included in the WHO classification.

### Hodgkin lymphoma subtypes

- Classical Hodgkin lymphoma
  - Nodular sclerosis
  - Mixed cellularity
  - Lymphocyte depletion
  - Lymphocyte rich.
- Nodular lymphocyte predominant Hodgkin lymphoma

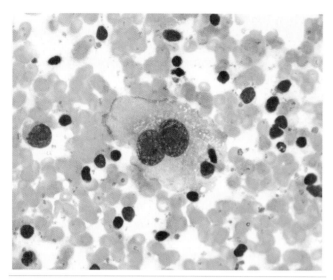

**Fig. 13.19** Hodgkin lymphoma. Note the large mirror-image binucleated lymphoid cell of Reed–Sternberg type with a mixed population of lymphoid cells in the background (MGG).

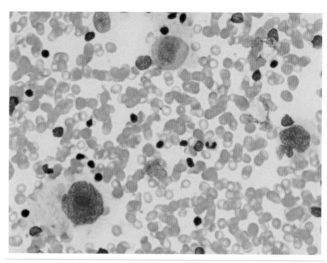

**Fig. 13.20** Hodgkin lymphoma. This field includes large mononuclear cells with abundant cytoplasm and prominent nucleoli. These are Hodgkin cells (MGG).

These subgroups can in most cases be identified in smears of aspirates by evaluation of the proportion of large atypical cells and reactive cells.[63–65,67]

The subtyping of Hodgkin lymphoma has clinical relevance with respect to prognosis. The nodular variant of the lymphocyte predominant Hodgkin lymphoma has an excellent prognosis sometimes even when untreated. Of the classical Hodgkin lymphoma subtypes, nodular sclerosis has been reported to have the best and lymphocyte depletion the worst prognosis.

It is important to realise that the histopathological identification of Hodgkin lymphoma can be difficult. Cases of non-Hodgkin lymphoma may be misdiagnosed as Hodgkin lymphoma. This problem seems to occur most often in the diffuse lymphocyte predominant and the lymphocyte depleted subgroups. If cases of non-Hodgkin lymphoma can be completely excluded, the prognostic difference between the subgroups of Hodgkin lymphoma diminishes. In addition, it has been shown that stage of disease, i.e. the extent of spread, rather than subtype, is the most important prognostic factor.[68] As a consequence, the current choice of treatment of classical Hodgkin lymphoma is often based on tumour extension, irrespective of histological subtype.

Several other neoplasms both of lymphoid and non-lymphoid origin may present with a morphological picture mimicking that of Hodgkin lymphoma. It is therefore important that the morphological diagnosis is confirmed by immunocytochemistry.

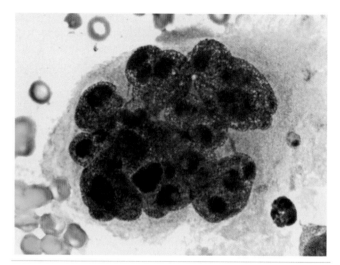

**Fig. 13.21** Hodgkin lymphoma. At the centre, there is a giant cell with a large multilobated nucleus with many huge nucleoli. This is a variant of the Reed–Sternberg cell (MGG).

### Cytological findings: Hodgkin lymphoma (Figs 13.19–13.23)

- Hodgkin cells are large mononuclear cells with a prominent nucleolus and abundant cytoplasm
- The Reed–Sternberg cell has a bilobed or multilobated nucleus with distinct nucleoli, and an abundant pale grey cytoplasm on MGG. The identification of both Hodgkin and Reed–Sternberg cells is highly suggestive of Hodgkin lymphoma

- In nodular sclerosis classical Hodgkin lymphoma the smears are often poorly cellular and contain fibroblasts, eosinophils and collagen fragments, in addition to the diagnostic Hodgkin and Reed–Sternberg cells
- Mixed cellularity classical Hodgkin lymphoma has a more complex cell pattern with lymphocytes, eosinophils, histiocytes and plasma cells along with a varying number of atypical cells
- The lymphocyte depleted subtype demonstrates a paucity of lymphocytes with a relative predominance of large atypical cells of Hodgkin and Reed–Sternberg type
- The nodular lymphocyte predominant form can be identified by the large number of small lymphocytes with few diagnostic atypical cells. True Reed–Sternberg cells are rarely seen but tumour cells with multilobulated nuclei (popcorn cell) can be found.

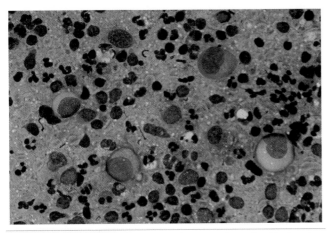

**Fig. 13.22** Hodgkin lymphoma. Scattered mononuclear cells with abundant cytoplasm and indistinct nucleoli can be seen. These are variants of the Hodgkin's cell (MGG).

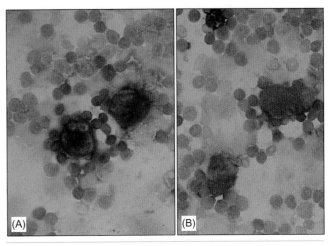

**Fig. 13.24** Hodgkin lymphoma. Immunocytochemistry on cytospin preparations of lymph node FNA. The large atypical cells are positive for: (A) CD30; (B) CD15 (alkaline phosphatase).

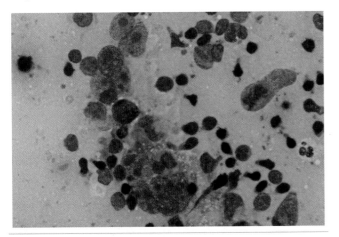

**Fig. 13.23** Infectious mononucleosis. Large atypical lymphoid cells with prominent nucleoli present. Cytologically, these cells are almost indistinguishable from those observed in Hodgkin lymphoma (MGG).

## Diagnostic pitfalls: Hodgkin lymphoma

The differential diagnosis includes several non-Hodgkin lymphomas, infectious mononucleosis and metastatic lymph node involvement. The greatest of these diagnostic dilemmas occurs with large cell anaplastic Ki-1 positive lymphomas, T-cell-rich B-cell lymphomas and peripheral T-cell lymphomas of mixed type. Each of these can present with large atypical cells, some of which are binucleate or multinucleated, in a background of lymphocytes and eosinophils. Using cytomorphology alone, these lymphomas can be indistinguishable from Hodgkin lymphoma. However, phenotyping will disclose their true nature. The importance of separating these disorders from Hodgkin lymphoma obviously lies in their differing clinical courses and treatment.

The cytological identification of infectious mononucleosis can be difficult. Immunocytochemistry and serology should therefore always corroborate the cytological diagnosis. Metastasis from non-lymphoid tumours such as melanomas, large cell carcinomas or seminomas can also cause diagnostic problems. However, knowledge of the existence and type of a primary malignancy will be helpful in selecting antibodies for immunological confirmation.

The rare suppurative variant of Hodgkin disease may pose diagnostic problems on FNA smears due to the paucity of tumour cells in a heavy background of granulocytes and cell débris.[69,70]

## Immunocytochemistry (Fig. 13.24)

### Classical Hodgkin lymphoma

Both Hodgkin and Reed–Sternberg cells are CD30 (Ki-1) and often CD 15 (Leu-M1) positive.[66] Both cells are negative for antibodies to CD45 as well as to pan-T and pan-B markers. It can sometimes be difficult to demonstrate the antigenic profile of the large atypical cells in cytospin preparations, because the Hodgkin and Reed–Sternberg cells are fragile and are often present in low numbers. Careful scrutiny of the immunological stains will however, reveal the phenotype of the diagnostic cells in a majority of cases.

### Nodular lymphocyte predominant Hodgkin lymphoma

The tumour cell is CD20, CD79a, CD45 and BCL6 positive. EMA can be detected in 50% of cases, while CD30 and CD15 are not expressed. Large cell anaplastic Ki-1 lymphomas are CD30 (Ki-1) and CD45 (LCA) positive but CD15 (Leu-M1) negative. They are also often positive for pan-T markers and EMA. The large atypical cells in T-cell-rich B-cell lymphomas are monoclonal B cells. They do not express CD15 (Leu-M1). In infectious mononucleosis the large atypical cells are either T-cells or polytypic B cells.

## Non-Hodgkin lymphoma

Non-Hodgkin lymphomas comprise 2–3% of all malignancies in developed countries. They represent a spectrum of neoplasms ranging from indolent to aggressive tumours, the latter having a rapidly fatal course. The age specific incidence increases throughout life. Their aetiology remains unknown but environmental factors, virus infections and genetic abnormalities are all considered of importance.

The clinical presentation of non-Hodgkin lymphoma shows an extremely variable pattern. Many patients seek medical advice because of a tumour mass which may be nodal or extranodal. General symptoms such as weight loss, fever, infections and lethargy are common and may be the initial complaint. Often, patients have widespread disease with bone marrow involvement at the time of diagnosis.

The histological diagnosis and method of classification have long been a matter of debate. Today pathologists use the WHO classification[54] which is summarised in Box 13.1. It is based both on morphology, immunophenotype and genetic features as well as clinical features. The subheadings used in this chapter in the descriptions of the different lymphomas refer to the WHO classification.

## B-cell neoplasms

### General cytological approach

Cytological evaluation of FNA smears from non-Hodgkin lymphomas includes:

- *Identification of the various cell types present.* To evaluate a lymph node smear it is essential to recognise normal lymphoid cells at all stages of development. Figure 19.1 depicts the lymphoid cell types as seen in an air-dried, MGG stained FNA smear from a benign lymph node

- *Estimation of the proportion of the various cell types.* A monotonous pattern is present when one cell type predominates but even so, additional cell types can be found in low numbers. Such a monotonous composition

indicates abnormal expansion of one, or at the most two subtypes of the lymphoid population. This pattern is seen in most follicular lymphomas and some large cell lymphomas. A mixture of lymphocytes of all types indicates stimulation of the entire lymphoid cell population. This suggests reactive lymphadenitis, but a few B-cell neoplasms and some T-cell lymphomas show a similar pattern

- *Evaluation of individual cell characteristics, such as size and nuclear atypia.* It should be pointed out that most lymphoma cells are faithful replicas of their normal counterparts. Distinct nuclear atypia is thus relatively rare and most often seen in large cell lymphomas

### Immunocytochemistry

As previously mentioned, it is important that the morphological assessment of a lymph node aspirate is accompanied by an immunological work-up. In the authors' laboratory, this approach has led to an improvement in the rate of conclusive diagnosis from approximately 70% to over 95%.

Cytospin preparations or suspensions for FCM are used for assessment of phenotype to establish whether the cells are T or B in origin, and whether clonal restriction of light chain production is present. In Western countries most lymphomas are of B-cell lineage with immunoglobulin light chain expression restricted to either kappa or lambda. Clonal expansion in T-cell lymphomas is more difficult to demonstrate. Loss of pan-T-cell subtype antigen or anomalous expression of T-cell subset antigens can be taken as evidence of clonality.

The initial immunological work-up should be based on a preliminary cytological evaluation. A diagnosis of reactive hyperplasia or B-cell lymphoma should entail a limited panel of antibodies to include pan-T and pan-B antibodies as well as antibodies to the light chains, Bcl-2 and CD10 (cALLa). A kappa:lambda ratio below 5:1 or lambda:kappa ratio not exceeding 3:1 strongly favours a polyclonal reactive B-cell population. Values exceeding these figures suggest a monoclonal malignant expansion of B cells. The subclassification of the B-cell lymphomas sometimes requires the additional staining with antibodies to CD5, CD23 and CD43.

The common acute lymphoblastic leukaemia antigen (cALLa or CD10) is expressed in some mixed cell lymphomas and large cell tumours. A majority of high-grade lymphomas are readily diagnosed as large cell neoplasms in cytological preparations, and in these cases immunocytochemistry is needed only to phenotype the neoplastic cells.

In contrast, a conclusive cytological diagnosis of many low-grade T-cell lymphomas is extremely difficult. The lack of strict immunological criteria for monoclonality further compounds this diagnostic dilemma. As in histopathology, in many cases it will require T-cell receptor (TCR) gene rearrangement analysis by PCR to prove that the process is neoplastic.

### Gene rearrangement analysis

Immunoglobulin (Ig) or TCR gene rearrangement is present in almost all lymphoid malignancies. Tumours which display an immunological B-cell phenotype most often show rearrangements of Ig genes. A pattern of TCR rearrangements is consistent with a T-cell lineage. FNA material from both B- and T-cell lymphomas has been used successfully for analysis of gene rearrangement.[71]

The sensitivity of these techniques allows the detection of a neoplastic population as low as 1–5% of the total cell sample.

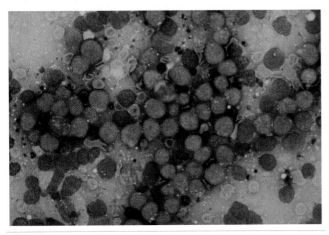

**Fig. 13.25** Precursor B-ALL/lymphoblastic lymphoma. Medium-sized blasts with irregular nuclei and scant rim of basophilic cytoplasm. Mitoses are present (MGG).

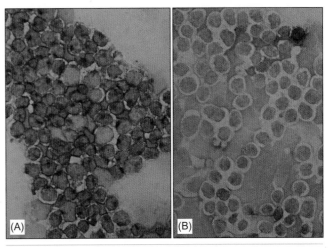

**Fig. 13.26** Precursor B-ALL/lymphoblastic lymphoma. Immunocytochemistry demonstrates CD19 positivity (A) and negative CD3 staining (B) (Alkaline phosphatase).

Such methods are thus important in the diagnosis of lymphoid malignancies and they should be part of the diagnostic armamentarium in laboratories that often evaluate patients with lymphoproliferative disorders.

In addition several subtypes of non-Hodgkin lymphomas are characterised by specific translocations which can be identified by FISH or PCR (see Ch. 34).

### Proliferation rate

The fraction of proliferating cells in non-Hodgkin lymphomas is related to prognosis and response to chemotherapy. Several methods are available to estimate the proliferation rate. Mitotic counting is time consuming and inaccurate. Flow cytometry is a rapid and an accurate technique but is not available in all laboratories. Staining with Ki-67 antibody or antibodies to proliferating cell nuclear antigen (PCNA) offers a highly sensitive procedure which can be performed in most laboratories. The Ki-67 antibody stains cells in late G, S, M and G2 phase.[72] It thus gives a figure which is approximately three times higher than methods which are selective for cells in S phase or mitosis.

### Diagnostic criteria for B-cell lymphomas (WHO classification)

#### Precursor B-lymphoblastic leukaemia/lymphoma

A majority of the patients are children under 6 years of age. Patients with the leukaemic form have blood and bone marrow involvement but CNS, gonads, liver and lymph nodes are frequent extramedullary sites. The lymphoma variant may present in lymph nodes, bone and soft tissue.

The prognosis is good for the leukaemic variant and a majority of patients are cured. The median survival is around 60 months for the lymphoma.

### Cytological findings: precursor B-lymphoblastic leukaemia/lymphoma (Fig. 13.25)

The blasts are rounded small to medium-sized cells with round often convoluted nuclei and a sparse grey-blue cytoplasm.

### Immunocytochemistry (Fig. 13.26)

The lymphoblasts express CD19, CD79a and CD10. TdT can be demonstrated in the early forms of B-precursor cells. There is no expression of surface immunoglobulin. The rate of proliferation is high.

### Genetics

Hypodiploid and hyperdiploid variants exist. There are several translocations reported the most common ones being t(1:19) and t(12;21).

### Chronic lymphatic leukaemia (CLL) and lymphocytic lymphoma

Most patients are over 50 years old. Bone marrow- (CLL) or lymph node- (lymphoma) involvement is typical. Most organs can however be involved. The 5-year survival is around 50%. This lymphoma is not curable.

### Cytological findings: chronic lymphatic leukaemia (CLL) and lymphocytic lymphoma (Fig. 13.27)

The smears are composed of small round lymphoid cells with a small rim of cytoplasm. The nucleus is somewhat larger than that of a mature lymphoid cell. The chromatin pattern is irregular and clumped. Mitoses are rare. A few prolymphocytes as well as blasts and macrophages may be present. Transformation to diffuse large B-cell lymphoma occurs and is characterised by a relative dominance of centroblasts and immunoblasts.

The differential diagnosis includes reactive hyperplasia, immunocytoma, CLL of T-cell type and follicular lymphoma with predominance of centrocytes. In patients without bone marrow involvement a correct diagnosis is often impossible without the aid of immunocytochemistry.

### Immunocytochemistry (Fig. 13.28)

The expression of B-cell antigens and light chain restriction are usually weak. CD5, CD23 and CD43 are positive. The fraction of proliferating cells is less than 10% as measured by Ki-67 antibody staining. Transformation results in a proliferation rate over 30%.

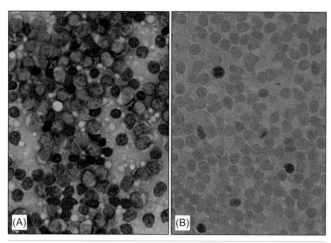

**Fig. 13.27** Chronic lymphocytic leukaemia. (A) Small- to medium-sized cells with round nuclei and sparse cytoplasm (MGG). (B) Ki-67 staining shows a low proliferation rate (immunoperoxidase).

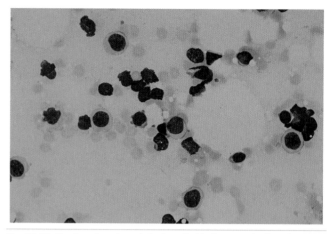

**Fig. 13.29** B-cell prolymphocytic leukaemia. Medium-sized cells with moderate amount of pale cytoplasm and round nuclei (MGG).

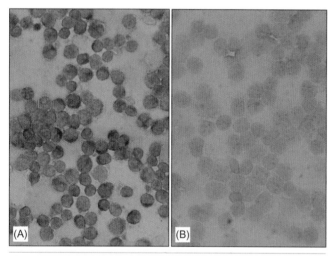

**Fig. 13.28** Chronic lymphocytic leukaemia. Immunocytochemistry on cytospin preparation from aspirate shown in Figure 13.27. (A) The cells are monoclonal for kappa. (B) No positivity for lambda staining (alkaline phosphatase).

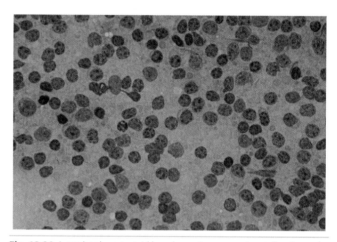

**Fig. 13.30** Lymphoplasmacytoid lymphoma/immunocytoma. Small monotonous cells with eccentric nuclei and typical chromatin pattern (MGG).

### Immunocytochemistry

The cells are CD19, CD20 and CD79a positive. CD5 is seen only in a minority of cases and CD23 is not expressed.

### Genetics

No constant translocation has been reported.

## Lymphoplasmacytic lymphoma

Elderly people are affected. Lymph node, bone marrow and spleen are often involved. The clinical course is usually indolent but the long-term prognosis is poor.

### Genetics

Almost all cases have abnormal karyotypes but no constant translocation has been reported.

## B-cell prolymphocytic leukaemia

Elderly patients predominate. Bone marrow and spleen involvement is typical but lymph node engagement occurs. This lymphoma responds poorly to chemotherapy and has a short survival.

### Cytological findings: B-cell prolymphocytic leukaemia (Fig. 13.29)

The prolymphocyte is medium-sized with a moderate amount of weakly basophilic cytoplasm and a round nucleus. A distinct central nucleolus is often seen.

Distinction from CLL and mantle cell lymphoma can be difficult.

### Cytological findings: lymphoplasmacytic lymphoma (Fig. 13.30)

The predominant cell is slightly larger than a mature lymphocyte. It has an eccentric nucleus with a plasma cell-like chromatin pattern. The cytoplasm is basophilic and more abundant than that seen in CLL. Additional cells such as plasma cells, mast cells and a few immunoblasts are regularly

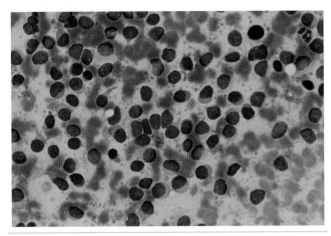

**Fig. 13.31** Hairy cell leukaemia. Small- to medium-sized cells with round to oval excentric nuclei and weakly basophilic rich cytoplasm (MGG).

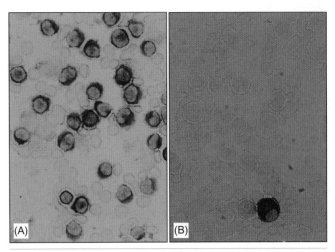

**Fig. 13.32** Hairy cell leukaemia. Immunocytochemistry on cytospin preparation from aspirate shown in Figure 13.31 demonstrating (A) kappa monoclonal cells and (B) a plasma cell positive for lambda (alkaline phosphatase).

observed. On morphology alone, this subtype is difficult to differentiate from some reactive conditions as well as CLL.

In some variants a substantial fraction of mature plasma cells are seen. The distinction from an extramedullary plasmacytoma can thus be difficult, but if more than 50% of the population consists of plasma cells it is likely to be a plasmacytoma.

### Immunocytochemistry
The expression of the B-cell antigens CD19, CD20 and CD79a is always seen and light chain restriction is readily demonstrated. CD5 and CD10 are not expressed. The fraction of proliferating cells varies from a few per cent to as high as 20%.

### Genetics
t(9;14) is detected in half of the cases.

## Hairy cell leukemia

The typical patient is a middle-aged male. The bone marrow and spleen are always involved but lymph node spread is relatively common. Long-term remissions are seen after chemotherapy.

### Cytological findings: hairy cell leukemia (Fig. 13.31)

The cells are small- to medium-sized with an oval nucleus with a smooth chromatin and without nucleoli. The cytoplasm is rich and has hairy projections in blood-smears. Such projections are, however, not seen in FNA smears from lymph nodes or spleen.[73]

### Immunocytochemistry
B-cell antigens such as CD19, CD20 and CD79a are expressed. In addition the cells are CD11c, CD25 and CD103 positive.

### Cytogenetics
No constant abnormality has been reported.

## Plasmacytoma/myeloma

Myeloma patients are often elderly while plasmacytoma patients are middle-aged. Bone marrow involvement with lytic bone destructions is typical for myeloma while plasmacytoma either

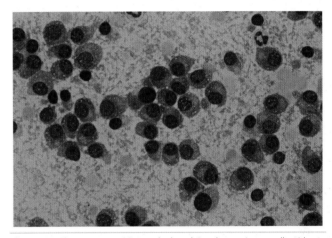

**Fig. 13.33** Plasmacytoma. Many naked nuclei and some intact cells with eccentric nucleus and distinct basophilic cytoplasm (MGG).

appear as a single lytic bone destruction or in the upper respiratory tract, although most extraosseous sites can be involved. Myeloma has a poor prognosis while plasmacytoma are potentially curable.

### Cytological findings: plasmacytoma/myeloma (Fig. 13.33)

The neoplastic cell may have a morphology almost identical to that of a normal plasma cell but usually shows atypia such as enlarged pleomorphic nuclei, double nuclei and large irregular cytoplasm.[74] The anaplastic variant is difficult to diagnose on cytology alone and immunocytochemistry must then be used to identify the cells.

### Immunocytochemistry (Fig. 13.34)
The cells lack expression of most B-cell antigens but show light chain restriction and are CD38, CD138 and often CD79a positive. EMA positivity is seen in some cases.

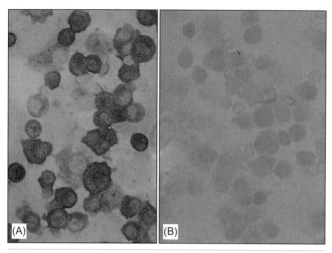

**Fig. 13.34** Plasmacytoma. (A) The cells are CD38 positive. (B) No positivity for CD20 (Alkaline phosphatase).

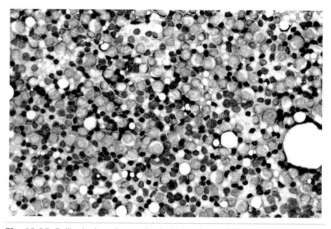

**Fig. 13.35** Follicular lymphoma Grade I. Mixed population of neoplastic lymphatic cells with dominance of medium-sized centrocytes and one centroblast. In addition some small mature lymphocytes (MGG).

## Cytogenetics

A number of genetic abnormalities have been described but no constant changes appear to exist.

## Nodal/extranodal (MALT) marginal zone B-cell lymphoma

Most patients are over 50 years old. The nodal variant affects lymph nodes mainly while the extranodal type involves the gastrointestinal tract and lung most often. Both subtypes run an indolent clinical course.

### Cytological findings: nodal/extranodal (MALT) marginal zone B-cell lymphoma

The tumour cell population is dominated by small- to medium-sized cells, the marginal zone cell which is centrocyte-like but with indistinct nucleoli and a more distinct cytoplasm. Some cases will have monocytoid-like cells due to an abundant cytoplasm.[75,76] In some MALT lymphomas the cells have distinct plasmacytic features. Plasma cells, centroblasts and some monocytoid B-cells are often present.

### Immunocytochemistry

The tumour cells are of B-phenotype and show light chain restriction but no expression of CD5, CD10, CD23 or CD43. The plasma cells are often monoclonal. The proliferation rate is usually low.

### Cytogenetics

The extranodal variant shows t(11;18) in half of the cases. The nodal type only rarely shows this abnormality.

## Follicular lymphoma

This subtype comprises one-third of all non-Hodgkin lymphomas. It usually affects middle-aged patients. Most patients have lymph node and bone marrow involvement. Extranodal spread is common. Grade I and II are indolent but not curable. In contrast, Grade III is aggressive but potentially curable.

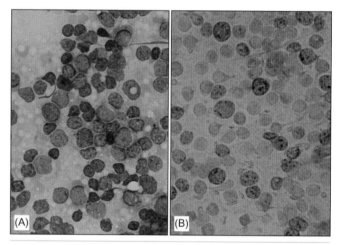

**Fig. 13.36** Follicular lymphoma Grade II. (A) There is a predominance of medium-sized cells with irregular cleaved nuclei. Some larger centroblasts are seen (MGG). (B) Ki-67 staining shows proliferation of both centrocytes and centroblasts (immunoperoxidase).

### Cytological findings: follicular lymphoma (Figs 13.35–13.37)

The predominating cell is the medium-sized centrocyte which has little cytoplasm and an irregular cleaved or angulated nucleus. These cells have a scant cytoplasm and may seem to form aggregates. Centroblasts are present but the proportion varies.[77–79] Follicular lymphomas are subdivided into Grade I, Grade II and Grade III based on the proportion of large cells present.[54] Thus Grade I has 0–5, Grade II 6–15 and Grade III >15 centroblast/high power field, respectively.

Other cell types present in follicular lymphomas are small mature non-neoplastic lymphoid cells, macrophages and epithelioid cells. A smear with a high number of non-neoplastic cells may be impossible to differentiate from reactive lymphadenopathy unless cytomorphology is complemented by immunocytochemical evaluation.

Follicular lymphomas show varying degree of follicular and diffuse growth pattern but a majority have a dominant follicular pattern. Obviously the growth pattern cannot be determined on FNA smears.

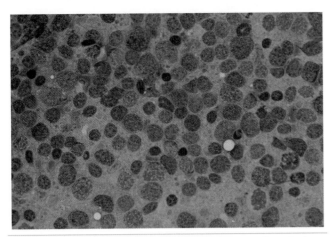

**Fig. 13.37** Follicular lymphoma Grade III. Mixed population of neoplastic immature centroblasts and immunoblasts (MGG).

## Immunocytochemistry (Fig. 13.38)

The B-cell lineage of these tumour cells is readily identified by expression of CD19, CD20 and CD79a. Light chain restriction can usually be demonstrated as well as positive staining for CD10. Expression of BCL-2 is seen in a majority of cases. Mature reactive T cells are present, and may constitute up to 50% of the lymphoid population. The proliferation fraction in the neoplastic B-cells varies considerably from case to case. Figures below 5% are seldom seen but in occasional cases up to 75% of the neoplastic population may react positively to proliferation markers (see Fig. 13.36B). Such cases show aggressive behaviour and should be treated as high-grade lymphomas irrespective of their cytological grading.

## Cytogenetics

A majority of these lymphomas show a t(14;18) translocation.

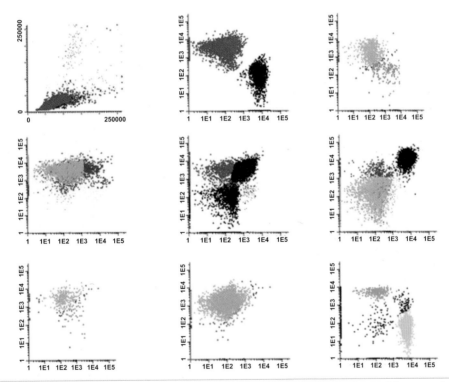

**Fig. 13.38** 8-colour flow cytometry analysis of fine needle aspirate from a lymph node with follicular lymphoma. The following antibody panel was used: Lambda FITC/ Kappa PE/CD19 PerCP-Cy5/ CD10 APC/ CD5 PE-Cy7/ CD4 APC-Cy7/ CD8 AM-Cyan/ CD3 Pacific Blue. Data were acquired using FACS-Canto and DIVA software (Becton Dickinson). Data analysis was done using Infinicyt (Cytognos, Salamanca, Spain) software. Upper row: Left: forward scatter/side scatter plot shows that most cells were in the lymphocyte area. Dead cells are excluded from analysis. Middle: CD19 vs CD3 plot shows 57% B cells (red) and 33% T cells (blue). Right: Kappa (orange)/Lambda (green) analysis in CD19/SSC gated B cells shows clonal excess of kappa with kappa/lambda ratio 12:1. Middle row: Left: CD19 vs CD5 plot within CD19/SSC gate shows a small population of CD5+ B-cells (5% of B cells). Middle: CD19 vs CD10 plot within CD19/SSC gate shows a large population of CD10+ B cells that correspond to germinal centre cells (80% of B cells). Right: CD3 vs CD5 plot shows that most T-cells were positive for both markers (blue). Lower row: Left: Kappa/lambda analysis of CD5+ B cells shows increased kappa/lambda ratio (6.5). Middle: Kappa/lambda analysis of CD10+ B cells shows monoclonal kappa+ population. Right: CD4 and CD8 expression in CD3-gated T-cell population. CD4/CD9 ratio was 5.5. (Courtesy of Professor A. Porwit, Hematopathology Division, Dept Pathology and Cytology, Karolinska University Hospital Solna, Stockholm, Sweden).

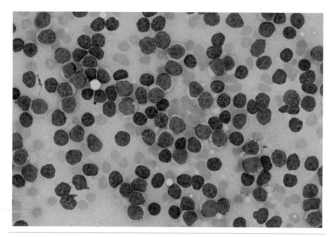

**Fig. 13.39** Mantle cell lymphoma. Small- to medium-sized cells with round nuclei and pale cytoplasm (MGG).

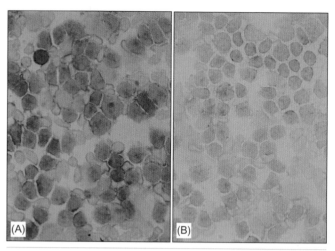

**Fig. 13.40** Mantle cell lymphoma. Immunocytochemistry. (A) The cells are CD5 positive. (B) No positivity is seen for CD10 (alkaline phosphatase).

## Mantle cell lymphoma

Most patients are over 60 years old. Lymph node involvement is common but bone marrow and extranodal spread occurs relatively often. Cure is not possible and the median survival is less than 5 years.

### Cytological findings: mantle cell lymphoma (Fig. 13.39)

The smears are monotonous composed of small- to medium-sized lymphoid cells, slightly larger than lymphocytes. The nuclei are cleaved and have a dispersed chromatin, inconspicuous nucleoli and a thin pale cytoplasm thus resembling centrocytes. [77,80,81]

In rare cases the cells are immature with larger nuclei and a high proliferation rate.[82] Two main variants are described. One shows a resemblance to lymphoblastic lymphoma and the term 'lymphoblastoid' has been proposed.[54] The second type shows a more heterogeneous population of cells with oval to cleaved nuclei and is referred to as the pleomorphic variant.

### Immunocytochemistry (Fig. 13.40)

The cells are of B phenotype (CD20) with light chain restriction. In addition the cells are consistently CD5 and CD43 positive and most often CD10 negative. All cases express Cyklin D1 and bcl-2. The fraction of proliferating cells is usually low, around 10% as measured by Ki-67 (Mib-1). The 'blastoid' variant has a high proliferation rate.

### Cytogenetics

Translocation t(11;14) is observed in a majority of cases as shown in Figure 13.41.

## Diffuse large B-cell lymphoma

Diffuse large B-cell lymphoma (DLBL) is mostly seen in elderly patients. Nodal presentation is common but extranodal manifestation is seen in around 1/2 of the cases. The clinical course is aggressive but some patients are cured.

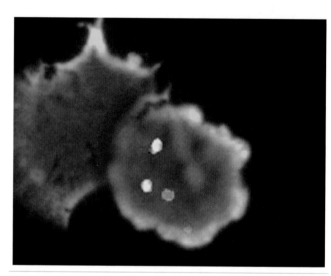

**Fig. 13.41** Mantle cell lymphoma. Interphase FISH using Vysis LSI IGH/CCND1 Dual Color, Dual Fusion Translocation Probe, detecting the translocation t(11;14)(q13;q32). In a normal cell two red (*CCND1*) and two green (*IGH*) signals can be seen (not shown). In the tumour cell the translocation splits the two genes and creates two red/green fusion signals. (Courtesy of Dr E. Blennow, Dept Clinical Genetics, Karolinska University Hospital Solna, Stockholm, Sweden).

### Cytological findings: diffuse large B-cell lymphoma (Figs 13.42–13.45)

The most common type of DLBL is composed of large round centroblasts (Fig. 13.42). The nuclei are only slightly irregular and show several small nucleoli, often at the nuclear membrane. The cytoplasm is scanty and may contain a few vacuoles. In addition, a number of other cells such as centrocytes, small mature lymphocytes and macrophages may be found.

Another type of DLBL is the polymorphic centroblastic lymphoma which contains immunoblasts in addition to centroblasts. Some centrocytes and small mature cells are regularly observed.

In some variants of DLBL the tumour cells are mostly of immunoblastic type (Fig. 13.43). These are large cells with an eccentric nucleus with unevenly distributed chromatin and

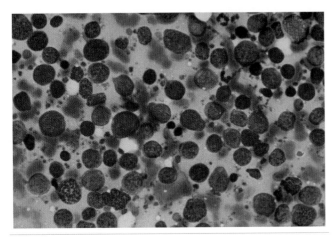

**Fig. 13.42** Diffuse large B-cell lymphoma. Centroblastic variant. Note the predominance of large rounded centroblasts (MGG).

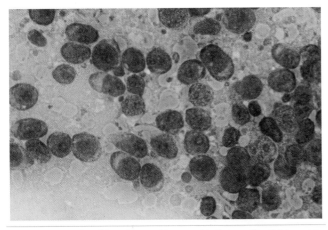

**Fig. 13.43** Large B-cell lymphoma of immunoblastic type. The field consists almost entirely of large cells with eccentric nuclei and strongly basophilic cytoplasm (MGG).

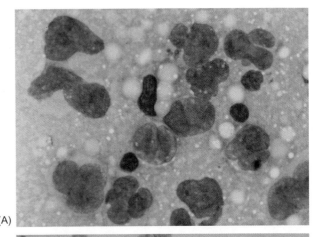

(A)

(B)

**Fig. 13.44** Diffuse large B-cell lymphoma of multilobated type. There are large cells with characteristic polymorphic multilobated nuclei. (A) MGG; (B) Papanicolaou.

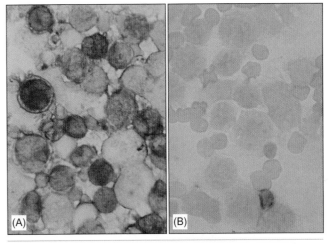

(A)　　　(B)

**Fig. 13.45** Diffuse large B-cell lymphoma of multilobated type (case shown in Figure 13.44. (A) Immunocytochemistry shows intense kappa expression in all cells. (B) One small mature lambda positive cell is seen (alkaline phosphatase).

a central distinct nucleolus. The cytoplasm is abundant with a greyish blue staining in MGG. Rarely, poorly differentiated carcinomas or melanomas may on cytomorphology be misdiagnosed as this variant of lymphoma.

An uncommon variant of DLBL is the multilobated centroblastic lymphoma, in which the cells are polymorphic with multilobated, sometimes bizarre nuclei (Figs 13.44, 13.45). Such cases may be difficult to identify as lymphoid in origin, and to distinguish from other high-grade neoplasms.

T-cell rich B-cell lymphomas are also included in the subgroup of DLBL (Figs 13.46, 13.47). They can morphologically be mistaken for Hodgkin lymphoma but immunological characterisation will identify the cells as monoclonal B-cells.[83,84]

## Immunocytochemistry (Figs 13.46, 13.47)

The cells in DLBL often express several B antigens such as CD19, CD20 and CD22. Kappa or lambda light chains are expressed in most cases and CD10 positivity is common in the centroblastic variants. A population of mature T cells is regularly present. The fraction of proliferating cells is usually around 50% or more, which predicts relatively aggressive clinical behaviour. The multilobated subtype often runs a rapid clinical course which is reflected in a proliferation fraction often exceeding 80%.

The immunoblasts are CD38 (OKT 10) negative, which differentiates them from a polymorphic myeloma (plasmacytosarcoma). The fraction of proliferating cells is usually above 75%.

## Cytogenetics

Approximately one-third of the cases show t(14;18) translocation.

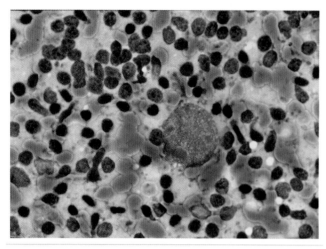

**Fig. 13.46** T-cell rich B-cell lymphoma. Numerous mature lymphocytes surrounding one large tumour cell with large nucleus and prominent nucleoli. The scanty cytoplasm is strongly basophilic (MGG).

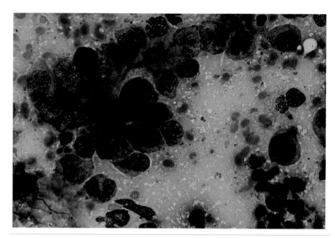

**Fig. 13.48** Mediastinal B-cell lymphoma. Polymorphic immature lymphoid cells with marked irregular nuclei and distinct relatively rich cytoplasm (MGG).

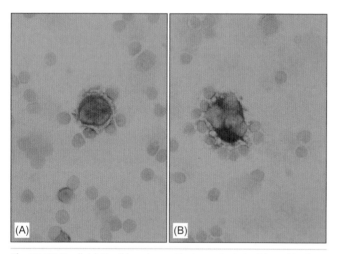

**Fig. 13.47** T-cell rich B-cell lymphoma. The large atypical cell is positive for (A) CD20 and (B) kappa (alkaline phosphatase).

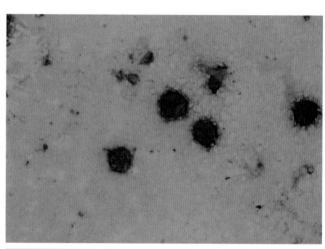

**Fig. 13.49** Mediastinal B-cell lymphoma. Immunocytochemistry of the case shown in Figure 13.48 shows that the large tumour cells are CD20 positive (alkaline phosphatase).

## Mediastinal large B-cell lymphoma

The typical patient is an adult female with massive involvement of mediastinal lymph nodes.[85] In early stages the response rate is good but long-term prognosis is uncertain.

> **Cytological findings: mediastinal large B-cell lymphoma (Fig. 13.48)**
>
> The tumour cells are large with round to irregular nuclei and a rich pale cytoplasm.[34] Small benign lymphocytes are often present. Fragments of sclerotic tissue are frequent findings.

### Immunocytochemistry (Fig. 13.49)

The B-phenotype can be demonstrated by positive staining for CD19 and CD20. Immunoglobulin expression is often absent. The cells are CD45 positive and may show weak positivity for CD30. There is no expression of CD10 and BCL-2.

### Cytogenetics

No specific translocation has been reported.

## Burkitt's lymphoma

Both the endemic and sporadic variant are most common in children. The endemic type often present with facial bone tumours but other extra nodal sites such as intestines, breast, ovaries and CNS can be involved. The sporadic variant most frequently presents as an abdominal mass but other extranodal sites are common. This highly aggressive lymphoma is often cured.

> **Cytological findings: Burkitt's lymphoma (Fig. 13.50)**
>
> The Burkitt cells are medium-sized with a low nuclear/cytoplasmic ratio. They have deep blue cytoplasm on MGG staining which contains many punched out vacuoles. The nuclei are round with clumped chromatin and central nucleoli. Mitotic figures are frequent as well as macrophages with apoptotic bodies.[86–88]

### Immunocytochemistry

The Burkitt lymphoma cells express CD19 and CD20. Light chain restriction can be demonstrated in all cases. The CD10 is

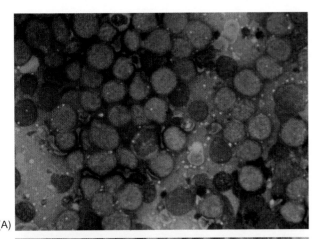

(A)

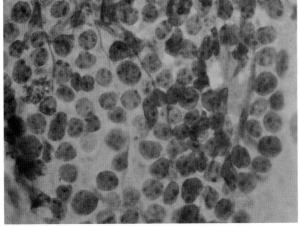

(B)

**Fig. 13.50** Burkitt's lymphoma. (A) Medium-sized round blast cells with scant cytoplasm which often contain small vacuoles (MGG). (B) Almost all cells are proliferating as shown by Ki-67 staining (immunoperoxidase).

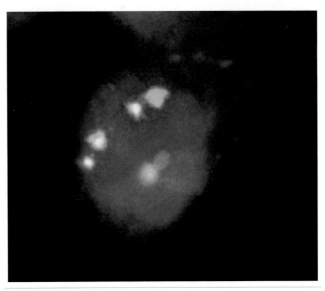

**Fig. 13.51** Burkitt's lymphoma. Interphase FISH using Vysis LSI IGH/MYC, CEP 8 Tri-color, Dual Fusion Translocation Probe, detecting the translocation t(8;14)(q24;q32). In a normal cell two red (*MYC*), two green (*IGH*) and two purple (centromere 8) signals can be seen (not shown). In the tumour cell the translocation splits the two genes and creates two red/green fusion signals. The centromere probe serves as control for possible *MYC* amplification and loss of der(8). (Courtesy of Dr E. Blennow, Dept Clinical Genetics, Karolinska University Hospital Solna, Stockholm, Sweden).

usually expressed but TdT can not be detected. The fraction of Ki-67 positive cells is above 90%.

## Cytogenetics (Fig. 13.51)

Most cases have a t(8;14) translocation but t(2;8) and t(8;22) translocations also occur.

### Post-transplant lymphoproliferative disorder

This mixed group of disorders is seen in patients on immunosuppressive regimens. EBV infection seems to play an important role in a majority of cases. Post-transplant lymphoproliferative disorder (PTLD) can be categorised into early lesions, polymorphic PTLD, monomorphic PTLD and other types.[54] The polymorphic PTLD usually responds to withdrawal of immunosuppression in contrast to the monomorphic PTLD, which is composed of a variety of lymphomas that should be treated accordingly.

### Cytological findings: post-transplant lymphoproliferative disorder

Smears from polymorphic PTLD show a mixed population of lymphoid cells ranging from mature small lymphocytes to immunoblasts and centroblasts. Plasma cells are frequent and necrosis is common. This complex picture will make a conclusive cytological diagnosis difficult without the aid of immunophenotyping.

The monomorphic PTLD group encompasses lymphomas such as diffuse large B-cell lymphoma, Burkitt/Burkitt-like lymphoma, myeloma or various T-cell lymphomas. The cytomorphology of these types are described separately in this chapter.

#### Immunocytochemistry

The polymorphic PTLD can be both poly- and monoclonal. The monomorphic PTLD is a monoclonal proliferation of T-cells or of T-phenotype which often show aberrant expression of T-cell antigens. The EBV associated antigen LMP-1 is expressed in most cases.

#### Genetics

The B-cell lymphomas show Ig gene rearrangement while the T-cell lymphomas have T-cell receptor gene rearrangement.

## Diagnostic criteria for T-cell lymphomas (WHO classification)

(Box 13.2)

### Precursor T-lymphoblastic leukaemia/ lymphoblastic lymphoma

Both the leukaemia and lymphoma are most frequent among adolescent males.[89] The leukaemia often presents with a mediastinal mass, which is also the site of predilection for the lymphoma.[90] A majority of the patients have long survival and many are cured.

## Box 13.2  WHO classification of T-cell lymphomas

### Leukaemic/disseminated

- Precursor T-lymphoblastic leukaemia/lymphoblastic lymphoma*
- T-cell prolymphocytic leukaemia
- T-cell large granular lymphocytic leukaemia
- Aggressive NK cell leukaemia
- Adult T-cell leukaemia/lymphoma*

### Cutaneous

- Mycosis fungoides*
- Sézary syndrome*
- Primary cutaneous anaplastic large cell lymphoma*
- Lymphomatoid papulosis

### Other extranodal

- Extranodal NK/T-cell lymphoma, nasal type*
- Enteropathy-type T-cell lymphoma
- Hepatosplenic T-cell lymphoma
- Subcutaneous panniculitis-like T-cell lymphoma

### Nodal

- Angioimmunoblastic T-cell lymphoma*
- Peripheral T-cell lymphoma, unspecified*
- Anaplastic large cell lymphoma*
- Neoplasm of uncertain lineage and stage of differentiation
- Blastic NK cell lymphoma

*Indicates lymphomas described here.

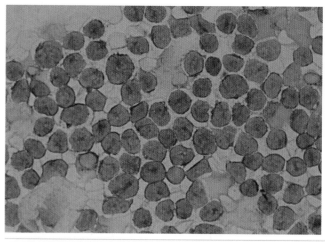

**Fig. 13.53** Precursor T-ALL/lymphoblastic lymphoma. Immunocytochemistry of the case shown in Figure 13.52. The blasts are CD3 positive (alkaline phosphatase).

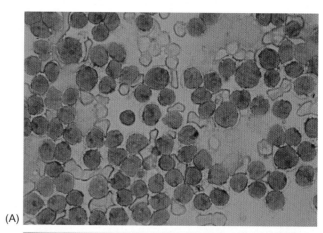

(A)

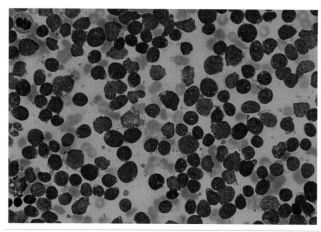

**Fig. 13.52** Precursor T-ALL/lymphoblastic lymphoma. Small- to medium-sized blasts with scant cytoplasm and irregular nuclei with coarse chromatin (MGG).

### Cytological findings: precursor T-lymphoblastic leukaemia/lymphoblastic lymphoma (Fig. 13.52)

The blasts are medium-sized with irregular nuclei and basophilic sparse cytoplasm often with vacuoles. Macrophages with tingible bodies are frequent.[31,32]

### Immunocytochemistry (Figs 13.53, 13.54)

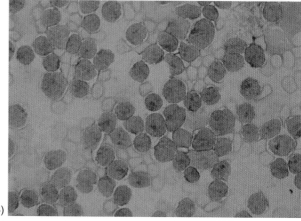

(B)

**Fig. 13.54** Precursor T-ALL/lymphoblastic lymphoma. Immunocytochemistry of the case shown in Figure 13.52. The blasts express CD8 (A) and CD10 (B) (alkaline phosphatase).

Most cells are CD3 and CD7 positive while other T-cell markers are variably expressed. TdT is expressed in all cases. CD10 may be expressed. The proportion of proliferating cells is high.

### Cytogenetics

Several variants of translocation have been described, the most common ones involving the T-cell receptor loci.

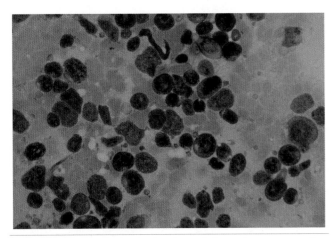

**Fig. 13.55** Adult T-cell leukaemia/lymphoma. Polymorphous tumour cells of varying size with marked irregular nuclei with multiple prominent nucleoli and coarse chromatin (MGG).

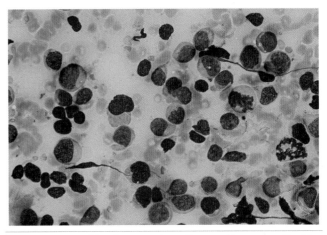

**Fig. 13.57** NK/T-cell lymphoma nasal type. Pleomorphic tumour cells with irregular nuclei and rich cytoplasm. Mitoses are frequent (MGG).

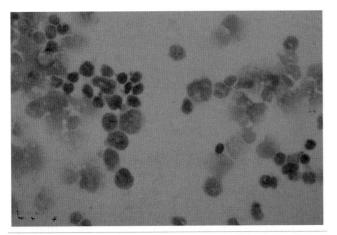

**Fig. 13.56** Adult T-cell leukaemia/lymphoma. Immunocytochemistry shows CD3 positivity of the tumour cells (Alkaline phosphatase).

## Adult T-cell leukaemia/lymphoma

This lymphoma is caused by the human retrovirus HTLV-1 and is endemic in Japan, the Caribbean and parts of Africa. Middle-aged patients present with lymph node and peripheral blood involvement. The acute form has a short survival time while the chronic type has a protracted clinical course.

### Cytological findings: adult T-cell leukaemia/lymphoma (Figs 13.55, 13.56)

The tumour cell is medium-sized to large and has a markedly irregular nucleus with distinct nucleoli. The cytoplasm is rich and deeply basophilic. Giant cells are often present.[91–93]

### Immunocytochemistry (Fig. 13.56)

The T-cell antigens CD2, CD3, CD4 and CD5 are expressed in most cases but there is no constant pattern. CD30 is often expressed. The rate of proliferation is high.

### Cytogenetics

The T-cell receptor genes are rearranged and the HTLV-1 virus is integrated.

## Extranodal NK/T-cell lymphoma, nasal type

Adult patients often present with extranodal tumours in the nasal cavity or nasopharynx. Other extranodal sites affected are skin and soft tissue. Lymph node spread can occur. The prognosis is poor in most cases.

### Cytological findings: extranodal NK/T-cell lymphoma, nasal type (Fig. 13.57)

The tumour cells are of variable size but in a majority of cases the cells are medium-sized to large. The nuclei are irregular and the cytoplasm pale grey (MGG).[94]

### Immunocytochemistry

Most cases are CD2 and CD56 positive. Other T-antigens are usually negative.

### Cytogenetics

The T-cell receptor is not rearranged. EBV is usually demonstrable.

## Mycosis fungoides/Sézary's syndrome

Elderly patients are affected. The skin is the main site for mycosis patients while patients with Sézary's syndrome have a generalised disease involving skin, blood and lymph nodes. Patients with limited mycosis fungoides have a good prognosis while patients with Sézary's syndrome have a short survival.

### Cytological findings: mycosis fungoides/Sézary's syndrome (Fig. 13.58)

In smears from lymph node aspirates the tumour cells are small- to medium-sized with 'cerebriform' nuclei. Some large atypical cells are usually present and may in fact predominate in cases of Sézary's syndrome.[95]

### Immunocytochemistry (Figs 13.59, 13.60)

The cells are positive for CD2, CD3, CD4 and CD5. The large cells may be CD30-positive.

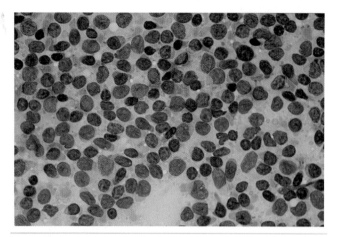

**Fig. 13.58** Mycosis fungoides. Small- to medium-sized cells with irregular nuclei (MGG).

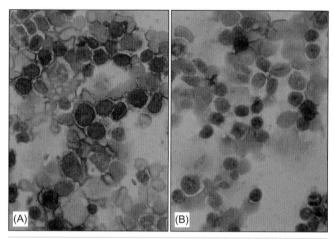

**Fig. 13.60** Mycosis fungoides. Immunocytochemistry from the case shown in Figures 13.58 and 13.59. (A). The tumour cells are of T helper phenotype. (B) Few T suppressor cells are present (alkaline phosphatase).

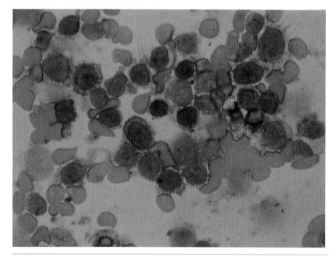

**Fig. 13.59** Mycosis fungoides. Immunocytochemistry on cytospin material from the aspirate shown in Figure 13.58. The neoplastic cells are of T phenotype as shown here with CD3 positive staining (alkaline phosphatase).

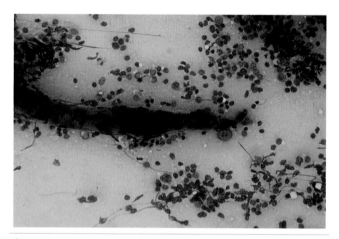

**Fig. 13.61** AILD. The smear shows a fragment of blood vessel with numerous lymphoid cells of varying size (MGG).

### Cytogenetics

The T-cell receptor genes are rearranged.

## Angioimmunoblastic T-cell lymphoma

Elderly patients predominate and usually present with peripheral lymphadenopathy, hepatosplenomegaly and bone marrow infiltration. Pruritus, pleural effusion and ascites are common symptoms. The prognosis is poor and few patients survive 5 years.

---

**Cytological findings: angioimmunoblastic T-cell lymphoma (Figs 13.61, 13.62)**

The cytology of this lymphoma is complex with a polymorphous population of small- to medium-sized neoplastic cells with pale cytoplasm. These cells are mixed with mature lymphoid cells, plasma cells, histiocytes and eosinophils. Fragments of small vessels can usually be seen.[96]

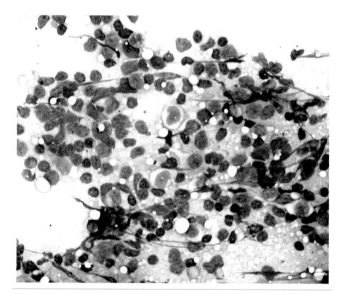

**Fig. 13.62** AILD. Polymorphous population of lymphoid cells of small to large size with irregular nuclei. Few cells have distinct pale and some have basophilic cytoplasm. There is an admixture of small mature lymphocytes and epithelioid cells (MGG).

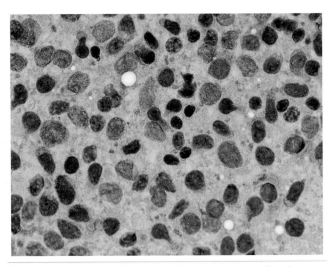

**Fig. 13.63** Peripheral T-cell lymphoma. The smear shows small- and medium-sized irregular lymphoid cells and several histiocytes (MGG).

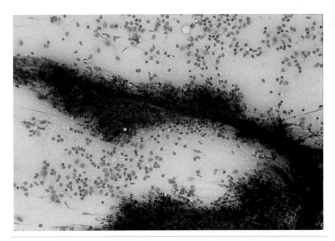

**Fig. 13.64** Peripheral T-cell lymphoma. The smear shows fragments of vessels in a background of lymphoid cells (MGG).

## Immunocytochemistry

Mature T-cells are mixed with CD4 and CD8 positive cells. The immunological findings are complex and seldom allows a conclusive diagnosis.

## Cytogenetics

The T-cell receptor genes are rearranged in a majority of cases.

## Peripheral T-cell lymphoma, unspecified

Most patients are adult but all ages can be affected. Generalised lymphadenopathy, bone marrow involvement and skin infiltration are the most common sites of presentation. The prognosis is dismal and few patients survive 5 years.

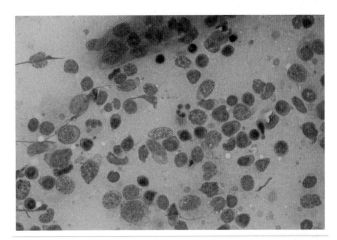

**Fig. 13.65** Peripheral T-cell lymphoma. Polymorphic lymphoid cells are seen together with a fragment of vessel (MGG).

> **Cytological findings: peripheral T-cell lymphoma, unspecified (Figs 13.63–13.65)**
>
> Aspirates from these lymphomas show a spectrum of atypical cells ranging from small to large. The cells have irregular nuclei often with marked nucleoli and coarse chromatin. Occasional large cells with multilobated or multiple nuclei are often seen. The cytoplasm of the atypical cells is also variable but the medium-sized and large cells have a rich cytoplasm which commonly stains pale grey in MGG preparations. Epithelioid cells, plasma cells and eosinophils are present in varying proportions. Fragments of vessels are often found. The cytological presentation of the individual subgroups seems to vary considerably. The rarity of these disorders also contributes to the difficulty of making a conclusive diagnosis on cytological smears alone.[97–99]

## Immunocytochemistry (Fig. 13.66)

A majority of the cases are CD4 (T helper) positive. Aberrant T-cell antigen expression and deletion of pan-T-antigens strongly indicate a neoplastic lymphoid population. The plasma cells, being reactive, are polyclonal. In keeping with their varying clinical behaviour of this process the proliferation rate varies between 10% and 50%.

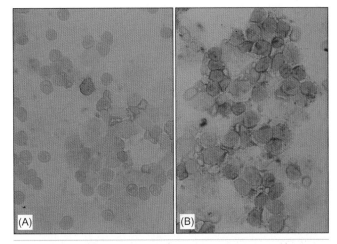

**Fig. 13.66** Peripheral T-cell lymphoma. This illustrates the immunocytochemistry on the aspirate shown in Figure 13.65. (A) One small B cell. (B) The larger polymorphic cells are of T phenotype with positivity for CD4 (alkaline phosphatase).

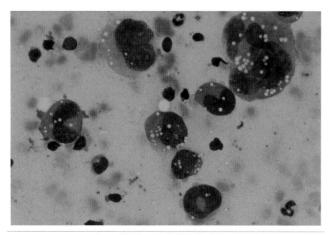

**Fig. 13.67** Anaplastic large cell lymphoma. Note the large pleomorphic cells with multilobated or ring-form nuclei and abundant vacuolated cytoplasm (MGG).

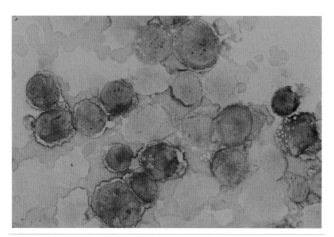

**Fig. 13.68** Anaplastic large cell lymphoma. Immunocytochemistry performed on the aspirate shown in Figure 13.67. The cells strongly express CD30/Ki-1 (Alkaline phosphatase).

## Cytogenetics

The TCR genes are rearranged in most cases.

## Anaplastic large cell lymphoma

Anaplastic large cell lymphoma (ALCL) is most frequent among children and young adults but it can occur at all ages. It is a systemic disease which involves lymph nodes and extranodal sites such as skin, bone, lung and soft tissue. Patients with ALK-positive tumour cells have high 5-year survival rate while that for ALK-negative cases is around 40%.

### Cytological findings: anaplastic large cell lymphoma (Fig. 13.67)

Two main morphological variants of ALCL exist: a large pleomorphic cell type and a small cell variant. The large cell type is characterised by pleomorphic tumour cells with multilobated, horseshoe- or ring-shaped nuclei. The ample cytoplasm is grey-blue (MGG) and often vacuolated. [100–103]

The small cell variant has small- to medium-sized cells with irregular nuclei and a moderate amount of cytoplasm. Often some large cells with distinct nuclear atypia can be found. [104,105]

**Table 13.1** Most frequent metastatic sites of commonest malignancies

| Lymph node metastasis in: | Primary tumour most likely in: |
| --- | --- |
| Supraclavicular fossa | Breast, lung, GIT, ovary, prostate |
| Neck (excl. supraclavicular fossa) | Oral cavity, pharynx, larynx, salivary glands, thyroid, lung, breast |
| Axilla | Breast, lung, ovary |
| Groin | Gynaecological tract, penis, prostate |

**Table 13.2** Cytokeratin primary site specificity

| Carcinoma CK profile | | Possible primary site |
| --- | --- | --- |
| CK 7+ | CK 20+ | Bladder, pancreas, ovary (mucinous) |
| CK 7+ | CK 20− | Breast, ovary, endometrium thyroid (papillary), lung (non small cell) |
| CK 7− | CK 20+ | Colorectal |
| CK 7− | CK 20− | Hepatocellular, prostate, renal, lung (squamous and small cell). |

## Immunocytochemistry (Fig. 13.68)

A strong membrane positivity for CD30 is present in all large tumour cells. The small cell variant is more weakly stained. The cells are often EMA positive and express T-cell antigens such as CD2 and CD4. ALK expression is seen in a majority of cases. The rate of proliferation is over 50%.

## Cytogenetics

The T-cell receptor genes are rearranged in most cases of ALCL. Translocation t(2;5) and t(1;2) can be detected in 70% and 20%, respectively.

## Metastatic lymph node disease

## Introduction

Lymph nodes enlarged by metastatic tumour spread often show diffuse involvement, therefore an FNA from an involved node will almost invariably result in diagnostic cells. Such 'foreign' cells are in most instances readily identified in a background of lymphoid cells. The diagnostic accuracy of FNA cytology in detecting lymph node metastasis is high and figures above 90% are usually quoted.

In previously healthy patients, the cytological identification of a lymph node metastasis results in a search for the primary tumour. This investigation will be focused on various organs depending on factors such as age, sex, clinical history, site of metastatic node and the cytological features. Table 13.1 summarises the most frequent metastatic sites for some of the most common malignancies.

The search for a primary tumour can be facilitated by immunological characterisation of the aspirated cells. In metastases from epithelial tumours the CK7, CK20 profile can often be helpful to focus on possible sites of the primary tumour (Table 13.2). Using an additional limited panel of antibodies,

**Table 13.3** Primary site information from an additional panel of antibodies

| Marker positivity | CK, EMA | | VIM | VIM | |
|---|---|---|---|---|---|
| Tumour | Carcinoma | | Melanoma | Sarcoma | |
| | *Marker* | *Subtype* | *Marker* | *Marker* | *Subtype* |
| | ER, PgR | Breast | HMB45, S100 | Desmin | Rhabdomyo |
| | Thyrog, TTF-1 | Thyroid | | NSE | Nerve sheet |
| | PSA, AR | Prostate | | CK | Epithelioid cell |
| | α-FETOP | Liver | | CD31 | Angio |
| | TTF-1 | Lung | | CD99 | Ewing/PNET |
| | CDX-2 | Colon | | CD34 | Dermatofibro |
| | Villin | Gastrointestinal | | | |
| | Uroplakin | Urinary tract | | | |
| | CA125, WTI | Ovary | | | |
| | Calcitonin | Medullary | | | |

AR, androgen receptor; CK, cytokeratin; EMA, epithelial membrane antigen; LC, leucocyte common; VIM, Vimentin; ER, oestrogen receptor; PgR, progesterone receptor; Thyrog, thyroglobulin; PSA, prostate specific antigen; α-FETOP, alpha-fetoprotein.

it is then often possible to obtain correct information about the primary site (Table 13.3). Unfortunately, some metastases defy all diagnostic efforts and their origin remains obscure. The cytological presentation of different tumours is relatively independent of metastatic site. Hence the following description of various metastases will focus on identification of tumour cell type.

## Metastatic epithelial tumours

### Cytological findings: metastatic epithelial tumours

#### Squamous carcinoma (Figs 13.69, 13.70)

Squamous carcinomas often yield a mixed pattern. In the well-differentiated type, keratinised cells with blue cytoplasm (MGG) are commonly seen. These cells have hyperchromatic nuclei and may show squamous pearl formation. The cellular atypia can be minimal and in such cases the diagnosis may rest on the knowledge that the cells were aspirated from a lymph node.

Some keratinising carcinomas show liquefaction and a yellow turbid thick material is aspirated from metastatic nodes of this kind. The smears consist largely of inflammatory cells and debris and malignant cells may be sparse, requiring careful search preferably in Papanicolaou stained smears. If such material is aspirated from a neck tumour the possibility of a branchial cleft cyst should be considered (Fig. 13.71). In an inflamed branchial cyst the epithelium can show some degree of atypia and thus mimic squamous cell carcinoma. In cases with slightly atypical squamous cells a repeat FNA from the periphery of the lesion may yield diagnostic cells.

FNA from poorly differentiated squamous carcinoma yield cohesive fragments of hyperchromatic polymorphic cells. Occasional small keratinised cells can point toward a diagnosis of squamous cell carcinoma but in their absence the cytological picture may be that of an undifferentiated malignant tumour which defies further categorisation.

#### Adenocarcinoma (Figs 13.72, 13.73)

These metastases will often disclose their nature by acinar structures or gland formation. The diagnosis of such typical metastases does not present significant problems, but their site of origin may be difficult to determine. In this process additional features might be helpful, for instance, mucin production is often seen in gastrointestinal and lung carcinomas. In metastases from lobular breast carcinomas, some cells may have cytoplasmiclumina with pinkish purple inclusions, magenta bodies on MGG staining. Cells with pale grey vacuolated large cytoplasm (MGG) and a nucleus with a central nucleolus are suggestive of a renal cell carcinoma.

Smears from FNA of metastatic colon carcinoma usually show fragments of palisading atypical cells in a necrotic background. In most cases this presentation, as well as CDx2 positivity, is enough to allow a conclusive diagnosis on cytology alone.

Metastases of papillary carcinoma usually have their origin in the ovary, thyroid, breast or lung. Psammoma bodies are most frequent in metastases originating from ovarian and thyroid carcinomas. Seropapillary ovarian carcinomas often spread to lymph nodes in the groin, lower axilla and supraclavicular fossa. In contrast a papillary carcinoma of the thyroid seldom spreads outside the regional nodes.

Smears of aspirates from poorly differentiated adenocarcinomas can be impossible to differentiate from other poorly-differentiated tumours and subtyping can only be made after immunocytochemistry.

#### Small cell carcinoma of undifferentiated type

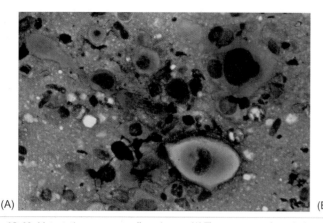

(A)

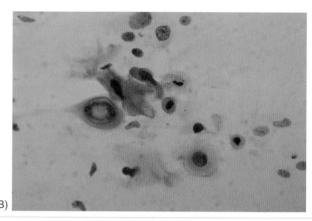

(B)

**Fig. 13.69** Metastatic squamous cell carcinoma. (A) There are several atypical squamous cells with hyperchromatic nuclei and blue cytoplasm (MGG). (B) Same aspirate alcohol fixed and Papanicolaou stained (MGG).

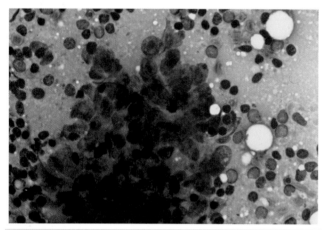

**Fig. 13.70** Lymph node metastasis from a poorly differentiated carcinoma of nasopharynx. Poorly cohesive cells with sparse indistinct cytoplasm (MGG).

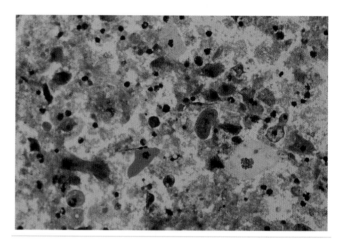

**Fig. 13.71** Branchial cleft cyst. Atypical squamous cells and inflammatory cells in a background of cell debris (MGG).

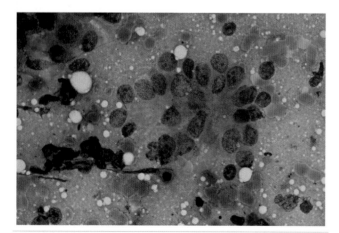

**Fig. 13.72** Metastatic adenocarcinoma. The glandular arrangement of the malignant epithelial cells is obvious. This is a deposit from a well-differentiated prostatic carcinoma (MGG).

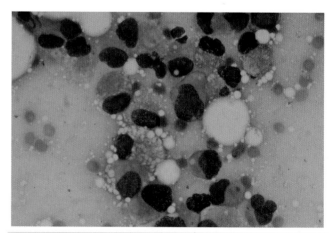

**Fig. 13.73** Metastatic adenocarcinoma. The tumour aspirate shows poorly differentiated adenocarcinoma cells which originated from a breast carcinoma (MGG).

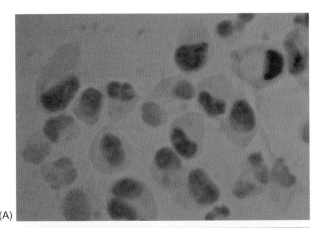

(A)

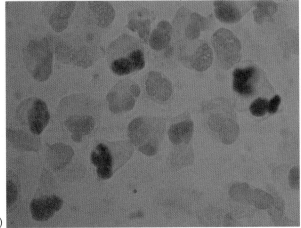

(B)

**Fig. 13.74** Breast carcinoma. (A) Oestrogen and (B) progesterone receptor staining of the aspirate shown in Figure 13.73 (immunoperoxidase).

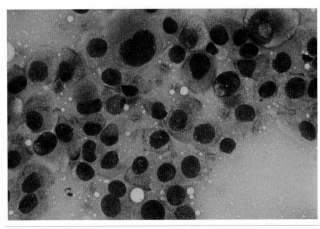

**Fig. 13.75** Metastatic malignant melanoma. The aspirate shows polymorphic dissociated cells containing pigment. Note the intranuclear inclusion, which is seen as a pale area within the nucleus of the cell in the top right corner (MGG).

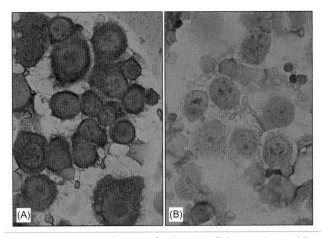

(A)  (B)

**Fig. 13.76** Immunocytochemistry of melanoma cells in cytospin material from aspirate shown in Figure 13.75. The tumour cells are HMB 45 positive (A) and cytokeratin negative (B), confirming their origin (alkaline phosphatase).

Metastases from small cell carcinoma of the lung yield crowded clusters of tumour cells showing moulding, with scanty cytoplasm, coarse chromatin, frequent mitoses and a background of necrosis. They may resemble lymphoma cells, but the presence of moulding in cohesive clumps of tumour cells and CD56 positivity, is strong evidence against a diagnosis of lymphoma. Paranuclear dots are commonly seen in MGG and CAM 5.2 stained smears from small cell carcinoma of undifferentiated type.[106–109]

## Immunocytochemistry

Epithelial markers are readily detected and cytokeratin can be used to confirm the epithelial nature of the tumour deposits. Evaluation of CK7 and CK20 expression can substantially reduce the number of possible primary sites (see Table 13.2).[110,111] Positive staining for prostate specific antigen (PSA), thyroglobulin or calcitonin will conclusively identify the primary site in appropriate cases. Carcinoid tumours show staining with chromogranin A and synaptophysin.

The presence of the oestrogen or the progesterone receptor strongly favours metastatic breast carcinoma (Fig. 13.74).

CA125 and WT1 positivity in combination with expression of oestrogen and progesterone receptors strongly favours an ovarian origin. Antibodies directed to other antigens such as CDX-2 and villin for gastrointestinal tract or uroplakin for bladder tumours and TTF-1 for lung cancer or thyroid are helpful in the identification of possible primary tumours (see Table 13.3).

Small cell undifferentiated carcinoma cells show positive staining with cytokeratin, albeit sometimes irregular or dot-like in distribution. They stain positively with some neural markers, such as N-CAM or UJ13A and CD56.

## Metastatic malignant melanoma

### Cytological findings: metastatic malignant melanoma (Figs 13.75, 13.76)

FNA from metastatic melanoma often have quite typical features, with polymorphic dissociated cells which may rarely contain fine pigment granules staining darkly on MGG. However, the cytoplasm often shows vacuoles only and this is referred to

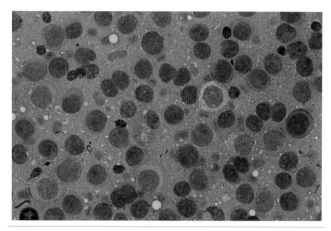

**Fig. 13.77** Metastatic malignant melanoma. In this case the aspirate consists of dissociated relatively monotonous round cells. This rare variant is difficult to differentiate from other round cell tumours (MGG).

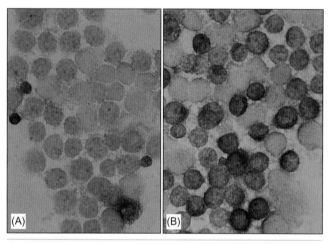

(A)          (B)

**Fig. 13.78** Immunocytochemistry of melanoma cells in cytospin material from the aspirate shown in Figure 13.77. The cells are leucocyte common antigen negative (A) and HMB 45 positive (B) (alkaline phosphatase).

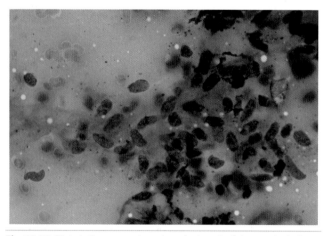

**Fig. 13.79** Metastatic sarcoma. Lymph node deposit of abnormal spindle cells from a Kaposi's sarcoma occurring in an HIV-positive patient (MGG).

as 'negative pigmentation'. The nuclei have large nucleoli which occasionally may be replaced by cytoplasmic invaginations into the nucleus. The cytology of metastatic melanoma can mimic either carcinoma or sarcoma, or even sometimes lymphoma.[112,113] Even if the patient has a history of melanoma it can be virtually impossible in some cases to arrive at a conclusive diagnosis based on cytomorphology alone.

### Immunocytochemistry (Figs 13.76, 13.78)

A limited panel of antibodies to epithelial and lymphoid antigens, S-100 and vimentin, together with antibody HMB-45, should be used. Positivity for vimentin, S-100 and HMB-45 will conclusively identify a metastatic melanoma. However, it is important to remember that positivity for HMB-45 is absent in approximately 20% of melanomas.

## Metastatic sarcomas

### Cytological findings: metastatic sarcomas (Fig. 13.79)

Sarcomas may occasionally spread to lymph nodes. The findings in FNA material mirror the diversity of histological appearances encountered in primary sarcomas of different types. Knowledge about the clinical history will allow a correct identification of a metastasis. However, in cases without a previously known sarcoma the exact subtyping of a lymph node metastasis can be difficult even with the use of immunocytochemistry. The possibility of a primary lymph node malignancy such as a histiocytic or dendritic cells sarcoma should be born in mind, since they mimic 'true' sarcomas. The importance lies in the fact that they are potentially curable in early stages.

### Immunocytochemistry

Antibodies to epithelial, melanocytic and lymphoid cells give negative staining reactions in sarcomatous metastases. Vimentin and markers for neural, vascular and myogenic differentiation will confirm the diagnosis of metastatic sarcoma.

# The role of the cytopathologist in patient management

With our greater understanding of lymph node pathology and the wide range and complexity of investigative techniques now available to cytopathologists, communication with the clinicians over the results of fine needle aspiration cytology has become essential for good patient management. It is important, therefore, that cytologists are able to attend the multidisciplinary meetings where decisions about further investigations and treatment are made, so as to explain their findings to the clinicians and ensure full clinicopathological correlation and optimal patient outcome (see Algorithm, p. 410).

## REFERENCES

1. Greig EDW, Gray ACH. Note on lymphatic glands in sleeping sickness. Lancet 1904;1:1570.

2. Guthrie CG. Gland puncture as a diagnostic measure. Bull Johns Hopkins Hosp 1921;32:266–69.

3. Morrison M, Samwick AA, Rubinstein J, et al. Lymph node aspiration. Clinical and hematologic observations in 101 patients. Am J Clin Pathol 1952;22:255–62.

4. Martin SE, Zhang HZ, Magyarosy E, et al. Immunologic methods in cytology: definitive diagnosis of non-Hodgkin's lymphoma using immunologic markers for T and B cells. Am J Clin Pathol 1984;80:666–73.

5. Tani EM, Christensson B, Porwit A, et al. Immunocytochemical analysis and cytomorphologic diagnosis on fine-needle aspirates of lymphoproliferative disease. Acta Cytol (Baltimore) 1988;32:209–15.

6. Oertel J, Oertel B, Kastner M, et al. The value of immunocytochemical staining of lymph node aspirates in diagnostic cytology. Br J Haematol 1988;70:307–16.

7. Tani E, Liliemark J, Svedmyr E, et al. Cytomorphology and immunocytochemistry of fine-needle aspirates from blastic non-Hodgkin's lymphomas. Acta Cytol (Baltimore) 1989;33:363–71.

8. Liliemark J, Tani E, Christensson B, et al. Fine-needle aspiration cytology and immunocytochemistry of abdominal non-Hodgkin's lymphomas. Leuk Lymphoma 1989;1:65–69.

9. Cafferty LL, Katz RL, Ordonez NG, et al. Fine-needle aspiration diagnosis of intra-abdominal and retroperitoneal lymphomas by a morphologic and immunocytochemical approach. Cancer 1990;65:72–77.

10. Skoog L, Tani E. The role of fine needle aspiration cytology in the diagnosis of non-Hodgkin's lymphoma. Diagn Oncol 1991;1:12–18.

11. Cartagena N, Katz RL, Hirsch-Ginsberg C, et al. Accuracy of diagnosis of malignant lymphoma by combining fine-needle aspiration cytomorphology with immunocytochemistry and in selected cases. Southern blotting of aspirated cells: a tissue controlled study of 86 patients. Diagn Cytopathol 1992;8:456–64.

12. Katz RL, Caraway NP. FNA lymphoproliferative diseases. myths and legends. Diagn Cytopathol 1995;12:99–100.

13. Leong ASY, Stevens M. Fine-needle aspiration biopsy for the diagnosis of lymphoma: a perspective. Diagn Cytopathol 1996;15:352–57.

14. Saddik M, el Dabbagh L, Mourad WA. Ex vivo fine-needle aspiration cytology and flow cytometric phenotyping in the diagnosis of lymphoproliferative disorders: A proposed algorithm for maximum resource utilisation. Diagn Cytopathol 1997;16:126–31.

15. Dunphy CH, Ramos R. Combining fine-needle aspiration and flow cytometric immunophenotyping in evaluation of nodal and extranodal sites for possible lymphoma: a retrospective review. Diagn Cytopathol 1997;16:200–6.

16. Clatch RJ, Foreman JR, Walloch JL. Simplified immunophenotypic analysis by laser scanning cytometry. Cytometry 1998;34:3–16. Review.

17. Horii A, Yoshida J, Hattori K, et al. DNA ploidy, proliferative activities, and immunophenotype of malignant lymphoma: application of flow cytometry. Head Neck 1998;20:392–98.

18. Liu K, Mann KP, Vitellas KM, et al. Fine-needle aspiration with flow cytometric immunophenotyping for primary diagnosis of intra-abdominal lymphomas. Diagn Cytopathol 1999;21:98–104.

19. Ravinsky E, Morales C, Kutryk E, et al. Cytodiagnosis of lymphoid proliferations by fine needle aspiration biopsy. Adjunctive value of flow cytometry. Acta Cytol 1999;43:1070–78.

20. Young NA, Al-Saleem TI, Ehya H, et al. Utilisation of fine needle aspiration cytology and flow cytometry in the diagnosis and subclassification of primary and recurrent lymphoma. Cancer (Cancer Cytopathol) 1998;84:252–61.

21. Young NA, Al-Salee MTI. Diagnosis of lymphoma by fine-needle aspiration cytology using the Revised European-American classification of lymphoid neoplasms. Cancer (Cancer Cytopathol) 1999;87:325–45.

22. Wakely PE. Aspiration cytopathology of malignant lymphoma. Cancer Cytopathology 1999;87:322–24.

23. Dong HY, Harris NL, Preffer FI, et al. Fine-needle aspiration biopsy in the diagnosis and classification of primary and recurrent lymphoma: a retrospective analysis of the utility of cytomorphology and flow cytometry. Mod Pathol 2001;14:472–81.

24. Mourad WA, Tulbah A, Shoukri M, et al. Primary diagnosis and REAL/WHO classification of non-Hodgkin's lymphoma by fine-needle aspiration: cytomorphologic and immunophenotypic approach. Diagn Cytopathol 2003;28:191–95.

25. Landgren O, Porwit Mac Donald A, Tani E, et al. A prospective comparison of fine-needle aspiration cytology and histopathology in the diagnosis and classification of lymphomas. Hematol J 2004;5:69–76.

26. Laane E, Tani E, Björklund E, et al. Flow cytometric immunophenotyping including Bcl-2 detection on fine needle aspirates in the diagnosis of reactive lymphadenopathy and non-Hodgkin's lymphoma. Cytometry B Clin Cytom 2005;64:34–42.

27. Vianello F, Tison T, Radossi P, et al. Detection of B-cell monoclonality in fine needle aspiration by PCR analysis. Leuk Lymphoma 1998;29:179–85.

28. Grosso LE, Collins BT. DNA polymerase chain reaction using fine needle aspiration biopsy smears to evaluate non Hodgkin's lymphoma. Acta Cytol 1999;43:837–41.

29. Lee LH, Cioc A, Nuovo GJ. Determination of light chain restriction in fine-needle aspiration-type preparations of B-cell lymphomas by mRNA in situ hybridisation. Appl Immunohistochem Mol Morphol 2004;12:252–58.

30. Safley AM, Buckley PJ, Creager AJ, et al. The value of fluorescence in situ hybridisation and polymerase chain reaction in the diagnosis of B-cell non-Hodgkin lymphoma by fine-needle aspiration. Arch Pathol Lab Med 2004;128:1395–403.

31. Reid AJ, Miller RF, Kocjan GI. Diagnostic utility of fine needle aspiration (FNA) cytology in HIV-infected patients with lymphadenopathy. Cytopathology 1998;9:230–39.

32. Stanley MW, Steeper TA, Horwitz CA, et al. Fine-needle aspiration of lymph nodes in patients with acute infectious mononucleosis. Diagn Cytopathol 1990;6:323–29.

33. Schnitzer B. Reactive lymphoid hyperplasia. In: Jaffe ES, editor. Surgical Pathology of the Lymph Nodes and Related Organs. Philadelphia: WB Saunders; 1985:22.

34. Rosai J, Dorfman RF. Sinus histiocytosis with massive lymphadenopathy. Arch Pathol 1969;87:63–70.

35. Schmitt F. Sinus histiocytosis with massive lymphadenopathy (Rosai-Dorfman Disease): cytomorphologic analysis on fine needle aspirates. Diagn Cytopathol 1992;8:596–99.

36. Stastny JF, Wilkerson ML, Hamati HF, et al. Cytologic features of sinus histiocytosis with massive lymphadenopathy. A report of three cases. Acta Cytol 1997;41:871–76.

37. Deshpande V, Verma K. Fine needle aspiration (FNA) cytology of Rosai Dorfman disease. Cytopathology 1998;9:329.

38. Das DK, Gulati A, Bhatt NC, et al. Sinus histiocytosis with massive lymphadenopathy (Rosai-Dorfman disease): report of two cases with fine-needle aspiration cytology. Diagn Cytopathol 2001;24:42–45.

39. Kikuchi M. Lymphadenitis showing focal reticulum cell hyperplasia with nuclear debris and phagocytosis. Nippon Ketsueki Gakkai Zasshi 1971;35:379–80.

40. Fujimoto Y, Kozima Y, Yamazuchi K. Cervical subacute necrotising lymphadenitis. A new clinicopathologic entity. Naika 1972;20:920–27.

41. Mannara GM, Boccato P, Rinaldo A, et al. Histiocytic necrotising lymphadenitis (Kikuchi-Fujimoto disease) diagnosed by fine needle aspiration biopsy. ORL J Ortorhinolaryngol Relat Spec 1999;61:367–71.

42. Flint D, Mahadevan M, Barber C, et al. Cervical lymphadenitis due to non-tuberculous mycobacteria: surgical treatment and review. Int J Pediatr Otorhinolaryngol 2000;53:187–94.

43. Baek CH, Kim SI, Ko YH, et al. Polymerase chain reaction detection of Mycobacterium tuberculosis from fine-needle aspirate for the diagnosis of cervical tuberculous lymphadenitis. Laryngoscope 2000;110:30–34.

44. Goel MM, Ranjan V, Dhole TN, et al. Polymerase chain reaction vs. conventional diagnosis in fine needle aspirates of

tuberculous lymph nodes. Acta Cytol 2001;45:333–40.

45. Pahwa R, Hedau S, Jain S, et al. Assessment of possible tuberculous lymphadenopathy by PCR compared to non-molecular methods. J Med Microbiol 2005;54:873–78.

46. Stanley MW, Horwitz CA, Burton LG, et al. Negative images of bacilli and mycobacterial infection: a study of fine-needle aspiration smears from lymph nodes in patients with AIDS. Diagn Cytopathol 1990;6:118–21.

47. Gupta SK, Kumar B, Kaur S. Aspiration cytology of lymph nodes in leprosy. Int J Lepr 1981;49:9–15.

48. Cavett JR III, McAfee R, Ramzy I. Hansen's disease (leprosy). Diagnosis by aspiration biopsy of lymph nodes. Acta Cytol 1986;30:189–93.

49. Tani EM, Franco M. Pulmonary cytology in paracoccidioidomycosis. Acta Cytol 1984;28:571–75.

50. Das DK, Bhatt NC, Khan VA, et al. Cervicofacial actinomycosis: diagnosis by fine needle aspiration cytology. Acta Cytol 1989;33:278–80.

51. Housini I, Dabbo DJ, Coyne L. Fine needle aspiration cytology of talc granulomatosis in a peripheral lymph node in a case of suspected intravenous drug abuse. Acta Cytol 1990;34:342–44.

52. Tabatowski K, Elson CE, Johnston WW. Silicone lymphadenopathy in a patient with a mammary prosthesis. Fine needle aspiration cytology, histology and analytical electron microscopy. Acta Cytol 1990;34:10–14.

53. Lukes RJ, Craver LF, Hall TC, et al. Report of the nomenclature committee. Cancer Res 1966;26:311.

54. Minimo C, Zakowski M, Lin O. Cytologic findings of malignant vascular neoplasms: a study of twenty-four cases. Diagn Cytopathol 2002;26:349–55.

55. Lennert K, Mohri N, Stein H, et al. The histopathology of malignant lymphoma. Br J Haematol 1975;31:193–203.

56. The non-Hodgkin's lymphoma pathological classification project. National Cancer Institute sponsored study of lymphomas: summary and description of a working formulation of clinical usage. Cancer 1982;49:2112–35.

57. Stansfeld AG, Diebold J, Kapanci Y, et al. Updated Kiel classification for lymphomas. Lancet 1988;i:292–93.

58. Harris N, Jaffe E, Stein H, et al. A revised European-American classification of lymphoid neoplasms: a proposal from the International Lymphoma Study Group. Blood 1994;84:1361–92.

59. Orell SR, Skinner JM. The typing of non-Hodgkin's lymphoma using fine needle aspiration cytology. Pathology 1982;14:389–94.

60. Young NA, Al-Saleem TI. Diagnosis of lymphoma by fine-needle aspiration cytology using the Revised European-American classification of lymphoid neoplasms. Cancer (Cancer Cytopathol) 1999;87:325–45.

61. Landgren O, Porwit Mac Donald A, Tani E, et al. A prospective comparison of fine-needle aspiration cytology and histopathology in the diagnosis and classification of lymphomas. Hematol J 2004;5:69–76.

62. Mourad WA, Tulbah A, Shoukri M, et al. Primary diagnosis and REAL/WHO classification of non-Hodgkin's lymphoma by fine-needle aspiration: cytomorphologic and immunophenotypic approach. Diagn Cytopathol 2003;28:191–95.

63. Fulciniti F, Vetrani A, Zeppa P, et al. Hodgkin's disease: diagnostic accuracy of fine needle aspiration; a report based on 62 consecutive cases. Cytopathology 1994;5:226–33.

64. Jimenez-Heffernan JA, Vicandi B, Lopez-Ferrer P, et al. Value of fine needle aspiration cytology in the initial diagnosis of Hodgkin's disease. Analysis of 188 cases with an emphasis on diagnostic pitfalls. Acta Cytol 2001;45:300–6.

65. Chieng DC, Cangiarella JF, Symmans WF, et al. Fine-needle aspiration cytology of Hodgkin disease: a study of 89 cases with emphasis on false-negative cases. Cancer 2001;93:52–59.

66. Frable WJ, Kardos TF. Fine needle aspiration biopsy: applications in the diagnosis of lymphoproliferative diseases. Am J Surg Pathol 1988;12:62–72.

67. Grosso LE, Collins BT, Dunphy CH, et al. Lymphocyte-depleted Hodgkin's disease: Diagnostic challenges by fine needle aspiration. Diagn Cytopathol 1998; 19:66–69.

68. Masik AS, Weisenburger DD, Vose JM, et al. Histologic grade does not predict prognosis in optimally treated advanced stage nodular sclerosing Hodgkin's disease. Cancer 1992;69:228–32.

69. Tani E, Ersoz C, Svedmyr E, et al. Fine-needle aspiration cytology and immunocytochemistry of Hodgkin's disease suppurative type. Diagn Cytopathol 1998;18:437–40.

70. Vicandi B, Jimenez-Heffernan JA, Lopez-Ferrer P, et al. Hodgkin's disease mimicking suppurative lymphadenitis: a fine-needle aspiration report of five cases. Diagn Cytopathol 1999;20:302–6.

71. Davey DD, Kamat D, Zaleski S, et al. Analysis of immunoglobulin and T-cell receptor gene rearrangement in cytologic specimens. Acta Cytol 1989;33:583–90.

72. Gedes J, Schwab U, Lemke H, et al. Production of a mouse monoclonal antibody reactive with a human nuclear antigen associated with cell proliferation. Int J Cancer 1987;31:13–20.

73. Kaw YT, Artymyshyn RL, Schichman SA, et al. Recurrent hairy cell leukemia presenting as a large mesenteric mass diagnosed by fine needle aspiration cytology. A case report. Acta Cytol 1994;38:267–70.

74. Tani E, Santos GC, Svedmyr E, et al. Fine-needle aspiration cytology and immunocytochemistry of soft-tissue extramedullary plasma-cell neoplasms. Diagn Cytopathol 1999;20:120–24.

75. Crapanzano JP, Lin O. Cytologic findings of marginal zone lymphoma. Cancer 2003;99:301–9.

76. Murphy BA, Meda BA, Buss DH, et al. Marginal zone and mantle cell lymphomas: assessment of cytomorphology in subtyping small B-cell lymphomas. Diagn Cytopathol 2003;28:126–30.

77. Rassidakis GZ, Tani E, Svedmyr E, et al. Diagnosis and subclassification of follicle center and mantle cell lymphomas on fine-needle aspirates: a cytologic and immunocytochemical approach based on the Revised European-American Lymphoma (REAL) classification. Cancer 1999;87:216–23.

78. Saikia UN, Dey P, Saikia B, et al. Fine-needle aspiration biopsy in diagnosis of follicular lymphoma: cytomorphologic and immunohistochemical analysis. Diagn Cytopathol 2002;26:251–56.

79. Sun W, Caraway NP, Zhang HZ, et al. Grading follicular lymphoma on fine needle aspiration specimens. Comparison with proliferative index by DNA image analysis and Ki-67 labeling index. Acta Cytol 2004;48:119–26.

80. Wojcik EM, Katz RL, Fanning TV, et al. Diagnosis of mantle cell lymphoma on tissue acquired by fine needle aspiration in conjunction with immunocytochemistry and cytokinetic studies. Possibilities and limitations. Acta Cytol 1995;39:909–15.

81. Gagneten D, Hijazi YM, Jaffe ES, et al. Mantel cell lymphoma: a cytopathological and immunocytochemical study. Diagn Cytopathol 1996;14:32–37.

82. Hughes JH, Caraway NP, Katz RL. Blastic variant of mantle-cell lymphoma: cytomorphologic, immunocytochemical, and molecular genetic features of tissue obtained by fine-needle aspiration biopsy. Diagn Cytopathol 1998;19:59–62.

83. Tani E, Johansson B, Skoog L. T-cell-rich B-cell lymphoma: fine-needle aspiration cytology and immunocytochemistry. Diagn Cytopathol 1998;18:1–4.

84. Tong TR, Lee KC, Chow TC, et al. T-cell/histiocyte-rich diffuse large B-cell lymphoma. Report of a case diagnosed by fine needle aspiration biopsy with immunohistochemical and molecular pathologic correlation. Acta Cytol 2002;46:893–98.

85. Hoda RS, Picklesimer L, Green KM, et al. Fine needle aspiration of a primary mediastinal large B-cell lymphoma. A case report with cytologic histologic and flow cytometric considerations.. Diagn Cytopathol 2005;32:370–73.

86. Stastny JF, Almeida MM, Wakely PE Jr, et al. Fine-needle aspiration biopsy and imprint cytology of small non-cleaved cell (Burkitt's) lymphoma. Diagn Cytopathol 1995;12:201–7.

87. Das DK, Sheikh ZA, Jassar AK, et al. Burkitt-type lymphoma of the breast: diagnosis by fine-needle aspiration cytology. Diagn Cytopathol 2002;27:60–62.

88. Geramizadeh B, Kaboli R, Vasei M. Fine needle aspiration cytology of Burkitt's lymphoma presenting as a breast mass. Acta Cytol 2004;48:285–86.

89. Tani E, Maeda S, Fröstad B, et al. Aspiration cytology with phenotyping and clinical presentation of childhood lymphomas. Diagn Oncol 1993;3:294–301.

90. Jacobs JC, Katz RL, Shabb N, et al. Fine needle aspiration of lymphoblastic lymphoma. A multiparameter diagnostic approach. Acta Cytol 1992;36:887–94.

91. Yao JL, Cangiarella JF, Cohen JM, et al. Fine-needle aspiration biopsy of peripheral T-cell lymphomas. A cytologic and immunophenotypic study of 33 cases. Cancer 2001;93:151–59.

92. Shimoyama M. Diagnostic criteria and classification of clinical subtypes of adult T-cell leukaemia-lymphoma. A report from the Lymphoma study Group. Br J Haematol 1991;79:428–37.

93. Oshima K, Tani E, Masuda Y, et al. Fine needle aspiration cytology of high-grade T-cell lymphomas in human T-lymphotropic virus type 1 carriers. Cytopathology 1992;3:365–72.

94. Ng WK, Lee CY, Li AS, et al. Nodal presentation of nasal-type NK/T-cell lymphoma. Report of two cases with fine needle aspiration cytology findings. Acta Cytol 2003;47:1063–68.

95. Galindo LM, Garcia FU, Hanau CA, et al. Fine-needle aspiration biopsy in the evaluation of lymphadenopathy associated with cutaneous T-cell lymphoma (mycosis fungoides/Sezary syndrome). Am J Clin Pathol 2000;113:865–71.

96. Ng WK, Ip P, Choy C, et al. Cytologic findings of angioimmunoblastic T-cell lymphoma:

analysis of 16 fine-needle aspirates over 9-year period. Cancer 2002;96:166–73.

97. Tani E, Masuda Y, Skoog L. Cytology and immunocytochemistry on fine-needle aspirates from peripheral T cell lymphomas. Diagn Oncol 1991;1:133–39.

98. Al Shanqeety O, Mourad WA. Diagnosis of peripheral T-cell lymphoma by fine-needle aspiration biopsy: a cytomorphologic and immunophenotypic approach. Diagn Cytopathol 2000;23:375–79.

99. Kocjan G. Lymph nodes. In: Kocjan G, editor. Clinical Cytopathology of the Head and Neck. London: Greenwich Medical Media; 2001.

100. Tani E, Löwhagen T, Nasiell K, et al. Fine needle aspiration cytology and immunocytochemistry of large cell lymphomas expressing the Ki-1 antigen. Acta Cytol 1989;33:359–62.

101. Bizjak-Schwarzbartl M. Large cell anaplastic Ki-1+ non-Hodgkin's lymphoma vs. Hodgkin's disease in fine needle aspiration biopsy samples. Acta Cytol 1997;41:351–56.

102. Mourad WA, al Nazer M, Tulbah A. Cytomorphologic differentiation of Hodgkin's lymphoma and Ki-1 + anaplastic large cell lymphoma in fine needle aspirates. Acta Cytol 2003;47:744–48.

103. Ng WK, Ip P, Choy C, et al. Cytologic and immunocytochemical findings of anaplastic large cell lymphoma: analysis of ten fine-needle aspiration specimens over a 9-year period. Cancer 2003;99:33–43.

104. Gatter KM, Rader A, Braziel RM. Fine-needle aspiration biopsy of anaplastic large cell lymphoma, small cell variant with prominent plasmacytoid features: Case report. Diagn Cytopathol 2002;26:113–16.

105. Kim SE, Kim SH, Lim BJ, et al. Fine needle aspiration cytology of small cell variant of anaplastic large cell lymphoma. A case report. Acta Cytol 2004;4825:4–8.

106. De Las Casas LE, Gokden M, Mukunyadzi P, et al. A morphologic and statistical comparative study of small-cell carcinoma and non-Hodgkin's lymphoma in fine-needle aspiration biopsy material from lymph nodes. Diagn Cytopathol 2004;31:229–34.

107. Skoog L, Schmitt FC, Tani E. Neuroendocrine (Merkel cell) carcinoma of the skin: immunocytochemical and cytomorphological analysis on fine needle aspirates. Diagn Cytopathol 1990;6:53–57.

108. Collins BT, Elmberger PG, Tani EM, et al. Fine-needle aspiration of Merkel cell carcinoma of the skin with cytomorphology and immunocytochemical correlation. Diagn Cytopathol 1998;18:251–57.

109. Dey P, Jogai S, Amir T, et al. Fine-needle aspiration cytology of Merkel cell carcinoma. Diagn Cytopathol 2004;31:364–65.

110. Wang NP, Zarbo RJ, Gown AM. Coordinate expression of cytokeratins 7 and 20 define carcinoma. Appl Immunohistochem 1995;3:99–107.

111. Miettinen M. Keratin 20: Immunohistochemical marker for gastrointestinal, urothelial, and Merkel cell carcinomas. Mod Pathol 1995;8:384–88.

112. Nasiell K, Tani E, Skoog L. Fine needle aspiration cytology and immunocytochemistry of metastatic melanoma. Cytopathology 1991;2:137–47.

113. Saqi A, McGrath CM, Skovronsky D, et al. Cytomorphologic features of fine-needle aspiration of metastatic and recurrent melanoma. Diagn Cytopathol 2002;27:286–90.

# Other lymphoreticular organs

Edneia Tani and Lambert Skoog

## Chapter contents

## Introduction

Lymph nodes form only part of the immunological system distributed throughout the body. Other organs and anatomical sites also harbour lymphoid tissue which participates in primary and secondary immune responses. The term 'extranodal lymphoid tissue' is used to refer to lymphoid tissue situated outside the lymph nodes. This tissue includes organs such as spleen, thymus and the nasopharyngeal lymphoid aggregations known as Waldeyer's ring. In addition, extranodal lymphoid tissue exists as mucosa associated lymphoid tissue (MALT) in the gastrointestinal tract, lung, salivary gland, thyroid and orbit.[1]

Inflammation, autoimmune disorders and malignant lymphomas can involve any of the extranodal collections of lymphoid tissue or lymphoreticular organs, as well as lymph nodes. However, in contrast, the extranodal lymphoid tissue is rarely the seat of metastatic tumour spread which is so frequently seen in lymph nodes.

This chapter will consider the main cytological findings in disease processes at the different anatomical sites of extranodal lymphoid tissue, highlighting any contrasting features with the conditions found in lymph nodes.

## Waldeyer's ring

Lymphoid tissue in the tonsils, base of the tongue and epipharynx compose Waldeyer's ring. These extranodal sites are often affected by inflammatory disorders, but are rarely the target of fine needle aspiration (FNA) sampling. Waldeyer's ring is a relatively frequent site for B-cell derived non-Hodgkin lymphomas, a high proportion arising particularly in the tonsils. In contrast, T-cell lymphomas and Hodgkin lymphoma are rarely encountered at this site.

All subtypes of B-cell neoplasms can occur in any part of Waldeyer's ring but follicular lymphomas and diffuse large B-cell lymphomas appear to be the most frequent. At the time of diagnosis, most patients have cervical node involvement as well.

The tonsil and epipharynx may also be the primary sites for poorly differentiated carcinomas. In these cases distinction from large cell lymphomas may pose a problem.

## FNA procedure

The aspiration technique is similar to that of most palpable lesions, but an 8 cm long 25 gauge (0.5 mm) needle will be necessary in most cases. Occasionally, a Franzén prostate needle guide is needed to reach targets not otherwise accessible. Aspiration with a 25 gauge needle usually gives sufficient material for both smears and immunological evaluation. Local anaesthesia is seldom required but when needed, it could be administered in spray form.

### Cytological findings: Waldeyer's ring (Figs 14.1, 14.2)

#### Reactive lymphoid hyperplasia

Reactive lymphoid hyperplasia is common in the lymphoid tissue of Waldeyer's ring, and is characterised by a spectrum of lymphoid cells ranging from small mature lymphocytes to immunoblasts. In addition, granulocytes, plasma cells and macrophages containing tingible body material are present.

#### Non-Hodgkin lymphomas

The cytological patterns of the different non-Hodgkin lymphomas are identical to those seen in lymph nodes as described in detail in the preceding chapter. Briefly, the smears are composed of a relatively uniform cell population apart from the mixed lymphomas which include neoplastic follicle centre cells as well as some benign lymphocytes. The most common high-grade lymphoma is the diffuse large B-cell lymphoma (Fig. 14.1). The cells have round nuclei with 1–4 small nucleoli often at the nuclear membrane. The cytoplasm is sparse and may contain small vacuoles.

#### Hodgkin lymphoma

Elderly patients may occasionally present with Hodgkin lymphoma in the tonsil. Akin to the situation in lymph nodes an immunological characterisation is needed to corroborate cytomorphology for a conclusive diagnosis.

#### Poorly differentiated carcinoma

Poorly differentiated carcinoma cells may superficially mimic those of a diffuse large B-cell lymphoma. However, carcinomas show a tendency to form aggregates in which the individual cells have poorly defined cytoplasm (Fig. 14.2).[1] In rare cases, a confident distinction is only possible by immunocytochemistry.

#### Metastases

Waldeyer's ring in particular, and also the tonsil, can be the site of metastases. Melanoma, renal cell carcinoma, synovial sarcoma and small cell undifferentiated lung carcinoma are examples of tumours we have seen metastasising to the tonsil.

### Immunocytochemistry

In reactive hyperplasia, polytypic B cells predominate. The vast majority of the lymphomas in this area are of B-cell phenotype,

*The authors gratefully acknowledge the debt to the late T. Löwhagen, whose contribution to the first edition of this chapter provided a substantial basis for the revised editions.*

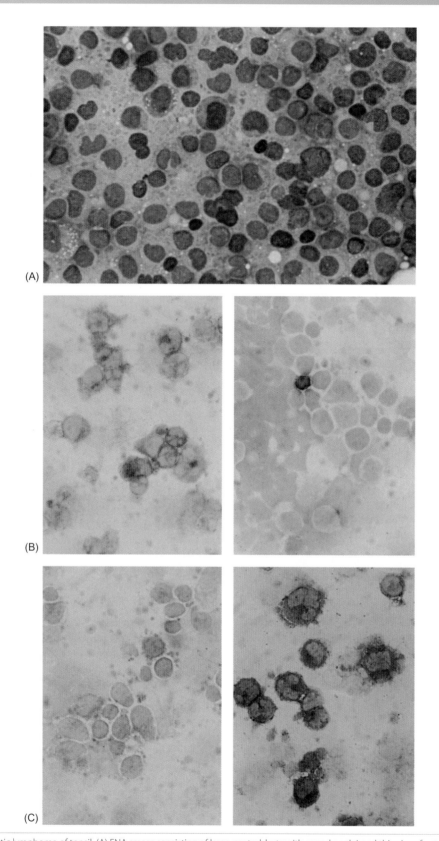

**Fig. 14.1** Centroblastic lymphoma of tonsil. (A) FNA smear consisting of large centroblasts with round nuclei and thin rim of cytoplasm (MGG). (B) Immunocytochemistry showing positive reactivity for a B-cell marker (CD20) in centroblasts (left) and one mature cell with T-phenotype (right). (C) Monoclonal lambda light chain expression in centroblasts (right) and negative staining for kappa chains (left).

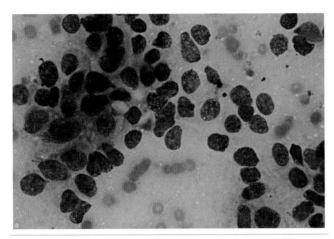

**Fig. 14.2** Poorly differentiated carcinoma of tonsil with pleomorphic tumour cells in loose clusters (MGG).

with readily detectable light chain restriction. Positive staining for cytokeratin (CK) or epithelial membrane antigen (EMA) will allow identification of an undifferentiated carcinoma. Nasopharyngeal carcinoma may also be LMP EBV positive.

## Thymus and mediastinum

The thymus is a lymphoepithelial organ that has a vital role in the development of T cells and natural-killer cells. It lies in the anterior part of the mediastinum and reaches its greatest size in childhood. In old age, the gland is almost indiscernible.

The thymus undergoes hyperplasia in the autoimmune disease myasthenia gravis, and is occasionally affected by primary neoplasms. These include thymomas, neuroendocrine tumours, lymphomas and germ cell tumours which arise in the epithelial, lymphoid or germinal crest tissue, respectively.[2]

The relative incidence of tumours differs in childhood and adult life. Thus, in childhood, lymphomas account for 50% of the neoplasms, while germ cell and mesenchymal tumours represent 20% each. In adults, thymomas are the most common neoplasm, representing approximately 50% of all primary tumours. Lymphomas are second and germ cell tumours third in frequency with a relative frequency of 25% and 15%, respectively. Carcinoids are rare as thymic tumours and are usually aggressive.

Tumours in the anterior mediastinum, such as thymomas, can be reached by puncture through the sternum or the intercostal space close to the sternum with the help of radiological guidance. However, endoscopic ultrasound-guided FNA cytology via the trachea or oesophagus is preferred and this technique has an excellent performance rate.

Chapter 2 also includes a discussion of mediastinal tumours.

## Lymphomas

The thymus appears to be the primary site for two types of lymphoma. The precursor T-cell lymphoblastic subtype occurs predominantly in young males. The second type is the mediastinal large B-cell lymphoma, which shows a predilection for women in the third or fourth decades.[3] The tumour cells, which resemble centroblasts or immunoblasts, are of B phenotype and are thought to be of thymic origin. With aggressive chemotherapy

this lymphoma has a relatively good prognosis. In addition to these two subtypes almost all other variants of lymphoma can affect the thymus in rare instances.

### Cytological findings: lymphomas (Figs 14.3, 14.4)

#### Precursor T-lymphoblastic lymphoma

The blasts vary in size; most are medium-sized cells with often vacuolated moderately rich basophilic cytoplasm and round to irregular nuclei (Fig. 14.3). The chromatin is fine and nucleoli are inconspicuous. There is usually a high mitotic rate. Eosinophils are common.[4–6]

#### Mediastinal large B-cell lymphoma

Aspirates show large atypical cells which vary considerably in size and shape (Fig. 14.4). There is usually an admixture of eosinophils and small benign lymphocytes. In addition, there are usually some small sclerotic tissue fragments in the smears. These features may raise suspicion of Hodgkin lymphoma.[7] Other tumours to be considered in the differential diagnosis include primary germ cell tumours of the mediastinum and seminoma. Immunophenotyping will be needed for a conclusive diagnosis.

### Immunocytochemistry

Precursor T-lymphoblastic lymphoma is a T-cell neoplasm with expression of the lymphoblastic marker terminal deoxynucleotidyl transferase (TdT). There is a variable expression of T-cell markers but CD3 and CD7 can often be detected. The fraction of proliferation cells as analysed by Ki-67 staining is often over 90%.

The mediastinal large B-cell lymphomas express the B-cell associated antigens CD19 and CD20. The tumour cells rarely express surface immunoglobulin. CD30 is often detected as well as CD45. This profile will allow a conclusive diagnosis in most cases.

## Germ cell tumours

In the mediastinum, these rare neoplasms are thought to arise in the primordial germinal crest of the thymus. The most common one is the benign teratoma, which accounts for over 80% of germ cell tumours. They often grow to a large size without symptoms and may be cystic. The malignant germ cell tumours such as seminomas, embryonal carcinomas and the rare yolk sac tumour are almost exclusively seen in males in the second and third decade of life.[2] In contrast, the choriocarcinoma is more frequent in girls. Most patients present with pain, cough and shortness of breath. In patients with these tumours it is important to exclude metastasis from a primary gonadal neoplasm, which, however, is extremely uncommon.

Teratomas are by definition benign and most patients are cured by resection. Pure seminomas have a favourable prognosis with over 90% 5-year survival. Embryonal carcinoma has a reported long-term survival of around 50%. Patients with choriocarcinoma have a poor prognosis.

### Cytological findings: germ cell tumours (Figs 14.5-14.7)

#### Benign teratoma

Aspirates from benign teratomas may contain stratified squamous epithelium, sebaceous material, hair and a variety of benign cells from all germinal layers.[8]

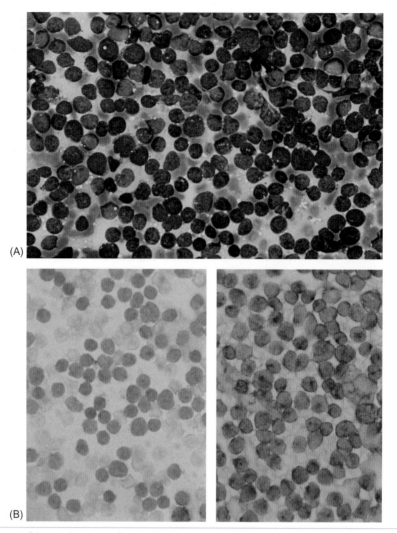

**Fig. 14.3** Lymphoblastic lymphoma of thymus. (A) Aspirate from mediastinum composed of small- to medium-sized blast cells (MGG). (B) Immunocytochemistry shows T-cell lineage with positive staining on the right and no reaction to the B-cell marker on the left (alkaline phosphatase).

### Seminoma

Smears from seminomas show dispersed fragile cells in a characteristic lacey or 'tigroid' background due to fragmentation of the glycogen-laden cytoplasm (Fig. 14.5). The tumour cell nuclei are pale, have evenly distributed chromatin and distinct nucleoli. Small lymphocytes may be present reflecting the histological presence of a lymphoid or granulomatous infiltrate in these neoplasms.[9,10]

### Embryonal carcinoma

Embryonal carcinoma is a pleomorphic tumour. The cells are usually in tight clusters and have a high nuclear/cytoplasmic ratio (Fig. 14.6). Individual cells may simulate immature lymphoid cells but their epithelial origin is identified by the finding of large nucleoli and the formation tight cell clusters, which can be adenocarcinoma like.[9,10]

### Yolk sac tumour and choriocarcinoma

The cytomorphology of the mediastinal variants has been reported to be similar to the gonadal tumors.[11] We have not aspirated any yolk sac tumour or choriocarcinoma in the mediastinum.

Metastases from any poorly differentiated carcinoma may be impossible to differentiate from embryonal carcinoma or teratocarcinoma by cytomorphology (Fig. 14.7).

## Immunocytochemistry

Seminomas are in most cases positive for placental alkaline phosphatase (PLAP), CD117 and vimentin. Some cells are weakly CK positive. Embryonal carcinomas show positivity for cytokeratin and CD30 and focal positivity for human chorionic gonadotrophin (HCG) and alpha-fetoprotein (AFP). These features allow differentiation between carcinomas of germ cell type and those of other origin.

Occasionally, mediastinal involvement by small cell undifferentiated carcinoma of lung may present diagnostic difficulties in distinguishing the cells from those of other poorly differentiated tumours involving the mediastinum. The neural cell adhesion molecule marker (N-CAM or UJ13 A) is usually positive in cells from small cell undifferentiated carcinoma as well as TTF-1 and CD56.

## Thymomas

These are tumours of middle-age and are exceedingly rare in children. Approximately half of the cases have symptoms related to the tumour mass but a substantial number of patients present with myaesthenia gravis. Most thymomas with spindle

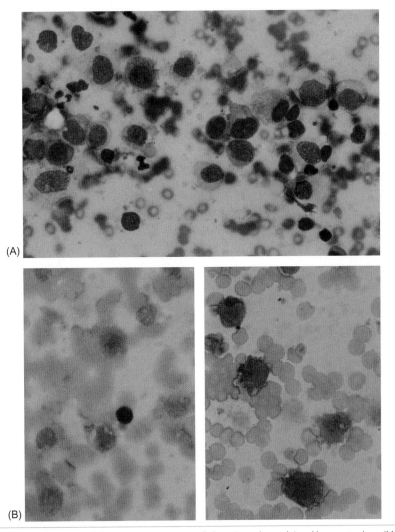

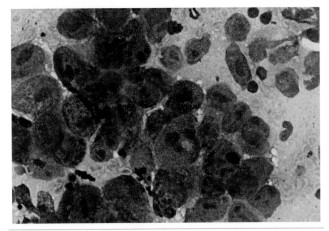

**Fig. 14.4** Large B-cell lymphoma of thymus. (A) The immature tumour cells have irregular nuclei and large cytoplasm (MGG). (B) Immunocytochemistry: B-cell positivity in tumour cells (right) and T-cell positivity in one mature T-cell (left) (alkaline phosphatase).

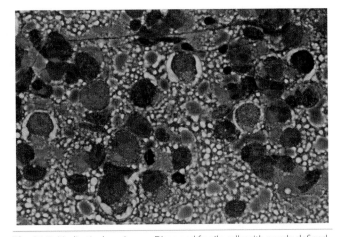

**Fig. 14.5** Mediastinal seminoma. Dispersed fragile cells with poorly defined cytoplasm in typical 'tigroid' background (MGG).

**Fig. 14.6** Embryonal carcinoma of mediastinum. Clusters of large malignant cells with distinct nucleoli (MGG).

or oval epithelial nuclei (type A) are benign but some may show invasive growth; however, metastases are exceedingly rare.[2] Malignant behaviour is usually reflected by an increased number of epithelial cells with round to polygonal nuclei (type B).[2] Tumour stage and tumour type are significant prognostic factors. Type A tumours have an excellent prognosis while type B tumours with advanced stage have a distinctly less favourable course.

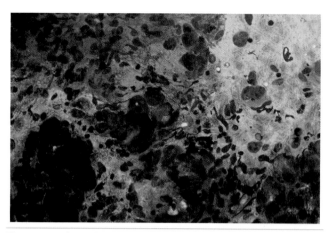

**Fig. 14.7** Mediastinal teratocarcinoma. Note the malignant epithelial cell cluster and fragment of undifferentiated mesenchymal tissue (MGG).

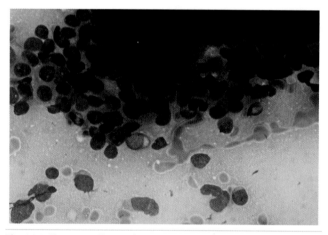

**Fig. 14.8** Thymoma. Cluster of monotonous epithelial cells with indistinct cytoplasm. Few lymphoid cells present (MGG).

### Cytological findings: thymomas (Fig. 14.8)

In type A, thymoma the epithelial cells are mostly oval to spindle shaped with homogeneous chromatin and indistinct cell borders. Type B tumours have round to polygonal nuclei with distinct nucleoli. These tumours have a component of mature lymphocytes.[12-14] The epithelial cells in both type A and type B are cohesive and rarely seen as isolated cells.

### Immunocytochemistry

The epithelial cells are strongly positive for various cytokeratins but CK20 is negative. In addition, there is often a focal CD20 positivity. The small lymphocytes are mainly CD3 or CD1a positive.

## Thymic carcinomas

These are rare tumours with an aggressive behaviour. They are distinguished from thymomas on the basis of marked cytological atypia. A variety of cell types such as squamous cell carcinoma, basaloid carcinoma, mucoepidermoid carcinoma and neuroendocrine carcinoma have been described. These variants are often difficult to separate from metastases.[12,15]

## Spleen

FNA of the spleen is usually requested for a patient with splenomegaly of unknown cause. If the enlargement is marked a palpable mass is found in the left upper quadrant. It then becomes an easy target for direct FNA biopsy. A non-palpable spleen can often be successfully sampled via a direct intercostal puncture but ultrasound guidance gives a distinctly higher success rate, with less risk of pneumothorax. In trained hands the complication rate is low.[16,17]

### Technical procedure

A few remarks concerning the technique may be useful. Infiltration of local anaesthetic is carried out as far as the peritoneum. This significantly reduces the risk of a vasovagal reaction. The biopsy needle preferred is a 25 gauge, 8 cm spinal needle with a stylet. The patient is instructed to maintain apnoea after several deep breaths. The needle is inserted, the stylet removed and the syringe attached. Suction of approximately 5 mL is applied and the needle moved back and forth. As soon as blood is seen in the needle hub the suction is stopped and the needle withdrawn.

After the biopsy, the patient should be supervised for approximately 1 hour to exclude complications. Patients with coagulopathies can be punctured but blood-typing and hospitalisation are obligatory.

## Non-neoplastic splenomegaly

Splenomegaly occurs in a number of aetiologically different conditions such as congestion, haematological disorders, storage diseases and inflammatory lesions. In the majority of such cases the underlying disorder is known and there is no need for diagnostic FNA biopsy. However, splenic cytology can be an important method of diagnosis for some disorders which primarily manifest themselves as splenomegaly.

### Haematophagocytic syndrome

This occurs in patients with immunosuppression resulting from a variety of disorders such as infections, most commonly of viral type, familial erythrophagocytic lymphohistiocytosis, AIDS and treatment with immunosuppressive drugs. The splenomegaly is usually marked.

### Cytological findings: haematophagocytic syndrome (Fig. 14.9)

A spectrum of lymphoid cells is present in a background of abundant blood and platelet aggregates. There are numerous histiocytic cells with abundant vacuolated cytoplasm. The histiocytes are cytologically benign but often contain phagocytosed erythrocytes.[18]

### Myeloid metaplasia

Myelofibrosis of the bone marrow and chronic myeloid leukaemia are accompanied by splenomegaly. This results from population of the spleen by blood forming cells normally confined to bone marrow, leading to the development of foci of extramedullary haemopoiesis.

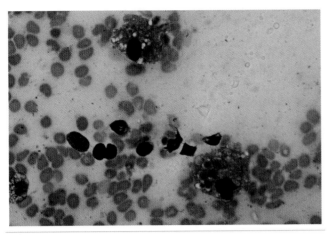

**Fig. 14.9** Haematophagocytic syndrome. Aspirate of the spleen with histiocytic cells containing phagocytosed erythrocytes and cell debris (MGG).

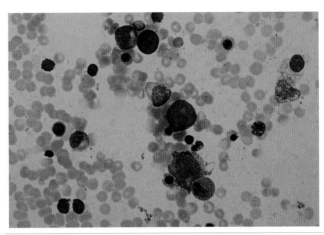

**Fig. 14.10** Myeloid metaplasia in myelofibrosis. Haemopoietic cells and some lymphoid cells (MGG).

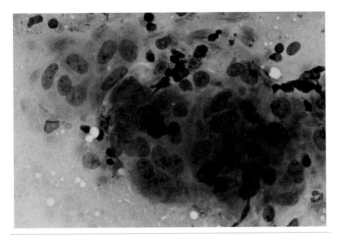

**Fig. 14.11** Granulomatous splenitis. Epithelioid cells in clusters from a patient with sarcoidosis (MGG).

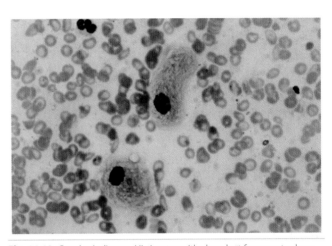

**Fig. 14.12** Gaucher's disease. Histiocytes with abundant foamy cytoplasm are typical of this storage disorder (MGG).

### Cytological findings: myeloid metaplasia (Fig. 14.10)

Normal splenic cells are in a minority, and haemopoietic cells dominate the smears.[19] Megakaryocytes may be mistaken for malignant cells by those not familiar with their appearance in cytological specimens.

## Granulomatous processes

The causes of granulomatous splenitis are numerous. The commonest of these are infections such as tuberculosis, but sarcoidosis and some malignant lymphomas produce a granulomatous reaction.

### Cytological findings: granulomatous processes (Fig. 14.11)

Numerous epithelioid histiocytes with ill-defined cytoplasm and pale elongated nuclei are present and often form granulomatous clusters. Multinucleated giant cells may be found in granulomas of any cause and are likely to be seen in sarcoidosis and tuberculosis. Caseation necrosis is sometimes identifiable in cases of tuberculosis as pale amorphous inflammatory debris. Mycobacteria are best identified by PCR

technique. In general the cytological presentation of splenic granulomatous disease is similar to that of lymph nodes (see Ch. 13). The diagnostic criteria for lymphomas associated with granulomatous splenomegaly are the same as those in node based disease and these have been described in the preceding chapter.

## Storage disorders

Massive splenomegaly results from pathological accumulation of macrophages laden with glucocerebrosides and sphingolipids in Gaucher's and Niemann-Pick's disease, respectively.

### Cytological findings: storage disorders (Fig. 14.12)

The smears contain numerous large histiocytes with foamy cytoplasm. The nuclei are monotonous and without nucleoli.

## Neoplastic splenomegaly

Metastases to the spleen are relatively rare and mostly seen in patients with widely disseminated disease.[20,21] In contrast, lymphomas frequently involve the spleen. Usually, splenic

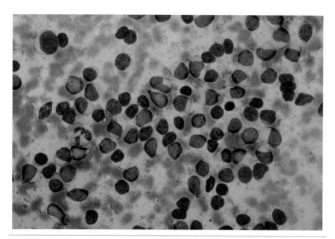

**Fig. 14.13** Hairy cell leukaemia. Small- to medium-sized lymphoid cells with pale distinct cytoplasm (MGG).

involvement reflects generalised disease, but primary lymphoma of the spleen does occur.[22–24]

## Non-Hodgkin lymphoma (NHL)

All types of NHL can affect the spleen and the cytological findings are identical to those of the lymphoma type in lymph node FNA. As in aspiration of lymphomatous nodes, the cytological diagnosis should be confirmed by immunocytochemistry. Splenic marginal zone lymphoma and hairy cell leukaemia are the most common lymphoma entities to cause splenomegaly.

### Cytological findings: non-Hodgkin lymphoma (Fig. 14.13)

Smears of splenic marginal zone lymphomas show small lymphocytes, medium-sized cells with abundant pale cytoplasm and occasional blast cells. Plasmacytic differentiation is often seen, and an admixture of epithelioid cells. Hairy cell leukaemia presents a monotonous cytological pattern. The cells are small but have relatively abundant pale cytoplasm, which typically show fine hair-like cytoplasmic processes in peripheral blood smears. In smears from lymph node aspirates these hairy projection are seldom seen. The nuclei are oval and typically lack nucleoli.

## Immunocytochemistry

Splenic marginal zone lymphoma expresses CD19 and CD20, CD5, CD10, CD43 and cyclin D1 are absent. Hairy cell leukaemia is positive for CD19, CD20, CD25 and CD103. The cells are CD5, CD10 and CD23 negative.

## Hodgkin lymphoma

The spleen is rarely the only site affected in cases of Hodgkin lymphoma and the diagnosis is therefore usually known prior to FNA. Suspicion of residual or recurrent disease can, however, lead to FNA. Involvement may be nodular, and when Hodgkin lymphoma is suspected multiple biopsies are recommended. Ultrasound guidance is of definite value in targeting involved areas.

### Cytological findings: Hodgkin lymphoma

The diagnosis rests on the identification of Hodgkin or Reed–Sternberg cells in a polymorphic cellular background. Epithelioid cells and granulomas may be present but should not lead to a diagnosis of Hodgkin lymphoma if the diagnostic cells are absent.

## Primary malignancies

Few primary malignant tumours have been documented by FNA cytology in the spleen.[25] The commonest of these are angiosarcomas and fibrosarcomas. Their cytological characteristics are the same as those seen at other sites.

## Mucosa associated lymphoid tissue (MALT)

Expansion of the MALT can be diffuse or tumorous. In both events it offers an easy target for FNA when present in the thyroid, orbit and salivary gland. Accordingly, this presentation will focus on disorders affecting MALT in these organs.

## Granulomatous disorders

In Western countries, sarcoidosis is probably the most common cause of a granulomatous process in MALT. The infiltrate is predominantly diffuse, consisting of noncaseating epithelioid granulomata, and is symptomatic only when massive enlargement has occurred. The salivary glands and orbit are more often affected than the thyroid.

### Cytological findings: granulomatous disorders

The normal tissue components are mixed with small mature lymphocytes and epithelioid cells in clusters. Giant cells are present in varying numbers. Necrosis is not seen. The rich admixture may raise the suspicion of a lymphoma and a conclusive diagnosis can only be given after immunological characterisation of the cells.

## Immunocytochemistry

A mixture of T cells and polyclonal B cells is found in these conditions.

## Autoimmune disorders

Sjögren's syndrome is an autoimmune disease affecting MALT, with multiple organ involvement. Dryness of the mouth and eyes are caused by lymphoid infiltration and atrophy of glandular tissue. Hashimoto's thyroiditis falls into the same category, with a diffuse or nodular infiltration of lymphocytes in the thyroid gland resulting in hypothyroidism accompanied by raised antibody titres in blood (see Ch. 17). Both of these conditions are more common in females.

### Cytological findings: autoimmune disorders (Fig. 14.14)

***Sjögren's sialadenitis***
Sjögren's sialadenitis is characterised by glandular atrophy and a spectrum of lymphoid cells including plasma cells. Small

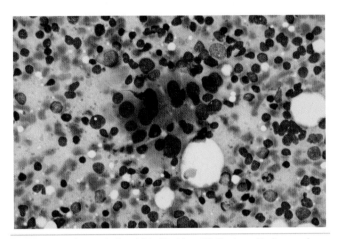

**Fig. 14.14** Hashimoto's thyroiditis. Hürthle cell follicular epithelium and mixed lymphoid cells (MGG).

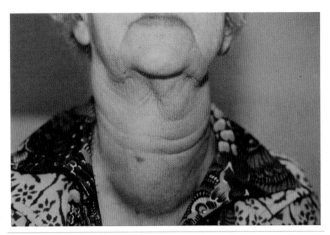

**Fig. 14.15** Lymphomatous goitre. Note the enormous asymmetrical enlargement of the thyroid gland in an elderly woman.

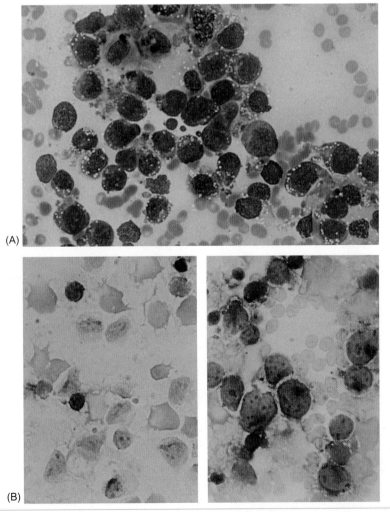

(A)

(B)

**Fig. 14.16** Aspirate from the patient in Figure 14.15. (A) Large atypical cells consistent with high-grade lymphoma (MGG). (B) Immunocytochemistry shows B cell lineage of the neoplastic cells (right). Few mature T cells present (left) (alkaline phosphatase).

mature lymphocytes predominate. Separation from a mono-morphic lymphoma infiltration requires immunocytochemistry.

### Hashimoto's disease

In Hashimoto's disease, thyroid follicular epithelium shows Hürthle cell transformation. The lymphoid population consists largely of small mature cells but centrocytes, centroblasts and plasma cells are also present (Fig. 14.14). When the follicular epithelial cells are few or without distinct Hürthle cell transformation, the possibility of a non-Hodgkin lymphoma must be considered. To differentiate conclusively between an autoimmune and a neoplastic lymphoid population can be impossible using cytomorphology alone and requires immunological characterisation of the cells.

## Immunocytochemistry

Marker studies on the lymphoid cells in Sjögren's disease and Hashimoto's thyroiditis will identify both T and polyclonal B cells.

## Malignant lymphomas (Fig. 14.15)

MALT can be the site of both primary and secondary malignant lymphomas. In general, lymphomas arising de novo in MALT tend to remain localised for many years, and therefore deserve special attention.[26–28] Orbital lymphomas usually do not show this behaviour and have a tendency to disseminate even though they are morphologically low grade. Node-based lymphomas which secondarily involve MALT are more aggressive than primary MALT lymphomas. The cytology and immunology of these initially node-based lymphomas are described in Chapter 13.

### Cytological findings: malignant lymphomas (Fig. 14.16)

MALT lymphomas are composed of small- to medium-sized cells resembling centrocytes and reactive B-cell follicles.[26–28] The tumour cells may show lymphoplasmacytoid features and

mature plasma cells are relatively frequent. Transformation into high-grade lymphoma may evolve from these low-grade neoplasms. Smears from low-grade MALT lymphomas are in most cases impossible to differentiate from reactive infiltrates using cytomorphology alone.

## Immunocytochemistry

The neoplastic cells are of B phenotype (CD20 positive) and show monotypic expression of immunoglobulin chains. The tumour cells are CD5 −, CD10 −, CD23 −, CD43 ±, CD11c ±. A high proportion of reactive cells in the aspirate will sometimes obscure identification of the monoclonal cell fraction.

## Cytogenetics

Trisomy 3 is present in the majority of cases. However, t(11;18) is found less frequently.

## Diagnostic value of FNA in assessment of extranodal lymphoid tissue

The contribution made by FNA cytology to the management of patients with diseases of extranodal lymphoid tissue can be expected to be similar to that of lymph node diseases. Thus, a conclusive cytological diagnosis, when possible corroborated by ancillary techniques, will in a majority of cases obviate the need for surgery for diagnostic purposes. There are, however, some tumours such as thymomas and thymic carcinomas which are very difficult to diagnose and subtype conclusively on FNA material and the cytological diagnosis will in such cases be more of advisory value to guide subsequent investigations. In common with the management of patients with lymphadenopathy, the cytopathologist today has an important role in clinical management through attendance at multidisciplinary meetings and by direct discussion of the cytological findings with the appropriate clinicians.

## REFERENCES

1. Kollur SM, El Hag IA. Fine-needle aspiration cytology of metastatic nasopharyngeal carcinoma in cervical lymph nodes: comparison with metastatic squamous-cell carcinoma, and Hodgkin's and non-Hodgkin's lymphoma. Diagn Cytopathol 2003;28:18–22.

2. Travis WD, Brambilla E, Müller-Hermelink HK, editorsTumors of the Thymus, et al. World Health Organization Classification of Tumors. Lyon: IARC Press; 2004. p. 145–247.

3. Banks PM, Warnke RA, Jaffe ES, Harris NL, Stein H, editors, et al. World Health Organization Classification of Tumors. Tumors of the Haematopoetic and Lymphoid Tissues. Lyon: IARC Press; 2001. p. 175–76.

4. Tani E, Maeda S, Fröstad B, et al. Aspiration cytology with phenotyping and clinical presentation of childhood lymphomas. Diagn Oncol 1993;3:294–301.

5. Jacobs JC, Katz RL, Shabb N, et al. Fine needle aspiration of lymphoblastic lymphoma. A multiparameter diagnostic approach. Acta Cytol 1992;36:887–94.

6. Wakely PE Jr., Kornstein MJ. Aspiration cytopathology of lymphoblastic lymphoma and leukemia: the MCV experience. Pediatr Pathol Lab Med 1996;15:243–57.

7. Hoda RS, Picklesimer L, Green KM, et al. Fine needle aspiration of a primary mediastinal large B-cell lymphoma. A case report with cytologic histologic and flow cytometric considerations. Diagn Cytopathol 2005;32:370–73.

8. Harun MH, Yaacob I. Congenital posterior mediastinal teratoma. A case report. Singapore Med J 1993;34:567–68.

9. Motoyama T, Yamamoto O, Iwamoto H, et al. Fine needle aspiration cytology of primary mediastinal germ cell tumors. Acta Cytol 1995;39:725–32.

10. Wakely PE Jr.. Cytopathology-histopathology of the mediastinum: epithelial, lymphoproliferative, and germ cell neoplasms. Ann Diagn Pathol 2002;6:30–43.

11. Yang GC, Hwang SJ, Yee HT. Fine-needle aspiration cytology of unusual germ cell tumors of the mediastinum: atypical seminoma and parietal yolk sac tumor. Diagn Cytopathol 2002;27:69–74.

12. Shin HJ, Katz RL. Thymic neoplasia as represented by fine needle aspiration biopsy of anterior mediastinal masses. A practical approach to the differential diagnosis. Acta Cytol 1998;42:855–64.

13. Chhieng DC, Rose D, Ludwig ME. Cytology of thymomas: emphasis on morphology and correlation with histologic subtypes. Cancer 2000;90:24–32.

14. Wakely PE Jr. Cytopathology of thymic epithelial neoplasms. Semin Diagn Pathol 2005;22:213–22.

15. Wakely PE Jr.. Fine needle aspiration in the diagnosis of thymic epithelial neoplasms. Hematol Oncol Clin North Am 2008;22:433–42.

16. Civardi G, Vallisa D, Bertè T, et al. Ultrasound-guided fine needle biopsy of the spleen: high clinical efficacy and low risk in a multicenter Italian study. Am J Hematol 2001;67:93–99.

17. Lal A, Ariga R, Gattuso P, et al. Splenic fine needle aspiration and core biopsy. A review of 49 cases. Acta Cytol 2003;47:951–59.

18. Zeppa P, Vetrani A, Ciancia G. Hemophagocytic histiocytosis diagnosed by fine needle aspiration cytology of the spleen. A case report. Acta Cytol 2004;48:415–19.

19. Sen R, Bhadani PP, Singh H, et al. Myeloid metaplasia in aspirates from enlarged spleens: a clue in the absence of peripheral blood findings characteristic of myelofibrosis. Acta Cytol 2006;50:379–83.

20. Lam KY, Tang V. Metastatic tumors to the spleen: a 25-year clinicopathologic study. Arch Pathol Lab Med 2000;124:526–30.

21. Cavanna L, Lazzaro A, Vallisa D, et al. Role of image-guided fine-needle aspiration biopsy in the management of patients with splenic metastasis. World J Surg Oncol 2007;5:13.

22. Campo E, Miguel R, Krenacs L, et al. Primary nodal marginal zone lymphomas of splenic and MALT type. Am J Surg Pathol 1999;23:59–68.

23. Zeppa P, Picardi M, Marino G. Fine needle aspiration biopsy and flow cytometry immunophenotyping of lymphoid and myeloproliferative disorders of the spleen. Cancer 2003;99:118–27.

24. Ramdall RB, Cai G, Alasio TM, et al. Fine needle aspiration biopsy for the primary diagnosis of lymphoproliferative disorders involving the spleen: one institution's experience and review of the literature. Diagn Cytopathol 2006;34:812–17.

25. Delacruz V, Jorda M, Gomez-Fernandez C, et al. Fine-needle aspiration diagnosis of angiosarcoma of the spleen: a case report and review of the literature. Arch Pathol Lab Med 2005;129:1054–56.

26. Stewart CJ, Jackson R, Farquharson M, et al. Fine-needle aspiration cytology of extranodal lymphoma. Diagn Cytopathol 1998;19:260–66.

27. Matsushima AY, Hamele-Bena D, Osborne BM. Fine-needle aspiration biopsy findings in marginal zone B cell lymphoma. Diagn Cytopathol 1999;20:190–98.

28. Crapanzano JP, Lin O. Cytologic findings of marginal zone lymphoma. Cancer 2003;99:301–9.

# Section 9

## Transplantation and Immunosuppression

# Organ transplantation

Eva von Willebrand and Irmeli Lautenschlager

## Chapter contents

## Introduction

Over the course of the last 20 years of the twentieth century, cytological methods and criteria for diagnosis established their role in the monitoring of organ transplants and are used today in transplantation centres around the world. Kidney and liver transplantation are the commonest procedures subjected to cytological monitoring but the techniques have been used for pancreas as well, and also for lung transplantation.

Cytological specimens from solid organ transplants are usually obtained either by fine needle aspiration (FNA), the method mostly used in monitoring kidney and liver transplants, or by collecting urine or bile for cytological analysis. In lung transplantation, bronchoalveolar lavage specimens are used for cytological assessment (see Ch. 2).

In modern clinical practice FNA was developed by Franzen in 1960[1] to diagnose urological malignancies and applied to renal transplants in humans for the first time in 1968 by Pasternack.[2] The cytology of allograft rejection was at the time practically unknown and during the following decade, experimental work on rat and human kidney allografts[3,4] helped to elucidate the immunological and cytological sequence of events in allograft rejection. This experimental work revealed that the inflammation indicative of activation of the immune system associated with rejection is seen earlier and is more specific in the transplanted organ than in the peripheral blood of the recipient.

The advantage of cytological methods is that the risk of complications to graft and patient as a result of the procedure is minimal, the specimens can be obtained daily if necessary, and the methods are quick to perform. In 1982, the FNA method was also applied in liver transplantation.[5,6] Experience of over 18 000 FNAs in kidney transplants and over 7000 FNAs in liver transplants has shown that cytological analysis of aspiration biopsies is well suited to monitoring the transplant during the early postoperative period when the risk of acute rejection is highest. The main limitation of cytology is that the information obtained is restricted in certain respects compared to histology, especially with regard to the architectural structure of the transplant.

In this chapter, we discuss the cytology of kidney and liver transplantation based on aspiration cytology methods and also summarise briefly the experiences of the technology in our hospital, as well in other transplant centres.

## Kidney transplant cytology

### Sampling and processing of cytological specimens

In renal transplantation the method most often used to obtain cytological specimens from the transplant is a modification of Franzen's FNA.[7]

FNAs are taken using a 20–22 gauge spinal needle connected to a 20 mL syringe which contains 5 mL of RPMI-1640 tissue culture medium supplemented with 5% human serum albumin, 50 IU/mL heparin and 1% Hepes buffer. An FNA pistol may be used, but is not necessary for the procedure. The transplant is usually located easily by palpation. When necessary, ultrasound guidance can be used.

The FNA is performed percutaneously without local anaesthesia in aseptic conditions. The needle is inserted into the renal cortex, full suction is applied and the needle is moved back and forth three or four times through a distance of 1–2 cm. In this way, the needle traverses the entire cortex and reaches several periglomerular and perivascular areas. Sampling is complete when the colour of cellular fluid can be seen in the needle hub. The needle is then rapidly withdrawn after releasing suction and the sample of 10–50 μL inside the needle is flushed immediately with tissue culture medium to get the whole sample into the syringe. The syringe with sample inside is then sent to the laboratory for immediate processing. If necessary, samples can be kept overnight in syringes containing culture medium in a refrigerator.

To compare the relative leucocyte distribution between peripheral blood and graft, simultaneous samples of blood, usually 2–3 drops, are taken from the fingertip into another syringe containing 5 mL of the same RPMI medium.

The FNA and blood samples are processed in parallel. The cells are centrifuged, resuspended, counted and 100–200 μL aliquots are spun onto microscope slides using a cytocentrifuge. The smears are air dried for routine diagnostic use and stained with May–Grünwald Giemsa (MGG). Parallel preparations can be used for other cytological stains or immunocytochemical staining techniques.

### Interpretation of cytological specimens

MGG-stained cytospin smears of the graft and blood are examined microscopically and the findings reported on a standard report form (Table 15.1), derived from the First International

**Table 15.1** FNA report evaluating specimen adequacy, leucocyte differential and morphological features of parenchymal cells

| Inflammatory cells | FNA | Blood | Increment | Correction factor | Corrected increment |
|---|---|---|---|---|---|
| Lymphoid blast cells | 3 | 0 | 3 | 1.0 | 3.0 |
| Activated lymphocytes | 4 | 0 | 4 | 0.5 | 2.0 |
| Lgl lymphocytes | 1 | 1 | | 0.2 | |
| Lymphocytes | 40 | 13 | 27 | 0.1 | 2.7 |
| PMN | | | | | |
| Juvenile forms | 0 | 0 | | 0.1 | |
| Neutrophils | 35 | 62 | | 0.1 | |
| Basophils | 0 | 2 | | 0.1 | |
| Eosinophils | 7 | 14 | | 0.1 | |
| Monoblast | 0 | 0 | | 1.0 | |
| Monocytes | 10 | 8 | 2 | 0.2 | 0.4 |
| Macrophages | 0 | 0 | | 1.0 | |
| Total corrected increment | | | | | 7.1 |
| Total blast cells/cytoprep | 22 | | | | |
| Parenchymal cells | Normal | Swelling | Swelling vacuolation | Necrosis |
| Morphology score | 1 | 2 | 3 | 4 |
| Parenchymal cells | | 2 | | |
| Parenchymal cells per 100 inflammatory cells | | | 20 | |

Workshop on Transplant Aspiration Cytology in Munich in 1982. The three most important features to be evaluated are specimen adequacy, the leucocyte differential and the morphological features of the parenchymal cells.

## Specimen adequacy

To be evaluated, the aspirate must be representative. The inevitable but variable contamination of renal and liver aspirates by blood makes assessment of specimen adequacy of utmost importance in interpretation of the findings.

Since the cellular infiltration of acute rejection is always most pronounced in the renal cortex, representative specimens must include sufficient cortical material. Cytological samples taken from the medulla are usually not diagnostic,[8] as is also the case in histology. The presence of glomeruli cannot be used as a criterion for adequacy since glomeruli do not always appear in aspirates and many of them are lost in processing. Instead, adequacy of representation is assessed by calculating the ratio of tubular cells to inflammatory leucocytes.

Cytological criteria for representative samples and reproducibility of transplant aspirate specimens have been established by analysing duplicate aspirates,[9] where a correlation coefficient of 0.95 was obtained if both specimens contained at least seven tubular cells per 100 inflammatory leucocytes. When the ratio of tubular cells to leucocytes in either sample fell below this, the correlation coefficient fell accordingly. Other groups have reported similar results for double aspirate biopsy analysis.[10]

## Inflammatory cells

- Small lymphocytes, activated lymphocytes, natural killer cells
- Lymphoid blast cells are mixed B and T cell types
- Monocyte-macrophage cells
- Eosinophils
- Platelets
- Neutrophils.

Most of the inflammatory leucocytes in cytological preparations can be identified readily according to standard haematological criteria[4,7] in routine MGG-stained smears (Fig. 15.1). These include small lymphocytes, activated lymphocytes with increased cytoplasmic basophilia, and large granular lymphocytes, which are the morphological form of natural killer cells.[11] The appearance of blast cells is diagnostic of acute rejection.

Lymphoid blast cells are characterised by their large size (15–25 μm in diameter), their large immature nuclei and intense cytoplasmic basophilia. Approximately 50% of the lymphoid blast cells are B blasts containing intracytoplasmic immunoglobulins, as identified by immunofluorescence staining. The other half of the blast cells are T blasts, characterised by T-cell surface antigens, and identified with monoclonal antibodies using immunoperoxidase staining.

Different forms of monocyte–macrophage cells can also be seen, including small monocytes, large monocytes with irregular, multilobed nuclei and macrophages in different stages of maturation. Macrophages are large cells, up to 60 μm in diameter, usually showing vacuolated cytoplasm and pyknotic

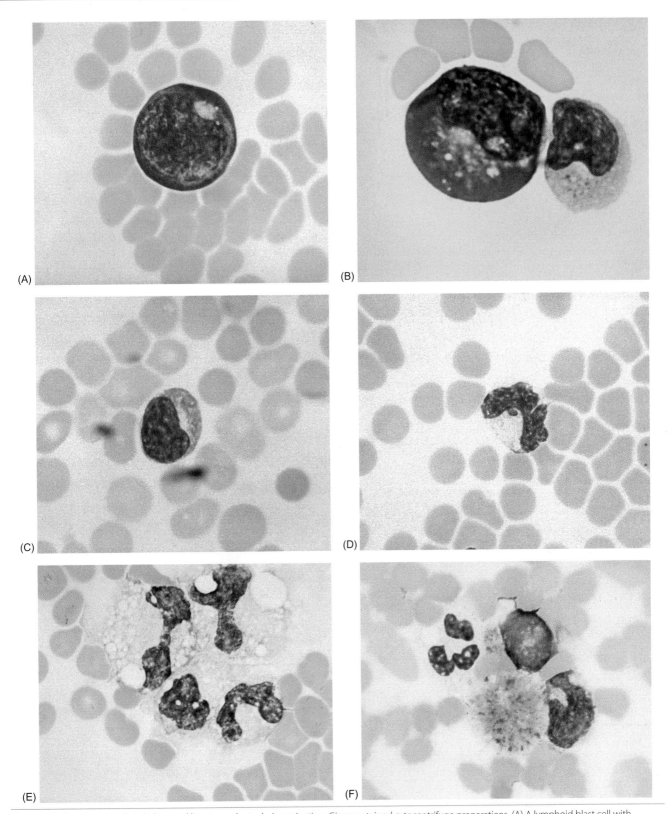

**Fig. 15.1** Inflammatory cells in kidney and liver transplants during rejection. Giemsa-stained cytocentrifuge preparations. (A) A lymphoid blast cell with immature nucleus and cytoplasmic basophilia; (B) a blast cell with plasmacytoid morphology and a large granular lymphocyte with cytoplasmic granulation; (C) an activated lymphocyte; (D) a monocyte with irregular nuclear contours; (E) macrophages with cytoplasmic vacuolation and elongated nuclei; (F) a thrombocyte aggregate with a monocyte.

elongated nuclei lying at the periphery of the cell. They are usually seen in abundance in the later phases of severe and irreversible rejection and in acute vascular rejection in the early phase.

Eosinophils are usually more frequent at the beginning of immunological reactivation, and are seen both in aspirates and in peripheral blood, indicating generalised immune response to the graft.[12] Platelets are also seen during rejection in excess in the graft.[13] Small loose platelet aggregates disappear during successful rejection treatment, but large aggregates on endothelial cells seem to indicate a worse prognosis.[13] Neutrophils are usually seen in excess in the graft only when there is irreversible rejection with necrotic changes. In cases with bacterial infection of the graft, neutrophil aggregates with intracellular bacteria can be seen.

## Cytological characteristics of renal parenchymal cells

- Usually single parenchymal cells
- Tubular fragments or glomeruli may be seen
- Endothelial cells
- Immunostaining confirms identification.

Aspiration biopsy specimens consist mainly of single parenchymal cells, although clumps of renal tubular cells or even parts of tubules and whole glomeruli may often be encountered in the specimens. The parenchymal cells most commonly seen are tubular cells from different parts of the nephron, and endothelial cells from the renal vascular endothelium, usually from capillary blood vessels (Fig. 15.2).

For more detailed characterisation of the parenchymal cells, immunocytochemistry can be used. With monoclonal antibodies different parenchymal cell types can be identified precisely. Cytokeratin antibodies are used for tubular cell characterisation, since these antibodies do not stain endothelial cells or leucocytes. Endothelial cells can be stained with antibodies to Factor VIII-related antigens or with vimentin antibodies, which do not stain tubular cells.[14]

## Morphological changes in parenchymal cells in different graft complications

- Non-specific cellular degeneration: in many conditions
- Acute tubular necrosis: degenerate cells, cytoplasmic vacuolation, frank necrosis
- Acute cyclosporin A (CyA) toxicity: degeneration with basophilia, isometric vacuolation
- Chronic CyA toxicity: tubular atrophy, degenerative changes, fibrosis
- Acute rejection: normal cells in early or short-lived rejections, degenerate/necrotic cells if severe
- Graft infarction: severe necrosis of tubular cells.

Changes in the parenchymal cells are scored from 1–4, 1 being normal and 4 representing necrosis, and this score is recorded in the report (Table 15.1). Although typical findings in parenchymal cells can be seen in several different graft complications, the findings are basically non-specific. Degenerative changes can be seen in tubular cells in acute tubular necrosis (Fig. 15.2), in advancing rejection, in CyA nephrotoxicity and also in urological complications. The information derived from graft parenchymal cell morphology is useful in the differential diagnosis of graft complications, but interpretation of the changes requires concomitant evaluation of the inflammation and also knowledge of the clinical data.

In acute tubular necrosis (ATN) the tubular cells are swollen, with cytoplasmic degeneration and irregular vacuolation. In very severe cases necrotic tubular cells may also be seen, but usually only a few. These changes are due to prolonged cold ischaemia

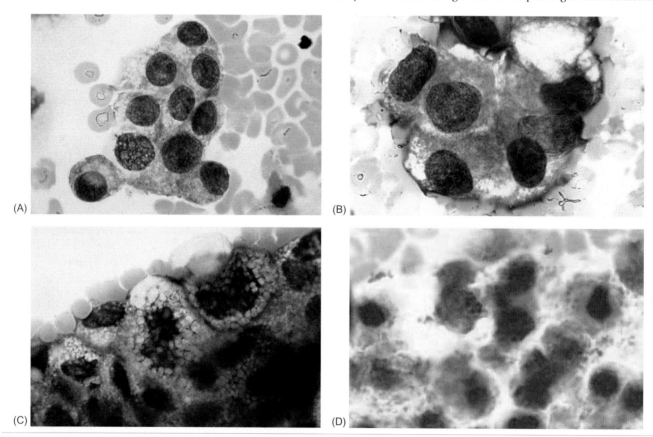

(A)

(B)

(C)

(D)

**Fig. 15.2** Renal parenchymal cells in Giemsa-stained cytopreparations. (A) A group of normal tubular cells; (B) swelling, degeneration and vacuolation in tubular cells in ATN; (C) pronounced isometric vacuolation and swelling in tubular cells during CyA toxicity; (D) necrotic tubular cells in graft necrosis.

and return to normal with improving graft function in 1–2 weeks. In pure ATN there are no signs of immunoactivation.

Similar, but more pronounced changes are seen in the tubular cells in acute CyA toxicity. The cells are swollen, with increased cytoplasmic basophilia and prominent isometric vacuolation.[15,16] Toxic isometric vacuolation is quite typical of acute CyA toxicity, although it is a non-specific phenomenon. It has also been reported in experimental kidney transplantation models.[17] The deposits of CyA and its metabolites can be demonstrated by specific monoclonal antibodies and immunofluorescence techniques.[18] Isometric vacuolation is not seen in chronic CyA toxicity, where tubular atrophy and degeneration with interstitial fibrosis are the dominating features. Today, with triple drug immunosuppressive treatment and rather low CyA doses, acute CyA toxicity is not a very common complication.

At the beginning of acute rejection, tubular and endothelial cells usually have normal morphology and also retain normal morphology in short, easily treated rejections. In severe and prolonged rejection, on the other hand, there are progressive degenerative changes in tubular cells and even necrosis in irreversible rejection.

Severe necrotic changes in tubular cells are also seen in graft infarction,[18] which is usually due to renal vein thrombosis. This clinical complication is often fulminant with rapidly progressing necrosis, but fortunately it is not a frequent event.

## Quantitation of inflammation in the transplant

### Incremental method

As all FNAs are contaminated with variable amounts of blood, inflammation in the graft is evaluated against the blood background by incremental analysis: differential counts of 100–200 leucocytes from the aspirate and blood specimens are performed and the blood values are subtracted from aspirate values to obtain the increment of inflammatory cells (Table 15.1). As all inflammatory cells in allograft rejection do not have equal diagnostic significance,[3,4] correction factors are used in calculating the corrected increment.[7] The cells with greatest significance in acute rejection, blast cells and macrophages, have a full correction factor of 1.0. Correction factors for all inflammatory cells are given in Table 15.1.

The sum of the corrected increment values, known as corrected increment units (CIU), represents the total corrected increment (TCI), which describes the intensity of inflammation in the graft. Usually, a TCI higher than 3.0 and a blast cell increment of 1.0 indicates acute rejection.[19,20] The presence of blast cells is in itself suggestive of immunological activation in the graft: therefore the total number of blast cells per cytopreparation is also counted. In a stable graft no blasts are seen, but during immune activation the number of blast cells rises up to 10–50 per cytopreparation and may be even higher.[19] In the analysis of Helderman et al.[21] a total count of >6 blast cells per slide proved representative of rejection independent of the TCI score. With the increment method it is possible to describe the FNA findings with a single numerical value instead of by description only, although the description is also important.

### Cytology in monitoring of the transplant

- Stable graft has minimal lymphocyte/monocyte infiltration
- Increase in blast cells and TCI with acute rejection

- Increase in macrophages has a poor prognosis
- Rejection reaction varies with the patient
- Acute vascular rejection shows monocytes and macrophages with few lymphocytes
- New treatment protocols reduce risk and severity of rejections.

Sequential follow-up of the transplant with regular aspiration biopsies and cytological samples permits definition of the course of intragraft events.

In a stable graft, lymphocytic/monocytic infiltration in the FNAs is either absent or minimal. When acute rejection begins increasing numbers of lymphoid and monocytic cells infiltrate the graft, and blast cells in particular appear in the aspirate. Lymphoid blast response is the hallmark of acute rejection together with an elevated TCI, usually also associated with deteriorating graft function. With successful rejection treatment inflammatory cells disappear from the graft and graft function improves. In unresponsive severe rejections macrophages begin to infiltrate the graft, tubular cell degeneration increases and graft necrosis ensues. Macrophage accumulation during rejection usually indicates a poor prognosis.

In most cases of acute cellular rejection, the inflammation follows the cytological pattern described above. However, individual patients may have different inflammatory profiles. Sometimes mild transient lymphocytic/monocytic infiltrates with some blast cells can be seen in the graft around 1 week after transplantation. These usually resolve without any further treatment and without deterioration in transplant function. In these cases of mild immunological activation the existing immunosuppressive treatment is efficient enough to keep the inflammation below the threshold of clinical rejection.[22]

Evidence of acute vascular rejection (AVR) is a major feature of rejections that do not respond to steroid treatment.[23] Diagnosis of AVR is always based on histology; however, characteristic cytological findings in acute vascular rejection have been defined.[23–25] These include accumulation of monocytes and macrophages in the graft. Lymphocytic infiltrates, especially of blast cells, are not prominent in AVR, at least not in the pure forms.[26] Combinations of ACR and AVR are also common[23,26] and are often resistant to ordinary steroid rejection treatment. Monoclonal or polyclonal antibodies, OKT3 or ATG and plasmapheresis are used in the treatment of these rejections.[23]

The immunosuppressive protocol used clearly modifies the FNA cytology profiles. Today, when most centres use modern immunosuppressive protocols based on cyclosporine, tacrolimus, mycophenolate mofetil or monoclonal antibodies and steroids, only approximately 20% of cadaver kidney grafts have any acute rejection episodes during the first postoperative month,[27] compared with 70% with the old treatment protocols using azathioprine and steroids.[28] The onset of rejection is also delayed and the inflammation is milder, with fewer blast cells. Regular monitoring by cytology thus also allows assessment of the impact of different immunosuppressive drugs on the graft.

## Immunocytochemistry

Using immunocytological techniques, such as immunoperoxidase or immunofluorescence staining with monoclonal antibodies, it is possible to evaluate in even greater detail the state of the transplant and the nature of the inflammatory infiltrates in the graft.[29–33] The different T and B lymphocyte subsets can be analysed, including their state of activation. Mononuclear phagocytes can be differentiated, as can parenchymal cells. Expression of adhesion molecules on parenchymal cells can also be evaluated with relevant monoclonal antibodies.

## Lymphocyte populations in graft rejections

In most acute cellular rejections CD8T lymphocytes outnumber CD4 cells in the graft, although at the beginning of the rejection episode CD4T cells seem to be frequent.[30] In severe irreversible rejections, persistence of CD4 dominance in the graft has been seen.[34]

Usually the sum of CD4 and CD8 cells in the transplant is greater than the total number of CD2 or CD3 positive T cells. A minority of lymphocytes are positive for both CD4 and CD8. The number of B lymphocytes is usually rather low during rejection, forming approximately 5–20% of the lymphocytes, but the number of B blast cells is relatively high; of the blast cells in rejection infiltrates approximately 50% are B blast cells and 50% T blast cells.

Different forms of mononuclear phagocytes can be stained and identified with relevant monoclonal antibodies. Lymphocyte subpopulations in grafts are, however, variable, both during different phases of rejection and also during viral infections, and cannot as such be used as diagnostic findings. Nevertheless, analysis of the different inflammatory subsets gives important additional information on the state of the transplant.

## Activation markers and adhesion molecules in acute rejection

Analysis of activation markers and the adhesion molecules of inflammatory cells infiltrating the graft and parenchymal cells has proved to be useful in rejection diagnosis. In acute rejection induction of interleukin-2 (IL-2) receptors (CD25) on activated lymphoid cells has been demonstrated[35] and HLA-class II antigens are induced on the tubular cells.[36,37] With successful rejection treatment CD25 positive lymphoid cells disappear rapidly and class II expression diminishes to background level.[35,38] In stable grafts there is no induction of activation markers.

Adhesion molecules are also induced during rejection on different transplant components. Constitutively normal kidneys express several adhesion molecules on the endothelial cells of vessels, such as intercellular adhesion molecule-1 (ICAM-1) and vascular cell adhesion molecule (VCAM-1).[39] Tubular cells do not normally express these molecules, or only in small quantities on the luminal surfaces, but during rejection these adhesion molecules are induced on cells of tubular origin. The induction of ICAM-1 on tubular cells occurs early in rejection and disappears rapidly with successful rejection treatment.[40] The role of these molecules as also the role of growth factors and their receptors in the rejection process is, at present, under intensive investigation.[41]

## Viral infections

Viral infections often cause differential diagnostic problems in transplant patients. Cytomegalovirus (CMV) infections (see Chs 12, 23) can induce generalised immunological activation in the patient; lymphoid blast cells, activated lymphocytes and large granular lymphocytes are found in the patient's blood and also

in the transplant aspirate.[42,43] CMV infections are also related to rejection, patients with frequent rejections having more CMV infections, while patients with CMV infection have more rejections. CMV infection has been shown to induce HLA class II antigens on kidney transplant tubular cells.[44] Apparently, this is the link to the rejection process. Specific virological methods, such as antigen detection, viral culture or PCR are, however, necessary to diagnose CMV or other viral infections.[45]

## Correlation with histology

The correlation between FNA cytology and histology in renal transplantation has been assessed in several studies.[7,10,24] A high concordance between simultaneous cytology and histology findings has been reported, particularly in acute cellular rejection, ATN, acute CyA toxicity and also when the graft situation is stable.[25,46–49] It has been shown that there is a relation between the histological severity of acute rejection, whether mild, moderate or severe, and the level of inflammation in cytology.[50] Diagnostic sensitivities and specificities of >90% have been reported in a prospective study comparing cytology and histology in monitoring of kidney transplant patients[21] and in a blind study comparing cytology and histology in 200 patients.[20]

Also a prospective, randomised study[51] compared cytology, histology and immunohistology in the rejection diagnosis, using clinical evaluation of rejection as the gold standard. The respective specificities were 96%, 87% and 80%, with sensitivities of 59%, 75% and 77%. In this analysis cytology had an increased tendency to miss clinical rejection episodes but proved most reliable in monitoring non-functioning or stable grafts.

Today the diagnosis of rejection in adult renal transplant recipients is usually based on histological findings scored according to the schema developed in the first meeting in Banff.[52] Monitoring of rejection and the response to treatment can be done with cytological samples and is especially used in children with renal transplants in order to minimise the number of core needle biopsies and the need of anaesthesia in small children.[53]

## Diagnostic value of cytology in organ transplant failure

The value of cytology in the differential diagnosis of graft complications of kidney transplants is presented in Box 15.1. The cytopathologist is an essential member of the team managing the care of transplant patients and plays an active role in interpreting the laboratory findings for the clinicians at the regular multidisciplinary-team meetings.

## Liver transplant cytology

As a result of experimental studies[5,54] and the experience gained in monitoring kidney allografts, FNA transplant cytology has also been applied to hepatic transplantation.[6,55,56] Liver FNA has been used as a routine clinical procedure since 1982.[6] It has proved to be a reliable method of diagnosing inflammation associated with acute liver rejection and for monitoring the response to antirejection therapy.[56–59] A good correlation with biopsy histology in the diagnosis of acute rejection has been reported from several centres.[60–64]

## Technical aspects

Liver allograft recipients are monitored with frequent FNAs from the day of transplantation, usually at 3–5 day intervals. Specimens should be obtained through the medial aspect of the right costal margin to minimise the risk of complications or contamination from the intraperitoneal cavity.[65] The technique for performing and processing FNAs of liver and corresponding blood specimens is similar to that described for renal allografts.[7] The quantitation of inflammation by the incremental method is also similar.[7]

### Cytological findings: acute liver allograft rejection

- Rejection is usually diagnosed by histology
- FNA is helpful in childhood transplants
- Emergence of lymphoid blast cells and increased lymphocytes at onset of rejection
- Macrophages predominate in irreversible rejection
- Combined clinical picture and all laboratory test results necessary for diagnosis
- Immunological activation marker analysis may help in assessment.

Diagnosis of liver allograft rejection is difficult, as clinical signs or biochemical markers are rather non-specific and the findings cannot be distinguished from conditions such as cholangitis, infections or cholestasis. Thus, invasive methods based on biopsy histology are necessary for the evaluation of liver rejection. However, as liver biopsy always creates some risk of complications, such as bleeding or infection, minimally invasive aspiration biopsy may provide an additional helpful method to visualise the intragraft immunological events. In paediatric transplantation,[66] the use of FNA technology has made it possible to minimise the number of core needle biopsies in children.

The liver biopsy histology is nowadays based on the Banff criteria[67] including the three main features of acute rejection: portal inflammation, bile duct inflammation/damage and venous endothelial inflammation. The hallmark of acute liver allograft rejection is infiltration of the portal areas by mononuclear cells. The inflammatory infiltrate consists mainly of lymphocytes and a few plasma cells. In addition, the cellular infiltrate often contains eosinophils, neutrophil polymorphs and mononuclear phagocytes. Portal inflammation with bile duct and vascular involvement, together with cholestasis, are characteristic histological findings in acute rejection.

In FNA material, the emergence of lymphoid blast cells and an increase in lymphocytes in the graft are typical findings at the beginning of acute liver rejection.[54,55] The first day on which FNA reveals inflammation with >3.0 CIU and the presence of lymphoid blast cells is considered as the onset of immune activation in the graft.[56] In the advanced stages of rejection the blastogenic response subsides and the cellular infiltrate becomes dominated by mononuclear phagocytes. Large numbers of macrophages are associated with irreversible rejection and parenchymal necrosis.[54,56] The neutrophil or eosinophil infiltration of the graft described in biopsy histology cannot usually be evaluated against the background blood in FNA material. However, blood eosinophilia correlates with immune activation in the graft.[56]

The clinical diagnosis of rejection is based not only on histological or FNA findings, but also on other laboratory parameters and clinical signs. It is well known from biopsy histology and FNA cytology that a few days after liver transplantation, some inflammatory infiltrate may appear in portal areas without tissue damage, and disappear without any clinical sign of rejection or additional immunosuppression.[68,69] This type of immune activation may be initiated by donor cells in the graft representing an *in situ* graft-versus-host (GVH) reaction, or alternatively could be an incomplete or subclinical form of the alloresponse under certain immunosuppressive conditions.[62] Thus, the typical findings on FNA or in biopsy histology, together with graft dysfunction are needed for the clinical diagnosis of acute liver allograft rejection.

Immunological activation marker analysis may be performed on the liver FNA specimens, as well. An increase in MHC class II positive lymphocytes and the appearance of IL-2 receptor expressing cells in the graft correlate with immune activation and blast response in the FNA.[70] Expression of class II antigens on liver parenchymal cells has also been shown to correlate with acute cellular rejection.[71,72] However, various infections, especially viral infections, also induce class II expression. Induction of adhesion molecules, such as in the graft ICAM-1, is an early marker for immune activation.[73,74] Induction of ICAM-1 on liver parenchymal cells can be regarded as even less specific than class II, since it is expressed on liver parenchymal cells not only during rejection and viral infections,[74,75] but also during bacterial infections.[75]

## Liver transplant cytology and infections

- Systemic bacterial and viral infections do not increase inflammation in the graft
- CMV shows mild lymphocyte activation and a few blasts on FNA
- Infection within the graft shows many neutrophils
- Graft lymphocytosis occurs with hepatitis C virus infection
- Full microbiology is necessary in monitoring grafts.

Systemic infections, such as bacterial sepsis or various viral infections, have practically no effect on FNA findings of intragraft inflammation.[76] In bacteraemia, a prominent neutrophilia is seen in the blood specimen, and characteristic findings in viral infections are either lymphocytosis or, after long-lasting viraemia, lymphopenia.

During CMV infection, which is the most common of the viral infections, mild lymphoid activation with a few lymphoid blasts is recorded in both FNA and the corresponding blood sample.[77] However, immune activation in the graft simply reflects the haematological changes in the background blood and the total inflammation seldom exceeds 3.0 CIU. Other characteristic findings for CMV infection are blood eosinophilia and increased numbers of large granular lymphocytes. This generalised immune response against CMV subsides with successful antiviral treatment.[77] Not only CMV, but also the other members of the herpesvirus family, such as human herpesvirus-6, are associated with lymphocyte dominated immune response, which can be falsely interpreted.[78]

Any infection located in the graft may lead to cellular changes in the FNA specimen. Large numbers of neutrophils in the aspirate, often with hypersegmented nuclei, indicate either a bacterial infection in the graft, an abscess or contamination from a wound infection. Intracellular bacteria are sometimes seen. Viral hepatitis may generate lymphocyte infiltration in the graft and cause differential diagnostic problems.[69] Hepatitis C virus (HCV) is common among liver transplant recipients, and recurrence of the infection is associated with graft lymphocytosis.[79] Because of the high incidence of infections in liver transplant patients, careful microbiological investigations, especially virological, should be included in patient monitoring.

## Liver parenchymal cell cytology

- FNA from normal transplants show hepatocytes, sometimes bile duct and endothelial cells
- Swelling and vacuolation of hepatocytes in early rejection
- Necrotic cells indicate severe rejection
- Degenerative changes without inflammation seen in vascular damage and drug toxicity
- CyA causes isometric vacuolation of hepatocytes
- Cholestasis with inflammation seen in rejection
- Cholestasis without inflammation suggest biliary tract or other complications.

Normal liver transplant FNAs contain hepatocytes in clusters and in single cell form (Fig. 15.3A) (see Ch. 8). The number of parenchymal cells is evaluated, and the specimens are considered representative according to the same principles as for renal FNAs.[9] In addition to hepatocytes, other parenchymal components such as bile duct cells (Fig. 15.3B) and endothelial cells are occasionally seen in FNA specimens.

Degenerative changes in hepatocytes with swelling and irregular vacuolation (Fig. 15.3C) are recorded in FNA during the inflammatory episodes of acute rejection.[56] Necrotic cells (Fig. 15.3D) in the FNA indicate severe tissue damage. Degeneration of hepatocytes without inflammation in the graft is due to other causes, such as vascular complications or drug toxicity. There are characteristic morphological changes associated with CyA hepatotoxicity[56,80] with isometric vacuolation of hepatocytes

(Fig. 15.3E). Deposits of CyA or its metabolites can be demonstrated in the cells by immunofluorescence.

Cholestasis is often recorded in association with an inflammatory episode or rejection (Fig. 15.3F). Bile droplets in hepatocytes or between the cells indicate either impaired graft function or extracellular cholestasis during rejection.[56] Cholestasis without inflammation indicates biliary complications or impaired graft function for reasons other than rejection.[56,58]

## The role of FNA cytology in liver transplantation

Although a close correlation between FNA and liver biopsy histology has been reported by several groups,[60–65] cytology is not intended to replace biopsy histology. In general, FNA is used for frequent monitoring, especially during the first 3–4 weeks after transplantation, when most acute liver rejections occur. During this time core needle biopsy is usually also obtained to confirm the diagnosis, to diagnose various complications other than rejection or to assess the degree of liver damage and need for retransplantation. After the first postoperative months, when chronic pathology of the liver graft supervenes, the diagnostic value of FNA decreases. If there is a suspicion of chronic rejection, as evidenced by the development of the vanishing bile duct syndrome or any other late complications, core needle biopsy histology is the only dependable diagnostic method.

Biochemical markers of graft dysfunction such as increased serum values of transaminases, alkaline phosphatase and bilirubin, correlate with inflammatory episodes in FNA, but the cytological diagnosis of acute rejection, based on lymphoid activation and blast response, can be recognised 1–3 days earlier by FNA. However, as has already been stated, graft dysfunction, together with cytological or histological findings are needed for the clinical diagnosis of liver rejection. However, monitoring of viral infections is necessary because of differential diagnostics.

In addition to diagnostic purposes, the FNA method can also be used for further studies on the mechanisms of liver allograft rejection and other intrahepatic immunological events.[81–87] Not only immunocytochemistry but also the modern molecular methods can be used for further analysis of the FNAB material, e.g. for the monitoring of gene expression profiles in the graft.[87] The scientific use of the FNA technology in transplantation might provide new applications in the future.

## The role of the cytopathologist in patient management

Cytological methods allow frequent monitoring of intragraft events in organ transplantation. FNA cytology can be performed daily if necessary, without risk to the graft or to the patient. Monitoring of the cytological and immunological sequence of events gives a dynamic picture of the progress of the graft and makes it possible to evaluate the effect of immunosuppressive treatment on the transplant.

The main limitation of the method is that cytology does not allow evaluation of the architectural structures of the transplant. Therefore, acute cellular rejection can be diagnosed

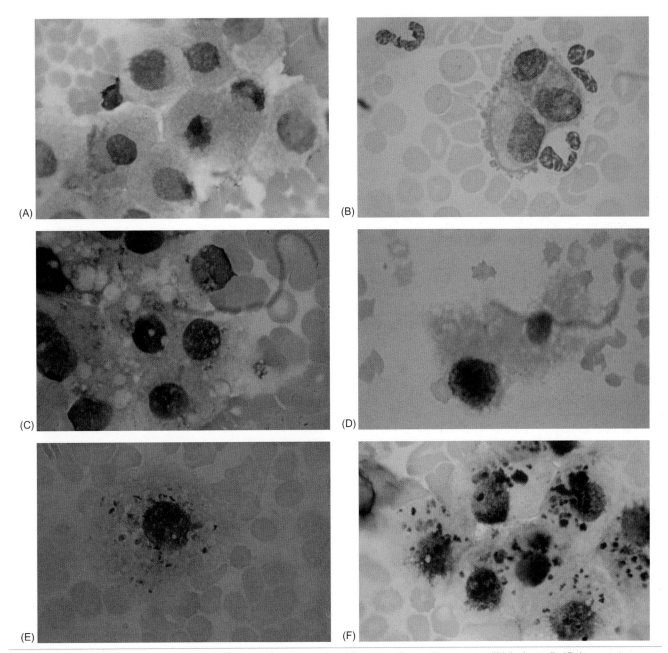

**Fig. 15.3** Liver parenchymal cells in Giemsa-stained cytocentrifuge preparations: (A) a group of normal hepatocytes; (B) bile duct cells; (C) degenerative changes in hepatocytes during rejection; (D) necrotic liver parenchymal cells; (E) fine isometric vacuolation in a hepatocyte during high dose CyA treatment; (F) accumulation of bile in hepatocytes indicating cholestasis.

with certainty, and in renal transplants, the identification of normal grafts or the presence of acute tubular necrosis or acute cyclosporin toxicity can be made. The most important conditions, in which cytology can only be suggestive, are acute vascular rejection in kidney transplants, chronic rejection, chronic cyclosporin toxicity and recurrent or de novo diseases in the transplant.

In liver transplantation, FNA cytology is a reliable method for diagnosing the immune activation of acute rejection. It also reveals cholestasis and parenchymal damage associated either with rejection or with biliary or vascular complications during the first months after transplantation. However, biopsy histology is desirable to confirm the results. The diagnosis of chronic rejection and other late complications is based on histology only. In addition to the diagnostic purposes the FNA technology has been applied in the scientific studies on mechanisms of intragraft immunological events.

In all transplant cytology, including pancreatic and lung transplantation, as well as liver and renal transplants, the cytopathologist is a vital part of the clinical team and should participate in the multidisciplinary team meetings. This ensures a full understanding between the clinicians and the pathologist, with maximum benefits to all including the patient.

# REFERENCES

1. Franzen S, Giertz G, Zaijcek J. Cytological diagnosis of prostatic tumors by transrectal aspiration biopsy. Br J Urol 1960;32:193–96.

2. Pasternack A. Fine-needle aspiration biopsy of human renal homografts. Lancet 1968;ii:82–84.

3. von Willebrand E, Häyry P. Composition and *in vitro* cytotoxicity of cellular infiltrates in rejecting human kidney allografts. Cell Immunol 1978;41:358–72.

4. von Willebrand E. Fine needle aspiration cytology of human renal transplants. Clin Immunol Immunopathol 1980;17:309–22.

5. Lautenschlager I, Höckerstedt K, Taskinen E, et al. Fine-needle aspiration cytology of liver allografts in pig. Transplantation 1984;38:330–34.

6. Lautenschlager I, Höckerstedt K, von Willebrand E, et al. Aspiration cytology of human liver allograft. Transplant Proc 1984;16:1243–46.

7. Häyry P, von Willebrand E. Practical guidelines for fine needle aspiration biopsy of human renal allografts. Ann of Clin Res 1981;13:288–306.

8. Belitsky P, Gupta R, Campbell J. Diagnosis of acute cellular rejection in kidney allografts by fine needle aspiration cytology. Transplant Proc 1984;16:1076–79.

9. von Willebrand E, Häyry P. Reproducibility of the fine needle aspiration biopsy. Analysis of 93 double biopsies. Transplantation 1984;38:314–16.

10. Belitsky P, Campbell J, Gupta R. Serial biopsy controlled evaluation of fine needle aspiration in renal allograft rejection. Lab Invest 1985;53:580–85.

11. Saksela E, Timonen T, Rank A, et al. Morphological and functional characterisation of isolated effector cells responsible for human natural killer cell activity to fetal fibroblasts and to cultured cell line targets. Immunol Rev 1979;44:71–123.

12. Lautenschlager I, von Willebrand E, Häyry P. Blood eosinophilia, steroids and rejection. Transplantation 1985;40:354–57.

13. von Willebrand E, Zola H, Häyry P. Thrombocyte aggregates in renal allografts. Analysis by the fine needle aspiration biopsy and monoclonal anti-thrombocyte antibodies. Transplantation 1985;39:258–62.

14. von Willebrand E, Lautenschlager I, Inkinen K, et al. Distribution of the major histocompatibility complex antigens in human and rat kidney. Kidney Int 1985;27:616–21.

15. von Willebrand E, Häyry P. Cyclosporin A deposits in renal allografts. Lancet 1983;ii:189–92.

16. Egidi F, De Vecchi A, Pagliari B, et al. Lack of relationship between blood cyclosporine levels and nephrotoxicity as assessed by fine needle aspiration biopsy of renal allografts. Transplant Proc 1985;17:2096–97.

17. Whiting PH, Thomson AW, Blair JT, et al. Experimental cyclosporin A nephrotoxicity. Br J Pathol 1982;63:88–94.

18. Hughes DA, Rapoport J, Roake JA, et al. Confirmation of renal allograft infarction using fine-needle aspiration cytology. In: Yussim A, Hammer C, editors. Contributions to Transplantation Medicine: Transplant Monitoring. Berlin: Wolfgang Pabst Verlag; 1992. p. 52–56.

19. von Willebrand E. Long-term experience with fine needle aspiration in kidney transplant patients. Transplant Proc 1989;21:3568–70.

20. Reinholt FP, Bohman S-O, Wilczek H, et al. Fine needle aspiration cytology and conventional histology in 200 renal allografts. Transplantation 1990;49:910–12.

21. Helderman JH, Hernandez J, Sagalowsky A, et al. Confirmation of the utility of fine needle aspiration biopsy of the renal allograft. Kidney Int 1988;34:376–81.

22. Häyry P, von Willebrand E. Transplant aspiration cytology. Transplantation 1984;38:7–12.

23. Salmela K, von Willebrand E, Kyllönen L, et al. Acute vascular rejection in renal transplantation, diagnosis and outcome. Transplantation 1992;54:858–62.

24. Cooksey G, Reeve RS, Wenham PW, et al. Comparison of fine needle aspiration cytology with histology in the diagnosis of renal allograft rejection. In: Kreis H, Droz D, editors Renal Transplant Cytology. Milan: Wichtig Editore; 1984. p. 73–78.

25. Reeve RS, Cooksey G, Wenham PW, et al. A comparison of fine needle aspiration cytology and Tru-Cut tissue biopsy in the diagnosis of acute renal allograft rejection. Nephron 1986;42:68–71.

26. von Willebrand E, Salmela K, Isoniemi H, et al. Induction of HLA class II antigen and interleukin 2 receptor expression in acute vascular rejection of human kidney allografts. Transplantation 1992;53:1077–81.

27. Isoniemi H, Ahonen J, Eklund B, et al. Renal allograft immunosuppression: early inflammatory and rejection episodes in triple drug treatment compared to double drug combinations or cyclosporin monotherapy. Transplant Int 1990;3:92–97.

28. Häyry P, von Willebrand E, Ahonen J, et al. Effects of cyclosporine, azathioprine and steroids on the renal transplant, on the cytological patterns of intra-graft inflammation and on concomitant rejection-associated changes in the recipient blood. Transplant Proc 1988;20:153–62.

29. Wood RFM, Bolton EM, Thompson JF, et al. Monoclonal antibodies and fine needle aspiration cytology in detecting renal allograft rejection. Lancet 1982;ii:278.

30. von Willebrand E. OKT 4/8 ratio in the blood and in the graft during episodes of human allograft rejection. Cell Immunol 1983;77:196–201.

31. Bolton EM, Thompson JF, Wood RF, et al. Immunoperoxidase staining of fine needle aspiration biopsies and needle core biopsies from renal allografts. Transplantation 1983;36:728–31.

32. Cooksey G, Reeve RS, Paterson AD, et al. Lymphocyte subpopulations in cytologic aspirates from human renal allografts. Transplant Proc 1985;17:630–32.

33. Hughes DA, Kempson MG, Carter NP, et al. Immunogoldsilver/Romanowsky staining: simultaneous immunocytochemical and morphological analysis of fine-needle aspirate biopsies. Transplant Proc 1988;20:575–76.

34. Lautenschlager I, von Willebrand E, Häyry P. Does T4 predominance in the graft signify severe rejection? Transplant Proc 1986;18:1311–13.

35. von Willebrand E, Häyry P. Relationship between cellular and molecular markers on inflammation in human kidney allograft rejection. Transplant Proc 1987;19:1644–45.

36. Hall BM, Duggin GG, Philips J, et al. Increased expression of HLA-DR antigens on renal tubular cells in renal transplants: relevance to the rejection response. Lancet 1984;ii:247–51.

37. Fuggle SV, McWhinnie DL, Chapman JR, et al. Sequential analysis of HLA-class II antigen expression in human renal allografts. Induction of tubular class II antigens and correlation with clinical parameters. Transplantation 1986;42:144–50.

38. Häyry P, von Willebrand E. The influence of the pattern of inflammation and administration of steroids on class II MHC antigen expression in renal transplants. Transplantation 1986;42:358–63.

39. Bishop GA, Hall BM. Expression of leucocyte and lymphocyte adhesion molecules in the human kidney. Kidney Int 1989;36:1078–85.

40. von Willebrand E, Loginov R, Salmela K, et al. Relationship between intercellular adhesion molecule-1 and HLA class II expression in acute cellular rejection of human kidney allografts. Transplant Proc 1993;25:870–71.

41. Savikko J, Kallio E, von Willebrand E. Early induction of platelet-derived growth factor ligands and receptors in acute rat renal allograft rejection. Transplantation 2001;72:31–37.

42. Hammer C. Diagnosis of inflammatory events. In: Hammer C, editor. Cytology in Transplantation. West Germany: Verlag RS Schulz; 1989. p. 127–54.

43. von Willebrand E, Lautenschlager I, Ahonen J. Cellular activation in the graft and in the blood during CMV disease. Transplant Proc 1989;21:2080–81.

44. von Willebrand E, Pettersson E, Ahonen J, et al. CMV infection, class II antigen expression, and human kidney allograft rejection. Transplantation 1986;42:364–67.

45. Van der Bij W, Toresma R, van Son WJ, et al. Rapid immunodiagnosis of active cytomegalovirus infection by monoclonal antibody staining of blood leucocytes. J Med Virol 1988;25:179–88.

46. Droz D, Campos H, Noel LH, et al. Renal transplant fine needle aspiration cytology: correlations to renal histology. In: Kreis H, Droz D, editors Renal Transplant Cytology. Milan: Wichtig Editore; 1984. p. 59–65.

47. Koller C, Hammer C, Gokel JM, et al. Correlation between core biopsy and aspiration cytology. Transplant Proc 1984;16:1298–300.

48. Egidi F, De Vecchi A, Banfi G, et al. Comparison of renal biopsy and fine needle aspiration biopsy in renal transplantation. Transplant Proc 1985;17:61–63.

49. Gupta R, Campbell J, Om A, et al. Serial monitoring of cellular rejection by simultaneous histology and fine needle aspiration cytology. Transplant Proc 1985;17:2123–24.

50. Hughes DA, McWhinnie DL, Sutton R, et al. Can incremental scoring of fine-needle aspirates predict histopathologic renal allograft rejection? Transplant Proc 1988;20:690–91.

51. Gray DWR, Richardson A, Hughes D, et al. A prospective, randomized, blind comparison of three biopsy techniques in the management of patients after renal transplantation. Transplantation 1992;53:1226–32.

52. Solez K, Axelsen RA, Benediktsson H, et al. International standardisation of criteria for the histologic diagnosis of renal allograft rejection: The Banff working classification of kidney transplant pathology. Kidney Int 1993;44:411–22.

53. Their M, von Willebrand E, Taskinen E, et al. Fine-needle aspiration biopsy allows early

detection of acute rejection in children after renal transplantation. Transplantation 2001;71:736–43.

54. Lautenschlager I, Höckerstedt K, Taskinen E, et al. Fine-needle aspiration biopsy in the monitoring of liver allografts I. Correlation between aspiration biopsy and core biopsy in experimental pig liver allografts. Transplantation 1988;46:41–46.

55. Vogel W, Margreiter R, Schmalzl F, et al. Preliminary results with fine needle aspiration biopsy in liver grafts. Transplant Proc 1984;16:1240–42.

56. Lautenschlager I, Höckerstedt K, Ahonen J, et al. Fine-needle aspiration biopsy in the monitoring of liver allografts II. Applications to human allografts. Transplantation 1988;46:47–52.

57. Hammerer P, Kraemer-Hansen H, Kremer B, et al. Aspiration cytology of liver transplants. Transplant Proc 1988;20:640–41.

58. Höckerstedt K, Lautenschlager I, Ahonen J, et al. Diagnosis of rejection in liver transplantation. J Hepatol 1988;2:217–21.

59. Greene CL, Fehrman I, Tillery GW, et al. Liver transplant aspiration cytology is a useful tool for identifying and monitoring allograft rejection. Transplant Proc 1988;20:657–58.

60. Kirby RM, Young JA, Hubscher SG, et al. The accuracy of aspiration cytology in the diagnosis of rejection following orthotopic liver transplantation. Transplant Int 1988;1:119–26.

61. Carbonnel F, Samuel D, Reynes M, et al. Fine needle aspiration biopsy of human liver allografts. Correlation with liver histology for the diagnosis of acute rejection. Transplantation 1990;50:704–7.

62. Schlitt J, Nashan B, Krick P, et al. Intragraft immune events after human liver transplantation. Correlation with clinical signs of acute rejection and influence of immunosuppression. Transplantation 1992;54:273–78.

63. Loderova A, Honsova E, Trunecka P, et al. Correlation of FNAB with histology in human liver allografts. Regional experience. Ann Transplant 2001;6:37–40.

64. Kwekkeboom J, Zondervan PE, Kuijpers MA, et al. Fine-needle aspiration cytology in the diagnosis of acute rejection after liver transplantation. Brit J Surg 2003;90:246–47.

65. Lautenschlager I, Höckerstedt K, Häyry P. Fine-needle aspiration biopsy in the monitoring of liver allografts. Review. Transplant Int 1991;4:54–61.

66. Their M, Lautenschlager I, von Willebrand E, et al. The use of fine-needle aspiration biopsy in detection of acute rejection in children after liver transplantation. Transplant Int 2002;15:240–47.

67. Banff schema for grading liver allograft rejection: an international consensus document. Hepatology 1997; 25:658–663.

68. Neuberger J, Adams DH. What is the significance of acute liver allograft rejection? J Hepatol 1998;29:143–50.

69. Schlitt HJ, Nashan B, Ringe B, et al. Differentiation of liver graft dysfunction by transplant aspiration cytology. Transplantation 1991;51:786–92.

70. Lautenschlager I, Höckerstedt K, Häyry P. Activation markers in acute liver allograft rejection. Transplant Proc 1988;20:646–47.

71. Zannier A, Faure JL, Neidecker J, et al. Monitoring of liver allografts using fine-needle aspiration biopsy: value of hepatocyte MHC-DR expression in the diagnosis of acute rejection. Transplant Proc 1987;19:3810–11.

72. Vogel W, Wohlfahrter P, Then P, et al. Longitudinal study of major histocompatibility complex antigen expression on hepatocytes in fine-needle aspiration biopsies from human liver grafts. Transplant Proc 1988;20:648–49.

73. Lautenschlager I, Höckerstedt K. ICAM-1 induction on hepatocytes as a marker for immune activation of acute liver allograft rejection. Transplantation 1993;56:1495–99.

74. Lautenschlager I, Höckerstedt K. Induction of ICAM-1 on hepatocytes precedes the lymphoid activation of acute liver allograft rejection and cytomegalovirus infection. Transplant Proc 1993;25:1429–30.

75. Steinhoff G, Wonigeit K, Pichlmayer R. Induction of ICAM-1 on hepatocyte membranes during liver allograft rejection and infection. Transplant Proc 1990;22:2308–9.

76. Höckerstedt K, Lautenschlager I, Ahonen J, et al. Differentiation between acute rejection and infection in liver transplant patients. Transplant Proc 1989;21:2317–18.

77. Lautenschlager I, Höckerstedt K, Salmela K, et al. Fine-needle aspiration biopsy (FNAB) in the monitoring of liver allografts; different cellular findings during rejection and CMV infection. Transplantation 1990;50:798–803.

78. Lautenschlager I, Höckerstedt K, Linnavuori K, et al. Human herpesvirus-6 infection after liver transplantation. Clin Infect Dis 1998;26:702–7.

79. Lautenschlager I, Nashan B, Schlitt HJ, et al. Different cellular patterns associated with hepatitis C virus reactivation, cytomegalovirus infection and acute rejection in liver transplant patients monitored with transplant aspiration cytology. Transplantation 1994;58:1339–45.

80. Ciardi A, Pecorella I, Rossi M, et al. Morphologic features in liver transplantation. Transplant Proc 1988;20:637–39.

81. Lautenschlager I, Nashan B, Schlitt HJ, et al. Early intragraft inflammatory events of liver allografts ending up with chronic rejection. Transplant Int 1995;8:446–51.

82. Kiuchi T, Schlitt HJ, Oldhafder KJ, et al. Backgrounds of early intragraft immune activation and rejection in liver transplant recipients. Impact of graft reperfusion quality. Transplantation 1995;60:49–55.

83. Martelius T, Mäkisalo H, Höckerstedt K, et al. A rat model of monitoring liver allograft rejection. Transplant Int 1997;10:103–8.

84. Martelius T, Salaspuro V, Salmi M, et al. Blockade of vascular adhesion protein-1 inhibits lymphocyte infiltration in rat liver allograft rejection. Am J Pathol 2004;165:1993–2001.

85. Lautenschlager I, Höckerstedt K, Meri S. Complement membrane attack complex and protectin (CD59) in liver allografts during acute rejection. J Hepatol 1999;31:537–54.

86. Kuijf ML, Kwekkeboom J, Kuijpers MA, et al. Granzyme expression in fine-needle aspirates from liver allografts is increased during acute rejection. Liver Transpl 2002;8:952–56.

87. Demirkiran A, Baan CC, Kok A, et al. Intrahepatic detection of FOXP3 gene expression after liver transplantation using minimally invasive aspiration biopsy. Transplantation 2007;83:819–23.

# Immunosuppression

Martin Young and Robert Miller

**Box 16.1  Conditions causing immune suppression**

AIDS (human immunodeficiency virus infection)

Chemotherapy

Steroid therapy

• Organ transplantation
• Collagen vascular diseases

Malignant disease

• Leukaemia
• Lymphoma
• Hodgkin lymphoma
• Myeloma

Congenital immunodeficiency syndromes

## Introduction

Immunosuppression is seen in a diverse group of patients as a result of a number of unrelated aetiologies. The underlying causes, shown in Box 16.1, include:

• HIV infection (presenting ultimately with acquired immunodeficiency syndrome – AIDS)
• Neoplastic disease, typically involving the bone marrow (leukaemia, lymphoma, Hodgkin lymphoma and metastatic disease)
• Organ transplant recipients and treated collagen diseases (medical immunosuppression)
• Congenital immunodeficiency syndromes.

This wide group of patients can present with a similar range of diseases which can be rapidly progressive, occurring in potentially very sick individuals. Illness in immunosuppressed individuals may be atypical in clinical presentation and not infrequently multifactorial. Under these circumstances speedy diagnosis can be life-saving; cytological investigation may provide invaluable clues towards diagnosis and subsequent management. AIDS accounts for a high percentage of immunosuppressed individuals and there are increasing numbers of immunosuppressed patients following medical treatment, such as organ transplantation.

In recent years, the clinical course of HIV infection in Europe, North America and Australasia has changed. Several factors are responsible for this, including an improved understanding of disease pathogenesis, the increasing use of prophylaxis against opportunistic infections and combination antiretroviral therapy (cART). Among populations with access to prophylaxis and cART there has been a significant reduction in AIDS-defining events due to opportunistic infections, hospital admissions, and all-cause HIV-associated mortality. Patients without access to these therapeutic interventions continue to present with advanced immunosuppression and with a variety of opportunistic infections and malignancies. This scenario continues to apply to many sub-Saharan and Asian populations among whom, for political and economic reasons, the HIV pandemic continues unabated. Following the introduction of cART in 1996, patients who are able to tolerate it live longer, have a dramatically lower incidence of opportunistic infections and Kaposi's sarcoma but remain at high risk of malignancy. This is reflected in a relative increase in AIDS-related malignancy, such as non-Hodgkin lymphoma.[1] Additionally, non-AIDS defining malignancies, including Hodgkin lymphoma and lung cancer, are observed with greater frequency than in the general population.[2]

This chapter specifically addresses the role of cytopathology in the management of patients with immunosuppression. However, the diagnostic problems encountered in such cases may also arise when there is no known background of immunodeficiency. The initial approach to diagnosis is similar in these patients, although the long-term management is likely to be different. It should not be forgotten that cytological examination is but one of many investigations and all findings should be discussed within a multidisciplinary team context.

## Technical aspects

The nature of the specimen relates to the clinical problem to be investigated.

## Bronchoalveolar lavage (BAL) and induced sputum (IS)

Respiratory problems are likely to be investigated by means of bronchoalveolar lavage, bronchial washings or induced sputum (see Ch. 2). These liquid samples are typically processed as cytospins, or possibly as ThinPrep (Hologic®) preparations depending on local practice. Rigorous attention should be paid to obtaining induced sputum samples. The patient should starve for several hours before the procedure, as it may provoke nausea and or vomiting. The patient should clean their mouth using a toothbrush and sterile water, then gargle using sterile water. This is to remove oral debris that may contaminate the sample. Expectoration is induced by 15–20 min inhalation of a mist of 3% saline from an ultrasonic nebuliser. Specimens are collected in sterile plastic containers for both cytology and microbiology. For diagnosis of *Pneumocystis* pneumonia (PCP), the highest yield is from specimens that are clear, and which resemble saliva; purulent specimens suggest PCP and/or a bacterial infection.

For BAL, a large volume (80–240 mL) of sterile saline is instilled in aliquots of 20–80 mL; aliquots are sequentially instilled and aspirated. Most clinicians collect the pooled 'return' and divide it up, with samples being sent for cytological, microbiological (including mycobacterial) and virological evaluation. Processing in the cytology laboratory is by standard techniques[3] but strict attention to safety precautions is mandatory. Because of the wide range of possible diagnoses and since more than one disease process may coexist, material should be stained by the Papanicolaou (PAP), Ziehl Neelsen (ZN) and Grocott methods and additional slides prepared and retained for May-Grünwald Giemsa (MGG), Gram, Perl's, immunocytochemistry or other special techniques.

## Lymph nodes

Enlarged lymph nodes or other solid lesions can be examined by means of fine needle aspiration (FNA) (see Ch. 13). If the lesion is small or deep seated the aspiration may be performed under ultrasound guidance. The sample may consist of direct spreads and liquid preparations taken from needle rinse samples according to local practice. Liquid samples are particularly important as they can be used for the preparation of further cytospins and/or cell block preparations for additional investigations such as flow cytometry, immunocytochemistry and *in situ* hybridisation. The FNA technique is straightforward and has been described elsewhere.[4] The capillary technique (without suction), using a 23G needle is recommended, A 20 mL syringe is usually attached in case of fluid samples to prevent spillage.

## Cerebrospinal fluid (CSF)

CSF is usually obtained following lumbar puncture for investigation of neurological disease. The volumes vary from 1 to 10 mL. The sample is typically prepared as a cytospin preparation and stained according to the methods of PAP and MGG. Additional special stains for fungi and other infective agents should be performed and ancillary studies including flow cytometry may be helpful. For further details please refer to Chapter 34.

## Health and safety issues

Health and safety precautions should be strictly observed with the use of protective gloves, masks, aprons and protective eye wear. Care should be taken when removing the needle; it is not recommended to re-sheath the needle before disposing of it. Instead it should be immediately placed together with the syringe in a suitable sharps container. It is important to follow local guidelines for decontamination and disposal of contaminated material with careful hand washing after the procedure. When taking FNA samples, a needle stick injury is a rare but significant hazard associated with this procedure. The risk of acquiring HIV infection following a percutaneous (needle-stick) exposure to HIV from a patient with known HIV infection in a healthcare setting is approximately 3/1000 injuries. Post-exposure prophylaxis (PEP) is recommended by both the Chief Medical Officers' Expert Advisory Group on AIDS in the UK and by the United States Public Health Service in the USA, if a healthcare worker has had a significant occupational exposure (from blood/other body fluid from a patient known to be HIV infected, or determined to be at high risk of HIV infection).[1,2] PEP should be started as soon as possible after the exposure (ideally within 1 hour) and continued for 28 days: PEP is not recommended beyond 72 hours post-exposure. The currently recommended regimen of PEP in the UK is Truvada (245 mg tenofovir and 200 mg emtricitabine [FTC], one tablet) OD and Kaletra [film coated tablets] (200 mg lopinavir and 50 mg ritonavir, two tablets) BD. In the UK, these recommendations are consistent with guidelines for PEP following non-occupational exposure to HIV.

# Opportunistic infection

## Bacterial infection

### Mycobacterial infection

Mycobacterial infection is strongly associated with immunosuppression. Worldwide HIV infection is the greatest risk factor for tuberculosis. Additionally immune suppressed patients are more likely to present with clinically significant infection with 'atypical' mycobacteria, which are rarely encountered as clinically important pathogens in the immune competent. This is exemplified by *Mycobacterium avium-intracellulare* (MAI), also known as *M. avium* complex (MAC), which in the context of profound HIV-associated immune suppression (CD4 count <100), may result in a disseminated infection. MAI may be identified by cytological examination of sputum, bronchoalveolar lavage fluid and lymph node FNA, by histological examination of liver, bone marrow and by culture of the above and of blood (Figs 16.1, 16.2).

### Cytological findings: MAI infection

- Little granulomatous reaction
- Epithelioid cells, giant cells or evidence of caseation are unlikely
- Numerous 'foamy' macrophages (filled with mycobacteria with ZN staining).

Patients who have recently commenced cART and who have an atypical mycobacterial infection, the so-called cART induced immune reconstitution inflammatory syndrome (IRIS) may confound the cytopathologist, as inflammatory responses may be modified, such that granulomatous response may be observed in response to *M. xenopi*, *M. kansasii* and MAC.[5] The organisms can also be visualised with MGG, Grocott and periodic acid-Schiff (PAS) stains. Culture is necessary to distinguish MAI from mycobacterium tuberculosis (MTB). More recently, the use of so-called Papanicolaou induced fluorescence (PIF) has been described to detect acid fast bacilli in Papanicolaou-stained preparations.[6]

*Mycobacterium* tuberculosis (MTB) occurs in persons other than immune suppressed, lung and lymph nodes being the commonest sites, although other organs are also affected. An account of the FNA diagnosis of 574 non-immunosuppressed cases is given by Das et al.[7] Evidence of epithelioid granulomata without necrosis was seen in 31.5% of FNAs and granulomata with necrosis in 31.9%. In the remaining cases (36.6%), the material consisted of acellular caseous debris. The sensitivity of FNA for diagnosing TB in the lymph nodes in other studies has been 62%, 38% of cases being false negative. Acid fast bacilli are found in less than half of the cases with classical morphology. In addition, morphology of mycobacterial infection in HIV-positive patients, particularly

those receiving antiretroviral treatment, may be altered and may not show typical granulomata and necrosis. Instead, an appearance of abscess, with prominent acute inflammation, may be present. In all cases of suspected mycobacterial infection and negative ZN stain, microbiological confirmation is required before treatment. Moreover, acid fast staining has been described in *Legionella pneumophila*.[8]

Respiratory disease remains the commonest clinical presentation in the imm|unosuppressed and the clinical distinction of *Pneumocystis jiroveci*, the causative agent for *Pneumocystis* pneumonia (PCP) from other fungal or bacterial infection is sometimes difficult. Extrapulmonary disease and disseminated MTB are not uncommon, and are frequently associated with lymphadenopathy, when FNA may be diagnostic.[9]

## Other bacterial infections

*Staphylococcus aureus, Haemophilus pneumoniae, Streptococcus pneumoniae, Pseudomonas aeruginosa* and *Legionella pneumophila* are all causes of pulmonary infection in immunosuppressed patients. In lung-allografted patients, such bacterial infections are a particular problem as those transplanted for cystic fibrosis may be colonized with multiple resistant *Pseudomonas aeruginosa* and *Burkholderia cepacia*.[10] None is amenable to cytological identification but must be considered in the differential diagnosis of pneumonia especially in cases where BAL is cytologically non-diagnostic. *Nocardia* can be morphologically recognised in BAL fluid,[11] but is uncommon (see Ch. 2).

## Viral infection

### Cytomegalovirus (Fig. 16.3)

Cytomegalovirus (CMV) is a DNA virus of the herpes virus group. It is a widely distributed opportunistic infectious agent in all classes of immunocompromised persons, particularly those with AIDS and organ transplant recipients, and usually presents with visceral manifestations, especially of the lung, brain, eye and gastrointestinal tract. CMV interstitial pneumonitis seen in bone marrow transplant patients is particularly aggressive compared with its counterpart in HIV infection[12]

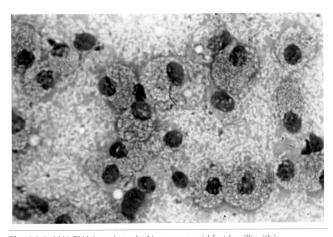

**Fig. 16.1** MAI: FNA lymph node. Numerous acid fast bacilli within macrophages (ZN).

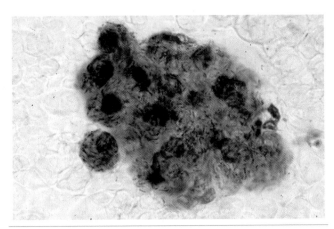

**Figure 16.2** MAI: FNA lymph node. Staining appearance of bacilli with MGG.

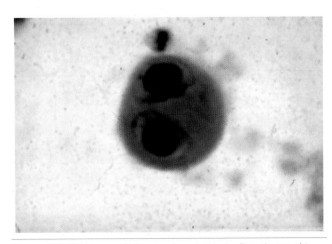

**Figure 16.3** CMV: Large cell showing characteristic 'owl's eye' cytopathic effect. BAL fluid (PAP).

and is associated with a high mortality rate.[13] It is the most common cause of opportunistic infection in lung allograft recipients in the 4–8 week postoperative period.[14] Indeed, in those who survive for two weeks or more, the prevalence of CMV infection may exceed 75%.[15] However, it is not always associated with a pneumonitis. PCR on BAL fluid and peripheral blood is a sensitive method of detecting active infection, but together with cytological investigations cannot distinguish between simple and pathological infection.

Among HIV-infected patients with *Pneumocystis jiroveci* pneumonia, CMV may be detected in bronchoalveolar lavage fluid or induced sputum. However, unless there is cytopathological evidence of active infection (intra-cytoplasmic and into nuclear inclusions) – this is often not clinically significant. By contrast, identification of CMV in these samples from a patient immunosuppressed following an organ transplant frequently has clinical significance. Culture of CMV for diagnostic purposes is slow and expensive and estimation of serological titres is not particularly helpful and has been superseded by PCR on blood, fluid and sputum (see Ch. 34). Early diagnosis and aggressive treatment improve survival.[16]

Identification of the characteristic viral cytopathic effects by light microscopy of histological or cytological material from the respiratory or gastrointestinal tract still provides the most rapid and certain means of diagnosis.[17–19]

## Cytological findings: CMV infection

- Papanicolaou-stained material: round or oval basophilic intranuclear inclusions, each surrounded by a clear halo due to margination of chromatin
- BAL fluid: pathognomonic 'owl's eye' viral inclusions can be identified in pneumocytes and macrophages
- Granular, occasionally eosinophilic, small inclusions sometimes seen in the cytoplasm.

Similar cells indicative of CMV oesophagitis have been identified in oesophageal brushings[20] and in FNA from the salivary glands.[21] Sensitivity of detection of CMV is enhanced by special techniques such as monoclonal antibody studies,[22] *in situ* hybridisation[23] and PCR, which is now a routine investigation in clinical practice.[24] *In situ* hybridisation has been successfully carried out on decolourised Papanicolaou-stained slides.[25]

### Herpes simplex and Herpes zoster

Recurrent *Herpes simplex* virus (HSV) types I and II infections are very troublesome to the immune suppressed, but are seldom life threatening. Mucocutaneous oral and facial lesions, oesophageal and cervical infection in women and anorectal involvement in homosexual men present similar clinical features to *H. simplex* infection in non-immunocompromised persons. In the earlier years of heart lung transplantation, 10% of patients were found to develop HSV pneumonia and ulcerative tracheobronchitis, but this has been minimised more recently by the introduction of prophylactic antiviral therapy with Acyclovir.[26,27] In the context of HIV infection, HSV is a very rare cause of pneumonitis (see Ch. 2).

## Cytological findings: Herpes simplex

- Multiple, moulded, 'ground glass' nuclei in squamous epithelial cells from any site including cervical smears, scrapings from cutaneous vesicles and oesophageal brushings
- Large bizarre multinucleated squamous cells can be found in sputum or bronchial brushings in herpetic tracheobronchitis.

The classical multiple moulded nuclei are particularly a feature of infections of squamous epithelium. Diagnosis by morphological appearance alone is therefore difficult on routine staining of BAL fluid. Additional investigation such as *in situ* hybridisation is helpful in suspected cases.[28]

Skin lesions due to *Herpes zoster* follow a dermatomal distribution and seldom present a clinical diagnostic problem. Scrapings from the vesicles contain the characteristic multinucleated squamous cells.

## Other viral infections

Both Epstein-Barr virus (EBV) and human papillomavirus (HPV) are associated with the condition of hairy leukoplakia, which produces a pearly-white raised lesion on the underside and lateral surface of the tongue.[29] Oesophageal lesions are also possible. Koilocytosis and herpetic-type nuclear inclusions are reported to occur. EBV is also associated with post-transplant lymphoproliferative disorders and possibly other malignant tumours, such as gastric carcinoma. The cytomorphological features are no different to those described in non-immunosuppressed individuals.

It is well established that genital HPV infection is linked with cervical pre-neoplasia and cervical cancer in women and anorectal and penile carcinoma in immunosuppressed men. Women who are immunosuppressed due to infection by HIV have a higher incidence and grade of cervical pre-cancer.[30] Pre-cancer in immunosuppressed men also follows a more aggressive course.[31] In a prospective cohort study Ellerbrock et al. reported that 20% of HIV-positive participants developed squamous intraepithelial lesion (SIL) compared with 5% of HIV-negative matched controls over a 30 month follow-up (incidence of 8.3 and 1.8 cases per 100 person-years, respectively).[32] It is interesting that enrolment in a well-managed cervical screening programme, such as the UK-NHSCSP, with contemporaneous access to cART, is associated with an incidence of invasive carcinoma no different from a non-HIV-positive cohort (see Chs 23, 25).[33]

Intranuclear inclusions due to *Polyoma virus* may occasionally be identified in exfoliated cells in urine from immunosuppressed patients, particularly transplant recipients. These are sometimes referred to as 'decoy' cells and can be mistaken for carcinoma-in-situ change (Fig. 16.4). JC virus (JCV) carries little clinical significance but BK viral infection is more likely to cause a viral nephropathy which can compromise graft survival.[34] In some units, urine cytology is employed as a means to detect recurrence of polyoma BK virus (BKV) infection with consequent modulation of the degree of immunosuppression.[35] Nested PCR is the most reliable means of diagnosis of polyoma virus in the urine and molecular biology remains the only means of distinguishing BK virus and JCV.[36]

*Hepatitis B* and *C* recurrent viral infections are common, especially in liver transplant patients allografted for *hepatitis B* (HBV) and *hepatitis C* (HCV) disease. Currently, antiviral therapy including lamivudine and its analogues may be effective in recurrent HBV disease, but therapy is not available for recurrent HCV.

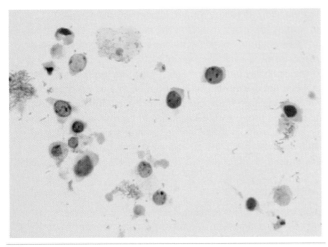

**Figure 16.4** Urine showing decoy cells from polyoma BK viral infection (PAP).

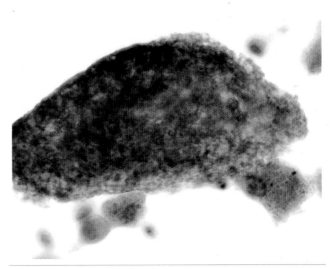

**Figure 16.5** PCP: Casts of PCP exudate showing outline of alveolus. Note foamy, honeycomb texture (PAP).

## Fungal infection

### *Pneumocystis* pneumonia (Figs 16.5, 16.6)

When it was first described, *Pneumocystis* was thought to be a protozoa and to be part of the life cycle of *Trypanosoma cruzi*. The organism is now known to be a fungus and it is apparent that different types of *Pneumocystis* infect individual hosts. The organism causing *Pneumocystis* pneumonia (PCP) in humans is now known as *Pneumocystis jiroveci*; the organism causing PCP in rats is called *P. carinii*. In populations with access to prophylaxis and or highly active antiretroviral therapy, PCP is now less frequently observed; presentation with PCP in the UK, N. America and Australasia largely occurs among patients unaware of their HIV serostatus, or who know their status but are unable or are unwilling to take prophylaxis and or cART.

Diagnosis of PCP requires demonstration of the organism from a clinically appropriate specimen, such as BAL fluid, hypertonic saline induced sputum, or lung tissue. Occasionally, *P. jiroveci* may be detected in sites other than the lung, e.g. head and neck lymph nodes, thyroid gland, pleural or ascitic fluid. Traditionally, detection of *P. jiroveci* in BAL fluid has been by light microscopy and routine stains such as Papanicolaou, Giemsa, Diff-Quik and Grocott (methenamine silver). Immunofluorescence staining may also be used. Despite the availability of specific prophylaxis and cART, PCP is the most common life-threatening opportunistic infection in HIV-infected individuals. Prior to the availability of cART, approximately 80% of patients had at least one episode of PCP. Recurrent disease is associated with a poor prognosis.[37] Among other immune suppressed groups, particularly transplant recipients, the incidence of PCP has been greatly reduced by the routine use of prophylactic trimethoprim-sulphamethoxazole.

Definitive diagnosis of PCP requires demonstration of *P. jiroveci* morphologically, as serological tests are not a reliable indicator of disease and culture of the organisms has not reliably been achieved. Diagnosis by cytological examination of induced sputum or bronchoalveolar lavage fluid is the technique of choice. Both methods of collection are safe, and cytology has the advantage of speed of assessment.

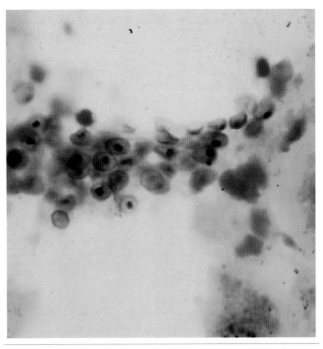

**Figure 16.6** PCP: Positive staining of cystic forms within alveolar cast (Grocott).

### Cytological findings: *Pneumocystis jiroveci*

- Characteristic foamy alveolar casts seen on Papanicolaou staining
- High-power examination of casts shows cystic forms with trophic forms giving a bubbly appearance to the exudate
- Grocott staining demonstrates cyst walls.

Examination of Papanicolaou-stained material is highly sensitive and specific for the detection of PCP, provided that lower respiratory tract sampling is adequate. The alveolar casts present can show a characteristic biphasic staining.[17,19] By focusing up and down on these casts, clear circular areas representing cystic forms of the organism and tiny dense staining specks indicative of the trophic form within are identifiable. With the Grocott stain, the walls of the cystic form stain black and characteristic clusters can be visualised within the casts.[18] Two 'mirror image' reniform structures are visible within intact cystic forms. Collapsed empty cystic forms are cup shaped. Fungal spores also stain with Grocott but they have thicker walls, may show budding and are not concentrated within foamy casts. The trophic forms of *P. jiroveci* stain weakly with Giemsa and Gram stains. Care should be taken not to over-interpret artefacts such as aggregates of red cells or air bubbles, as being PCP (Figs 16.7, 16.8).

The sensitivity of induced sputum examination using light microscopy is in the region of 56%.[38] Sensitivity of detection of PCP by BAL is higher, ranging from 79% to 98%.[39–41] Transbronchial biopsy (TBB) is now rarely performed in HIV-infected patients presenting with a pneumonitis and who undergo diagnostic bronchoscopy. The yield from TBB for PCP and other infections is equivalent to that from BAL and complications, including haemorrhage and pneumothorax occur with greater frequency in HIV-infected patients undergoing TBB, when compared with the general population. There is apparent overlap between qPCR results from patients with PCP and from those with other equally immune suppressed individuals with diagnoses other than PCP, e.g. bacterial pneumonia. This observation currently limits the diagnostic utility of qPCR.

Percutaneous FNA of the lungs also yields diagnostic material[42] but is generally considered to be associated with an unacceptable level of complications, especially pneumothorax.

In lung allograft recipients and other transplant patients, immunosuppression modifies the morphological response to PCP infection. Characteristically, there is a granulomatous response with small numbers of cystic forms, and so very few organisms may be seen on TBB.[43] If neither induced sputum nor BAL are diagnostic, open lung biopsy is an option. Imprint smears prepared from the tissue can be helpful and are quick to process, representing a useful technique when examination is required out of routine laboratory hours, provided trained staff are available to interpret the findings. Extrapulmonary dissemination of *P. jiroveci* is documented[44] but is very unusual.

## Candidosis

The commonest species (Fig. 16.9) are *Candida albicans, C. tropicalis* and *C. parapsilosis*. All appear similar morphologically and culture is necessary for speciation but *C. albicans* is encountered most frequently in clinical practice. Mucocutaneous and genital candidosis are widespread in the community and many healthy people harbour saprophytic oral *Candida* spp. Candidosis of the gastrointestinal,[45] respiratory and urinary tracts as well as disseminated infection occur in debilitated and immunosuppressed patients. Although invasive oesophageal candidosis is an indicator disease of AIDS and 'oral thrush' very common, systemic candidosis occurs in only a small percentage of cases. Invasive fungal infections, including candidosis, are among the most common life-threatening opportunistic infections in transplant recipients and in patients with leukaemia, lymphoma and allied conditions. Drug regimes that lead to bone marrow depletion or steroid and immunosuppressive drug therapy also predispose to invasive candidosis.

| **Cytological findings: candidosis** |
| --- |

- Small discrete oval spores
- Filamentous pseudohyphae
- No dichotomous branching or true septation (a useful distinguishing feature from aspergillus)
- Budding spores arising at points of constriction along the pseudohyphae are a helpful morphological feature.[19]

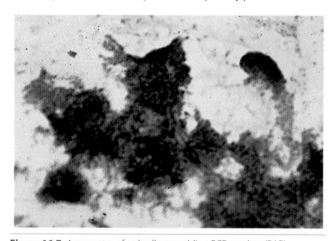

**Figure 16.7** Aggregates of red cells resembling PCP exudate (PAP).

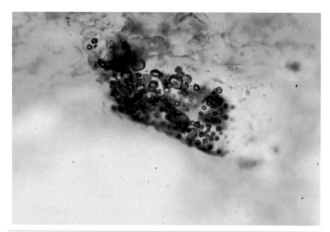

**Figure 16.8** Air artifact resembling PCP exudate (Grocott).

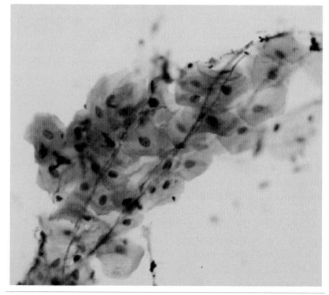

**Figure 16.9** Cytospin preparations from oesophageal brushings: filamentous pseudohyphae (PAP).

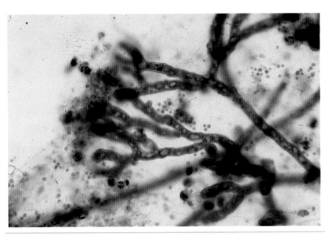

**Fig. 16.10** BAL fluid: *Aspergillus* spp. Grocott's methenamine silver-stained preparation in the bronchoalveolar lavage demonstrates *Aspergillus* fungi with septate hyphae and 45 degree branching.

## Aspergillus

*Aspergillus* spp. (Fig. 16.10) are responsible for several different forms of illness, including tracheobronchitis, bronchocentric granulomatosis, non-invasive aspergillosis (mycetoma) and invasive aspergillosis leading to pneumonia or abscess formation and granulomatous manifestations in any part of the body. Disseminated invasive infection is a potentially lethal complication of immunosuppression in transplant recipients and patients with lymphoma. It is relatively uncommon in AIDS. Clinically, *Aspergillus* infection may be a problem in lung-allografted patients, especially at the donor-recipient bronchial anastomosis, where ischaemic cartilage predisposes to invasion.[46]

*Aspergillus fumigatus*, *A. flavus* and *A. niger* are usually indistinguishable in cytological and histological preparations as the characteristic conidiophore vesicles are uncommonly present[47] and culture is necessary for speciation. *Aspergillus* is seldom a saprophyte and the finding of hyphae in sputum, BAL[47] or PCFNA[48,49] specimens is highly suggestive of clinical infection.

### Cytological findings: aspergillosis

- Hyphae of *Aspergillus* spp. are larger than those of *Candida* spp.
- Septate hyphae
- Dichotomous branching: two equal divisions at approximately 45 degrees.

## *Cryptococcus*

Infection with *Cryptococcus neoformans* (Figs 16.11, 16.12) generally presents with meningitis or pneumonitis but in disseminated disease, cryptococci can be identified in lymph nodes, genitourinary tract and liver. The gastrointestinal tract is very seldom involved. *Cryptococcus* can be detected in BAL fluid or sputum. The diagnosis can also be established from FNA of lymph nodes or from CSF, peripheral blood and even from skin biopsy. The use of mucicarmine staining or India ink may assist in the diagnosis in CSF specimens.[50] In patients who present with cryptococcal meningitis and who have recently commenced cART, there may be an over-exuberant inflammatory response in CSF, with both lymphocytes and plasma cells being identified, which may confound cytological diagnosis.

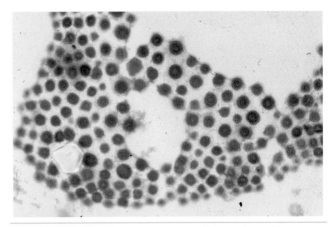

**Fig. 16.11** CSF *Cryptococcus*. Numerous yeast like organisms with magenta-stained capsule (mucicarmine).

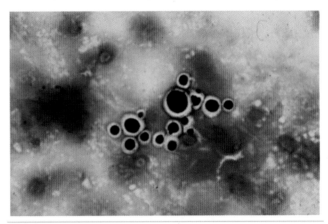

**Fig. 16.12** Sputum *Cryptococcus*. Pale translucent capsule (Grocott).

### Cytological findings: *Cryptococcus*

- Spherical budding yeasts
- Mucoid capsule, although non-encapsulated strains do occur, particularly in AIDS patients
- The capsule is pale and translucent with Papanicolaou[19,51] or MGG stains but a diagnostic bright magenta with Mayer's mucicarmine
- 'Central nuclei' stain with Grocott and periodic acid-Schiff.

Non-encapsulated forms can be mistaken for spores of *Candida* spp. The single buds are attached by a narrow isthmus to the parent cell, which distinguishes them from *Blastomyces dermatitidis*, in which the connection is broader. In cytological laboratories, cryptococci are most likely to be encountered in cerebrospinal fluid (CSF) or FNA of the lung.[51]

## Histoplasma

*Histoplasma capsulatum* is a dimorphic fungus, the yeast phase of which is the invasive form. Distribution is worldwide, but is most prevalent in the southern states of N. America and portions of Central and South America. Disseminated histoplasmosis (Fig. 16.13) may be due to reactivation of a latent infection as a result of the onset of immunocompromised status, or may arise from new acquisition. Many of the clinical features of the disease resemble tuberculosis. The yeast forms are

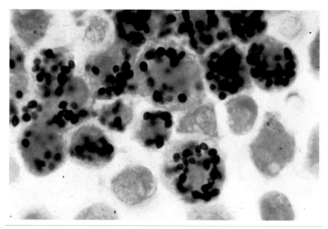

**Fig. 16.13** Histoplasma. Intracellular yeast forms within macrophages (BAL Gomori).

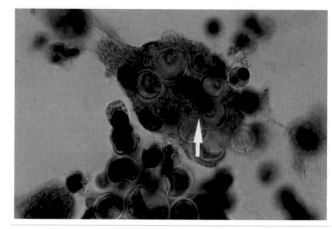

**Fig. 16.14** Paracoccidiomycosis. Large thick-walled cyst with endospores (arrow). Sputum (PAP).

intracellular and have been reported in alveolar macrophages in BAL,[52] in sputum[19] and in FNA of lymph nodes.[53]

## Other fungal Infections

Morphological identification of other types of fungi is possible from cytological material,[54] although precise speciation is not always feasible. Those described below are illustrated in Chapter 2.

The class *Zygomycetes* includes many genera, which are morphologically indistinguishable. All have broad non-septate hyphae, which stain lightly with Grocott and resemble 'tangled cellophane ribbons'. *Mucor* spp. is the commonest form.

*Blastomycosis* is very uncommon in Europe. Disseminated disease can occur in immune suppressed individuals, but is rare outside endemic areas – *Blastomyces dermatitidis* (N. America) and *B. brasiliensis* (S. America). The mother and daughter yeast cells of *B. dermatitidis* and *B. brasiliensis* are attached to each other by a broader base than those of *C. neoformans* (see Figs 2.41A, B, 2.37). *Paracoccidiodes brasiliensis* is a soil-borne fungus found mainly in south and central America and Mexico. Disseminated paracoccidioidomycosis occasionally follows pulmonary disease in non-immunosuppressed individuals but is uncommon in endemic areas. Acute paracoccidioidal pneumonia occurs in immunocompromised patients and is generally followed by disseminated infection. It is unlikely to be seen in Europe. Diagnosis is made by identification of large thick-walled spherules containing endospores (Figs 16.14, 16.15).[19,55]

## Parasitic infestation

### Toxoplasmosis

Infection with *Toxoplasma gondii* can present perinatally as a congenital infection or in childhood in the absence of immune suppression but otherwise is uncommon except in association with HIV infection or lymphoma and allied conditions. Infection can give rise to enlarged lymph nodes which typically show reactive lymphoid hyperplasia, clusters of epithelioid cells and many tingible body macrophages. The demonstration of toxoplasma pseudocysts by immunocytochemistry can be achieved by FNA.[56] The positive diagnosis of toxoplasma-related changes

(A)

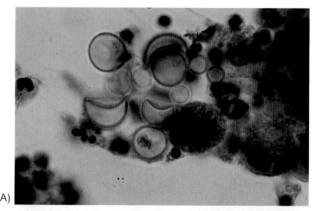

(B)

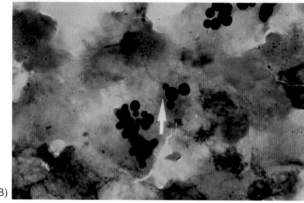

**Fig. 16.15** Paracoccidioidomycosis in bronchoalveolar lavage fluid: round yeasts, many of them with several peripheral buds fitting the pattern of *Paracoccidioides brasiliensis*. (A) PAP; (B) Grocott.

in lymph nodes also requires the exclusion of other causes of granulomatous lymphadenopathy. The central nervous system (CNS) is involved in most cases. Extracerebral *T. gondii* infection is unusual but disease in lungs, gastrointestinal tract, heart or other sites may be found at autopsy.[57] Toxoplasmosis was common in heart transplantation until the advent of prophylaxis. Since then it has become very rare. Diagnosis of cerebral toxoplasmosis is by identification of the characteristic cysts filled with tiny organisms in CSF, brain biopsy or stereotactic FNA material.[58] Serological investigation is helpful but raised titres occur in subclinical infection.

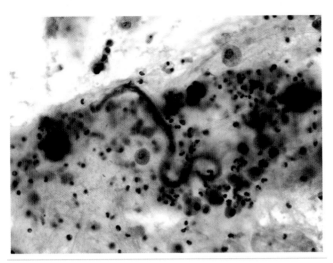

**Fig. 16.16** Strongyloidiasis. Larvum of *S. stercoralis*. Bronchoalveolar lavage (PAP).

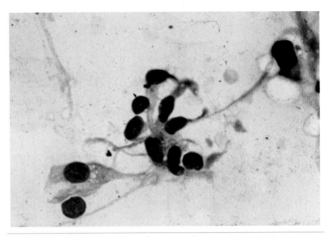

**Fig. 16.17** Kaposi sarcoma. Spindle cell proliferation (FNA, MGG).

## Intestinal protozoal infections

Diarrhoea is a common clinical presentation in HIV-infected patients who have CD4 counts <100. In the immune competent *Cryptosporidium parvum* produces self-limiting diarrhoea. In HIV-infected patients and very low (<50 CD4 counts) *Cryptosporidium* may cause chronic high volume diarrhoea.[59] The small protozoal organisms, 2–4 μm in diameter, cling to the mucosal brush border of the intestine. They stain with Grocott, which is excellent on biopsy material but not very suitable for stool specimens as the organisms are difficult to distinguish from fungal spores. Modified Ziehl Neelsen or auramine-phenol stains are preferable for the identification of oocysts in faeces.[59] Endoscopic sampling for cytological diagnosis is sometimes helpful. Other protozoa include *Entamoeba histolytica* and *Giardia lamblia* and *Strongyloides stercoralis*, which are recognisable in routine cytologically stained specimens (Fig. 16.16). *Isospora belli* is another unusual cause of enteritis. The differential diagnosis of *I. belli* and *Cryptosporidium* are summarised by Strigle et al.[60]

## Neoplastic disease

### Kaposi sarcoma (Fig. 16.17)

Kaposi sarcoma (KS) occurs in various forms but is particularly associated with HIV infection and its presence is an AIDS-defining illness. It is most frequently encountered among men who have sex with other men and is relatively rare in patients whose risk for HIV infection is haemophilia. It is also uncommon in patients with other forms of immunosuppression, such as transplant recipients. The lesion is strongly associated with human herpes virus (HHV8 or KSHV).[61] The skin is involved in 75% of patients but visceral lesions are present in many cases especially the lungs (see Chs 2, 28), gastrointestinal tract and lymph nodes. The clinical presentation of pulmonary KS is with tracheo-bronchial disease, parenchymal lesions, which may mimic or coexist with an opportunistic infection, or pleural disease (effusions). Antemortem identification is difficult, as bronchial brushings or biopsies are seldom reliably diagnostic,

given the sub-mucous location of the KS lesions. Even open lung biopsy may fail to reveal focal lesions.[62]

In the alimentary tract, as KS is a subepithelial tumour, cytological sampling of endoscopically visible lesions is also seldom diagnostic (see Ch. 7).

Several reports describe the diagnostic appearance of KS in FNA.[55,63–65]

---

**Cytological findings: Kaposi sarcoma**

- Smears moderately cellular and bloody
- Cellular fragments
- Numerous cells with spindle-shaped and hyperchromatic nuclei
- Many 'trapped' red blood cells between the spindle cells
- Mild pleomorphism
- No mitotic figures
- Some tumour cells show fibrillary cytoplasmic processes.

Since morphological appearances are non-specific, given the appropriate clinical context, the diagnosis can be made with greater confidence if immunocytochemical marking for KSHV (HHV8) and CD34 can be demonstrated as distinction from granulation tissue, reparative processes and other spindle cell tumours is difficult (Figs 16.17, 16.18).

---

### Lymphoproliferative disorders

Patients with both congenital and acquired immunodeficiency have an increased incidence of lymphoproliferative disorders (Fig. 16.19), particularly transplant recipients[66] and AIDS patients.[67,68] Any organ may be involved but the CNS, lymph nodes and gastrointestinal tract are the most common sites. Cytological diagnosis is most likely to be required from examination of CSF,[58] serous fluids, FNA of lymph nodes[55,64] or other sites. Definitive diagnosis from gastric brushings is seldom possible due to the mainly submucosal nature of the lesions and the likelihood that only Papanicolaou-stained material will be available.[60]

Transplant patients, in particular heart/lung recipients, who receive relatively large amounts of immunosuppression may develop a spectrum of post-transplant lymphoproliferative disorders (PTLD).[69] These range from the benign hyperplastic

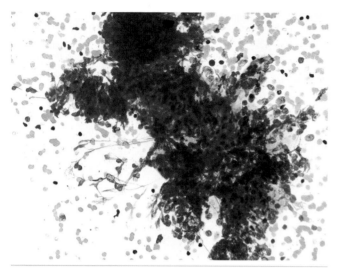

**Fig. 16.18** Castleman disease mimicking Kaposi sarcoma (FNA lymph node, MGG).

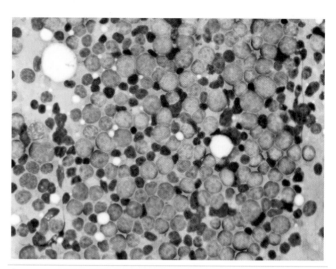

**Figure 16.20** Atypical appearing lymphoid cells in PGL Note mixed nature of the population (MGG).

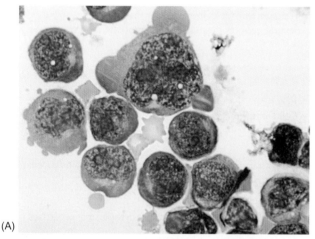

(A)

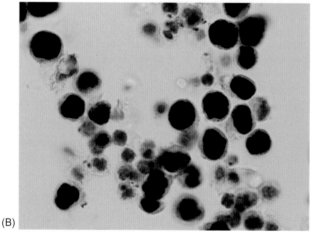

(B)

**Fig. 16.19** Non-Hodgkin lymphoma. Primary effusion lymphoma. Ascitic fluid from a patient with AIDS. (A) MGG; (B) KSHV.

conditions, which are likely to regress with reduction in immunosuppression, through polyclonal and oligoclonal proliferations to overt non-Hodgkin lymphoma, which may not respond to withdrawal of immunosuppression (see Fig. 34.5).

The PTLD may occur either within the graft or elsewhere, with gastrointestinal involvement being common. Both T and B cell types may be associated with EBV infection.[69]

Non-Hodgkin lymphoma in the immunosuppressed is usually high grade, such as diffuse large B-cell lymphoma or Burkitt lymphoma with or without plasmablastic differentiation. Strigle et al.[55] identified a lymphoproliferative lesion in 186 of 396 (46%) FNA specimens obtained from HIV-positive patients. They diagnosed by immunocytochemistry B-cell lymphoma in 22 of 186 (11%) aspirates. The remaining 141 (35%) showed evidence of persistent generalised lymphadenopathy (PGL) (Fig. 16.20). A more recent study by Lowe et al. looked at 73 FNA investigations from 62 patients who were HIV-positive and taking HAART, performed over a period from 1998 to 2006.[2] In this series, PGL again was the most common diagnosis at 34.3%. Malignant diagnoses were made in 12.3% cases and included non-Hodgkin lymphoma (5.4%) and Kaposi sarcoma (5.4%). Some 15% cases showed infection and most of these were mycobacterial in nature; 31% of cases were found to be non-diagnostic due to insufficient sampling. The use of ancillary techniques including flow cytometry and immunocytochemistry may be required for confirmation of diagnosis. The cytomorphological features of lymphomas are similar to those seen in non-immunosuppressed individuals (see Chs 13, 14).

## Other malignant tumours

A wide range of tumours other than Kaposi sarcoma and lymphoma are seen in individuals with AIDS and those on immunosuppressive therapy. Patients with lymphoma, leukaemia and allied conditions are also at risk of secondary malignancy. Aetiology is multifactorial but it is probable that the high incidence of infection with HPV and hepatitis B and C virus are contributory factors in the development of squamous neoplasia and hepatocellular carcinoma respectively. In the study by Strigle et al.,[55] 12 of 396 FNA specimens showed malignant processes other than lymphoma or Kaposi sarcoma. These included three cases of metastatic melanoma.

In a paediatric HIV population, Michelow et al., in addition to non-Hodgkin lymphoma, found cases of nephroblastoma, rhabdomyosarcoma, myeloma and melanotic progonoma that could be diagnosed by FNA.[70] Cervical cytology and the cellular appearances of carcinoma, melanoma and other tumours are similar to those of the non-immunosuppressed population and descriptions will be found elsewhere in this book (see Ch. 23).

## Associated conditions and pitfalls: immunosuppression due to miscellaneous conditions

Drug therapy and irradiation can induce marked cytological alterations, which at times may produce changes virtually indistinguishable from malignant transformation.[71] Knowledge of the history of irradiation and/or the administration of antineoplastic drugs in particular is vital for the cytopathologist if correct interpretation is to be achieved.

Toxic iatrogenic effects causing diagnostic difficulties are most likely to be encountered in the examination of BAL fluid.[72] In addition to drugs and irradiation, graft versus host disease, rejection of lung allograft and non-specific pneumonitis may all cause exfoliation of bizarre cells. Nuclei are frequently greatly enlarged, hyperchromatic and contain macronucleoli but commonly also display degenerative changes with patchy chromatin and discontinuous nuclear membranes. Multinucleation is prominent. Cytoplasm may be dense or show evidence of vacuolation. Affected bronchial epithelial cells may retain their cilia, which is a helpful feature and militates against an erroneous diagnosis of adenocarcinoma. Cells, arising from areas of atypical squamous metaplasia, however, can show cytomorphological changes almost identical to squamous cell carcinoma and are a particular pitfall.[71] Bizarre squamous cells may be seen in obliterative bronchiolitis of the lung allograft,[46] especially following total lymphoid irradiation.

Other pulmonary lesions listed in Box 16.2 include alveolar haemorrhage, when numerous haemosiderin-laden Perls' positive macrophages are found. Occult alveolar haemorrhage has been described in association with Kaposi's sarcoma.[73] Small numbers occur in other conditions and diagnosis again requires correlation with clinical history.

Lipoproteinosis may very occasionally be associated with PCP and sudanophilic macrophages are then recovered in the BAL fluid. Lymphocytic interstitial pneumonia (LIP) is a common complication of HIV infection in children but is much less common in adults. The clinical presentation is similar to PCP.[74] The aetiology is unknown but it is believed to be a tissue response to EBV and HIV infection, or both. High levels of CD8 T cells have been reported in BAL fluid[75] but this finding is not diagnostic as a CD8 lymphocytosis is typical of AIDS even in the absence of LIP. Open biopsy is usually necessary for diagnosis.[73]

The urinary tract is the other system that is most likely to give rise to interpretive problems. Post-radiation effect and alterations due to chemotherapy are extensively reviewed by Koss.[76] Cyclophosphamide-induced atypia in exfoliated cells in urine can be particularly severe. Bizarre cells with hyperchromatic nuclei can be numerous and give rise to false suspicion of malignancy if the history of chemotherapy is unknown. Long-term follow-up of patients who have received cyclophosphamide is

---

### Box 16.2 Principal causes of pulmonary dysfunction in the immune suppressed

**Infection**

- Bacterial
  - *Staph. aureus*
  - *Strep. pneumoniae*
  - *H. influenzae*
  - *P. aeruginosa*
  - *L. pneumophila*
  - *M. tuberculosis*
  - *M. avium-intracellulare*
- Viral
  - *Cytomegalovirus*
  - *Herpes simplex*
  - *Adenovirus*
- Fungal
  - *P. jiroveci*
  - *Candida* spp.
  - *Aspergillus* spp.
  - *C. neoformans*
  - *H. capsulatum*
  - *C. immitis*
- Parasitic
  - *T. gondii*
  - *S. stercoralis*

**Neoplasia**

- Lymphoproliferative disorders
- Leukaemia
- Hodgkin lymphoma
- Myeloma
- Kaposi sarcoma
- Bronchial carcinoma
- Secondary carcinoma

**Iatrogenic processes**

- Irradiation
- Drug toxicity
- Oxygen toxicity
- Graft versus host disease
- Rejection of lung allograft

**Idiopathic and miscellaneous processes**

- Lipoproteinosis
- Alveolar haemorrhage
- Lymphocytic interstitial pneumonia
- Non-specific interstitial pneumonia

---

prudent, however, as there is an associated risk of transitional and squamous cell carcinoma. Immunosuppression can activate polyoma virus infection and the morphological effects of this, combined with other iatrogenic changes can be pronounced.[76]

## The role of cytology in management of the immunosuppressed patient (Fig. 16.21)

Cytology has an important role in the diagnosis of opportunistic infections and tumours in immune suppressed patients.

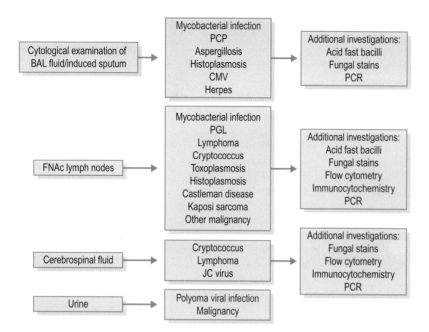

The most frequently encountered investigations are induced sputum/BAL fluid for diagnosis of respiratory episodes and FNA of lymph nodes for diagnosis of lymphadenopathy. FNA is a worthwhile procedure and in most instances allows a rapid diagnosis, obviating the need for surgery and enabling swift treatment to be undertaken where necessary. Ancillary studies form an important diagnostic component. Universal safety precautions must be strictly adhered to (Fig. 16.21). The multidisciplinary team meeting is the ideal forum to exchange clinical and pathological information for optimum patient management.

# REFERENCES

1. Grogg KL, Miller RF, Dogan A. HIV infection and lymphoma. J Clin Pathol 2007;60:1365–72.

2. Lowe SM, Kocjan GI, Edwards SG, et al. Diagnostic yield of fine-needle aspiration cytology in HIV-infected patients with lymphadenopathy in the era of highly active antiretroviral therapy. Int J STD & AIDS 2008;19:553–56.

3. Young JA. Pulmonary cytology. ACP Broadsheet. J Clin Pathol 1993;46:589–95.

4. Reid AJC, Miller RF, Kocjan GI. Diagnostic utility of fine needle aspiration (FNA) cytology in HIV-infected patients with lymphadenopathy. Cytopathology 1998;9:230–39.

5. Lawn S, Bekker L, Miller R. Immune reconstitution disease associated with mycobacterial infections in HIV-infected individuals receiving antiretrovirals. Lancet Infect Dis 2005;5:361–73.

6. Jungare A, Gadkari R, Lele VR, et al. Utility of Papanicolaou stain-induced fluorescence in the cytodiagnosis of extrapulmonary tuberculosis. Acta Cytologica 2005;49:600–6005.

7. Das DK, Bhambhani S, Pant JN, et al. Superficial and deep-seated tuberculous lesions: fine needle aspiration cytology diagnosis of 574 cases. Diagn Cytopathol 1992;8:211–15.

8. Bentz JS, Carroll K, Ward JH, et al. Acid-fast-positive Legionella pneumophila a possible pitfall in the cytologic diagnosis of mycobacterial infection in pulmonary specimens. Diagn Cytopathol 2000;22:45–48.

9. Barnes PF, Bloch AB, Davidson DT, et al. Tuberculosis in patients with human immunodeficiency virus infection. N Engl J Med 1991;324:1644–50.

10. Maurer JR, Frost AE, Estenne M, et al. International guidelines for the selection of lung transplant candidates. J Heart-Lung Transpl 1998;17:703–9.

11. Rodriquez JL, Barrio JL, Pitchenik AE. Pulmonary nocardiosis in the acquired immunodeficiency syndrome. Chest 1986;90:912–14.

12. Barry SM, Johnson MA, Janossy G. Cytopathology or immunopathology? The puzzle of cytomegalovirus pneumonitis revisited. Bone Marrow Transplant 2000;26:591–97.

13. de Medeiros CR, Moreira VA, Pasquini R. Cytomegalovirus as a cause of very late interstitial pneumonia after bone marrow transplantation. Bone Marrow Transplant 2000;26:443–44.

14. Dawber JH, Paradis IL, Dummer JS. Infectious complications in pulmonary allograft recipients. Clin Chest Med 1990;11:291–308.

15. Duncan SR, Paradis IL, Yousein SA, et al. Sequelae of CMV pulmonary infections in lung allograft recipients. Am Rev Respir Dis 1992;146:1419–25.

16. Ljungman P, Englehard D, Link H, et al. Treatment of interstitial pneumonitis due to cytomegalovirus with ganciclovir and intravenous immune globulin: experience of European Bone Marrow Transplant Group. Clin Infectious Dis 1992;14:831–35.

17. Young JA, Hopkin JM, Cuthbertson WP. Pulmonary infiltrates in immunocompromised patients: diagnosis by cytological examination of bronchoalveolar lavage fluid. J Clin Pathol 1984;37:390–97.

18. Nassar A, Zapata M, Little JV, et al. Utility of reflex Gomori methenamine silver staining for Pneumocystis jirovecii on bronchoalveolar lavage cytologic specimens: A review. Diagn Cytopathol 2006;34:719–23.

19. Young JA. Colour Atlas of Pulmonary Cytology. London: Harvey Miller and Oxford University Press; 1985 37–51.

20. Teot LA, Ducatman BS, Geisinger KR. Cytologic diagnosis of cytomegaloviral oesophagitis: a report of three acquired immunodeficiency syndrome related cases. Acta Cytologica 1993;37:93–96.

21. Santiago K, Rivera A, Cabanas D, et al. Fine needle aspiration of cytomegalovirus sialadenitis in a patient with acquired immunodeficiency syndrome: pitfalls of Diff-Quik staining. Diagn Cytopathol 2000;22:101–3.

22. Martin WJ, Smith TF. Rapid detection of cytomegalovirus in bronchoalveolar lavage specimens by a monoclonal antibody method. J Clin Microbiol 1986;23:1006–8.

23. Hilborne HL, Nieberg RK, Chen L, et al. Direct in situ hybridization for rapid detection of cytomegalovirus in bronchoalveolar lavage. Am J Clin Pathol 1987;87:766–69.

24. Olive DM, Simek M, Al-Mufti S. Polymerase chain reaction assay for detection of

human cytomegalovirus. J Clin Microbiol 1989;27:1238–42.

25. Iwa N, Sasaki M, Yutani C, et al. Detection of cytomegalovirus DNA in pulmonary specimens: confirmation by in situ hybridization in two cases. Diagn Cytopathol 1992;8:357–60.

26. Smyth RL, Higenbottom TW, Scott JP, et al. Herpes simplex virus infection in heart-lung transplant recipients. Transplantation 1990;49:735–39.

27. Smyth RL, Higenbottom TW, Scott JP, et al. Herpes simplex virus infection in heart-lung transplant recipients. Transplantation 1990;49:735–39.

28. Grosby JH, Pantazis CG, Stigall B. In situ hybridization for confirmation of herpes simplex virus in bronchoalveolar smears. Acta Cytologica 1991;35:248–50.

29. Fraga FJ, Chaves BMA, Burgos LE, et al. Oral hairy leucoplakia, a histopathologic study of 32 cases. Am J Dermatopathol 1990;12:571–78.

30. Danso D, Lyons F, Bradbeer C. Cervical screening and management of cervical intraepithelial neoplasia in HIV-positive women. Int J STD AIDS 2006;17:579–84.

31. Sheherd NA. Anal intraepithelial neoplasia and other neoplastic precursor lesions of the anal canal and perianal region. Gastroenterol Clin North Am 2007;36:969–87.

32. Ellerbrock TV, Chiasson MA, Bush TJ, et al. Incidence of cervical squamous intraepithelial lesions in HIV-infected women. JAMA 2000;283:1031–37.

33. Massad LS, Seaberg EC, Watts DH, et al. Low incidence of invasive cervical cancer among HIV-infected US women in a prevention program. AIDS 2004;18:109–13.

34. Randhawa P, Uhrmacher J, Pasculle W, et al. A comparative study of BK and JC virus infections in organ transplant recipients. J Med Virol 2005;77:238–43.

35. Hirsch HH, Brennan DC, Drachenberg CB, et al. Polyomavirus-associated nephropathy in renal transplantation: interdisciplinary analyses and recommendations. Transplantation 2005;79:1277–86.

36. Boldorini R, Zarini EO, Vigano P, et al. Cytologic and biomolecular diagnosis of HIV-positive patients. Acta Cytologica 2000;44:205–10.

37. Mitchell DM, Johnson MA. Treatment of lung disease in patients with the acquired immunodeficiency syndrome. Thorax 1990;45:219–24.

38. Metersky ML, Aslenzadeh J, Stelmach P. A comparison of induced and expectorated sputum for the diagnosis of Pneumocystis carinii pneumonia. Chest 1998;113:1555–59.

39. Broaddus C, Daka MD, Stulbarg MS, et al. Bronchoalveolar lavage and transbronchial biopsy for the diagnosis of pulmonary infections in the acquired immunodeficiency syndrome. Ann Intern Med 1985;102:747–52.

40. Orenstein M, Webber CA, Cash M, et al. Value of bronchoalveolar lavage in the diagnosis of pulmonary infection in acquired immune deficiency syndrome. Thorax 1986;41:345–49.

41. Golden JA, Holland H, Stulbarg MS, et al. Bronchoalveolar lavage as the exclusive diagnostic modality for Pneumocystis carinii pneumonia. Chest 1986;90:18–21.

42. Wallace JM, Batra P, Gong H, et al. Percutaneous needle lung aspiration for diagnosing pneumonitis in patients with acquired immunodeficiency syndrome. Am Rev Respir Dis 1985;131:382–92.

43. Travis WD, Pithluga S, Lipschick GY, et al. Atypical pathologic manifestation of Pneumocystis carinii pneumonia in the required immune deficiency syndrome. Am J Surg Pathol 1990;14:615–25.

44. Radin DR, Baker EL, Klatt EV, et al. Visceral and nodal calcification in patients with AIDS-related Pneumocystis carinii infections. AJR 1990;154:27–31.

45. Young JA, Elias E. Gastro-oesophageal candidiasis; diagnosis by brush cytology. J Clin Pathol 1985;38:293–96.

46. Stewart S. Lung Transplantation in Practical Pulmonary Pathology. London: Edward Arnold; 1995 88–109.

47. Stanley MW, Davies S, Deike M. Pulmonary aspergillosis: an unusual cytologic presentation. Diagn Cytopathol 1992;8:585–87.

48. McCalmont TH, Silverman JF, Geisinger KR. Fine needle aspiration cytology. Application in cardiac transplantation for the diagnosis of pulmonary aspergillosis. Arch Surg 1991;126:394–96.

49. Stanley MW, Deike M, Knoedler J, et al. Pulmonary mycetomas in immunocompetent patients: diagnosis by fine needle aspiration. Diagn Cytopathol 1992;8:577–79.

50. Kocjan G, Miller R. The cytology of HIV-induced immunosuppression. Changing pattern of disease in the era of highly active antiretroviral therapy. Cytopathology 2001;12:281–96.

51. Young JA. Lung, pleura and chest wall. In: Young JA, editor. Fine Needle Aspiration Cytopathology. Oxford: Blackwell; 1993. p. 97–121.

52. Blumenfeld W, Gan GL. Diagnosis of histoplasmosis in bronchoalveolar lavage fluid by intracytoplasmic localization of silver-positive yeast. Acta Cytologica 1991;710–12.

53. Strigle SM, Rarwick MV, Cosgrove MM, et al. A review of fine-needle aspiration cytology findings in human immunodeficiency virus infection. Diagn Cytopathol 1992:41–42.

54. Johnston WW. Cytopathology of mycotic infections. Lab Med 1971;2:34–40.

55. Strigle SM, Rarwick MV, Cosgrove MM, et al. A review of fine-needle aspiration cytology findings in human immunodeficiency virus infection. Diagn Cytopathol 1992:41–42.

56. Zaharopoulos P. Demonstration of parasites in toxoplasma lymphadenitis by fine-needle aspiration cytology: report of two cases. Diagn Cytopathol 2000;22:11–15.

57. Miller RF, Lucas SB, Bateman NT. Disseminated Toxoplasma gondii infection presenting with a fulminant pneumonia. Genitourin Med 1996;72:139–43.

58. Strigle SM, Gal AA. Review of central nervous system cytopathology in human immunodeficiency virus infection. Diagn Cytopathol 1991;7:387–401.

59. Casemore DP, Sands RL, Curry A. Cryptosporidium species: a 'new' human pathogen. J Clin Pathol 1985;38:1321–36.

60. Strigle SM, Gal AA, Martin SE. Alimentary tract cytopathology in human immunodeficiency virus infection: a review of experience in Los Angeles. Diagn Cytopathol 1990;6:409–20.

61. Hengge UR, Ruzicka T, Tyring SK, et al. Update on Kaposi's sarcoma and other HHV8 associated diseases. Part 2: pathogenesis, Castleman's disease, and pleural effusion lymphoma. Lancet Infect Dis 2002;2:344–52.

62. Ognibene FP, Shelhamer JH. Kaposi's sarcoma. In: White DA, Slover DE (eds) Pulmonary effects of AIDS. Clin Chest Med 1988; 9:459–465.

63. al-Rikabi AC, Haidar Z, Arif M, et al. Fine-needle aspiration cytology of primary Kaposi's sarcoma of lymph nodes in an immunocompetent man. Diagn Cytopathol 1998;19:451–54.

64. Martin-Bates E, Tanner A, Suvarna SK, et al. Use of fine needle aspiration cytology for investigating lymphadenopathy in HIV positive patients. J Clin Pathol 1993;46:564–66.

65. Wilkinson AH, Smith JL, Hunsicker LG, et al. Increased frequency of post-transplant lymphomas in patients treated with cyclosporine, azathioprine, and prednisone. Transplantation 1989;47:293–96.

66. Wilkinson AH, Smith JL, Hunsicker LG, et al. Increased frequency of post-transplant lymphomas in patients treated with cyclosporine, azathioprine, and prednisone. Transplantation 1989;47:293–96.

67. Levine AM. Reactive and neoplastic lymphoproliferative disorders and other miscellaneous cancers associated with HIV infection. In: DeVita VT, Hellman S, Rosenberg SA, editors AIDS: aetiology, treatment and prevention. Philadelphia: JB Lippincott; 1988. p. 263–75.

68. Raphael M, Gentilhomme O, Tulliez M, et al. Histopathologic features of high-grade non-Hodgkin's lymphomas in acquired immunodeficiency syndrome. Arch Pathol Lab Med 1991;155:15–20.

69. Swerdtow S. Post-transplant lymphoproliferative disorders; a morphologic, phenotypic and genotypic spectrum of disease. Histopathology 1992;20:73–385.

70. Michelow P, Meyers T, Dubb M, et al. The utility of fine needle aspiration in HIV positive children. Cytopathology 2008;19:86–93.

71. Walloch JL, Hong HY, Bibb LM. Effects of therapy on cytologic specimens. In: Bibbo M, editor. Comprehensive Cytopathology. Philadelphia: WB Saunders; 1991. p. 860–77.

72. Huang M-S, Colby TV, Goellner JR, et al. Utility of bronchoalveolar lavage in the diagnosis of drug-induced pulmonary toxicity. Acta Cytol 1989;33:533–38.

73. Hughes-Davies., Kocjan G, Spittle MF, et al. Occult alveolar haemorrhage in bronchopulmonary Kaposi's sarcoma. J Clin Pathol 1992;45:536–37.

74. Das S, Miller RF. Lymphocytic interstitial pneumonitis in HIV infected adults. Sex Transm Infect 2003;79:88–93.

75. Teirstein AS, Rosen MJ. Lymphocytic interstitial pneumonia. Clin Chest Med 1988;9:467–71.

76. Koss LC. The urinary tract in the absence of cancer. In: Diagnostic Cytology and its Histopathology Bases. 4th edn Philadelphia: JB Lippincott; 1992. p. 890–933. 76. . . 4th edn.

# Section 10

## Endocrine System

# Thyroid gland

Ian D. Buley

## Chapter contents

## Anatomy and physiology

The thyroid is a bilobed endocrine organ situated on either side of the trachea and oesophagus. The lobes are joined anteriorly by an isthmus extending over the trachea. Each lobe is about 5 cm in length and extends from the oblique line of the thyroid cartilage to the sixth tracheal ring. The gland's relationship to other neck structures is indicated in Figure 17.1. It is invested by the pretracheal fascia, which is firmly attached posteriorly to the second to fourth tracheal rings. For this reason, the gland and tumours arising from it characteristically move with the larynx on swallowing.

The gland produces thyroxine under the control of thyroid stimulating hormone (TSH) secreted by the pituitary. It also contains neuroendocrine parafollicular cells, which produce calcitonin. The thyroid is derived embryologically as a downgrowth from the base of the tongue. A tubular evagination of endodermally derived cells, the thyroglossal duct, extends inferiorly in front of the laryngeal cartilage and the trachea. The distal end proliferates, forming the thyroid lobes and the path of descent should be obliterated. The calcitonin secreting cells are thought to arise as a separate contribution to the embryonic thyroid gland from the fourth and fifth pharyngeal pouches (ultimobranchial body).

Histologically, the gland consists of numerous follicles (Fig. 17.2), which are the functional units capable of synthesising, storing and secreting triiodothyronine and tetraiodothyronine ($T_3$ and $T_4$); hormones having a wide range of actions stimulating metabolism. The follicles are spheroidal structures lined by a single layer of cuboidal follicular cells. The cells have microvillous processes embedded in the central store of

thyroglobulin or colloid, which is a large iodinated glycoprotein from which $T_3$ and $T_4$ are subsequently split after endocytosis. In the euthyroid state the follicles vary in size but average 200 μm in diameter. Secretion of thyroid hormones takes place

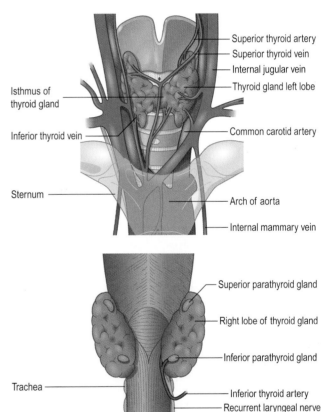

Superior thyroid artery
Superior thyroid vein
Internal jugular vein
Thyroid gland left lobe

Isthmus of thyroid gland

Inferior thyroid vein

Common carotid artery

Sternum

Arch of aorta

Internal mammary vein

Superior parathyroid gland

Right lobe of thyroid gland

Inferior parathyroid gland

Trachea

Inferior thyroid artery
Recurrent laryngeal nerve

**Fig. 17.1** The anterior and posterior relationships of the thyroid.

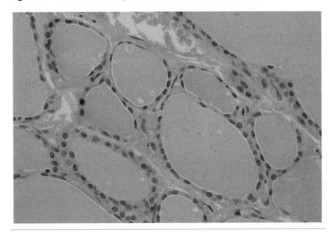

**Fig. 17.2** Normal thyroid histology (H&E).

directly into the rich network of capillaries seen in this vascular organ. Longstanding stored thyroglobulin may accumulate calcium oxalate crystals and ageing follicular cells accumulate lipofuscin.

The parafollicular or C cells are part of the diffuse neuroendocrine system. Although termed parafollicular, these cells are incorporated into follicles. They secrete calcitonin. This hormone has a hypocalcaemic action but its physiological importance in man is unclear. The C cells are immunoreactive to other peptides, including somatostatin, and it is possible that these substances are involved in local paracrine control of $T_3$ and $T_4$ production and secretion. These cells are extremely difficult to distinguish from follicular cells using conventional histological stains. The cells are slightly larger, paler and spindle or polyhedral in shape with a faintly granular cytoplasm. They are preferentially localised in the thyroid to the central regions of the lateral lobes and are particularly seen in proximity to solid cell nests, which are thought to be ultimobranchial body remnants.

## Historical perspective

Fine needle aspiration (FNA) of the thyroid was documented in the Martin and Ellis paper of 1934.[1] It was further developed in papers by Tempka et al. and Piaggio-Blanco et al. in 1948 (cited in Grunze and Spriggs[2]) and the use of the technique was established subsequently by Scandinavian workers.[3,4] FNA is now recognised to be the first-line investigation for a solitary or dominant thyroid nodule, has a valuable role in the diagnosis of the diffuse non-toxic goitre and can be used to confirm the diagnosis of clinically obvious malignancy, enabling the separation of treatable lymphomas from poor prognosis anaplastic carcinomas. FNA superseded core biopsy of the thyroid. Core biopsy was associated with an increased risk of patient discomfort and complications with little difference in diagnostic value. Modern narrow-bore single action needle devices are believed to be safer and may have a role in selected patients who have had previous inadequate needle aspiration or where FNA findings are discordant with clinical findings.[5] At present the thyroid is one of the organs most frequently sampled by means of FNA.[6]

## Clinical indications for FNA of thyroid nodules, the influence of thyroid imaging and mode of FNA guidance

The most frequent indication for thyroid FNA is in the evaluation of a solitary thyroid nodule or dominant nodule in the context of a nodular goitre. Prior to consideration of needle aspiration, the history, examination, biochemical and imaging findings need to be considered. Findings of significance for possible thyroid malignancy include a family history of thyroid cancer or adrenal phaeochromocytoma, previous head and neck irradiation, rapid growth, hardness or adherence of the lump to surrounding structures and the presence of associated lymphadenopathy. The minimum piece of biochemical data needed is the TSH level. Serological information and thyroid autoantibody levels can also be helpful in some circumstances. Imaging would usually be by ultrasound. If the TSH level is depressed suggesting thyroid overactivity, a radionuclide

scan may be helpful. If the nodule is 'hot' indicating localised increased thyroid hormone production, FNA can be avoided as the incidence of malignancy is very low so long as there are no suspicious ultrasound or clinical findings.[7]

Thyroid nodules are now frequently first detected during the course of an imaging study. The management of these 'incidentalomas' depends on the type of imaging and in the case of ultrasound detection on the detailed high resolution characteristics. Focal nodules detected by fluorodeoxyglucose-positron emission tomography, FDG-PET scans, have a significant risk of malignancy. They are often primary thyroid cancers even when scanning is for staging another malignancy and warrant FNA.[7,8] Focal hot nodules detected on technetium-99m methoxyisobutylisonitrile scintigraphy, sestamibi scans and confirmed to be discrete on ultrasound require aspiration as they are frequently neoplasms rather than functional nodules.[7] Nodules first detected sonographically are frequently small. Modern high resolution and Doppler ultrasound has allowed the definition of suspicious features over and above description as solid or cystic and whether there is associated lymphadenopathy. These features include microcalcifications, the irregularity of the nodule margin and intra-lesional vascularity. Lesions of any size with suspicious features should be aspirated. Some of these lesions may be microcarcinomas of uncertain clinical significance but diagnosis and surgical removal is appropriate as a minority behave aggressively. Incidental ultrasonically detected thyroid nodules lacking suspicious radiological or clinical features and less than 10 mm in diameter are usually not aspirated as they have a low risk of malignancy. Larger nodules may be aspirated unless they are clearly cystic and ultrasound follow-up is feasible. Thyroid nodules are seen in at least 16% of patients undergoing neck CT or MRI. They do not automatically warrant needle aspiration. They should be evaluated by ultrasound and the decision to proceed to FNA should be made by the clinician on the basis of those findings.[7]

FNA using palpation alone for guidance is more rapid and less expensive than ultrasound guidance. It is particularly applicable to larger discrete nodules that are clearly within the thyroid. The ultrasonic features of these lesions give useful information as to their nature and allow assessment of the rest of the thyroid and local lymph nodes. If ultrasound is to be carried out then ultrasound guidance should be considered. It allows accurate placement of the needle in less well circumscribed or small nodules, it allows preferential sampling of solid areas in mixed solid-cystic abnormalities, is useful where previous palpation guided FNA has failed, where the anatomy is distorted by prior surgery, where lesions are close to major blood vessels or if the patient has a bleeding diathesis. While ultrasound guidance has advantages in certain circumstances, the adequacy and accuracy of thyroid FNA in large unselected series may be more dependant on the skills and technique of the operator rather than the mode of guidance.[9]

## Technique

Aspiration by the pathologist with immediate staining and interpretation allows the preparation of optimal specimens and the best appreciation of the clinical history, examination findings and the results of biochemical, serological and imaging data. The procedure should be preceded by clinical examination of the neck from the front and behind the seated patient.

The differential diagnostic possibilities of lumps in the neck should be considered (Table 17.1). Patient consent should be obtained. This may be verbal or written depending on local or national policies. The FNA procedure, risks and complications, particularly haematoma formation, should be described. The possibility of a non-contributory, false negative or false positive result should be mentioned.

Thyroid FNA should be carried out with the patient lying flat, positioned with a pillow beneath the shoulders and neck. This enables the head to fall back in a relaxed position, which separates the sternomastoid muscles, uncovering more of the lateral lobes of the thyroid. Patients will need reassurance as needle aspiration of the neck is one of the more alarming sites for aspiration cytology. They should also be asked not to speak or swallow during the procedure to avoid movement of the gland. A wipe with an alcohol swab is usually sufficient skin cleansing. Routine local anaesthetic injection is not recommended. When aspiration is performed in children topical anaesthetic cream is valuable but its use requires forethought, as the cream must be applied under an occlusive dressing for at least an hour to ensure anaesthesia. The vascularity of the thyroid means that a 23, 25 or 27 gauge bevelled needle should be used. For the majority of thyroid lesions at most only three passes of the needle in a single plane should be carried out; persisting beyond this results in blood contamination of the sample and the dilution or loss of diagnostic features. An exception is in sclerosing malignancies where multiple passes may be necessary to obtain sufficient material. Traversing the sternomastoid should be avoided as it is painful, obscures the depth of the lesion and muscle spasm makes directional control of the needle difficult. Use of a syringe holder allows comfortable single-handed operation of the syringe, freeing the other hand to localise the target.[10] A syringe holder is particularly useful in cystic lesions where the fluid can be drained in a single needle pass.

With ultrasound guided FNA, use of plastic tubing between the needle and syringe allows an assistant to operate the syringe facilitating manipulation of the ultrasound probe. Ultrasonic localisation of the lesion and needle usually results in more bleeding and delay in preparation of slides which diminishes the quality of the specimen. Ultrasound guidance should be restricted to cases where it is advantageous for lesion localisation. The operator should not allow ultrasound gel to contaminate the specimen.[5]

Needle puncture without the use of an aspirating syringe, the capillary technique, may be advantageous for both palpation and ultrasound guided FNA. Holding the needle alone allows fine and controlled passes. Numerous studies have shown that this technique is particularly valid in the thyroid[11–13] and achieves adequate specimens at least as often as conventional aspiration. In the experience of the author and other workers, blood contamination is reduced but the yield of diagnostic material can be reduced.[14] The technique does not facilitate the diagnostic and therapeutic aspiration of cysts in the thyroid but is particularly recommended where previous aspirates have been heavily blood contaminated.

The careful sampling necessary in the thyroid, because of its vascularity, means that at least two aspirates should be taken at any one time from lesions to reduce the risk of false negative diagnosis. Larger nodules should be aspirated in different areas. In the author's practice, a minimum of four aspirates are taken during the course of initial presentation and subsequent clinical follow-up before a lesion is assumed to be benign and the patient discharged. Where a thyroid tumour coexists with regional adenopathy, both the thyroid and lymph node should be aspirated to rule out coexisting pathology and to allow preoperative staging in the case of thyroid malignancy. Following aspiration, manual pressure should be applied to the site for approximately 1 minute. After the procedure the patient should be advised to sit up slowly and rest for a while before getting up. Most patients experience a little dizziness after having the neck extended backwards during the FNA procedure.

## Specimen preparation

Material can be spread by a conventional one step technique but a two stage spreading technique may be used where there is heavy blood contamination.[15] Cyst fluid should have both direct smear preparations and subsequent centrifuge, cytospin or thin-layer preparations made from the remaining fluid. May–Grünwald Giemsa (MGG) or a rapid Romanowsky-type stain such as Diff-Quik is recommended as this allows the visualisation of colloid and can be used alone in thyroid FNA. Alcohol wet-fixation and Papanicolaou (PAP) staining can provide complementary information in a minority of cases. Liquid-based cytology (LBC) preparations can facilitate examination of poor-quality blood-stained specimens and may partially compensate for poor aspiration or spreading technique. The technique is more expensive and time-consuming, however, and the definition of specimen adequacy has yet to be established.[16] Comparisons between series of conventional and LBC specimens have given variable results and it is not yet clear whether this technique allows the level of diagnostic accuracy possible with good quality conventional preparations. Cytological features appreciated less often in LBC preparations include diffuse colloid, lymphocytes and in papillary carcinoma fewer nuclear

**Table 17.1** Fine needle aspiration of lumps in the neck

| Structure | Pathology |
| --- | --- |
| Thyroid | Multinodular goitre and colloid nodules |
| | Thyroiditis and hyperplasia |
| | Neoplasms |
| Lymph nodes | Reactive |
| | Malignant – lymphomas and metastases |
| Salivary gland | Sialadenitis |
| | Neoplasms |
| Branchial arch remnant | Branchial cyst |
| Carotid bifurcation | Carotid body tumour and aneurysm |
| Lymphatics | Cystic hygroma |
| Pharynx | Pharyngeal pouch |
| Thymus | Ectopic thymoma |
| Bone | Cervical rib, hyoid bone |
| Skin and soft tissues | Skin tumours including dermoid cysts, lipoma, haemangioma, sarcomas, fasciitis and fibromatosis |
| Parathyroid | Cyst or carcinoma |

grooves and pseudoinclusions. These preparations have also been reported to show loss of cellular preservation in groups, more cell shrinkage and disruption.[17–22] Material collected into liquid preservatives for cytospins, cell blocks or commercial LBC fluids can be a useful adjunct to direct preparations particularly where ancillary studies are needed.

## Contraindications and complications

There are no absolute contraindications to needle aspiration of the thyroid in cooperative patients. Overall FNA of the thyroid is a very safe procedure. The main risk is haematoma formation causing tracheal compression in those with large goitres or malignant tumours. There are a few reported cases of acute airway obstruction requiring surgical decompression after thyroid FNA.[23] Care should be exercised in those who are anticoagulated using the smallest needle calibre possible with accurate and controlled needle passes. Clotting status should be checked prior to neck aspiration in those taking therapeutic doses of warfarin or heparin. FNA is usually possible in those taking standard doses of aspirin, non-steroidal anti-inflammatory drugs, antiplatelet drugs and prophylactic doses of heparin. Where it is safe to do so it would be preferable to suspend heparin treatment at least 8 h and antiplatelet therapy 3–5 days prior to aspiration. When there is a particular risk of haemorrhage, patients should be warned to seek medical attention if there is swelling or persisting pain after aspiration. Ultrasound guidance can facilitate the avoidance of larger vessels. Puncture of the carotid requires the aspirator to occlude the puncture site for 5 minutes. Puncture of the trachea may lead to transient coughing. Temporary laryngeal nerve paresis has been recorded post-aspiration,[24] as has haemorrhagic necrosis of thyroid tumours, particularly adenomas.[25] Needle track implantation by a thyroid malignancy is extraordinarily rare.[26,27] Infection following FNA is also rare.[28] Worrisome histological alterations such as regenerative nuclear changes, vascular proliferations, metaplasias and capsular pseudo-invasion may occur in approximately 10% of thyroid excisions following FNA but awareness of these artefacts by histopathologists avoids misdiagnosis. Cytopathologists need to be aware that reaspiration within a few weeks of a previous aspirate can show changes resulting from haematoma formation and healing.[29]

## Normal cytological findings

Aspiration of normal thyroid tissue yields colloid and sheets of follicular cells together with similar dissociated cells (Fig. 17.3). The colloid stains blue/mauve with MGG or the Diff-Quik stain and is seen as a wash of background colour. The Papanicolaou method does not stain colloid well. If the aspirate is contaminated by blood, the diluted colloid may be difficult to distinguish from serum. Follicular cells are relatively small with regular round or slightly oval nuclei of a similar size to those of lymphocytes. The chromatin pattern is even and single small nucleoli are just discernible. Where aspirated in a sheet, the nuclei appear evenly spaced in a honeycomb pattern, each with a small amount of pale, poorly defined, cytoplasm. The cytoplasm of dissociated cells is disrupted and the cells usually appear as bare nuclei. Occasionally whole follicles may

be aspirated and these appear as pseudo-giant cells in three-dimensional clusters. The central colloid is usually inapparent (Fig. 17.4).

The follicular cells may contain deep blue intracytoplasmic paravacuolar granules (Fig. 17.5). These consist of lysosomal accumulations of lipofuscin and haemosiderin. These granules

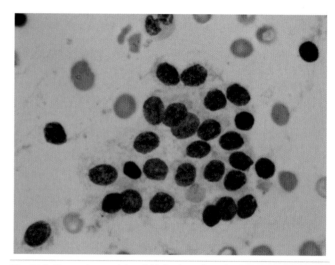

**Fig. 17.3** Sheet of normal thyroid follicular cells with a background 'wash' of colloid (MGG).

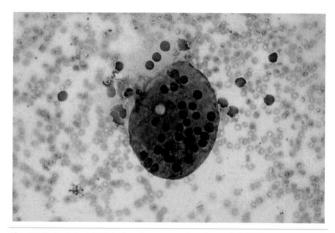

**Fig. 17.4** An intact follicle forming a pseudo-giant cell (MGG).

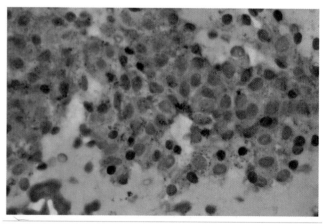

**Fig. 17.5** Paravacuolar granules in follicular cells (MGG).

can occur in normal thyroid but are more frequently seen in functional pathology, such as in a multinodular goitre where there are cystic and haemorrhagic changes. They also occur occasionally in neoplasms.[30] Other pigments may accumulate in the thyroid and prolonged use of minocycline for acne results in a black thyroid with accumulation of lipofuscin and a pigment derived from the breakdown of the antibiotic.[31]

Extraneous cells can be obtained by the passage of the needle through the strap muscles of the neck or sternomastoid muscle. Striated muscle fibres stain a characteristic deep blue colour and cross-striations can be seen. Puncture of the trachea yields respiratory epithelial cells, mucus and occasionally fragments of cartilage. Adipose tissue is not usually obtained except in the very obese and its presence should raise the possibility of a lipoma of the neck,[32] although there are other possibilities including aspiration of a thyrolipoma[33] and adipose metaplasia in a nodular goitre.

## Developmental abnormalities

### Lingual, subhyoid and retrosternal thyroid

Failure of descent of the organ leads to the formation of a lingual thyroid, the presence of mature functional thyroid tissue at the base of the tongue. Presentation may be with dysphonia, dysphagia or respiratory obstruction. This may necessitate surgical removal but the nature of the tongue mass can be diagnosed by needle aspiration, hence avoiding untreated postoperative hypothyroidism in the 70% of cases who have no thyroid tissue at the normal site. Incomplete descent leads to thyroid tissue placed high in the neck and this subhyoid thyroid presents as a mass in the neck. Some 40% of normal individuals have a persistence of the distal extremity of the thyroglossal duct and this pyramidal lobe extends superiorly from the isthmus and lies over the second and third tracheal rings. It may lie slightly to the left of the midline. Excessive descent of thyroid tissue into the superior mediastinum forms a retrosternal thyroid which may manifest as a mediastinal mass with compression symptoms, particularly if the gland becomes nodular.

### Thyroglossal cyst

Should the thyroglossal duct persist, a thyroglossal cyst or sinus may form. This is a characteristically midline swelling most often present immediately below the hyoid bone. Presentation typically occurs in children or young adults with a history of a painless mass of long duration. The cyst may become infected, inflamed and then prone to spontaneous rupture through the skin with sinus formation. Histologically, the cyst is lined by respiratory-type or squamous epithelium with lymphoid tissue in the wall. There may be small amounts of adjacent thyroid tissue. FNA yields clear or mucoid fluid with degenerate foamy cells and respiratory or squamous cells. The possibility of skin or tracheal contamination should be considered. Some reactive lymphoid tissue may be obtained. Inflammatory cells predominate in infected cysts. The presence of thyroid follicular cells or recognisable colloid is less common. Cholesterol crystals may be seen. Rarely, carcinomas arise in a thyroglossal cyst or duct. These are usually papillary in type and follicular tumours are exceptionally rare. Squamous carcinoma and anaplastic

carcinoma have been recorded but medullary carcinomas are unknown and this is thought to be a consequence of the embryological derivation of the parafollicular cells.[34]

---

**Cytological findings: thyroglossal cyst**

- Clear or mucoid fluid on aspiration
- Respiratory epithelial and/or squamous cells are present
- Reactive lymphoid cells may be seen
- Follicular cells or colloid are less frequently seen
- Inflammatory cells in infected cysts.

---

### Lateral aberrant thyroid

Lateral aberrant thyroid was once thought to represent developmental inclusions of thyroid tissue positioned lateral to the jugular veins. It is now recognised that most if not all such cases represent follicular pattern metastases in cervical lymph nodes arising from occult papillary carcinomas of the thyroid.

### Thymus

The thymus develops from the third pharyngeal pouch and a thymoma may arise in ectopic tissue incorporated into the lower pole of the thyroid, mimicking a thyroid mass.[35]

## Acquired non-neoplastic conditions

### Multinodular goitre, colloid nodules and cysts

The thyroid gland is in a state of constant but varying activity, becoming more active at puberty, in pregnancy and with physiological stress. It even changes in size and activity during the normal menstrual cycle. These changes may lead to a sporadic goitre. Whether the goitre is sporadic or due to a well-defined cause (Box 17.1), with persistence of a goitrogenic stimulus the gland may cease to behave in an homogeneous fashion. While the patient is usually euthyroid, parts of the gland are hyperplastic whereas other areas are inactive and accumulate colloid. The latter areas form enlarged colloid nodules and the structure of these may break down, particularly after spontaneous haemorrhage, to form cysts. Radioiodine studies show the enlarged inactive follicles and cysts as radioactively cold areas, a characteristic shared with most thyroid neoplasms. Occasionally,

---

**Box 17.1  Goitres – diffuse enlargement of the thyroid**

Simple non-toxic goitre

- Physiological (including endemic, due to dietary iodine deficiency)
- Dietary goitrogens, goitrogenic drugs and chemicals
- Dyshormonogenetic: inborn errors of thyroxine synthesis

Multinodular goitre; syn: colloid goitre, nodular goitre, adenomatous goitre

Toxic goitre

Thyroiditis

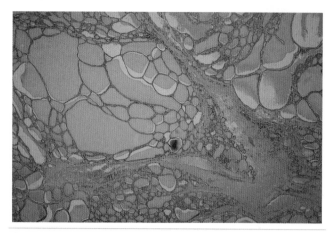

**Fig. 17.6** Nodular goitre (H&E).

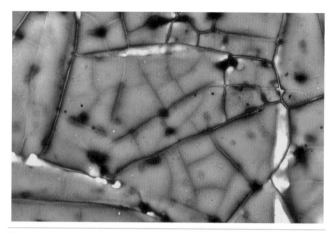

**Fig. 17.7** Thick varnish-like coat of colloid with 'crazy paving' pattern (MGG).

a hyperplastic focus within a nodular goitre may cause clinical hyperthyroidism. Autoimmune thyroiditis or hyperplasia may supervene on a multinodular goitre and these cases become respectively hypo- or hyperthyroid.

Histologically, a multinodular goitre is characterised by nodularity with fibrosis, calcification and deposition of haemosiderin and cholesterol as evidence of previous haemorrhage (Fig. 17.6). Within the areas of fibrosis and haemorrhage, groups of follicular cells may show regenerative and degenerative changes.

Multinodular goitre presents clinically in approximately 5% of the population and the female to male ratio is at least 3:1. It presents as a mass in the neck, which may cause tracheal or oesophageal compression. Haemorrhage into a colloid nodule causes the sudden and painful appearance or enlargement of a mass in the neck. A dominant nodule in the context of a multinodular goitre is the most frequent indication for FNA and correct diagnosis of a colloid nodule or cyst with the exclusion of malignancy allows the avoidance of surgery in most cases.

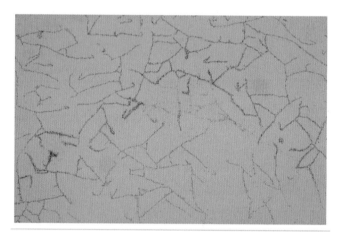

**Fig. 17.8** Ghost-image of colloid formed by red blood cells (MGG).

### Cytological findings: multinodular goitre

- Abundant colloid
- Debris-containing histiocytes
- Cystic degeneration results in aspirates of brown fluid containing degenerate red blood cells, cholesterol crystals, debris-containing histiocytes and degenerate follicular cells
- Follicular cells often with paravacuolar bodies
- Follicular cells may show degenerative and regenerative changes
- Fragments of fibrous stroma
- Hürthle cells, hyperplastic changes and lymphoid cells may be seen.

FNA of a small colloid goitre with little nodularity may yield normal findings. Aspiration of a colloid nodule yields abundant colloid and this may be recognised macroscopically as a thick transparent yellow fluid. It forms a varnish-like coat over the slide and tends to develop a crazy paving pattern of cracks (Fig. 17.7). This thick coat of colloid may be lost on staining if the slide has not been allowed to dry thoroughly. This can occur in a FNA clinic setting where immediate staining and interpretation is carried out and in this circumstance drying the slide in a stream of air, e.g. from a fan, is particularly recommended. Loss of colloid may result in a ghost image of the colloid being

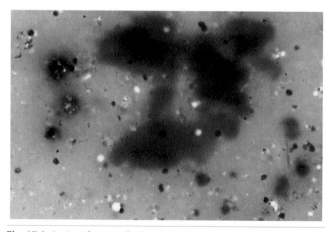

**Fig. 17.9** Aspirate from a colloid nodule with degenerate foamy cells (MGG).

formed by red blood cells in the aspirate (Fig. 17.8). The colloid consistency is variable and may appear thin and diffuse but inspissated dense fragments of colloid may also be seen.

Degenerate foamy cells containing both haemosiderin and lipofuscin will be seen scattered among the colloid (Fig. 17.9). Conventionally, these are considered to be histiocytes, although some may be degenerate follicular cells. Follicular cells are also seen. These vary from being few in number to being numerous and most frequently occur in monolayered sheets. Follicular cells in multinodular goitre more frequently contain paravacuolar bodies. An appreciation of the ratio between the quantities of colloid and follicular cells is crucial to the distinction of the benign functional abnormality in a multinodular goitre from a potentially malignant follicular neoplasm. The presence of abundant colloid indicates a low likelihood of neoplasia. A high cellularity raises the suspicion of neoplasia. This assessment of the cell to colloid ratio is subjective and relies on optimal specimen preparation. In particular, a heavy admixture of blood dilutes the follicular cells and obscures the colloid. Blood clot, on occasion, may also give a false impression of increased cellularity by trapping groups of follicular cells. Repeat FNA by an experienced operator may be helpful and if the problem cannot be resolved excision biopsy should be recommended.

The number of follicular cells is likely to be increased where a hyperplastic nodule has been included in the aspiration and the cytological features of hyperplasia need to be searched for. These may be florid with the formation of marginal fire flares (see Fig. 17.13 and Hyperplasia, below), or may be more subtle with an increase in the amount of cytoplasm and mild patchy nuclear enlargement resulting in anisonucleosis with visible small single nucleoli. These changes are seen in cells originating from smaller, more active, follicles and foci of microfollicular architecture may be recognised in such cases. Features of hyperplasia are suggestive of a functional abnormality but occasionally well-differentiated tumours may show similar features including marginal 'fire flares'. Reactive lymphocytes and oncocytic (Hürthle cell) change in follicular cells may be seen particularly where there is coexisting thyroiditis (see Thyroiditis, below). In a multinodular goitre, degenerative and regenerative changes in follicular epithelium may be marked (Fig. 17.10) and care must be taken not to mistake these cells for anaplastic carcinoma cells either of the spindle cell or giant cell form. The clinical and cytological context of these cells, which are usually few in number and show degenerative changes, must be taken into account.

Aspiration may also yield small fragments of loose fibrous stroma containing groups of follicular cells (Fig. 17.11). Fragments of calcification can be seen and some mimic Psammoma bodies. Nuclear grooves or nuclear inclusions, which are also regarded as indicative of papillary carcinoma, may be seen rarely as isolated findings in multinodular goitre.[36]

Where haemorrhage has occurred into a colloid nodule the aspirate is of chocolate-brown fluid with disappearance or shrinkage of the mass. The fluid requires centrifugation for proper examination. Degenerate red blood cells are present and in longstanding cysts cholesterol crystals are seen. Debris-containing foamy histiocytes may be numerous and follicular cells tend to be few and appear degenerate. The main differential diagnosis is with cystic degeneration in a tumour, particularly papillary carcinoma. If there is a residual mass this should be aspirated and the thyroid adjacent to a cyst should also be sampled. Almost half of benign cysts are cured by the first aspiration. Recurrent cysts should be excised for cure and to exclude an underlying neoplasm.[37] Other differential diagnoses include thyroglossal cyst and parathyroid cyst.

## Hyperplasia

Primary hyperplasia of the thyroid, or Graves' disease, results from the presence of autoantibodies to the TSH receptor on

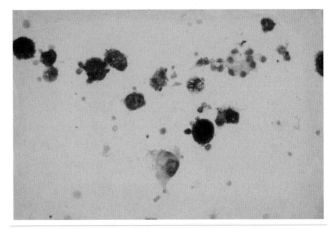

**Fig. 17.10** Aspirate from a nodular goitre with debris-laden macrophages and follicular cells, one of which shows marked regenerative and degenerative change (MGG).

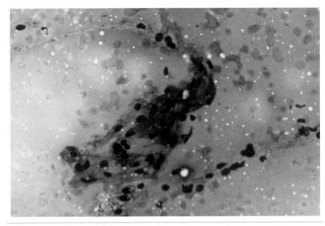

**Fig. 17.11** Aspirate from a nodular goitre showing a fragment of fibrous stroma (MGG).

follicular cells. These IgG antibodies mimic the action of TSH at the receptor site. Separate antibodies, which stimulate the cellular hyperplasia of the thyroid, are also present. Thyroid hyperplasia is one component of the syndrome of Graves' disease which also includes exophthalmos and pretibial myxoedema. The condition affects females at least five times as often as males and has a peak age distribution in the third and fourth decades. The clinical features are a consequence of the hypermetabolic state induced by excess thyroxine and are summarised in Table 17.2.

Histologically, there is diffuse hyperplasia with small follicles containing pale-staining colloid. The follicular cells appear crowded and may protrude as papillary projections into the follicle. The cells are enlarged and columnar with pale cytoplasm and scalloping of the adjacent colloid. Foci of Hürthle cell change may be seen and the thyroid interstitium may contain a reactive lymphoid infiltrate (Fig. 17.12).

Diagnosis is achieved by clinical examination, biochemical and serological tests. FNA is not necessary for primary diagnosis. Hyperplastic changes can be seen in other clinical situations (Box 17.2) and particularly as a focal change in multinodular

**Table 17.2** Manifestations of Graves' disease

| Psychological | Nervousness, emotional lability, heat intolerance, tiredness |
|---|---|
| Nervous system | Tremor, eye changes |
| Cardiovascular | Arrhythmias, tachycardia, cardiomegaly |
| Gastrointestinal | Good appetite, weight loss, diarrhoea |
| Musculoskeletal | Weakness (proximal myopathy), osteoporosis |
| Skin | Hot and sweaty |

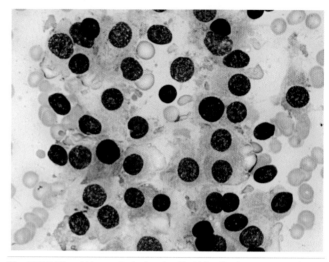

**Fig. 17.13** Thyroid hyperplasia showing florid 'fire flare' appearances (MGG).

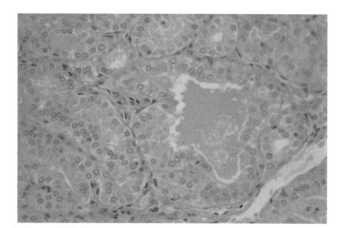

**Fig. 17.12** Thyroid hyperplasia (H&E).

---

**Box 17.2  Causes of hyperthyroidism**

Common

- Graves' disease (diffuse toxic goitre)
- Toxic multinodular goitre
- Toxic adenoma

Uncommon

- Acute phase of thyroiditis
- Hyperfunctioning thyroid carcinoma
- Choriocarcinoma, hydatidiform mole (TSH like activity)
- TSH secreting pituitary tumour
- Neonatal thyrotoxicosis (mother with Graves' disease)
- Struma ovarii (ovarian teratoma – no thyroid hyperplasia)
- Iatrogenic (exogenous – no thyroid hyperplasia)

---

goitre and in the initial stages of autoimmune thyroiditis (see below).

**Cytological findings: hyperplasia**

- Blood-stained aspirates
- Thin, often barely visible, colloid
- Moderate cellularity
- Dispersed follicular cells with an enlarged round nucleus and single nucleolus, mild anisonucleosis
- Cytoplasmic marginal vacuolation ('fire flares').

Aspiration of the thyroid yields blood-stained material due to the vascularity of the gland. Colloid may not be recognised

and where it is seen it appears as a thin pink wash with MGG stains. Among the blood is a dispersed population of thyroid follicular cells of moderate cellularity with enlarged round nuclei and an easily discernible single nucleolus. There may be some variation in nuclear size. The cytoplasm is increased in amount and is fragile with a faintly frothy texture. It stains pale blue/grey with MGG stains. Bare nuclei may be present. Flat sheets of cells may be seen and in these groups the characteristic marginal vacuolation of cells is present. These pink soap bubble, colloid suds, flame or fire flare appearances (Fig. 17.13) are a manifestation of the active pinocytosis of thyroglobulin from the small follicles found in thyroid hyperplasia. They are found in the majority but not all cases of hyperplasia. Occasional small follicular structures and papillary formations may be seen. Small numbers of lymphocytes may be recognised, although these are often inapparent due to dilution by blood. The pathogenic overlap between Graves' disease and Hashimoto's thyroiditis results in the recognition of Hürthle cell changes, epithelioid histiocytes and multinucleate giant histiocytes in some cases.[38]

Caution needs to be exercised in the interpretation of aspirates from Graves' disease which has failed to respond to medical therapy. The drugs used, which interfere with thyroid hormone biosynthesis, can cause marked nuclear atypia as can the previous use of ablative radioactive iodine. This can lead to confusion with anaplastic or even papillary carcinoma.[39] Dyshormonogenetic goitres similarly show florid hyperplastic features often with papillary architecture and also show nuclear atypia.

## Thyroiditis

Inflammation of the thyroid can be subdivided into lymphocytic and autoimmune (Hashimoto's) thyroiditis, de Quervain's thyroiditis, Riedel's thyroiditis and acute bacterial thyroiditis. FNA in this situation is usually carried out to exclude neoplasia as rapid enlargement of the gland, firmness, nodularity and fixation to surrounding structures may occur in inflammatory conditions. Ultrasound and isotope scans can be misleading and suggest neoplasia. Additionally, thyroiditis may coexist with a neoplasm such as papillary carcinoma and indeed primary lymphoma of the thyroid is predisposed to by underlying autoimmune thyroiditis. FNA can also contribute to the primary diagnosis of Hashimoto's thyroiditis, particularly in the minority of cases which do not have classical serological changes.

## Lymphocytic and autoimmune thyroiditis

A non-specific lymphocytic infiltrate may be found focally in the thyroid adjacent to neoplasms (focal lymphocytic thyroiditis) but the majority of cases of lymphocytic thyroiditis are due to autoimmune disease. A lymphocytic infiltrate and even germinal centre formation may occur in Graves' disease but the classical destructive autoimmune thyroiditis is Hashimoto's thyroiditis. In 95% of cases the patient is female and typically middle-aged, although the disease can occur in other age groups including children. The disease is often familial and may be associated with other organ-specific autoimmune disorders. The patient usually presents with a smooth and moderately enlarged painless goitre. In the acute initial phase of the disease there may be mild thyrotoxicosis (Hashitoxicosis). The majority of patients progress to hypothyroidism over a period of a few years, although the time course may be much longer and such low-grade thyroiditides account for the idiopathic myxoedema of the elderly. Microsomal antibodies are present in high titre in 95% of cases. Hashimoto's thyroiditis is a clinicopathological diagnosis depending on clinical, serological and morphological findings.

The typical gross pathology is a diffuse firm enlargement of the thyroid gland with a pale grey lobulated cut surface. Occasionally the proliferation is nodular and peripherally placed nodules containing lymphoid and epithelial cells may be mistaken for malignancy in a cervical lymph node. Histologically (Fig. 17.14), there is a lymphoplasmacytic infiltrate with germinal centre formation. This is associated with destruction of the follicles and fibrosis. Occasional epithelioid histiocytes and multinucleate histiocytes are seen. The residual follicular cells show an oxyphilic metaplastic change termed oncocytic, Askanazy or Hürthle cell change. These cells may also show mixed hyperplastic features and form papillary infoldings. They show nuclear enlargement and variability in size and shape. Squamous metaplasia may be seen. In a minority of cases, Hashimoto's thyroiditis may be predominantly a fibrosing process and can be confused clinically with malignancy.

### Cytological findings: autoimmune thyroiditis

- Reactive lymphoid cells including follicle centre cells and plasma cells
- Oncocytic (Hürthle) cells
- Multinucleate and epithelioid histiocytes
- Usually little colloid.

Aspiration cytology yields numerous lymphoid cells. These appear reactive and polymorphous with a mixed cell population of lymphocytes, centrocytes, centroblasts, immunoblasts, plasma cells, follicular dendritic cells and occasional tingible-body macrophages (Fig. 17.15). Large multinucleate histiocytes (Fig. 17.16) and small groups of epithelioid histiocytes (Fig. 17.17) may be seen. The latter can be distinguished from epithelial cells by the more delicate quality of their cytoplasm and the presence of footprint-shaped nuclei. The lymphoid cells may be seen admixed within groups of epithelial cells. The epithelial cells show oncocytic (Hürthle

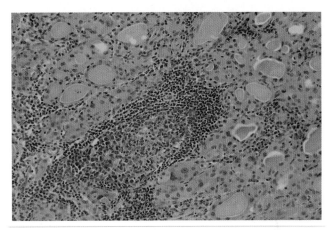

**Fig. 17.14** Hashimoto's thyroiditis: histological appearances (H&E).

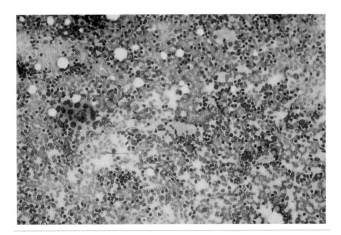

**Fig. 17.15** Hashimoto's thyroiditis: cytological appearances with reactive appearing lymphoid cells, histiocytes and groups of Hürthle cells (MGG).

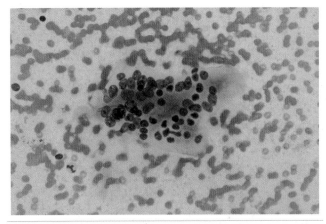

**Fig. 17.16** Hashimoto's thyroiditis. Multinucleate histiocyte (MGG).

cell) change manifested by an increase in the size of the cell and nucleus. The cytoplasm is moderately dense and blue-grey (MGG stain) with a fine granularity better appreciated on the Papanicolaou stain. Cell-to-cell boundaries within the groups are not particularly well-defined. Some of the cell groups may have a vaguely papillary outline. The nuclei appear enlarged, sometimes grossly so. They are hyperchromatic and may appear atypical with variation in size and shape particularly

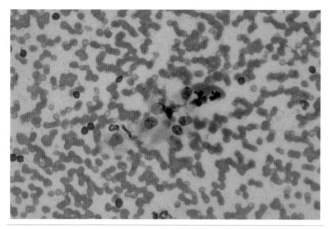

**Fig. 17.17** Hashimoto's thyroiditis. Epithelioid histiocytes (MGG).

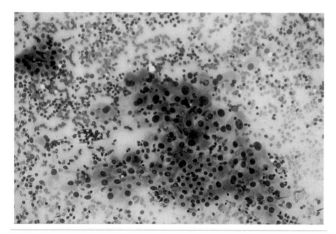

**Fig. 17.18** Hashimoto's thyroiditis. Oncocytic (Hürthle) cells (MGG).

in longstanding disease. Nucleoli can be prominent. Rarely, intranuclear inclusions are seen. In Hashimoto's thyroiditis mixed Hürthle cell and hyperplastic appearances are commonly seen within individual cells (Fig. 17.18). The exact appearances in an aspirate are dependent on the phase of the disease. Early in the disease abundant lymphocytes are present and later Hürthle cell change and fibrosis predominate.[40]

### Diagnostic pitfalls: autoimmune thyroiditis

Hürthle cell groups can be confused with those of papillary carcinoma; points of distinction include the granular quality of the cytoplasm in the former and the presence of more distinct cell-to-cell boundaries in the latter. This distinction is particularly relevant as there is an association between papillary carcinoma and autoimmune thyroiditis. The other main differential diagnostic problem is the distinction from a Hürthle cell neoplasm. Hürthle cell nodules with a less intense inflammatory component may occur in later phase Hashimoto's thyroiditis and the appearances may mimic a neoplasm both histologically and cytologically.[41] Paradoxically, the extent of nuclear variability may be less in a Hürthle cell neoplasm. The groups of cells in neoplasms may show a more papillary or trabecular architecture and are not usually associated with a reactive lymphoid infiltrate. The mixed Hürthle cell-hyperplasia appearance rarely occurs in neoplasms.

There is an increased risk of lymphoma in Hashimoto's thyroiditis and recognition of this coexisting pathology relies upon the appreciation of a monomorphic pattern among the lymphoid cells (see Lymphoma, below). In addition, Hürthle cells are likely to be sparse or absent. Clinical follow-up and repeat FNA is required to avoid false negative diagnosis of coexisting lymphoma. The lymphomas are most often high grade and of B cell type. Immunocytochemistry and flow cytometry to demonstrate monoclonality of light chain expression may be helpful particularly in the low-grade lymphomas which can be more difficult to diagnose.[42]

## de Quervain's thyroiditis (granulomatous thyroiditis)

This condition is a rare form of thyroid inflammation probably due to viral infection in genetically predisposed individuals. Mumps, measles, adenovirus, Epstein–Barr virus, Coxsackie and influenza viruses have been implicated. Typically, it presents in adults following an upper respiratory infection with fever and diffuse tender enlargement of the thyroid. Thyroid pain may be referred to the jaw or ears. There is a female predominance. The usual time course of the illness is a few months. There may be initial mild hyperthyroidism but this is followed by hypothyroidism, which is usually transient. Asymmetric involvement of the gland may raise the question of neoplasia and hence cases come to cytological attention. Histopathologically, there is an initial infiltration of the follicles by mixed inflammatory cells. This appears to result in damage and the release of thyroglobulin to which there is a foreign-body granulomatous reaction. Subsequently there is follicular regeneration and interfollicular fibrosis.

### Cytological findings: de Quervain's thyroiditis

- Numerous multinucleate histiocytes
- Mixed inflammatory cells including epithelioid histiocytes and lymphocytes
- Degenerative changes in follicular cells, cell debris and colloid.

The cytological findings (Fig. 17.19) are of numerous multinucleate histiocytes together with mixed inflammatory cells. These include epithelioid histiocytes forming granulomas and lymphocytes. Degenerating follicular cells may be seen together with a 'dirty' background including cell debris and colloid. Ingested colloid can occasionally be seen within the multinucleate histiocytes. The presence of apparent necrosis and degenerative atypia in follicular cells may lead to an inappropriate suspicion of malignancy.[43]

Granulomatous changes may also arise in the thyroid as a histiocytic response to haemorrhage, as a reaction to spilled colloid adjacent to a neoplasm following clinical examination (palpation thyroiditis), with mycobacterial[44] or fungal infections, in sarcoidosis, in some forms of vasculitis and as a foreign body reaction. The latter has been recorded in a case of Teflon injection into the vocal cord with contamination of the adjacent thyroid.[45] All of these conditions might mimic the appearances of de Quervain's thyroiditis on FNA. Multinucleate giant cells are also seen in autoimmune thyroiditis and aspiration of intact follicles (pseudo-giant cells) should not be confused with multinucleate histiocytes. Osteoclast-like giant cells may occur as a reactive population in anaplastic carcinoma of the thyroid. If these cells predominate in an aspirate they may cause diagnostic confusion with a granulomatous process.[46]

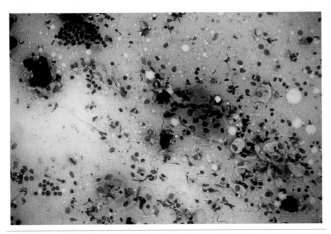

**Fig. 17.19** de Quervain's thyroiditis: thyroiditis: cytological appearances with multinucleate histiocytes, acute and chronic inflammatory cells, cell debris, colloid and follicular cells with degenerative changes (MGG).

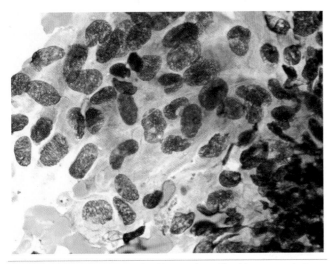

**Fig. 17.20** Riedel's thyroiditis. Fibroblasts and myofibroblasts may mimic malignancy (MGG).

## Riedel's thyroiditis

This is a very rare inflammatory fibrosis of unknown aetiology involving the thyroid and infiltrating adjacent tissues of the neck. It presents with a very firm (ligneous) mass, which appears to be fixed to surrounding structures and hence mimics malignancy clinically and radiologically. It occurs in adults and shows a female predominance. There may be pressure symptoms with dysphagia or stridor. The gland can be focally involved or totally involved, and in the latter case there may be hypothyroidism. Histologically, fibrous tissue replaces the gland. The follicles are obliterated and appear atrophic. Hürthle cell change is not seen. The fibrosis is dense and hyaline but may also contain an inflammatory infiltrate chiefly of lymphocytes and plasma cells. The inflammatory infiltrate has a perivascular distribution and vasculitis, particularly affecting veins, may be seen.

### Cytological findings: Riedel's thyroiditis (Fig. 17.20)

- Usually low cellularity with fragments of fibrous tissue
- Fibroblasts and myofibroblasts
- Occasional lymphocytes, plasma cells and polymorphs
- Absence of necrosis, germinal centre cells, oncocytic cells, multinucleate and epithelioid histiocytes.

---

**Box 17.3  Thyroid neoplasms**

Primary neoplasms
Benign

- Adenoma
- Atypical adenoma

Malignant

- Angioinvasive follicular carcinoma
- Follicular carcinoma
- Papillary carcinoma
- Mixed follicular and medullary carcinoma
- Medullary carcinoma
- Anaplastic carcinoma
- Lymphoma
- Sarcomas

Secondary neoplasms

---

The findings on FNA may be non-specific. The aspirate is often poorly cellular and may include only a few fibroblasts and inflammatory cells. The appearances resemble those seen in fibromatosis and aspirates can be of moderate cellularity with fragments of fibrous tissue including single and small clusters of spindle cells. These cells vary from bland fibroblasts with a uniform pale nucleus to more active appearing myofibroblastic cells with more basophilic cytoplasm, larger nuclei and visible nucleoli. The cells do not show a raised nuclear to cytoplasmic ratio and lack mitoses. There may be scattered inflammatory cells including lymphocytes, plasma cells, neutrophils and rare eosinophils. There is no necrosis in the background. Germinal centre cells and oncocytic cells are not seen in contrast to the fibrosing variant of Hashimoto's thyroiditis. Multinucleate and epithelioid histiocytes are not seen in contrast to de Quervain's thyroiditis. Where there is clinical suspicion biopsy will be necessary to exclude a sclerosing malignancy of the thyroid, particularly the spindle cell variant of anaplastic carcinoma.[47]

## Other forms of thyroiditis

Infection by mycobacteria, fungi and viruses have been mentioned in the context of granulomatous or de Quervain's thyroiditis. In addition cytomegalovirus and *Pneumocystis jirovecii (carinii)* infection of the thyroid are recorded in the immunocompromised.[48] Microfilaria of various species have been visualised as incidental findings in aspirates from cystic degeneration in multinodular goitres.[49] Acute bacterial infection also occurs, particularly in the debilitated, with resultant acute inflammation and abscess formation.

## Thyroid neoplasms

Thyroid neoplasms (Box 17.3) show great differences in their epidemiology, pathogenesis, presentation, natural history, management and prognosis depending upon the histological subtype. Overall thyroid cancer is more common in females with an approximate predominance of 2.5:1. It also shows marked geographical variation but accounts for approximately 0.5% of cancer deaths in the UK. Known risk factors include irradiation to the head and neck area and residence in an endemic goitre region.

## Follicular neoplasms

### Follicular adenoma

Follicular adenomas are the most common of thyroid neoplasms. Autopsy series have shown an incidence of the order of 3% of the adult population. They are slow-growing and show morphological and biochemical evidence of follicular cell differentiation. There is a range of appearances with microscopic features recapitulating the embryology and functional states of the thyroid. Hence, there are embryonal, fetal, normofollicular and macrofollicular histological subtypes. Adenomas may also demonstrate various metaplasias and degenerative changes and hence there are Hürthle cell, clear cell, signet-ring cell adenomas, the adenolipoma showing adipose metaplasia in its stroma and the adenochondroma with cartilaginous metaplasia. Atypical adenomas show nuclear atypia. Common to these tumours, however, are the presence of a well circumscribed and complete fibrous capsule with compression of the surrounding thyroid gland and a relatively uniform appearance of the tumour within the capsule which differs from the surrounding thyroid (Fig. 17.21). Adenomas are usually solitary masses in contrast to colloid nodules in a multinodular goitre. Larger tumours may show degenerative changes with areas of fibrosis and calcification. They may undergo cystic degeneration. Irrespective of their histological pattern they are benign and usually asymptomatic. Occasionally, haemorrhage occurs into an adenoma and the patient presents with a painful and tender mass. A small minority of adenomas behave autonomously and cause hyperthyroidism. The majority of adenomas are hypofunctional and appear as cold nodules on radioisotope scanning.

### Follicular carcinoma

Follicular carcinoma is the second most common type of thyroid carcinoma, constituting approximately 25% of the total. It shows a female predominance in the ratio of 2.5:1 and presents most commonly in the 40–60 age range. The tumour characteristically metastasises haematogenously with secondaries predominantly in the skeleton and lungs.

These malignant thyroid epithelial tumours show evidence of follicular differentiation with no features to suggest any of the other subtypes. They range from well-differentiated to poorly differentiated (Figs 17.22, 17.23). Well-differentiated carcinomas may be cytologically bland and resemble adenomas; indeed well-differentiated follicular carcinoma may appear cytologically less atypical than the benign atypical adenoma. Follicular carcinoma is characterised by the architectural features of local and vascular invasion. Some carcinomas appear totally encapsulated and are so defined on the basis of vascular invasion in capsular vessels. Such lesions can be difficult to diagnose, requiring the examination of multiple histological blocks of the capsule. Treatment for encapsulated or minimally invasive lesions can be by lobectomy and isthmusectomy; widely invasive lesions require total thyroidectomy followed by ablative radioactive [131]I and thyroxine replacement therapy. The overall prognosis gives a 5-year survival of approximately 70%, dependent on the grade, invasiveness and stage of the tumour.

Well-differentiated skeletal metastases can be very indolent with survival for many years. Hürthle cell or oncocytic variants of follicular carcinoma constitute approximately 5% of the total. They show different genetic alterations to usual follicular carcinomas. These have been thought to be intrinsically more aggressive than other follicular carcinomas but the consensus view is that these lesions behave similarly according to their invasiveness, grade and stage. They do not take up radioactive iodine well and hence treatment may be less successful. Hürthle cell tumours may undergo clear cell change caused by swelling of

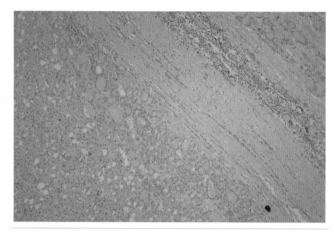

**Fig. 17.21** Follicular adenoma with capsule and adjacent compressed and atrophic thyroid follicles (H&E).

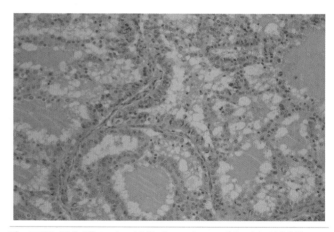

**Fig. 17.22** Well-differentiated follicular carcinoma of the thyroid (H&E).

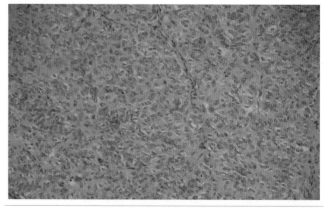

**Fig. 17.23** Poorly differentiated follicular carcinoma of the thyroid (H&E).

the numerous mitochondria which they contain and this is one of the derivations of clear cell variants of follicular carcinoma.

## Fine needle aspiration of follicular neoplasms

FNA serves as a screening tool for the diagnostic triage of follicular lesions. It should exclude those with a non-neoplastic diagnosis and select follicular neoplasms. The non-neoplastic cases do not require surgery but may require clinical and/or cytological follow-up to avoid false negative diagnosis. The neoplasms require surgical excision and histological examination to make the definitive diagnosis of an adenoma or carcinoma on the basis of the architectural features. The triage relies primarily on the appreciation of the degree of cellularity of the specimen and its relationship with the amount of colloid present. These observations are dependent on the technical quality of the smear; reliable diagnosis requires good quality specimens from a consistent aspirator. Approximately 25% of aspirates designated as possible follicular neoplasia will be malignant histologically and will include follicular pattern papillary carcinomas as well as follicular carcinomas.[50]

### Cytological findings: follicular neoplasms

- Cellular aspirates with little, usually thick, colloid, i.e. a high cell to colloid ratio
- Cells groups arranged in microfollicles with central colloid
- Cytological features of hyperplasia usually absent
- Atypical features may be present: nuclear crowding, increased nuclear size, frequency and number of nucleoli raised, nuclear membrane irregularity and irregular chromatin distribution. These do not necessarily imply malignancy.

Aspirates from follicular neoplasms are apt to be blood-stained due to the vascularity of the tumour. With the exception of thyroid hyperplasia, most neoplasms are more cellular than functional abnormalities and also contain less colloid. Colloid, where present, may occur as small inspissated globules within follicular arrangements which can superficially resemble psammoma bodies (Fig. 17.24). The follicular cells, which occur dispersed and in groups, may appear cytologically bland and similar to those seen in aspirates from a multinodular goitre. The cells tend to show less variation of appearance in follicular neoplasms with a repetitive pattern of cell groups. Cytological features of hyperplasia are usually absent in neoplasms. The presence of numerous microfollicular aggregates (Fig. 17.25) implies a follicular neoplasm as such structures are uncommon in nodular goitre aspirates. There may be nuclear enlargement and crowding in the cell groups. The presence of one or more nucleoli may be appreciated.[51–53]

### Diagnostic pitfalls: follicular neoplasms

The cytological appearances of a benign hyperplastic nodule in a multinodular goitre and the appearances of a follicular neoplasm can overlap. Hence, one diagnostic problem is the distinction between a macrofollicular follicular neoplasm and a nodule in a multinodular goitre. With the exception of the rare macrofollicular pattern papillary carcinoma few of the former are malignant and this is an uncommon though potential source of false negative diagnosis in practice. The clinical context may be helpful and the policy of clinical follow-up and repeat FNA minimises the possibility of a missed well-differentiated malignancy.

The distinction between a follicular adenoma and a well-differentiated follicular carcinoma cannot, at present, be made reliably on a needle aspirate sample. The presence of cytological atypia is common to many benign endocrine tumours including thyroid adenomas. This is exemplified by the aspirate illustrated in Figure 17.26 from an atypical adenoma. Methods used to try to resolve this difficulty have included nuclear DNA content and nuclear morphometry.

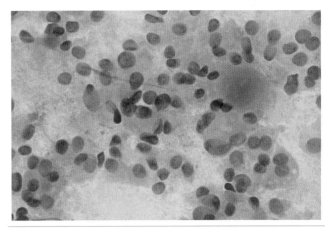

**Fig. 17.24** Aspirate from a follicular neoplasm including an inspissated globule of colloid (Papanicolaou).

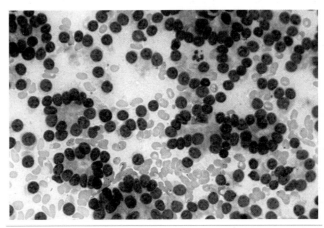

**Fig. 17.25** Aspirate from a follicular neoplasm including microfollicular aggregates (MGG).

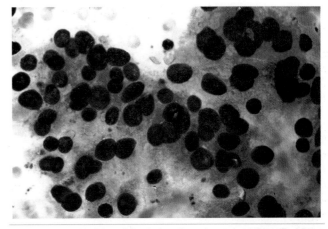

**Fig. 17.26** Aspirate from a follicular neoplasm showing cytological atypia. The subsequent histology showed a benign atypical adenoma (MGG).

Adenomas can be diploid, aneuploid or polyploid in common with follicular carcinoma and hence DNA content does not appear helpful. The results of nuclear morphometry studies to distinguish well-differentiated follicular carcinoma from adenoma have been conflicting. The proportion of cells with nucleoli and the number of nucleoli per cell appear helpful but do not discriminate absolutely, three or more nucleoli per cell being rare in follicular adenomas and occurring in occasional cells in 70% of follicular carcinomas.[54] A study showed that the combination of nuclear diameter, percentage of nucleolated cells and numbers of nucleoli improves the distinction between adenoma and carcinoma above that achieved by subjective evaluation.[55] Silver staining nucleolar organiser region area and number have also been investigated but there is overlap between benign lesions and the higher values seen with malignancies.[56] A wide range of cell surface antigens, enzymes and molecular genetics have also been investigated as potential discriminants. These include CD44, Galectin-3, the antibody HBME-1 and telomerase.[57,58] Loss of genetic heterozygosity and molecular profiling microarray analysis are also under investigation.[59–61] Distinction between a follicular adenoma and follicular carcinoma remains problematical and a report of 'follicular neoplasm' should be given in appropriate cases. It must be ensured that the physician or surgeon understands the meaning of the phrase and the need for excision in all such cases. A comment may be added as regards the presence of atypia. The most discriminant atypical features are high cellularity, crowding in cell groups, increased nuclear size, more than 75% of cells with nucleoli, cells with three or more nucleoli, nuclear membrane irregularity and irregular chromatin distribution. The presence of necrotic debris also supports the suspicion of malignancy.[62] In a minority of cases where the clinical findings suggest malignancy and the aspirates show marked cytological atypia, it is appropriate to diagnose malignancy just as one may with the anaplastic carcinomas. Intraoperative frozen section has a limited role in separating widely invasive follicular carcinomas requiring total thyroidectomy from follicular adenomas and minimally invasive carcinomas which can be managed by local resection. This is because preoperative imaging allows this distinction to be made in most cases.

## Variant follicular neoplasms

### Insular carcinoma

The insular carcinoma is a poorly differentiated follicular carcinoma. Histologically, it consists of well-defined nests of fairly uniform cells and small follicles. These cells often show prominent mitotic activity and the tumour is infiltrative and aggressive in behaviour. Cytologically, smears are hypercellular with sheets of cells, occasional microfollicular aggregates and dispersed cells. The sheets of cells typically show nuclear crowding. The cells are relatively uniform with no gross pleomorphism. Intracytoplasmic vacuoles containing thyroglobulin may be seen. Necrosis may be present. The nuclear to cytoplasmic ratio is high with mild to moderate anisokaryosis and nuclear atypia. Intranuclear inclusions and nuclear grooving can be seen together with a papillary configuration to some of the cell groups and this can cause confusion with papillary carcinoma.[63–64]

### Clear cell tumours

Clear cell and signet-ring cell variants of follicular neoplasms may cause diagnostic difficulty. Clear cell change can occur in

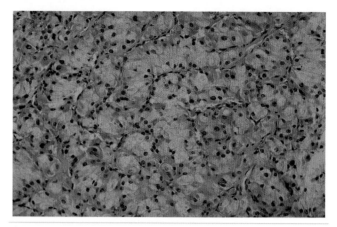

**Fig. 17.27** Hürthle cell adenoma with focal clear cell change (H&E).

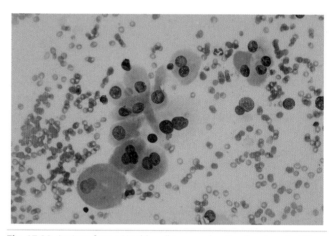

**Fig. 17.28** Aspirate from a Hürthle cell tumour showing the characteristic appearances together with the central binucleate cell which shows clear cell change (MGG).

nodular goitre, follicular neoplasms, papillary carcinoma and medullary carcinoma.[65] Frequently it represents clear cell metaplasia in a Hürthle cell neoplasm (Fig. 17.27). This change may be focal or extensive. Cytologically (Fig. 17.28) there is abundant pale diffusely vacuolated cytoplasm superimposed on the features of the underlying neoplasm. Where the clear cell change is extensive the possibility of a non-thyroid neoplasm should be considered, in particular a parathyroid tumour or metastatic carcinoma of the kidney.[66]

### Hürthle cell tumours

Hürthle (oncocytic) cell tumours present particular difficulties. The differential diagnoses are with autoimmune thyroiditis and nodular goitre. FNA samples are cellular and lack an associated chronic inflammatory infiltrate. There is not the polymorphic cell population seen in thyroiditis or in nodular goitre. The tumour cells have the characteristic abundant finely granular blue-grey cytoplasm in large polygonal or oval cells. The cells may be single, in loose groups or may have a papillaroid/trabecular architecture where tumour cells are arranged around 'transgressing' blood vessels. The characteristic nuclear enlargement and pleomorphism of Hürthle cells is seen with prominent nucleoli. Binucleation is common (Figs 17.28–17.30). Intranuclear inclusions may be present though Hürthle cell tumours with nuclear features of papillary carcinoma may actually be oncocytic

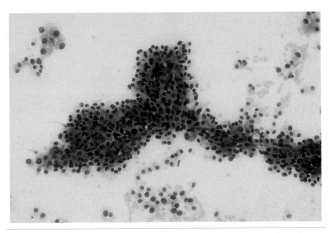

**Fig. 17.29** Aspirate from a Hürthle cell tumour illustrating a papillaroid architecture (MGG).

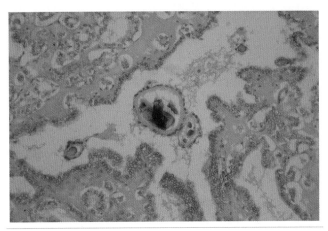

**Fig. 17.31** Papillary carcinoma of the thyroid illustrating the characteristic overlapping 'ground-glass' nuclei and psammoma bodies (H&E).

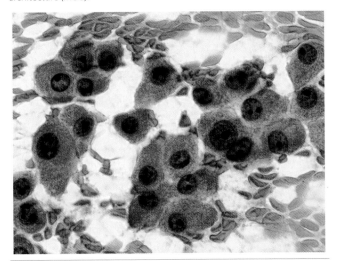

**Fig. 17.30** Hürthle cell tumour aspirate showing nuclear enlargement, pleomorphism and prominent nucleoli (PAP).

papillary carcinoma variants. Though nuclear pleomorphism, crowding and dyscohesion are more frequent in carcinoma the distinction between adenoma and carcinoma is unreliable and the diagnosis of a Hürthle cell neoplasm requiring surgical excision should be made.[67,68] Molecular studies may contribute to this distinction in the future.[69]

## Papillary carcinoma

Papillary carcinoma is the most common malignancy of the thyroid and constitutes 70% of the clinically apparent carcinomas. There is a female predominance of approximately 3:1. It can occur at any age but presents most commonly in the 30–50 age range. Cases in young adults and children are not uncommon. Thorough postmortem studies and examination of thyroids removed for functional abnormalities have shown a high incidence, of between 6% and 35% of the population, of clinically unsuspected, occult, papillary carcinoma. These are small tumours of less than 1 cm diameter. The significance of this finding and the metastatic potential of such cases is, as yet, unknown. A well-established risk factor for papillary carcinoma is exposure of the thyroid to irradiation during childhood either therapeutically or due to radioactive fall-out. The region surrounding Chernobyl in the Ukraine, which sustained

a nuclear accident in 1986, has shown a significant increase in childhood cases.[70]

Patients present with a lump in the thyroid or adjacent neck, the latter due to cervical node metastases. This carcinoma generally has a better prognosis than follicular carcinoma, with a 10-year survival of the order of 80%. The majority of cases can be managed by a total thyroidectomy. Spread of the tumour is by local invasion and by lymphatics. Early blood vessel spread is uncommon. As long as involved lymph nodes can be excised, lymphatic spread does not significantly worsen the prognosis.

Histologically, most cases lack a capsule and intraglandular metastases (multicentricity) are seen in one-quarter of cases. The tumour consists of papillae with a central fibrovascular core covered by cuboidal or columnar cells. These cells have distinctive nuclear features. The nuclei are large and pale staining with a ground glass appearance due to peripheral displacement of the chromatin. Typically the nuclei overlap. Small nucleoli are seen peripherally. A proportion of nuclei show cytoplasmic inclusions and longitudinal nuclear grooving. Some papillae in approximately 50% of cases contain concentrically laminated calcified concretions or psammoma bodies (Fig. 17.31).

These tumours are not exclusively papillary: trabecular and follicular areas are common. Indeed, purely follicular variants of papillary carcinoma are recognised, diagnosis being dependent on the nuclear characteristics. Such tumours have been shown to have the behaviour and prognosis of typical papillary carcinomas. Papillary carcinoma is the most common of several conditions in which focal squamous metaplasia may occur in the thyroid. There are some subtypes of papillary carcinoma, which carry a poorer prognosis. These include the diffuse sclerosing variant, which may present as a diffuse painful enlargement of the gland mimicking thyroiditis, the tall cell and columnar cell variants. The tall cell variant where cell height is at least 2–3 times cell width is the most common of the aggressive subtypes and diagnosis has serious prognostic and management implications. Other variants include oncocytic (Hürthle cell) forms, clear cell forms, the Warthin-like tumour and papillary carcinoma with a nodular fasciitis-like stromal component.[71]

## Cytological findings: papillary carcinoma

- Cellular aspirate with little colloid
- Papillary fronds and sheets of cells

- Dense blue-grey cytoplasm with well-defined cell boundaries
- Intranuclear inclusions
- Nuclear grooves
- Psammoma bodies
- Multinucleate histiocytes particularly where there is cystic degeneration
- 'Chewing-gum' colloid.

Cytologically, papillary carcinoma is the least difficult of the thyroid malignancies to diagnose. Aspirates are cellular and the tumour is characterised by the presence of papillary fronds. These are of varying shapes and sizes but show a smooth surface contour and peripheral palisading of the surface cells (Fig. 17.32). The core, which is less often visualised, is made up of a small amount of fibrous tissue and a small blood vessel. More often the connective tissue core is not aspirated and only papillaroid groups of epithelial cells are seen. Monolayered sheets and ovoid single cells may be seen. The cells in the sheets are relatively large with a polygonal shape. The cytoplasm appears dense and blue-grey with Giemsa stains, it is indistinct in Papanicolaou-stained material. The cytoplasm has characteristically well-defined cell-to-cell boundaries with scalloped borders unlike groups of Hürthle cells, with which there may be a superficial resemblance. The nuclei are enlarged and oval with mild to moderate nuclear pleomorphism. The chromatin pattern may or may not be coarsened. Multiple small nucleoli are usually evident. Intranuclear cytoplasmic inclusions are found without difficulty in 90% of cases (Fig. 17.33). Characteristically, these are well-defined, empty-looking round or oval holes in the nucleus. They usually occupy at least one-third of the nuclear area. Nuclear grooves traversing the entire longitudinal axis of the nucleus and shorter clefts are present in a similar proportion but are a little more difficult to visualise on air-dried and MGG-stained preparations (Fig. 17.34).

Psammoma bodies are seen in approximately one-third of aspirates from papillary carcinomas. They appear as variably blue staining (MGG) refractile laminated structures in the tips of the papillary fragments (Fig. 17.35). Aspirates from approximately half of the cases of papillary carcinoma also contain large multinucleate histiocytes (Fig. 17.36). They are inapparent on histological examination but originate from the interpapillary space particularly where the tumour has a cystic component. In some cases dense chewing-gum colloid may be present but this is not a particularly constant or specific feature in the author's experience (Fig. 17.37).[72–75]

## Papillary carcinoma variants

An infiltrate of lymphocytes may be seen due to non-specific focal thyroiditis in association with a papillary carcinoma but lymphoid cells may be prominent in the diffuse sclerosing and Warthin-like variants of papillary carcinoma.[76,77] Cytological findings have been described for the columnar cell variant which shows elongated cells with hyperchromatic and ovoid nuclei in the absence of intranuclear inclusions and nuclear grooves.[78] The tall cell variant has elongated cells with dense cytoplasm and typical nuclear features of papillary carcinoma.[79] The diffuse sclerosing variant which as well as a chronic inflammatory element is characterised by abundant psammoma bodies and squamous metaplasia.[80] The features of the variant with a nodular fasciitis-like stroma have been described.[81] Aspirates

from the follicular and macrofollicular variants tend to show more colloid and a follicular architectural pattern. The characteristic nuclear features, particularly inclusions and grooves may be infrequent and the aspirate may be misclassified as a follicular neoplasm or even as a benign hyperplastic nodule.

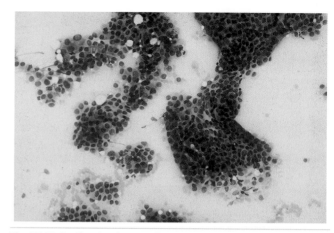

**Fig. 17.32** Papillary fronds in papillary carcinoma (MGG).

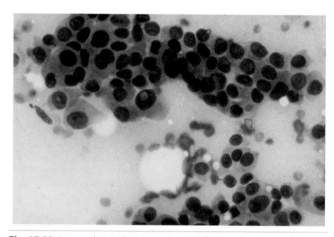

**Fig. 17.33** Intranuclear inclusions and well-defined cell boundaries in papillary carcinoma (MGG).

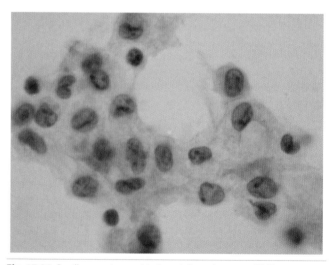

**Fig. 17.34** Papillary carcinoma. Nuclear clefts and grooves (PAP).

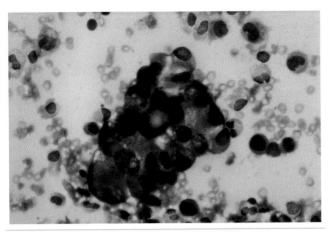

**Fig. 17.35** Papillary carcinoma. Psammoma body (MGG).

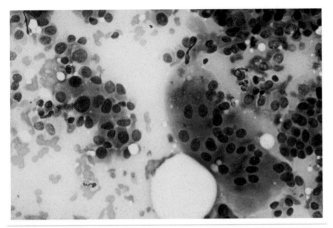

**Fig. 17.36** Papillary carcinoma. Multinucleate histiocyte (MGG).

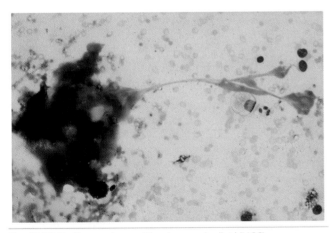

**Fig. 17.37** Papillary carcinoma. 'Chewing-gum' colloid (MGG).

Nuclear membrane thickening and the characteristic dense cytoplasm are usually present.[82,83]

### Diagnostic pitfalls: papillary carcinoma

In practice, the papillary architecture, nuclear inclusions, abundant nuclear grooves, the quality and definition of the cytoplasm are found to be of most use in diagnosis. These are all strong indicators of papillary carcinoma but it should be remembered that rarely intranuclear inclusions and nuclear grooves can be seen in other lesions including multinodular goitre, Hashimoto's thyroiditis, hyalinising trabecular

adenoma, Hürthle cell tumours, follicular tumours, including insular carcinoma, and medullary carcinoma.[63,72] Psammoma bodies are a very valuable finding but are seen in only one-third of cases. Their presence in any thyroid aspirate is always suspicious of papillary carcinoma and an indication for surgery. They can nonetheless very rarely be seen in thyroid hyperplasia, multinodular goitre, Hashimoto's thyroiditis and in hyalinising trabecular adenoma[84] and can also be confused with inspissated colloid. Papillae are valuable but may be absent if a predominantly follicular area of the tumour is sampled[82,83] and can also occur in hyperplasia and in a nodular goitre. Accurate diagnosis of papillary carcinoma, therefore, depends upon recognition of the combination of the most common features.

Cystic degeneration in a papillary carcinoma alters the cytological appearance. These cases are generally less cellular and show degenerative features with a background of debris and macrophages. The tumour cells may show cytoplasmic foamy vacuolation. Three-dimensional tight clusters of cells may be seen. Such cases may require centrifugation of the fluid aspirate in order to distinguish the findings from cystic degeneration in a colloid nodule.[85] Cystic change is particularly common in metastatic papillary carcinoma in neck lymph nodes and aspiration typically of brown-tinged fluid from a neck node requires careful examination to exclude this diagnosis.

A range of ancillary studies are being investigated as aids to the diagnosis of papillary carcinoma. These include preferential expression of cytokeratin 19, detection of BRAF mutation and RET/PTC chromosomal rearrangements. They have yet to find a place in routine diagnostic practice.[42,60,61]

## Hyalinising trabecular tumour

A tumour, which causes difficulties in cytological diagnosis, is the hyalinising trabecular tumour. This is usually a benign tumour described as an adenoma but a malignant variant has been described. On molecular genetic grounds it appears to be a variant of papillary carcinoma.[86] Histologically, the tumour is well circumscribed and encapsulated with polygonal or spindled cells arranged in trabeculae and small islands. Scattered follicles containing thyroglobulin are present. Occasionally, small papillary projections occur into cystic spaces. The trabeculae are surrounded by hyaline fibrosis and basement membrane material. This eosinophilic material may mimic amyloid, although it is Congo red negative. Elongated epithelial cells may be arranged radially around the basement membrane material. Prominent vascular sinusoids are present within the stroma. Intranuclear inclusions and nuclear grooving can be seen. Calcification and the occasional formation of psammoma bodies may be present (Fig. 17.38). The tumour cells stain immunocytochemically for thyroglobulin and are negative for calcitonin. Histologically and cytologically,[87] these tumours can be mistaken for both papillary carcinoma by virtue of the nuclear characteristics and medullary carcinoma due to the eosinophilic stroma and the paragangliomatous appearance of the islands of cells. Figure 17.39 illustrates such a case,[88] which was misdiagnosed as suspicious of papillary carcinoma, on the basis of the nuclear characteristics with numerous cytoplasmic inclusions and grooves, but differed from a typical papillary carcinoma aspirate by the poor cellularity, a haemorrhagic aspirate, the lack of clear

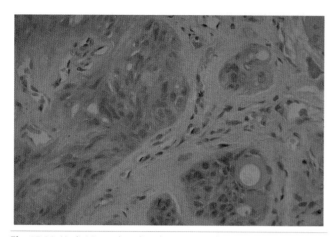

**Fig. 17.38** Hyalinising trabecular adenoma. Histology (H&E).

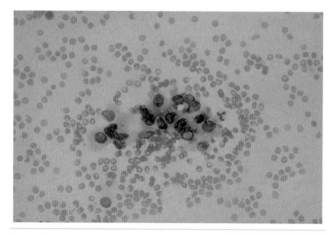

**Fig. 17.39** Hyalinising trabecular adenoma. Cytological appearances with intranuclear inclusions (MGG).

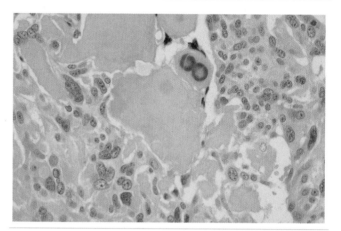

**Fig. 17.40** Medullary carcinoma. Amyloid showing calcification (H&E).

papillae and viscous colloid, and the spindling of some of the cells. Fragments of hyaline material may also be seen. The rarity of this tumour and its misleading cytological features mean that correct diagnosis on FNA is unlikely.

## Medullary carcinoma

Medullary carcinoma of the thyroid is a malignant epithelial tumour showing parafollicular cell differentiation. It constitutes 5–10% of thyroid carcinomas. Seventy-five per cent of the cases are sporadic, the peak of the age distribution being in the fifth decade. The remaining 25% occur in a younger population, particularly in the third and fourth decades, in the context of the multiple endocrine neoplasia syndromes (Box 17.4). There is a slight female preponderance. The tumour invades locally and tends to metastasise early to local lymph nodes. Bloodstream spread is common. Treatment is primarily surgical and prognosis is dependent upon the stage and completeness of excision. There is an overall 5-year survival of approximately 70%.

The tumour usually lacks a capsule and is clearly infiltrative histologically with frequent blood vessel and lymphatic invasion. The tumour occurs in the central and upper parts of the thyroid lobes. It is characterised by amyloid deposition (Fig. 17.40) but this is not invariable, occurring in 80% of cases. The amyloid shows some positivity with antibodies to

calcitonin and is derived from this secretory product. The amyloid may calcify and metaplastic bone formation can occur. The carcinoma cells are tremendously variable. They are usually polyhedral in shape but may show spindling, be small ovoid carcinoid-like cells or may mimic small cell carcinoma. Giant cell, clear cell, melanotic, mucinous and oncocytic forms are also recognised. Architecturally common patterns are trabecular and an alveolar paragangliomatous arrangement. Rarer patterns include the angiomatous, tubular and papillary forms. The cells contain neurosecretory granules and immunocytochemically 80% of cases stain positively for calcitonin. There is a rare group of tumours, which show features of both medullary and follicular differentiation with immunocytochemical positivity for both calcitonin and thyroglobulin.

### Cytological findings: medullary carcinoma

- Dispersed cellular aspirate
- Variable cell size and shape
- Cytoplasmic granularity
- Amyloid
- Calcitonin positivity.

Cytologically, the aspirates are moderately to highly cellular depending on the degree of stromal fibrosis and amyloid deposition. The cells are poorly cohesive often with a dispersed pattern and vary from case to case in size and shape as would be expected from the histological description given. Most commonly the cells are polygonal, ovoid or spindled in shape (Fig. 17.41). There may be pleomorphism of cell size and shape within a single aspirate and the presence of a mixed cell population is a diagnostic pointer to medullary carcinoma. The nuclei in the polygonal or ovoid cell types are often eccentrically placed within the cytoplasm, giving a plasmacytoid appearance. Multinucleate cells and nuclear pleomorphism may be present with occasional bizarre giant cells. Nucleoli are small and inconspicuous. Occasional nuclear grooves and intranuclear cytoplasmic inclusions may be present. The chromatin pattern is typically speckled. Mitoses are rare. MGG staining shows a proportion of the cells to have a fine, typically pink, cytoplasmic granularity (Fig. 17.42). This granularity may also be recognised in Papanicolaou stained smears but with less ease. Immunocytochemical staining, which substantiates the diagnosis, confirms that the granules contain calcitonin (Fig. 17.43).

Other special techniques which may be helpful, particularly for the minority of cases that are calcitonin negative, are immunocytochemical positivity for chromogranin A, synaptophysin and carcinoembryonic antigen with negativity for thyroglobulin. These techniques avoid confusion of the cytoplasmic granularity with that seen in Hürthle cell neoplasms. Other points of distinction are the denser cytoplasm and presence of prominent nucleoli in Hürthle cell tumours. Amyloid appears as amorphous or fibrillar blue-magenta material (Fig. 17.44). With Papanicolaou staining it is pink/orange. It can be confused with small fragments of loose connective tissue or colloid, is often present in small amounts and may be absent in up to 50% of cases. Occasionally it may appear in discrete blobs surrounded by tumour cells giving a follicular pattern. Congo red staining, which can be carried out on spare or destained material, helps confirm its nature. Rarely, fragments of calcification and even psammoma bodies may be seen.[89] It should also be noted that amyloid can also be seen in thyroid aspirates from the rare amyloid goitre.[90] Mixed follicular and medullary carcinomas are defined by the presence of calcitonin positivity. Their cytological appearances may be very misleading and the diagnosis of a follicular neoplasm may be made. The author has experience of one case[88] misdiagnosed as a papillary carcinoma due to the presence of abundant intranuclear inclusions a nd the confusion of amyloid with chewing-gum colloid. The cytological appearances of mucinous[91] and melanotic[92] variants of medullary carcinoma have been described. Measuring the patients serum calcitonin may help in cases where cytological diagnosis is difficult.

## Anaplastic carcinoma

Anaplastic carcinomas are a group of tumours that include at least a component of undifferentiated carcinoma. They constitute approximately 5% of thyroid carcinomas and occur in the elderly with a female predominance. They are highly aggressive tumours presenting with a rapidly advancing hard mass in the thyroid. At presentation there is often hoarseness, stridor and dysphagia. Death is usually as a result of local invasion,

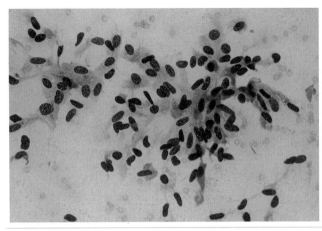

**Fig. 17.41** Medullary carcinoma. Spindled cells with pink granules in the cytoplasm (MGG).

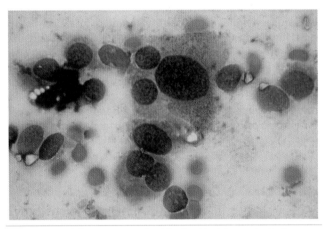

**Fig. 17.42** Medullary carcinoma. Ovoid cells with pink granules in the cytoplasm (MGG).

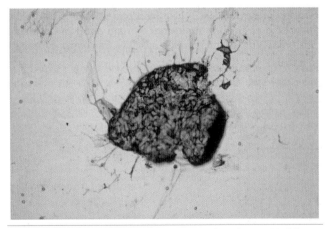

**Fig. 17.43** Immunoalkaline phosphatase staining for calcitonin. Medullary carcinoma aspirate.

although nodal and haematogenous spread also occurs. Most cases are inoperable at presentation; radiotherapy and chemotherapy are generally ineffective. Survival in most cases is limited to a few months.

Histologically, the appearances are variable with principally giant cell, spindle cell and squamoid forms. Anaplastic carcinomas are highly pleomorphic with a high mitotic index. Foci of necrosis may be present. About 10% of cases contain admixed osteoclast-like giant cells. The spindle cell form may be associated with a prominent stromal response and can mimic a variety of sarcomas. With the exception of angiosarcoma in endemic goitre regions, true sarcomas of the thyroid are extremely rare. Occasionally foci of well-differentiated thyroid carcinomas may be observed amongst the anaplastic carcinoma suggesting that these tumours arise by dedifferentiation of all the major subtypes of carcinoma. Immunocytochemically, there is usually low-molecular-weight cytokeratin expression, although this may be lost during the course of dedifferentiation. Thyroglobulin expression is frequently lost. Vimentin expression and coexpression with cytokeratins is common, particularly in spindle cell areas.[93]

FNA has a particularly valuable role enabling the confirmation of what is usually clinically obvious malignancy without recourse to needle core biopsy or surgery. This enables the immediate adoption of appropriate management. Most importantly, however, FNA allows the identification of treatable thyroid lymphomas, which may present in an identical fashion to anaplastic carcinoma.

## Cytological findings: anaplastic carcinoma

- Elderly patients with a rapidly advancing hard mass in the neck
- Bizarre giant, squamoid or spindle cells
- Necrosis may be present.

Aspirates show bizarre giant or spindle cells (Figs 17.45, 17.46) which may be isolated or in small clusters. The cellularity of the specimen is variable: the spindle cell variant may be paucicellular due to the fibrosis associated with this subtype. The cells have pleomorphic nuclei and may be multinucleate. Multiple nucleoli are usually present. The chromatin pattern is coarse and clumped. Necrosis and neutrophil polymorphs may be observed and this material may predominate. Osteoclast-like giant cells may be seen. Occasionally elements of better-differentiated areas are present and if sampling is poor only these areas might be aspirated, giving a tumour diagnosis which may be at odds with the aggressive clinical behaviour. In the differential diagnosis pleomorphic and spindle cells may also be seen in medullary carcinoma. Occasional bizarre cells may be seen as a degenerative change in multinodular goitre, in follicular adenomas and following irradiation or chemotherapy but in the appropriate clinical and cytological setting there should be no difficulty with diagnosis. The possibility of a metastatic carcinoma should also be considered.[94–96]

## Lymphoma

Lymphomas of the thyroid may either originate in that site or affect the thyroid secondarily as a manifestation of systemic disease. Primary lymphoma constitutes approximately 5% of thyroid malignancies. This tumour occurs predominantly in middle-aged and elderly women presenting with a rapidly enlarging firm mass. Local compression effects with dysphagia, stridor and voice change are not uncommon and hence the mode of presentation is very similar to that of anaplastic carcinoma. There is a strong association, described in some series

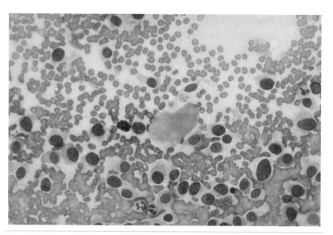
**Fig. 17.44** Amyloid in a medullary carcinoma (MGG).

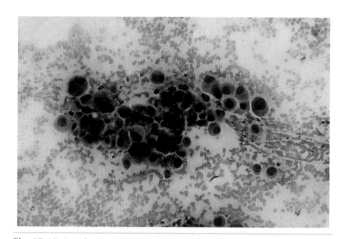
**Fig. 17.45** Anaplastic carcinoma. Giant cell form (MGG).

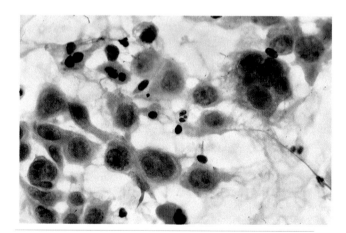
**Fig. 17.46** Anaplastic carcinoma. Spindle cell form with necrosis (MGG).

as being up to 94%,[97] between primary thyroid lymphoma and preceding Hashimoto's thyroiditis.

The lymphomas are predominantly B-cell non-Hodgkin lymphomas (NHL). The morphology and behaviour of these neoplasms suggests that they arise as tumours of the mucosa associated lymphoid tissues (MALT lymphomas). Hodgkin's disease presenting in the thyroid is rare and always associated with cervical or mediastinal lymphadenopathy.[98] Plasmacytomas and Langerhans cell histiocytosis occasionally affect the thyroid.

Lymphoma cells diffusely infiltrate the thyroid parenchyma and, after involving the entire gland, then affect the surrounding soft tissues. The lymphoid cells characteristically invade the lumina of thyroid follicles giving rise to lymphoepithelial lesions. Blood vessel wall invasion may also be seen. NHL can be divided broadly into low-grade and high-grade types. At presentation the majority of cases are high-grade diffuse large B-cell lymphomas often seen together with low-grade marginal zone lymphoma. Low-grade NHL are small cell in type and predominantly marginal zone B-cell lymphomas (MALT type) though occasional primary follicular lymphomas are seen. In most cases a background of autoimmune thyroiditis can be seen. Treatment is usually by radiotherapy and surgical decompression if necessary. If there is evidence of dissemination, chemotherapy is appropriate. The prognosis for localised disease is good with approximately 75% 10-year survival.

### Cytological findings: lymphoma

Cytologically, high-grade NHL consists of a population of dissociated large blastic lymphoid cells usually with the typical background of pale-blue fragments of cytoplasm (lymphoglandular bodies) (Fig. 17.47). These appearances usually present no difficulty in distinguishing anaplastic carcinoma and lymphoma but, given the very different prognosis and treatment, immunostaining for leucocyte common antigen and the absence of cytokeratin staining is usual for confirmation.

The low-grade lymphomas are more difficult to diagnose, particularly if the aspirates also harvest cells from the surrounding autoimmune thyroiditis. There may, therefore, be a mixed cell population of reactive and neoplastic lymphoid cells together with Hürthle cells. Multiple aspirates may be necessary to clarify the situation. Low-grade NHL can be recognised by the more monotonous lymphoid population with a predominance of small centrocyte-like cells. Plasmacytic differentiation may be seen. If a mixture of reactive and neoplastic elements is obtained the cytological appearances may only be suspicious. In this circumstance immunocytochemistry for light chain restriction may be difficult to interpret; flow cytometry on a dedicated sample in an appropriate medium can be helpful and polymerase chain reaction (PCR) may demonstrate a clonal proliferation but final diagnosis often require biopsy. The small malignant cells are usually readily recognisable as lymphoid in type. The differential diagnostic possibilities of a small cell medullary carcinoma and the poorly differentiated insular carcinoma should be considered. The author's own practice is to recommend biopsy confirmation of the diagnosis of low-grade NHL in the thyroid in view of the diagnostic difficulties prior to radiotherapy whereas this is generally not necessary for high-grade lymphomas[99](see Ch. 14).

## Metastatic malignancies

Careful postmortem examination reveals metastatic carcinoma in the thyroid in approximately 10% of cases of malignancy. The most common sites of origin are breast, kidney, lung, the gastrointestinal tract and squamous carcinomas of the head and neck region. Metastatic melanoma also occurs. Clinical presentation with a secondary malignancy in the thyroid is, however, rare. One series of nearly 25 000 FNA of the thyroid revealed only 25 cases of metastases. Eleven of these cases had

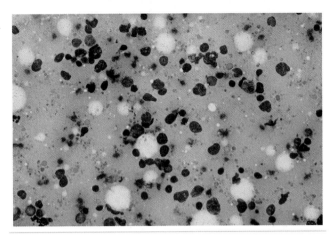

**Fig. 17.47** High-grade non-Hodgkin lymphoma aspirate from the thyroid. Note the 'lymphoglandular bodies' (MGG).

a known history of previous malignancy and in the absence of such a history only five cases were identified as metastatic.[100] Secondary malignancies cause difficulty in diagnosis, as they may be confused with primary thyroid neoplasms.

Clear cell carcinoma of the kidney mimics clear cell tumours of the thyroid. A clear cell tumour in the thyroid is more likely to be a secondary than a primary thyroid neoplasm, particularly if there is a past history or current radiological evidence of a renal tumour. Thyroglobulin immunostaining is generally unreliable, as a renal secondary aspirate may be contaminated by thyroglobulin from the surrounding thyroid and some clear cell tumours of the thyroid are thyroglobulin negative.[101] More discriminant staining is provided by immunocytochemical positivity for TTF-1 and CD117 in primary thyroid carcinoma and CD10 positivity in renal adenocarcinoma.[66] Carcinomas from the breast or lung may mimic anaplastic or papillary carcinoma of the thyroid. Pure squamous carcinomas of the thyroid are rare and are more likely to represent local spread from an oesophageal, pharyngeal, laryngeal or tracheal primary or metastasis from the bronchus. Cases of carcinoid and amelanotic melanoma metastatic to the thyroid simulating medullary carcinoma have been recorded. In general, when a neoplasm is recognised in an aspirate from the thyroid of a patient with a history of a cancer elsewhere in the body, the possibility that it is a metastasis rather than a second primary should be strongly considered. Biopsy confirmation should be considered where there is any cytological or clinical doubt to avoid unnecessarily poor prognostication in those with previous malignancy and to ensure appropriate treatment of a primary thyroid neoplasm.[102,103]

## Specimen adequacy and diagnostic accuracy

Detailed analysis of thyroid cytology diagnostic accuracy is hampered by the numerous techniques used and differences in subsequent cytological and histological categorisation.[104] The majority of aspirates are benign and there is no subsequent histological correlation. The success of FNA is a function of a low false negative rate and a high true positive rate allowing appropriate selection of patients for subsequent surgical excision. The false negative rate is particularly dependant on sample adequacy with an appropriate quantity of good-quality material presented for staining and interpretation. Adequate interpretive skills are also required and particularly so in maximising the true positive rate.

**Table 17.3** Royal College of Pathologists guidance on reporting of thyroid cytology FNA specimens[122]

| | | |
|---|---|---|
| Thy1 | | Insufficient for cytological diagnosis. To be considered of adequate epithelial cellularity, samples from solid lesions should have at least six groups of thyroid follicular epithelial cells across all the submitted slides, each with at least 10 well-visualised epithelial cells. |
| | | The reason for sample insufficiency should be clearly stated in the cytology report. |
| | Thy1c | Cyst-fluid specimens which do not reach the epithelial cell adequacy criterion above and which contain mostly macrophages but without abundant colloid. |
| | | *Comment:* There is a recognised risk of non-representative sampling, especially in cystic papillary thyroid carcinomas. It is important not to offer false reassurance on suboptimal epithelial cellularity. Careful assessment is needed, possibly with MDM discussion. |
| Thy2 | | Non-neoplastic. Samples in this category should achieve the epithelial cellularity adequacy criterion described above .This non-neoplastic category therefore includes: normal thyroid tissue, thyroiditis, hyperplastic nodules, colloid nodules; these samples will contain easily identifiable colloid with cytologically bland follicular epithelial cells reaching the cellular adequacy criteria outlined above. |
| | Thy2c | Cyst specimens which consist predominantly of colloid and macrophages, even when too few follicular epithelial cells are present to meet the adequacy criteria outlined above, can be considered to be 'consistent with a colloid cyst' in the appropriate clinical setting. |
| Thy3 | | Neoplasm possible. The majority of the lesions in this category are follicular neoplasms. Due to the limitations of FNA cytology, the nature of these lesions cannot be determined solely by FNA cytology and MDM discussion is needed to decide further management. |
| | Thy3a | Samples which exhibit cytological atypia or other features which raise the possibility of neoplasia, but which are insufficient to categorise otherwise with confidence into any other category. These should form only a small minority of Thy3 cases. This group is to be classed as Thy3a ('a' for 'atypia'). For further details as to clinical scenarios in which category 3a applies, see ref. 122. |
| | Thy3f | Samples suggesting follicular neoplasms. These should form the majority of the Thy3 category. The histological possibilities therefore include hyperplastic or other cellular but non-neoplastic nodules, as well as neoplasms, including follicular adenomas and follicular carcinomas. Follicular variants of papillary thyroid carcinoma without clear nuclear features of papillary thyroid cancer may fall into this category. These cannot be reliably distinguished on cytology alone. This group is to be classed Thy3f ('f' for 'follicular'). Samples consisting almost inclusively/exclusively of Hürtle cells are also included here. |
| Thy4 | | Suspicious of malignancy. Those samples which are suspicious of malignancy, but which do not allow confident diagnosis of malignancy. This includes specimens of low cellularity and mixed cell types (normal and atypical). The tumour type suspected should be clearly stated, and will often be papillary carcinoma. This category should not be used for samples that exhibit mild atypia, which should be categorised as Thy3a. Cases of definite malignancy, but where a specific diagnosis cannot be made (e.g. lymphoma vs anaplastic carcinoma), should be in the Thy5 category. |
| Thy5 | | Malignant. These samples are those that can be confidently diagnosed as malignant. The tumour type should be clearly stated, e.g. papillary thyroid carcinoma, medullary thyroid carcinoma, anaplastic thyroid carcinoma, lymphoma, other malignancy, including potentially non-thyroid/metastatic malignancy. |

FNA, fine needle aspiration; MDM, multidisciplinary meeting.

Some consideration must be given to what constitutes an adequate aspirate. The evidence available is difficult to assess[5] but it has been proposed, on the basis of reviewing large numbers of known false negative cases, that the minimum criteria for adequacy in the examination of thyroid nodules and exclusion of neoplasia should be the presence of at least five or six clusters of 10 cells or more on each of at least two slides taken from separate aspirates. Even with these criteria, false negatives will still occur and a further reduction in that rate will result from further aspirations.[5,105] Clearly, even very scanty aspirates can be diagnostic where there are characteristic features, for example of a papillary carcinoma or Hashimoto's thyroiditis. If atypia is present it should be described and interpretation attempted even if little material is present. Colloid-rich specimens with scanty follicular cells can, in the appropriate clinical and radiological context, be regarded as diagnostic. Cyst fluid samples where there is no residual mass after aspiration can also be regarded as adequate even if of low cellularity.

The unsatisfactory and false negative rate is, of course, dependent on the underlying pathology and upon the skills of the aspirator and interpreter. Inadequate samples in most studies account for approximately 10–15% of the total. Inadequate rates of less than 5% have been described in studies including palpation guided, ultrasound guided and thin-layer prepared samples.[106–108] Improved performance of the technique is achieved where a limited number of individuals both aspirate and interpret the specimens. Aspiration by the pathologist with access to all of the clinical information together with immediate staining and interpretation reduces false negative rates and allows the best judgement as to whether an aspirate is adequate or not and whether further aspirates are advisable.[109–111] Failing immediate diagnosis an on-site evaluation of specimen adequacy by a cytopathologist or cytotechnologist can decrease the percentage of unsatisfactory specimens and limit the number of needle passes required.[112–114] Use of ultrasound-guidance where palpation-guided FNA has failed and in indistinct, impalpable, deeply placed and mixed solid-cystic lesions improves adequacy rates.[9]

The most important role of thyroid FNA is in the diagnosis of solitary or dominant nodules. Fewer than 5% of palpable nodules are malignant. The use of needle aspiration reduces the use of surgery by approximately one-third, doubles the proportion of malignancies among surgical resections and increases cost-effectiveness.[115] Serious diagnostic delay due to false negative FNA is uncommon where there is an appreciation of the false negative rate for a single aspirate and adequate clinical follow-up and/or repeat FNA of apparently benign lesions before patients are discharged from clinic.[116] The published false negative rate of thyroid FNA varies between 1% and 10%.[5] The highest rates are associated with cystic carcinomas. False positive diagnoses are rare, less than 1% of cases, where the convention of diagnosing follicular neoplasia rather than always attempting to specify adenoma or carcinoma is used. The use of clear and consistent reporting categories with defined follow-up or therapeutic actions decreases errors and ensures appropriate interpretation of needle aspiration results by clinical colleagues.[117–119]

**Table 17.4** The Bethesda system for reporting thyroid cytopathology with RCPath equivalents of implied risk of malignancy

| Diagnostic category | Risk of malignancy (%) |
|---|---|
| Non-diagnostic or unsatisfactory/Thy1/Thy1c | 0–10 |
| Benign/Thy2/Thy2c | 0–3 |
| Atypia of undetermined significance or follicular lesion of undetermined significance/Thy3a | 5–15 |
| Follicular neoplasm or suspicious for a follicular neoplasm/Thy3f | 15–30 |
| Suspicious for malignancy/Thy4 | 60–75 |
| Malignant/Thy5 | 97–99 |

**Table 17.5** The Bethesda system for reporting thyroid cytopathology: recommended diagnostic categories and RCPath equivalents

| Bethesda | RCPath |
|---|---|
| **I. Non-diagnostic or unsatisfactory** | **Thy1** |
| Cyst fluid only | Thy1c |
| Virtually acellular specimen | |
| Other (obscuring blood, clotting artifact, etc.) | |
| **II. Benign** | **Thy2** |
| Consistent with a benign follicular nodule (includes adenomatoid nodule, colloid nodule, etc.) | |
| Consistent with lymphocytic (Hashimoto) thyroiditis in the proper clinical context | |
| Consistent with granulomatous (subacute) thyroiditis | |
| Other | Thy2c |
| **III. Atypia of undetermined significance or follicular lesion of undetermined significance** | Thy3a |
| **IV. Follicular neoplasm or suspicious for a follicular neoplasm** | Thy3f |
| Specify if Hürthle cell (oncocytic) type | |
| **V. Suspicious for malignancy** | **Thy4** |
| Suspicious for papillary carcinoma | |
| Suspicious for medullary carcinoma | |
| Suspicious for metastatic carcinoma | |
| Suspicious for lymphoma | |
| Other | |
| **VI. Malignant** | **Thy5** |
| Papillary thyroid carcinoma | |
| Poorly differentiated carcinoma | |
| Medullary thyroid carcinoma | |
| Undifferentiated (anaplastic) carcinoma | |
| Squamous cell carcinoma | |
| Carcinoma with mixed features (specify) | |
| Metastatic carcinoma | |
| Non-Hodgkin lymphoma | |
| Other | |

## Integrated management schemes for thyroid cytology

Several classification and integrated management schemes have been proposed and are in use (Tables 17.3, 17.4).[120,121] Other schemes include the *Bethesda Atlas of Terminology* and the Royal College of Pathologists guidance on the reporting of thyroid cytology specimens (Table 17.5).[122] To ensure effective use of thyroid cytology pathologists should agree with local surgeons, endocrinologists, radiologists and oncologists on the use of any particular terminology and ideally meet to discuss individual cases at multidisciplinary-team meetings. The various management schemes differ in the terminology used and in follow-up protocols but in common they prescribe a surgical referral for suspicious or definite differentiated thyroid cancer and appropriate further investigation, radiotherapy and/or chemotherapy for anaplastic carcinoma, lymphoma or metastatic malignancy. The distinction between follicular adenoma and carcinoma remains problematic and suspected follicular neoplasms warrant a surgical referral and lobectomy for diagnosis. In recognition of the risk of false negative cytology non-neoplastic aspirates should have a degree of follow-up by ultrasound imaging and usually a repeat FNA prior to discharge of the patient. When there is strong clinical or radiological suspicion the decision to proceed to lobectomy may be made despite a benign cytological diagnosis. The management schemes also recognise the crucial importance of the quality of thyroid FNA specimens and include stipulations as to adequacy and actions to be taken, including the use of image guidance, where samples are non-diagnostic.

## REFERENCES

1. Martin HE, Ellis EB. Aspiration biopsy. Surg Gynaecol Obstet 1934;59:578–89.
2. Grunze H, Spriggs AI. History of Clinical Cytology: A Selection of Documents. 2nd edn. Darmstadt: G-I-T Verlag Ernst Giebeler; 1983 132.
3. Söderström N. Puncture of goiters for aspiration biopsy. A preliminary report. Acta Med Scand 1952;144:237–44.
4. Einhorn J, Franzén S. Thin-needle biopsy in the diagnosis of thyroid disease. Acta Radiol 1962;58:321–36.
5. Kocjan G, Feichter G, Hagmar B, et al. Fine needle aspiration cytology: a survey of current European practice. Cytopathology 2006;17:219–26.
6. Pitman MB, Abele J, Ali SZ, et al. Techniques for thyroid FNA. A synopsis of the National Cancer Institute thyroid fine-needle aspiration state of the science conference. Diagn Cytopathol 2008;36:407–24.
7. Cibas ES, Alexander EK, Benson CB, et al. Indications for thyroid FNA and pre-FNA requirements. A synopsis of the National Cancer Institute thyroid fine-needle aspiration state of the science conference. Diagn Cytopathol 2008;36:390–99.

8. Are C, Hsu JF, Schoder H, et al. FDG-PET detected thyroid incidentalomas: need for further investigation? Ann Surg Oncol 2007;14:239–47.

9. Ljung B-ME, Langer J, Mazzaferri EL, et al. Training, credentialing and re-credentialing for the performance of thyroid FNA. A synopsis of the National Cancer Institute thyroid fine-needle aspiration state of the science conference. Diagn Cytopathol 2008;36:400–6.

10. Buley ID, Roskell DE. Fine-needle aspiration cytology in diagnosis: uses and limitations. Clin Oncol (R Coll Radiol) 2000;12:166–71.

11. Haddadi-Nezhad S, Larijani B, Taranger SM, et al. Comparison of fine-needle-nonaspiration with fine-needle-aspiration technique in the cytologic studies of thyroid nodules. Endocr Pathol 2003;14:369–73.

12. Rivsa SA, Husain M, Khan S, et al. A comparative study of fine needle aspiration cytology versus non-aspiration technique in thyroid lesions. Surgeon 2005;3:273–76.

13. Pothier DD, Narula AA. Should we apply suction during fine needle cytology of thyroid lesions? A systematic review and meta-analysis. Ann R Coll Surg Engl 2006;88:643–45.

14. Mair S, Dunbar F, Becker PJ, et al. Fine needle cytology – is aspiration suction necessary? A study of 100 masses in various sites. Acta Cytol 1989;33:809–13.

15. Abele JS, Miller TR, King EB, et al. Smearing techniques for the concentration of particles from fine needle aspiration biopsy. Diagn Cytopathol 1985;1:59–65.

16. Michael CW, Pang Y, Pu RT, et al. Cellular adequacy for thyroid aspirates prepared by ThinPrep: How many cells are needed? Diagn Cytopathol 2007;35:792–97.

17. Scurry JP, Duggan MA. Thin layer compared to direct smear in thyroid fine needle aspiration. Cytopathol 2000;11:104–15.

18. Malle D, Valeri RM, Pazaitou-Panajiotou K, et al. Use of thin-layer technique in thyroid fine needle aspiration. Acta Cytol 2006;50:23–27.

19. Frost AR, Sidawy MK, Ferfelli M, et al. Utility of thin-layer preparations in thyroid fine-needle aspiration: diagnostic accuracy, cytomorphology, and optimal sample preparation. Cancer 1998;84:17–25.

20. Afify AM, Liu J, Al-Khafaji BM. Cytologic artefacts and pitfalls of thyroid fine needle aspiration using ThinPrep: a comparative retrospective review. Cancer 2001;93:179–86.

21. Cochaud-Priollet B, Pratt JJ, Polivka M, et al. Thyroid fine needle aspiration: the morphological features on ThinPrep slide preparations. Eighty cases with histological control. Cytopathology 2003;14:343–49.

22. Stamataki M, Anninos D, Brountzos E, et al. The role of liquid based cytology in the investigation of thyroid lesions. Cytopathology 2008;19:11–18.

23. Hor T, Lahiri SW. Bilateral thyroid hematomas after fine-needle aspiration causing acute airway obstruction. Thyroid 2008;18:491–92.

24. Tomoda C, Takamuva Y, Ito Y, et al. Transient vocal cord paralysis after fine-needle aspiration biopsy of thyroid tumor. Thyroid 2006;16:697–99.

25. Gordon DL, Gattuso P, Castelli M, et al. Effect of fine needle aspiration biopsy on the histology of thyroid neoplasms. Acta Cytol 1993;37:651–54.

26. Karwowski JK, Nowels KW, MacDougall IR, et al. Needle track seeding of papillary thyroid cancer from fine needle aspiration biopsy. A case report. Acta Cytol 2002;46:591–95.

27. Panunzi C, Palliotta DS, Papini E, et al. Cutaneous seeding of a follicular thyroid cancer after fine-needle aspiration biopsy? Diagn Cytopathol 1994;10:156–58.

28. Nishihara E, Miyauchi A, Matsuzuka F, et al. Acute suppurative thyroiditis after fine needle aspiration causing thyrotoxicosis. Thyroid 2005;15:1183–87.

29. Pandit AA, Phulpager MD. Worrisome histologic alterations following fine needle aspiration of the thyroid. Acta Cytol 2001;45:173–79.

30. Sidawy MK, Costa M. The significance of paravacuolar granules of the thyroid: a histologic, cytologic and ultrastructural study. Acta Cytol 1989;33:929–33.

31. Keyhani-Rofagha S, Kooner DS, Landas SK, et al. Black thyroid: a pitfall for aspiration cytology. Diagn Cytopathol 1991;7:640–43.

32. Butler SL, Oertel YC. Lipomas of anterior neck simulating thyroid nodules: diagnosis by fine-needle aspiration. Diagn Cytopathol 1992;8:528–31.

33. Rollins SD, Flinner RL. Thyrolipoma: diagnostic pitfalls in the cytologic diagnosis and review of the literature. Diagn Cytopathol 1991;7:150–54.

34. Shahin A, Burroughs FH, Kirby JP, et al. Thyroglossal duct cyst: a cytopathologic study of 26 cases. Diagn Cytopathol 2005;33:365–69.

35. Oertel YC. Thymoma mimicking papillary carcinoma; another pitfall in fine needle aspiration. Diagn Cytopathol 1997;17:61–63.

36. Harach HR, Zusman SB, Day ES. Nodular goiter: a histocytological study with some emphasis on pitfalls of fine-needle aspiration cytology. Diagn Cytopathol 1992;8:409–19.

37. Sarda AK, Bal S, Gupta SD, et al. Diagnosis and treatment of cystic disease of the thyroid by aspiration. Surgery 1988;103:593–96.

38. Anderson SR, Mandel S, LiVolsi VA, et al. Can cytomorphology differentiate between benign nodules and tumours arising in Graves' disease? Diagn Cytopathol 2004;31:64–67.

39. Granter SR, Cibas ES. Cytologic findings in thyroid nodules after 131I treatment of hyperthyroidism. Am J Clin Pathol 1997;107:20–25.

40. MacDonald L, Yazdi HM. Fine needle aspiration biopsy of Hashimoto's thyroiditis. Sources of diagnostic error. Acta Cytol 1999;43:400–6.

41. Carson HJ, Castelli MJ, Gattuso P. Incidence of neoplasia in Hashimoto's thyroiditis: a fine needle aspiration study. Diagn Cytopathol 1996;14:38–42.

42. Filie AC, Asa SL, Geisinger KR, et al. Utilisation of ancillary studies in thyroid fine needle aspirates. A synopsis of the National Cancer Institute thyroid fine-needle aspiration state of the science conference. Diagn Cytopathol 2008;36:438–41.

43. Shabb NS, Salti I. Subacute thyroiditis: Fine needle aspiration cytology of 14 cases presenting with thyroid nodules. Diagn Cytopathol 2006;34:18–36.

44. Mondal A, Patra DK. Efficacy of fine needle aspiration cytology in the diagnosis of tuberculosis of the thyroid gland: a study of 18 cases. J Laryngol Otol 1995;109:36–38.

45. Wilson RA, Gartner WS Jr. Teflon granuloma mimicking a thyroid tumor. Diagn Cytopathol 1987;3:156–58.

46. Berry B, MacFarlane J, Chan N. Osteoclastoma-like anaplastic carcinoma of the thyroid: diagnosis by fine needle aspiration cytology. Acta Cytol 1990;34:248–50.

47. Harigopal M, Sahoo S, Recant WM, et al. Fine needle aspiration of Riedel's disease: report of a case and review of the literature. Diagn Cytopathol 2004;30:193–97.

48. Walts AE, Pitchon HE. Pneumocystis carinii in FNA of the thyroid. Diagn Cytopathol 1991;7:615–17.

49. Maheswari V, Khan L, Mehdi G, et al. Microfilariae in thyroid aspiration smear – an unexpected finding. Diagn Cytopathol 2008;36:40–41.

50. Mihai R, Parker AJC, Roskell D, et al. One in four patients with follicular thyroid cytology (THY3) has a thyroid carcinoma. Thyroid 2009;19:33–37.

51. Kaur A, Jayaram G. Thyroid tumours: cytomorphology of follicular neoplasms. Diagn Cytopathol 1991;7:469–72.

52. Baloch ZW, Fleisher S, LiVolsi VA, et al. Diagnosis of 'follicular neoplasm.' A gray zone in thyroid fine needle aspiration cytology. Diagn Cytopathol 2002;26:41–44.

53. Renshaw AA, Wang E, Wilbur D, et al. Interobserver agreement on microfollicles in thyroid fine-needle aspirates. Arch Pathol Lab Med 2006;130:148–52.

54. Montironi R, Braccischi A, Scarpelli M, et al. The number of nucleoli in benign and malignant thyroid lesions: a useful diagnostic sign in cytological preparations. Cytopathol 1990;1:153–61.

55. Montironi R, Braccischi A, Scarpelli M, et al. Well-differentiated follicular neoplasms of the thyroid: reproducibility and validity of a decision tree classification based on nucleolar and karyometric features. Cytopathol 1992;3:209–22.

56. Solymosi T, Toth V, Sapi Z, et al. Diagnostic value of AgNOR method in thyroid cytopathology: correlation with morphometric measurements. Diagn Cytopathol 1996;14:140–44.

57. Sanabria A, Carvalho AL, Piana de Andrade V, et al. Is galectin-3 a good method for the detection of malignancy in patients with thyroid nodules and a cytologic diagnosis of 'follicular neoplasm'? A critical appraisal of the evidence. Head Neck 2007;29:1046–54.

58. Aogi K, Kitahara K, Buley I, et al. Telomerase activity in lesions of the thyroid: application to diagnosis of clinical samples including fine needle aspirates. Clin Cancer Res 1998;4:1965–70.

59. Carroll NM, Carty SE. Promising molecular techniques for discriminating among follicular thyroid neoplasms. Surg Oncol 2006;15:59–64.

60. Hunt J. Molecular testing in solid tumours: an overview. Arch Pathol Lab Med 2008;132:164–67.

61. Schmitt FC, Longatto-Filho A, Valent A, et al. Molecular techniques in cytopathology. J Clin Pathol 2008;61:258–67.

62. Harach HR, Zusman SB. Necrotic debris in thyroid aspirates: a feature of follicular carcinoma of the thyroid. Cytopathol 1992;3:359–64.

63. Oertel YC, Miyahara-Felipe L. Cytologic features of insular carcinoma of the thyroid: a case report. Diagn Cytopathol 2006;34:572–75.

64. Nguyen GK, Akin MR. Cytopathology of insular carcinoma of the thyroid. Diagn Cytopathol 2001;25:325–30.

65. Harach HR, Virgili E, Soler G, et al. Cytopathology of follicular tumours of the

thyroid with clear cell change. Cytopathol 1991;2:125–35.

66. Ambrosiani L, Declich P, Bellone, et al. Thyroid metastases from renal clear cell carcinoma: a cytohistological study of two cases. Adv Clin Path 2001;5:11–16.

67. Elliott DD, Pitman MB, Bloom L, et al. Fine needle aspiration biopsy of Hürthle cell lesions of the thyroid gland. A cytomorphologic study of 139 cases with statistical analysis. Cancer 2006;108:102–9.

68. Nguyen GK, Husain M, Akin MR. Cytodiagnosis of benign and malignant Hürthle cell lesions by fine-needle aspiration biopsy. Diagn Cytopathol 1997;20:261–65.

69. Wu HH-J, Clouse J, Ren R. Fine-needle aspiration cytology of Hürthle cell carcinoma of the thyroid. Diagn Cytopathol 2008;36:149–54.

70. Furmanchuk AW, Averkin JI, Egloff B, et al. Pathomorphological findings in thyroid cancers of children from the Republic of Belarus: a study of 86 cases occurring between 1986 (post-Chernobyl) and 1991. Histopathol 1992;21:401–8.

71. Baloch ZW, LiVolsi VA. Pathology of thyroid gland. In: LiVolsi VA, Asa SL, editors Endocrine Pathology. Philadelphia: Churchill Livingstone; 2002. Ch. 4.

72. Baloch ZW, LiVolsi VA, Asa SL, et al. Diagnostic terminology and morphologic criteria for cytologic diagnosis of thyroid lesions. A synopsis of the National Cancer Institute thyroid fine-needle aspiration state of the science conference. Diagn Cytopathol 2008;36:425–37.

73. Kaur A, Jayaram G. Thyroid tumours: cytomorphology of papillary carcinoma. Diagn Cytopathol 1991;7:462–68.

74. Bhambhani S, Kashyap V, Das DK. Nuclear grooves: valuable diagnostic feature in May-Grünwald-Giemsa-stained fine needle aspirates of papillary carcinoma of the thyroid. Acta Cytol 1990;34:809–12.

75. Miller TR, Bottles K, Holley EA, et al. A stepwise logistic regression analysis of papillary carcinoma of the thyroid. Acta Cytol 1986;30:285–93.

76. Pai RR, Lobo FD, Upadhyay K, et al. Warthin-like tumour of the thyroid – the fine needle aspiration cytology features. Cytopathol 2001;12:127–29.

77. Fadda G, Mule A, Zannoni GF, et al. Fine needle aspiration of a Warthin-like thyroid tumour. Report of a case with differential diagnostic criteria vs other lymphocyte rich thyroid lesions. Acta Cytol 1998;42:998–1002.

78. Ylagen LR, Dehner LP, Huethner PC, et al. Columnar cell variant of papillary thyroid cancer. Report of a case with cytologic findings. Acta Cytol 2004;48:73–75.

79. Das DK, Mallik MK, Sharma P, et al. Papillary thyroid cancer and its variants in fine needle aspiration smears. A cytomorphologic study with particular reference to tall cell variant. Acta Cytol 2004;48:325–36.

80. Triggiani V, Ciampollilo A, Maiorana E. Papillary thyroid cancer , diffuse sclerosing variant with abundant psammoma bodies. Acta Cytol 2003;47:1141–43.

81. Us-Krasovec M, Golouh R. Papillary carcinoma with exuberant nodular fasciitis-like stroma in a fine needle aspirate. A case report. Acta Cytol 1999;43:1101–4.

82. Baloch ZW, Gupta PK, Yu GH, et al. Follicular variant of papillary carcinoma. Cytologic and histologic correlation. Am J Clin Pathol 1999;111:216–22.

83. Chung D, Ghossein RA, Lin O. Macrofollicular variant of papillary carcinoma: a potential thyroid FNA pitfall. Diagn Cytopathol 2007;35:560–64.

84. Ellison E, Lapuerta P, Martin SE. Psammoma bodies in fine needle aspirates of the thyroid predictive value for papillary carcinoma. Cancer 1998;84:169–75.

85. Castro-Gomez L, Cardova-Ramirez S, Duarte-Torres R, et al. Cytologic criteria of cystic papillary carcinoma of the thyroid. Acta Cytol 2003;47:590–94.

86. Cheung CC, Boerner SL, MacMillan CM, et al. Hyalinising trabecular tumour of the thyroid: a variant of papillary carcinoma proved by molecular genetics. Am J Surg Pathol 2000;24:1622–26.

87. Casey MB, Sebo TJ, Carney JA. Hyalinizing trabecular adenoma of the thyroid gland; cytologic features in 29 cases. Am J Surg Pathol 2004;28:867–69.

88. Kulacoglu S, Ashton-Key M, Buley I. Pitfalls in the diagnosis of papillary carcinoma of the thyroid. Cytopathol 1998;9:193–200.

89. Papaparaskevac K, Nagel H, Droese M. Cytologic diagnosis of medullary carcinoma of the thyroid gland. Diagn Cytopathol 2000;22:351–58.

90. Nijhawan US, Marwaha RK, Sahoo M, et al. Fine needle aspiration cytology of amyloid goiter. A report of 4 cases. Acta Cytol 1997;41:830–34.

91. Haleem Akthar M, Ali MA, Iqbal Z. Fine needle aspiration biopsy of mucus producing medullary carcinoma of the thyroid. Report of a case with cytologic, histologic and ultrastructural correlations. Diagn Cytopathol 1990;6:112–17.

92. de Lima MA, Dias Medeiros J, Rodrigues Da Cunha L. Cytological aspects of melanotic variant medullary thyroid carcinoma. Diagn Cytopathol 2001;24:206–8.

93. Ordonez N, Baloch ZW, Matias-Guin X, et al, et al. Undifferentiated (anaplastic) carcinoma. In: DeLellis RA, Lloyd RV, Heitz PU, editors Pathology and genetics of tumours of endocrine organs. WHO classification of tumours. Lyon: IARC press; 2004. p. 77–81.

94. Fortson JK, Durden FL, Patel V, et al. The coexistence of anaplastic and papillary carcinomas of the thyroid: a case presentation and literature review. Am Surg 2004;70:1116–19.

95. Luze T, Tötsch M, Bangerl I, et al. Fine needle aspiration cytodiagnosis of anaplastic carcinoma and malignant haemangioendothelioma of the thyroid in an endemic goitre area. Cytopathol 1990;1:305–10.

96. Us-Krasovec M, Golouh R, Auersperg M, et al. Anaplastic thyroid carcinoma in fine needle aspirates. Acta Cytol 1996;40:953–58.

97. Derringer GA, Thompson LD, Frommelt RA, et al. Malignant lymphoma of the thyroid gland: a clinicopathologic study of 108 cases. Am J Surg Pathol 2000;24:623–39.

98. Wang SA, Rahemtullah A, Faquin WC, et al. Hodgkin's lymphoma of the thyroid; a clinicopathologic study of 5 cases and review of the literature. Mod Pathol 2005;18:1577–84.

99. Sangalli G, Serio G, Zampatti C, et al. Fine needle aspiration cytology of primary lymphoma of the thyroid. A report of 17 cases. Cytopathol 2001;12:257–63.

100. Schmid KW, Hittmair A, Öfner C, et al. Metastatic tumours in fine needle aspiration biopsy of the thyroid. Acta Cytol 1991;35:722–24.

101. Rikabi ACA, Young AE, Wilson C. Metastatic renal clear cell carcinoma in the thyroid gland diagnosed by fine needle aspiration cytology. Cytopathol 1991;2:47–49.

102. Aron M, Kapila K, Verma K. Role of fine-needle aspiration cytology in the diagnosis of secondary tumours of the thyroid – twenty years experience. Diagn Cytopathol 2006;34:240–45.

103. Michelow PM, Leiman G. Metastases to the thyroid gland. Diagnosis by aspiration cytology. Diagn Cytopathol 1995;13:209–13.

104. Poller DN, Stelar EB, Yiangou C. Thyroid FNAC cytology: can we do it better. Cytopathology 2008;19:4–10.

105. Hamburger JI, Husain M, Nishiyama R, et al. Increasing the accuracy of fine-needle biopsy for thyroid nodules. Arch Pathol Lab Med 1989;113:1035–41.

106. Raab SS, Vrbin CM, Grzybicki DM, et al. Errors in thyroid gland fine-needle aspiration. Am J Clin Pathol 2006;125:873–82.

107. Ravetto C, Colombo L, Dottorini ME. Usefulness of fine-needle aspiration in the diagnosis of thyroid carcinoma: a retrospective study in 37,895 patients. Cancer 2000;90:357–63.

108. Yang GC, Liebeskind D, Messina AV. Ultrasound-guided fine needle aspiration cytology of the thyroid assessed by ultrafast Papanicolaou stain. Data from 1135 biopsies with two to six years follow-up. Thyroid 2001;11:581–89.

109. Kocjan G. Evaluation of the cost effectiveness of establishing a fine needle aspiration cytology clinic in a hospital outpatient department. Cytopathology 1991;2:13–18.

110. Mayall D, Denford A, Chang AD. Improved FNA cytology results with a near patient diagnosis service for non-breast lesions. J Clin Pathol 1998;51:541–44.

111. Singh N, Ryan D, Berney M, et al. Inadequate rates are lower when FNAC samples are taken by cytopathologists. Cytopathology 2003;14:327–31.

112. Nasuti JF, Gupta PK, Baloch ZW. Diagnostic value and cost-effectiveness of on-site evaluation of fine needle aspiration specimens: a review of 5,688 cases. Diagn Cytopathol 2002;27:1–4.

113. Zhu W, Michael CW. How important is on-site adequacy assessment for thyroid FNA? An evaluation of 883 cases. Diagn Cytopathol 2007;35:183–86.

114. Redman R, Zalazwick H, Mazzaferri EL, et al. The impact of assessing specimen adequacy and number of needle passes for fine-needle aspiration biopsy of thyroid nodules. Thyroid 2006;16:55–60.

115. Hamberger B, Gharib H, Melton LJ, et al. Fine-needle aspiration biopsy of thyroid nodules: impact on thyroid practice and cost of care. Am J Med 1982;73:384–831.

116. Dwarakanathon AA, Staren ED, D'Amore MJ, et al. Importance of repeat fine-needle biopsy in the management of thyroid nodules. Am J Surg 1993;166:350–52.

117. Raab SS, Grzybicki DM, Sudilovski D, et al. Effectiveness of Toyota process redesign in reducing thyroid gland fine-needle aspiration error. Am J Clin Pathol 2006;124:585–92.

118. Jing X, Michael CW, Pu RT. The clinical and diagnostic impact of using standardised criteria of adequacy assessment and diagnostic terminology on thyroid nodule fine needle aspiration. Diagn Cytopathol 2008;36:161–66.

119. Orell SR, Phillips J. The role of fine needle biopsy in the investigation of thyroid disease

and its diagnostic accuracy. In: The thyroid, fine needle biopsy and cytological diagnosis of thyroid lesions. Monographs in Clinical Cytology, Vol. 14. Basel: Karger; 1997. Ch. 3.

120. Layfield LJ, Abrams J, Cochand-Priollet., et al. Post thyroid FNA testing and treatment options: a synopsis of the National Cancer Institute thyroid fine-needle aspiration state of the science conference. Diagn Cytopathol 2008;36:442–48.

121. British Thyroid Association and Royal College of Physicians. Fine-needle aspiration cytology. Section 3, Guidelines for the Management of Thyroid Cancer, 2nd edn. London: British Thyroid Association and Royal College of Physicians; 2007. Also online. Available at: www.british-thyroid-association.org.

122. The Royal College of Pathologists. Guidance on the reporting of thyroid cytology specimens. 2009. http://www.rcpath. org/resources/pdf/g089guidanceonthere-portingofthyroidcytologyfinal.pdf

# Other endocrine organs

Ian D. Buley

## Chapter contents

## The parathyroid glands

### Anatomy and physiology

There are usually four parathyroid glands arranged as two pairs. The upper pair, which develop as a dorsal diverticulum of the fourth pharyngeal pouch, are present at the posterolateral border of the thyroid just beneath the upper poles. The lower pair, derived from the third pharyngeal pouch, are located at the lower poles of the thyroid. They are situated within the pretracheal fascia either on the surface or just within the thyroid tissue. Anomalies of position in the neck and anterior mediastinum may occur. A fifth supernumerary gland occurs in approximately 5% of individuals and is usually present in thymic tissues inferior to the thyroid. Rarely, more than five glands may occur. The glands are ovoid in shape. The weights of individual glands are variable but in the adult the total glandular weight averages 120 mg in males and 142 mg in females. Any single gland weighing more than 60 mg is likely to be abnormal. The average maximal dimension is 5 mm, although the normal range of size extends up to 1 cm.

Histologically, the parathyroid cells are arranged in cords and sheets set within a richly vascular stroma. Small follicles containing colloid-like material may be seen and the appearances can mimic those of the thyroid gland. During puberty and early adult life the glands accumulate adipose tissue, fat cells insinuating themselves amongst the endocrine cells. The endocrine cells have two main histological subtypes: the chief cell and the oxyphil cell. The former predominate and are rounded cells with pale granular or vacuolated cytoplasm. They are rich in glycogen and lipid. Oxyphil cells increase in number with age and may form discrete nodules. These cells are larger with abundant eosinophilic cytoplasm containing numerous mitochondria. Transitional forms between chief cells and oxyphil cells also occur.

The parathyroid glands produce and secrete parathyroid hormone (PTH). This single chain polypeptide contributes to the maintenance of calcium ion homeostasis together with vitamin D metabolites. A fall in the level of extracellular calcium ion concentration cause the release of PTH which promotes the renal excretion of the phosphate ion, enhances renal tubular reabsorption of calcium, stimulates bone resorption and stimulates the synthesis of the active metabolite of vitamin D, 1,25 dihydroxycholecalciferol. The latter promotes intestinal calcium absorption and increases its release from bone. The resulting increase in extracellular calcium ion has a negative feedback action on the parathyroid, decreasing the release of PTH.

## Parathyroid disease and histopathology

### Primary hyperparathyroidism

The most common pathology of the parathyroid is primary hyperparathyroidism. This is a common cause of hypercalcaemia, occurring in approximately 0.25% of the population. It is more common in middle-aged and elderly women. It occurs sporadically, can also be familial and may be associated with the multiple endocrine neoplasia syndromes (see Box 17.4). The disease may be detected incidentally on routine laboratory tests or may present clinically with painful bones, renal stones, abdominal pain from peptic ulceration or pancreatitis and with fatigue and depression. The underlying pathology is either parathyroid hyperplasia, which affects all of the glands, or an adenoma or carcinoma, which nearly always affects only a single gland. The most common pathology is an adenoma, which gives rise to approximately 80% of cases. Treatment is surgical removal of the affected gland. Hyperplasia requires the removal of three glands and partial removal of the fourth gland. As the histological appearances of a single hyperplastic gland and a gland containing an adenoma may be similar, distinction may require perioperative frozen section examination of two glands. In the case of an adenoma, the second gland will be normal or atrophic whereas in hyperplasia the glands will show similar changes.

### Parathyroid adenoma

Parathyroid adenomas usually weigh between 200 mg and 1 g. The weight of the gland correlates with the clinical symptomatology and in patients with severe hyperparathyroid bone disease adenomas frequently weigh 10 g or more. Some 90% of adenomas occur in the upper or lower parathyroids, with the lower glands more frequently involved, and 10% occur in other sites in the neck and mediastinum. They are brown in colour and may show areas of haemorrhage, cystic degeneration, fibrosis or calcification. Microscopically, the adenoma (Fig. 18.1) is a well-circumscribed proliferation of cells within a thin fibrous capsule. Usually, residual compressed atrophic parathyroid is seen adjacent to the adenoma. This is most commonly seen at the vascular hilum of the gland. The cell population of the adenoma may consist of dark granular or pale vacuolated chief cells, oxyphil cells or transitional-type cells. Some chief cells show extreme vacuolation and form 'water-clear' cells. Frequently, the cell population is mixed. Adenomatous chief cells contain less cytoplasmic lipid than normal or atrophic chief cells. Architecturally, the

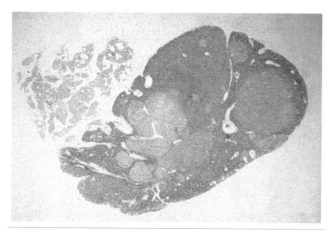

**Fig. 18.1** Parathyroid adenoma with adjacent normal parathyroid tissue (H&E).

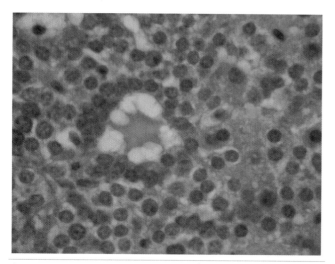

**Fig. 18.2** Parathyroid adenoma. Chief cells on the left side with a follicular arrangement. Oxyphilic cells on the right (H&E).

cells may be arranged in sheets, nodules, nests, cords, in rosettes or follicles and may even form a papillary pattern (Fig. 18.2). Adenomas contain few stromal fat cells except in the case of the rare lipoadenoma. In common with many other benign endocrine tumours parathyroid adenomas may show marked nuclear pleomorphism. Mitoses are, however, rare. In the follicular pattern, calcification of the intraluminal secretion gives rise to structures resembling psammoma bodies.

## Parathyroid hyperplasia

Parathyroid hyperplasia affects the chief cells of all of the glands giving rise to the common chief cell hyperplasia and the rare water-clear cell hyperplasia. Involvement of the glands is often uneven both between and within glands, giving rise to nodular proliferations, which may be difficult to distinguish from an adenoma if only a single gland is available for examination. The parenchyma is dense with closely packed cells and a decrease in the number of stromal fat cells. There is no compressed rim of normal parathyroid tissue. Hyperplastic chief cells show a decrease in their content of lipid. The cells in hyperplasia also show variable architecture, being arranged in sheets, trabeculae, alveoli or in follicles. Cystic change may occur rarely. Marked nuclear pleomorphism is rare.

## Parathyroid carcinoma

Parathyroid carcinoma is rare, causing only approximately 1% of cases of primary hyperparathyroidism. Most cases have severe hypercalcaemia and the parathyroid tumour is large and may be palpable. Classically, at operation the tumour is hard and invasive with adherence to surrounding structures. Histologically, there is a thick fibrous capsule, which may be invaded by the malignant cells. Fibrous bands often extend into the parenchyma of the tumour. Blood vessel invasion may be seen. The diagnostic features of malignancy are mainly architectural. The tumour cells are usually of chief cell type, although oxyphil carcinomas have been described. The cells are arranged in sheets or trabeculae. They show some nuclear enlargement, coarsening of the chromatin pattern and prominent nucleoli, but paradoxically lack the bizarre pleomorphism, which may be seen in some adenomas. Mitoses are usually seen. The prognosis depends on successful surgical removal, as the tumour is not very sensitive to radiotherapy or current chemotherapy.

## Parathyroid cysts

Parathyroid cysts are rare. They may develop as a result of degeneration of a hyperplastic or adenomatous gland but most are pharyngeal pouch remnants. Those arising from adenomatous or hyperplastic glands may be associated with hyperparathyroidism. Very rarely they may cause vocal cord paralysis. They usually occur in relation to the inferior parathyroids and can measure up to 10 cm in diameter. They are lined by a layer of chief cells and the wall may contain nodules of parathyroid, thymic or lymphoid tissue. Needle aspiration of those arising from pharyngeal pouch remnants is frequently curative. The remainder may require surgical removal.[1]

### Cytological findings: hyperplasia, adenoma, carcinoma and cysts

No absolute cytological criteria for the distinction between hyperplastic and adenomatous parathyroid cells have been defined. Aspirates from parathyroids yield thick, crowded cell groups with irregular borders sometimes clustering around branching vascular cores giving a papillary appearance. The cells are usually monomorphic. A moderate amount of finely granular cytoplasm is present and occasional small vacuoles are seen. Around the cell groups numerous bare nuclei are present. Nuclei are round and hyperchromatic with granular chromatin. Small nucleoli may be present (Fig. 18.3). In adenomas, occasional larger pleomorphic nuclei may occur and cell groups may be less cohesive.[2] Oxyphil cells have abundant granular cytoplasm and variable nuclear size resembling thyroid Hürthle cells.[3] Fragments of hyaline colloid-like material may be seen together with follicular arrangements particularly in some parathyroid adenomas.[4] Intranuclear inclusions, mast cells, lymphocytes and amyloid are occasional features.[5–8]

As might be expected from the histological appearances, the cytological findings in parathyroid carcinoma do not enable reliable distinction from an adenoma or even hyperplasia but with the appropriate clinical and radiological information the identification of parathyroid cells enables the diagnosis of primary[9,10] or secondary[11,12] malignancy to be suggested. FNA may be particularly helpful in distinguishing between a bony metastasis and bone changes, resulting from hyperparathyroidism.[13]

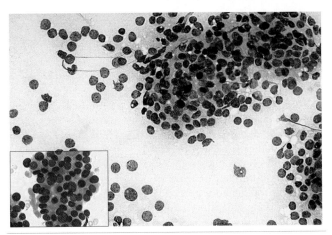

**Fig. 18.3** Aspirate from a parathyroid adenoma showing crowded cell groups of monomorphic cells with granular cytoplasm and round nuclei. There is a background of bare nuclei (MGG). Inset: high-power view of parathyroid adenoma. Courtesy of Dr Knezevic-Obad.

A parathyroid cyst aspiration characteristically yields clear watery fluid but occasionally cloudy golden-brown fluid is obtained, resembling that aspirated from thyroid cysts. The fluid is often poorly cellular. Follicular and papillary cell arrangements which may be seen can cause further diagnostic confusion. Most parathyroid cysts are clinically 'non-functional' but assay of the fluid for parathyroid hormone as well as immunocytochemical staining of the aspirated cells for Chromogranin A and PTH may be useful in diagnosis[14,15] facilitating resolution of the differential diagnosis with thyroid, branchial, thymic or thyroglossal cysts.

### Cytological findings: parathyroid lesions

- Crowded cell groups showing nuclear overlapping and moulding with surrounding bare nuclei
- Branching vessels may be seen in cell groups
- Monomorphic cells with granular cytoplasm
- Round hyperchromatic nuclei
- Occasional pleomorphic cells especially in adenomas
- Mitoses suggest carcinoma
- Oxyphil cells, colloid-like material and follicular arrangements may be seen
- Cysts yield watery clear fluid of low cellularity. Follicular or papillary fragments may be seen. PTH assay or immunostaining may aid diagnosis

## The role of FNA of the parathyroid and diagnostic pitfalls

Parathyroid lesions may be aspirated as masses in the neck clinically believed to be of thyroid origin and earlier reports of parathyroid cytology indicated the difficulty in distinguishing the findings from thyroid lesions.[16] These include follicular lesions, papillary carcinoma, medullary carcinoma[17] and lymphocytic thyroiditis.[18] The distinction may be complicated as parathyroid lesions may be intrathyroidal and by the observation that parathyroid tumours and thyroid carcinomas may coexist as they share the common aetiological factor of radiation to the neck.[19] Distinguishing between thyroid and parathyroid cells may require the use of special techniques to identify the neurosecretory

granules in the parathyroid cells. These include immunocytochemistry for PTH or chromogranin A together with a lack of immunostaining for thyroglobulin or calcitonin as appropriate. Immunoassay for PTH can be carried out on material obtained by FNA[20] and reverse transcriptase polymerase chain reaction detection of PTH gene mRNA in needle aspirates has been described.[21] The morphological distinguishing features are dense nuclear chromatin and lack of a regular architecture in the cell groups of parathyroid lesions. The absence of characteristic features of thyroid tissue, colloid, macrophages and follicular structures may also be helpful,[22] although all of these features may be seen in parathyroid lesions.[15] In one comprehensive survey colloid-like material was seen in 21%, macrophages in 10% and follicular arrangements in 15% of parathyroid smears.[8]

The refinement of ultrasonography and other imaging techniques including CT, MRI and technetium-99m sestamibi (Tc99 MIBI) scanning has enabled planned FNA of the enlarged parathyroid gland.[2] FNA and PTH estimation has been used as an adjunct to imaging prior to minimally invasive parathyroidectomy.[23] It can be particularly helpful in Tc99 MIBI negative parathyroids and where imaging is complicated by coexisting thyroid nodules.[24] As well as distinguishing parathyroid from thyroid masses the nature of any coexisting thyroid nodules is determined and this may be an indication for open thyroidectomy and parathyroidectomy rather than minimally invasive parathyroid surgery alone. Combined FNA and PTH estimation is also helpful where parathyroids are ectopic[25] and in postoperative recurrent or persistent hyperparathyroidism.[26] Non-surgical destructive techniques for parathyroid adenomas also rely on accurate identification of parathyroid tissue. FNA can also contribute to diagnosis of parathyroid cysts and carcinomas.

## Complications

Complications of parathyroid FNA are rare. Parathyroid tissue is readily engraftable and can be autotransplanted. Inadvertent capsular rupture when removing parathyroid tissue, benign or malignant, can result in seeding and growth of numerous foci of parathyroid cells in the operative field or parathyromatosis. A potential complication of FNA, particularly applicable to parathyroid tissue, is needle tract implantation. This has not been associated with aspiration of benign parathyroid lesions[27] but cutaneous and needle track spread after FNA of parathyroid carcinomas has been recorded.[28,29] Needle aspiration of parathyroid lesions can result rarely in damage to the gland. Autoinfarction, with resolution of hypercalcaemia, is recorded after aspiration of a cystic hyperplastic gland.[30] FNA induced fibrosis in and around parathyroid adenomas can mimic the histological appearances of parathyroid carcinoma[31] and complicate subsequent surgery. One study noted a doubling of operative time removing previously aspirated glands.[32] Avoiding excessive numbers of needle passes and the use of 25–27 gauge needles may limit this potential complication.

## The adrenal glands

### Anatomy and physiology

The adrenal glands are situated superomedially to each of the kidneys. On the right side, the adrenal capsule is usually fused with the overlying liver capsule and occasionally the gland may be embedded within the liver. Each adrenal weighs between 5 g and 6.5 g and measures approximately 4×3×0.5 cm.

The adrenal gland is composed of two distinct parts. The medulla is derived from the neural crest and is a sympathetic paraganglion responsible for the secretion of adrenaline and noradrenaline. The cortex, which constitutes 90% of the gland, is mesodermally derived. It is divided into three concentric regions. The outer zona glomerulosa secretes mineralocorticoids, which are responsible for the conservation of sodium ions and water and the excretion of potassium ions. The inner zona fasciculata and reticularis secrete glucocorticoids, which have a wide range of effects on carbohydrate, protein and lipid metabolism, and sex hormones.

Histologically (Fig. 18.4), the zona glomerulosa consists of clumps of endocrine cells surrounded by a delicate but richly vascular connective tissue stroma. The cytoplasm has a poorly staining, clear cell appearance due to the presence of abundant lipid and smooth endoplasmic reticulum. The zona fasciculata consists of cords of secretory cells with abundant clear and foamy appearing cytoplasm. The cells of the zona reticularis are arranged in a network of branching cords and are smaller with a more compact cytoplasm, which may contain lipofuscin granules. The cells, phaeochromocytes, of the adrenal medulla are arranged in clumps in a vascular stroma of sinusoids and larger venous channels. They have abundant granular basophilic cytoplasm and large nuclei. Some sympathetic ganglion cells are also present.

## The role of FNA of the adrenal

Adrenal cells may be encountered by chance in attempted aspirates of surrounding structures such as the liver and kidney. Imaging techniques with CT and ultrasound guided aspiration enables planned investigation of adrenal masses. Both adrenals particularly the left adrenal are amenable to sampling by transgastric endoscopic ultrasound directed FNA.[33] Interpretation of an aspirate must be with full knowledge of the clinical, radiological and where appropriate the biochemical findings, e.g. the cytological findings from an adrenal adenoma may be identical to those from a normal adrenal, diffuse hyperplasia or nodular hyperplasia. The findings may be very similar in adrenocortical carcinoma and even in a renal clear cell adenocarcinoma. FNA allows the diagnosis of metastases in the adrenal, adrenocortical tumours, phaeochromocytomas, ganglioneuromas and

neuroblastomas. Collection of cell block or liquid based cytology specimens can be helpful for immunostaining. FNA can also be of use in the diagnosis of some infections affecting the adrenal such as tuberculosis and histoplasmosis, allows confirmation of the presence of a simple adrenal cyst and the diagnosis of myelolipoma of the adrenal.

Approximately 3% of those having abdominal CT or MRI show adrenal cortical nodules, either adenomas or nodular hyperplasia, of greater than 1 cm in diameter. Consequently the principal indication for adrenal FNA is the need to investigate incidental adrenal masses ('incidentalomas') in patients who have had abdominal imaging as part of their staging investigations for malignancy particularly bronchogenic carcinomas. Adrenal FNA is a highly specific and safe technique for the diagnosis of carcinoma metastatic to the adrenal gland. In some studies the probability of such masses being metastatic cancer or a primary adrenal lesion are approximately equal.[34–38] Several large studies have shown greater than 90% accuracy in the diagnosis of adrenal masses.

Clinically symptomatic functional adrenal masses for example adrenal adenomas and phaeochromocytomas are usually removed without prior FNA. For incidentally detected adrenal lesions where there is no prior history of malignancy there is a case for removing all larger lesions (over 4 cm diameter) without preceding FNA as both a diagnostic and therapeutic procedure. Radiological findings should exclude the diagnosis of myelolipoma and biochemical findings phaeochromocytoma. These are usually adrenocortical neoplasms and larger size as well as any atypical cytological features is an indication for excision. Smaller such nodules may warrant FNA to aid the decision as to whether surgery is necessary.

## Complications of adrenal FNA

These include pneumothorax, haemorrhage, abscess formation and needle track tumour implantation. Where aspiration is carried out without prior biochemical testing for phaeochromocytoma, there is also a small risk of provoking a hypertensive crisis.[39]

## Normal findings

- Needle aspiration yields cortical cells and medulla cells are seen only occasionally
- Cortical cells are present in loose aggregates and cords
- The cytoplasm is delicate, foamy and pale staining
- Occasional cells from the zona reticularis with denser cytoplasm containing lipofuscin are seen
- The nuclei are small and round with an even chromatin pattern and a small nucleolus
- Intranuclear cytoplasmic inclusions may be seen
- Occasional small spindle-shaped stromal cells are present
- Similar appearances are seen in aspirates from diffuse or nodular hyperplasia.

## Adrenal cyst

Adrenal cysts are increasingly detected as radiological incidental findings, although they may present with a mass or with flank

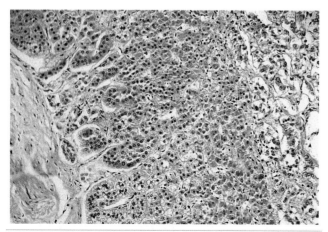

**Fig. 18.4** Adrenal gland. Normal histology (H&E).

pain. Their aetiology is unclear. They may arise as a result of adrenal haemorrhage, or may arise from lymphangiomas, haemangiomas or vascular malformations. Occasionally they are bilateral. Histologically, they are lined by fibrous tissue which may show calcification.

### Cytological findings: adrenal cyst

- Clear, turbid or bloody fluid is aspirated
- The samples are poorly cellular with occasional inflammatory cells and debris
- Occasional adrenal cortical cells are seen
- If haemorrhage has occurred into the cyst erythrocytes and haemosiderin-containing macrophages are present
- The possibility of cystic degeneration in an adrenal tumour should be considered and the appropriate cytological features sought
- In endemic areas hydatid cyst is a possible differential diagnosis.

## Adrenal myelolipoma

This is a rare benign tumour of the adrenal which is usually asymptomatic and an incidental finding in up to 0.8% of autopsies. Occasionally, it presents clinically with abdominal pain or a mass. Increasingly, small tumours are being detected in staging CT scans in patients with malignancy. They are usually detected in the middle-aged and elderly and can measure up to 34 cm in diameter and weigh more than 5 kg. The tumour has been associated with hypertension, atherosclerosis, diabetes mellitus, adrenal cortical tumours and hyperplasia, chronic inflammatory states and various malignancies. It may be, however, that the presence of some of these conditions merely increases the chance of detection of the lesion. The radiographic appearances are of a low-density mass with areas of punctate calcification. These features are usually diagnostic with no need for FNA. Surgical excision is unnecessary unless the lesion is symptomatic. The radiographic differential diagnosis, however, lies between myelolipoma, metastatic carcinoma, adenoma, granulomatous disease, renal angiomyolipoma and for larger tumours would include retroperitoneal liposarcoma. Where there is doubt as to the diagnosis FNA should be carried out.[40]

### Cytological findings: myelolipoma

- Adipose tissue with haemopoietic elements
- Granulocytic elements and megakaryocytes are readily identified.

## Granulomatous infectious disease

Tuberculosis of the adrenal gland is the classical cause of adrenal insufficiency, Addison's disease (Box 18.1). Aspiration of the bilaterally enlarged adrenals yields granulomatous material together with caseous necrosis. Material can be aspirated for culture. Ziehl Neelsen staining often reveals mycobacteria. Disseminated histoplasmosis has also been diagnosed by needle aspiration of the adrenal with recognition of the silver-staining intracytoplasmic yeasts in clusters of histiocytes.[41] Cases of North American *blastomycosis* and *cryptococcosis* diagnosed by adrenal FNA are also recorded.[42,43]

## Adrenal adenomas

Adrenal adenomas are benign adrenocortical tumours. Some may be functional, leading to Cushing's syndrome or Conn's syndrome if glucocorticoids or mineralocorticoids, respectively, are being secreted (Boxes 18.2 and 18.3). If sex hormones are secreted, these tumours may cause precocious puberty or virilism.

---

**Box 18.1  Addison's disease**

Aetiology
Primary adrenal

1. Autoimmune
2. Tuberculous
3. Congenital adrenal hypoplasia
4. Adrenal haemorrhage. Waterhouse–Friederichsen syndrome
5. Others: amyloidosis, sarcoidosis, haemochromatosis, metastatic carcinoma, surgical, other infections

Features

- Chronic: weakness, hypoglycaemia, weight loss, hyperpigmentation, vitiligo (in autoimmune cases), anorexia, nausea, salt and water depletion
- Acute: adrenal crisis: circulatory collapse, vomiting and abdominal pain

---

**Box 18.2  Cushing's syndrome**

Aetiology

1. Pituitary basophil adenoma
2. Benign and malignant adrenocortical tumours
3. Exogenous ACTH secretion by other tumours, e.g. oat cell carcinoma of the bronchus
4. Bilateral adrenal hyperplasia
5. Iatrogenic, i.e. steroid therapy

Features

- Truncal obesity, 'moon face', 'buffalo hump'
- Muscle wasting and weakness, osteoporosis, thin skin, striae, bruising, acne, low resistance to infection
- Diabetes, hypertension, amenorrhoea, hirsutism, steroid psychosis

---

**Box 18.3  Conn's syndrome**

Aetiology

1. Approximately 80% of cases are due to an adrenal adenoma. Rarely, adrenocortical carcinoma causes pure hyperaldosteronism
2. Multinodular adrenal hyperplasia

Features

- Hypertension, polydipsia, nocturia, muscle weakness, cramps and tetany
- Biochemically, there is a hypokalaemic alkalosis with a high aldosterone level and low renin and angiotensin

Clinically unsuspected 'non-functioning' adenomas are found in approximately 2% of adult autopsies. Typical adrenal adenomas weigh less than 50 g and measure up to 5 cm in diameter. They are well-circumscribed solitary tumours and are usually bright yellow due to their lipid content. They may be brown or black if they have accumulated lipofuscin. Histologically, they consist of a proliferation of clear and compact type cells similar or identical to their normal counterparts. Occasional enlarged nuclei are present but atypia and mitotic activity are very rare.

Aspiration yields numerous adrenal cortical cells with small regular round nuclei and abundant lipid-containing foamy cytoplasm. Cells with more compact cytoplasm and cells containing lipofuscin may be seen. They are arranged in sheets, cords and as dispersed single cells. Binucleate cells may be seen. The chromatin pattern is dispersed and only occasional small nucleoli are seen. There is occasional nucleomegaly but no or only minimal atypia. Intranuclear inclusions are seen occasionally. Necrosis and mitotic activity are absent (Fig. 18.5).[34,35,44,45] The fragility of the cytoplasm may lead to its disruption and the presence of numerous bare nuclei on a foamy background of disrupted cytoplasm. This appearance may resemble that of a small round cell tumour or even small cell carcinoma as an appearance resembling nuclear moulding may be seen.[46]

## Adrenocortical carcinoma

Adrenocortical carcinomas are rare. They usually present in middle age and show an equal sex distribution. Approximately half of the cases have hormonal abnormalities, principally due to an excess of glucocorticoids, and this abnormal secretion is not suppressed by high-dose dexamethasone therapy. The tumour may also present with an abdominal mass, abdominal pain, fever and weight loss.

Carcinomas are larger than adenomas, usually weighing more than 100 g and having a diameter of at least 5 cm. Macroscopically, there may be areas of haemorrhage and necrosis. Microscopically, the appearances may closely resemble those of an adenoma but atypia, mitotic activity and necrosis can be seen. The tumour is often poorly circumscribed with an infiltrative margin and invasion of large veins may be present. In well-differentiated carcinomas the size and weight of the tumour are of great importance in the prediction of malignancy. Overall this carcinoma has a poor prognosis, is often recurrent after surgery and responds poorly to radiotherapy or chemotherapy.

Cytologically, aspirates are cellular and show loss of cohesion. The appearances of a well-differentiated tumour are similar to those of an adenoma but some nuclear enlargement, atypia, mitoses and necrosis may be seen (Fig. 18.6). Less-differentiated tumours show increasing atypia with coarsened chromatin, a thickened nuclear membrane and the presence of prominent nucleoli. The cytoplasm tends to contain less lipid. Poorly differentiated carcinomas show extreme cellular pleomorphism with often bizarre multinucleated cells.[47] Spindle cell forms may be seen.[48] The distinction of adrenocortical carcinomas from adenomas has been investigated by special techniques including flow cytometry for ploidy, proliferation index and differential expression of cytokeratins and vimentin but these appear to be of limited diagnostic utility.

### Cytological findings: adrenal cortical tumours

- Sheets, cords and dispersed cells
- Abundant foamy fragile cytoplasm giving a bubbly lipid-rich background
- Abundant round or ovoid bare nuclei
- Uniform small nuclei with occasional nucleomegaly in benign adrenal nodules and adenomas. Intranuclear inclusions may be seen
- Larger tumours >5 cm, nuclear atypia, necrosis, mitoses and spindled cells suggest malignancy.

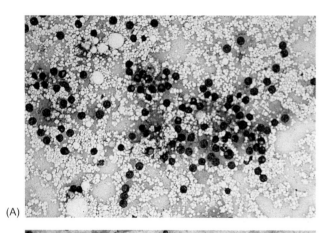

(A)

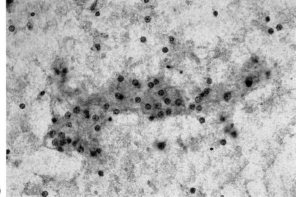

(B)

**Fig. 18.5** Aspirate from an adrenal adenoma showing loose sheets of cells with abundant fragile foamy cytoplasm and uniform bare nuclei (A: MGG; B: PAP).

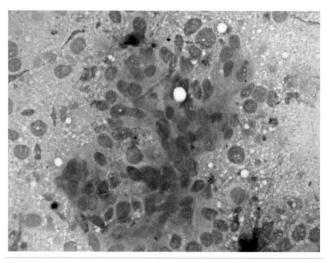

**Fig. 18.6** Recurrent adrenocortical carcinoma showing similar appearances to an adenoma but with nuclear atypia and necrosis in the background (MGG).

## Metastatic malignancy

Of all of the endocrine organs the adrenal is the most frequently affected by metastatic tumour. The most common metastasis to the adrenal is from bronchogenic carcinoma. Metastases from the breast, kidney, stomach, pancreas, ovary, colon, melanoma and lymphoma are also not uncommon. Metastases are more frequently bilateral and particularly with an appropriate history may present no diagnostic difficulty. However, some metastases may mimic an adrenal tumour cytologically and where initial presentation is with the adrenal mass, diagnosis may be problematic.[49] The differential diagnostic problem can usually be resolved by clinical and biochemical data with appropriate use of immunostains as indicated in the diagnostic pitfalls section. CK7, CK20 and TTF-1 staining may be particularly helpful in identifying the primary site when metastatic carcinoma has been identified.[50]

## Tumours of the adrenal medulla

### Neuroblastoma, ganglioneuroblastoma and ganglioneuroma

Neuroblastoma arises from primitive neuroblasts. Some 70% of cases occur in children under 4 years of age and the majority of cases arise in the adrenal, although they may also arise elsewhere in the retroperitoneum, in the chest and in the neck. Approximately 70% of cases have metastases at presentation. Catecholamines and breakdown products may be found in the urine but hypertension is rare. Histologically, the tumour consists of a diffuse growth of uniform small cells which focally show the formation of rosette structures arranged around a central zone of neurofibrils (Fig. 18.7). Treatment is primarily chemotherapy and prognosis is generally poor but dependent on the age of the patient, stage and grade of tumour. Particularly in younger patients, the tumour may spontaneously regress or mature to a ganglioneuroma.

> **Cytological findings: neuroblastoma (Fig. 18.8)**
>
> - Cellular aspirate with numerous loosely cohesive small oval tumour cells with little cytoplasm
> - Bipolar cells with cytoplasmic processes may be seen

- The nuclei appear hyperchromatic with a granular chromatin pattern
- Small nucleoli are visible
- Occasional rosette arrangements can be seen
- Characteristically, a fine pink (with MGG) fibrillar background is present due to the production of neurofibrils.

The differential diagnosis is that of small round cell tumours of childhood including Wilms' tumour, Ewing's sarcoma, embryonal rhabdomyosarcoma and lymphoblastic lymphoma. The differential diagnosis between these tumours can be aided by glycogen staining, electron microscopy, immunocytochemistry and cytogenetic analysis and hence, in appropriate cases, some material should be reserved for these investigations. In the context of an adrenal neuroblastoma the differential diagnosis with a Wilms' tumour (nephroblastoma) may arise. Morphologically, the nephroblastoma differs by the presence of three elements representing blastemal cells, epithelial differentiation with tubular and glomeruloid arrangements and spindle cells originating from the stromal element. Electron microscopy reveals neurosecretory granules, neurofilaments and microtubules in neuroblastoma and immunocytochemically there is positivity for neurone specific enolase, chromogranin A, synaptophysin, neural cell adhesion molecule (CD56) and neurofilaments. Approximately 70% of neuroblastomas have cytogenetically visible deletions in the short arm of chromosome 1.[51,52]

Ganglioneuroblastomas are partially differentiated neuroblastomas. They have a better prognosis than neuroblastomas

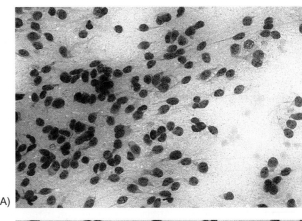

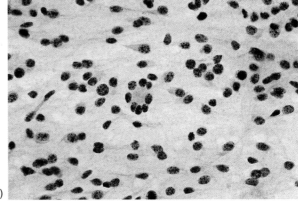

(A)

(B)

**Fig. 18.8** Aspirate from a neuroblastoma showing oval cells in a fibrillary background with occasional rosettes (A: MGG; B: PAP).

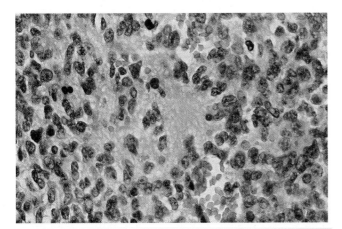

**Fig. 18.7** Neuroblastoma (H&E).

and occur more frequently in the retroperitoneum than in the adrenal. Histologically, they show gangliocytic differentiation and this is reflected in the aspiration cytology findings where neuroblasts are seen admixed with large ganglion cells. These have abundant granular cytoplasm and large eccentrically placed nuclei with prominent nucleoli. The cells may be bi- or multinucleate. Intermediate cell forms between the neuroblast and ganglion cell are also present.[53,54]

The ganglioneuroma is a benign tumour occurring most frequently in adults. The tumour is usually found in the retroperitoneum or posterior mediastinum though may occur in the adrenal. Aspiration yields groups of spindle cells with narrow undulating nuclei, similar to those found in peripheral nerve sheath tumours (neurilemmomas and neurofibromas), together with occasional ganglion cells.[55]

## Phaeochromocytoma

Paraganglia consist of scattered collections of neuroendocrine cells thought to be derived from the neural crest. They exist in proximity to branches of both the sympathetic and parasympathetic autonomic nervous system. The adrenal medulla is an example of a sympathetic paraganglion and the carotid body is a parasympathetic paraganglion.

The phaeochromocytoma is a paraganglionoma of the adrenal medulla. It is a rare tumour that may occur at any age. The peak age distribution is between the ages of 20 and 50. The sex distribution is approximately equal. The tumour occurs sporadically but in as many as 30% of cases is associated with familial disorders. This is chiefly the MEN II syndrome but there are also associations with neurofibromatosis, Von Hippel–Lindau syndrome and Sturge–Weber syndrome. Familial cases are frequently bilateral, arise on a background of hyperplasia of the medulla in MEN II, and present in a younger age group.

Phaeochromocytomas secrete catecholamines, giving rise to the classical clinical features of paroxysmal hypertension with associated headache, sweating, anxiety, tremor, fatigue, nausea and vomiting, abdominal pain and visual disturbance. Paroxysms may be precipitated by stress, exercise, posture changes or even abdominal palpation. In practice, paroxysmal features are often absent and patients may present with sustained hypertension only. A small minority of tumours may be clinically non-functional. Diagnosis is by the measurement of urinary catecholamines and their metabolites, vanillylmandelic acid and metadrenalines. Surgical handling and removal of phaeochromocytomas is associated with a risk of precipitating massive secretion of catecholamines and a hypertensive crisis. Accordingly, patients are treated with alpha and beta adrenoceptor blocking drugs preoperatively.

Macroscopically, the tumour is well circumscribed and yellow or brown in colour. Larger tumours show areas of haemorrhage, necrosis and cystic degeneration. Histologically, the tumour is highly vascular with numerous vascular sinusoids surrounding tumour cells. The tumour cells are arranged in nests, although these may be poorly defined and may form sheets or cords of cells (Fig. 18.9). The cells have well-defined granular cytoplasm and nuclei with prominent nucleoli. There may be marked nuclear pleomorphism. Approximately 10% of phaeochromocytomas behave in a malignant fashion. The diagnosis of malignancy, which is often retrospective, depends ultimately on the demonstration of local invasion and metastasis and

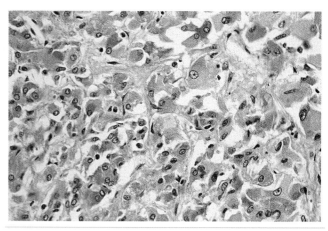

**Fig. 18.9** Phaeochromocytoma (H&E).

cannot be made definitively on the basis of cytological features. Histologically, a diffuse growth pattern, confluent tumour necrosis, high cellularity, cellular monotony, spindle cells and an increased proliferative index show some association with malignant behaviour. Phaeochromocytomas can show gangliocytic differentiation and mixed phaeochromocytomas and ganglioneuromas or ganglioneuroblastomas occur.

Diagnosis of phaeochromocytoma depends on clinical features, imaging techniques and measurements of catecholamines and their metabolites. FNA should not be carried out where these parameters suggest the diagnosis in view of the risk of provoking a hypertensive crisis or haemorrhage. Nonetheless, phaeochromocytomas are aspirated as part of the investigation of an adrenal or retroperitoneal mass and the risks appear to be small. Radiologists have been recommended to use no larger than a 22 gauge needle, to restrict the number of needle passes to minimise haemorrhage and to be aware of the emergency treatment of severe changes in blood pressure.[39]

Aspiration produces bloody but cellular smears with numerous poorly cohesive cells. Groups of cells are arranged in loose alveolar clusters. Large bizarre nuclei may be seen with bi- and multinucleate forms. Intranuclear inclusions are usually easily found. Mitoses are rare. Nucleoli are often prominent and the chromatin appears hyperchromatic but even. There is a variety of cell shapes including polygonal, pleomorphic and occasional spindle cells. The larger cells show some resemblance to ganglion cells. The cytological pleomorphism provides no information as to the likely benignity or malignancy of the tumour. Characteristically for this neuroendocrine tumour there is abundant cytoplasm in which red granules (MGG) can be seen (Fig. 18.10). The cytoplasm appears fragile with poor definition of its boundaries. Lipid may accumulate in the cytoplasm in this tumour and on occasion there may be difficulty in distinguishing the findings from those of an adrenal cortical tumour. This problem may be resolved by the histochemical, immunocytochemical or electron microscopic demonstration of neurosecretory granules.[56] Chromogranin A is positive: it should be noted that synaptophysin is positive in both adrenal cortical tumours and phaeochromocytoma. Rarely, phaeochromocytomas may accumulate lipofuscin or a melanin like pigment, which may cause confusion with malignant melanoma.[57] Ganglioneuromatous differentiation in a phaeochromocytoma yields ganglion cells and spindle cells in addition to phaeochromocytes.[58]

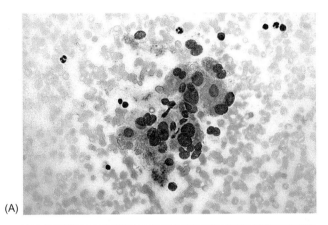

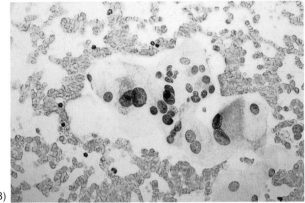

Fig. 18.10 Aspirate from a phaeochromocytoma with poorly cohesive pleomorphic cells, some are multinucleate and the MGG stain shows red granularity. (A: MGG; B: PAP).

### Cytological findings: paraganglionomas

- Haemorrhagic aspirates
- Acinar groups of cells with some dissociation
- Cells may be pleomorphic with prominent nucleoli especially in phaeochromocytoma
- Intranuclear inclusions
- Abundant poorly defined cytoplasm with red granularity (MGG)
- Cellular pleomorphism does not imply malignancy but necrosis and mitotic activity does.

### Diagnostic pitfalls: FNA adrenal

Adrenal aspirates can be contaminated by cells from adjacent organs including the liver and kidneys. This can cause diagnostic confusion. Some adrenal tumours can have similar cytological appearances. These include adrenocortical carcinoma, adenomas, clear cell carcinoma of the kidney, hepatocellular carcinoma, phaeochromocytoma, melanoma and metastases of other carcinomas. Oncocytic adrenocortical and renal neoplasms can appear identical.[59] Further investigations may help to resolve these diagnostic pitfalls. Clinical or biochemical evidence of steroid secretion should be ascertained. Neurosecretory granules are present in phaeochromocytomas and they may be visualised by electron microscopy or their presence demonstrated by their argentaffin properties or immunocytochemically by positivity for chromogranin A. Glycogen and mucin stains

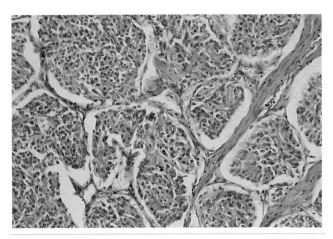

Fig. 18.11 Carotid body tumour (H&E).

may also contribute to the distinction between adrenocortical carcinoma and renal cell carcinoma or another secondary carcinoma, respectively.

Clear cell carcinoma of the superior pole of the kidney may mimic radiologically an adrenal neoplasm, and ipsilateral or contralateral adrenal metastases of renal adenocarcinoma are not uncommon. Cytologically, renal adenocarcinoma cells mimic an adrenocortical neoplasm. The adherence of cells to capillaries and fragments of basement membrane and the presence of papillary or tubular structures suggests a renal tumour. Adrenocortical carcinomas have been cited as having certain features more frequently than renal adenocarcinomas. These include focal dramatic anisonucleosis and crushed spindled fragments.[60] Adrenocortical cells are not glycogen-rich and are negative immunocytochemically for epithelial membrane antigen (EMA), CD10 and the RCC antigen unlike renal carcinomas, which are usually positive. Positivity for Melan A clone A103, alpha inhibin, calretinin and synaptophysin favour the diagnosis of an adrenocortical tumour.[61–64]

## Other paraganglionomas including carotid body tumours

Paraganglionomas may also arise in the retroperitoneum or pelvis and in these sites have been termed extraadrenal phaeo-chromocytomas. Paraganglionomas associated with the para-sympathetic nervous system are usually non-functional and most frequently present in the neck as a carotid body tumour. Jugulotympanic paraganglionomas have been termed glomus jugulare and glomus tympanicum tumours according to their sites of origin within the temporal bone. Similar tumours occa-sionally occur in the mediastinum.

Carotid body tumours are located at and firmly attached to the carotid bifurcation. Classically on examination they can be moved horizontally but not vertically. They are extremely vas-cular and may pulsate. They occur in patients of all ages with a slight preponderance in females. Some cases are familial and these cases are more likely to be bilateral. Patients present with a mass in the neck which may cause local compression and hence hoarseness, dysphagia or carotid sinus syndrome. The majority are benign, but approximately 10% behave in a malignant fash-ion. Histologically (Fig. 18.11), they consist of well-defined nests of cuboidal cells separated by vascular fibrous septa. Wrapped around the cuboidal cells are occasional spindle-shaped sustentacular cells. There are no absolutely reliable histological features to separate benign from malignant tumours. The cuboidal cells contain neurosecretory granules, are argyrophil, weakly argentaffin and immunostain positively for chromogranin A.

Jugulotympanic paraganglionomas usually arise within the temporal bone and present as a mass in the middle ear, external auditory meatus or as a mass at the base of the skull. They may occur at any age and there is a strong female predilection. Some cases are familial, may be bilateral and may coexist with carotid body tumours. These slow growing tumours may produce auditory disturbances and cranial nerve palsies. They rarely metastasise but may cause death if intracranial extension occurs.

## The role, cytological findings and diagnostic pitfalls of FNA of carotid body tumours

A carotid body tumour is part of the differential diagnosis of a mass in the neck (see Table 17.1). Ideally it should be diagnosed clinically and by imaging studies. Preoperative diagnosis is important to forewarn the surgeon of the possibility of severe haemorrhage and damage to the carotid artery at diagnostic excisional biopsy of what might be assumed to be a cervical lymph node. FNA should be carried out cautiously in view of the risk of haemorrhage and the small possibility of precipitating compression or thrombosis of the underlying carotid artery.

The cytological findings in jugulotympanic and carotid body paragangliomas are identical and very similar to those of a phaeochromocytoma. Aspiration yields blood-stained samples with tumour cells both singly and in loose clusters. Blood contamination may be severe with relatively few tumour cells. There may be an acinar or follicular arrangement. There is abundant poorly defined cytoplasm with a red granularity. Nuclei vary from round to spindle shaped; the chromatin pattern appears uniform, although there may be some variation in

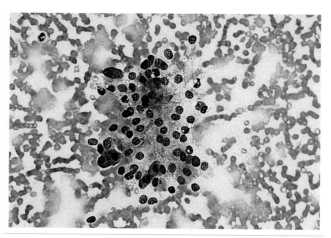

**Fig. 18.12** Aspirate from a carotid body tumour showing haemorrhagic material including loosely cohesive mildly pleomorphic cells with granular cytoplasm (MGG).

nuclear size, and intracytoplasmic nuclear inclusions may be present. Single or multiple nucleoli may be present (Fig. 18.12). Nuclear pleomorphism, as in most endocrine tumours, does not signify malignancy, which is defined by architectural features, although the presence of necrosis and frequent mitoses is suspicious.

The presence of acinar or follicular structures, cytoplasmic granularity and intranuclear inclusions may cause confusion with a range of thyroid pathologies. Immunocytochemical or histochemical methods can demonstrate the presence of neurosecretory granules enabling distinction from metastatic follicular or papillary carcinoma. There still may be confusion with medullary carcinoma of the thyroid and the clinical presentation and location of the lesion should be considered together with the immunocytochemical absence of calcitonin.[65-68] Rarely ectopic parathyroid glands can also be located at the carotid bifurcation causing diagnostic confusion.[8]

## REFERENCES

1. Ippolito G, Palazzo FF, Sebag F, et al. A single institution 25 year review of the parathyroid cysts. Langenbecks Arch Surg 2006;391:13–18.

2. Tseng FY, Hisao YL, Chang TC. Ultrasound-guided fine needle aspiration cytology of parathyroid lesions. A review of 72 cases. Acta Cytol 2002;46:1029–36.

3. Giorgadze T, Stratton B, Baloch ZW, et al. Oncocytic parathyroid adenoma: problem in cytologic diagnosis. Diagn Cytopathol 2004;31:276–80.

4. Lin F, Gnepp DR, Pisharodi LR. Fine needle aspiration of parathyroid lesions. Acta Cytol 2004;48:133–36.

5. Goellner JR, Candill JL. Intranuclear holes (cytoplasmic pseudoinclusions) in parathyroid neoplasms or 'holes happen'. Cancer (Cancer Cytopathol) 2000;90:41–46.

6. Davis Davey D, Glant MD, Berger EK. Parathyroid cytopathology. Diagn Cytopathol 1986;2:76–80.

7. Mincione GP, Borrelli D, Cicchi P, et al. Fine needle aspiration cytology of parathyroid adenoma: a review of seven cases. Acta Cytol 1986;30:65–69.

8. Bondeson L, Bondeson A-G, Nissborg A, et al. Cytopathological variables in parathyroid lesions: a study based on 1,600 cases of hyperparathyroidism. Diagn Cytopathol 1997;16:476–82.

9. Hara H, Oyama T, Kimura M, et al. Cytologic characterisation of parathyroid carcinoma: a case report. Diagn Cytopathol 1998;18:192–98.

10. Nasser G, Loberant N, Salameh A, et al. Oxyphil cell carcinoma of the parathyroid: a rare cause of hyperparathyroidism. Clin Oncol 1995;7:323–24.

11. Saikia B, Dey P, Saikia UN, et al. Fine needle aspiration of metastatic scalp nodules. Acta Cytol 2001;45:537–41.

12. Ikeda K, Tate G, Suzuki T, et al. Cytologic comparison of a primary parathyroid cancer and its metastatic lesions: a case report. Diagn Cytopathol 2006;34:50–55.

13. Sulak LE, Brown RW, Butler DB. Parathyroid carcinoma with occult bone metastases diagnosed by fine needle aspiration cytology. Acta Cytol 1989;33:645–48.

14. Layfield LJ. Fine needle aspiration cytology of cystic parathyroid lesions: a cytomorphologic overlap with cystic lesions of the thyroid. Acta Cytol 1991;35:447–50.

15. Absher KJ, Truong LD, Khurana KK, et al. Parathyroid cytology: avoiding diagnostic pitfalls. Head Neck 2002;24:157–64.

16. Löwhagen T, Sprenger E. Cytologic presentation of thyroid tumors in aspiration biopsy smear: a review of 60 cases. Acta Cytol 1974;18:192–97.

17. Friedman M, Shimaoka K, Lopez CA, et al. Parathyroid adenoma diagnosed as papillary carcinoma of thyroid on needle aspiration smear. Acta Cytol 1983;27:337–40.

18. Auger M, Charbonneau M, Huttner J. Unsuspected intrathyroidal parathyroid adenoma: mimic of lymphocytic thyroiditis in fine needle aspiration specimens – a case report. Diagn Cytopathol 1999;21:276–79.

19. Beecham JE. Coexistent disease as a complicating factor in the fine needle aspiration diagnosis of papillary carcinoma of the thyroid. Acta Cytol 1986;30:435–38.

20. Abati A, Skarulis MC, Shawker T, et al. Ultrasound-guided fine-needle aspiration of parathyroid lesions: a morphological and

immunocytochemical approach. Hum Pathol 1995;26:338–43.

21. Covaco BM, Torrinha F, Mendonca E, et al. Preoperative diagnosis of suspicious parathyroid adenomas by RT-PCR using mRNA extracted from leftover cells in a needle used for ultrasonically guided fine needle aspiration cytology. Acta Cytol 2003;47:5–12.

22. Tseleni-Balafonta S, Gakiopoulou H, Kavantzas N, et al. Parathyroid proliferations: a source of diagnostic pitfalls in FNA of thyroid. Cancer 2007;111:130–36.

23. Abraham D, Sharma PK, Bentz J, et al. Utility of ultrasound-guided fine-needle aspiration of parathyroid adenomas for localisation before minimally invasive parathyroidectomy. Endocr Pract 2007;13:333–37.

24. Erbil Y, Salmaslioglu A, Kabul E, et al. Use of preoperative parathyroid fine-needle aspiration and parathormone assay in the primary hyperparathyroidism with concomitant thyroid nodules. Am J Surg 2007;193:665–71.

25. Stephen AE, Milas M, Garner CN, et al. Use of surgeon-performed office ultrasound and parathyroid fine needle aspiration for complex parathyroid localisation. Surgery 2005;138:1143–51.

26. Maser C, Donovan P, Santos F, et al. Sonographically guided fine needle aspiration with rapid parathyroid hormone assay. Ann Surg Oncol 2006;13:1690–95.

27. Kendrick ML, Charboneau JW, Curlee KJ, et al. Risk of parathyromatosis after fine needle aspiration. Am Surg 2001;67:290–94.

28. Spinelli C, Bonadio AG, Berti P, et al. Cutaneous spreading of parathyroid carcinoma after fine needle aspiration cytology. J Endocrinol Invest 2000;23:255–57.

29. Agarwal G, Dhingra S, Mishra SK, et al. Implantation of parathyroid carcinoma along fine needle aspiration track. Langenbecks Arch Surg 2006;391:625–26.

30. Ing SW, Pelliteri PK. Diagnostic fine-needle aspiration biopsy of an intrathyroid parathyroid gland and subsequent eucalcaemia in a patient with primary hyperparathyroidism. Endocr Pract 2008;14:80–86.

31. Alwaheeb S, Rambaldini G, Boerner S, et al. Worrisome histologic alterations following fine-needle aspiration of the parathyroid. J Clin Pathol 2006;59:1094–96.

32. Norman J, Politz D, Browarsky I. Diagnostic aspiration of parathyroid adenomas causes severe fibrosis complicating surgery and final histologic diagnosis. Thyroid 2007;17:1251–55.

33. Stelow EB, Debol SM, Stanley MW, et al. Sampling of the adrenal glands by endoscopic ultrasound-guided fine-needle aspiration. Diagn Cytopathol 2005;33:26–30.

34. Katz RL, Patel S, Mackay B, et al. Fine needle aspiration cytology of the adrenal gland. Acta Cytol 1984;28:269–82.

35. Saboorian MH, Katz RL, Charnsangarej C. Fine needle aspiration cytology of primary and metastatic lesions of the adrenal gland. A series of 188 biopsies with radiologic correlation. Acta Cytol 1995;39:843–51.

36. Wu HHJ, Cramer HM, Kho J, et al. Fine needle aspiration cytology of benign adrenal cortical nodules: a comparison of cytologic findings with those of primary and metastatic adrenal malignancies. Acta Cytol 1998;42:1352–58.

37. De Augustin P, Lopez-Rios F, Alberti N, et al. Fine needle aspiration biopsy of adrenal glands: a ten year experience. Diagn Cytopathol 1999;21:92–97.

38. Fassina AS, Borsato S, Fedeli U. Fine needle aspiration cytology (FNAC) of adrenal masses. Cytopathology 2000;11:302–11.

39. Casola G, Nicolet V, van Sonnenberg E, et al. Unsuspected pheochromocytoma: risk of blood-pressure alterations during percutaneous adrenal biopsy. Radiology 1986;159:733–35.

40. Hasan M, Siddiqui F, Al-Ajmi M. FNA diagnosis of adrenal myelolipoma: a rare entity. Diagn Cytopathol 2008;36:925–26.

41. Deodhare S, Sapp M. Adrenal histoplasmosis: Diagnosis by fine needle aspiration biopsy. Diagn Cytopathol 1997;17:42–44.

42. Heaston DK, Handel DB, Ashton PR, et al. Narrow gauge needle aspiration of solid adrenal masses. Am J Radiol 1982;138:1143–48.

43. Kawamura M, Miyazaki S, Mashiko S, et al. Disseminated cryptococcosis associated with adrenal masses and insufficiency. Am J Med Sci 1998;316:60–64.

44. Dusenbery D, Dekker A. Needle biopsy of the adrenal gland: retrospective review of 54 cases. Diagn Cytopathol 1996;14:126–34.

45. Wadih GE, Nance KV, Silverman JF. Fine needle aspiration cytology of the adrenal gland. Fifty biopsies in 48 patients. Arch Pathol Lab Med 1992;116:841–46.

46. Min K-W, Song J, Boesenberg M, et al. Adrenal cortical nodule mimicking small round cell malignancy on fine needle aspiration. Acta Cytol 1988;32:543–46.

47. Ren R, Guo M, Sneige N, et al. Fine needle aspiration of adrenocortical carcinoma; cytologic spectrum and diagnostic challenges. Am J Clin Pathol 2006;126:389–98.

48. Nance KC, McLeod DL, Silverman JF. Fine needle aspiration cytology of spindle cell neoplasms of the adrenal gland. Diagn Cytopathol 1992;8:235–41.

49. Mitchell ML. Ryan FP Jr, Shermer RW. Pulmonary adenocarcinoma metastatic to the adrenal gland mimicking normal adrenal cortical epithelium on fine needle aspiration. Acta Cytol 1985;29:994–98.

50. Rosai J. Special techniques in surgical pathology. In: Rosai S, Ackermans S, editors. Surgical Pathology. 9th edn, Vol. 1. London: Mosby; 2004: 55–61.

51. Pohar-Marinsek Z. Difficulties in diagnosing small round cell tumours of childhood from fine needle aspiration cytology samples. Cytopathology 2008;19:67–79.

52. Heim S, Mitelman F. Cytogenetics of solid tumours. In: Recent Advances in Histopathology. Edinburgh: Churchill Livingstone; 1992: 37–67.

53. Kumar PV. Fine needle aspiration cytologic diagnosis of ganglioneuroblastoma. Acta Cytol 1987;31:583–86.

54. Otal-Salaverri C, González-Cámpora R, Hevia-Vazquez A, et al. Retroperitoneal ganglioneuroblastoma: report of a case diagnosed by fine needle aspiration cytology and electron microscopy. Acta Cytol 1989;33:80–84.

55. Yen H, Cobb CJ. Retroperitoneal ganglioneuroma: a report of diagnosis by fine needle aspiration cytology. Diagn Cytopathol 1998;19:385–87.

56. Jimenez-Heffernan JA, Vicandi B, Lopez-Ferrer P, et al. Cytologic features of pheochromocytoma and retroperitoneal paraganglioma: a morphologic and immunohistochemical study of 13 cases. Acta Cytol 2006;50:372–78.

57. Handa U, Khullar U, Mohan H. Pigmented pheochromocytoma: report of a case with diagnosis by fine needle aspiration. Acta Cytol 2005;49:421–23.

58. Layfied LJ, Glasgow BJ, Du Puis MH, et al. Aspiration cytology and immunohistochemistry of a pheochromocytoma-ganglioneuroma of the adrenal gland. Acta Cytol 1987;31: 33–39.

59. Wragg T, Nguyen GK. Cytopathology of adrenal cortical oncocytoma. Diagn Cytopathol 2001;24:222–23.

60. Sharma S, Singh R, Verma K. Cytomorphology of adrenal carcinoma and comparison with renal cell carcinoma. Acta Cytol 1997;41:385–92.

61. Shin SJ, Hoda RS, Ying L, et al. Diagnostic utility of the monoclonal antibody A103 in fine needle aspiration biopsies of the adrenal. Am J Clin Pathol 2000;113:295–302.

62. Fetsch PA, Powers CN, Zakowski MF, et al. Anti alpha inhibin: marker of choice for the consistent distinction between adrenocortical carcinoma and renal cell carcinoma in fine needle aspiration. Cancer 1999;87:168–72.

63. Rosai J. Adrenal gland and other paraganglia. In: Rosai S, Ackerman S, editors. Surgical Pathology. 9th edn, Vol 1 London: Mosby; 2004:1123.

64. Jalali M, Krishnamurthy S. Comparison of immunomarkers for the identification of adrenocortical cells in cytology specimens. Diagn Cytopathol 2005;33:78–82.

65. Engzell U, Franzén S, Zajicek J. Aspiration biopsy of tumours of the neck II. Cytologic findings in 13 cases of carotid body tumour. Acta Cytol 1971;15:25–30.

66. González-Cámpora R, Otal-Salaverri C, Panea-Flores P, et al. Fine needle aspiration cytology of paraganglionic tumors. Acta Cytol 1988;32:386–90.

67. Fleming MV, Oertel YC, Rodriguez ER, et al. Fine-needle aspiration of six carotid body paragangliomas. Diagn Cytopathol 1993;9:510–15.

68. Jacobs DM, Waisman J. Cervical paraganglioma with intranuclear vacuoles in a fine needle aspirate. Acta Cytol 1987;31:29–32.

# Section 11

## Male Genital Tract

# Prostate gland

Aasmund Berner and Svante R. Orell

## Chapter contents

## Introduction

Transrectal fine needle aspiration biopsy (FNA) was introduced in Sweden in 1960 by Franzén, Giertz and Zajicek as a minimally invasive cytological method to confirm a clinical diagnosis of carcinoma of the prostate. It has now been in use for nearly 50 years and has proved to be a simple, safe and accurate method of investigation of palpable lesions in the prostate gland.[1,2]

## Epidemiology of prostatic cancer

Prostate cancer accounts for 9.7% of malignant tumours in men and is the most common cancer among males in the Western world.[3] It is one of the leading causes of cancer death in men, second only to lung cancer, and an increasing number of men are being diagnosed with prostate cancer worldwide. Autopsy studies have shown invasive carcinoma in 8% of men in their 20s, rising to 80% for men in their 70s.[4] It has been estimated that four-fifths of these cancers are truly occult but that one-fifth have the potential to become clinically manifest and eventually lethal. This malignancy is, however, not invariably lethal and may have a prolonged natural history, being now diagnosed at earlier stages due to widespread serum prostate-specific antigen (PSA) testing.

Thus, a large proportion of clinically significant cancers remain undetected. At the time of diagnosis, almost half of the cancers are advanced and a little over half are localised and potentially curable. These data emphasise the need for improvement in the diagnosis and detection of prostatic cancer. Some improvement may already have occurred. Rietbergen et al. found that among cancers detected by screening, 78% had organ-confined disease.[5]

## Aetiology and pathogenesis

The aetiology and pathogenesis of prostatic cancer are not known. The majority of prostate cancers are sporadic, and only 5–15% of cases are hereditary.[6]

## Clinical features

Clinical symptoms develop only late in the disease. They are mainly related to bladder outlet obstruction. Such symptoms are non-specific and may be caused by prostatic enlargement of whatever nature, including benign prostatic hyperplasia and some forms of prostatitis. Haematuria or haemospermia are sometimes the first symptoms. However, most cancers are asymptomatic and detected by routine rectal palpation, abnormal transrectal ultrasound examination or by a raised serum PSA. Not infrequently, secondary deposits cause the presenting symptoms, for example, supraclavicular lymph node enlargement or pain from bone secondaries, while the primary tumour is silent.

## Diagnostic procedure

Three clinical methods are currently available for the detection and diagnosis of carcinoma of the prostate: digital rectal examination (DRE), measurement of serum PSA levels and transrectal ultrasonography (TRUS). Each method alone has limited sensitivity and specificity, but combination of the three has significantly improved the cancer detection rate. If there is no palpable abnormality, a serum PSA level over 4 ng/mL in combination with an abnormal TRUS, or a PSA level over 10 ng/mL alone, are highly suggestive of clinically significant cancer.[3,7] If cancer is suggested by one or more of these diagnostic methods, preoperative morphological confirmation of the diagnosis is the next step. Other indications are palpable abnormality in a patient who is not a candidate for radical surgery; patients with disseminated disease and long waiting lists for core needle biopsy (CNB). This can be done by needle biopsy, either by transrectal FNA for cytological diagnosis, or by transrectal or transperineal CNB for histological examination. The diagnostic accuracy of FNA is comparable with that of CNB.[2,8]

CNB needles in use today are usually 18 gauge or less. Some workers claim that with needles of this size, the complication rate is similar to that of FNA.[9] Others find that the risk of complications is higher and patient discomfort is greater with CNB and recommend it be used selectively.[10] Tumour implantation in the needle track has not been reported for prostatic FNA but does occur, albeit rarely, following transrectal CNB.[11]

Transrectal FNA remains the simplest, quickest and least expensive method to confirm clinically palpable cancer.[1,3] Ultrasound directed CNB is more appropriate in the investigation of non-palpable malignancy suggested by either a high serum PSA or by an abnormal transrectal ultrasonogram.[12–14]

## Technique of transrectal FNA of prostate

FNA is guided by transrectal palpation. The Franzén guide cannula was designed to make it possible to position the needle accurately in the abnormal area felt with the fingertip. It is secured by a metal ring fixed to the fingertip and a plate in the palm of the hand. A rubber fingerstall is pulled over it. The needles are 23 gauge or 25 gauge and the results are comparable with CNB of the prostate.[8,15,16] Up to six passes can be made in one session but two to four are usually sufficient.

FNA of the prostate is an out-patient procedure that needs no patient preparation. Prophylactic administration of antibiotics should be considered in patients at increased risk of infection since septic reactions can occur. Post biopsy haematuria is a not infrequent occurrence but significant haemorrhagic complications do not occur even in patients on anticoagulant treatment.[17]

Whether to use air-dried smears stained with a Romanowsky stain, such as May–Grünwald Giemsa (MGG) or Diff-Quik, or wet-fixed smears for Papanicolaou (PAP) or haematoxylin and eosin (H&E) staining, is a matter of personal preference. Air-dried smears are more dependent on correct smearing technique. Highly cellular smears from a cancer make good air-dried preparations. The thin liquid aspirate often obtained from benign prostatic hyperplasia is more suitable for a liquid-based technique or alcohol fixation.

Special stains are rarely used in prostatic cytology. Staining for PSA and for prostate-specific acid phosphatase (PSAP) is helpful in confirming a primary prostatic adenocarcinoma and in the distinction between adenocarcinoma and transitional cell carcinoma. Staining for high-molecular-weight cytokeratins, which are present in the prostate only in basal cells, has been found helpful in differentiating benign proliferative processes from well-differentiated adenocarcinoma.[18,19] A recent study has shown that detection of p504S is a sensitive and specific marker for prostatic carcinoma.[20] Immunohistochemical analysis is essential in the recognition of small cell carcinoma of neuroendocrine type. Finally, macrophage markers and PSA/PSAP can be used in distinguishing granulomatous prostatitis from poorly differentiated carcinoma, which is occasionally also a problem histologically.

## Causes of prostatic enlargement

The purpose of FNA is to confirm a clinical suspicion of cancer and to decide the nature of a palpable abnormality. Any condition that can cause prostatic enlargement, firmness and irregularity therefore enters the differential diagnosis. The most common cause is nodular benign prostatic hyperplasia. Prostatitis may also cause a palpable abnormality, in particular granulomatous prostatitis can clinically mimic cancer. An enlarged seminal vesicle can occasionally feel suspicious.

Most prostatic neoplasms are adenocarcinomas. A few uncommon types such as prostatic duct (endometrioid) adenocarcinoma and mucinous adenocarcinoma can be separated from the usual acinar adenocarcinoma. Neuroendocrine tumours and transitional

---

**Box 19.1 Neoplasms of the prostate**

Epithelial neoplasms

- Adenocarcinoma
  - Usual type
  - Prostatic duct (endometrioid/papillary) type
  - Mucinous type
- Neuroendocrine (small cell) tumours
- Transitional cell carcinoma
- Others
  - Squamous cell carcinoma
  - Adenosquamous carcinoma
  - Adenoid cystic carcinoma
  - Basal cell carcinoma

Carcinosarcoma

Non-epithelial tumours

- Benign
  - Leiomyoma
  - Haemangioma, etc.
- Sarcoma
  - Rhabdomyosarcoma
  - Leiomyosarcoma
  - Cystosarcoma phyllodes
- Malignant lymphoma
- Germ cell tumours

---

cell carcinomas are uncommon and so are mesenchymal tumours. A classification of prostatic tumours modified from Murphy[21] is presented in Box 19.1.

## Benign prostatic hyperplasia

It is usually not difficult to obtain cellular material from a case of benign prostatic hyperplasia (BPH). However, the cells may be diluted by a large amount of thin secretion and may need to be concentrated by two-step smearing. Admixture with blood is rarely a problem. In general, smears of BPH aspirates contain many fewer cells than smears from adenocarcinoma.

### Cytological findings: benign prostatic hyperplasia

- Monolayered sheets of bland glandular epithelial cells
- Abundant pale cytoplasm, sometimes with red (MGG) cytoplasmic granules
- Distinct cell membranes producing a honeycomb pattern
- Uniformly distributed round or oval nuclei
- Bland granular chromatin, inconspicuous nucleoli
- Background of abundant thin and thick secretion
- Inflammatory cells variable.

Benign glandular epithelial cells are cohesive without overlapping or crowding and occur mainly as large monolayered sheets, reflecting the relatively large size of the glands in BPH. The cells are polygonal with central round nuclei and abundant pale cytoplasm, and cell membranes are distinctly visible, giving the epithelial sheets a honeycomb pattern. Single cells are uncommon unless too much pressure at smearing has caused the sheets to break up. However, it has been pointed out

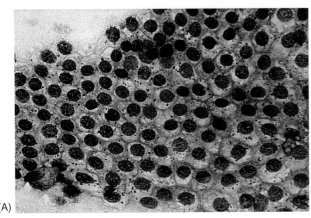

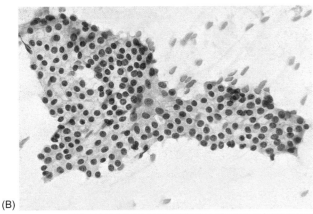

**Fig. 19.1** Benign prostatic glandular epithelium. Monolayered sheets with regular distribution of nuclei, visible cell membranes and coarse red cytoplasmic granules visible in (A) (A: MGG; B: PAP).

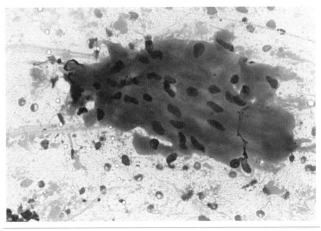

**Fig. 19.2** Fragment of smooth muscle stroma in smear from case of BPH (MGG).

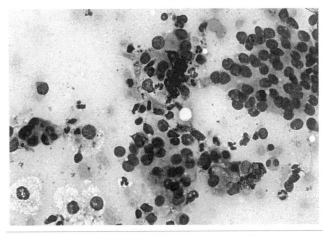

**Fig. 19.3** Chronic prostatitis. Note irregular distribution and some overlapping of nuclei in glandular epithelium (MGG).

that small groups of cells suggestive of loss of cohesion occur in prostatic smears from men younger than 40 years.[22]

The nuclei of benign epithelial cells have inconspicuous nucleoli and finely granular chromatin (Fig. 19.1). In MGG-stained smears, coarse dark red cytoplasmic granules are commonly present (Fig. 19.1A). The granules are a strong indicator of benignity, although they can occasionally be found also in well-differentiated carcinoma.

Smears may have a thin and watery background of secretion, with a high protein content condensed to dark staining clumps, amyloid bodies or concretions. A small number of histiocytes, lymphocytes and neutrophils are frequently seen in the absence of prostatitis. Fragments of spindle smooth muscle cells and stroma are rarely seen (Fig. 19.2).

Other elements that may be found in BPH are metaplastic or mature squamous epithelial cells from the mucosa of the bladder neck or urethra, and mucin-secreting columnar cells from the rectal mucosa, and cells from the seminal vesicles. The metaplastic cells are cytologically bland and should not raise a suspicion of malignancy.

## Prostatitis

### Cytological findings: prostatitis

- Numerous inflammatory cells including neutrophils
- Benign glandular epithelial cells which may show mild atypia.

Inflammatory cells should be present in large numbers before a cytological diagnosis of prostatitis is made. The glandular epithelial cells may appear mildly atypical. The nuclei may be irregularly distributed, cell membranes may be less distinct and there may be a slight reduction in cell cohesion with more frequent single cells. No multilayering of cells in aggregates or microacinar groupings of epithelial cells are seen, the chromatin is bland and nucleoli remain inconspicuous (Fig. 19.3).

## Granulomatous prostatitis

### Cytological findings: granulomatous prostatitis

- Large multinucleated histiocytic giant cells
- Many histiocytes, some of epithelioid type
- Various inflammatory cells
- Degenerate or mildly atypical glandular epithelium.

When present, large multinucleated histiocytic giant cells, which often contain clumps of phagocytosed secretion, render the diagnosis of granulomatous prostatitis obvious.

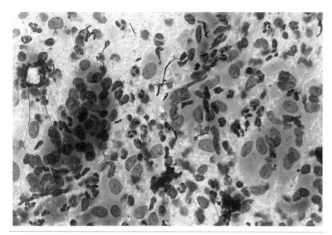

**Fig. 19.4** Granulomatous prostatitis. Characteristic large multinucleated giant cells not shown; note epithelioid histiocytes, inflammatory cells in background and fragment of mildly atypical glandular epithelium (MGG).

Cytological diagnosis is important since there is often a high level of suspicion of cancer clinically. Histiocytes are frequent, most are of epithelioid type and may form granulomatous clusters. There is a dirty background of secretion, debris and various inflammatory cells.

The diagnosis may be less obvious if spindled histiocytes predominate and giant cells are absent (Fig. 19.4). In the presence of granulomatous prostatitis, mild epithelial atypia should not be a cause for concern. Histiocytes may sometimes appear atypical, particularly in MGG smears. If this causes diagnostic problems, immunocytochemical staining for macrophage markers are helpful.

## Seminal vesicle

### Cytological findings: seminal vesicle

- Glandular epithelial cells with atypical, pleomorphic nuclei
- Coarse intracytoplasmic pigment granules
- Spermatozoa in the background.

The epithelial cells of the seminal vesicle often display a degree of nuclear atypia and pleomorphism. Nuclei may be huge, of irregular shape, hyperchromatic and have large nucleoli, and may be indistinguishable from malignant cells. The clue to the correct diagnosis lies in the presence of coarse lipofuscin pigment granules, which stain dark black/green with MGG and brown with Papanicolaou staining (Fig. 19.5). Other helpful features are the presence of heads of spermatozoa in the background and a knowledge that the biopsy derives from the upper lateral corner of the prostate.

## Adenocarcinoma

Prostate cancer is an heterogeneous disease with considerable variation in clinical course. Tumour grading is performed in an effort to predict behaviour and choice of treatment.[3,5,22] However, all grading systems are subjective and difficult to reproduce. Several

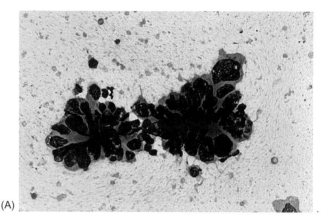

(A)

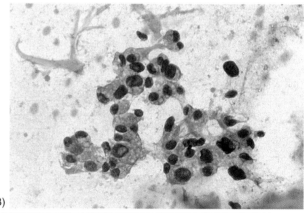

(B)

**Fig. 19.5** Seminal vesicle epithelial cells. Note nuclear pleomorphism and the presence of coarse cytoplasmic pigment (A: MGG; B: PAP).

architectural criteria apply in the diagnosis of adenocarcinoma of the prostate. The smears are usually highly cellular and mixtures of benign and malignant cells are commonly seen. A large number of atypical cells is suggestive of cancer and may be one of the most important signs in very well-differentiated tumours.

### Cytological findings: adenocarcinoma

- Multilayered aggregates of cells showing nuclear crowding and overlapping and loss of visible cell borders
- Cells have a tendency to form multiple microacinar groupings
- Usually a mixture of benign and malignant cells in the malignant smear
- Loss of cell cohesion and dissociation of cell aggregates
- Increase in nuclear size and in nucleolar size
- Chromatin coarseness and prominent nucleoli
- Cytoplasm of adenocarcinoma cells pale and poorly defined, sometimes vacuolated
- Cell borders are indistinct.

The orderly monolayered sheets of benign glandular epithelium are replaced by multilayered aggregates of cells showing nuclear crowding, overlapping and loss of visible cell borders. Within the aggregates, the cells have a tendency to form multiple microacinar groupings (Fig. 19.6). This feature is generally so characteristic that a prostatic origin may be suggested when it is seen in a metastasic site. Loss

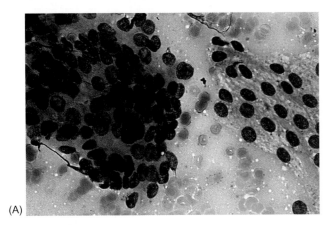

(A)

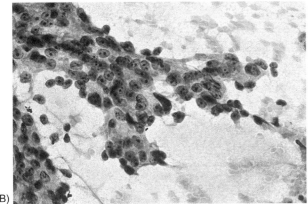

(B)

**Fig. 19.6** Moderately differentiated adenocarcinoma (Grade II). Note nuclear enlargement, crowding and overlapping and contrasting benign epithelium in (A); nucleolar enlargement and chromatin clumping in (B); microacinar pattern in both (A: MGG; B: PAP).

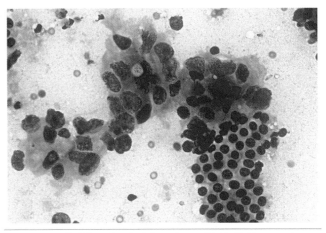

**Fig. 19.7** Poorly differentiated adenocarcinoma (Grade III). Note severe nuclear atypia and striking contrast with benign epithelium (MGG).

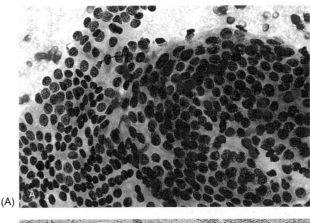

(A)

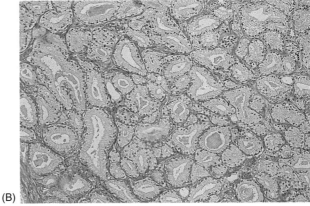

(B)

**Fig. 19.8** Well-differentiated adenocarcinoma (Grade I). Abundance of cells showing nuclear crowding and mild enlargement but a bland chromatin (A: MGG; B: tissue section, H&E).

of cell cohesion and dissociation of cell aggregates increases with decreasing differentiation, except perhaps in young patients.[22] Standard cytological criteria of malignancy such as nuclear pleomorphism and chromatin abnormalities are obvious in less well-differentiated carcinoma (Fig. 19.7). In well-differentiated tumours, nuclear abnormalities are more subtle (Fig. 19.8). The two most important criteria are increases in nuclear size and in nucleolar size. Chromatin coarseness and nucleoli are clearly shown in Papanicolaou stained smears (Fig. 19.9). The cytoplasm of adenocarcinoma cells is pale and poorly defined and cell borders are indistinct. Sometimes the cytoplasm is finely vacuolated, resembling that of renal cell carcinoma; sometimes it is dispersed in the background leaving the nuclei stripped. There is usually a mixture of benign and malignant cells in the malignant smear. The contrast between the orderly, monolayered sheets of benign glandular epithelium and the irregular, multilayered aggregates and dispersed cells of carcinoma is readily appreciated (Figs 19.6–19.8). In addition to an appropriate pattern and a sufficient degree of dyskaryosis, the diagnosis of cancer requires the absence of basal cells. This can be confirmed by using a cocktail of immunostains comprising P504S/34βE12/p63.[23] In metastases, the cytological pattern described above is usually suggestive enough to raise this possibility[16] which can be confirmed by immunostaining for PSA and PSAP[24] and P504S.[21]

## Cytological grading of prostatic carcinoma

Most workers have found cytological grading to be less reliable than histological grading. This is one reason why most urologists prefer CNB to FNA in the diagnosis of prostatic cancer. However, a simple three-grade system based on cell cohesion/dissociation and nuclear atypia proposed by Esposti in 1971 has shown a good correlation with survival.[25] Gleason grading is fundamentally an architectural rather than cytological

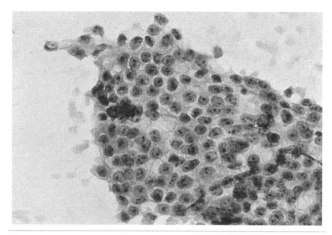

**Fig. 19.9** Relatively well-differentiated adenocarcinoma (Grades I–II). Note cohesive monolayered sheet and fairly regular distribution of nuclei but also nuclear enlargement, prominent nucleoli and mild chromatin irregularity (PAP).

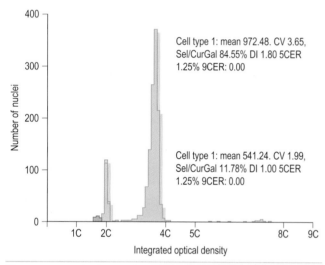

Cell type 1: mean 972.48. CV 3.65, Sel/CurGal 84.55% DI 1.80 5CER 1.25% 9CER: 0.00

Cell type 1: mean 541.24. CV 1.99, Sel/CurGal 11.78% DI 1.00 5CER 1.25% 9CER: 0.00

**Fig. 19.10** Aneuploid stem cell population in a case of clinically localised prostate cancer. A similar pattern can be seen even when cytologically, the aspirate is difficult to distinguish from a non-cancerous prostatic FNA.

system,[26] making it difficult to apply directly to FNA specimens, although estimations of Gleason scores have been reported on cytological matherial.[8,27] Gland size roughly determines Gleason pattern. Small, regular, and intermediate-size glands correspond to Gleason acinar patterns 1 or 2; irregular glands to Gleason acinar pattern 3; and very small, highly irregular or abortive glands to Gleason acinar pattern 4. Undifferentiated carcinoma is either solid or dissociated.

FNA cell material is eminently suitable for DNA analysis, such as flow cytometry or static image analysis (Fig. 19.10), molecular studies and proteomics (see also Ch. 4).[28,29] Ploidy levels have been found to be superior to morphological grading and clinical stage as a prognostic indicator, particularly on small localised tumours, in combination with proliferation index.[30,31] In order to enhance the predictive information a number of other biomarkers have been studied. However, so far only a few are currently employed in clinical practice, i.e. p53, AMACR, hepsin and SIM2.[27,32,33] Recently Berg and colleagues documented the association between the presence of disseminated prostatic carcinoma cells and increasing Gleason score,

which should alert clinicians and patients discussing treatment options at time of diagnosis.[34]

## Diagnostic pitfalls: adenocarcinoma

Technical limitations such as specimen adequacy or non-representative sampling are the main causes of false negative diagnosis. Well-differentiated adenocarcinoma may not show any obvious cytological criteria of malignancy and is often difficult to distinguish from atypical small acinar proliferation (ASAP) which refers to the spectrum of lesions most commonly comprising post-atrophic hyperplasia, adenosis, atypical adenomatous hyperplasia and high-grade prostatic intraepithelial neoplasia (HGPIN).[8] In the absence of a cancer diagnosis histological confirmation may be necessary.

False positive cytological diagnoses are often due to morphological patterns that can be confused with carcinoma such as ASAP, HGPIN, inflammation and seminal vesicle contamination. FNAs lack the context of 'tissue patterns' that are helpful in distinguishing between these lesions in histological material.[8,35] HGPIN is a non-destructive intraductal pre-neoplastic epithelial proliferation (Fig. 19.11). This condition is not easily distinguished from cells of a well-differentiated adenocarcinoma, but in HGPIN specimens ducts are often seen as sheets of several hundred nuclei spread side-to-side *en face*. In doubtful or borderline cases, CNB for histological examination should be performed.

Distinguishing poorly differentiated adenocarcinoma from transitional cell carcinoma and neuroendocrine tumours can cause problems.[35] This distinction is of clinical importance since the latter tumours are unresponsive to hormonal treatment. The differential diagnosis may require the use of immunocytochemical markers. Epithelial cells from the rectal mucosa can occur as small glandular structures and may raise a suspicion of adenocarcinoma. However, the cells are tall, columnar and palisading, with goblet cell forms, and there is usually abundant mucus in the background (Fig. 19.12).

FNA prostate has an important place not only in diagnosis, but also in predicting prognosis and choice of treatment. Hormone and irradiation therapy induce morphological changes both in the non-malignant and malignant residual prostatic tissue.[36–38] Irradiation- and cytotoxic drug-induced changes in benign glandular epithelium may mimic malignant cells and the carcinoma cells, when present, are frequently bizarre. The effects of hormone therapy include atrophic cells, shrunken and pyknotic nuclei, squamous metaplasia and cytoplasmic vacuolation (Fig. 19.13). An adenocarcinoma responding well to hormonal treatment may no longer be recognisable as malignant in smears taken after commencement of treatment.[37,38] Tumour grading is not recommended after hormonal or irradiation therapy.[38]

## Subtypes of adenocarcinoma

### Ductal (endometrioid) adenocarcinoma

Ductal adenocarcinoma of the prostate has also been termed endometrioid, endometrial, papillary or papillary ductal adenocarcinoma.[39,40] Recently, the very existence of prostatic ductal adenocarcinoma as a discrete clinicopathological entity has been questioned.[41] Cytological atypia may be subtle, the

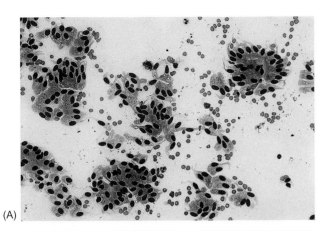

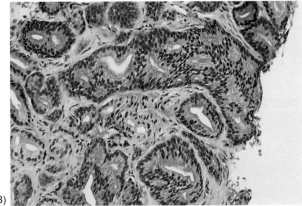

**Fig. 19.11** Prostatic intraepithelial neoplasia (PIN). Cellular smear of moderately atypical columnar epithelial cells. Intraglandular cribriform atypical epithelial proliferation seen in sections (A: MGG; B: tissue section, H&E).

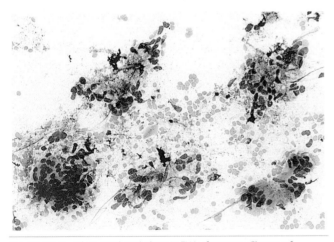

**Fig. 19.12** Rectal mucosal epithelium in FNA of prostate. Clusters of columnar epithelial cells, some goblet cells. Prostatic glandular epithelium lower left (MGG).

diagnosis being based on the presence of abnormal papillary fragments. One of the reports describes longitudinal nuclear grooves similar to those of papillary carcinoma of thyroid.

The hypothesis that these tumours are of Müllerian origin has been abandoned since the tumour cells are strongly positive for PSA and PSAP, in both primary and metastatic sites. However, there are differences between ductal and acinar adenocarcinomas in the 34βE12 and AMACR immunoprofiles.

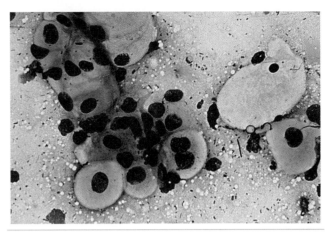

**Fig. 19.13** Hormonal effects. Case of adenocarcinoma showing good response clinically. Note glycogenisation and squamous metaplasia and absence of clearly malignant cells (MGG).

34βE12 is absent in acinar adenocarcinomas, while the presence of a few 34βE12 positive basal cells may be seen in the intraductal component of ductal adenocarcinoma. The tumour appears to arise from the larger periurethral ducts. Whether its clinical behaviour differs from that of the usual adenocarcinoma is not clear and it has been suggested this is not a separate entity but a growth pattern of typical adenocarcinoma spreading into periurethral ducts.[40]

## Mucinous adenocarcinoma

Some mucin is not uncommonly seen in prostatic adenocarcinoma. A predominantly mucinous pattern is rare. In such a case the possibility of an adenocarcinoma invading the prostate from the bowel or the bladder must be considered. The problem can be solved by immunohistochemical studies since primary mucinous carcinoma of the prostate stains positively for PSA, PSAP and P504S.

## Neuroendocrine (small cell) carcinoma

Neuroendocrine cells are not infrequently found in prostatic adenocarcinoma in variable numbers. In some cancers, a small cell anaplastic pattern is seen focally or throughout the tumour. The cells stain positively for chromogranin, synaptophysin and other neuroendocrine markers, but are negative for PSA and P504S. On the other hand, prostate carcinoma metastases may mimic small cell carcinoma.[42] Small cell carcinomas are highly malignant and do not respond to hormonal treatment. The smear pattern is similar to neuroendocrine small cell cancers at other sites. The tumour cells are partly dispersed and partly seen in tight clusters with nuclear moulding. The cytoplasm is scanty and nuclei are hyperchromatic with inconspicuous nucleoli and tend to be elongated (Fig. 19.14). Part of the tumour cell population may show the usual adenocarcinoma pattern.

## Transitional cell carcinoma

Transitional cell carcinoma (TCC) in the prostate is usually associated with a primary urinary bladder or urethral urothelial

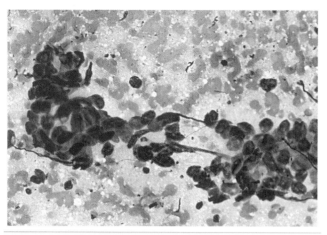

**Fig. 19.14** Small cell (neuroendocrine) carcinoma of prostate. Cluster of closely packed cells with scanty cytoplasm, ovoid hyperchromatic nuclei with some moulding; nucleoli not visible. Confirmed by TURP, staining for chromogranin positive, PSA negative (MGG).

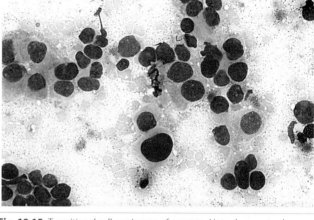

**Fig. 19.15** Transitional cell carcinoma of prostate. Note dense cytoplasm, pleomorphic hyperchromatic nuclei and lack of architectural pattern (MGG).

carcinoma and constitutes less than 3% of prostatic cancers. It is often difficult to know with certainty the primary site of origin and so prostatic urethral and periurethral prostatic ductal sites are often lumped together.[43] Prostatic urothelial carcinoma is diagnosed in the absence of urinary bladder urothelial carcinoma. Its distinction is important because treatment is different from that of adenocarcinoma. Since it is infiltrating the glandular tissue, the malignant cells are mixed with benign cells in FNA smears and may constitute only a minority of the cells.

### Cytological findings: transitional cell carcinoma

- Malignant cells single and in multilayered aggregates, no obvious microacinar pattern
- Single cells with dense (squamoid) cytoplasm and distinct cell borders
- Prominent nuclear pleomorphism and hyperchromasia
- Negative staining for PSA and PSAP.

TCC of the prostate is usually high grade and solid. The neoplastic cells are single or form irregular multilayered aggregates without obvious papillary or glandular structures. Sometimes, palisading of cells at the periphery of solid cords can give an impression of glandular groupings. Cell borders are indistinct in cell aggregates but are well defined in single cells. The cytoplasm is also denser than that of adenocarcinoma cells and may appear squamoid. Variation in nuclear size is much more prominent than that in adenocarcinoma and nuclear chromatin is also more variable; some nuclei are intensely hyperchromatic (Fig. 19.15). Immunoperoxidase staining for PSA, PSAP and p504S is helpful in difficult cases.

## Rare epithelial tumours

### Squamous cell carcinoma

Squamous cell carcinoma of the prostate is rare, forming less than 1% of prostatic cancer.[44] It may be pure squamous or mixed adenosquamous. It is highly aggressive and responds

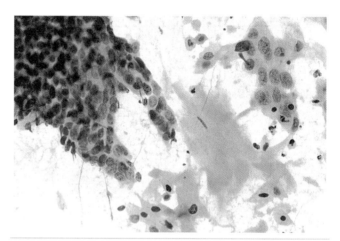

**Fig. 19.16** Squamous cell carcinoma of prostate. The fragment to the left shows no obvious squamous differentiation, to the right keratinising atypical cells (PAP).

poorly to treatment. Some patients have a history of hormonal treatment, radiotherapy or schistosomiasis. Like TCC, it arises from the bladder or urethral mucosa or from periurethral ducts. Cytological criteria are the same as for squamous carcinoma at other sites (Fig. 19.16). Squamous metaplasia, for example occurring in relation to infarcted adenomatous nodules, lacks nuclear atypia and should not cause any suspicion of malignancy.

### Adenoid cystic carcinoma

This tumour rarely occurs in the prostate. It is histologically and cytologically similar to adenoid cystic carcinoma of salivary glands and may be associated with adenocarcinoma of the usual type. PSA is negative in these tumours, which have a better prognosis than the common adenocarcinoma.

### Sarcomatoid carcinoma

Sarcomatoid carcinoma is a rare biphasic tumour in the prostate. Fewer than 60 cases have been reported in the literature.[40]

The two elements of sarcomatoid carcinoma are a malignant epithelial component and a malignant mesenchyme-like (sarcomatous) component.

## Non-epithelial neoplasms

Only embryonal rhabdomyosarcoma[45] and leiomyosarcoma (Fig. 19.17)[46] occur with some frequency, the former mainly in young patients, the latter in older patients. Malignant lymphoma, whether a manifestation of systemic disease or rarely primary, may present as a prostatic tumour. All subtypes, non-Hodgkin or Hodgkin lymphoma, may occur. Diagnostic criteria are the same as at other sites. The main differential diagnoses are small cell carcinoma of neuroendocrine type and embryonal rhabdomyosarcoma.

## The role of cytology in management of prostate cancer

The ideal method to detect prostate cancer should have a high sensitivity to significant cancers while failing to find insignificant tumours. It has been shown in patients with clinical cancer that tumour volume and histological Gleason grade are strong predictors of tumour stage and progression, and may be helpful in choice of treatment.[2] However, prostate cancer is heterogeneous and frequently multifocal and only 20% of tumours are clinically significant.[4] Most urologists prefer prostate CNB using automated biopsy devices. In recent years new automated CNB devices have been introduced, and the use of an increasing number of core needles results in an increase in the detection rate of prostate cancer.[13,47] Consequently, most pathologists who were trained after 1990 have little opportunity to examine prostate FNAs. Prostate FNAs lack the context of 'tissue patterns' that are the basis of the Gleason system, although estimated gland size in cytological smears roughly determines Gleason pattern and a sensitivity of 90–95% is achieved with either method.[8]

When applying immunocytochemistry on FNAs, a major limitation is the lack of positive controls and the frequent

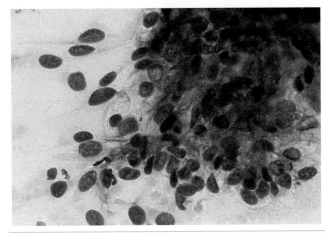

**Fig. 19.17** Leiomyosarcoma of prostate. Tissue fragment of atypical spindle cells separated by intercellular collagen. Note attenuated strands of grey (eosinophilic) cytoplasm (MGG).

background staining. To overcome this, different ancillary methods are used, such as cultured anaplastic cell lines with known immunophenotype as positive controls,[48] cell block preparation, cytospins or liquid monolayer preparation.[49] FNA material is eminently suitable for DNA analysis (Fig. 19.10), molecular studies and proteomics,[28,29] and molecular testing has recently been used with promising results.[29,32,33] Given the non-invasive nature of FNA and recent progress in molecular biology techniques, one might expect further utilisation of this biopsy material, perhaps even in targeted molecular forms of therapy of prostate cancer.[34,50,51]

Ideally FNA and CNB should not be mutually exclusive but should be applied in a selective manner. Transrectal FNA is the method of choice in patients with a palpable prostatic lesion whereas CNB is recommended by most urologists on patients with an elevated serum PSA and clinically suspicious prostatic tumour. Palpable and deep-seated metastases should preferentially be examined by FNA with ultrasound guidance, due to the non-invasive nature of the FNA procedure. As with all cytological methods, good communication between clinician, radiologist and pathologist at regular multidisciplinary team meetings is essential for achieving full benefit for the patient.

## REFERENCES

1. Perez-Guillermo M, Acosta-Ortega J, Garcia-Solano J. The continuing role of fine-needle aspiration of the prostate gland into the 21st century: a tribute to Torsten Løwhagen. Diagn Cytopathol 2005;32:315–20.

2. al-Abadi H. Fine needle aspiration biopsy vs. ultrasound-guided transrectal random core biopsy of the prostate. Comparative investigations in 264 cases. Acta Cytol 1997;41:981–86.

3. Gronberg H. Prostate cancer epidemiology. Lancet 2003;361:859–64.

4. Sakr WA, Grignon DJ, Haas GP, et al. Age and racial distribution of prostatic intraepithelial neoplasia. Eur Urol 1996;30:138–44.

5. Rietbergen J, Hoedemaeker R, Boeken Kruger A, et al. The changing pattern of PC at the time of diagnosis: characteristics of screen detected PC in a population based screening study. J Urol 1999;161:1192–98.

6. Bratt O. Hereditary prostate cancer: clinical aspects. J Urol 2002;168:906–13.

7. Otto SJ, De Koning HJ. Update on screening and early detection of prostate cancer. Curr Opin Urol 2004;14:151–56.

8. Maksem JA, Berner A, Bedrossian C. Fine needle aspiration biopsy of the prostate gland. Diagn Cytopathol 2007;35:778–85.

9. al-Abadi H. Fine needle aspiration biopsy vs. ultrasound-guided transrectal random core biopsy of the prostate. Comparative

investigation in 246 cases. Acta Cytol 1997;41:981–86.

10. Dearnaley DP, Kirby RS, Malone P, et al. Diagnosis and management of early prostatic cancer. Report of a British Association of Urological Surgeons Working Party. BJU Int 1999;83:18–33.

11. Vaghefi H, Magi-Galluzzi C, Klein EA. Local recurrence of prostate cancer in rectal submucosa after transrectal needle biopsy and radical prostatectomy. Urology 2005;66:881–82.

12. Hautmann SH, Conrad S, et al. Detection rate of histologically insignificant prostate cancer with systematic sextant biopsies and fine needle aspiration cytology. J Urol 2000;163:1734–38.

13. Guichard G, Larre S, Gallina A, et al. Extended 21-sample needle biopsy protocol for diagnosis of prostate cancer in 1000 consecutive patients. Eur Urol 2007;52:430–35.

14. Stamatiou K, Alevizos A, Karanasiou V, et al. Impact of additional sampling in the TRUS-guided biopsy for the diagnosis of prostate cancer. Urol Int 2007;78:313–17.

15. Deliveliotis C, Stauropoulos NJ, Macrychoritis C, et al. Transrectal needle aspiration verusus transperineal needle biopsy in diagnosis of prostate carcinoma. Int Urol Nephrol 1995;27:173–77.

16. Bøcking A. Cytopathology of the prostate. Patologe 1998;19:53–58.

17. Lee G, Attar K, Laniado M, et al. Safety and detailed patterns of morbidity of transrectal ultrasound guided needle biopsy of prostate in a urologist-led unit. Int Urol Nephrol 2006;38:281–85.

18. Hammerich KH, Ayala GE, Wheeler TM. Application of immunohistochemistry to the genitourinary system (prostate, urinary bladder, testis, and kidney). Arch Pathol Lab Med 2008;132:432–40.

19. Humprey PA. Diagnosis of adenocarcinoma in prostate needle biopsy tissue. J Clin Pathol 2007;60:35–42.

20. Beach R, Gown AM, De Peralta-Venturina MN, et al. P504S immunohistochemical detection in 405 prostatic specimens including 376 18-gauge needle biopsies. Am J Surg Pathol 2002;26:1588–96.

21. Murphy WM. Urological Pathology. Philadelphia: Saunders; 1989.

22. Howell LP, Arnott TR, de Vere-White R. Aspiration biopsy cytology of the prostate in young adult men. Diagn Cytopathol 1990;6:89–94.

23. Herawi M, Epstein JI. Immunohistochemical antibody cocktail staining (p63/HMWCK/AMACR) of ductal adenocarcinoma and Gleason pattern 4 cribriform and noncribriform acinar adenocarcinomas of the prostate. Am J Surg Pathol 2007;31:889–94.

24. Reyes CV, Thompson KS, Jensen JD, et al. Metastasis of unknown origin: the role of fine-needle aspiration cytology. Diagn Cytopathol 1998;18:319–22.

25. Esposti PL. Cytologic malignancy grading of prostatic carcinoma by transrectal aspiration biopsy. Scand J Urol Nephrol 1971;5:119–209.

26. Humprey PA. Gleason grading and prognostic factors in carcinoma of the prostate. Mod Pathol 2004;17:292–306.

27. Willems JS, Löwhagen T. Transrectal fine needle aspiration biopsy for cytologic diagnosis and grading of prostatic carcinoma. Prostate 1981;2:381–95.

28. Rapkiewicz A, Espina V, Zujewski JA, et al. The needle in the haystack: application of breast fine-needle aspirate samples to quantitative protein microarray technology. Cancer 2007;25:173–84.

29. DeMarzo AM, Nelson WG, Isaacs WB, et al. Pathological and molecular aspects of prostate cancer. Lancet 2003;361:955–64.

30. Azua J, Romeo P, Valle J, et al. Cytologic differentiation grade and malignancy DNA index in prostatic adenocarcinoma. Anal Quant Cytol Histol 1997;19:102–6.

31. Ahlgren G, Falkmer U, Gadaleanu V, et al. Evaluation of DNA ploidy combined with a cytometric proliferation index of imprints from core needle biopsies in prostate cancer. Eur Urol 1999;36:314–19.

32. Halvorsen OJ, Oyan AM, Bo TH, et al. Gene expression profiles in prostate cancer: association with patient subgroups and tumor differentiation. Int J Oncol 2005;26:329–36.

33. Halvorsen OJ, Rostad K, Oyan AM, et al. Increased expression of SIM2s protein is a novel marker for aggressive prostate cancer. Clin Cancer Res 2007;13:892–97.

34. Berg A, Berner A, Lilleby W, et al. Impact of disseminated tumor cells in bone marrow at diagnosis in patients with nonmetastatic prostate cancer treated by definitive radiotherapy. Int J Cancer 2007;120:1603–9.

35. Perez-Guillermo M, Acosta-Ortega J, Garcia-Solano J. Pitfalls and infrequent findings in fine-needle aspiration of the prostate gland. Diagn Cytopathol 2005;33:126–37.

36. Roznovanu SL, Radulescu D, Novac C, et al. The morphological changes induced by hormone and radiation therapy on prostate carcinoma. Rev Med Chir Soc Med Nat Iasi 2005;109:337–42.

37. Tomic R, Angstrom T, Ljungberg B. Cellular changes in prostatic carcinoma after treatment with orchidectomy, estramustine phosphate and medroxyprogesterone acetate. Scand J Urol Nephrol 1997;31:255–58.

38. Goldstein NS, Martinez A, Vicini F, et al. The histology of radiation therapy effect on prostate adenocarcinoma as assessed by needle biopsy after brachytherapy boost. Am J Clin Pathol 1998;110:765–75.

39. Humphrey PA. Prostate Pathology Chs 17, 18. Chicago: ASCP Press; 2003 354–390.

40. Young RH, Srigley JR, Amin MB, et al. Tumors of the Prostate Gland, Seminal Vesicles, Male Urethra, and Penis, Third series, Chs 5, 6, Fascicle 28. Washington DC: Armed Forces Institute of Pathology; 2000 217–288.

41. Bock BJ, Bostwick DG. Does prostatic ductal adenocarcinoma exist? Am J Surg Pathol 1999;23:781–85.

42. Parwani AV, Ali SZ. Prostatic adenocarcinoma metastases mimicking small cell carcinoma on fine-needle aspiration. Diagn Cytopathol 2002;27:75–79.

43. Greene FL, Page DL, Fleming ID, et al. Urethra. In: AJCC, editors. Cancer Staging Manual, 6th edn. New York: Springer Verlag; 2002: 341–343.

44. Parwani AV, Kronz JD, Genega EM, et al. Prostate carcinoma with squamous differentiation: an analysis of 33 cases. Am J Surg Pathol 2004;149:137–39.

45. Moroz K, Crespo P, de las Morenas A. Fine needle aspiration of prostatic rhabdomyosarcoma. A case report demonstrating the value of DNA ploidy. Acta Cytol 1995;39:785–90.

46. Cookingham CL, Kumen NB. Diagnosis of prostatic leiomyosarcoma with fine needle aspiration cytology. Acta Cytol 1985;29:170–73.

47. Hautmann SH, Conrad S, Henke RP, et al. Detection rate of histologically insignificant prostate cancer with systematic sextant biopsies and fine needle aspiration cytology. J Urol 2000;163:1734–38.

48. Wiatrowska BA, Berner A, Torlakovic G, et al. Cultured anaplastic cell lines as immunocytochemistry controls: a comparison of ThinPrep-processed smears and conventional air-dried cytospins. Diagn Cytopathol 2001;25:303–8.

49. Munoz de Toro M, Maffini MV, Giardina RH, et al. Processing fine needle aspirates of prostate carcinomas for standard immunocytochemical studies and in situ apoptosis detection. Pathol Res Pract 1998;194:631–36.

50. Luo J, Isaacs WB, Trent JM, et al. Looking beyond morphology: cancer gene expression profiling using DNA microarrays. Cancer Invest 2003;21:937–49.

51. Bucca G, Carruba G, Saetta A, et al. Gene expression profiling of human cancers. Ann NY Acad Sci 2004;1028:28–37.

# Testis and scrotum: cytology of testicular and scrotal masses and male infertility

Ika Kardum-Skelin and Paul J. Turek

## Chapter contents

## Introduction

Enlargement of the male external genitalia implies any one of various events within and around the scrotum, while the testes themselves may or may not be enlarged. The condition occurs in all age groups, is usually associated with pain, as with haematocele after surgical procedures, testicular torsion and similar events and may be accompanied by other local or general symptoms. A number of causes may lead to either unilateral or bilateral scrotal enlargement. Any testicular enlargement, oedema or pain requires a thorough diagnostic work-up to exclude the possibility of carcinoma of the testis.

## Diagnostic work-up of testicular and scrotal masses

### Inspection and palpation

The appearance, size and symmetry of the scrotum and contents are determined by inspection. This may reveal the hypoplastic appearance of an undescended testicle. Consistency of the scrotum is determined by palpation: a 'bag of worms' sensation signifies a varicocele and when the patient assumes a supine position, venous blood flows out, thus reducing the swelling; palpable enlargement caused by a testicular mass; the findings typical of torsion of the spermatic cord, or the 'blue dot' sign, which indicates torsion of the appendix testis or appendix of epididymis.[1]

### Transillumination

Transillumination is performed in a dark room using a light source. If the light passes through the scrotum, it is very probably filled with fluid. Unlike spermatocele and hydrocele both of which can generally be transilluminated, light passage through a haematocele is not possible due to the dark colour of the blood.

## Ultrasound

Ultrasound is a proven and safe diagnostic procedure. Ultrasound showed 100% accuracy in the evaluation of hydroceles, haematoceles and paratesticular masses, but was less informative in testicular abscesses (80%) and epididymo-orchitis (77%).[2] Ultrasound was able to distinguish accurately between the normal and a pathological scrotum. Extratesticular lesions were readily differentiated from testicular lesions. Abnormal testicular echo patterns were usually associated with tumours, whereas orchitis, granulomas and haematomas were found to have a similar appearance. Ultrasound may also be useful in post-orchiectomy follow-up examinations to exclude tumour in the contralateral testis.[3]

Advances in ultrasound technology in recent years have made ultrasound the examination of choice for imaging scrotal pathology, whether acute or chronic in nature. Doppler technology has increased the radiologist's ability to assess flow within the prepubertal testicle, thus allowing for assessment of viability in the undescended testis as well as in neonatal torsion. Ultrasound is a readily available, non-invasive examination without radiation exposure, which provides excellent anatomical detail and serves as an important and very helpful imaging modality in all types of paediatric scrotal pathology.[4]

## Fine needle aspiration cytology

Fine needle aspiration (FNA) of the testis and scrotum is a simple, rapid, minimally invasive and painless out-patient procedure. The sample obtained is more representative than biopsy as several separate punctures can be made, and there is no local scarring.[5] FNA has become increasingly popular for evaluating both superficial and deep-seated lesions.[6] Testicular FNA offers valuable prognostic parameters in selected patients with varicocele scheduled for sclerotherapy.[7] The cytopathological pattern of neoplasia is highly characteristic, indicating the diagnosis with high precision. FNA is the technique of choice for the study of the pathology of scrotal contents, and it should be employed on the patient's very first visit. The main advantage of FNA is avoiding delay in the diagnosis.[8] No local seeding of tumour has been observed by the FNA procedure.[9] FNA can also be a useful method to evaluate clinically suspect testicular infiltration in children with acute lymphoblastic leukaemia,

To Iva, Matko, Vlado, Ashley, Sophia and Vanessa. We would like to acknowledge the help of Professor I Crepinko and all the staff of the Laboratory of Cytology and Hematology, Merkur University Hospital in Zagreb and The Turek Clinic in San Francisco.

and can be considered as an alternative procedure to surgical biopsy for screening testicular recurrence of childhood acute lymphoblastic leukaemia.[10]

## Biopsy

Testis biopsy was first reported by Hotchkiss and Engle at the New York Hospital, Cornell Medical Center in the late 1930s. The primary purposes of testicular biopsy are to distinguish between obstructive azoospermia and primary seminiferous tubular failure and to differentiate malignant from benign testicular lesions. Until standards for the evaluation of aspirated material are well established, open testis biopsy is the diagnostic procedure of choice.[11] The procedure can be performed as core needle biopsy (CNB), testis-sparing biopsy, or open surgical biopsy. There are four main clinical scenarios when CNB testicular biopsy is performed: (1) lesions with equivocal malignant ultrasound features; (2) discrepancy between radiological and clinical findings; (3) suspected malignant process where orchiectomy is unnecessary, e.g. lymphoma; and (4) atrophic testes, where it is frequently difficult to differentiate malignancy from the heterogeneous echo pattern.[12] Testis-sparing surgery may be required if a benign lesion is considered highly likely. If frozen section analysis is equivocal, then radical orchiectomy is required. Testis-sparing surgery proved feasible in highly selected cases.[13]

## Tumour markers

Determination of tumour markers in the blood can be useful in the diagnosis of testicular tumours. Proteins secreted by particular tumours of the testis, such as alpha-fetoprotein (AFP) or beta-human chorionic gonadotrophin (β-hCG), can be demonstrated in 90% of patients with embryonal carcinoma of the testis and 10% of patients with seminoma.[14]

## Benign lesions of the scrotum

Pathological processes of the scrotum are numerous. They include a few common and well-known diseases and a large spectrum of rare lesions. The testis may also be involved by some systemic diseases (Table 20.1).[15]

Epididymal nodules are not infrequently encountered in surgical practice. These are generally small and slippery and FNA is not easy. But as it is rapid and less traumatic than a biopsy, FNA has an important role in the differential diagnosis of epididymal nodules because it can detect malignancy and benign conditions such as tuberculosis and acute and chronic epididymo-orchitis. Gupta et al. found that the lesions most commonly diagnosed by FNA were as follows: tuberculous epididymitis (30.7%), non-specific inflammation (4.4%), microfilaria (0.9%), hydrocele (11.4%), spermatocele (18.4%), spermatic granulomas (5.3%), adenomatoid tumour (1.3%), leiomyosarcoma (0.4%) and lipoma (0.4%).[16] They found FNA to be useful in the diagnosis of 90.3% of cases, thereby avoiding surgical biopsy and other investigations.

Symptoms such as a 'pulling' sensation in the testis, oedema, painful ejaculation, blood in the semen, palpable nodules, or

**Table 20.1** Conditions leading to scrotal enlargement

| Non-neoplastic disorders | Inflammation and systemic diseases | Orchitis |
| --- | --- | --- |
| | | Epididymitis |
| | | Retention lesions |
| | Cystic lesions | Hydrocele |
| | | Varicocele |
| | | Spermatocele |
| | | Haematocele |
| | Trauma and surgical procedure sequels | Torsion |
| | | Trauma |
| | | Surgical procedure of the testis |
| | | Surgical procedure in the inguinal region |
| | Hernia | |
| Testicular tumours | Germ cell tumours | Seminoma |
| | | Embryonal carcinoma |
| | | Yolk sac tumour |
| | | Teratoma |
| | | Choriocarcinoma |
| | Sex cord stromal cell tumours | Granulosa cell tumour |
| | | Sertoli cell tumour |
| | | Leydig cell tumour |
| | | Androblastoma |
| | | Gynandroblastoma |

change in the colour or structure of the scrotal skin may also occur due to a number of other benign diseases and conditions.

## Inflammatory conditions

These conditions mostly develop in association with epididymitis, although inflammation may occasionally involve only one of these organs. Inflammation can be caused by viruses or microorganisms. Specific types of inflammation, such as tuberculosis, are quite common.

### Cytological findings: inflammatory conditions

Cytological appearances depend on the cause of the inflammation. Bacterial inflammation leads to polymorphonuclear (neutrophilic granulocyte) infiltration in the acute stage of disease. Disease progression from the subacute to subchronic form is associated with accumulation of monocytes and macrophages, along with numerous degenerate acute inflammatory cells, whereas in the chronic stage there is accumulation of lymphocytes and plasma cells. Viral inflammation is characterised by mononuclear (lymphocytes and plasma cells) infiltration. In granulomatous lesions, characteristic multinucleated histiocytic cells of Langhans type and epithelioid histiocytes are found along with lymphocytic and plasma cell infiltration. Tuberculosis is the most common granulomatous lesion in the testis and epididymis, characterised by the above features and necrosis.[17]

## Spermatic granuloma

Spermatic granuloma is a granulomatous lesion that presents clinically as a nodular lesion in the region of the epididymis. There are only a few documented cases of spermatic granuloma cytology in the literature. FNA reveals mixed inflammatory cells consisting of plentiful macrophages along with lymphocytes and scattered polymorphs in a fluidy background containing many spermatozoa and sperm heads. Sperm heads are also noted within macrophages. Ill-formed to well-formed granulomas were seen in all the cases. FNA has an important role in the differential diagnosis of epididymal nodules as it can rule out malignancy and other benign cytological diagnoses like tuberculosis, acute and chronic epididymo-orchitis. Distinction of spermatic granulomas from the more common tuberculous granulomatous infection is important from the cytopathologist's point of view.[18]

## Cystic lesions

Cystic lesions include hydrocele, haematocele and spermatocele.[5] Testicular enlargement due to the accumulation of fluid, blood or seminal fluid may mimic tumour findings.

## Hydrocele and haematocele

Accumulation of fluid or blood in the scrotum occurs due to trauma, surgical procedures of the testis or inguinal region associated with compromised testicular supply with blood and/or increased vascular permeability. Any systemic disorder leading to impaired regulation of body fluid may also lead to oedema in the scrotal region. The nature of the disorder determines whether testicular enlargement will be bilateral (e.g. heart failure, liver decompensation, anasarca), or unilateral.

### Cytological findings: hydrocele and haematocele

In hydrocele cases, fluid is obtained by cytological puncture, yielding scant cellularity in the sediment, consisting of some mesothelial cells and lymphocytes (Fig. 20.1A). In addition to previously described cellular elements, polymorphonuclear granulocytes, typical and reactive mesothelial cells, histiocytes and cellular detritus are found in persistent hydroceles. Microbiological cultures are sterile. In haematocele, the specimen contains blood and/or phagocytosed erythrocytes and siderophages, depending on the duration of haematocele (Fig. 20.1B).

## Spermatocele

A cystic growth in the epididymal region occurs due to seminal duct distension caused by inflammation or some other disorder (obstruction by adhesions, tumour, etc.), and is mostly painless (Fig. 20.1C).

### Cytological findings: spermatocele

Milky fluid is obtained by puncture, and spermatozoa lacking motility are found in the smear. Histiocytes and epididymal lining cells are found in persistent spermatoceles.[5]

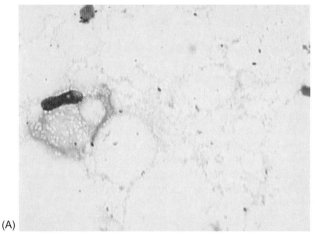

(A)

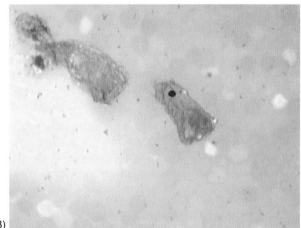

(B)

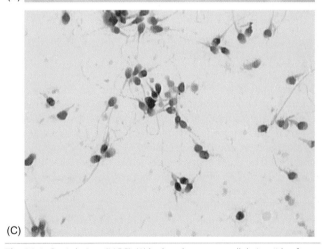

(C)

**Fig. 20.1** Cystic lesions (MGG): (A) hydrocele – sparse cellularity with a few histiocytes and erythrocytes; (B) haematocele – note the background of erythrocytes and fibrin; (C) spermatocele with numerous spermatozoids.

## Varicocele

Varicocele occurs due to varicosity of the vascular plexus conveying venous blood from the testis. The condition develops as a consequence of pressure upon outflow veins, for example by a kidney tumour. The cause, however, usually remains unknown, and it has not yet clear why it more frequently occurs on the left side. On palpation, the scrotum feels like a 'bag of worms'. The diagnosis is generally made by ultrasound, while cytological puncture is not indicated.

## Epidermal cysts

Epidermal cysts are located intradermally; they can be small yet they may cause great enlargement of the scrotum.

### Cytological findings: epidermal cysts

Similar to the samples obtained at other locations, cytological samples contain squames and superficial squamous epithelial cells. These growths are very susceptible to infection, therefore numerous neutrophilic granulocytes are observed in addition to the previously mentioned cell types. Histiocytic cells and a variable number of lymphocytes and plasma cells can also be found in subacute or subchronic states, depending on the duration of the lesion.

## Hernia

This disorder is characterised by impaired communication between the abdominal cavity and scrotum, when a segment of the omentum or intestine slips into the scrotal sac. History data reveal the enlargement to be more pronounced on standing, coughing, carrying heavy objects, or with strain on examination.

### Cytological findings: hernia

Cytological puncture is not indicated in unambiguous cases. However, when cytological puncture is performed in unrecognised cases, besides adipose tissue elements the samples contain mesothelial cells or intestinal epithelium, and occasionally even intestinal content (faeces or microbiological intestinal flora).

## Tumours of the testis

The histopathology of testicular tumours, emphasising new, unusual, or underemphasised aspects is presented in an excellent review by Young.[19] Because of the good prognosis for some testicular tumours and early detection of the disease, any scrotal enlargement should be considered a tumour until proved otherwise. The pathogenesis of testicular tumours is unknown. A higher incidence of testicular tumours has been reported in patients with cryptorchidism or Klinefelter's syndrome, as a post-traumatic condition or based on a positive family history. In spite of numerous studies demonstrating the usefulness of FNA cytology in the diagnosis of testicular enlargement, both for differentiation between non-neoplastic and malignant tumours and for tumour typing, there remains a dose of scepticism among urologists as to whether to approach a primary tumour by FNA or orchiectomy followed by histopathology. However, the wisdom of removing the testis for what may turn out to be a benign lesion has to be questioned. Therefore, FNA testis as a minimally invasive procedure should be the first diagnostic method following imaging techniques (mostly ultrasound, and less frequently computed tomography or magnetic resonance imaging).

Tumours of the germinal epithelium account for 95% of all malignant tumours of the testis; sex cord stromal tumours are very rare, generally are Sertoli cell or Leydig cell tumours, and are usually benign.

## Germ cell tumours

Testicular carcinoma is a rare malignant tumour, mainly affecting the 15–40 age group. It is a serious malignancy as it affects boys and young men. Tumours of the germinal epithelium include seminoma, embryonal carcinoma, yolk sac tumour and choriocarcinoma. The tumours may be mixed and only one component may be present in an FNA sample.

### Seminoma

Seminomas, along with ovarian dysgerminoma and other germinomas of extragonadal sites are classified in the group of germinomas. Seminoma is the most common tumour type in dysgenetic gonads and retained testis.[20] Histologically, it is classified as typical, anaplastic or spermatocytic seminoma.

### Cytological findings: seminoma

- Discohesive tumour cells
- Well-defined, vacuolated cytoplasm
- Prominent nucleolus
- Background lymphocytes
- 'Tigroid' background in some cases.

The cytological picture depends on the histological type of seminoma. Seminoma cells are found isolated (atypical seminoma), isolated or in loose clusters (typical seminoma), or arranged in clusters as in an adenocarcinoma in spermatocytic seminoma. Typical seminoma cells are larger than lymphoid cells, with spherical or oval nuclei, finely granulated chromatin with multiple tiny nucleoli, and basophilic, frequently vacuolated cytoplasm. Atypical seminoma is characterised by cellular pleomorphism, pronounced anisonucleosis and coarsely granular, unevenly distributed chromatin. In spermatocytic seminoma, cells are mostly of medium size and mononuclear; however, binucleated forms may also be found. Besides seminoma cells, lymphocytes and granulomatous reaction with epithelioid cells, and occasionally multinucleated giant cells may be found in typical seminoma, and some lymphoid cells are seen in atypical seminoma. In spermatocytic seminoma, cytological smears are clear, free from lymphoid cells and granulomatous reaction. Seminoma cells are positive for placental alkaline phosphatase (PLAP), and occasionally for CD30. Positivity for $\beta$-hCG can be recorded in case of differentiation from choriocarcinoma, and for AFP in the presence of embryonal carcinoma components (Fig. 20.2).

### Embryonal carcinoma

Embryonal carcinoma is a highly malignant tumour, occurring frequently in association with other tumours of the germinal epithelium.[21]

### Cytological findings: embryonal carcinoma

Unlike seminoma, where cells are mostly individually distributed (except for in the spermatocytic form), in embryonal carcinoma, cells are more frequently found in loose clusters varying in size, sometimes in papillary or glandular configuration. Cell pleomorphism is observed, with large

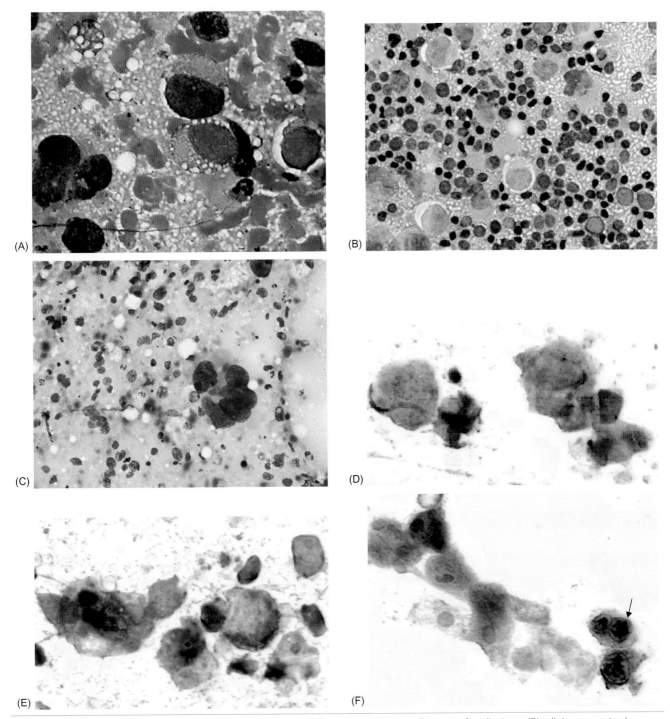

**Fig. 20.2** Seminoma: (A) typical seminoma cells; (B) 'tigroid' background of seminoma; (C) germ cell tumour of mediastinum; (D) cells immunostained for placental alkaline phosphatase (PLAP); (E) cells immunostained for CD30; (F) seminoma cells negative for leucocyte common antigen (LCA) (leucocyte immunostained – arrow).

vesicular nuclei and irregular nucleoli. The cytoplasm is pale and basophilic, but usually poorly preserved. Cells are positive for CD30, PLAP and AFP (Fig. 20.3).

## Teratoma

Teratoma is composed of all three germ layers. Macroscopically, teratoma can be solid or cystic, and microscopically mature or immature, depending on the presence of well-differentiated

tissues such as brain, skin, bone, etc., or of an embryonic component along with mature tissue elements.

### Cytological findings: teratoma

The cytological picture depends on the type of tissue found in the tumour. An epithelial, fibroblastic or cartilaginous component is most frequently present. Teratoma is quite frequently associated with seminoma, embryonal carcinoma or choriocarcinoma.

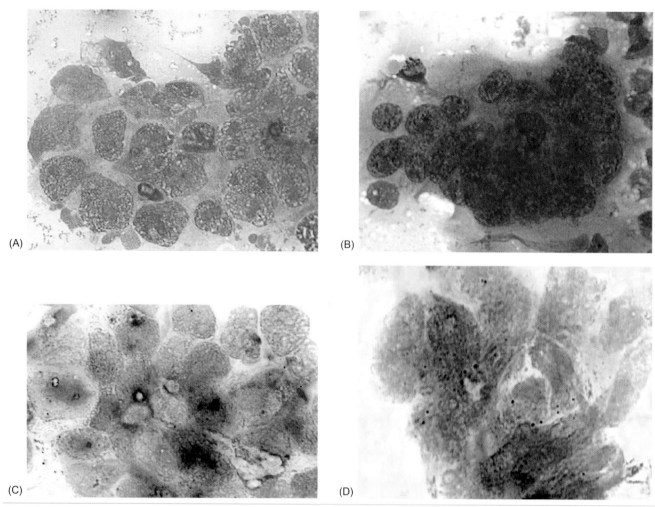

**Fig. 20.3** Embryonal anaplastic carcinoma: (A) MGG stain; (B) trophoblastic component (MGG); (C) anaplastic cells positive for placental alkaline phosphatase (PLAP); (D) cells positive for CD30.

## Yolk sac tumour

Yolk sac tumour is the most common tumour of germinal epithelium in children, although accounting for only 1% of all malignant tumours of the testis. It occurs as a testicular tumour or at some extragonadal localisation.

### Cytological findings: yolk sac tumour

- Papillary fragments of tumour cells
- Metachromatic basement membrane-like material in the fragments.

In yolk sac tumour, there are clusters of large cells resembling adenocarcinoma, which on immunocytochemistry are positive for AFP and have PAS positive diastase-resistant cytoplasmic staining. Hyaline globules contain ferritin and possibly some $\alpha_1$-antitrypsin (Fig. 20.4).[22]

## Sex cord stromal tumours

Sex cord stromal tumours develop from the gonadal stroma and are a type of testicular or ovarian tumour. They account for 5% of all testicular neoplasms. Sex cord stromal tumours, which arise from the supporting tissues of the testis, include granulosa,

Leydig and Sertoli cell tumours, androblastoma (Sertoli and Leydig cells) and gynandroblastoma (granulosa and Sertoli cells).

### Cytological findings: sex cord stromal tumours

Leydig cell tumours yield highly cellular aspirates of isolated cells with a granular background of cytoplasmic material. The nuclei are naked and round, with marked variability in size, and with one to three nucleoli. Chromatin is finely granular and well distributed. Leydig cell tumour cells show abundant grey-blue cytoplasm with spherical or oval nuclei in May–Grünwald Giemsa-stained smears. In FNA cytology, it may occasionally show numerous intranuclear and intracytoplasmic Reinke's crystals, some of them found in-between the cells.[23,24]

In tumours of Sertoli cell origin, FNA smears show large polygonal tumour cells with abundant, finely granular or vacuolated eosinophilic cytoplasm and eccentric nuclei with one distinct nucleolus. A variable amount of amorphous calcification is described as a constant feature.[25] Malignant Sertoli cell tumours of the testis are extremely rare. The aspirate shows tissue fragments and isolated discohesive tumour cells with characteristic testicular Sertoli cells.[26]

Testicular granulosa cell tumours are rare gonadal stromal tumours showing single or cohesive groups of vimentin,

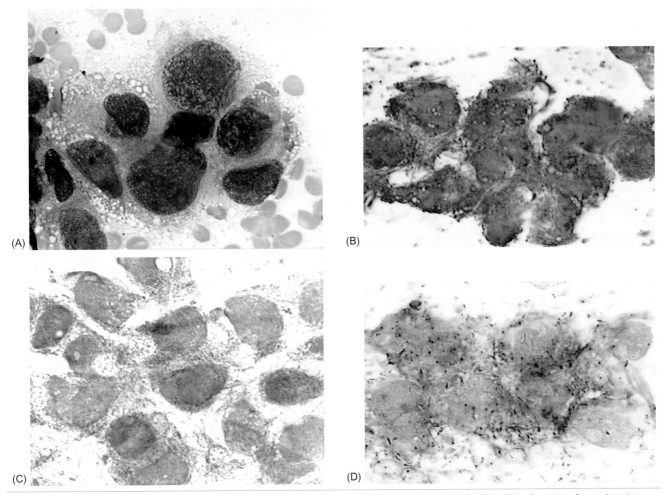

**Fig. 20.4** Yolk sac tumour: (A) MGG stain; (B) strong cell positivity for alpha-fetoprotein (AFP); (C) cells negative for CD30; (D) cells positive for cytokeratin.

α-inhibin and S-100 positive spindle cells with regular nuclei, fine chromatin and inconspicuous nucleoli.[27] Typically, neoplastic cells have oval nuclei with a longitudinal groove, giving a 'coffee bean' appearance. On immunohistochemistry, there is strong staining for vimentin, variable results for cytokeratin, and a negative reaction for epithelial membrane antigen. Oestrogen and progesterone receptors can also be helpful in the diagnosis because they are expressed in this neoplasm. Immunostaining with the Müllerian inhibiting substance can be useful for distinguishing between granulosa and Leydig cell tumours.[28]

## Other primary and secondary tumours of the testis

Primary non-Hodgkin lymphoma of the testis (PTL) accounts for 9% of testicular neoplasms and 1–2% of all non-Hodgkin lymphomas. It is the most common testicular malignancy in elderly men. An association of PTL with trauma, chronic orchitis, cryptorchidism and filariasis has been reported; however, there are no case-control studies confirming the aetiological role of these conditions. Diffuse large B-cell lymphoma (DLBCL) is the most common histotype in primary forms (Fig. 20.5); aggressive histological types, especially Burkitt's lymphoma, are prevalent

in cases of secondary involvement of the testis.[29] Besides PTL, the testis may also be involved in leukaemias, mostly in acute lymphoblastic leukaemia of childhood, when testicular involvement may be found at the time of the first diagnosis or during clinical relapses after treatment (Fig. 20.6A,B).[30] Cases of testicular granulocytic sarcoma (Fig. 20.6C,D) as a form of relapse in a patient with acute megakaryoblastic leukaemia (Fig. 20.6E, F),[31] and of acute myeloid leukaemia relapse as isolated bilateral testicular granulocytic sarcoma[32] have also been described.

## Epididymal tumours

Adenomatoid tumour is a benign tumour, probably of mesothelial origin, which shows a typical cytological picture with isolated cells, and nests and sheets of cells. The cells without atypia have eccentric nuclei, inconspicuous nucleoli and well-defined, clear and vacuolated cytoplasm.[33]

## Testicular cytology for infertility

The clinical investigation of male infertility or scrotal masses often involves the use of cytopathology. Male infertility occurs

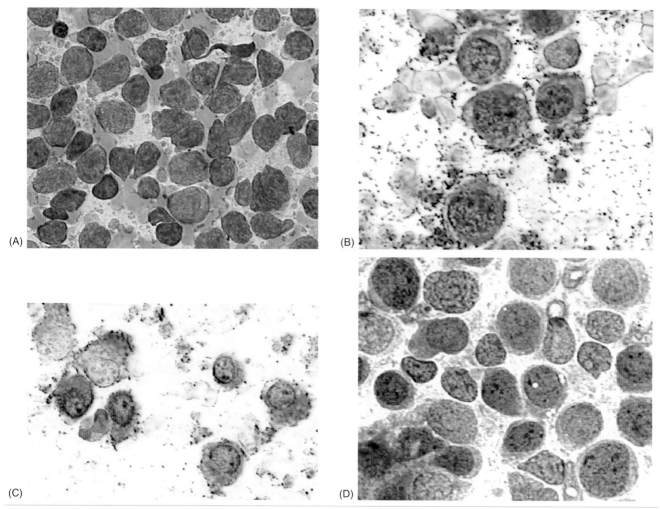

**Fig. 20.5** Diffuse large B-cell lymphoma: (A) MGG stain; (B) cells positive for CD20; (C) cells positive for CD30; (D) cells negative for CD3.

in 10–15% of reproductive age couples worldwide and in approximately 5% of affected couples, the infertility is due to a lack of sperm in the ejaculate, termed azoospermia. Testicular cytopathology plays a significant role in the expert evaluation of this diagnosis in the same way that cytopathology can provide accurate diagnoses for many testicular and scrotal masses with their myriad causes, both benign and malignant.

## History of testis cytology for infertility

FNA cytology has been used to examine pathological human tissue from various organs for over 100 years.[34] As an alternative to open testicular biopsy, for the last 40 years, it has helped to characterise states of human male infertility due to defective spermatogenesis.[35] Although recognised as a reliable and informative technique,[36,37] testis FNA has not been widely used to evaluate male infertility. Recently, however, testicular FNA has gained popularity as both a diagnostic and therapeutic tool for the management of clinical male infertility for several reasons:

- The testis is an ideal organ for evaluation by FNA because of its uniform cellularity and easy accessibility

- The trend toward minimally invasive procedures and cost-containment favours FNA compared to surgical testis biopsy
- The realisation that the specific histological abnormality observed on testis biopsy has no definite correlation to either the aetiology of infertility or to the ability to find sperm for assisted reproduction
- Assisted reproduction has undergone dramatic advances such that testis sperm are routinely used for biological pregnancies, thus fueling the development of novel FNA techniques to both locate and procure sperm.

For these reasons, there has been a resurgence of FNA as an important, minimally invasive tool for the evaluation and management of male infertility.

## How has infertility medicine changed?

Advances in assisted reproductive technology (ART) have revolutionised the ability to help men with even the severest forms of male infertility to become fathers. This field began in earnest in 1978 when the first successful *in vitro* fertilisation (IVF) cycle was performed (Fig. 20.7). This technique involves controlled ovarian stimulation followed by egg retrieval, *in vitro*

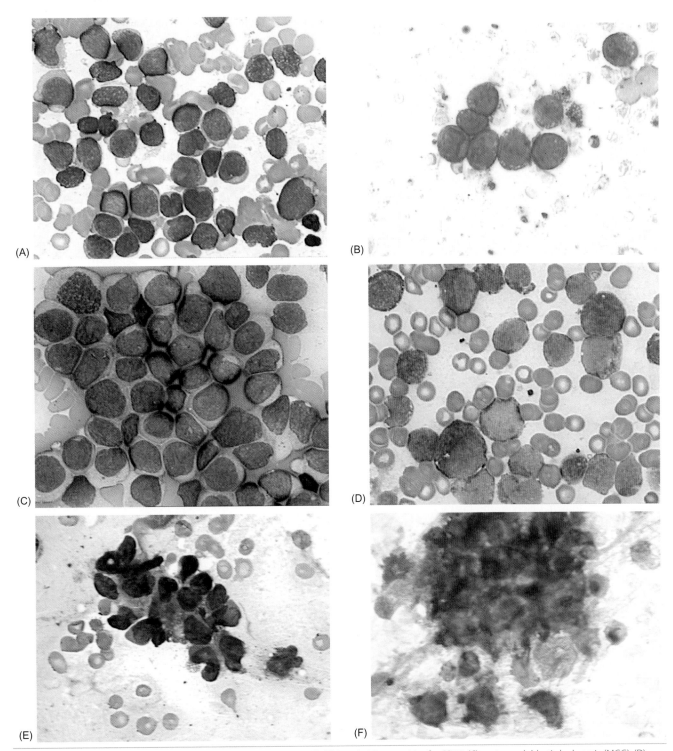

**Fig. 20.6** Relapse of acute leukaemia: (A) lymphoblastic leukaemia (MGG); (B) lymphoblasts positive for CD10; (C) acute myeloblastic leukaemia (MGG); (D) myeloperoxidase positive blasts; (E) acute megakaryoblastic leukaemia (MGG); (F) megakaryoblasts positive for CD61.

fertilisation and embryo transfer to the uterus. In the USA, the number of babies born to infertile couples with IVF has risen logarithmically from 260 babies in 1985 to almost 50 000 in 2003. Another significant advance in ART was the development of intracytoplasmic sperm injection (ICSI) in 1992.[38] Performed in conjunction with IVF, ICSI involves the injection of a single viable sperm directly into the egg cytoplasm *in vitro* to facilitate fertilisation in cases of low sperm numbers (Fig. 20.7). ICSI has

decreased the numerical sperm requirement for egg fertilisation from hundreds of thousands of sperm for each egg with IVF to a single sperm. In addition, ICSI allows sperm with limited intrinsic fertilising capacity to fertilise eggs reliably, including 'immature' sperm obtained from the reproductive tract of men with no sperm in the ejaculate. Indeed, ICSI has become so popular that more than 56% of IVF cases performed in US clinics routinely use it.

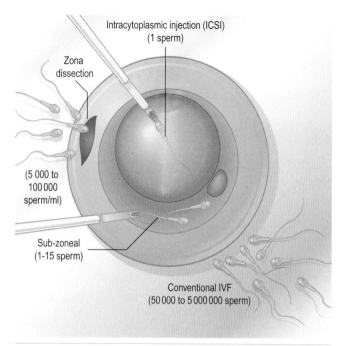

Intracytoplasmic injection (ICSI)
(1 sperm)

Zona
dissection

(5 000 to
100 000
sperm/ml)

Sub-zoneal
(1-15 sperm)

Conventional IVF
(50 000 to 5 000 000 sperm)

**Fig. 20.7** Evolution of *in vitro* fertilisation (IVF) and adjunctive micromanipulation methods. Among the techniques illustrated, IVF and intracytoplasmic sperm injection (ICSI) are currently the most commonly used.

germ cell types that is very detailed and relatively laborious for routine clinical use.

Regardless of the methodology, the analysis of testis biopsy histology lacks clinical value in cases of infertility because there is no clear correlation between histological patterns or Johnsen score and the underlying aetiology of infertility. That is to say, the clinical utility of understanding the histological pattern is low, because biopsy patterns do not correlate well with specific and correctable diseases. In addition, the interobserver variability in testis biopsy readings for infertility is significant. This was aptly demonstrated in a study by Cooperberg et al. in which the histology readings from two independent pathological reviews were prospectively compared from 113 testis biopsies undertaken for infertility.[44] Importantly, in 28% of cases preparation artifact or insufficient biopsy size rendered the sample suboptimal for interpretation. In addition, in 46% of cases, the two reviews disagreed and this discordance resulted in significant changes in clinical care in 27% of cases. The most common error in pathological review was the under-appreciation of mixed histological patterns that are common and characteristic of infertile men with no sperm counts. Thus, although commonly used to evaluate male infertility, the classical testis biopsy has little or no correlation with specific diseases, is associated with significant variability in interpretation and can miss mixed patterns of spermatogenesis that may qualify infertile men for assisted reproduction.

## How does FNA cytology compare with testis histology for infertility?

In many countries, testicular FNA cytology is preferable to surgical biopsy for the evaluation of male infertility. In addition to accurately demonstrating the presence or absence of sperm and mature sperm with tails, FNA provides tubular cells for cytological analysis, also informative for the diagnosis in infertility. Unlike testis biopsy histology, however, FNA cytology has not been rigorously evaluated for the ability to distinguish *in situ* neoplasia and testicular cancer. Despite this caveat, the correlation of FNA cytology to testis biopsy histology is very high (84–97%) in comparative studies comprising almost 400 patients (Table 20.2).

Similar to the issue with biopsy histology, although several excellent descriptions of testis seminiferous epithelium cytology have been reported, no individual classification method has been uniformly adopted by cytologists as a standard approach. Papic et al. quantified each cell type and calculated various cell indices and ratios and found that cytological smears correlated well with histological diagnoses.[45] Verma et al. also determined differential cell counts in patients with normal spermatogenesis; however, the reported ratios differ dramatically differed from those of Papic.[46] Batra et al. have also published a cytological schema in which the spermatic index, Sertoli cell index, and sperm-Sertoli cell indices are categorised into various histological groups.[47] Using this system, they reported that differences in cell counts and indices could predict histological categories. Among the different classification systems for testis FNA, those that attempt to correlate cytological findings with biopsy histology hold the most promise to replace histology.

With the goal of replacing the more invasive biopsy histology with FNA cytology, we also developed a simple working classification schema for testis FNA cytology that is based on pattern recognition.[48] The identified patterns represent histological diagnoses but are based on relative numbers of three

The success of ICSI has also encouraged reproductive clinicians to look beyond the ejaculate and into the male reproductive tract to find sperm. Currently, sources of sperm routinely used for ICSI include sperm from the vas deferens, epididymis and testicle. Interestingly, as ART has evolved, so too have novel FNA techniques to help diagnose and treat severe male infertility. An example of this is the use of testicular FNA 'mapping' to systemically assess and localise sperm for ART in men with azoospermia (no sperm count) and testis failure characteristically associated with 'patchy' or 'focal' spermatogenesis.[39] Indeed, this combination of techniques has allowed men with even the severest forms of infertility, including men who are azoospermic after chemotherapy for cancer, to become fathers.[40]

## How accurate is testis biopsy for infertility?

From a contemporary search of the English literature, it is apparent that diagnostic testicular biopsy has been used to study the pathological basis of male infertility for 60 years.[41] The surgical biopsy accurately describes the testicular architecture and is the best technique for detecting *in situ* neoplasia or cancer. It also allows the overall assessment of the interstitium (Leydig cell number and hypertrophy). Levin described a qualitative method of assessing testicular histological patterns that is commonly used clinically to assess testis pathology in male infertility. Recognised patterns include: normal spermatogenesis, hypoplasia or hypospermatogenesis, complete or early maturation arrest Sertoli cell-only or germ cell aplasia, incomplete or late maturation arrest and sclerosis.[42] Johnsen proposed a more quantitative analysis of testis cellular architecture based on the concept that testicular damage causes a successive disappearance of the most mature germ cell type.[43] The Johnsen scoring system involves a quantitative assessment of individual

**Table 20.2** Literature that correlates testicular FNA cytology to biopsy histology

| Study | Patients (*n*) | Agreement (%) |
|---|---|---|
| Persson et al. 1971[58] | 42 | 86 |
| Gottschalk-Sabag et al. 1993[36] | 47 | 87 |
| Mallidis and Gordon Baker 1994[37] | 46 | 94 |
| Craft et al. 1997[59] | 19 | 84 |
| Odabas et al. 1997[60] | 24 | 90 |
| Mahajan et al. 1999[61] | 60 | 97 |
| Rammou-Kinia et al. 1999[62] | 30 | 87 |
| Meng et al. 2000[55] | 87 | 94 |
| Qublan et al. 2002[63] | 34 | 96 |
| Arïdo an et al. 2003[64] | 40 | 90 |
| Mehrotra and Chaurasia 2008[65] | 58 | 94 |

easily identified germ cell types on cytological assessment: primary spermatocytes, spermatids and spermatozoa. The various germ and Sertoli cells are not precisely counted but are loosely quantified by assessing the relative number of cells present. For example, with normal spermatogenesis, 10–20 sperm are visualised per high power cytological field. Figure 20.8A shows the FNA cellular pattern in normal spermatogenesis, in which the numbers of primary spermatocytes, round spermatids, and spermatozoa are normalised to one. This does not imply that there are equal cell numbers of each of these cell types, but represents a standard ratio of cell types for comparison with other FNA categories. The FNA patterns for hypospermatogenesis (Fig. 20.8B), Sertoli cell-only (Fig. 20.8C), early maturation arrest (Fig. 20.8D) and late maturation arrest (Fig. 20.8E) show different ratios of these three cell types relative to normal spermatogenesis and are relatively easy to categorise in this way. An example of a normal testis biopsy with a paired cytology from the same normal testis is given in Figure 20.9A and paired histology and cytology from a case of hypospermatogenesis is given in Figure 20.9B. In a review of 87 patients with paired FNA maps and biopsy, we observed this cytological classification to be reproducible and accurate. Histological categories determined by FNA patterns correlated well with open biopsy histology across all patterns in 94% of cases.[48] FNA cytology was also able to describe completely the mixed histologies of 12 out of 14 cases. Thus, the determination of histology by FNA cytology pattern is accurate and suggests that the more invasive testicular biopsy is unnecessary for diagnosing states of infertility. Alternatively, it is possible that newer processing methods can be applied to testis FNA cytology specimens to concentrate and prepare seminiferous tubules for sectioning similar to classic histological preparations.[49] Either way, testis cytology is a viable alternative to histology in the evaluation of male infertility.

## Newer concepts: FNA 'mapping' of sperm for infertility

It has become clear to reproductive urologists who regularly perform testis sperm retrieval in azoospermic men for IVF-ICSI that spermatogenesis varies geographically within the testis. This underscores the limitation and inadequacy of a single, localised testis biopsy or a single FNA specimen to reflect the biology of the entire organ accurately. In fact, the current clinical challenge is to determine which infertile men with azoospermia harbour sperm for IVF-ICSI and to locate the areas of sperm production precisely within atrophic, non-obstructed testes. This clinical need led to the development of testis FNA 'mapping' in male infertility. In a pilot study of 16 men from 1997, we initially proposed using testis FNA to 'map' the organ for mature sperm.[50] The concept of mapping testis for sperm was inspired by the work of Gottschalk-Sabag and colleagues[36] and modelled on the approach to prostate biology in which multiple prostate biopsies are used to detect foci of prostate cancer. Similarly, FNA was applied systematically to detect the presence or absence of sperm in varied geographical areas of the testis. In this study, azoospermic men underwent simultaneous testicular biopsies and site-matched FNA, and FNA was found to be more sensitive in detecting sperm, as several men had sperm found by FNA but not on biopsy.[50] Additionally, in one-third of patients, localised areas of sperm were detected by FNA in areas distant from biopsy sites without sperm. These data confirmed intratesticular heterogeneity with respect to sperm distribution and suggested the potential of FNA to localise patches of active spermatogenesis in failing testes.

Testicular FNA mapping is performed using a classical FNA technique.[46] Under local anaesthesia in the office, the testis and scrotal skin are fixed relative to each other with a gauze wrap posteriorly (Fig. 20.10). The 'testicular wrap' is a convenient handle to manipulate the testis and also fixes the scrotal skin over the testis for the procedure. Percutaneous aspiration sites are marked on the scrotal skin, 5 mm apart according to a template (Fig. 20.11). The number of aspiration sites varies with testis size and ranges from four (to confirm obstruction) to 15 per testis (for non-obstructive azoospermia). FNA is performed with a sharp-bevelled, 23 gauge, 1-inch needle using the established suction cutting technique.[51] Precise, gentle, in-and-out movements, varying from 5 mm to 8 mm, are used to aspirate tissue fragments. Ten to 30 needle excursions are made at each site. Suction is released and the tissue fragments expelled onto a slide, gently smeared, and immediately fixed in 95% ethyl alcohol. Pressure is applied to each site for haemostasis. A routine Papanicolaou stain is performed. Smears are reviewed by experienced cytologists for: (1) specimen adequacy, defined as at least 12 clusters of testicular cells or at least 2000 well-dispersed testis cells and (2) the presence or absence of mature sperm with tails. For immediate interpretation, fixed slides are stained with undiluted toluidine blue and read with brightfield microscopy after 15 seconds. Patients take an average of two analgesic pills after the procedure. Complications in over 800 patients have included one episode of haematospermia and another patient with postoperative pain for 7 days.

In another study, we applied systematic testis FNA to determine which men were candidates for IVF-ICSI and to guide sperm-retrieval procedures.[52] Sperm retrieval guided by prior FNA maps were proposed as an alternative to other methods of sperm retrieval, which are generally performed on the same day as IVF and that are associated with a significant chance of sperm retrieval failure. In 19 azoospermic men, sperm retrieval guided by prior FNA maps found sufficient sperm for all eggs at IVF in 95% of cases. In addition, FNA-directed procedures enabled simple percutaneous FNA sperm retrieval in 20% of cases, and minimised the number of biopsies (mean 3.1) and volume

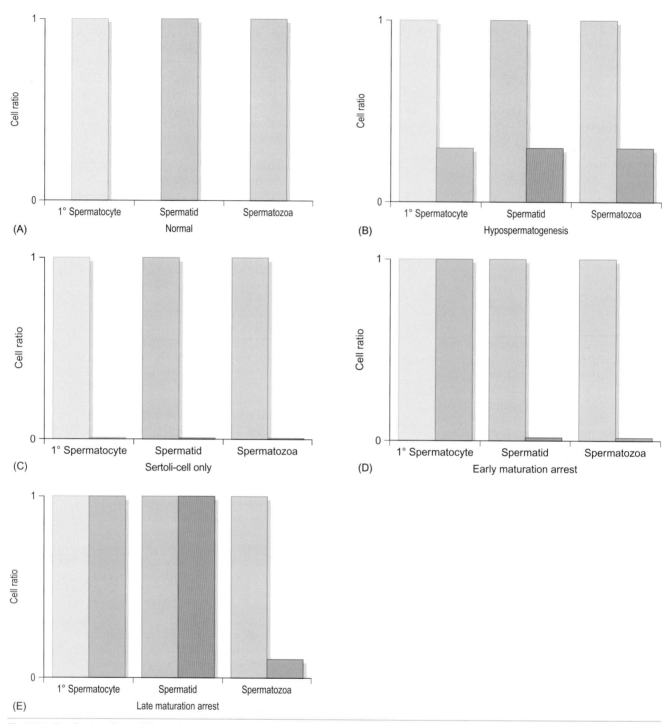

**Fig. 20.8** Classification of testis FNA cytology into histological categories using pattern recognition. (A) Schematic graph of the cellular pattern in normal spermatogenesis. (B) Graph of the cellular pattern in hypospermatogenesis (grey columns). (C) Graph of the cellular pattern in Sertoli-cell only (grey columns). (D) Graph of the cellular pattern in early maturation arrest (grey columns). (E) Graph of the cellular pattern in late maturation arrest (grey columns). (Adapted from: Meng MV, Cha I, Ljung B-M et al. Testicular fine needle aspiration in infertile men: Correlation of cytologic pattern with histology on biopsy. Am J Surg Path 2001; 25:71–79.)

of testicular tissue (mean 72 mg) taken when open biopsies were required. Testis sparing procedures are particularly important in men with atrophic or solitary testes and sperm retrieval guided by information from prior FNA maps can conserve testicular tissue. Thus, this study confirmed that FNA maps can accurately identify azoospermic patients who are candidates for sperm retrieval and ICSI. In addition, it demonstrated that FNA maps can provide crucial information with respect to precise

location of sperm in the testis and minimise the invasiveness of sperm retrieval procedures.

Currently, two kinds of maps are performed in the evaluation of azoospermic infertile men. A compound map (>four sites/testis) is typically performed as a diagnostic test to find sperm in failing testes (Fig. 20.11). This procedure is indicated for men who have testicular atrophy, an elevated serum follicle stimulating hormone (FSH) level, or a prior biopsy revealing

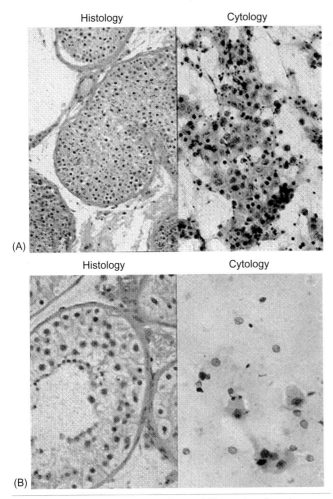

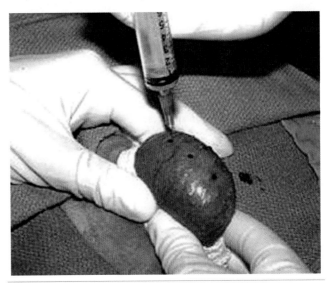

**Fig. 20.10** Technique of testicular FNA under local anesthesia. Scrotal skin is fixed over the anterior testis by placing a gauze wrap behind it. After aspiration sites are marked on the scrotal skin, FNA is performed with a separate, sterile needle and syringe at each site and the cytological material smeared, fixed in alcohol and stained by Papanicolaou method.

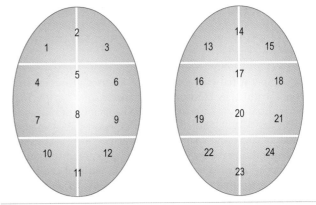

**Fig. 20.9** Matched testis biopsy histology and FNA cytology from the same patient. (A) Normal spermatogenesis. Note the presence of numerous small, darkly stained cells consistent with mature sperm (histology, H&E; cytology, PAP) and (B) hypospermatogenesis. Note that substantially fewer mature sperm are observed in both specimens (histology, H&E; cytology, PAP).

**Fig. 20.11** Extended FNA mapping template for men with non-obstructive azoospermia used to define the presence or absence of testicular sperm. This example shows 12 individual FNA sites per testis.

abnormal or absent spermatogenesis. A simple map (<four sites/testis) is used to confirm the clinical expectation of sperm production in men who may be obstructed and azoospermic. Simple FNA maps are offered to those planning reconstructive procedures (e.g. vasovasostomy) or sperm aspiration from the epididymis who desire more complete information about spermatogenesis before proceeding with reconstruction or sperm retrieval. Regardless of the type of map, these procedures are generally diagnostic in nature because an experienced cytologist using high-resolution microscopy has a much better chance of finding sperm on a differentially stained testicular tissue specimen than does an andrology laboratory technician looking at the same tissue for sperm as part of a sperm-retrieval procedure in an unstained specimen with a phase contrast microscope.

## The biology of sperm production: lessons from FNA mapping

From a comprehensive study of 118 consecutive azoospermic, infertile men who underwent FNA mapping, we have learned much about the geography of spermatogenesis in both normal

(obstructed) and abnormal (non-obstructed) testes.[39] In men with obstructive azoospermia, sperm was found in all sites and in all locations on the FNA map. However, in men with non-obstructive azoospermia, sperm was found in just under 50% of cases. In the subgroup of men with no sperm on a prior testis biopsy, FNA maps revealed sperm in 27% of cases. This increased sensitivity in sperm detection is probably due to sampling of a larger volume of the testis. Confirming the heterogeneity of spermatogenesis in the infertile testis, we observed intratesticular (site-to-site within the same testis) variation in sperm presence in 25% of cases and an intertesticular (side-to-side in the same individual) discordance rate of 19%. This is consistent with the FNA findings from other investigators and suggests that bilateral examination is crucial to fully informing men with non-obstructive azoospermia about opportunities for fatherhood.[53,54] We have also analysed FNA mapping results to determine whether particular geographic sites were more likely to have sperm than others.[39] Individual testis maps from each side were pooled, and from this analysis all FNA sites showed sperm at about the same frequency; there was no suggestion of sperm 'hot spots' in non-obstructive testes. Thus, FNA mapping is a valuable diagnostic tool that not only guides the treatment of infertile men but also provides a wealth of phenotypic information about the infertility condition.

Although the correlation of testis FNA cytology to testis biopsy histology is clear in the literature (Table 20.1), we asked how the global organ findings from testis FNA mapping compared with biopsy histology. In other words, what is the chance of finding sperm on the map with each specific biopsy pattern? In a study of 87 patients, in whom a mean of 1.3 biopsies and 14 FNA sites were taken per patient, we found striking correlations between FNA and histological results (Fig. 20.6).[55] Overall, sperm was found by FNA mapping in 52% of non-obstructive azoospermic patients. Pure histological patterns of Sertoli cell-only and early maturation arrest were associated with a very poor likelihood of sperm detection (4–8%). In contrast, patients with other pure pattern histologies or mixed patterns had high rates of FNA sperm detection (77–100%). (Fig. 20.12). Thus, sperm detection with FNA showed wide variation depending on testis histology. In addition, certain histological patterns may reflect a more global testicular dysfunction due to underlying genetic causes, and thus a poorer likelihood of sperm identification.

## FNA 'mapping' in the treatment of severe male factor infertility

Surgical sperm retrieval for IVF-ICSI in cases of infertility due to non-obstructive azoospermia is successful 40–60% of the time, without prior knowledge of the geography of testis sperm production.[56] With the addition of diagnostic FNA mapping, the rate of successful sperm retrieval can be increased substantially. In addition, based on sperm quantity and distribution in the testes as assessed by the map, sperm retrieval can proceed from the least invasive to the most invasive methods. From a

review of cases ($n = 159$) of non-obstructive azoospermia, we observed that 44% of mapped cases required sperm retrieval by needle aspiration, 33% required open, directed surgical biopsies and 23% needed microsurgically assisted dissection of the entire testis parenchyma for successful sperm retrieval. In addition, the majority (78%) of these cases required only unilateral sperm retrieval to get sufficient sperm for IVF-ICSI. Overall, sufficient sperm for all oocytes retrieved was possible in 95% of cases with prior maps, ranging from 100% in simple aspiration cases to 80% of microdissection cases. In addition, among men who underwent a second sperm retrieval procedure, sperm was successfully retrieved in 91% of attempts, and in all patients who had a third sperm retrieval. This suggests that knowledge of sperm location with FNA mapping can simplify and streamline sperm retrieval procedures in very difficult cases of non-obstructive azoospermia.

## Role of FNA cytology in testicular and scrotal lesions and male infertility

Handa et al. performed a study of the role of FNA in male infertility and in non-neoplastic lesions of the testis and scrotum and found inflammatory lesions (31.7%), non-inflammatory lesions (25.6%), infertility cases (26.2%) and inconclusive findings in 16% of cases, the latter mainly derived from epididymal lesions.[57] Among the inflammatory lesions, the most frequent was non-specific inflammation, followed by granulomatous epididymo-orchitis, spermatic granuloma and microfilaria. Non-inflammatory lesions included spermatocele, haematoma/torsion, hydrocele, benign epididymal cyst and calcinosis cutis. Among patients investigated for infertility, 53% had normal spermatogenesis, 14% had Sertoli cells only, 19% had maturation arrest, 14% showed hypospermatogenesis and 7% showed an atrophic pattern. FNA of the testis and scrotum are simple, quick, minimally invasive out-patient procedures. The sample obtained is equivalent to that of a biopsy and several multiple separate punctures can be made safely, with minimal local scarring.

## Summary of testis FNA and male infertility

- FNA cytology plays an important role in the diagnosis of a wide variety of testicular and scrotal lesions
- FNA can help avoid unnecessary surgery in men of reproductive age
- Testis FNA cytology correlates well with testis biopsy histology in the evaluation of male infertility
- Testis FNA cytology is rapid and safe and provides information not only on the presence or absence of sperm but, when applied in multiple areas as a 'map', can precisely localise sperm production
- Testis FNA cytology can direct sperm retrieval procedures and minimise the amount of testicular tissue removed
- With wider sampling of the testis achieved with FNA cytology, the heterogeneity of sperm production can be more accurately defined and sperm-retrieval procedures improved

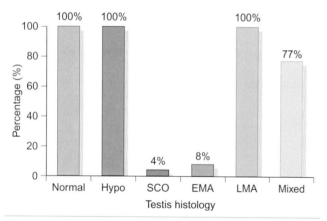

**Fig. 20.12** Correlation between biopsy histology and FNA mapping. Sperm presence was determined by FNA map and histological patterns by surgical biopsy. Hypo, hypospermatogenesis; SCO, Sertoli cell-only; EMA, early maturation arrest: LMA, late maturation arrest. (Adapted from Meng MV, Cha I, Ljung B-M et al. Relationship between classic histological pattern and sperm findings on fine needle aspiration map in infertile men. Hum Reprod 2000; 15:1973–1977.)

- Although assessment of architecture and the basement membrane is not possible with FNA, whole organ cytological examination of seminiferous tubule patterns with mapping provides useful phenotypic information about severe male factor infertility.

In summary, FNAC is a valuable tool for the evaluation of both scrotal masses and male infertility.

## REFERENCES

1. Zornow DH, Landes RR. Scrotal palpation. Am Fam Physician 1981;23:150–54.

2. Gutman H, Golimbu M, Subramanyam BR. Diagnostic ultrasound of scrotum. Urology 1986;27:72–75.

3. Scott RF, Bayliss AP, Calder JF, et al. Indications for ultrasound in the evaluation of the pathological scrotum. Br J Urol 1986;58:178–82.

4. Munden MM, Trautwein LM. Scrotal pathology in pediatrics with sonographic imaging. Curr Probl Diagn Radiol 2000;29:185–205.

5. Handa U, Bhutani A, Mohan H, et al. Role of fine needle aspiration cytology in nonneoplastic testicular and scrotal lesions and male infertility. Acta Cytol 2006;50:513–17.

6. Almeida MM, Mendonça ME, Sousinha M, et al. Application of aspiration cytology in the diagnosis of tumour lesions in children. Acta Med Port 1991;4:71–75.

7. Bettella A, Merico M, Spolaore D, et al. Needle aspiration testicular cytology as diagnostic parameter in the assessment with varicocele. Arch Ital Urol Androl 2001;73:3–13.

8. Pérez-Guillermo M, Sola Pérez J. Aspiration cytology of palpable lesions of the scrotal content. Diagn Cytopathol 1990;6:169–77.

9. Verma K, Ram TR, Kapila K. Value of fine needle aspiration cytology in the diagnosis of testicular neoplasms. Acta Cytol 1989;33:631–34.

10. de Almeida MM, Chagas M, de Sousa JV, et al. Fine-needle aspiration cytology as a tool for the early detection of testicular relapse of acute lymphoblastic leukemia in children. Diagn Cytopathol 1994;10:44–46.

11. Cornell University. What's New in Male Infertility Treatment at Cornell Testis Biopsy. Cornell University Weill Medical College Cornell Institute for Reproductive Medicine. New York: Cornell. Online. Available at: http://www.maleinfertility.org/new-biopsy.html.

12. Soh E, Berman LH, Grant JW, et al. Ultrasound-guided core-needle biopsy of the testis for focal indeterminate intratesticular lesions. Eur Radiol 2008;18:2990–96.

13. Passman C, Urban D, Klemm K, et al. Testicular lesions other than germ cell tumours: feasibility of testis-sparing surgery. BJU Int 2008;103:488–91.

14. Emerson RE, Ulbright TM. The use of immunohistochemistry in the differential diagnosis of tumors of the testis and paratestis. Semin Diagn Pathol 2005;22:33–50.

15. Roy C, Tuchmann C. Scrotal ultrasonography. Part I: common non-cancerous pathologies. J Radiol 2003;84:581–95.

16. Gupta N, Rajwanshi A, Srinivasan R, et al. Fine needle aspiration of epididymal nodules in Chandigarh, north India: an audit of 228 cases. Cytopathol 2006;17:195–98.

17. Sah SP, Bhadani PP, Regmi R, et al. Fine needle aspiration cytology of tubercular epididymitis and epididymo-orchitis. Acta Cytol 2006;50:243–49.

18. Tewari R, Mishra MN, Salopal TK. The role of fine needle aspiration cytology in evaluation of epididymal nodular lesions. Acta Cytol 2007;51:168–70.

19. Young RH. Testicular tumors – some new and a few perennial problems. Arch Pathol Lab Med 2008;132:548–64.

20. Caraway NP, Fanning CV, Amato RJ, et al. Fine-needle aspiration cytology of seminoma: a review of 16 cases. Diagn Cytopathol 1995;12:327–33.

21. Gupta R, Mathur SR, Arora VK, et al. Cytologic features of extragonadal germ cell tumors: a study of 88 cases with aspiration cytology. Cancer 2008;114:504–11.

22. Erlandson RA. Endodermal sinus (yolk sac) tumour. In: Erlandson RA, editor. Diagnostic Transmission Electron Microscopy of Tumours. New York: Raven Press; 1994. p. 346–48.

23. Vielh P, Borghesi R, Validire P, et al. Leydig cell tumour of the testis: a case diagnosed by fine-needle sampling without aspiration with histologic, immunohistologic, and electron microscopic analysis. Diagn Cytopathol 1991;7:601–5.

24. Jain M, Aiyer HM, Bajaj P, et al. Intracytoplasmic and intranuclear Reinke's crystals in a testicular Leydig-cell tumor diagnosed by fine-needle aspiration cytology: a case report with review of the literature. Diagn Cytopathol 2001;25:162–64.

25. Pettinato G, Insabato L, De Chiara A, et al. Fine needle aspiration cytology of a large cell calcifying Sertoli cell tumour of the testis. Acta Cytol 1987;31:578–82.

26. Kronz JD, Nicol TL, Rosenthal DL, et al. Metastatic testicular Sertoli-cell tumour: cytopathologic findings on fine-needle aspiration. Diagn Cytopathol 1998;19:127–30.

27. Barroca H, Gil-Da-Costa MJ, Mariz C. Testicular juvenile granulosa cell tumour: A case report. Acta Cytol 2007;51:634–36.

28. Hisano M, Souza FM, Malheiros DM, et al. Granulosa cell tumour of the adult testis. Report of a case and review of the literature. Clinics 2006;61:77–78.

29. Vitolo U, Ferreri A, Zucca E. Primary testicular lymphoma. Crit Rev Oncol Hematol 2008;65:183–89.

30. Koss LG, Melamed MR, editors. Koss' Diagnostic Cytopathology and its Histologic Bases, 5th edn. Philadelphia: Lippincott Williams and Wilkins; 2006.pp. 1274–1285.

31. Sastre JL, Ulibarrena C, Armesto A, et al. Testicular granulocytic sarcoma as a form of relapse in a patient with acute megakaryoblastic leukemia. Sangre (Barc) 1998;43:248–50.

32. Ghadiany M, Attarian H, Hajifathali A, et al. Relapse of acute myeloid leukemia as isolated bilateral testicular granulocytic sarcoma in an adult. Urol J 2008;5:132–34.

33. Manjunath GV, Nandini NM, Sunila. Fine needle aspiration cytology of adenomatoid tumour – a case report with review of literature. Indian J Pathol Microbiol 2005;48:503–4.

34. Posner C. Die diagnostische Hodenpunktion. Berl Klin Wochenschr 1905;42b:1119–21.

35. Hendricks FB, Lambird PA, Murph GP. Percutaneous needle biopsy of the testis. Fertil Steril 1969;20:478–81.

36. Gottschalk-Sabag S, Glick T, Weiss DB. Fine needle aspiration of the testis and correlation with testicular open biopsy. Acta Cytol 1993;37:67–72.

37. Mallidis C, Gordon Baker HW. Fine needle tissue aspiration biopsy of the testis. Fertil Steril 1994;61:367–75.

38. Palermo G, Joris H, Devroey P, et al. Pregnancies after intracytoplasmic injection of single spermatozoon into an oocyte. Lancet 1992;340:17.

39. Turek PJ, Ljung B-M, Cha I, et al. Diagnostic findings from testis fine needle aspiration mapping in obstructed and non-obstructed azoospermic men. J Urol 2000;163:1709–16.

40. Damani MN, Master V, Meng MV, et al. Post-chemotherapy ejaculatory azoospermia: fatherhood with sperm from testis tissue using intracytoplasmic sperm injection. J Clin Oncology 2002;20:930–36.

41. Firket J, Damian-Gillet M. Value and importance of testicular biopsies in Klinefelter's syndrome. Acta Clin Belg 1951;6:80–81.

42. Levin HS. Testicular biopsy in the study of male infertility: its current usefulness, histologic techniques, and prospects for the future. Hum Pathol 1979;10:569–84.

43. Johnsen SG. Testicular biopsy score count – a method for registration of spermatogenesis in human testes: normal values and results in 335 hypogonadal males. Hormones 1970;1:2–25.

44. Cooperberg MR, Chi T, Jad A, et al. Variation in testis biopsy interpretation: implications for male infertility care in the era of intracytoplasmic sperm injection. Fertil Steril 2005;84:672–77.

45. Papic Z, Katona G, Skrabalo Z. The cytologic identification and quantification of testicular cell subtypes. Acta Cytol 1988;32:697–706.

46. Verma AK, Basu D, Jayaram G. Testicular cytology in azoospermia. Diagn Cytopathol 1993;9:37–42.

47. Batra VV, Khadgawat R, Agarwal A, et al. Correlation of cell counts and indices in testicular FNAC with histology in male infertility. Acta Cytol 1999;43:617–23.

48. Meng MV, Cha I, Ljung B-M, et al. Testicular fine needle aspiration in infertile men: Correlation of cytologic pattern with histology on biopsy. Am J Surg Path 2001;25:71–79.

49. Stock D, Misir V, Johnson S. Optimising FNA processing – a collection fluid allowing Giemsa, PAP and H&E staining, and facilitating thinprep, cytospin and direct smears and ancillary tests. Cytopathology 2000;11:523–24.

50. Turek PJ, Cha I, Ljung B-M. Systematic fine-needle aspiration of the testis: correlation to biopsy and results of organ 'mapping' for mature sperm in azoospermic men. Urology 1997;49:743–48.

51. Ljung B-M. Techniques of aspiration and smear preparation. In: Koss LG, Woyke S, Olszewski W, editors. Aspiration Biopsy: Cytologic Interpretation and Histological Bases, 2nd edn. New York: Igaku-Shoin; 1992. p. 12–34.

52. Turek PJ, Givens C, Schriock ED, et al. Testis sperm extraction and intracytoplasmic sperm injection guided by prior fine needle aspiration mapping in nonobstructive azoospermia. Fertil Steril 1999;71:552–57.

53. Weiss DB, Gottschalk-Sabag S, Bar-On E, et al. Seminiferous tubule cytologic pattern in infertile, azoospermic men in diagnosis and therapy. Harefuah 1997;132:614–18.

54. Samli M, Sariyuce O, Basar M, et al. Evaluation of nonobstructive azoospermia with bilateral testicular biopsy. J Urol 1999;161:342.

55. Meng MV, Cha I, Ljung BM, et al. Relationship between classic histological pattern and sperm findings on fine needle aspiration map in infertile men. Hum Reprod 2000;15:1973–77.

56. Tournaye H, Liu J, Nagy PZ, et al. Correlation between testicular histology and outcome after intracytoplasmic sperm injection using testicular spermatozoa. Hum Reprod 1996;11:127–32.

57. Handa U, Bhutani A, Mohan H, et al. Role of fine needle aspiration cytology in nonneoplastic testicular and scrotal lesions and male infertility. Acta Cytol 2006;50:513–17.

58. Persson PS, Ahern C, Obrant KO. Aspiration biopsy smear of testis in azoospermia. Scand J Urol Nephrol 1971;5:22–26.

59. Craft I, Tsirigotis M, Courtauld E, et al. Testicular needle aspiration as an alternative to biopsy for the assessment of spermatogenesis. Hum Reprod 1997;12:1483–87.

60. Odabas O, Ugras S, Aydin S, et al. Assessment of testicular cytology by fine-needle aspiration and the imprint technique: are they reliable diagnostic modalities? Br J Urol 1997;79:445–48.

61. Mahajan AD, Imdad Ali N, Walwalkar SJ, et al. The role of fine-needle aspiration cytology of the testis in the diagnostic evaluation of infertility. Br J Urol 1999;84:485–88.

62. Rammou-Kinia R, Anagnostopoulou I, Tassiopoulos F, et al. Fine needle aspiration of the testis. Correlation between cytology and histology. Acta Cytol 1999;43:991–98.

63. Qublan HS, Al-Jader KM, Al-Kaisi NS, et al. Fine needle aspiration cytology compared with open biopsy histology for the diagnosis of azoospermia. J Obstet Gynaecol 2002;22:527–31.

64. Arïdo an IA, Bayazït Y, Yaman M, et al. Comparison of fine-needle aspiration and open biopsy of testis in sperm retrieval and histopathologic diagnosis. Andrologia 2003;35:121–25.

65. Mehrotra R, Chaurasia D. Fine needle aspiration cytology of the testis as the first-line diagnostic modality in azoospermia: a comparative study of cytology and histology. Cytopathology 2008;19:363–68.

# Section 12

## Female Genital Tract

# Vulva, vagina and cervix: normal cytology, hormonal and inflammatory conditions

Tanya Levine and Winifred Gray

## Chapter contents

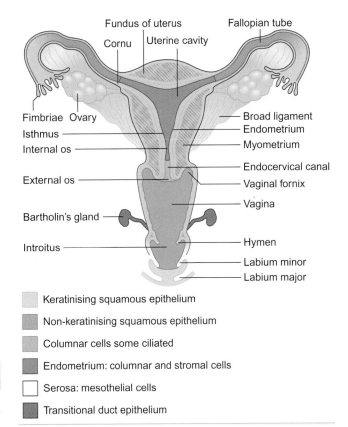

Keratinising squamous epithelium

Non-keratinising squamous epithelium

Columnar cells some ciliated

Endometrium: columnar and stromal cells

Serosa: mesothelial cells

Transitional duct epithelium

**Fig. 21.1** Diagram of the female genital tract demonstrating the main structures and the types of epithelium covering the surface accessible to sampling directly or indirectly by exfoliative cytology. (Courtesy of Professor D. Coleman and Mrs P. Chapman, with permission from Butterworths, London.)

## Introduction

The foundations for the success of cytological screening for cervical cancer were laid by two publications; Bales in 1927 and Papanicolaou in 1928 in which the morphology of cervical cancer cells in vaginal samples was described.[1] Since then, the morphological spectrum of squamous and glandular abnormalities in cervical cytology has expanded to include pre-cancerous and invasive cervical tumours as well as tumours with origin elsewhere in the female genital tract and metastases from extragenital sites. Crucial to the recognition of these cells is an understanding of normal vulval, vaginal, cervical and endometrial cytology, including hormonal and inflammatory/reactive conditions. The morphology of these cells is similar whether assessing conventional direct smears or newer liquid-based cytology preparations. Cytological findings in cervical neoplasia and other genital tract neoplasms are covered in Chapters 23–27.

## Gross and microscopic anatomy

The basic structure of the female genital tract is depicted diagrammatically in Figure 21.1, illustrating the different types of lining epithelium that may be seen in cytological samples from various sites.

## Vulva

The labia majora and minora of the vulva are covered by keratinising squamous epithelium (Fig. 21.2) which undergoes very little hormonal change during the menstrual cycle. The outer surfaces of the labia majora are hair-bearing. The inner surfaces have many sebaceous glands and apocrine sweat glands, the secretions of which provide protection against infection and local damage to the skin.

*The authors dedicate this chapter to Dr E. Hudson and Professor D. Coleman who have done so much for gynaecological cytology; and we thank Dr M. Boon for her contribution to the chapter in previous editions of this book.*

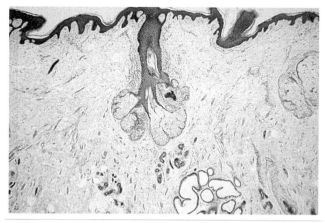

**Fig. 21.2** Vulval skin showing stratified squamous keratinising epithelium with skin appendages (H&E).

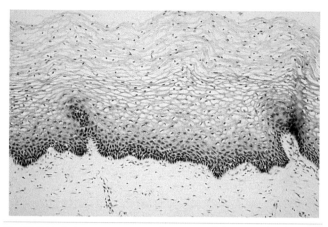

**Fig. 21.3** Vaginal squamous mucosa is not normally keratinised and is hormone sensitive, in contrast to vulval skin. The squamous cell cytoplasm is clear in this section due to the presence of glycogen (H&E).

The labia show pigmentation from the age of puberty, diminishing on the inner aspect of the labia minora where only a thin layer of keratin is present. This epithelium extends to cover the vestibule as far as the hymen. The vagina and the urethra open onto the vestibule of the vulva. Mucin secreting glands are present on either side of the vaginal introitus, including Bartholin's glands, which are situated in the lower vaginal wall, providing protection and lubrication.

## Vagina

Developmentally, the upper two-thirds of the vagina is formed by fusion of the two mullerian ducts *in utero*. The tube thus formed differentiates into the uterus and cervix above and unites distally with the urogenital sinus to form the vagina. Thus the lower third of the vagina has a different embryological origin from the upper two-thirds. The importance of this dual derivation lies in the fact that the mullerian epithelium in the upper two-thirds is initially columnar in type, but undergoes metaplasia in utero to squamous mucosa on exposure to the acid pH of the vagina. Normally the change to squamous epithelium is complete, but the process may be interrupted, leading to persistence of glandular tissue in the adult vagina, a condition known as vaginal adenosis (see Fig. 21.99).

Under normal conditions, the vagina is lined by stratified squamous non-keratinising epithelium throughout (Fig. 21.3), usually showing no hair follicles, sweat glands or sebaceous glands to weaken its surface. The mucosa is subject to cyclical changes under the influence of the sex hormones.

## Cervix

The cervix is a cylindrical fibromuscular structure of variable length, within which lies the endocervical canal connecting the body of the uterus at the internal os with the vagina at the external os. The lower portion of the cervix protrudes into the vagina, forming the anterior, posterior and two lateral fornices in the upper vagina where pooling of secretions and exfoliated cells occurs. The outer aspect of the cervix, known as the ectocervix or portio vaginalis, is covered by squamous mucosa in continuity with vaginal epithelium distally and with the lining of the endocervix at or near the external os (Fig. 21.4).

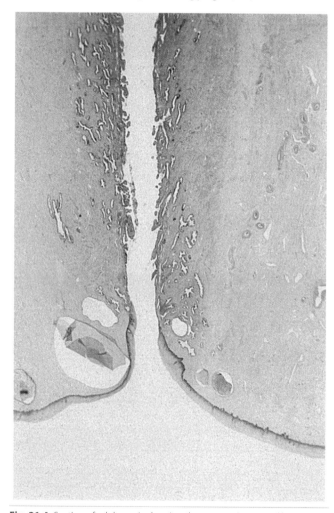

**Fig. 21.4** Section of adult cervix showing the ectocervix covered by non-keratinising squamous epithelium, the external os and the endocervical canal running towards the body of the uterus. Endocervical crypts face downwards and are lined by a single layer of columnar epithelial cells (H&E).

The endocervical canal is not exposed to the vaginal pH and therefore retains its glandular lining of tall columnar epithelium, with an inconspicuous layer of reserve cells beneath, resting on basement membrane. The glandular mucosa forms branching crypts that extend into the stroma of the cervix in

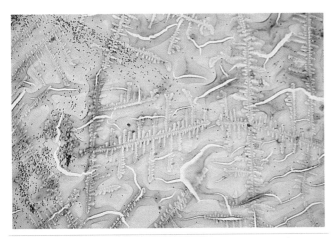

**Fig. 21.5** Cervical mucus in a conventional/direct cervical smear taken at midcycle showing a ferning pattern due to the effects of oestrogen.

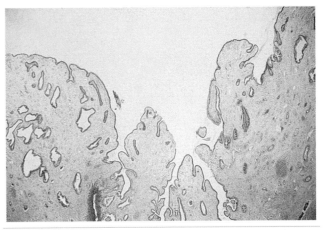

**Fig. 21.6** Ectropion. At menarche and during certain phases of reproductive life, the squamocolumnar junction is everted so that the endocervical glands come to lie on the outer aspect of the cervix, producing an ectropion (H&E).

a racemose pattern for a distance of up to 5 mm; the orifices facing distally. The canal itself is narrow, being only a few millimetres wide, and in health, is filled by a plug of mucus. During the menstrual cycle the physical properties of the cervical mucus change. Prior to ovulation the mucus is dilute, and when spread on to a slide and dried, it forms a fern-like pattern (Fig. 21.5). After ovulation, the mucus becomes thicker and no longer demonstrates ferning.

It will be apparent from the above description that there is a point of junction between the squamous epithelium of the ectocervix and the lining of the endocervical canal. This meeting point is referred to as the squamocolumnar junction. The changes that occur in this area are of crucial significance in cervical pathology.

## Squamocolumnar junction and transformation zone

Major changes in the size and shape of the cervix take place during reproductive life. Before puberty, the squamocolumnar junction forms the outer boundary of the endocervical glands, known as the 'original' squamocolumnar junction, coinciding with the site of the external os.

After puberty, the location of the squamocolumnar junction changes as the cervix alters in shape. The endocervical mucosa of the lower canal, including the underlying crypts, is everted and comes to lie on the ectocervical aspect of the cervix, resulting in an ectropion or ectopy (Fig. 21.6). An ectropion is clinically visible as a reddened zone extending out from the external os. It is sometimes mistakenly called an erosion, although no actual ulceration is present and the condition is physiological.

Endocervical eversion is followed by progressive metaplasia of the exposed mucosa to more protective squamous epithelium under the influence of the vaginal pH, the term metaplasia referring to a change from one type of epithelium to another. The metaplastic process arises in the reserve cell population that normally replenishes the columnar epithelium. Instead, these reserve cells differentiate as immature squamous metaplastic cells beneath the single layer of columnar cells on the surface (Fig. 21.7A).

The metaplastic layers increase and mature progressively to form a new normal squamous mucosa indistinguishable from the original squamous epithelium of the ectocervix. The underlying endocervical crypts remain facing on to the ectocervix as a permanent marker of the site of the original squamocolumnar

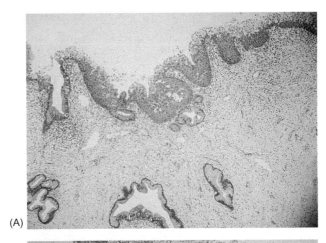

(A)

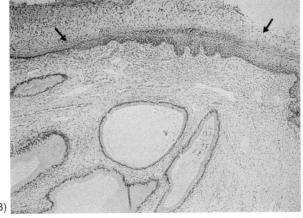

(B)

**Fig. 21.7** (A) Reserve cell hyperplasia is seen beneath everted columnar epithelium. The cells are starting to show multilayered immature squamous metaplasia, forming a transformation zone. (H&E). (B) The transformation zone (between arrows) is now maturing but its site of origin is marked by the position of the first endocervical gland. Note the plug of mucus covering the surface (H&E).

junction and this can be recognised colposcopically as well as in histological section (Fig. 21.7B). Glands with orifices obstructed by the metaplastic process are prone to distend with mucus, even becoming visible macroscopically as rounded nodules on the ectocervix, known as nabothian follicles.

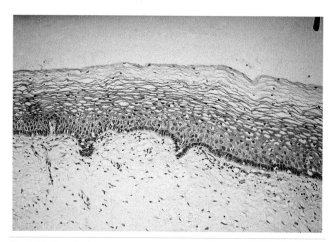

**Fig. 21.8** Stratified squamous mucosa from the cervix during reproductive life shows a distinct row of primitive basal cells resting on a thin basement membrane. Above this there is progressive maturation from 3 to 4 parabasal cell layers to an intermediate cell layer with more cytoplasm and preserved nuclear structure, while the uppermost superficial cells have condensed pyknotic nuclei and voluminous cytoplasm (H&E).

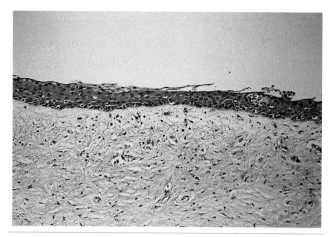

**Fig. 21.9** Postmenopausal atrophy of ectocervical squamous mucosa. The epithelium is thinned, with crowding of squamous cells due to their reduced cytoplasm. The basal layer is still distinct and polarisation of cells is visible (H&E).

The extent to which eversion of the endocervix occurs varies in different women and the new junction may be asymmetrical in relation to the external os, with ectropion covering one or both sides of the ectocervix, even extending on to the vaginal walls. Ectropion is liable to recur with certain hormonal events. The most obvious of these is pregnancy, during which ectopy is a common finding due to enlargement of the cervix under the influence of progesterone. Some types of oral contraceptive therapy have a similar effect. After the menopause the cervix shrinks and the squamocolumnar junction migrates into the endocervical canal.

The area of metaplastic epithelium proximal to the original squamocolumnar junction is referred to as the transformation zone since it is an area of epithelial instability. Immature metaplastic cells appear to carry an extra risk of neoplastic change.

### Structure of stratified squamous epithelium (Figs 21.8, 21.9)

The germinal layer is composed of a single row of small regular cells adhering to a basement membrane and showing signs of active growth. These undifferentiated cells are referred to as the basal cells. Above this layer it is possible to distinguish parabasal cells, immature and crowded, lying two to three cells deep. These cells mature into an intermediate layer of variable thickness in which the cells have more cytoplasm, the nuclei still show a recognisable chromatin pattern and the cells are bound to each other by intercellular cytoplasmic bridges.

In fully mature cervical squamous mucosa there is a superficial layer consisting of cells that do not normally mature any further. Intercellular bridges are not highly developed at this level so that the cell bonds are weaker. Superficial cells are actually dead or dying and exfoliate spontaneously. Sometimes a thin upper layer of cells with dark cytoplasmic keratohyaline granules may be present in histological sections, formed of the cells that precede keratinisation, but a keratinised layer is not seen under normal conditions.

Mucosal thickness depends upon hormonal status as the parabasal, intermediate and superficial layers are all hormonally responsive. Under the influence of oestrogen a superficial layer develops in about 4 days. This multilayered epithelium provides a barrier against external injuries and stores nutrients in the form of glycogen.

## Cytological identification of epithelial cells

Identification of squamous cells from the various layers described above is a basic step in the interpretation of cervical smears. The Papanicolaou stain is ideally suited for this purpose, having been devised originally to assess hormonal status according to the degree of cytoplasmic maturation in vaginal squamous cells. Columnar and metaplastic cells are identified by a combination of morphology and staining reactions.

Two of the components of the Papanicolaou stain are cytoplasmic stains: eosin, which stains superficial cells pink or orange, and light green, which is taken up by the cytoplasm of all of the less mature cells. Because the stains are alcohol-based, the cytoplasmic staining is particularly delicate and translucent, unless keratinisation is present, when the staining becomes densely orangeophilic. Thus the full range of squamous cells can be identified by a combination of morphological and tinctorial features. The nuclei are stained by haematoxylin. Good fixation is an essential prerequisite for successful use of the Papanicolaou stain, particularly for revealing nuclear detail. The samples illustrated in this chapter are all stained by the Papanicolaou method except where otherwise stated. As far as possible, liquid-based cytological preparations have been used.

## Basal cells

These small primitive cells are parent to all the cells in the squamous mucosa that migrate to the surface, die and exfoliate. They are difficult to recognise in a smear with confidence and are likely to be sampled only rarely due to their deep position in the mucosa and their firm attachment to the basement membrane. They are said to occur in short rows of small regular cells with sparse green cytoplasm, oval nuclei and a high nuclear/cytoplasmic (N:C) ratio. The chromatin pattern is fine and several chromocentres may be present.[2]

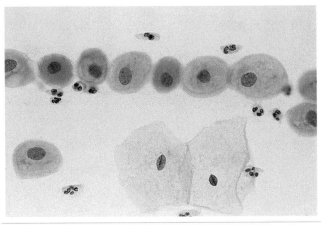

**Fig. 21.10** A row of parabasal cells, rounded or polygonal in shape, dissociated and in small groups. The cytoplasm is dense and cyanophilic, the nuclei stain darkly and the nuclear/cytoplasmic ratio is high compared with the intermediate cells at lower edge.

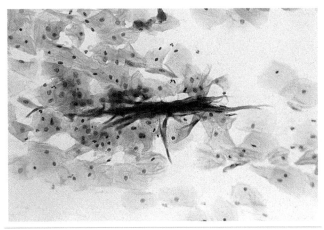

**Fig. 21.12** An epithelial spike/raft of parakeratotic squamous cells.

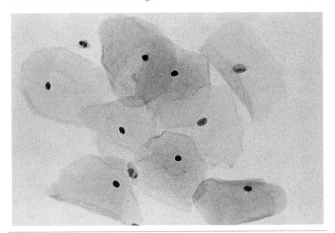

**Fig. 21.11** Intermediate and superficial squamous cells. The former have translucent green cytoplasm with a tendency to fold at the periphery; the nuclei show a vesicular chromatin pattern and the nuclear/cytoplasmic ratio is low. The superficial cells are large, flat, polygonal and dissociated, with pinkish orange cytoplasm. The tiny dark nuclei have lost their chromatin pattern.

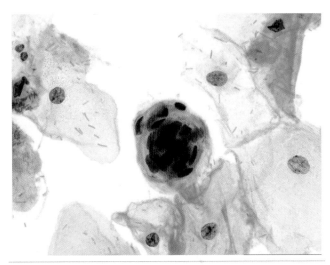

**Fig. 21.13** Concentric epithelial pearls can be seen in normal cervical cytology samples.

## Parabasal cells (Fig. 21.10)

- Round to oval cells with fairly dense green cytoplasm
- Nuclei occupy about one half of the cell and have a fine chromatin pattern
- Immature parabasal cells lie in sheets while more mature cells are usually dissociated.

Parabasal cells may predominate in atrophic smears from postmenopausal women. In younger women postnatal atrophy or high dose progesterone oral contraception produce similar changes. With poor fixation and in some inflammatory states parabasal cytoplasm may be amphophilic, taking up eosin staining centrally with peripheral cyanophilia.

## Intermediate cells (Fig. 21.11)

- Large polygonal cells, ample pale green filmy cytoplasm often folded at periphery
- Nucleus round or ovoid, vesicular, fine chromatin pattern
- Cytoplasmic disintegration (cytolysis) may be present.

The cells lie in tight groups or discretely in the smear, depending upon the hormonal state. In the second half of the cycle, when cell clumping is greatest, the cytoplasm becomes ragged and may disintegrate altogether, leaving bare nuclei. Under the influence of high levels of progesterone, intermediate cells tend to accumulate glycogen, forming an irregular central deposit of pale yellow stained material.

## Superficial cells (Fig. 21.11)

- Large polygonal cells, pink to orange flat cytoplasm, rarely folded
- Nuclei small condensed or pyknotic; no visible internal structure
- Cells are usually discrete, in contrast to intermediate cells.

Cells from the granular layer, if formed, display small dark blue keratohyaline granules evenly distributed in the cytoplasm. Nests and aggregates of benign squamous cells known as epithelial pearls and rafts are sometimes seen in normal smears (Figs 21.12, 21.13).

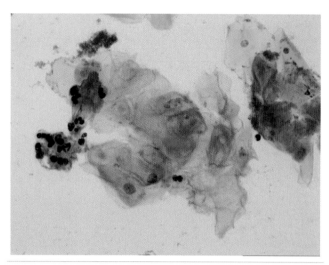

**Fig. 21.14** Vulval contamination of a cervical smear is suggested by these yellowish orange anucleate squames. They are also seen in direct vulval scrapes.

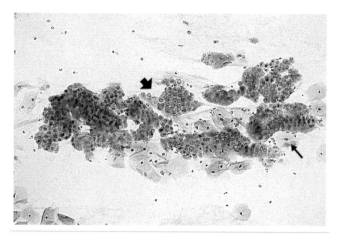

**Fig. 21.15** Endocervical cells in sheets and groups, their columnar form giving a picket-fence (arrow) or honeycomb appearance (arrowhead). The cytoplasm is delicate and nuclei are rounded with a vesicular chromatin pattern.

## Anucleate squames

- Mature superficial squamous cells with loss of nuclei
- Stain with eosin producing orange or yellow stained cytoplasm (Fig. 21.14)
- Site of nucleus may be recognisable as a lighter central area or nuclear ghost.

Anucleate squames are often present in combination with granular cells, indicating completion of keratinisation. The cells are a normal finding in vulval scrapes. Numerous anucleate squames in a smear from the cervix suggests an area of keratinisation (hyperkeratosis) due to irritation from, for instance, prolapse or the wearing of a pessary. Hyperkeratosis also occurs in human papillomavirus infection, leukoplakia and in some cases of cervical carcinoma. The presence of anucleate squames is, however, of low predictive value for these conditions. Less mature cells from the deeper layers may also become anucleate, usually in association with degenerative changes.

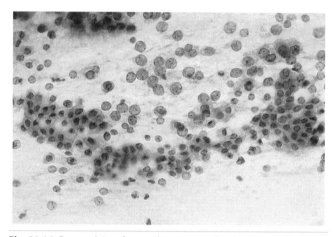

**Fig. 21.16** Bare nuclei are frequently seen around endocervical cell groups. The nuclei become swollen and flattened like a fried egg when unsupported by cytoplasm, with pale but uniform chromatin. These nuclei may be of reserve cell origin.

## Endocervical cells (Fig. 21.15)

- Columnar cells with basal nuclei, in flat variable sized sheets or loosely associated
- Cyanophilic translucent cytoplasm or vacuolated
- Viewed from above, sheets have a honeycomb appearance
- In profile, cells in 'picket-fence' palisades with basal nuclei and columnar cytoplasm
- From above, nuclei rounded, from the side the nuclei are oval
- Fine chromatin pattern, one or more small nucleoli often near the nuclear membrane
- Bare nuclei may accompany groups of degenerate endocervical cells (Fig. 21.16).

Sometimes cilia are visible, staining pink with eosin, attached to the terminal bar at the luminal pole of the cell (Fig. 21.17). Cilia are more commonly seen postmenopausally but may also arise with tuboendometrioid metaplasia which can occur in the

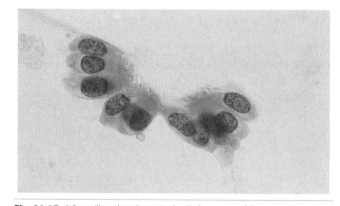

**Fig. 21.17** A few ciliated endocervical cells form part of the normal glandular epithelium of the cervix but the cilia are not often seen as they are prone to undergo degenerative changes.

process of healing of the cervical mucosa after injury such as post-conisation.

Occasionally endocervical cell cytoplasm may become distended by mucus producing a goblet cell appearance. Care

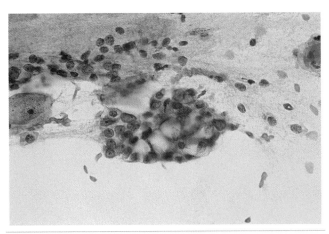

**Fig. 21.18** Endocervical cells with goblet cell morphology due to distension with mucin.

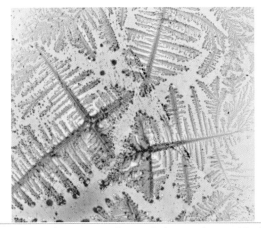

**Fig. 21.20** Cervical mucus spread in a cervical smear taken at midcycle showing a ferning pattern due to the effects of oestrogen (× MP).

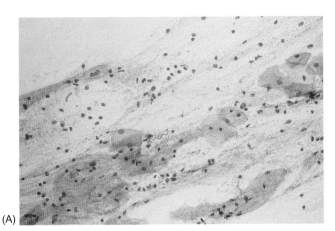

(A)

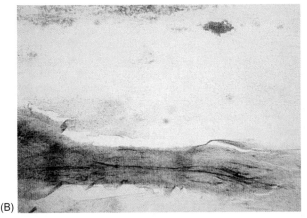

(B)

**Fig. 21.19** (A) Background mucus stained pale pink or green is a useful indicator of sampling from the cervix. Vaginal and vulval smears usually contain little or no mucus. (× MP) (B) The mucous plug of the cervix may be spread on a smear largely intact. The plug contains inflammatory cells but the remainder of the smear will be clean, in contrast to a genuine infection (× LP).

should always be taken to examine the overall morphology of these cell groups to exclude the rare possibility of intestinal-type glandular intraepithelial neoplasia (see Ch. 24) (Fig. 21.18) Background mucus from endocervical cells stains variably, either faintly green or tinged with pink. The amount of mucus present

in a sample, its quality and distribution also vary considerably (Fig. 21.19). With conventional smears a 'ferning' effect may be evident at the time of ovulation (Fig. 21.20). This pattern is not seen with liquid-based cytology preparations.

Endocervical cells may show considerable variation in nuclear size within a group, although the polarity is maintained (Fig. 21.21).

## Metaplastic cells

- Cells the size of parabasal or early intermediate cells in small sheets
- Detached cells have cytoplasmic projections resulting from loosened connecting bridges to adjacent cells
- Delicate or dense cyanophilic cytoplasm or prematurely keratinised
- Nuclei vary in size, having vesicular chromatin and a high nuclear:cytoplasmic ratio.

These cells are a normal constituent of smears from the cervical os once the transformation zone has developed (Fig. 21.22). While immature, they do not exfoliate spontaneously but can be lifted from the surface of the cervix by the abrading action of a spatula or brush. With progressive maturation, the cells increasingly resemble intermediate and superficial cells from the original ectocervix and therefore cannot be recognised as a separate cell population in cervical samples.

The cytoplasmic projections that give a spidery contour to the single cells result from their forcible removal during sample taking. In metaplastic cell sheets the cytoplasmic projections may appear as fine intercellular bridges (Fig. 21.23). In the unstable environment of the transformation zone, premature keratinisation of these cells may occur and the cytoplasm is then a deep orange colour. Other degenerative changes such as vacuolation and the presence of intracytoplasmic polymorphs may be seen, even in the absence of significant inflammation. Degenerative nuclear changes may also occur if maturation of the transformation zone is arrested; these include pyknosis, referring to condensation of the entire nucleus, and fragmentation or dissolution of chromatin, referred to as karyorrhexis and karyolysis, respectively.

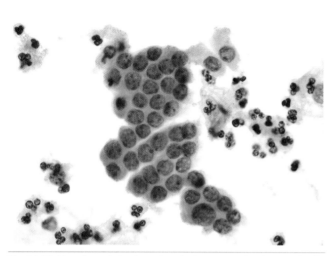

**Fig. 21.21**  Note the variation in nuclear size in occasional endocervical cells (most prominent at the bottom), but polarity is maintained.

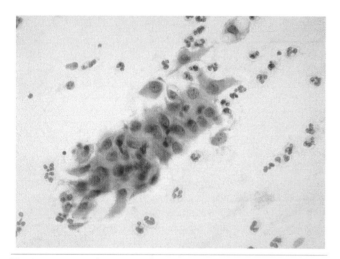

**Fig. 21.22**  A metaplastic group showing angular and polygonal cells with dense blue-green cytoplasm and nuclei resembling those of endocervical cells.

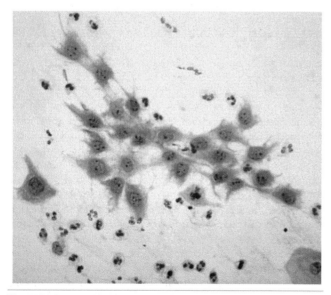

**Fig. 21.23**  Immature squamous metaplasia showing spidery cytoplasmic projections due to forceful removal of the cells from the mucosa.

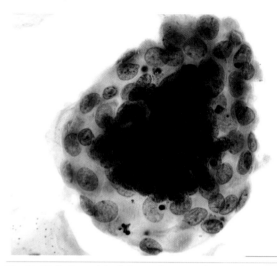

**Fig. 21.24**  Endometrial cells in a well-preserved group showing a central core of compact stroma surrounded by a looser regimented layer of small dark epithelial cells. This is the characteristic appearance of endometrial cells shed early in menstruation.

## Other epithelial and inflammatory cells in cervical and vaginal smears

### Endometrial cells

Endometrial cells may be seen normally in cervical samples up to 12 days from the onset of menstruation. Factors influencing their presence beyond this may reflect underlying endometrial pathology in a woman over 40 years of age or could be due to exogenous hormonal manipulation such as hormone replacement therapy or oral contraceptive use; tamoxifen use, intrauterine device carriage and dysfunctional bleeding are further potential sources of endometrial cells outside the allowed phase of the cycle.

The appearance of endometrial cells varies with the stage of the cycle and their degree of preservation. During and shortly after menstruation they are grouped in well-formed tight three-dimensional clusters with a peripheral rim of epithelial cells and a central core of stromal cells (Fig. 21.24). Degenerative changes quickly supervene, with crumpling of the nuclei and disorganisation of the cells. These then stand out as small clusters of densely hyperchromatic crowded cells (Fig. 21.25), in contrast to the larger, more regular and better-preserved groups of endocervical cells. Neutrophil polymorphs are often seen within endometrial clusters. Endometrial cells of both epithelial and stromal origin can be very well preserved in liquid-based preparations reflecting prompt fixation at the time of sample taking. Loose aggregates and single histiocytes are often associated with shed endometrial cells and may be confused with severely dyskaryotic cells if their reniform nuclei and delicate cytoplasm are overlooked.

The cellular changes in endometrial cells in cervical smears in pathological states, such as endometrial hyperplasia or neoplasia, are described in Chapter 26.

### Reserve cells

Subcolumnar reserve cells are infrequently identified in cervical smears as they do not exfoliate. Possibly they are represented

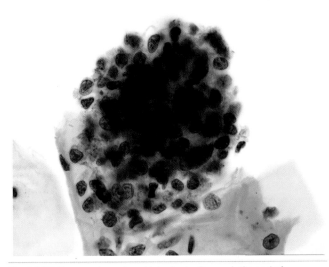

**Fig. 21.25** Degenerate endometrial cells shed towards the end of menstruation are darkly stained and maybe associated with histiocytes and debris. Cell detail can be difficult to make out at this stage and awareness of the timing of smear collection in the cycle is important.

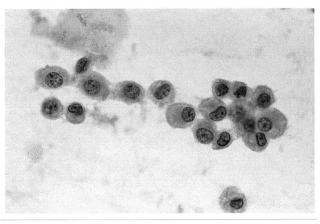

**Fig. 21.27** Macrophages are dissociated cells, varying greatly in size and appearance but often small in cervical smears. This collection includes several with bean-shaped nuclei and foamy cytoplasm, features typical of macrophages.

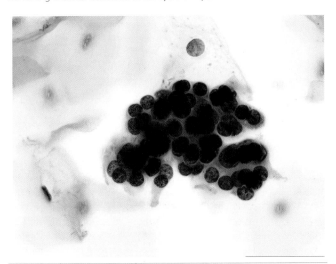

**Fig. 21.26** Reserve cell hyperplasia in a cervical smear. This crowded group of glandular cells includes a population of smaller darker nuclei, presumed to represent reserve cells.

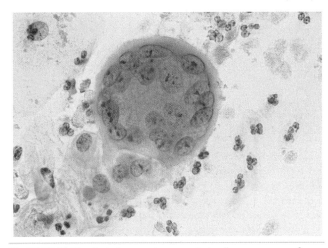

**Fig. 21.28** Multinucleated macrophages or giant cells are a non-specific finding, especially after the menopause. They are also seen in granulomatous inflammation or repair and after radiotherapy.

by some of the bare nuclei seen in the vicinity of some endocervical groups. When reactive reserve cell hyperplasia has occurred the cells can sometimes be identified as syncytial groups of small crowded cells with indistinct cell borders and round darkly stained nuclei which often overlap (Fig. 21.26). They may be distinguished from the cell groups of glandular dyskaryosis by the lack of architectural abnormalities, the smaller size and uniform chromatin pattern of their nuclei and by the presence of associated bare nuclei and normal endocervical cells in conventional smears.

## Neutrophil polymorphs

These are the commonest of the non-epithelial cells found in normal smears, their presence being physiological within the mucous plug of the cervix. They can be found in large numbers without necessarily implying significant infection, although they are usually increased in cases of cervicitis or vaginitis and also in established malignant disease of the cervix. The clinical context and the overall cytological findings are important

in evaluating their significance. There may be problems in the interpretation of a sample if the epithelial cells are largely obscured by polymorphs. This problem is overcome to a considerable extent by the use of liquid-based methods of preparation (see Fig. 21.57).

## Macrophages

Macrophages are sometimes seen as part of the inflammatory cell population, especially following menstruation and in postmenopausal women. They are extremely variable in size and appearance, but can generally be distinguished from parabasal or columnar cells by their ill-defined foamy cytoplasm, their eccentric bean-shaped nuclei, and the presence of ingested particulate material in some instances. However, many of them have small round central nuclei and do not contain phagocytosed particles, making identification less certain. It is helpful when in doubt to examine neighbouring cells as these frequently include other macrophages with more typical features (Fig. 21.27).

Macrophages, although usually dissociated cells, may be loosely aggregated especially in postmenstrual smears. They may become multinucleated and very large, forming giant cells, a phenomenon most often seen in postmenopausal women (Fig. 21.28).

## Lymphocytes

These cells are usually scanty, forming a minor component of the inflammatory cell population in some normal women. They are present in larger numbers in follicular cervicitis, in association with tingible-body macrophages (see Fig. 21.67).

## Other inflammatory cells

Eosinophils, basophils (mast cells) and plasma cells (see Fig. 21.58) are occasionally seen in samples, recognisable by their characteristic morphology.

## Cells other than inflammatory and epithelial cells

### Spermatozoa

Spermatozoa are seen in postcoital smears, even several days after intercourse (Fig. 21.29).

### Contaminants

Cytological specimens can be contaminated at any stage in the collection, transmission or laboratory preparation of the sample. Liquid-based cytology preparations are less prone to contamination from these sources. In addition, cervical samples may include extraneous material from the vagina or vulva, even including parasites or their ova from the digestive tract, especially in those parts of the world where parasitic infestations are common.[3] Even outside such endemic areas parasites are encountered from time to time in cervical smears and their identification is important in patient management.

Ova of the threadworm *Enterobius vermicularis*[4] (Fig. 21.30) are not infrequently seen in smears from infected patients, especially if there is poor personal hygiene. The eggs are oval and are smaller than schistosome ova, with a smooth double-walled shell, often with one side flipped over. The larva can usually be recognised within. Occasionally adult forms can be identified (Fig. 21.31).

Descriptions of *Ascaris lumbricoides*, *Taenia coli*,[5] *Trichuris trichura*, *Hymenolepis nana*[6] and the microfilaria of *Wuchereria bancrofti*[7,8] have been recorded. *Schistosoma haematobium*, *S. japonicum* and *S. mansoni* ova can be identified in smears as elliptical ova, larger than those of the threadworm *E. vermicularis*. The first two are the common types of schistosome ova found in cervical smears and are distinguished by the presence of either a terminal or lateral spine, respectively (Fig. 21.32).[9] The trophozoites of *Balantidium coli* may be seen in patients with intestinal infestation by this uncommon protozoal organism (Fig. 21.33).

*Pediculus humanus*, the body louse, and the pubic louse, *Phthirus pubis*, are seen occasionally in cervical smears (Fig. 21.34). The louse may be damaged during smear preparation, with fragmentation of the tail part from head and legs.

Many external contaminants have been described, including pollen and insects due to atmospheric contamination, and

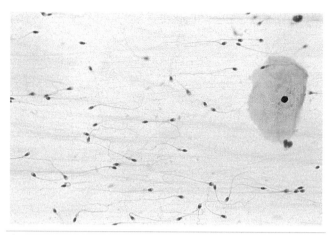

**Fig. 21.29** Spermatozoa are a common finding in cervical samples. They show darkly stained ovoid sperm heads with some preserved tails.

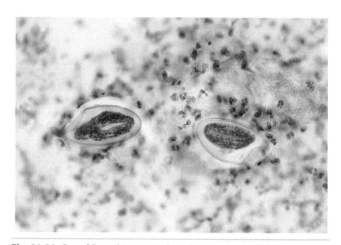

**Fig. 21.30** Ova of *Enterobius vermicularis*, showing the thick glassy eosinophilic capsule and larva within.

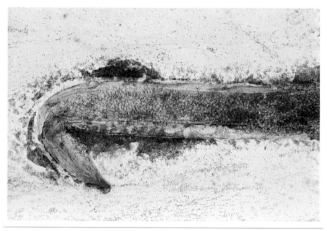

**Fig. 21.31** Adult *Enterobius vermicularis* worm in a conventional cervical smear.

also various fungi, either from contaminated laboratory solutions, the water supply or from the atmosphere (Fig. 21.35). Particulate material from sources such as tampons or glove powder is usually easily identified (Fig. 21.36).[10]

A refractile brown deposit overlying the central portion of the cytoplasm, known as 'cornflake artefact', may be seen

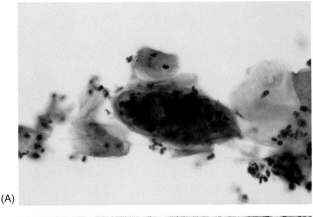

(A)

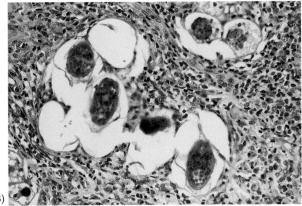

(B)

**Fig. 21.32** (A) *Schistosoma haematobium* ovum in a conventional/direct cervical smear taken from a patient with vulval schistosomiasis. Note the size of the ovum compared with the squamous cells, and the terminal spine. (B) Vulval biopsy from the same patient showing numerous ova within the dermis and a surrounding foreign body reaction (H&E).

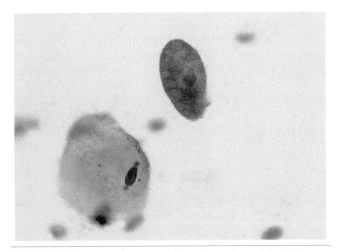

**Fig. 21.33** *Balantidium coli*, a protozoal organism pathogenic in the large bowel, is a rare finding in smears and may not signify infection. In this asymptomatic patient only occasional trophozoites were seen. No treatment was given.

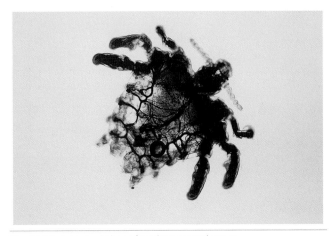

**Fig. 21.34** Pubic (crab) louse found in a cervical smear.

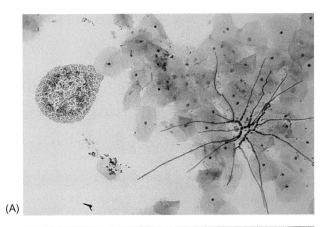

(A)

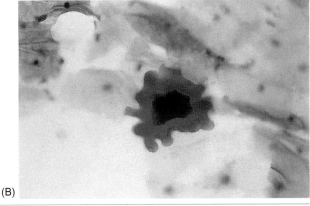

(B)

**Fig. 21.35** (A) Contamination of a cervical sample by fungal spores and hyphae, probably from the atmosphere. (B) A plant particle (scleroid) seen occasionally in smears due to atmospheric contamination.

in samples – particularly on direct smears and may obscure nuclear detail (Fig. 21.37). This is thought to result from the trapping of air on the surface of cells during mounting, especially in thickly spread direct smears. Inadequate removal of spray fixative containing Carbowax may cause similar problems.

The artefact may be so marked as to require a further sample for accurate assessment.

Lubricant contamination may occasionally be seen with some liquid-based cytology preparations. The morphological appearances are variable and include amorphous blue deposits and stringy eosinophilic background material.[11]

Carryover of cellular material from one sample to another may occur during sample preparation, including staining, posing difficulty in assessing the findings. The contaminant cells are often distributed along the upper or side edge of the slide in direct smears and may be in a slightly different plane of focus

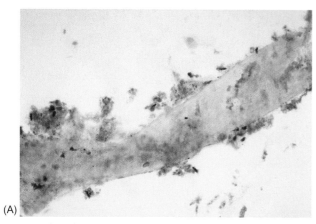

(A)

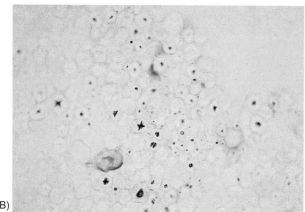

(B)

**Fig. 21.36** (A) Cotton fibres in a conventional/direct cervical smear. (B) Glove powder can often be seen in conventional/direct smears. Even without polarised light, the characteristic Maltese cross structure can be seen at the centre of some of the starch particles.

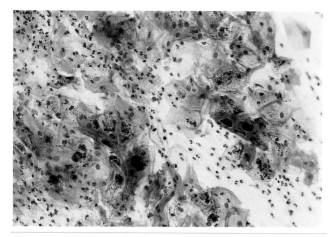

**Fig. 21.37** 'Cornflake' artifact refers to a brown slightly refractile deposit overlying the nuclei, sometimes obscuring nuclear detail completely.

from the rest of the cells. If there is any abnormality in the carryover it is confined to cells at this site and does not appear to relate to the morphology of other cells present.

## Assessment of quality of smears

The question of adequacy of cervical samples is central to the success of cervical screening in the prevention of cervical cancer

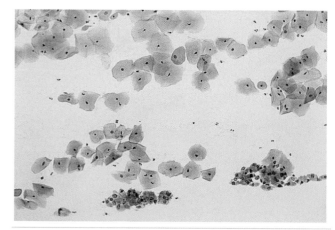

**Fig. 21.38** A good-quality sample consists of well-displayed cells with representative sampling of both squamous and endocervical or metaplastic epithelium.

death (see Chs 22–24). The problem of establishing exactly what constitutes an adequate sample has received increasing attention in recent years, culminating in broad guidelines from various sources, including the British Society for Clinical Cytology (BSCC), which has issued criteria for acceptability of smear quality[12] (currently on direct conventional smears only). In North America, the Bethesda system (TBS) of terminology advocates a minimum threshold for sample adequacy.[13] While there is by no means unanimity over these criteria, it is important that cytologists have a degree of confidence about the threshold of acceptability of sample quality.

The feature of paramount importance in assessing sample quality is that there should be adequate numbers of epithelial cells on the slide, with evidence that they are from the appropriate area of the cervix (Fig. 21.38). In theory, the latter requirement can only be satisfied if squamous metaplastic cells, endocervical cells and mucus are present to indicate transformation zone origin and if the sample taker has visualised the cervix and sampled the entire circumference of the transformation zone at the external os.[14] Clearly, however, metaplastic cells will not be firmly identifiable once the transformation zone is fully mature, and endocervical cells will not always be sampled, especially after the menopause. Recognition of a representative sample therefore requires knowledge of the woman's age and menstrual status and of any hormonal treatment.

Formal training in cervical sample taking is essential if the test is to be reliable and such training is increasingly available. As a quality assurance measure, the proportion of inadequate or unsatisfactory cervical samples in relation to the entire sample workload of a laboratory provides a valuable indication of the standard of reporting and of the level of expertise of the sample takers. The National Health Service Cervical Screening Programme (NHSCSP) has set up a system in England and Wales monitoring laboratory reporting against national targets to ensure that laboratories fall within acceptable ranges for all reporting categories.[12]

In the UK, to reduce the possibility of incorrect assessment by the laboratory, quality control screening procedures are mandatory for all negative and inadequate samples prior to report authorisation. These samples must be read by two independent screeners – one of whom will perform a full in-depth screen with overlapping fields of view and covering the entire sample. The second screener will perform a more rapid assessment of the sample. This may occur after the initial full-screening – so-called 'rapid review' or prior to the full-screen: 'rapid preview'. These abbreviated quality assurance screening methods have been found to detect abnormalities missed on initial primary screening.[15–17]

## Criteria for assessing smear quality

- As a working principle, in conventional/direct samples, the cervical smears should consist of clearly displayed cellular material covering at least one-third of the area under the coverslip, and preferably over one-half. The mere inclusion of columnar or metaplastic cells, or both, does not necessarily confirm that the entire circumference of the transformation zone has been fully sampled. The smear taker has to be relied upon for confirming the thoroughness of the sampling procedure
- Squamous cells of cervical origin are usually distributed in loosely cohesive streaks along the lines of spread of the smear. This is helpful in attempting to determine whether squamous cells are cervical or vaginal in origin, the latter usually lying in a flat dispersed pattern due to the lack of background mucus. However, postmenopausal smears with little or no mucus may, misleadingly, appear to be vaginal in origin
- Whether smears without any endocervical cells or recognisable metaplastic cells should be accepted as representative is debatable. The presence of these cells is determined largely by the position of the squamocolumnar junction and the state of maturation of the transformation zone, factors that are hormone dependent. Thus it may not be possible to include endocervical cells or identify metaplastic cells at all times. An additional factor is the nature of the sampling device (Fig. 21.39), the Aylesbury spatula giving a greater yield from within the canal than the Ayre spatula. Brushes and broom devices provide the largest endocervical component. There are many reports of comparative trials of the different smear taking instruments,[18–22] the general conclusion being that devices with an extended arm give a more representative sample and have a greater likelihood of including abnormalities
- An excess of leucocytes obscuring epithelial cells (Fig. 21.40A) may require investigation for a treatable cause, especially if a discharge is present. Recommendation to repeat the smear at midcycle often provides a better sample than at other times of the cycle. Similarly, unsatisfactory smears taken postnatally should be repeated when normal menstrual cycles are re-established
- Blood-stained smears are often poorly fixed or obscured by the blood (Fig. 21.40B). Contact bleeding on smear taking may be due to an ectropion, requiring treatment before a satisfactory smear can be obtained
- Postmenopausal atrophy leads to scanty or inflamed smears, often with no endocervical cells. The threshold of acceptance of smears from these women must be adjusted, but if there is cause to doubt the adequacy of sampling, a short course of local oestrogen cream prior to smear taking usually ensures better sampling (Figs 21.41A,B).[23]

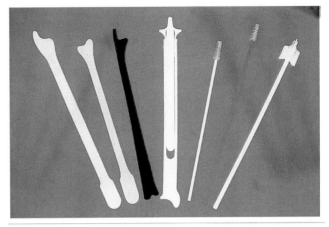

**Fig. 21.39** A sample of the variety of spatulas and brushes available for smear taking. The original Ayre spatula (second from left) is shaped without a prolongation to increase endocervical sampling. The Aylesbury spatula (far left) is in widespread use in the UK. Brushes are recommended for liquid-based cytology.

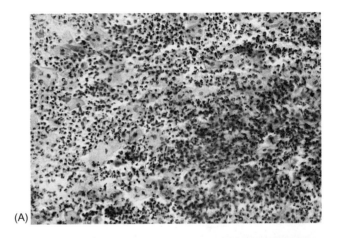

(A)

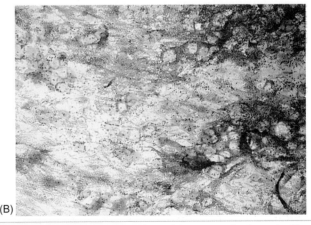

(B)

**Fig. 21.40** Unsatisfactory samples due to: (A) an excess of polymorphs. (B) An excess of blood in a direct/conventional smear.

## Liquid-based cytology samples

Liquid-based thin layer cytological preparations (LBC), usually collected by brush sampling, reduce the rate of obscured and inadequate samples by removing much of the inflammatory debris and blood and providing a representative sample of all

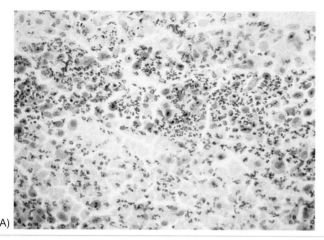
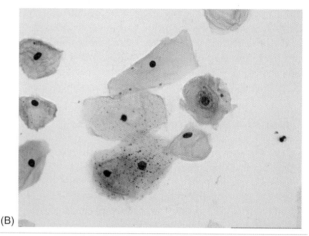

(A)   (B)

**Fig. 21.41** (A) Postmenopausal samples are sometimes unsatisfactory due to a combination of low cellularity and an excess acute inflammatory cell exudate obscuring the underlying epithelial cell morphology. (B) Interpretation can be improved by the use of local oestrogen cream for 1–2 weeks, then repeating the smear; the findings are then usually easily assessed.

of the material from the spatula, most of which is usually discarded in routine smear preparation. Since 2008, the entire UK NHSCSP has adopted LBC preparations. The Bethesda System in America has adopted 5000 cells per sample as a minimum threshold for adequacy.[13] With its 3–5 yearly routine screening interval, the UK NHSCSP's more stringent criteria are considered more appropriate than those adopted by TBS, but none have yet been agreed nationally, and sample adequacy is the subject of a Health Technology Assessments (HTA) study which has yet to report (see Ch. 22).

## Influence of sex hormones on squamous epithelium

The diagnostic potential of cytohormonal evaluation using vaginal smears was reported as early as 1925 by Papanicolaou.[24] Hormonal cytology is a bioassay, which means that it is not a measurement of the concentration of circulating hormone; rather it is the effect of the hormone on the target organ, in this case the stratified squamous epithelium, that is evaluated and this may reflect the combined effect of several hormones. The ratio of superficial cells with pyknotic nuclei to less mature cells with vesicular nuclei was estimated at intervals, giving a karyopyknotic index (KPI). Other indices included counting cells with eosinophilic cytoplasm, so providing an eosinophilic index (EI). Such techniques have now been replaced by direct measurement of serum hormone levels.

## Oestrogens

Oestrogens promote growth and maturation of stratified squamous epithelium up to and including the superficial layer. Smears contain many superficial epithelial cells when the oestrogen level is high and unopposed by progesterone, as in the first half of the menstrual cycle. These cells lie quite flat and are generally discrete; the smear background is noticeably free of polymorphs (Fig. 21.41B).

A small dose of oestrogen can cause atrophic squamous epithelium to develop into epithelium with several layers of

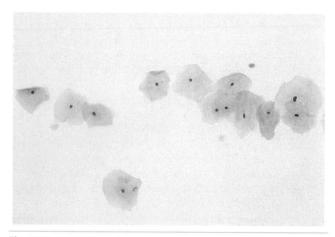

**Fig. 21.42** Oestrogenic effects are manifested by the appearance of large, flat dissociated eosinophilic superficial squamous cells in a clean background.

intermediate cells. When the dose of oestrogen is increased or prolonged, intermediate cells mature into superficial cells.

## Progesterone

Once the stratified squamous epithelium has matured under the influence of oestrogen, progesterone causes rapid desquamation of the topmost layers. The intermediate cells develop curled edges giving a folded appearance, and the cytoplasm often contains glycogen, staining yellow at the centre of the cell. Exfoliation occurs in compact clusters of cells in which the margins of individual cells are indistinct.

Many Döderlein's bacilli (lactobacilli) and leucocytes appear in the smear. They bring about cytolysis of the intermediate cells, causing dissolution of the cell cytoplasm (Fig. 21.43). As a result, numerous naked vesicular nuclei are present and the smear may appear hypocellular. Further progesterone induces the appearance of boat-shaped navicular cells (Fig. 21.44).

When there is mild oestrogen deficiency, as may be encountered at the time of the menopause, the cytological pattern is difficult to distinguish from that of progesterone or androgen

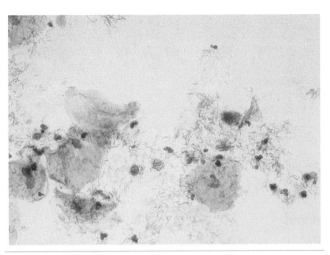

**Fig. 21.43** Progesterone effects include maturation of squamous cells to intermediate level, with increased glycogen content; proliferation of lactobacilli and cytolysis follow further exposure to progesterone.

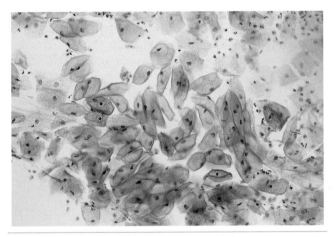

**Fig. 21.44** Navicular cells containing yellow stained glycogen are characteristically boat-shaped with the nucleus pushed to the periphery of the cell and the cytoplasm folded at the cell margins.

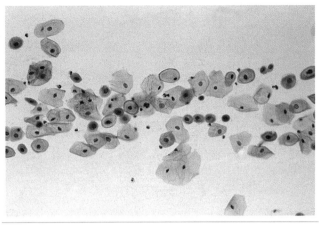

**Fig. 21.45** Androgenic effects include maturation of an atrophic smear to intermediate cell level. The background is usually clean, lacking the cytolysis seen with progesterone activity.

stimulation. The clusters are, however, usually slightly smaller, often containing no more than 10 cells.

If progesterone is administered to patients with an atrophic mucosa, maturation of the squamous epithelium including the superficial layers is the initial result. Administration of progesterone to patients with pre-existing mature epithelium leads to disappearance of the superficial layer and no superficial cells are found in the smear.

## Androgen

Administration of this hormone when the stratified squamous epithelium is atrophic and smears are composed exclusively of parabasal cells results in a predominance of intermediate cells (Fig. 21.45).[25] The smears are particularly rich in cells.[25] If androgens are administered to patients with fully mature stratified squamous epithelium, the opposite effect is seen: superficial cells disappear, to be replaced by intermediate cells. Prolonged administration of androgens produces a smear pattern with cytolysis.

## Physiological cytohormonal patterns

These are best revealed in vaginal smears taken from the lateral vaginal wall, preferably sequentially; but the changes are mirrored by the findings in cervical smears. Vulval tissues are much less responsive to cyclical hormonal fluctuations, although subject to hormonally determined development and atrophy at the menarche and the menopause, respectively.

### Birth–7 days

Maternal sex hormones penetrate the placenta during pregnancy and exert an influence on the epithelial cells of the genital tract of the fetus *in utero*. The vaginal epithelium of a newborn female baby is therefore fully mature.

### From the 1st week to puberty

In this period, production of sex hormones is low. Vaginal smears normally manifest atrophy with many parabasal cells.

### Puberty

With cyclical production of the sex hormones the squamous mucosa slowly reaches maturity. At first, many intermediate epithelial cells are seen; when menstrual cycles begin, many superficial cells are also present. In the second half of these cycles, however, a true progesterone pattern is not apparent as the cycles are initially anovulatory. In the cervix the squamocolumnar junction at this stage coincides with the site of the most distal endocervical gland.

### Sexual maturity

When menstrual cycles become ovulatory, the following consecutive patterns can be expected (see Fig. 21.46):

- Menstrual phase (1st–5th day). The smear contains erythrocytes, leucocytes, endometrial cells, and superficial and intermediate epithelial cells
- Proliferative or follicular phase (6th–10th day). First a large number of histiocytes appear, often in loose aggregates. These are mainly derived from endometrial stromal cells shed in a process known as 'the exodus'. There are also many early intermediate squamous epithelial cells lacking

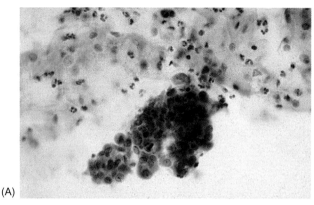

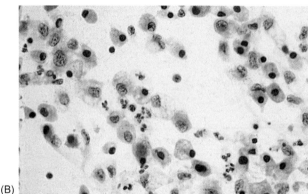

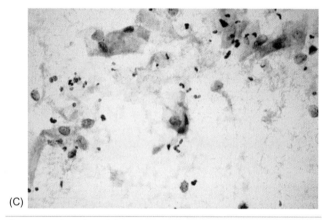

**Fig. 21.46** These three fields show some of the characteristic features of cervical samples at different stages of the menstrual cycle. (A) Menstrual phase with endometrial cells. (B) Early proliferative phase with stromal histiocytes ('exodus'). (C) Late secretory phase with marked cytolysis.

the folding seen under the influence of progesterone. Polymorphs and endometrial cells are present, the latter decreasing in number up to the 10th–12th day. Towards the end of the proliferative phase superficial squamous cells increase in number

- Ovulation (11th–13th day). During this phase there are numerous superficial epithelial cells lying flat and obviously discrete. The pattern is 'clean', that is, practically without leucocytes and with very few bacteria. In some conventional smears the endocervical mucus creates a pattern of ferning on the slide (see Fig. 21.20)
- Secretory or luteal phase (14th–21st day). The pattern changes abruptly after ovulation: now intermediate

squamous cells predominate. Within several days the characteristic progesterone pattern appears, with folding and clustering of intermediate cells, the reappearance of polymorphs and many lactobacilli

- Towards the end of the cycle, marked cytolysis develops, accompanied by a further increase in polymorphonuclear leucocytes. Just before menstruation, the proportion of mature epithelial cells increases once again. A few women also shed endometrial cells several days before menstruation. In some women with normal ovulatory cycles, the characteristic progesterone pattern is absent and only the midcycle peak of oestrogenic effects points to ovulation.

## Pregnancy

In the event of pregnancy, the corpus luteum does not involute but instead grows larger, producing increasing amounts of progesterone and oestrogen. The cytological pattern of pregnancy is that of heightened progesterone activity, with clustering and folding of intermediate cells and the presence of navicular cells. These boat-shaped cells are distended with yellow glycogen, having a rim of folded cytoplasm and the nucleus pushed to the periphery (Fig. 21.44). The changes are most pronounced in the third trimester, when numerous lactobacilli are seen and the accompanying cytolysis is at its height.

About 3 months after conception, the placenta takes over the task of producing progesterone and oestrogens from the corpus luteum. Arias-Stella changes, seen in the endometrium in some pregnancies, may also develop in endocervical glands and have been described as a rare finding in cervical or vaginal smears.[26,27] The cells have an exaggerated secretory pattern as seen in the endometrial glands, and show enlarged degenerate hyperchromatic nuclei with intranuclear inclusions. The association with pregnancy and lack of any preserved abnormal chromatin pattern, combined with awareness of this entity, should ensure correct assessment of the findings.

Syncytiotrophoblastic cells are multinucleated cells from the outer surface of the chorionic villi and hence are foetal in origin, occurring only rarely in cervical cytology samples, for instance from patients with placenta praevia or in the presence of a threatened miscarriage. The cells are large, with an average of 50 nuclei per cell and a characteristic coarse-grained chromatin pattern resembling coarsely ground pepper. The number of nuclei is large in relation to the amount of cytoplasm. The cytoplasm is granular, in contrast to that of a histiocytic giant cell.

Cytotrophoblastic cells also cover the villi. They are cuboidal cells with central nuclei. Cytologically, these cells cannot be firmly identified and may mimic neoplastic cells due to their prominent nucleoli, coarse chromatin pattern and high N:C ratio (Fig. 21.47).

Intact placental villi have occasionally been identified in samples taken postpartum[28] As illustrated in Figure 21.48, a villus may be recognised by its size and form, with degenerate trophoblastic cells and inflammatory debris coating a long three-dimensional structure which has a translucent quality internally.

Decidual cells are modified endometrial stromal cells responding to the high circulating progesterone levels in pregnancy or to high progesterone content oral contraceptives. Decidual changes may also occur in the stromal cells of the cervix and are occasionally sampled in smears taken during or shortly after pregnancy. The cells are swollen and pale due to their content of glycogen. They have abundant clear, sometimes vacuolated cytoplasm and

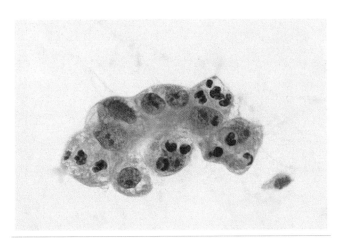

**Fig. 21.47** Trophoblastic cells are difficult to identify with confidence. This group of degenerate cuboidal cells with enlarged hyperchromatic nuclei is presumed to be of cytotrophoblastic origin. The cells were present in a smear taken 2 weeks after a miscarriage. Follow-up samples have been normal.

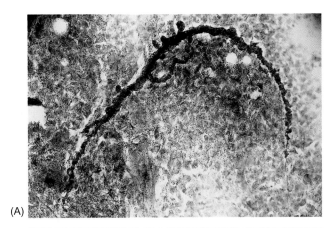

(A)

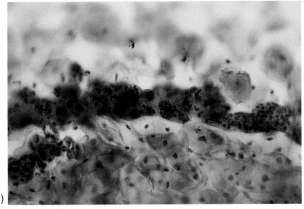

(B)

**Fig. 21.48** (A) Placental villus in a conventional/direct cervical smear taken 6 weeks after delivery. The structure appears three-dimensional on low power. (B) High-power magnification shows degenerate trophoblasts on the outer surface with a few adherent inflammatory cells.

central large nuclei. The chromatin is often smudged and ill-defined and nucleoli are prominent. Decidual cells can be recognised by the fact that, in contrast to squamous epithelial cells, they are not flat but convex; the cells are round to oval and the cytoplasm appears to be less dense than that of epithelial cells (Fig. 21.49).[29]

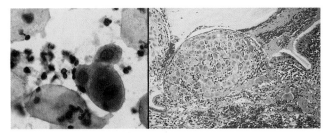

**Fig. 21.49** (A,B) Decidual cells seen in a postnatal cervical sample taken at the same time as the accompanying biopsy. In the sample the cells have dense rather convex cytoplasm with bland nuclei, as in the biopsy (H&E).

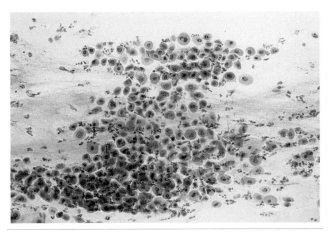

**Fig. 21.50** Postnatal atrophy/lactational change. Note the darkly stained nuclei in some of these small atrophic cells. These changes can be difficult to assess and may require a further smear after menstrual cycles are re-established, for accurate interpretation.

## Postpartum

With expulsion of the placenta, the most important source of progesterone and oestrogen disappears. The smear pattern changes to one chiefly composed of parabasal epithelial cells, which are somewhat angular and contain glycogen or may undergo keratinisation (Fig. 21.50). Such cells are called lactational or postpartum cells. They are derived from the parabasal epithelial layer, which becomes hyperplastic during pregnancy and exfoliates after delivery. These cells may appear in the smear until the normal ovarian cycle has resumed.

One-third of women in the postpartum period do not show these typical postpartum cells; highly divergent patterns may be seen, including inflammatory and repair changes if there has been damage to the cervix in labour.

## Lactation

During breast-feeding, the postpartum pattern described above may persist for as long as the ovarian cycle is suppressed. This picture can pose problems in recognition of precancerous changes since the cells are small and active, with a relatively high N:C ratio. For this reason the postnatal period is best avoided for routine cervical screening, deferring smear taking in well-screened women until normal menstrual cycles have returned.

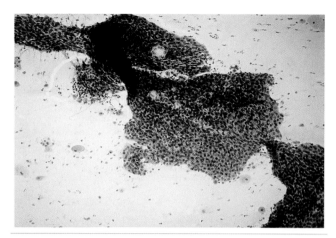

**Fig. 21.51** Postmenopausal atrophy is usually more pronounced than postnatal atrophy, resulting ultimately in sheets of undifferentiated parabasal cells.

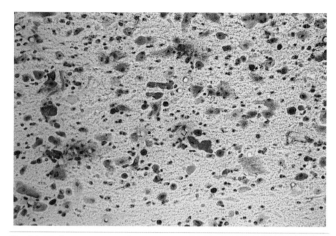

**Fig. 21.52** Postmenopausal atrophic samples may show altered staining of cytoplasm producing the picture referred to as 'red atrophy'. This degree of atrophy may be difficult to assess.

## Premenopausal phase

Just before the onset of the menopause, the cycles often become anovulatory and irregular. In this period persistent ovarian follicles may be encountered when ovulation fails to occur. Unopposed oestrogen production replaces the pro-gestogenic phase of the cycle and smears show a predominance of superficial cells or sometimes intermediate cells without glycogen storage: oestrogen withdrawal bleeding takes place after a variable interval. When both ovulatory and anovulatory cycles occur, a mixed picture is often seen, either due to pro-gesterone effects with many Döderlein's bacilli and cytolysis, or due to early atrophy.

## Postmenopausal state

Following the menopause, when ovarian cycles no longer occur, the stratified squamous epithelium undergoes no further cyclical changes. A highly variable cellular pattern may then be seen. In the early postmenopausal phase, there are many flat dispersed intermediate epithelial cells. Alternatively, a 'mixed pattern' with no single cell type predominating can be found.

With advancing age, progressive atrophy usually occurs but at an unpredictable rate. Eventually in most women, para-basal cells predominate. They are arranged singly or in variable sized sheets of undifferentiated cells with scanty cytoplasm (Fig. 21.51). Endocervical cells may be absent, partly because the squamocolumnar junction has retreated into the canal out of reach of sampling; also because they are less easily dis-tinguished from parabasal cells in sheets. The emergence of many dissociated parabasal cells with dense reddish orange cytoplasm and pyknotic nuclei is aptly termed 'red atrophy' (Fig. 21.52).

Atrophic direct smears may contain cyanophilic bodies known as 'blue blobs' (Fig. 21.53). They are similar in size and shape to parabasal cells. Their origin is disputed, some claim-ing they are degenerate cells, while others have found them to be derived from inspissated mucus. It is likely that both mechanisms are valid. Ultimately, they disintegrate into gran-ular background material. They differ from tumour nuclei in their lack of internal structure and they evoke no inflammatory reaction.[30]

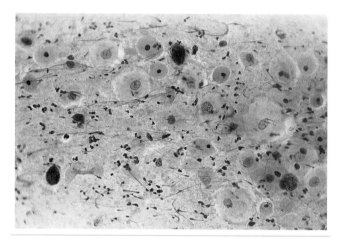

**Fig. 21.53** Round or oval darkly stained bodies known as 'blue blobs' can be a feature of atrophic postmenopausal direct/conventional smears. They must be distinguished from bare nuclei and may raise concern about dyskaryosis, but they lack any defined chromatin pattern.

## Other hormonal effects

Some ovarian neoplasms such as hilus cell and Sertoli-Leydig cell tumours may secrete male sex hormones and granulosa cell tumours frequently produce oestrogens. Vaginal or cervical smears from postmenopausal women who have a granulosa cell tumour may show many superficial cells, and also small groups of endometrial cells (see Ch. 27).

Oestrogen-containing drugs can produce oestrogenic effects, and similarly many superficial cells are found when therapeutic compounds such as digitalis and anticoagulant drugs are taken.

In postmenopausal women, the adrenal glands are the main source of oestrogen. Stimulation of the adrenals, for instance in anxiety states, may result in high levels of all adrenal hormones, resulting in an increase of superficial cells. Similarly, obesity is associated with persistence of oestrogen effects since adipose tissue acts as a depot for steroid hormone production.

## Inflammation and infection of the vagina and cervix

The squamous mucosa of the vagina and cervix are in continuity. Both are therefore exposed to similar risks of infection and have similar protective mechanisms. The vulva shares certain of these risks, although the presence of a surface layer of keratin ensures resistance to some of the infections seen in the adjacent vagina.

The natural protection of the vagina and cervix against infections is determined by the general state of health,[31] a competent immune system,[32] the presence of intact stratified squamous epithelium, the acid pH of the vagina and an equilibrium between the various microorganisms normally present as commensals. These organisms do not cause infection in normal women since they create a stable polymicrobial vaginal milieu. If this equilibrium is disturbed, one type may overgrow the others and the vaginal milieu then becomes monomicrobial. Thus locally, the chance of invasion by microorganisms from outside or of a commensal organism causing inflammation depends upon whether one or more of the following has occurred:

- Damage to the squamous epithelium by mechanical or chemical factors
- An ectropion is present with its thin covering of endocervical columnar epithelium, which is more easily penetrated by bacteria
- A decrease in thickness of squamous epithelium as seen in atrophic mucosa with only a few cell layers
- A change in vaginal pH from acidic to neutral or to an alkaline environment: in the course of the menstrual cycle the pH varies from 6.8 during menstruation to 3.9 during the second half of the cycle
- A rapid increase in or abundance of microorganisms.

## Non-specific cervicitis/vaginitis

Most patients with vaginitis or cervicitis complain of an excessive vaginal discharge, which may be white (leucorrhoea), discoloured or blood-stained. It cannot be assumed that this is always due to infection. Spread of infection is determined to a large extent by the nature of the organism. Various mechanisms by which infectious agents travel from the lower to the upper genital tract include the possibility that trichomonads or spermatozoa act as vectors for the infectious agents, or that passive transport occurs.[33] An ascending infection may ultimately cause endometritis and salpingitis.

Histologically, an acute inflammatory process develops in the stroma, consisting of hyperaemia, exudation of fluid and migration of neutrophil polymorphs from the bloodstream to the site of infection (Fig. 21.54), where they are involved in phagocytosis of organisms and cell debris. Eosinophils are found particularly when the inflammation is due to allergy or parasites. When inflammation persists, it becomes chronic in type, with lymphocytes, plasma cells and histiocytes predominating (Fig. 21.55). Some inflammatory processes are chronic in type from the outset due to the nature of the factors

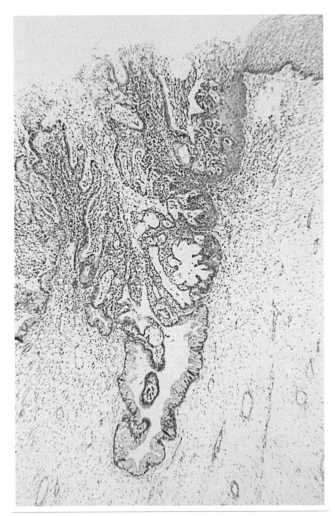

**Fig. 21.54** Acute cervicitis is present in this histological section which shows many neutrophil polymorphs infiltrating the glands and stroma (H&E).

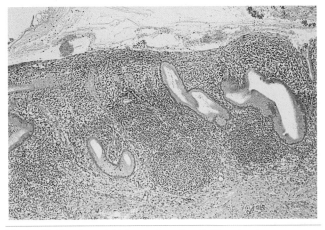

**Fig. 21.55** Chronic cervicitis in a section of cervix. There is a dense infiltrate of chronic inflammatory cells in the submucosa and some lymphoid aggregates with germinal centres have formed, indicating follicular cervicitis (H&E).

inducing the inflammation. Granulomata composed of epithelioid histiocytes, giant cells and lymphocytes may form, particularly with certain specific infecting organisms. Eventually, scarring may ensue.

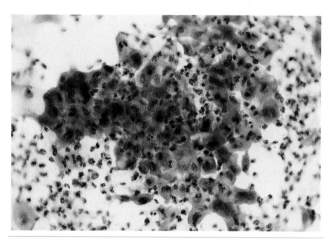

**Fig. 21.56** Acute cervicitis changes in a sample from a patient with vaginal discharge. There is an acute inflammatory exudate of polymorphs around and within the epithelial group. The cells show nuclear enlargement and variable staining.

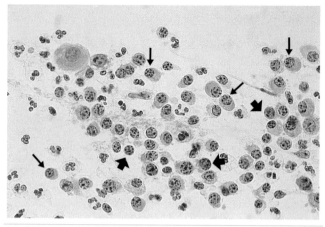

**Fig. 21.58** Lymphocytes and plasma cells mingle together in this smear from a patient with chronic cervicitis. The lymphocytes (arrowheads) have smaller nuclei than the plasma cells,

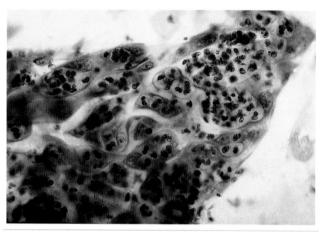

**Fig. 21.57** Acute cervicitis in a sheet of vacuolated metaplastic cells permeated by neutrophil polymorphs, indicating active inflammation.

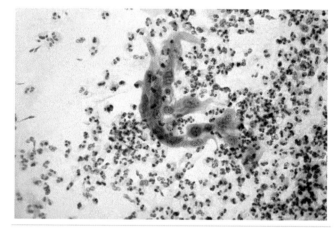

**Fig. 21.59** Metaplastic cells in an inflammatory background, showing marked nuclear reactive and degenerative changes with amphophilic cytoplasmic staining.

## Cytological findings: non-specific cervicitis/vaginitis

### Background findings in inflammatory smears:

- A marked increase in acute inflammatory cells, beyond the physiological mild to moderate leucocytosis seen in normal women
- Epithelial cells covered by an exudate of polymorphs, and polymorphs may be seen permeating the cytoplasm of epithelial cells (Figs 21.56, 21.57)
- Lymphocytes may be present, with or without plasma cells (Fig. 21.58)
- Reactive and degenerative changes in epithelial cells with altered maturity of cells
- Fibrinous and proteinaceous material may form a granular or smooth, usually eosinophilic, background in the smear.

### Cytoplasmic changes in squamous cells include:

- Vacuolation
- Perinuclear haloes
- Altered staining
- Abnormal keratinisation.

Small vacuoles may appear in the cytoplasm, sometimes merging into a single large vacuole pushing the nucleus to one side. The residual thin border of cytoplasm can usually be identified as that of a squamous cell because it retains its compact appearance. Leucocytes may be seen within vacuoles in the epithelial cells, a process known as leucophagocytosis or emperipolesis (Fig. 21.57). Condensation or thinning of cytoplasm may occur (Figs. 21.59, 21.60). The cytoplasm immediately surrounding the nuclear membrane is often lighter in colour, forming a narrow zone of clearing (Fig. 21.61). The boundary of this halo is often vague.

Changes in staining reaction are seen with certain types of inflammation. Intermediate, parabasal and metaplastic cells show eosinophilia. In senile vaginitis when there is inflammation of atrophic squamous mucosa parabasal cells may stain deep orange to red with eosin and the cytoplasm appears more dense than normal (see Fig. 21.52). Premature or excessive keratinisation of squamous cells may occur. The former involves individual cell keratinisation and is referred to as dyskeratosis (Fig. 21.62). Surface keratinisation may retain nuclear remnants forming layers of parakeratosis (see Fig. 21.12) or may consist of pure keratin (Fig. 21.63). Although non-specific, these changes are most often seen in association with human papillomavirus infection.

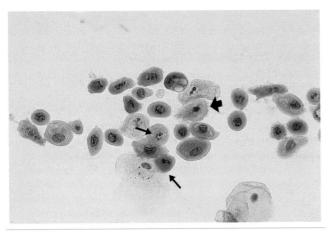

**Fig. 21.60** Metaplastic cells showing variable preservation of cytoplasm with karyorrhexis (arrows) and pyknosis (arrowhead) of nuclei due to degenerative changes in response to inflammation

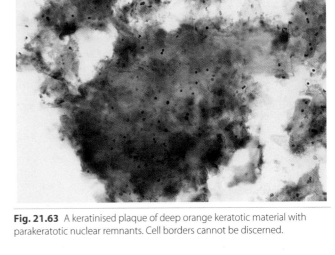

**Fig. 21.63** A keratinised plaque of deep orange keratotic material with parakeratotic nuclear remnants. Cell borders cannot be discerned.

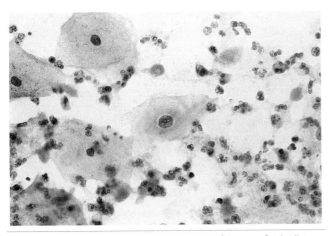

**Fig. 21.61** Perinuclear haloes can be seen in two of the superficial cells, forming a narrow zone of pallor around the nucleus. This is a non-specific inflammatory response most often seen in *Trichomonas vaginalis* infection, as here, or due to *Candida* infection.

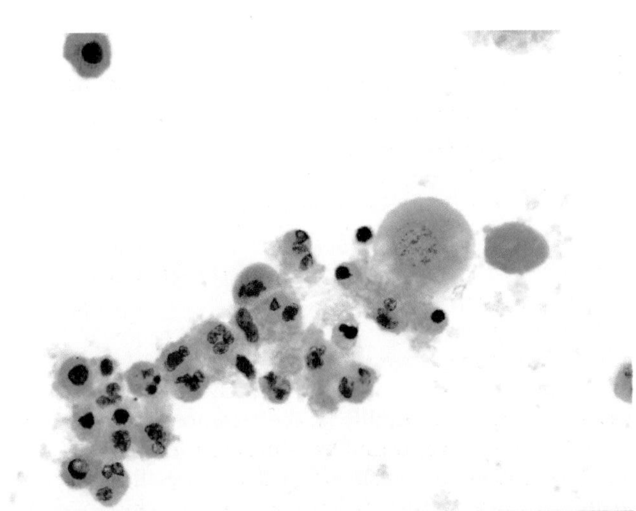

**Fig. 21.62** Dyskeratosis in immature squamous cells with dense green and occasional orangeophilic cytoplasm. The nuclei show degenerative changes, including ghost nuclei on the right.

### Nuclear abnormalities in squamous cells include:

- Swelling/anisonucleosis
- Wrinkling of nuclear membranes
- Multinucleation
- Chromatin degeneration.

The nucleus commonly enlarges, with pale staining chromatin due to fluid absorption. This results in considerable variation in nuclear size. Wrinkling of the nuclear membrane may occur, with selective condensation of chromatin at the nuclear margin and clearing of the nucleus centrally (Fig. 21.60) but nuclear symmetry is retained. Multinucleation is common. Condensation of the chromatin, known as pyknosis, may occur in dying cells, or the nucleus may disintegrate and fragment in a process known as karyorrhexis (Fig. 21.61). Dissolution of the nucleus or karyolysis is sometimes seen in inflamed smears. Nucleoli may be prominent and multiple or may disappear altogether.[34]

### Endocervical cell inflammatory changes include:

- Cytoplasmic degeneration
- Variation in nuclear size
- Ciliocytophthoria.

Sometimes, the delicate cytoplasm loses definition and lies in tatters around the nucleus or is permeated by polymorphs (Fig. 21.64). Nuclei vary markedly in size, but the shape remains round to oval. Nucleoli may be enlarged or multiple. The chromatin is often somewhat coarsened but never markedly so. Nuclear overlapping due to cell crowding, as seen in dyskaryotic columnar cells, does not occur apart from when due to multinucleation, which is common in individual cells. When regeneration supervenes, mitotic figures are seen in the endocervical epithelium, but the mitoses are always morphologically normal.

Occasionally anucleate small ciliated tufts are found, consisting of the terminal plate and pink or red cilia (Fig. 21.65), mingling with vacuolated endocervical cells without cilia resembling histiocytes. Pyknotic nuclear remnants are usually also seen. This phenomenon, ciliocytophthoria (CCP), was originally thought to be due solely to viral damage, but is now recognised as a non-specific degenerative change.[35]

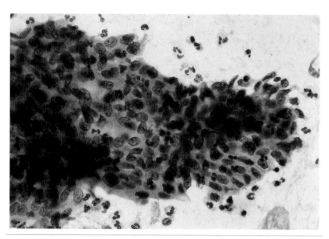

**Fig. 21.64** A sheet of endocervical cells showing polymorphs within the cell group. There is loss of the regular honeycomb pattern with some nuclear irregularity and ragged cytoplasmic borders.

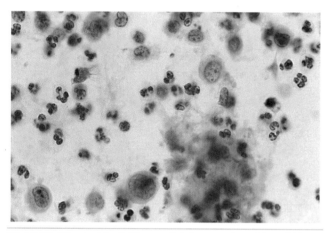

**Fig. 21.65** Ciliocytophthoria. The sample is from a patient with cervicitis associated with an IUCD. A tuft of pink cilia can be seen (left) with cell debris and pyknotic nuclear remnants on the right.

## Diagnostic pitfalls: non-specific cervicitis

Although several studies have shown that inflammatory changes in smears are associated with isolation of pathogenic organisms in around 40% of cases,[36,37] the overall significance of inflammatory changes in smears from asymptomatic women has been called into question by other work showing lack of correlation between smear findings and identification of pathogens. One practice-based study in Canada[38] found a virtually equal rate of positive cultures (48% and 47%, respectively) in women with and without cytological inflammatory changes. The authors conclude that inflammatory smears are a poor predictor of cervical infection.

Readers experienced in cytology will be aware that there are some inflammatory and degenerative characteristics shared with dyskaryotic squamous cells. These include nuclear enlargement, chromatin condensation, hyperchromasia and altered cytoplasm. Dyskaryotic cells, however, usually exhibit

coarse chromatin granularity, uneven chromatin clumping causing irregular nuclear contours, or other abnormalities of chromatin pattern, in contrast to the empty-looking nucleus with marginal chromatin condensation seen in the presence of inflammation. Nevertheless, diagnostic problems in this area should not be underestimated.

Caught between uncertainty about the significance of an inflammatory picture, the risk of under-reporting a potentially serious abnormality and the desire not to engender unnecessary anxiety for the patient, the cytologist must interpret inflammatory smear findings in the light of clinical details and the degree of confidence in establishing the absence of dyskaryosis, given that the sample is of appropriate quality. National policies on management of smears with inflammatory changes and possible dyskaryosis vary widely, but should be based on the following principles:

- In the UK, samples in which there are nuclear changes that might be dyskaryotic are reported as showing 'borderline nuclear changes' ('atypical squamous cells of undetermined significance' (ASCUS) in TBS[13]), and repeated after a short interval. Referral for colposcopy is indicated if the nuclear changes persist. UK guidelines have been published[39,40] for distinguishing borderline changes from minor reactive changes and from dyskaryosis
- Minor inflammatory changes that are clearly not dyskaryotic and which show no evidence of a specific pathogen can be reported as 'within normal limits'
- In the presence of a vaginal discharge or clinical evidence of cervicitis, a borderline smear picture should encourage the clinician to undertake microbiological investigations prior to repeating the smear
- In some cases, inflammatory changes may mimic high-grade dyskaryosis. In such instances, changes are reported as 'borderline/high-grade dyskaryosis cannot be excluded'. Because the patients given such a grade are referred directly to colposcopy and biopsy, this category should be used sparingly (see Ch. 25).

Examples of findings from a case with simple reactive changes not requiring early repeat smears, a case with more marked nuclear abnormality reported as showing borderline nuclear changes necessitating a follow-up smear in 3–6 months and an example of definite dyskaryosis requiring referral for colposcopy are shown in sequence in Figure 21.66. The diagnosis of dyskaryosis is the subject of the following chapters and the use of the term 'borderline change' is explored further in Chapter 25.

## Special types of cervicitis and vaginitis

### Follicular cervicitis

This condition, also known as chronic lymphocytic cervicitis, is characterised histologically by the presence of a submucosal infiltrate of lymphocytes forming lymphoid follicles with active germinal centres (see Fig. 21.55). Although usually an incidental finding in postmenopausal women, in younger women there is some association with chlamydial infection. In the presence of ulceration or if the cervix is scraped firmly, elements of a follicle may be found in smears.

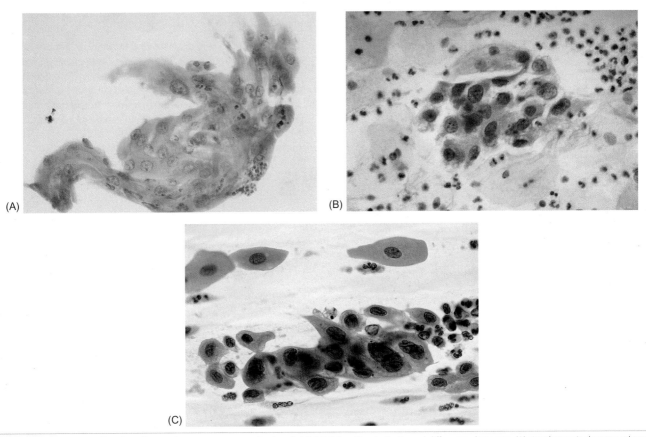

**Fig. 21.66** A spectrum of nuclear changes in squamous metaplastic cells highlighting the similarity and differences between: (A) simple repair changes where there is bland nuclear enlargement in a group of immature metaplastic cells; (B) Borderline changes in metaplastic cells with some nuclear hyperchromasia but the group also includes normal nuclei (see cells on left of group) and (C) dyskaryotic nuclear changes in partially mature cells, in which the enlarged irregular nuclei show coarsely granular chromatin.

### Cytological findings: follicular cervicitis (Fig. 21.67)

- Small and large lymphocytes
- Tingible body macrophages
- Other inflammatory cells.

Small mature lymphocytes are characterised by a thin eccentric rim of cytoplasm, round hyperchromatic nuclei with uniformly dense chromatin and no obvious nucleoli. Larger immature lymphocytes, several times the size of the small lymphocytes and with paler nuclei are also present.

Tingible body macrophages from the germinal centre of the lymphoid follicles confirm the diagnosis. These cells have pale nuclei and prominent nucleoli, with vague but voluminous cytoplasm, typically containing ingested cellular debris. Mitotic figures may be observed among these cells. Plasma cells and polymorphonuclear leucocytes are sometimes present.

### Diagnostic pitfalls: follicular cervicitis

Follicular cervicitis may prompt a false positive diagnosis of severe dyskaryosis if the small dispersed lymphoid cells are not correctly identified in liquid-based cytology samples. Helpful pointers include recognition of clusters of lymphoid cells including tingible body macrophages.[41]

The findings may also be mistaken for malignant lymphoma (see Ch. 13). In malignant lymphoma, the pattern is usually rather monotonous, consisting predominantly of one type of cell with no tingible body macrophages, whereas a great variety of cells is seen in chronic lymphocytic cervicitis.

## Atrophic vaginitis

Senile or atrophic vaginitis implies inflammation of the atrophic epithelium of the vagina and cervix associated with hormonal deprivation, as occurs in many postmenopausal women. This smear picture may not be accompanied by any clinical symptoms.

### Cytological findings: atrophic vaginitis

- Poorly preserved parabasal cells, usually dissociated
- Numerous polymorphs covering other cells.

The parabasal cells are often poorly stained with dense irregular or pyknotic or fragmented nuclei. There is often a marked acute inflammatory cell infiltrate reflecting the thinned epithelium which is prone to damage. Although much of this inflammatory cell exudate can be removed with newer liquid-based cytology techniques, if the morphology of the underlying epithelial cells is still obscured by inflammation that sample should be considered inadequate for further evaluation. A change in the staining reaction of the cytoplasm of the majority of cells in the smear from green to deep orange is sometimes seen, producing appearances known as 'red atrophy' (Figs 21.52, 21.68). There may also be a tendency for cells to form syncytia.[42] In conventional smears, with loss of cytoplasm the nuclei may appear as dark purple nuclear streaks due to the spreading and 'blue blobs' may be noted.

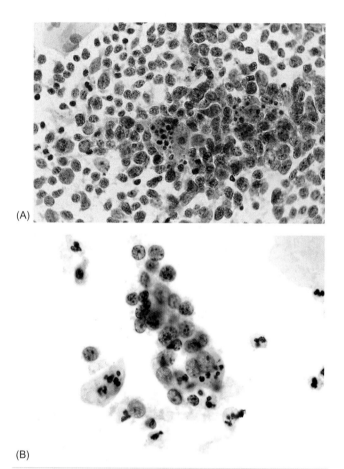

(A)

(B)

**Fig. 21.67** (A) Follicular cervicitis. An aggregate of lymphoid cells at the centre is surrounded by scattered lymphocytes of variable size. Several tingible body macrophages are present at the centre, with ingested particulate material in the cytoplasm. (B) High power of follicular cervicitis in which single lymphoid cells may mimic severe dyskaryosis.

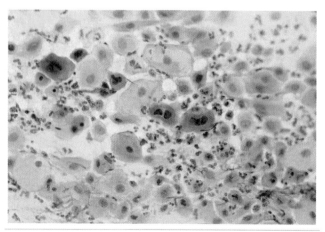

**Fig. 21.68** This atrophic smear is from a postmenopausal woman aged 59 and shows several partially keratinised orange cells with hyperchromatic and irregular nuclei. They appear degenerate and chromatin detail cannot be seen. Subsequent direct smears reverted to normal after use of local oestrogen cream.

## Diagnostic pitfalls: atrophic vaginitis

The cytological picture of senile vaginitis may be difficult to interpret as pyknotic nuclei in particular cause problems in evaluation. It is essential to note that these nuclei are dark and homogeneous without a clearly defined chromatin pattern (see Fig. 21.52). When interpretation of a smear from a patient with senile vaginitis is difficult, the clinician can be requested to treat the patient with oestrogen, either applied locally or taken orally. A smear test 1–2 weeks later will have a clean background with more mature epithelial cells that are usually easily assessed (see Fig. 21.41A,B). If dyskaryotic cells are present they should be recognisable because they do not mature.[43]

## Bacterial microorganisms of the vagina and cervix

In routine smears it is only possible to establish the shape and distribution of bacteria. These features may suggest a particular organism but definitive identification must be made by microbiological culture. It is essential to be fully aware of the endogenous flora of the vagina to understand the role of bacteria in vaginitis and cervicitis.

## Endogenous flora of the vagina

Döderlein's bacilli or lactobacilli are rod-shaped organisms 3–6 μm in length, arranged singly or in chains (Fig. 21.69). Their enzymes are able to dissolve the cell wall of intermediate cells by cytolysis, freeing the glycogen content.

Lactobacilli are not found in cervical samples when the pH is alkaline, as they are dependent on an acid pH. Lactobacillus overgrowth with extreme cytolysis can occur during pregnancy, in the second half of the menstrual cycle, when progesterone containing contraceptive drugs are used, and sometimes at the menopause, especially in diabetics.

Corynebacteria are Gram-positive bacilli that can theoretically be distinguished from lactobacilli by their arrangement in

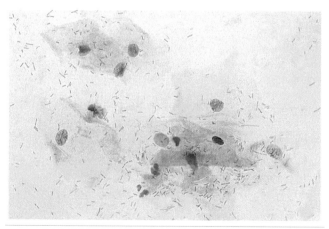

**Fig. 21.69** Lactobacilli. The background of this smear shows numerous rod-shaped organisms, arranged singly and in short chains. Cytolysis of intermediate cells is also apparent, leaving bare nuclei and wisps of cytoplasm.

groups. However, identification is almost impossible to achieve in a cervical smear. These bacteria can proliferate in the vagina because the mucous membrane functions as a culture medium, breakdown of the epithelial cells ensuring a continuous supply of nutrients in the form of amino acids and glycogen.

Leptothrix are non-pathogenic thread-like bacteria lying in loops or sometimes in pairs (Fig. 21.70). They are much longer than Döderlein's bacilli and the latter never lie in loops. Leptothrix are sometimes found together with trichomonads. The presence of Leptothrix in a smear is of no clinical importance and their precise microbiological identity is unclear.

## Exogenous bacteria

Bacteria from the surrounding environment can be introduced into the vagina. If the endogenous flora is poorly developed, for instance before puberty when the epithelium is thin and contains no glycogen, local organisms from outside the vagina proliferate and may eventually dominate the field.

In adults, microorganisms from without are most commonly introduced during coitus from the skin of the vulva, perineum or penis. Semen, too, can contain pathogenic microorganisms from the urethra or prostate gland of the sexual partner in cases of urethritis or prostatitis. Other sources of extrinsic infection include spread of organisms from the upper genital tract and blood-borne spread.

### Coccoid overgrowth

The perineal skin flora forms a heterogeneous group of organisms consisting of short rods and cocci. Staphylococci in groups and streptococci in chains are included in this coccoid flora and may gain access to the vagina or cervix. They are only pathogenic in the vagina when the epithelium is damaged.

Coitus influences the pH and protein concentration in the vagina since semen is alkaline and the ejaculate is rich in protein. Both factors can affect bacterial growth: coccoid organisms, in particular, need an alkaline environment for an overgrowth to occur, while the altered pH inhibits the growth of lactobacilli. The presence of coccoid bacteria is not usually reported.

### Gardnerella vaginalis

*Gardnerella vaginalis* is a small rod-shaped bacterium. It is transmitted by sexual intercourse and can be cultured in 20% of asymptomatic women. The significance of this finding is not well understood,[44] but the organism can be associated with the symptomatic condition bacterial vaginitis,[45] also known as bacterial vaginosis.[46] Patients with symptoms due to bacterial vaginosis have pruritus and leucorrhoea. The vagina contains a mixed population of microorganisms, including *Gardnerella vaginalis, Bacteroides* spp., anaerobic cocci, *Mobiluncus* spp. and *Mycoplasma hominis*. A pH above 4.5 and interaction between *Gardnerella* and various *Bacteroides* organisms are factors in the production of symptoms.

Since the exact aetiology and pathogenesis of bacterial vaginosis is still unclear, the definition of bacterial vaginosis proposed at an international meeting held in Stockholm in 1984 is followed: 'A replacement of Döderlein bacteria by characteristic groups of bacteria accompanied by changed properties of the vaginal fluid'. Clinically, the diagnosis is based on the presence of a thin homogeneous discharge with a pH above 4.5 and a fishy amine odour, more manifest when the pH is further raised by KOH. Diagnosis is particularly important in pregnancy, as there is a risk of chorioamnionitis and preterm delivery if the condition is untreated.[47,48]

### Cytological findings: *Gardnerella vaginalis*

- Clue cells
- Mixed bacteria, mainly coccoid
- Absence of polymorphs.

In a routine smear, coccoid bacteria are seen mainly on squamous epithelial cells which, as a result, stain darkly and appear cloudy (Fig. 21.71). In the North American literature these cells are called 'clue cells', but the term 'glue cell' may be more apt since the *Gardnerella* organisms seem to be glued to squamous cells. Examination of these cells under oil immersion allows detection of the different organisms present; small rods which are *Gardnerella vaginalis*, cocci and curved bacilli, *Mobiluncus spp*[49] The range of organisms present can be confirmed by Gram-stain.[50]

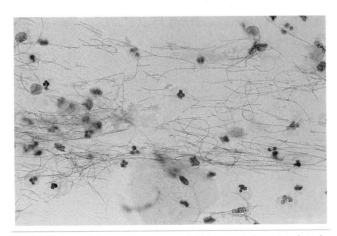

**Fig. 21.70** Leptothrix organisms are seen in this smear in long strands and loops. Note the absence of any significant inflammatory infiltrate.

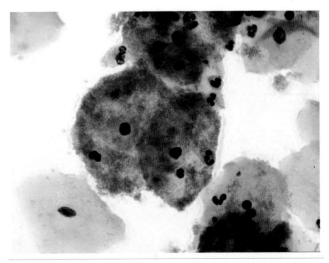

**Fig. 21.71** Coccoid overgrowth creating a bacterial haze over a superficial cell.

## Actinomyces spp.

*Actinomyces* organisms are 'higher bacteria', capable of forming colonies, and commonly found in the cervical smears of women using various types of intrauterine devices (IUDs),[51] particularly plastic devices. The organisms are usually saprophytic and cause no symptoms. They are also found in association with vaginal pessaries, and in the presence of foreign bodies such as forgotten tampons. They are frequently present in the tonsillar crypts of the pharynx, and may therefore be transmitted to the vagina by orogenital contact. Gupta[52] reports that actinomycotic infection can cause clinical symptoms of lower genital tract inflammation, including a malodorous brownish discharge in some cases. Dissemination of *Actinomyces* spp. to distant sites has also been documented.[53]

---

### Cytological findings: *Actinomyces* spp.

- Colonies of filamentous organisms staining dark blue
- Variable inflammatory exudate
- Variable inflammatory changes in epithelial cells.

---

With Papanicolaou staining, actinomycotic colonies appear as dark 'bales of wool', stained blue with haematoxylin. Thin radiating filaments protrude outwards from the central tangled mass (Fig. 21.72A). The diagnostic sulphur granules seen macroscopically in sputum are seldom found in cervicovaginal smears. Special stains, such as the Gram-stain or Gomori's methenamine silver, may be of help in confirming the diagnosis and in differentiating these bacteria from other organisms forming radiating colonies (Fig. 21.72B).[52] Lactobacilli are usually absent, having been replaced by a coccoid flora.

Non-specific inflammation frequently accompanies the organisms, whether or not there are any symptoms. The epithelial cells may show inflammatory changes; particularly endocervical and endometrial cells. In the latter the endometrial groups may appear slightly enlarged with vacuolated cytoplasm. Dispersed discrete single cells may be identified too – either shed from the endometrial clusters or representing inflamed/metaplastic changes in endocervical cells. Actinomycotic organisms are usually commensal. However, some gynaecologists advocate removal of the IUD and treatment with antibiotics because in rare instances certain *Actinomyces* spp. may cause pelvic inflammatory disease with subsequent infertility or ectopic pregnancy. The presence of actinomycotic organisms in a smear is usually reported to enable interpretation of the finding in the light of any clinical abnormalities, but the mere presence of the organism cannot be equated with infection.

## Neisseria gonorrhoeae

Gonorrhoea is caused by gonococci *Neisseria*. In women, the epithelial cells of the urethra and endocervix are infected. Infection may extend to the vestibular glands causing bartholinitis and to the endometrium causing endometritis or salpingitis if the fallopian tubes are involved. Involvement of the peritoneal cavity may lead to pelvic inflammatory disease.

In cervical samples the bacteria are shaped like coffee beans in a characteristic pattern of pairs (diplococci), whereby the round sides of the two beans face outward. They are slightly larger than the cocci of the perineal flora and have occasionally been identified in routine Papanicolaou stained cervical smears.[54] The mainstay of diagnosis is by microbiological culture or by RNA–DNA *in situ* hybridisation.

## Mycobacterium tuberculosis

Tuberculous endometritis or cervicitis is almost always secondary to tuberculosis of the fallopian tubes, which in turn results from blood-borne infection due to primary tuberculosis of lung

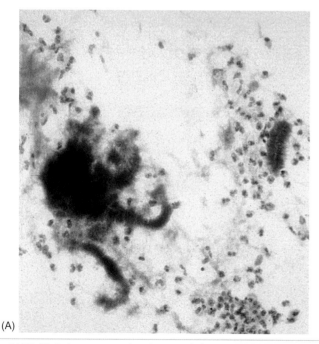 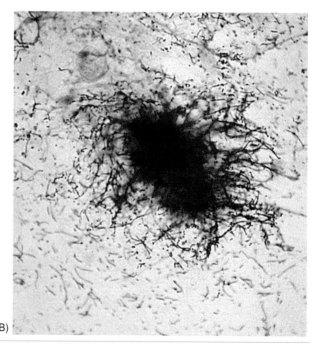

(A)        (B)

**Fig. 21.72** (A) *Actinomyces* organisms in a sample from an asymptomatic woman with an IUCD *in situ*. The organisms form a tangled mass of filamentous bacteria projecting irregularly from the margins. (B) Gram-staining of a destained sample shows the filamentous structure of the organisms and reveals many organisms in the background.

or intestine. The infection is relatively rare in Western society, but is more common in developing countries.

Tuberculosis cervicitis or endometritis histologically is characterised by granulomatous inflammation with caseation necrosis. Acid fast bacilli may be demonstrated by Ziehl Neelsen staining. Cervical cytology samples, from these patients, may be unaffected or contain exfoliated acute and chronic inflammatory cells as well as cells from the granulomatous inflammation including histiocytes, giant cells and even granular amorphous background matrix material indicating caseation necrosis.[55] Correlation with the clinical picture and microbiological culture is mandatory.

The pattern of tuberculous cervicitis must be distinguished from tissue repair and ulceration, either of which may accompany the infection. Samples then show ragged sheets of reactive epithelial cells with enlarged nuclei and prominent nucleoli as well as non-specific background inflammation.

### Calymmatobacterium (Donovania) granulomatosis

This bacterium causes granuloma inguinale (donovaniasis), a venereal infection common in tropical and subtropical climates, being rare in Europe and the USA. It induces granulomatous inflammation with caseous necrosis mainly in the skin of the external genitalia and perianal region. Scrapings from ulcerated lesions of the vulva, vagina or cervix show histiocytes with multiple vacuoles containing straight or curved dumbell-shaped rods. They have prominent bipolar granules known as Donovan bodies.[56,57] Donovan bodies can be visualised with Warthin–Starry silver staining method as well as by Giemsa staining.

### Treponema pallidum

The spirochaetal organism *Treponema pallidum*, causative agent of syphilis, usually infects the vulva initially but may produce a primary chancre on the cervix. The organisms cannot be identified in Papanicolaou stained smears, although demonstrable by silver stains such as the Warthin–Starry method. The overall picture in a cervical sample is that of non-specific inflammation.

## Protozoa

### Trichomonas vaginalis

*Trichomonas vaginalis* is a protozoan organism found in the vagina, either as a saprophyte or as a pathogenic organism.[58] In the male, the organism can be found in the prostate gland. Infection is regarded as venereal in origin,[59] requiring treatment of both partners for complete eradication. *Trichomonas vaginalis* infection can produce a variety of symptoms including a foamy or white discharge, vaginal dryness, postcoital and intermenstrual bleeding. Punctate haemorrhagic spots may develop in the mucosa, an appearance known as 'strawberry vagina'.

*Trichomoniasis* is usually but not invariably associated with inflammation. The vaginal pH is often alkaline, and a coccoid flora is frequently seen.

### Cytological findings: *Trichomonas vaginalis* (Figs 21.73–21.75)

- Unicellular pear-shaped organisms 8–20 μm in diameter
- Pale grey-green cytoplasm with eosinophilic granules centrally

- Oval or crescentic vesicular nuclei, lightly stained
- Inflammatory changes in cells often pronounced.

Trichomonads vary in size and shape, sometimes even occurring as giant forms measuring over 150 μm. There is some correlation between size and pathogenicity: the smaller organisms are more likely to be symptomatic. They vary from oval or triangular to comma or tadpole-shaped and move by means of trailing flagella, which are rarely seen in Papanicolaou-stained smears. They multiply by binary fission and the organisms can be found in mitosis.

With a pronounced inflammatory reaction, the sample shows a characteristic purple colour caused by the pinkish red colour of mature epithelial cells and the darkly stained polymorphs. The latter are often arranged as an agglomeration around an organism. A web of fibrinous exudate may be seen in the background. Leptothrix organisms may be present as well.

Trichomonads sometimes attach to the surface of squamous cells to form a ring around the margin. They may even invade the epithelial cell cytoplasm. The nuclei of squamous epithelial cells are enlarged and hyperchromatic; the chromatin pattern can be irregular and perinuclear haloes are common.[60] Secondary orangeophilia of cell cytoplasm may be seen.

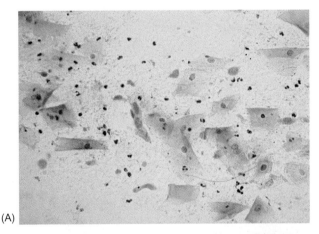

(A)

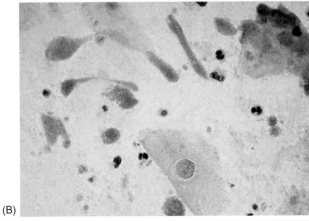

(B)

**Fig. 21.73** (A) *Trichomonas vaginalis* organisms are rounded or ovoid cyanophilic organisms, larger than polymorphs but smaller than the parabasal cells at centre. (B) This closer view of the protozoa shows their variable shapes. The cytoplasmic granules and outline of a nucleus can just be discerned. Note the halo around the intermediate cell nucleus.

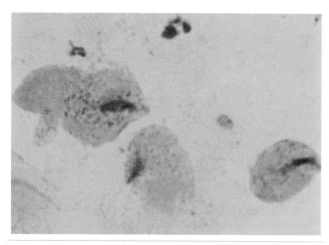

**Fig. 21.74** Giant trichomonads showing obvious vesicular crescentic nuclei stained lightly by haematoxylin.

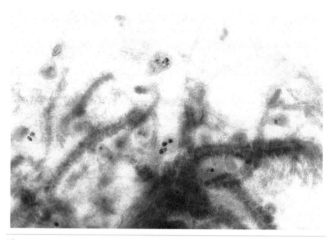

**Fig. 21.76** *Entamoeba gingivalis* organisms can be seen at the margins of this colony of actinomycotic organisms in a smear from a patient with an IUCD. The protozoa have ingested fragments of leucocytes.

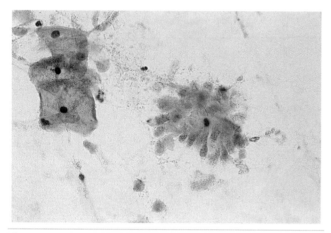

**Fig. 21.75** Trichomonads attached to the margin of a squamous cell. Many free organisms are also seen.

### Diagnostic pitfalls: *Trichomonas vaginalis*

In atrophic smears mucus, cell fragments and parabasal cells with karyolysis can be mistaken for trichomonads. Although similar in size and staining, they lack the crescentic nucleus and cytoplasmic granules of *T. vaginalis*.

## Entamoeba gingivalis

*Entamoeba gingivalis* has been reported in 10% of patients with an IUD colonised by actinomycotic organisms.[61] This protozoan parasite is often found in the oral cavity if teeth and gums are in poor condition. Spread to the genital tract probably occurs by orogenital contact. *Entamoeba gingivalis* is unlikely to be pathogenic in this setting.

### Cytological findings: *Entamoeba gingivalis*

- Rounded amoeboid organisms 10–40 μm in diameter
- Pale cyanophilic cytoplasm with eccentric nuclei
- Ingested polymorphs within cytoplasm.

The organism is virtually always found in combination with actinomycotic colonies at the borders of the tangled organisms where it attaches itself to the filaments ( Fig. 21.76). *E. gingivalis* can usually be differentiated from the more pathogenic *E. histolytica*. Trophozoites of the former show ingestion of polymorphs, a coarser karyosome, less delicate pattern of peripheral chromatin and multidirectional pseudopodia; *E. histolytica* trophozoites contain ingested erythrocytes, a fine central karyosome, delicate peripheral chromatin and unidirectional pseudopodia.[62]

## Entamoeba histolytica

*Entamoeba histolytica* infection, also known as *amoebiasis*, is widespread in subtropical and tropical areas. Infection begins when trophozoites invade the colonic mucosa and may remain localised for many years, or may extend to the liver and other organs, including the female genital tract. The majority of patients with genital amoebiasis have simultaneous amoebic colitis, suggesting that protozoa reach the genital tract by direct contamination due to poor hygiene.

Cytological diagnosis is based on identification of the protozoa. These small round or oval organisms have cytoplasm staining faintly with the light green component of the Papanicolaou stain. Erythrophagocytosis is frequently seen. With the aid of the PAS stain, the parasite can be readily identified because of its high glycogen content.[63] The background of the smear may contain many polymorphs and necrotic granular material.

Most European laboratories do not encounter *E. histolytica* in smears, but sporadic cases do occur in developed countries, usually imported from endemic areas.

## Fungi

Most of the fungal infections in the vagina are caused by *Candida albicans*, sometimes still known as monilia. A few cases are due to *Geotrichum candidum* or *Torulopsis glabrata*, which is now classified with candida. Other fungal elements seen are usually contaminants.

## Candida albicans

This dimorphic fungus is a common cause of symptomatic infection, with a white curdy non-odorous vaginal discharge and pruritus vulvae. *Candida* infections are prone to occur when the progesterone level is high, as in pregnancy or when contraceptive hormones are used. Infections are also common when bacterial equilibrium is disturbed, for example by broad-spectrum antibiotics or chemotherapeutic drugs.

In symptomatic infections, the organisms invade the squamous cells. When saprophytic, as in 20% of cases, spores and pseudohyphae are sparse in the sample, lying between or on top of the squamous cells.

### Cytological findings: *Candida albicans* (Figs 21.77, 21.78)

- Double-contoured pale pink hyphae and pseudohyphae
- Pseudohyphae appear septate
- Spores are eosinophilic, measuring 2–4 μm
- Inflammatory changes are variable.

In Papanicolaou stained smears, the filaments of *Candida* stain faintly with eosin, sometimes with haematoxylin. They are usually pseudohyphae, formed by branching chains of elongated buds, giving an appearance of septation likened to a bamboo cane.

The epithelial cells, often lying in plaques due to progesterone effects, are entangled with the candidal pseudohyphae that run between the cells. There is usually an associated inflammatory exudate as well as reactive/inflammatory changes in epithelial cell cytoplasm including perinuclear haloes.

### Diagnostic pitfalls: *Candida albicans*

Degenerate red blood cells may be mistaken for spores and streaks of mucus for hyphae. They do not show the typical structure of *Candida*. Contaminant fungi are occasionally a source of confusion.

There is often little or no inflammatory exudate and the *Candida* may then not be relevant clinically, especially if there are no symptoms and only spores are found. The fungus should be reported, stating the extent and whether in the form of spores or hyphae, to enable clinical assessment to be made.

The squamous cells may show reactive changes such as nuclear enlargement, orange staining of cytoplasm and perinuclear haloes.

## Candida glabrata

Vaginal infection by this organism, formerly known as *Torulopsis glabrata*, is much less common than *Candida albicans* infection. Slight pruritus or burning can occur but discharge is slight and

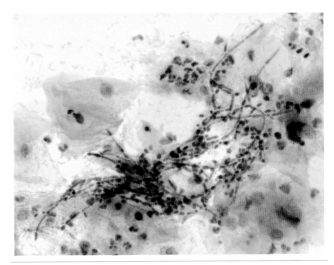

**Fig. 21.77** Budding yeasts and pseudohyphae of saprophytic *Candida albicans* in a lightly inflamed cervical smear.

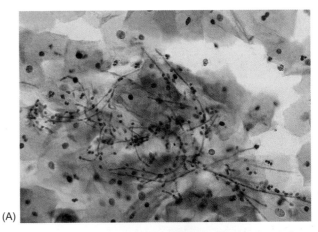

(A)

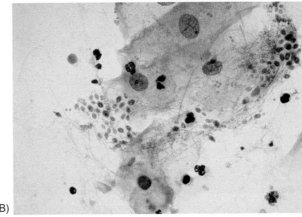

(B)

**Fig. 21.78** (A) *Candida* hyphae forming a tangled mass overlying a plaque of squamous cells. Some spores can be seen between the hyphae. (B) Spore forms of *Candida* are often seen in smears, as illustrated. They do not necessarily signify active infection in the absence of hyphae.

there may be no symptoms. Spores of variable size (2–8 μm) with unilateral gemmation in small groups with absence of filaments. Lactobacilli are often present. Cell changes are slight apart from eosinophilia.[64]

## Viruses

### *Herpes simplex* virus

*Herpes simplex* type II virus (HSV II) or *herpes genitalis* and the related *herpes simplex* type I virus (HSV I) or *herpes labialis* belong to the neurodermotropic herpesviruses. These have a predilection for tissues of ectodermal origin such as skin or mucosa and also for nervous tissue. *Herpes labialis* causes blisters on the lips. HSV infection of the genital tract, caused chiefly by HSV II and occasionally by HSV I, is acquired by sexual contact.

Primary genital HSV infection is manifested by the appearance of multiple widespread vesicles or ulcerative lesions on the external genitalia. Small pustular lesions may coalesce into large areas of ulceration. The ulcers persist from 4 to 15 days until crusting and healing occur.

Primary genital herpes is associated with HSV cervicitis in 90% of patients,[65] and is frequently accompanied by systemic symptoms such as fever, headache, malaise and muscle pain. In addition, there are local symptoms of pain, itching, dysuria, vaginal or urethral discharge, and tender swollen inguinal lymph nodes. The disease is self-limiting. After an attack the virus assumes a state of latency, usually in the dorsal root ganglia of the lumbosacral plexus.

In some women, recurrent episodes of infection occur. Because antibodies to the virus have already been produced, recurrences are of short duration and have much milder symptoms. HSV may affect the cervix alone, without involving the external genitalia and these patients may be asymptomatic. Immunosuppressed patients are predisposed to more frequent and more severe recurrent episodes.

### Cytological findings: *herpes simplex* virus (Fig. 21.79)

- Swollen nuclei with multinucleation
- Ground glass chromatin with prominent nuclear membranes
- Nuclear inclusions.

The cytopathic effects evolve in three stages. In the first stage there is increased granularity in epithelial nuclei with fine intranuclear vacuolation. It may be difficult to distinguish these changes from those seen in degenerate cells due to other causes. The second stage is marked by further change in the chromatin pattern, which becomes indistinct, giving a so-called 'ground glass' appearance to the nucleus. This is caused by swelling of the viral material in the nucleus.[66] A distinct nuclear membrane is visible. The cytoplasm becomes dense and basophilic. In the third stage the nucleus contains an acidophilic inclusion body, which is surrounded by a clear zone.[67] The inclusion bodies have been described by virologists as 'tombstones' because they reveal the death of the cell.

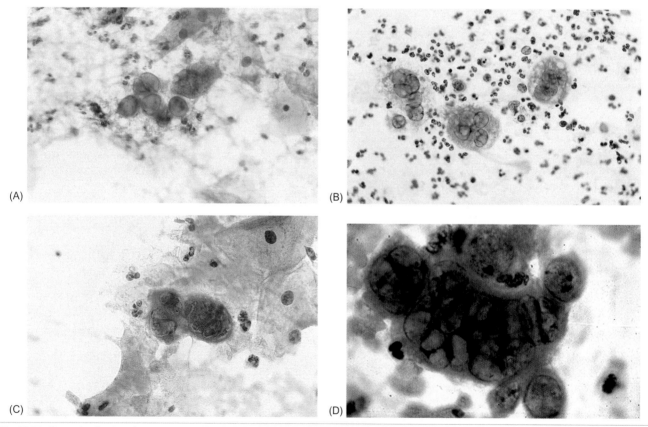

(A)

(B)

(C)

(D)

**Fig. 21.79** *Herpes simplex* virus changes in cervical epithelial cells. (A) Initially there is swelling of the nuclei, followed by degeneration of chromatin leading to a ground glass pattern. (B) Multinucleation is a prominent feature. (C) Inclusion bodies appear as the cells start to die. (D) High-power view of multinucleated cell with ground glass nuclei and nuclear inclusions.

In the second and third stages many multinucleated cells are found. They may contain 20 or more nuclei lying close together, moulding against each other without overlapping – a point of contrast with those in reactive multinucleated endocervical cells or histiocytes. The nuclei show ground glass changes and inclusion bodies as described above. These multinucleate cells are characteristic of herpetic infection at any site.

The virus infects cells from the ectocervical and endocervical epithelium. The cell shape is usually distorted and may make identification of cell type difficult. Immunoperoxidase techniques have proved reliable for the confirmation of HSV II.[68] More recently, specific probes have become available for the demonstration of HSV II by means of DNA *in situ* hybridisation.

### Diagnostic pitfalls: herpes simplex virus

Multinucleation and nuclear swelling are reactive features common to various other inflammatory and repair processes, although usually lesser in degree than in herpes simplex infection. Ground glass nuclear changes are more specific, as are intranuclear inclusions.

The risk of over-diagnosis of HSV in endocervical brush samples in particular has been stressed by Stowell et al., who found multinucleation and margination of nuclear chromatin to be of limited value in diagnosis compared with the presence of a ground glass chromatin pattern, which had a sensitivity and specificity of 95%.[69]

The diagnosis of herpetic infection should also prompt screening for other sexually transmitted infections. If unsuspected, ulcerated and necrotic herpetic lesions of the cervix may mimic invasive cancer macroscopically. Finally, there is a risk, albeit low, that maternal herpesvirus infection may be transmitted to the foetus during vaginal delivery; this infection is potentially fatal.

## Human papillomavirus (HPV): wart virus infection

Genital warts or condylomata acuminata are caused by infection with human types of papillomaviruses (see Ch. 25). The viruses are epidermotropic, infecting first the basal layer of cells and inducing proliferation of the infected epithelium. Productive growth with viral shedding from the surface of the lesion occurs later.

Virus infection of the cervix does not always lead to morphological changes detectable by light microscopy. Furthermore, if present in a cervical cytology sample the HPV infection cannot be subtyped, this requires *in situ* hybridisation or PCR. The virus produces characteristic cytopathic effects in squamous cells, recognisable in tissue sections and in cervical samples. Two major types of condylomatous lesions can be distinguished histologically, namely the papillary type, which is clinically visible as a genital wart or condyloma acuminatum, and the flat wart or condyloma planum, which may only be detectable by colposcopy or, in the male, by peniscopy (Fig. 21.80). Condylomata acuminata are usually multiple and may be present on the vulva or vagina as well as the cervix.[70]

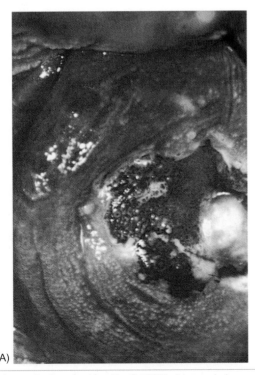

(A)

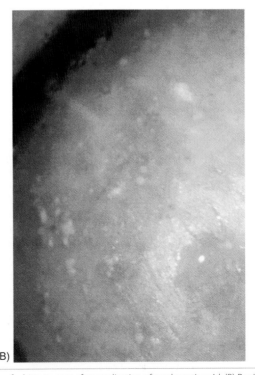

(B)

**Fig. 21.80** (A) Colposcopic view of cervix with a flat HPV lesion revealed as an area of white mucosa after application of weak acetic acid. (B) Peniscopy of partner of the above patient with HPV infection. Note multiple flat lesions.

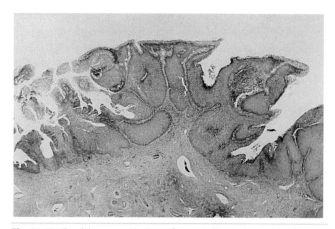

**Fig. 21.81** Condyloma acuminatum of cervix in histological section. The form is that of a raised excrescence of folded hyperplastic epithelium, with a layer of keratinisation on the surface and some non-specific inflammation in the underlying stroma.

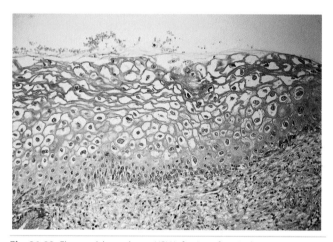

**Fig. 21.82** Flat condyloma due to HPV infection of cervical mucosa. The mucosa is thickened. Koilocytosis is present in the upper layers, with dyskeratosis, enlarged crumpled or pyknotic nuclei, binucleation and a few normal mitoses.

## Histological features of HPV infection

Condylomata are composed of thickened squamous epithelium, often keratinised, arranged in numerous papillary folds supported by projecting cores of fibrovascular tissue (Fig. 21.81). Cytopathic viral effects can be seen in histological sections, consisting of a broad empty zone around the nucleus with a thick rim of residual cytoplasm at the periphery. The nucleus is enlarged, hyperchromatic and crumpled. Cells with these changes are called koilocytes, derived from the Greek word *koilos*, meaning 'hollow'. Multinucleation, normal mitotic figures and premature keratinisation of individual cells (dyskeratosis) are also seen.

Flat condylomas or condylomata plana can only be identified with the aid of the colposcope.[71] Histologically, they lack the classical exophytic papillary epithelial proliferation of condylomata acuminata, the mucosa being only slightly thickened, but the cytopathic changes in individual cells can be seen, enabling a diagnosis of HPV infection to be made with some confidence (Fig. 21.82).

Whereas condylomata acuminata occur predominantly in the native stratified squamous epithelium of the vulva, vagina and ectocervix, flat condylomas are most commonly found in the metaplastic epithelium of the transformation zone.[72] The condylomatous metaplastic epithelium may grow into endocervical glandular necks, replacing pre-existing columnar epithelium. The lesion is referred to as an inverted or endophytic condyloma.

Papillomavirus particles can be visualised in the cell nuclei of infected squamous cells by electron microscopy. They were first described in the papillary lesion in 1968[73] and in the flat lesion in 1978.[74] Their appearance proved to be identical to the viral particles found in skin warts. Application of DNA *in situ* hybridisation has made it clear that cervical condylomata and skin warts are caused by different HPV subtypes.[75]

Since these initial reports, much progress has been made in the field of papillomavirus research, with the help of molecular biological techniques. Of the 200 or more different HPV strains capable of infecting mucosa or skin, approximately 40 HPV subtypes infect the female genital tract.[76] HPV 6 and 11 are preferentially found in benign condylomatous lesions of the cervix (usually >90% of genital warts) and low-grade cervical intraepithelial neoplasia (CIN I).[77] They are termed 'low-risk' HPV. 'High-risk' HPV subtypes include 16, 18 and close relatives 31, 33, 35, 52, 39, 45, 59, 66, 51. They are the cause of virtually all cervical cancers.[78] Approximately 80% of CIN II-III lesions contain high-risk HPV sequences on DNA analysis.[79] Some 70% of all women who develop squamous cell carcinoma in the UK have evidence of HPV 16 or 18 infection[76] – underscoring the importance of the UK HPV vaccination programme against high-risk subtypes in teenage girls starting from 2008.

Most genital warts, and the changes in smears induced by the infection, regress after about 2 years and in general can be managed conservatively by close cytological surveillance[80] or by ablative therapy in the first place. If evidence of high-grade dyskaryosis supervenes in the cytological sample, colposcopic examination and appropriate treatment are required. Policies on the management of HPV infection in the absence of dyskaryosis vary a great deal, however, reflecting uncertainty about its exact significance for an individual woman (see Ch. 30).

HPV subtyping of infected cervical squamous cells has been proposed as an alternative to routine cervical screening, women carrying high-risk subtypes of the virus being then investigated by colposcopy (see Chs 29, 30 and 31).[81]

It remains to be seen whether primary HPV testing is a cost-effective alternative to cytological screening. Recent UK studies are currently assessing the use of integrating high-risk HPV triage within the national screening programme in the management of women with low-grade (borderline or mildly dyskaryotic) cervical cytology and as a 'test of cure' following conisation for CIN.[82]

### Cytological findings: human papillomavirus

- Koilocytosis
- Enlarged hyperchromatic nuclei
- Bi- and multinucleation
- Cytoplasmic keratinisation.

In cervical samples, the presence of koilocytic cells provides the most reliable evidence of HPV infection. Koilocytes were first described by Koss and Durfee in 1956.[83] They are defined as squamous cells with a large well-demarcated clear perinuclear zone surrounded by a dense peripheral

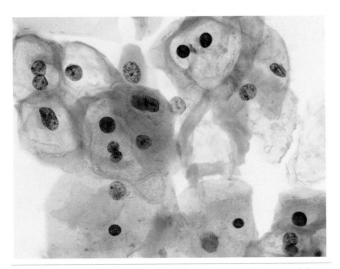

**Fig. 21.83** Koilocytes with well-defined clearing of cytoplasm around the nuclei and variable nuclear enlargement. The cell arrowed is considered to show mild dyskaryotic changes. Note how some cells are bi-nucleate.

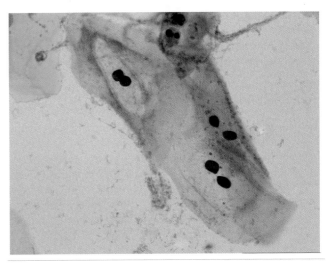

**Fig. 21.84** Koilocytes showing borderline nuclear changes in which the nuclei appear near normal with minimal enlargement and change in chromatin.

cytoplasmic rim. The shape of the clear zone may be oval, rounded or scalloped (Fig. 21.83). Superficial and intermediate cells are the cells most frequently showing koilocytic changes, but parabasal and metaplastic cells can also be affected.

The nucleus is enlarged and may appear crumpled or wrinkled at the margins, with loss of nuclear detail, producing a smudged effect. Some degree of hyperchromasia is usual and pyknosis or karyorrhexis is often seen. Binucleation is extremely common and sometimes multinucleation is evident.

Hyperkeratosis and parakeratosis are frequently observed: superficial cells stain intensely orange and are arranged in plaques of variable size and shape described as pearls, rafts or spikes. Anucleate squames are often present but are not a specific finding.[84] Dissociated dyskeratotic cells may also be present.

Tanaka et al. reported the cytological findings in cervical smears in relation to HPV subtype in 150 cases positive for HPV by Southern blot analysis.[85] Their results indicate that all of the above criteria correlate well with the presence of HPV, but koilocytosis, dyskeratosis, parakeratosis and karyorrhexis are the most specific. Using the presence of two out of these three criteria alone, a diagnostic specificity of 100% was achieved, with a sensitivity of 36%.

A further study found that cytology samples from women with HPV infection proved by PCR technique contained koilocytes in only 3% of cases, demonstrating that HPV is underdiagnosed when koilocytosis is the sole cytological criterion used.[86] Hyperkeratosis was the most frequent morphological change in these smears (66%), followed by parakeratosis (34%). Detection of HPV by DNA hybridisation on reprocessed routine Papanicolaou smears[87] has shown that up to 21% of normal smears without koilocytosis contain HPV.

## Diagnostic pitfalls: human papillomavirus

Koilocytosis must be distinguished from vacuolation of cells from other causes such as glycogen content, non-specific degenerative changes or the perinuclear haloes associated with inflammation. The nuclei of koilocytes differ from those of other cells, being enlarged, wrinkled and often lacking in

nuclear detail, appearing smudged or pyknotic. The koilocytic zone is large and fairly empty, in contrast to the yellow staining of glycogen storage in the cytoplasm or the small neat area of pallor seen in perinuclear halo formation.

Multinucleation is not specific for wart virus infection as it can be seen in many reactive processes, including after irradiation. Nevertheless, it is a common feature in HPV infection, adding weight to the overall picture especially when extensive in superficial and intermediate cells. Nuclear moulding does not occur, in contrast to herpetic multinucleation.

Nuclear enlargement, chromatin disturbance and irregular nuclear contours are among the nuclear features of dyskaryosis. It is often extremely difficult or impossible to establish with certainty whether dyskaryosis, especially mild dyskaryosis, has developed in the presence of HPV changes. Such cases should be managed according to the suspected grade of dyskaryosis.

Some koilocytes may contain virtually near normal-appearing nuclei along with perinuclear clearing and dense peripheral cytoplasmic staining (Fig. 21.84). In this situation the HPV infected squamous cell is classified as 'borderline nuclear changes' according to current UK terminology. In the Bethesda system koilocytic HPV changes are classified with mild dyskaryosis as a low-grade squamous intraepithelial lesion (SIL), whereas nuclear abnormalities of viral type without koilocytosis generally fall into the ASCUS category. Following a UK terminology conference in 2002, the BSCC has recommended merging koilocytic changes with mild dyskaryosis as low-grade dyskaryosis, approximating to the two tier American Bethesda System.[40] This has still to be adopted by the NHSCSP. Koilocytes are a striking finding in samples from flat lesions, but in some samples from visible genital warts only anucleate squames and parakeratotic cells from the surface may be found. Thus cytology is a more sensitive test for identifying flat condylomata than macroscopically visible genital warts. Attempts at subtyping HPV by morphological changes in smears has proved to be unreliable on criteria known at present.[85] HPV subtyping can be performed on liquid-based cytology samples in conjunction with screening of the thin layer preparation to establish whether high-risk subtypes of HPV are present when low-grade abnormalities are found in the sample. This adjunctive test allows rational management of the sample findings.

## Cytomegalovirus

The endocervical epithelium is susceptible to cytomegalovirus (CMV) infection[88,89] but in spite of this, infection is uncommon and is often asymptomatic. Reactivation of latent CMV occurs in 2–4% of pregnant women, probably due to disturbance of steroid metabolism and altered immunity and also in immunosuppressed patients for other reasons, and can be recognised in transplant patients.

### Cytological findings: cytomegalovirus

Small irregular nuclear inclusion bodies are observed at first. Later the enlarged nuclei contain a very large single eosinophilic inclusion body surrounded by a narrow halo which gives the cells an 'owl's eye' appearance (Figs 21.85, 21.86).[89] The cytoplasm may contain finely granular basophilic inclusions. Electron microscopy or immunocytochemistry can be used to verify the presence of the virus.

Cervical screening is not a practical way of detecting cytomegalovirus. The number of affected cells is often very low.[90] If inclusion-bearing cells are detected in pregnancy, however, it is important to investigate the possibility of active cytomegalovirus infection because this may threaten the health of the developing foetus.

## Molluscum contagiosum

This pox virus produces crops of hyperplastic skin nodules which may infect the vulval area. Large inclusion bodies fill the squamous cells at the core of the lesion, pushing the nucleus to the outer rim of the cell (Fig. 21.87). Eventually the material at the core is discharged on to the skin surface. The diagnosis can be made on scrapings from these lesions, and occasionally molluscum bodies are found in cervical smears.

## Adenovirus

Cells with features suggesting adenovirus infection can be of endocervical, metaplastic or parabasal type. Early in the infection they contain three or four small eosinophilic nuclear inclusions with halos; later a large eosinophilic nuclear inclusion with an irregularly lobulated contour develops. Some chromatin deposition on the nuclear membrane may be found. Multinucleation is not seen.[91]

## Chlamydia trachomatis

Although they are in fact bacteria, chlamydiae are placed between bacteria and viruses because of their properties and characteristics. They contain DNA and RNA, have discrete cell walls and are sensitive to tetracycline and sulphonamides, like bacteria. On the other hand, they are obligatory intracellular organisms that multiply within the host cell by binary fission, like viruses.

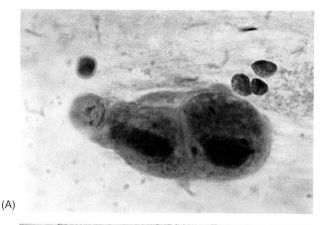

(A)

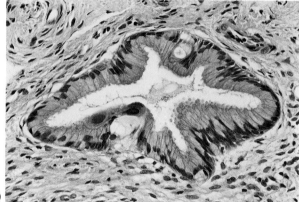

(B)

**Fig. 21.85** (A) Cytomegalovirus infection in a renal transplant patient. The sample showed several groups of cells with enormous dense inclusion bodies surrounded by a large halo giving the characteristic 'owl's eye' appearance. Note the granular area in the cytoplasm representing viral particles. (B) Histological section shows isolated cells in endocervical cells with similar features.

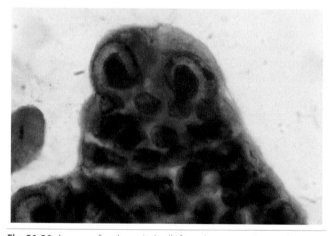

**Fig. 21.86** A group of endocervical cells from the same patient as shown in Figure 21.85, demonstrating the 'owl's eye' appearance very clearly.

Within the genus *Chlamydia*, two species are recognised namely *Chlamydia trachomatis* and *Chlamydia psittaci*. By serological methods different types of *Chlamydia trachomatis* can be identified. Serotypes A–C are associated with endemic blinding trachoma, serotypes D–K with sexually transmitted oculogenital infections and serotype L with lymphogranuloma venereum.

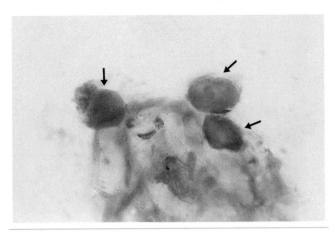

**Fig. 21.87** Molluscum bodies (arrows) are seen among anucleate keratinised squames, filling the cells with dense orange inclusion material. This vulval direct/conventional smear was from a patient with Molluscum contagiosum infection. (Courtesy of Professor B. Naylor, Michigan, USA).

*Chlamydia trachomatis* infection is the commonest sexually transmitted disease (STD) in the USA and Western Europe. Diagnosis is important, since infection can lead to infertility in the female many years after primary exposure. Epidemiological studies have shown that sexually active teenagers and women with other venereal disease, such as gonorrhoea, are high-risk groups for cervical chlamydial infection. The prevalence of infection in patients attending STD clinics can range up to 17.5% for men and 13.5% for women.[92]

In women, the infection is often asymptomatic. Since columnar epithelium and metaplastic cells are the target cells for *Chlamydia trachomatis*, the cervix is the most commonly infected site in the female genital tract. Ascending infection may lead to salpingitis and pelvic inflammatory disease, both important causes of infertility and ectopic pregnancy. Pregnancy and the use of oral contraceptives promote the risk of infection because there is often an ectropion, providing an increased surface area lined by endocervical columnar cells. Follicular cervicitis may be associated with *Chlamydia trachomatis* infection in younger premenopausal women.

Different types of 'diagnostic' inclusion bodies have been described.[93] Studies of the accuracy of cytological diagnosis of chlamydial infection based on the detection of various inclusion bodies, however, reveal an average sensitivity of only 27% and specificity of 79%, with large numbers of false positive and false negative results.[94] The most reliable cytological evidence of chlamydial infection is the presence of so-called indicator cells.[95] It must be stressed that the mainstay of diagnosis for this infection rests with microbiology and not cytology.

### Cytological findings: *Chlamydia trachomatis*

Indicator cells are metaplastic cells with altered cytoplasmic staining due to the presence of small ill-defined nebular inclusions, giving the cytoplasm a freckled, mottled appearance. Other inclusions and vacuoles in metaplastic cells cannot be regarded as evidence of chlamydial infection. The cytoplasmic changes can be found in endocervical cells and may also be seen in dyskaryotic cells. Follicular cervicitis may be present.

Definitive diagnosis of *Chlamydia trachomatis* requires confirmation by immunofluorescence,[96] immunoperoxidase

staining methods,[97] isolation techniques using cultured HeLa cells[98] or PCR.[99]

## Iatrogenic lesions

Cell patterns in cervical smears are influenced by a variety of medical treatments including the use of oral contraceptives. Surgical procedures involving the cervix may also influence the findings in smears. Some aspects of these iatrogenic influences will be considered in more detail below.

## Changes induced by hormones

### Hormonal contraceptives

Oral contraceptives influence both the squamous and glandular epithelium. Different formulations vary in their effects clinically and cytologically, depending on the balance of oestrogenic and progesterone activity and whether or not an ovulatory peak is induced. High-dose progesterone oral contraception is more commonly used today than the formulations with a high level of oestrogen.

### Cytological findings: hormonal contraceptives

- Scanty samples with cytolysis
- Atrophic changes after long-term use
- Endometrial cells due to breakthrough bleeding at midcycle.

Cytolysis is a prominent feature in high progesterone regimes and may, at times, be so extreme that the sample is rendered inadequate for further assessment.

The oral contraceptive pill, by 'dampening' normal ovarian function, may lead to an atrophic pattern in samples; this is seen particularly with the injectable progesterone compound Depo-Provera.

Inhibition of the hypothalamus may be so marked that when oral contraception is discontinued normal cycles are not resumed. A vaginal or cervical sample then shows an atrophic pattern. Midcycle breakthrough bleeding, during oral contraceptive use, will lead to shedding of normal morphology endometrial cells in cervical samples taken.

### Hormone replacement treatment (HRT)

Hormone replacement can be used to treat menopausal symptoms and to protect against the long-term risks of postmenopausal osteoporosis and heart disease. The therapy may be sequential, based on a combination of oestrogen counterbalanced by the inclusion of cyclical progesterone, thus re-creating the hormonal environment of the premenopausal woman, or may consist of a continuous low dose of either or both hormones, which is not usually associated with any withdrawal bleeding.

In either case, cervical samples usually contain superficial and intermediate cells but may not show a fully oestrogenised picture in all women, depending on the type of hormonal preparation used. It is important to remember that regular menstruation occurs when sequential therapy is given and that groups of endometrial cells may therefore be found within the first 12 days of the cycle, or later if breakthrough bleeding occurs. Some women experience bleeding while receiving continuous HRT.

The risk of atypical endometrial hyperplasia and development of endometrial carcinoma is increased in women on HRT,[100] particularly if the oestrogen content is not counterbalanced by progesterone administration. The cytological recognition of clusters of atypical endometrial cells outside the normal time of endometrial shedding should lead to appropriate investigation to exclude these complications.

Local administration of oestrogen per vaginam is used as intermittent HRT for short-term effect, providing, among other benefits, a helpful method of obtaining a mature cervical smear in cases where an atrophic sample has been difficult to interpret.

## Tamoxifen therapy

Tamoxifen is a synthetic compound with anti-oestrogenic properties used with increasing frequency in the treatment of breast carcinoma in postmenopausal women and also in premenopausal patients if the tumour cells are shown to have oestrogen receptors.[101] Paradoxically, the effect of Tamoxifen on the female genital tract includes a weak oestrogenic action so that postmenopausal cytology samples show increased squamous maturation in a high proportion of cases.[102] Oestrogen associated changes can be seen in the endometrium in up to 30% of women receiving the hormone, usually after several years of therapy.[103] In general, the samples have a clean background and a modestly oestrogenic picture, developing early after starting treatment[104] (Fig. 21.88A).

Tamoxifen therapy carries a heightened risk of endometrial hyperplasia and carcinoma, particularly in postmenopausal women.[105] Other tumours, including benign polyps ± in situ carcinomatous changes[106] and sarcomatous tumours of uterus and cervix[107] are also associated with its use. Vaginal adenosis[108] has also been described secondary to Tamoxifen use.

Cytology samples from these patients require careful screening for the detection of abnormal glandular cells (Fig. 21.88B), with appropriate investigation and treatment if needed.

## Other drugs with hormonal activity

Various non-hormonal preparations exert an influence on the maturation and exfoliation of squamous epithelium. Digitalis is known to stimulate mucosal maturation. Tetracyclines cause accelerated exfoliation, so that in some cases only parabasal cells are found in smears soon after starting therapy.[109]

### Intrauterine devices (IUDs)

IUDs are made from a variety of materials, the commonest being plastic or copper. They may be used premenopausally as a form of contraception or in pre- and postmenopausal women to administer HRT locally. Different designs are available. All types are prone to induce changes in the cervical mucosa and superficial endometrium, leading to changes in cervical cytology samples.

### Cytological findings: intrauterine devices

- Endometrial shedding at any stage of the cycle
- Single and clustered enlarged vacuolated glandular cells
- Neutrophilic inflammatory cell exudate
- Actinomycotic colonies.

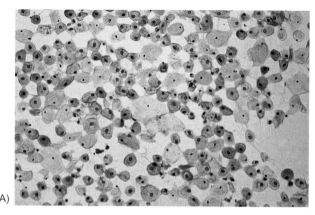

(A)

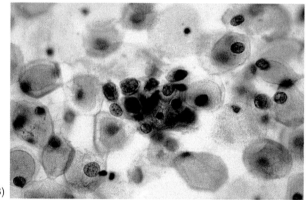

(B)

**Fig. 21.88** (A) Tamoxifen therapy induces squamous maturation in cervical sample in some postmenopausal women. The samples tend to have a clean background as seen here. Maturation of the smear is dose related. (B) A cluster of hyperchromatic glandular cells is seen at the centre, in a smear from a patient with early endometrial carcinoma who had received Tamoxifen therapy for 3 years.

Endometrial cells may be seen at any stage of the menstrual cycle, outside the usual cyclical timespan. Occasionally, groups of atypical endometrial cells display swollen nuclei and coarse vacuolation of the cytoplasm, accompanied by inflammatory debris.[110] An erroneous diagnosis of endometrial adenocarcinoma may be made in such cases. Endocervical cells may show pronounced enlargement, prominent nucleoli and mitotic figures. They occur as single rounded cells associated with cell debris or in clusters (Fig. 21.89). The cytoplasm is often vacuolated and polymorphs can be seen in the cytoplasm or in vacuoles. In addition small metaplastic cells maybe exfoliated that may simulate severely dyskaryotic squamous cells if the IUD history is not included on the sample request form and associated atypical glandular cells not recognised (Fig. 21.90).[111]

The samples frequently show many polymorphs, to the extent that the epithelial cells may be obscured. Histiocytes with phagocytosed spermatozoa, foreign body giant cells and even fibroblasts can also be seen.[112] Actinomycotic colonies are common, particularly with plastic devices.[113] Saprophytic amoebae may also be found,[114] together with a coccoid flora. Removal of the IUD in these circumstances should rarely be necessary, especially if the woman is asymptomatic. Symptoms of pelvic inflammatory disease in the presence of an IUD warrant investigation and treatment. Calcification around particles from the IUD can result in the presence of psammoma bodies in the smear (Fig. 21.91).[115,116]

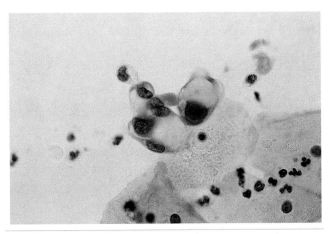

**Fig. 21.89** IUCD changes in endocervical cells, showing enlarged pleomorphic cells with vacuolated cytoplasm and hyperchromatic nuclei. Repeat samples are indicated if interpretation is problematical.

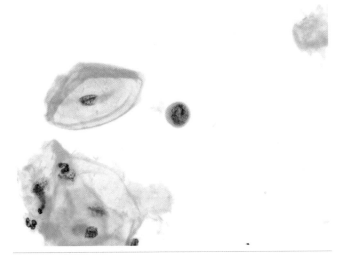

**Fig. 21.90** Single atypical endometrial cell mimicking severe dyskaryosis. The smear is from a woman using IUD contraception.

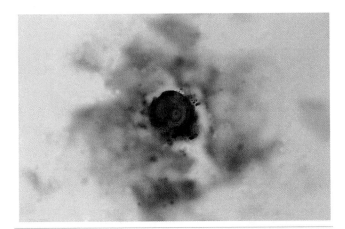

**Fig. 21.91** Psammoma body in cervical sample associated with IUCD use. This was an isolated finding and there was no evidence of malignancy.

## Surgical intervention: repair and regeneration

In the healing stages after surgical procedures such as conisation, subtotal hysterectomy or curettage, cervical samples

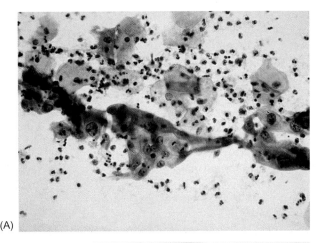

(A)

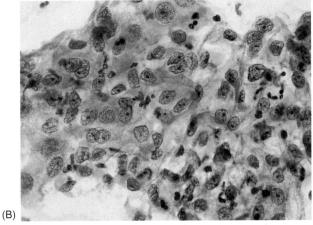

(B)

**Fig. 21.92** (A) Repair changes. This group of metaplastic cells shows ill-defined cell boundaries, some nuclear variation and prominent nucleoli. (B) A sheet of immature metaplastic cells showing repair changes with irregular pleomorphic nuclei and prominent nucleoli.

usually show evidence of inflammation and repair. More limited procedures such as electrocoagulation, laser vaporisation, cryotherapy and excision of cervical lesions by diathermy loop excision (DLE) are associated with similar changes.

The repair process is affected by regeneration of residual epithelium to cover the area of excision. This may take several weeks depending on the extent of the procedure, the presence or absence of local infection and the general health of the patient. Smear findings are also influenced by these factors.

### Cytological findings: surgical intervention – repair and regeneration

- Repair changes
- Inflammation
- Metaplasia.

Repair cells are usually metaplastic in origin and are found in ragged, flat sheets of rather pleomorphic cells with ill-defined cell boundaries (Fig. 21.92). They may show slight or even marked nuclear atypia due to coarsening of the chromatin with condensation at the nuclear membrane, and frequently have large active or multiple nucleoli.[117] Distinction from dyskaryosis and invasive carcinoma because of the large nucleoli, may be difficult without a full history, but the architectural regularity, preserved N:C ratio and the lack of significant abnormality of chromatin distribution usually leads to a correct diagnosis. In cases of doubt the smear should be reported as having 'borderline changes/high-grade dyskaryosis cannot be excluded'.

In most cases, atypical cells are found within the first 4 weeks following cryosurgery or DLE and smears return to normal within 8 weeks.[118] The healing process may lead to changes in squamous cells which mimic neoplasia.[119,120] It is therefore not prudent to take follow-up cervical samples before at least 6 months after treatment has lapsed.

## Tubal and tuboendometrioid metaplasia (TEM)

Follow-up cytology samples after surgery to the cervix may contain sheets of glandular cells with crowded hyperchromatic nuclei, which may show gross anisonucleosis, giving an initial impression of endocervical dyskaryosis. These cells have been shown to arise from areas of tubal or tuboendometrioid metaplasia in the vicinity of the external os of the cervix at the site of previous surgical treatment (Fig. 21.93). The incidence of this

regenerative phenomenon in histological sections of cervix following surgery for reactive or neoplastic conditions varies from 30% to 70% in different series (see Ch. 25).[121,122]

Hyperchromatic and crowded groups of small cells in TEM may be mistaken for dyskaryosis in glandular cells.[123,124]

### Cytological findings: tubal and tuboendometrioid metaplasia (Fig. 21.93)

- Sparse groups of crowded dark epithelial cells
- Lack of architectural features of endocervical dyskaryosis
- Ciliated or regular non ciliated luminal borders may be seen
- An appropriate history.

At low magnification, occasional groups of darkly stained cells are readily seen in both spatula and brush samples. The groups are two or three-dimensional, consisting of small crowded cells with central hyperchromatic nuclei and very little cytoplasm. The presence of cilia or a terminal bar is not a dependable finding as these structures are prone to degenerative changes, but if found, these provide reassurance that the cell groups are likely to be metaplastic rather than neoplastic in type. No feathering or other architectural abnormalities typical of glandular neoplasia are seen in tubal or tuboendometrial metaplasia and there are no mitoses or enlarged nucleoli.

The three-dimensional groups lack the central stromal core of endometrial cell clusters shed physiologically. However, some postoperative follow-up cases contain large casts of glands in the absence of tuboendometrioid metaplasia. The glandular structures are composed of uniform cells with regular nuclei and small nucleoli; mitoses may be seen and sometimes a few stromal cells or capillary fragments may be seen along the outer border of the gland. These intact glands are thought to come from the isthmic region of the endometrial cavity especially if the endocervical canal has been shortened by excisional treatment. They are referred to as lower uterine segment sampling and are commoner in brush samples than in spatula smears (Fig. 21.94).[125]

Endometriosis of the cervix is also found in a few cases following surgery, with foci of endometrial glands set in endometrial stroma (see Chs 24, 25). Cells from these lesions have the same appearances as groups from the endometrial

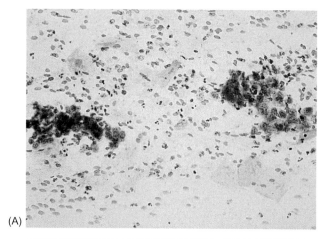

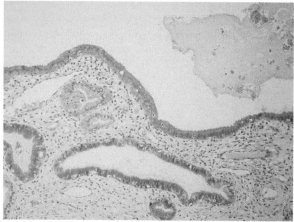

(A)

(B)

**Fig. 21.93** (A) Tubal metaplasia. Irregular clusters of glandular cells in a follow up sample after excisional treatment of CIN. The cells appear crowded and irregular and include occasional larger cells with clear cytoplasm. The findings suggest tubal metaplasia, given the clinical setting. (B) Section from the cervix of this patient shows tubal metaplasia in several of the glands and also in the surface epithelium.

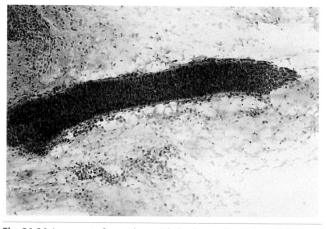

**Fig. 21.94** Large cast of an endometrial gland, one of several in a follow-up endocervical brush smear after cervical surgery.

cavity, although usually better preserved and present at times unrelated to the normal menstrual cycle.

## Radiation changes

Radiotherapy has been used in the treatment of malignant tumours of the female genital tract, notably carcinoma of the cervix, for over a century.[126] Under the influence of ionising radiation, benign as well as malignant cells change markedly and interpretation of these samples raises particular problems. The changes have been well documented by Shield et al.[127]

### Cytological findings: radiation changes (Figs 21.95, 21.96)

- Swelling of cells and nuclei with preserved N:C ratio
- Bizarre cell shapes
- Altered cytoplasmic staining
- Nuclear degenerative changes.

General cellular enlargement is seen, affecting both nucleus and cytoplasm so that the N:C ratio remains largely within normal limits. Bizarre cell shapes are seen, with altered cytoplasmic staining affinity to light green at the periphery and to eosin around the nucleus, giving the two-tone effect of amphophilia. Cytoplasmic vacuolation is a prominent feature, either fine and uniformly distributed or coarse and variable in distribution. The nuclei acquire a peculiar wrinkled appearance. They are hyperchromatic, with a coarse but uniformly dense chromatin pattern. Multinucleation is common and vacuolation of nuclei may be seen. The nucleoli are often enlarged and even pleomorphic but the ratio of nucleolus to nucleus remains low. Nuclear degeneration with karyorrhexis is often seen.

During radiotherapy treatment, cytology samples are characterised by numerous leucocytes, with much cellular debris and blood. Many histiocytes and multinucleated giant cells may be seen, as well as repair and radiation changes. Radiosensitive malignant cells generally disappear during the course of the radiotherapy. Shortly after irradiation, samples become atrophic even in premenopausal women. Epithelial cells are shed in large fragments due to the fragility of the mucosa and stromal cells may be noted. As many as 20 years after radiotherapy an effect may still be apparent in the

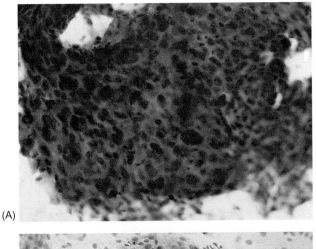

(A)

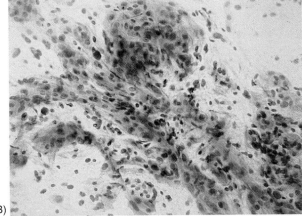

(B)

**Fig. 21.95** Radiotherapy changes (A) Radiation repair. Vaginal direct smear 6 months after radiotherapy for carcinoma of the cervix. The sheet of immature epithelium shows some features of repair but there is more marked nuclear swelling and the staining is variable. (B) Vaginal direct smear taken 5 years after radiotherapy for endometrial carcinoma. There is pronounced atrophy and the fragile cells are in sheets. Some nuclear enlargement persists.

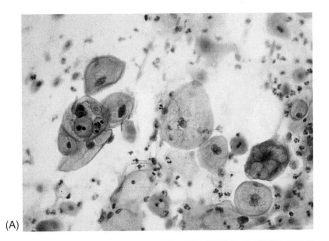

(A)

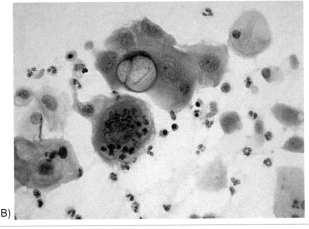

(B)

**Fig. 21.96** (A,B) Radiation damage in vaginal direct smear from a postmenopausal woman treated for carcinoma of the ovary by surgery and radiotherapy. The cells and nuclei are swollen and deeply stained but the nuclear/cytoplasmic ratio is normal. Fine and coarse vacuolation of cytoplasm has occurred and degenerate polymorphs are seen within cells. Note also some binucleation and the prominent nucleoli.

epithelial cells; usually, however, the changes subside over a period of time. It should be noted that current UK guidelines discourage vault cytology as a means of follow-up for women treated with radiotherapy for cervical cancer.

## Diagnostic pitfalls

Residual malignant cells may undergo any or all of the above changes but in addition they should also fulfil the nuclear criteria of malignancy and represent a separate population from the majority of cells in the smear. Helpful features pointing to a recurrence include an irregular chromatin distribution in the nucleus, a high N:C ratio and a resemblance to the original tumour. Differentiation of radiation effects from dyskaryosis is not, however, always possible by cytology alone. A detailed clinical history, colposcopic examination of the vaginal vault or cervix and biopsy of any visible lesion may be necessary to resolve the problem.

There are other conditions that may be confused with radiotherapy effects in treated patients. These include atrophy caused by hormonal treatment, inflammation from causes other than the radiotherapy, and the effect of cytotoxic agents given in conjunction with the radiotherapy. Folic acid deficiency during radiotherapy specifically affects the maturation of cell nuclei. In some of these conditions there may be cytomegaly, nuclear enlargement and hyperchromasia, vacuolation of cytoplasm, multinucleation and abnormal nuclear shapes.[128] Differentiation from radiation effects and from dyskaryosis may require colposcopy and biopsy of any abnormality.

### Radiation dysplasia

Samples from patients who have received radiotherapy may in time develop cellular abnormalities morphologically resembling those of neoplasia (Fig. 21.97). This condition, known as radiation dysplasia, can develop after a latent period varying from several months to 20 years. According to the literature,[127] radiation dysplasia of the vagina develops in 18.7–26% of patients who have received radiotherapy, usually within 3 years of treatment. Approaching 30% of cases have been found to regress,[129] but the natural history of these lesions is not fully known. The majority are believed either to persist or progress.

The dyskaryotic cells may be found either as isolated cells or in sheets. The shapes of the cells vary from polygonal to oval or round. The cytoplasm is usually eosinophilic but may also stain an indefinite colour.[127] The nuclei are often slightly enlarged, and oval or round. Hyperchromatism and coarsening of the chromatin are common but macronucleoli are not a feature.[130]

Radiation dysplasia must be differentiated from acute radiation changes and from a new or recurrent carcinoma. The likelihood of progression of radiation dysplasia to *in situ* carcinoma is twice that of the equivalent lower grades of CIN arising without any preceding irradiation. A distinction should be made between radiation dysplasia developing within 3 years of treatment and one that develops later, which has a considerably better prognosis.[130]

Most studies have given a diagnostic sensitivity approaching 50% for detection of tumour recurrence in follow-up cytology, with a range of 11.5–85%, probably reflecting dif-

ferences in access to the recurrence for sampling. In about one-quarter of cases the cytological detection precedes any clinical evidence of recurrent carcinoma.[127] False negative results are common, due to a high level of inadequate samples and also problems of access.[131] For these reasons, cytological follow-up of patients treated for cancer of the female genital tract is not generally used.

## Drug therapy effects

### Cytotoxic drugs

Cytotoxic agents are used in the primary treatment of certain tumours such as haematological malignancies, and also as palliative treatment for advanced inoperable cancers. Their use leads to cellular changes similar to those seen in the epithelium as a result of radiotherapy. Busulfan therapy, for example, gives rise to cells with markedly enlarged abnormal nuclei and abundant cytoplasm.[132] Multinucleation is common. The histology and cytological patterns in these drug reactions may be hard to distinguish from intraepithelial neoplasia (Fig. 21.98).

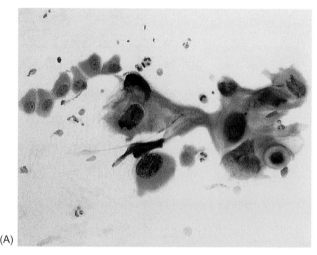

(A)

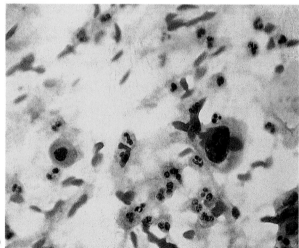

(B)

**Fig. 21.97** (A,B) Radiation dysplasia. This patient had radiotherapy for endometrial carcinoma 4 years previously. A follow-up vault smear showed immature squamous cells with a high nuclear/cytoplasmic ratio and intense hyperchromasia. A vault biopsy showed severe dysplasia consistent with radiation induced dysplasia.

An early study on the effects of prolonged cyclophosphamide administration showed enhanced development of neoplasia.[133] The finding of atypical cells associated with cytotoxic drug therapy warrants close cytological surveillance.

## Immunosuppressive drugs

Drugs inhibiting the immunological defence mechanisms of the body are used increasingly as treatment for a wide range of medical conditions and also to prevent organ rejection in transplant patients. The state of immunosuppression induced by these agents increases the risk of HPV infection, precancerous changes in the cervix[134] and progression to cervical cancer. Women who are immunosuppressed due to infection by the human immunodeficiency virus (HIV) also have a higher incidence of cervical precancer, although if enrolled in a well-managed cervical screening programme with contemporaneous access to antiretroviral drugs, the incidence of invasive carcinoma is not significantly raised over a non-HIV positive cohort (see Ch. 18).[135]

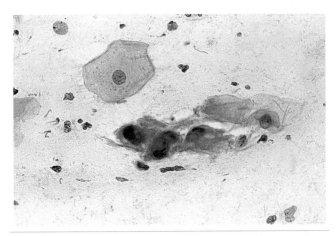

**Fig. 21.98** Cytotoxic therapy effects seen in a smear from a patient with non-Hodgkin lymphoma treated with cyclophosphamide. The cells show enlarged hyperchromatic nuclei with possible dyskaryosis. Close follow-up is necessary since the risk of CIN is increased in these patients.

## Diethylstilboestrol exposure *in utero*

The hormone diethylstilboestrol (DES) was used in the USA and some European countries in the mid-part of the twentieth century to maintain pregnancy in cases of threatened or habitual abortion. By the 1970s, it was noted that daughters of such pregnancies showed persistence of columnar epithelium in the vagina, known as vaginal adenosis which had a higher risk of malignant change, particularly clear cell carcinoma, compared to usual stratified squamous epithelium.[136] The glandular metaplasia falls into three types; mucinous, tubo-endometrial and embryonic and overlap may occur within these groups. Exact classification of these glandular cells may be difficult in cervical/vaginal cytology samples (see Fig. 21.99). With the cessation of DES use the incidence of this condition has dramatically decreased, although spontaneous vaginal adenosis can occur and may be related to oral contraceptive use.[137]

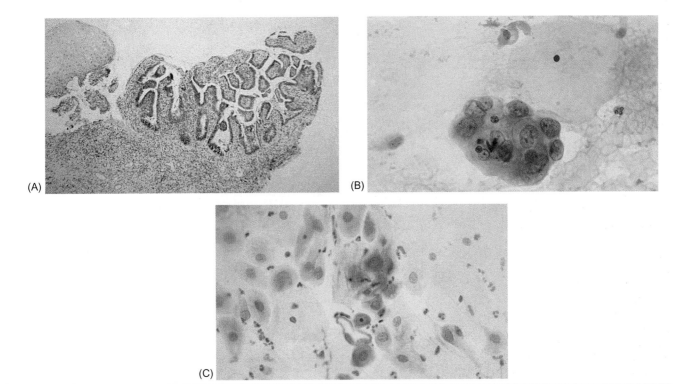

(A)

(B)

(C)

**Fig. 21.99** Vaginal adenosis. (A) Vaginal biopsy from a 12-year-old girl whose mother was given diethylstilboestrol in pregnancy. The normal squamous mucosa is partly replaced by columnar epithelium, which has failed to undergo metaplasia *in utero* to mature squamous epithelium. (B) Conventional vaginal smear taken directly from an area of vaginal adenosis showing a cluster of hyperplastic glandular cells with reactive nuclei. (C) Conventional vaginal smear with immature metaplastic epithelium from an area of persistent metaplasia in the vagina of the daughter of a woman given DES in pregnancy.

# REFERENCES

1. Grunze H, Spriggs AI. Cytology in gynaecology. In: History of Clinical Cytology, 2nd edn. G-I-T: Verlag Ernst Giebeler; 1983. p. 86–93.

2. Boon ME, Suurmeijer AJH. The Pap Smear, 3rd edn. Amsterdam: Harwood Academic; 1996.

3. Yassin SM, Garret M. Parasites in cytodiagnosis. Acta Cytol 1980:539–44.

4. Bhambhani S, Milner A, Pant J, et al. Ova of Taenia and Enterobius vermicularis in cervicovaginal smears. Acta Cytol 1985;29:193–94.

5. Bhambhani S. Egg of Ascaris lumbricoides in cervicovaginal smear. Acta Cytol 1984;28:92.

6. Gupta PK. Microbiology, inflammation and viral infections. In: Bibbo M, editor. Comprehensive Cytopathology. Philadelphia: WB Saunders; 1991. p. 115–52.

7. Chandra K, Annousamy R. An unusual finding in the vaginal smear. Acta Cytol 1975;19:403.

8. Vargese R, Raghuveer CV, Pai MR, et al. Microfilariae in cytological smears: a report of six cases. Acta Cytol 1996;40:299–301.

9. Learmonth GM, Murray MM. Helminths and protozoa as an incidental finding in cytology specimens. Cytopathology 1990;1:163–70.

10. Van Hoeven KH, Bertolini PK. Prevalence, identification and significance of fiber contaminants in cervical smears. Acta Cytol 1996;40:489–95.

11. Holton T, Smith D, Terry M, et al. The effect of lubricant contamination on ThinPrep® (Cytyc) cervical cytology. Cytopathology 2008;19:236–43.

12. Patnick J, Johnson J. Achievable standards, Benchmarks for reporting and criteria for evaluating cervical cytopathology. Cytopathology 2000;11:212–42.

13. Solom D, Davey D, Kurman R, et al. The Bethesda System. Terminology for reporting results of cervical cytology. JAMA 2002;287:2114–19.

14. Vooijs PG, Elias A, van der Graaf Y, et al. Relationship between the diagnosis of epithelial abnormalities and the composition of cervical smears. Acta Cytol 1985;29:323–28.

15. Baker A, Melcher D, Smith RS. Role of rescreening of cervical smears in internal quality control. J Clin Pathol 1995;48:1002–4.

16. Cross P. Rapid screening in cervical cytology – a simple method with a big impact. Cytopathology 2004;15:71–73.

17. Arbyn M, Schenck U, Ellison E, et al. Meta-analysis of the accuracy of rapid pre-screening relative to full-screening of pap smears. Cancer Cytopathol 2003;99:9–16.

18. Wolfendale MR, Howe-Guest R, Usherwood MM, et al. Controlled trial of a new cervical spatula. BMJ 1987;294:33–35.

19. Alons-van Kordelaar JJM, Boon ME. Diagnostic accuracy of squamous cervical lesions studied in spatula-cytobrush smears. Acta Cytol 1988;32:801–4.

20. Waddell CA, Rollason TP, Amarilli JM, et al. The cervix: an ectocervical brush sampler. Cytopathology 1990;1:171–81.

21. Williamson SLH, Hair T, Wadhera V. The effects of different sampling techniques on smear quality and the diagnosis of cytological abnormalities in cervical screening. Cytopathology 1997;8:188–95.

22. Jarvi K. Cervex brush v. vaginal-cervical-endocervical (VCE) triple smear techniques in cervical sampling. Cytopathology 1997;8:282–88.

23. Waddell CA. The influence of the cervix on smear quality: 1. Atrophy: an audit of cervical smears taken post-colposcopic management of intraepithelial neoplasia. Cytopathology 1997;8:274–81.

24. Papanicolaou GN. The diagnosis of early human pregnancy by the vaginal smear method. Proc Soc Exp Biol Med 1925;22:436.

25. Boschann HW. Zytologische untersuchungen uber die wirkung von androgenen am atrofischen vagina-epithel in abhangigkeit von dosierung und applikationsakt. Arch Gynak 1956;187:139.

26. Yates WA, Persad RV, Stanbridge CM. The Arias-Stella reaction in the cervix: a case report with cervical cytology. Cytopathology 1997;8:40–44.

27. Kobayashi TK, Okamoto H. Arias-Stella changes in cervico-vaginal specimens (letter). Cytopathology 1997;8:289–90.

28. Quincey C, Persad RV, Stanbridge CM. Chorionic villi in post partum cervical smears. Cytopathology 1995;6. 149–55.

29. Murad TM, Terhart K, Flint A. Atypical cells in pregnancy and postpartum smears. Acta Cytol 1981;25:623–30.

30. Ziabkowski TA, Naylor B. Cyanophilic bodies in cervico-vaginal smears. Acta Cytol 1976;20:340–42.

31. Larsen B, Galask RP. Vaginal microbial flora: composition and influences of host physiology. Ann Intern Med 1982;96(Suppl 6):926–30.

32. Henry-Stanley MJ, Simpson M, Stanley MW. Cervical cytology findings in women infected with the human immunodeficiency virus. Diagn Cytopathol 1993;9:508–9.

33. Keith LG, Berger GS, Edelman DA, et al. On the causation of pelvic inflammatory disease. Am J Obst Gynecol 1984;149:215–24.

34. Gondos B. Cell degeneration: light and electron microscopic study of ovarian germ cells. Acta Cytol 1974;18:504–10.

35. Muller Kobold-Wolterbeek AC, Beyer-Boon ME. Ciliocytophthoria in cervical cytology. Acta Cytol 1975;19:89–91.

36. Kelly BA, Black AS. The inflammatory cervical smear: a study in general practice. Br J Gen Pract 1990;40:238–40.

37. Wilson JD, Robinson AJ, Kinghorn S, et al. Implications of inflammatory changes on cervical pathology. BMJ 1990;300:638–40.

38. Parsons WL, Godwin M, Robbins C, et al. Prevalence of cervical pathogens in women with and without inflammatory changes on smear testing. BMJ 1993;306:1173–74.

39. BSCC/NCN Working Party report. Borderline changes in cervical smears. J Clin Pathol 1994;47:481–92.

40. Denton KJ, Herbert A, Turnbull LS, et al. The revised BSCC terminology for abnormal cervical cytology. Cytopathology 2008;19:137–57.

41. Halford J. Cytological features of chronic follicular cervicitis in liquid-based specimens: a potential diagnostic pitfall. Cytopathology 2002;13:364–70.

42. Smolka H, Soost HJ. Grundriss und Atlas der Gynakologischen Zytodiagnostik. Stuttgart: Thieme; 1971 111–116, 138–143.

43. Kashimura M, Baba S, Nakamura S, et al. Short-term estrogen test for cytodiagnosis in postmenopausal women. Diagn Cytopathol 1987;3:181–84.

44. Giacomini G, Reali D, Vita D, et al. The diagnostic cytology of non specific vaginitis. Diagn Cytopathol 1987;3:198–204.

45. Gardner HL, Dukes CD. Haemophilus vaginalis vaginitis: a newly defined specific infection previously classified as 'nonspecific' vaginitis. Am J Obstet Gynecol 1955;69:962–76.

46. Spiegel CA, Eschenbach DA, Amsel R, et al. Curved anaerobic bacteria in bacterial (nonspecific) vaginosis and their response to antimicrobial therapy. J Infect Dis 1983;148:817–22.

47. Brennan JP, Silverman N, van Hoeven KH. Association between a shift in vaginal flora on Papanicolaou smear and acute chorioamnionitis and preterm delivery. Diagn Cytopathol 1999;21:7–9.

48. Michael CW. The Papanicolaou smear and the obstetric patient: a simple test with great benefits. Diagn Cytopathol 1999;21:4–6.

49. Schnadig VJ, Davie KD, Shafer SK, et al. The cytologist and bacteriosis of the vaginal-ectocervical area. Clues, commas, and confusion. Acta Cytol 1989;33:287–97.

50. Prey M. Routine Pap smears for the diagnosis of bacterial vaginosis. Diagn Cytopathol 1999;21:10–13.

51. Gupta PK, Hollander DH, Frost JK. Actinomycetes in cervicovaginal smears: an association with IUD usage. Acta Cytol 1976;20:295–97.

52. Gupta PK. Intrauterine contraceptive devices: vaginal cytology, pathologic changes and clinical implications. Acta Cytol 1982;26:571–613.

53. De la Monte SM, Gupta PK, White III CL. Systemic Actinomyces infection: a potential complication of intrauterine contraceptive devices. JAMA 1982;248:1876–77.

54. Arsenault GM, Kalman CF, Sorensen KW. The Papanicolaou smear as a technique for gonorrhea detection: a feasibility study. J Am Vener Dis Ass 1976;2:35–38.

55. Angrish K, Verma K. Cytologic detection of tuberculosis of the uterine cervix. Acta Cytol 1981;25:160–62.

56. De Boer AL, de Boer F, van der Merwe JV. Cytologic identification of Donovan bodies in granuloma inguinale. Acta Cytol 1984;28:126–28.

57. Naib ZM. Exfoliative Cytopathology, 3rd edn. Boston: Little Brown; 1985.

58. Bridland R. Trichomoniasis. Tskr Norske Laegoforg 1962;82:441.

59. Gupta PK, Frost JK. Human urogenital trichomoniasis epidemiology, clinical and pathological manifestations. Acta Univ Carol 1988;30:399–410.

60. Frost JK. Trichomonas vaginalis and cervical epithelial changes. Ann NY Acad Sci 1962;97:792–99.

61. De Moraes-Ruehsen M, McNeill RE, Frost JK, et al. Amoebae resembling Entamoeba gingivalis in the genital tracts of IUD users. Acta Cytol 1980;24:413–20.

62. Rachman R, Rosenberg M. Distinction between Entamoeba gingivalis and Entamoeba histolytica, revisited. Acta Cytol 1986;30:82.

63. Fentanes de Torres E, Benitez-Bribiesca L. Cytologic detection of vaginal parasitosis. Acta Cytol 1973;17:252–57.

64. Boquet-Jiminez E, Alvarez San Cristobal A. Cytologic and microbiological aspects of vaginal Torulopsis. Acta Cytol 1978;22:331–34.

65. Corey L, Adams HG, Brown ZA, et al. Genital herpes simplex virus infection: clinical manifestations, course and complications. Ann Int Med 1983;98:958–72.

66. Langley FH, Crompton AC. Epithelial Abnormalities of the Cervix Uteri. Berlin: Springer; 1973.

67. Ng ABP, Reagan JW, Lindner E. The cellular manifestations of primary and recurrent herpes genitalis. Acta Cytol 1970;14:124–29.

68. Anderson GH, Matisic JP, Thomas BA. Confirmation of herpes simplex viral infection by an immunoperoxidase technique. Acta Cytol 1985;29:695–700.

69. Stowell SB, Wiley CM, Powers CM. Herpesvirus mimics: a potential pitfall in endocervical brush specimens. Acta Cytol 1994;38:43–50.

70. Marsh M, Brooklyn NY. Papilloma of the cervix. Am J Obstet Gynecol 1952;64:281–91.

71. Meisels A, Fortin R. Condylomatous lesions of the cervix and vagina I. Acta Cytol 1976;20:64–71.

72. Metzelaar-Venema A. Correlation Study between Macroscopy and Cytology of Condylomatous Lesions of the Cervix. The Eighth European Congress of Cytology, Szczecin, 1978.

73. Dunn AEG, Ogilvie MM. Intranuclear virus particles in human genital wart tissue: observations on the ultrastructure of the epidermal layer. J Ultrastruct Res 1968;22:282–95.

74. Laverty CR, Russel P, Hills E, et al. The significance of non-condylomatous wart virus infection of the cervical transformation zone: a review with discussion of two illustrative cases. Acta Cytol 1978;22:195–201.

75. Zur Hausen H, Meinhof W, Schreiber W, et al. Attempts to detect virus-specific DNA sequences in human tumors. I. Nucleic acid hybridisations with complementary RNA of human wart virus. Int J Cancer 1974;13:650–56.

76. Stanley M. Prophylactic HPV vaccines. J Clin Pathol 2007(60):961–65.

77. Greer CE, Wheeler CM, Ladner MB, et al. Human papillomavirus (HPV) type distribution and serological response to HPV type 6 virus-like particles in patients with genital warts. J Clin Microbiol 1995;33:2058–63.

78. Cogliano V, Baan R, Straif K, et al. Carcinogenicity of human papillomaviruses. Lancet Oncol 2005;6:204.

79. Clifford GM, Smith JS, Aguado T, et al. Comparison of HPV type distribution in high-grade cervical lesions and cervical cancer. A meta-analysis. Br J Cancer 2003;89:101–5.

80. Dudding N, Sutton J, Lane S. Koilocytosis: an indication for conservative management. Cytopathology 1996;7:32–37.

81. Kitchener HC, Alomonte M, Wheeler P, et al. HPV testing in routine cervical screening; cross-sectional data from the ARTISTIC trial. Br J Cancer 2006;95:56–61.

82. Smith J. The future of cytology laboratories. Cytopathology 2007;s1:18:5–186.

83. Koss LG, Durfee GR. Unusual patterns of squamous epithelium of the uterine cervix: cytologic and pathologic study of koilocytic atypia. Ann NY Acad Sci 1956;63:1245–61.

84. Kern S. Significance of anucleated squames in Papanicolaou stained cervicovaginal smears. Acta Cytol 1991;35:89–93.

85. Tanaka H, Chua K-L, Lindh E, et al. Patients with various types of human papilloma virus: covariation and diagnostic relevance of cytological findings in Papanicolaou smears. Cytopathology 1993;4:273–83.

86. Burrows DA, Howell LP, Hinrichs S, et al. Cytomorphologic features in the diagnosis of human papillomavirus infection of the uterine cervix. Acta Cytol 1990;34:737–38.

87. Rakoczy P, Hutchinson L, Kulski JK, et al. Detection of human papillomavirus in reprocessed routine Papanicolaou smears by DNA hybridisation. Diagn Cytopathol 1990;6:210–14.

88. Vesterinen E, Leinikki P, Saksela E. Cytopathogenicity of cytomegalovirus to human ecto- and endocervico-epithelial cells in vitro. Acta Cytol 1975;19:473–81.

89. Huang AC, Naylor B. Cytomegalovirus infection of the cervix detected by cytology and histology: a report of five cases. Cytopathology 1993;4:237–41.

90. Morse AR, Coleman DV, Gardner SD. An evaluation of cytology in the diagnosis of herpes simplex virus infection and cytomegalovirus infection of the cervix uteri. J Obstet Gynec Br Commonw 1974;81:393–98.

91. Laverty CR, Russell P, Black J, et al. Adenovirus infection of the cervix. Acta Cytol 1977;21:114–17.

92. Beato CV. Progress Review: Sexually Transmitted Diseases. Healthy People 2010. Online. Available at: www.healthypeople.gov/document/html/volume2125stds.htm.

93. Gupta PK, Lee EF, Erozan YS, et al. Cytologic investigations in Chlamydia infection. Acta Cytol 1979;23:315–20.

94. Bernal JN, Martinez MA, Dabacens A. Evaluation of proposed cytomorphologic criteria for the diagnosis of Chlamydia trachomatis in Papanicolaou smears. Acta Cytol 1989;33:309–13.

95. Boon ME, Hogewoning CJA, Tjiam KH, et al. Cervical cytology and Chlamydia trachomatis infection. Arch Gynecol 1983:131–40.

96. Tam H, Stamm W, Handsfield H, et al. Culture-independent diagnosis of Chlamydia trachomatis using monoclonal antibodies. N Engl J Med 1984;310:1146–50.

97. Crum CP, Mitao M, Winkler B, et al. Localizing Chlamydia infection in cervical biopsies with the immunoperoxidase technique. Int J Gynec Pathol 1984;3:191–97.

98. Kuo CC, Wang SP, Wentworth BB, et al. Primary isolation of TRIC organisms in HeLa 229 cells treated with DEAE dextran. J Infect Dis 1972;125:665–68.

99. Claas HC, Melchers WJ, de Bruijn IH, et al. Detection of Chlamydia trachomatis in clinical specimens by the polymerase chain reaction. Eur J Clin Microbiol Inf Dis 1990;9:864–68.

100. Sturdee D. Endometrial carcinoma and HRT. Reviews in Gynaecologic Practice 2005;5:51–56.

101. Legha S. Tamoxifen in the treatment of breast cancer. Ann Int Med 1988;109:219–28.

102. Eells TP, Alpern HD, Grzywacz C, et al. The effect of tamoxifen on cervical squamous maturation in Papanicolaou stained cervical smears of postmenopausal women. Cytopathology 1990;1:263–68.

103. Neven P. Tamoxifen and endometrial lesions (editorial). Lancet 1993;342:452.

104. Bertolissi A, Carter G, Turrin D, et al. Behaviour of vaginal epithelial maturation and sex hormone-binding globulin in postmenopausal breast cancer patients during the first year of Tamoxifen therapy. Cytopathology 1998;9:263–70.

105. Jordan VC, Assiki VJ. Endometrial carcinoma and tamoxifen; clearing up a controversy. Clinical Cancer Research 1995;1:467–72.

106. McCluggage WG, Sumathi VP, McManus DT. Uterine serous carcinoma and endometrial intraepithelial carcinoma arising in endometrial polyps: Report of 5 cases including 2 associated with tamoxifen treatment. Human Pathol 2003;34:939–43.

107. Lavie O, Barnett-Griness O, Narod SA. The risk of developing uterine sarcoma after tamoxifen use. Int J of Gynaecol Cancer 2007;18:352–56.

108. Ganesan R, Ferryman S, Waddell CA. Vaginal adenosis in a patient on Tamoxifen therapy: a case report. Cytopathology 1999;10:127–30.

109. Koss LG. Diagnostic Cytology and its Histopathologic Bases, 4th edn. Philadelphia: Lippincott; 1992.

110. Fornari ML. Cellular changes in the glandular epithelium of patients using IUCD – a source of cytologic error. Acta Cytol 1974;18:341–45.

111. Dela Gaza E, De La Gaza S. Cervico-vaginal cytology In women with intra-uterine devices. Patologica 1980;18:183–91.

112. Sagiroglu N, Sagiroglu E. The cytology of intrauterine contraceptive devices. Acta Cytol 1970;14:58–65.

113. Gupta PK, Hollander DH, Frost JK. Actinomycetes in cervicovaginal smears: an association with IUD usage. Acta Cytol 1976;20:294–98.

114. Arroyo G, Quinn JA Jr.. Association of amoebae and Actinomyces in an intrauterine contraceptive device user. Acta Cytol 1989;33:298–300.

115. Highman WJ. Calcified bodies and the intrauterine device. Acta Cytol 1971;15:473–76.

116. Boon ME, Kirk RS, de Graaff Guilloud JC. IUD pathology; psammoma bodies and some opportunistic infections detected in cervical smears of women fitted with an IUD. Contracept Deliv Syst 1981;2:231–36.

117. Bibbo M, Keebler CM, Weid GL. The cytologic diagnosis of tissue repair in the female genital tract. Acta Cytol 1971;15:133–37.

118. Hasegawa T, Tsutsui F, Kurihara S. Cytomorphologic study on the atypical cells following cryosurgery for the treatment of chronic cervicitis. Acta Cytol 1975;19:533–38.

119. Butler EB. The Cytology of the Cervix After Cryosurgery. The Sixth European Congress of Cytology, Weimar, 1976.

120. Bukovsky A, Zidovsky J. Cytologic phenomena accompanying uterine cervix electrocoagulation. Acta Cytol 1985;30:353–62.

121. Suh KS, Silverberg SG. Tubal metaplasia of the uterine cervix. Int J Gynecol Pathol 1990;9:122–28.

122. Ismail SM. Cone biopsy causes cervical endometriosis and tuboendometrioid metaplasia. Histopathol 1991;18:107–14.

123. Ducatman BS, Wang HH, Jonasson JG, et al. Tubal metaplasia: a cytologic study with comparison to other neoplastic and non-neoplastic conditions of the endocervix (Leiman G, editorial comment). Diagn Cytopathol 1993;9:98–105.

124. Hirschowitz L, Eckford SD, Philpotts B, et al. Cytological changes associated with tubo-endometrioid metaplasia of the uterine cervix. Cytopathology 1994;5:1–8.

125. Lee KR. Atypical glandular cells in cervical smears from women who have undergone cone biopsy: a diagnostic pitfall. Acta Cytol 1993;37:705–9.

126. Cleaves MA. Radium with a preliminary note on radium rays in the treatment of cancer. J Adv Ther 1903:667–82.

127. Shield PW, Daunter B, Wright RG. Review. Post-irradiation cytology of cervical cancer patients. Cytopathology 1992;3:167–82.

128. Van Niekerk WA. Cervical cytological abnormalities caused by folic acid deficiency. Acta Cytol 1966;10:67–73.

129. Mclennan MT, Mclennan LE. Significance of cervicovaginal cytology after radiation therapy for cervical cancer. Am J Obstet Gynecol 1975;121:96–100.

130. Patten SF, Reagan JW, Obenauf M, et al. Postirradiation dysplasia of uterine cervix and vagina: an analytical study of the cells. Cancer 1963;16:173–82.

131. Muram D, Curry RH, Drouin P. Cytologic follow-up of patients with cervical carcinoma treated by radiotherapy. Am J Obstet Gynecol 1982;142:350–54.

132. Gureli N, Denham SW, Root SW. Cytologic dysplasia related to busulfan (myleran) therapy. Obstet Gynec 1963;21:466–70.

133. Walker SE, Bole GG. Augmented incidence of neoplasia in female New Zealand black/New Zealand white mice treated with long-term cyclophosphamide. J Lab Clin Med 1971;78:978–79.

134. Gupta PK, Pinn VM, Taft PD. Cervical dysplasia associated with azathioprine (Imuran) therapy. Acta Cytol 1969;13:373–77.

135. Massad LS. Low incidence of invasive cervical cancer among HIV infected US women in a prevention programme. AIDS 2004:109–13.

136. Herbst AL, Kurman RJ, Scully RE. Vaginal and cervical abnormalities after exposure to stilboestrol in utero. Obstet Gynecol 1972;40:287–98.

137. Kranl TC, Zelger B, Kopfler H, et al. Vulval and vaginal adenosis. Br J Dermatol 1998;139:128–31.

# Cervical screening programmes

Karin J. Denton and Mina Desai

## Chapter contents

## Introduction

In the middle of the twentieth century, screening for cervical cancer was heralded as the solution to a type of cancer that had hitherto been almost invariably fatal. Yet it has taken the best part of the latter half of that century to see falls in incidence and mortality in those countries that have well organised screening programmes. This chapter will address the problems and some of the solutions to running a cervical screening programme and will explore some of the recent developments that could be used to enhance the screening procedure.

## Principles of screening

Screening can be defined as the testing of people who do not have any recognisable signs of the condition in question, with the purpose of reducing risk for that individual of future ill health due to disease. Screening encompasses the whole system and is a programme not a test.[1]

Screening for disease in a population might seem to offer obvious benefits, but as Raffle and Gray have stated, 'All screening programmes do harm. Some do good as well and, of these, some do more good than harm at a reasonable cost'.[1] The aim of any screening programme is to detect disease at an earlier stage than it could have been detected by symptomatic presentation, but clearly the disease is only suitable for screening if the benefits outweigh the harms in this equation.

In order to give benefit, the test must be effective in detecting the disease. This is the sensitivity of the test. It must detect disease at a stage where intervention and treatment lead to a better outcome than if the disease had been left to present symptomatically and obviously there must be an effective treatment. In terms of harm, the screening test and follow-up investigations for those who screen positive must not confer more harm than good and this confers an ethical dilemma – is it acceptable to harm the many for the benefit of the few? Finally, the screening programme must be economically viable, and this needs to be addressed in terms of competition for resources and health priorities, albeit very different in different settings.

Cervical screening in the UK meets these criteria, and is an excellent example of a successful screening programme. However, this has not always been the case.

## History of cervical screening in the UK

George Papanicolaou had described cytological changes in cervical smears in 1928[2] but his technique was not widely implemented for many years. It was not until the 1950s that cervical smears were first taken in the UK, but there was no properly organised programme. Screening tended to concentrate on young women attending for contraceptive and antenatal care, predominantly from higher socioeconomic groups. These women were at low risk of cervical carcinoma and women continued to die of the disease in undiminished numbers. It became apparent, however, that in areas where a well-organised programme was in place, for example Scotland,[3] mortality began to fall.

This prompted the establishment of a true national screening programme, which by 1998 was producing guidance documents to standardise and improve procedures throughout the country. A national computer system (The Exeter system) was procured, which is still in use today. Computerised call and recall of women started in 1998. A national coordinating team was appointed and continued to produce documents on all aspects of the screening programme.

However, although the programme was much improved it became apparent that there were still a number of problems. A series of errors were highlighted in very critical reports, culminating in the investigation into screening services at Kent and Canterbury which was published in 1997.[4] This defined the need for robust quality assurance (QA), which is one of the main features of the programme today.

There is now abundant evidence that the UK cervical screening programmes have greatly reduced the incidence of cervical cancer[5–7] and this reduction appears to be continuing, although the rate of improvement may be decreasing. There is also evidence that without screening, the incidence of cervical cancer would be increasing dramatically, so that it is now calculated that 75% of cases are prevented, saving thousands of lives per year in England and Wales (Figs 22.1, 22.2).[5]

## The UK cervical screening programmes

There are three separate screening programmes in the UK, in England, Scotland and Wales, all very similar with slight differences in governance and details of policy. The information given here relates to the English programme, the National Health Service Cervical Screening Programme (NHSCSP).

Cervical screening is led by the National Screening Office, headed by a director of screening who is accountable at a high level within the Department of Health. The National Screening Office has a coordinating role, to seek expert opinion, produce national specification documents, coordinate the evaluation of all the local programmes and to assess the introduction of new technologies and screening strategies.

Delivery at a local level involves many individuals and organisations whose roles are described in Box 22.1.

## Quality assurance and governance

The responsibility for commissioning cervical screening lies with the local Primary Care Trust (PCT), and the overseeing and performance management of this role rests with the Strategic

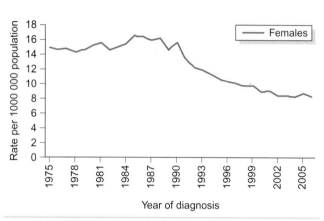

Fig. 22.1 Age standardised (European) incidence rates, cervical cancer, Great Britain 1975–2006.

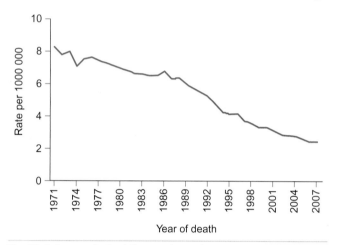

Fig. 22.2 Age standardised (European) mortality rates, cervical cancer, Great Britain 1975–2007.

---

### Box 22.1 Roles of organisations in the English cervical screening programme

**Primary care trust (PCT)**
- Responsible for commissioning services for their registered population
- Hold population database
- Operate call and recall, generating list of women to be invited
- Operate fail-safe processes
- Public health lead role is key to local coordination
- Responsibility for governance of sample takers, some as direct employees, others through normal governance routes for general practitioners
- Participate in audit of cases of invasive cervical cancer

**Cytology laboratory**
- Receive and report cervical samples
- Adhere to all quality standards
- Transmit results to sample taker and PCT
- Operate fail-safe procedures
- Work with histology and colposcopy to correlate cases
- Participate in audit of cases of invasive cervical cancer

**Colposcopy**
- Investigation and treatment of women with abnormal cervical samples according to national quality standards
- Communicate results to women
- Communicate to GPs and call recall databases
- Operate fail-safe processes
- Participate in audit of cases of invasive cervical cancer

**Histology laboratory**
- Report cervical histology according to national quality standards
- Histology/cytology correlation
- Provide information to cancer registries
- Liaise with colposcopy
- Participate in audit of cases of invasive cervical cancer

**Sample takers**
- Provide appointments for women to have samples
- Take samples according to national quality standards
- Explain to women what the screening programme is, gain informed consent to participate
- Ensure women receive the result in writing and arrange any further investigations (these responsibilities are often delegated)

Health Authority (SHA) for that Region. Responsibility for performance of parts of the service delivered within hospitals rests with the NHS Trust concerned, ultimately with its Chief Executive. All professionals working within the programme have a responsibility to ensure they have been adequately trained and are conversant with the programme.

Each region has a quality assurance team reporting to the Regional Director of Public Health. This is a team led by a senior individual who monitors the quality of all parts of the programme, including visits to the service at least once every 4 years. The QA process monitors procedural and outcome measurements, comparing performance to national quality specifications, and to national outcome statistics. The QA team also aims to recognise and disseminate good practice. Ultimately the purpose of the QA process is to identify potential problems early so that they can be resolved before women come to harm.

Large scale 'look back' exercises when mistakes emerge are very damaging to morale within the service and to uptake of screening by women, for whom there is often considerable distress. The greatest success of the QA process is that since this was fully established in 1996/1967, these enquiries have largely been avoided. Key outcome measures reviewed by the QA process are summarised in Table 22.1.

In conclusion, the NHSCSP is a process which is specified in detail[9] and fully quality assured. It is a national, lifelong process for women, interlinking all disciplines with fail-safe processes at every stage where intervention is required.

## Litigation

Cervical screening is a screening test and therefore cannot and does not prevent all cases of cervical cancer. This inevitably leads to the possibility of women or their families taking legal action for perceived failure to prevent the adverse effects of cervical cancer in cases where the system has not protected a patient adequately. These adverse effects range from loss of fertility, to postoperative morbidity and of course sometimes to death.

In the UK there are a significant number of such cases involving cervical screening each year, although the exact number is not published. The vast majority are either dropped or a settlement is reached out of court; very few have reached trial, when the details become public.

In the past, legal attention has focused on cytology laboratories but, increasingly, all parts of the programme are coming under review. It is highly likely that issues such as failure to invite women, failure to act on non-responder notifications, fail-safe failures and inadequate treatment at colposcopy could for example be the basis for litigation.

The legal principle used in the UK in many such cases is the Bolam test, which states that a course of action is not negligent if it would have been followed by a substantial body of responsible medical opinion at the time. Unfortunately, the Bolam test has proved difficult to apply to cervical cytology on those occasions where a sample reported as negative is found on review to contain abnormal cells. Although it has to be accepted that all competent screeners will occasionally miss an abnormality, this has not proved to be an acceptable defence and such cases nearly always lead to a settlement.

Since 2007, all cases of cervical cancer diagnosed in England have been subjected to a full audit, including review of the previous cytology, the histology, colposcopy and recall history. Results

**Table 22.1** Outcome measures in cervical screening quality assurance

| Outcome measure | Description | Acceptable value |
|---|---|---|
| Coverage | Eligible population having an adequate sample in the last 5 years | 80% |
| Laboratory sensitivity | Abnormal samples recognised as such (detected by rapid re/preview) | 90% all grade; 95% high-grade dyskaryosis |
| Positive predictive value (PPV) | Proportion of women with cytology result of moderate dyskaryosis or worse who have CIN 2 or worse on histology | 10th–90th centiles of all laboratories; 70.7–88.9% (2007–2008)[6] |
| Detection rates for abnormalities | Proportion of samples taken in a primary care setting reported as abnormal by each laboratory | 10th–90th centiles of all laboratories; Low grade 3.6–7.4%; High grade 0.7–1.4%[8] |

of this audit are offered to women. It is unclear at the time of writing whether this will result in an increase in litigation.

## Comparison with other national cervical screening programmes

The NHSCSP is reputed to be one of the best screening programmes in the world but it was not the first, and is not the only successful programme. In terms of international comparison, however, the NHSCSP does have several distinguishing features.

- It is based on national specifications which are very detailed, and it is fully quality assured
- Cervical screening is free to all eligible women because this is a publicly funded programme provided entirely through state health services
- There is a national call/recall database. In most national settings, for example the USA, there is no national call/recall database. Other organisations, such as health maintenance organisations or private insurers may operate such a system but only to their own members
- Quality assurance by peer review is fully open. Elsewhere, many laboratories providing screening services are privately operated and peer review may be less open because of commercial sensitivities
- Laboratories are not remunerated per adequate sample. Elsewhere, because laboratories are paid per sample, there is no incentive to reduce the number of samples taken. Some European countries have a very high frequency of screening partly for this reason
- There is less pressure on laboratories in the UK to avoid an inadequate report, because unlike other settings, this will not affect reimbursement, and sample-takers are not able to move their work to a laboratory with a lower inadequate rate. The threshold for an inadequate report is higher in the

UK than elsewhere. For example, in the USA, a threshold of 5000 cells on a liquid-based cytology sample is taken as adequate, which would not be acceptable in the UK and may be responsible for failure to detect disease in some women[10]

- In the UK there tend to be close relationships between cytology laboratories, histology laboratories and colposcopy clinics, so that most women will follow the same routes of referral. This is not the case in many countries, which must make the 'joined up' approach to cervical screening more difficult

- In countries where health is seen as an individual responsibility, public health initiatives such as defining starting age and screening interval are difficult to apply, and few countries have the same kind of outcome information as the UK, nationally recorded and accessible

- Colposcopy is similar in many countries and efforts have been made to standardise nomenclature,[11,12] but often the way in which colposcopy is used is quite different to the UK. If there is no primary care system, there may be little difference between a colposcopy appointment and an appointment for a cervical cytology sample. Colposcopy is not always seen as the highly specialised field that it is in the UK; most gynaecologists consider it within their core work

- Terminology of cervical cytology varies in different countries but most terminologies are fairly easily translated. Recently it has been proposed that the terminology used in the UK should be modified to relate more closely to that of the Bethesda System which is in use in the USA and many other parts of the world (see Ch. 25). The correlation between different terminologies is shown in Table 22.2 (see Ch.23).

**Table 22.2** Comparison of terminology classifications in common usage

| BSCC 1986 | BSCC (proposed new terminology) | Bethesda system 2001 | ECTP terminology | NHMRC terminology |
|---|---|---|---|---|
| Negative | Negative | Negative for intraepithelial lesion or malignancy | Within normal limits | Negative |
| Inadequate | Inadequate | Unsatisfactory for evaluation | Unsatisfactory due to: | Unsatisfactory |
| Borderline nuclear change | 1. Borderline change, high-grade dyskaryosis not excluded<br>2. Borderline change in endocervical cells<br>3. Borderline change, squamous, but not otherwise specified | 1. Atypical squamous cells ASC-US (undetermined significance) ASC-H (cannot exclude HSIL)<br>2. Atypical endocervical/ endometrial/glandular cells: not otherwise specified (NOS) or favour neoplastic | 1. Koilocytes (without changes suggestive of intraepithelial neoplasia)<br>2. Squamous cell changes (not definitely neoplastic but merit early repeat)<br>3. Atypical glandular cells (qualify) | 1. Low-grade epithelial abnormality (LGEA)<br>2. Minor non-specific changes of HPV<br>3. Inconclusive (HGEA cannot be excluded) |
| Mild dyskaryosis | Low-grade dyskaryosis (includes all cases of Koilocytosis provided that no high-grade dyskaryosis is present) | Low-grade squamous intraepithelial lesion (LSIL) | Mild dysplasia (CIN1) | LGEA: cervical intraepithelial neoplasia 1 |
| Moderate dyskaryosis | High-grade dyskaryosis | High-grade squamous intraepithelial lesion (HSIL) | Moderate dysplasia (CIN2) | HGEA: cervical intraepithelial neoplasia 2 |
| Severe dyskaryosis | High-grade dyskaryosis | HSIL | 1. Severe dysplasia (CIN3)<br>2. Carcinoma *in situ* (CIN3) | HGEA: cervical intraepithelial neoplasia 3 |
| Severe dyskaryosis ?invasive | High-grade dyskaryosis ?invasive | Squamous cell carcinoma | 1. Severe dysplasia ?invasive<br>2. Invasive squamous cell carcinoma | Carcinoma |
| ?Glandular neoplasia | ?Glandular neoplasia Endocervical Non-cervical | Endocervical carcinoma *in situ* Adenocarcinoma Endocervical Endometrial Extrauterine NOS | Adenocarcinoma AIS Endocervical Endometrial Extrauterine NOS | HGEA Adenocarcinoma *in situ* Carcinoma |

BSCC: British Society for Clinical Cytopathology; ECTP: European Community Training Project; NHMRC: the National Health and Medical Research Council. (Modified from Denton 2008.[13])

Finally, it must be remembered that the vast majority of cases of cervical cancer worldwide do not occur in developed countries with cervical screening programmes. There is a huge burden of disease in resource-poor settings and screening there is difficult both practically and ethically. Should scarce resources be spent on cervical screening when maternal and infant mortality are very high? Can a national programme be implemented, especially outside big cities? Can high coverage be achieved? Is adequate treatment available for disease detected by screening? In practical terms, it has been the experience of several countries that training sample-takers and laboratory staff to a high enough level to provide a quality service and to retain such staff is difficult. Overall, effective cervical screening in resource-poor settings is extremely challenging and it may be that other means of disease prevention ultimately prove more effective.

## New methods in cervical screening

Despite the fall in cervical cancer incidence and mortality with the introduction of organised, quality-assured screening, there is some evidence that a plateau may have been reached with the traditional method of screening.[14,15] It appears that the conventional smear test is not sufficiently sensitive, specific or consistent in reliably detecting cervical intraepithelial neoplasia (CIN).[16,17] A meta-analysis of European studies[18] has shown that the median sensitivity of conventional cytology is only 50%, but with marked variation in sensitivity in different national settings.[19]

The issue of specificity is also important in an organised screening programme. To decrease the false negative rate, there is a tendency to increase inadequate and false positive rates. This approach leads to unnecessary colposcopy and treatment-associated morbidity. Low-grade abnormality has shown spontaneous regression rates of up to 60%.[20] This has economic, social and psychological consequences.

In the developing world, where the major burden of disease is due to failure to screen, improvement in screening coverage is important, while in the developed world, where coverage is 80% or more, the move towards new technologies is essential. A number of new technologies are available, some of which have already been introduced in various screening programmes in the developed world. The main procedures currently available are as follows:

- Liquid-based cytology (LBC)
- Automated scanning devices
- Computer-assisted microscopy
- Digital colposcopy with automated image analysis
- Human papillomavirus (HPV) testing
- Molecular markers
- HPV vaccine.

### Liquid-based cytology

Conventional cervical smears are directly spread on a glass slide: therefore the cells of interest are mixed with debris, blood and exudate. Major disadvantages of this technique are the suboptimal preservation of cells and cellular obscuring by unwanted material, leading to a high proportion of cases reported as inadequate or suboptimal for assessment. In UK, the rate of inadequate smears with conventional technology was as high as 10%.

LBC technique preserves cells in a liquid medium and removes most of the debris, blood and exudate either by filtration or density gradient centrifugation. The advantages are: improved cellular details for assessment, reduction in inadequate and suboptimal rates, availability of residual material for HPV and other molecular tests and linkages with an automated screening device.

The cervical screening programme in the UK is fully converted to LBC technology using two widely available systems, the ThinPrep® (HOLOGIC) and SurePath® (BD) systems. There are major differences in preparation techniques and presentation on glass slides between these two systems. However, initial data from the UK screening programme have not shown any significant difference in inadequate rate, high-grade dyskaryosis pick-up rate or positive predictive value between these systems.

In many countries in Europe and worldwide, LBC has not been introduced completely into screening programmes due to the higher cost compared with conventional cytology. In the UK, an analysis by the National Institute for Clinical Excellence (NICE) concluded that the increased cost of consumables could be offset by changes elsewhere in the screening programme, particularly the reduction in inadequate samples.[21] These findings are likely to be unique to the UK. A recent meta-analysis concluded that there was no significant improvement in the sensitivity for the detection of high-grade CIN with LBC technology compared with conventional cytology.[22]

Many new generation LBC systems are emerging from the developed and developing worlds. These systems are being evaluated in different countries. The developing world is looking into a low-cost system for collection of material for HPV testing, while the developed world is seeking a system linked with an automated scanning system giving sensitivity and specificity superior to the HPV test. A project is underway in the UK to evaluate all available LBC systems.

## Automated scanning devices and computer-assisted microscopy

The introduction of LBC in UK laboratories provides a platform for automation in the cervical screening process. Attention has focused on this by the decision of the UK government to set a turnaround time target, of 14 days from the sample being taken to the result being received by the woman, to be achieved by 2010. This target gives laboratories only 7 days to process and report cervical samples. Currently, two FDA-approved semi-automated machines are available, which can expedite the microscopic analysis of the process; however, the available data on effectiveness and cost-effectiveness are not sufficient for the UK screening programme to make a decision regarding its introduction in cytology laboratories. The Health Technology Authority (HTA) funded MAVARIC (Manual Assessment Versus Automated Reading In Cytology)[23] trial is assessing each system. It is also designed to provide a head-to-head comparison of both systems. The trial is due to report in 2009, and if favourable, the UK screening programme will look into at the practicality of introducing these technologies in cytology laboratories.

## Details of currently available systems

Currently, no machines are available to provide fully automated screening by computers without human intervention. There are two FDA-approved semi-automated slide scanning devices consisting of a highly automated microscope and a field of view computer that interprets the images. However, the final decision is made by the human eye in the majority or all cases. These systems are the BD FocalPoint GS Imaging System (formerly known as TriPath AutoPap System) and the HOLOGIC ThinPrep ImagingSystem (formerly known as Cytyc ThinPrep Imaging System). There are major differences between these two systems. Details of the devices are beyond the scope of this book and it is likely that considerable modifications will have been made before either of these or other automated screening devices are in regular use. However, at this stage, laboratories and screening programmes should be aware of the following long-term and short-term implications of introducing any type of automated scanning device.[24]

## Short-term implications

- Decision on which system of automation
- Calculation of minimum workload required for cost-effective implementation of the machine:
  - 35K recommended by ScHARR report[25] in the UK will be too low
  - Reconfiguration of laboratories into fewer larger centres
  - Re-examine viability of the hub and spoke arrangement, where samples are processed on one site but returned to a distant site for screening
- Space and environment requirement of the machine
- Continuous processing of the machine will be more cost-effective; but requires extended working hours and changes to working practices
- Calculation of the new minimum and maximum workload for screening staff
- Reduction in the workforce
- Sharing of expensive, motorised microscopes with a shift system of work for screeners
- Re-training of all staff
- Changing cultural beliefs: machines are not better than human beings
- Cultural dilemma: can a machine give results without human eye intervention?
- Which quality control (QC) method? Rapid rescreening versus pre-screening versus double screening
- Re-visiting quality assurance (QA) criteria for performance data of individual screeners and laboratory as a whole
- QA/QC procedures for the machine
- Drawing up the protocol for troubleshooting for the machine and for the machine reject rates and reasons
- Decision on whether to perform QC on slides designated as not for further review (NFR) by the FocalPoint GS Imaging System
- Revision of the report format to include how the slide was prepared and screened and decision about who signs reports for archiving without human eye intervention
- Revision of patient information leaflet.

## Long-term implications

- Risk of litigation: human versus machine errors
- Who takes the medico-legal responsibility for machine error?
- Effect on workload of machine (total volume and pattern) following the introduction of HPV testing and HPV vaccination.

## Summary

The technological development in semi-automated screening devices for cervical screening is very rapid. There are two Food and Drug Administration (FDA)-approved systems in the market. Both are designed to perform computer-assisted analysis of cell images followed by location guided screening of limited 'Fields Of View'. There are major differences between these two systems.

There are several publications and two systemic reviews on the subject; however, the HTA funded MAVARIC trial in UK is the only trial which is designed to do a head-to-head comparison of these two technologies in a large prospective randomised trial. If the results of this trial, due in 2009, are favourable, the NHSCSP will have to give careful consideration to the short and long-term implications associated with the introduction of this technology.

## Automated image analysis of digital colposcopy

In many developing countries, it is difficult to introduce a screening programme dependent on cervical smears and colposcopic examination. Due to poor resources, a single visit approach with screening, diagnosis and treatment carried out in the same session has been evaluated. Visual inspection with acetic acid (VIA) and visual inspection with Lugol's iodine (VILI) as an affordable and effective alternative screening policy have been evaluated in several cross-sectional studies.[26] The results of these studies show acceptable sensitivity and specificity as a viable alternative screening policy if performed by trained professionals. A multispectral digital colposcope (MDC) acquires reflectance images of the entire cervix with white light before and after acetic acid application. The image analysis is performed after developing the classifiers for local image regions. Further work is required for fully automatic image interpretation.[27] The machine requires minimal training, therefore it has the potential to provide an alternative to VIA and VILI in resource-poor settings if the equipment can be produced at a lower cost. Studies are required to validate the results in a screening population.

## HPV testing

Infection with certain types of human papillomavirus (HPV) is universally accepted as the principal causative factor in the development of cervical cancer and its precursor lesions.[28,29] Detection of high-risk anogenital HPV types has shown clinical utility within cervical screening programmes.

## Proposed clinical utility of HPV testing

- As a primary screening tool
- For triage of low-grade abnormality ASCUS (borderline changes) and LSIL (mild dyskaryosis)
- For follow-up of patients after treatment for CIN as test of cure
- For evaluation of regression, persistence or progression of disease
- As a QA measure for evaluation of cytology, histology and colposcopy mismatch.

## Role of the HPV test as a primary screening tool

Several studies have demonstrated that HPV testing has a higher sensitivity and negative predictive value (NPV) for the detection of high-grade cervical intraepithelial neoplasia (CIN) compared with repeat cytology with conventional smears.[30] However, the specificity and positive predictive value (PPV) of HPV testing are lower than those of cytology.

In Europe, several population-based randomised controlled trials have been established to compare cytology alone with cytology and HPV testing in primary cervical screening. The results of these trials will provide evidence for deciding whether HPV testing should be used within programmes as a primary screening tool complementing cervical cytology or replacing it. Initial results of two of these trials indicate that HPV testing in combination with cytology is more sensitive than conventional cytology alone in detecting high-grade CIN at an earlier stage.[31,32] The ARTISTIC (A Randomized Trial In Screening To Improve Cytology)[33] trial in UK and NTCC (New Technology in Cervical Cancer)[34] trial in Italy are the only randomised trials comparing liquid-based cytology with HPV testing and the results of these trials will be important to compare as LBC has also demonstrated increased sensitivity.[35] Early results of ARTISTIC trials have already shown that, although there was a reduced incidence of CIN3+ in the second screening round in the combined LBC and HPV tests arm, over two rounds there was no difference and combined testing would not be cost-effective.

For cost-effectiveness, the higher sensitivity of HPV testing may allow the screening interval to be extended safely to 5 years or longer. Screening algorithms have already been produced by several investigators demonstrating the use of primary testing with HPV followed by cytology for HPV-positive women only or primary screening with HPV and cytology. If both tests are negative, a repeat test after 5 years or longer can be advised.

Several new molecular markers and seroimmunological assays are being introduced which may improve management algorithms for HPV-positive women and may completely replace the need for cytology. HPV genotyping techniques are readily available. This may help because the majority of CIN3+ lesions are associated with types 16/18.[36] Potential screening algorithms for primary screening with HPV instead of cytology are being investigated in various countries.

## HPV test for the triage of low-grade abnormality and as test of cure

Following the successful introduction of LBC techniques which gave a platform for HPV testing, the UK has introduced this test for the triage of both ASCUS (borderline changes) and LSIL (mild dyskaryosis) abnormalities at six sentinel sites, with a view to roll-out nationally if successful. In the United States,

HPV testing is approved for the triage of women with ASCUS cytology[37,38] only. The value of the HPV test in this setting is due to its high negative predictive value and added sensitivity to detect high-grade CIN, which will reduce unnecessary repeat cytology testing and the associated anxiety for women. The difference in the algorithm of management of patients between the UK and the USA is historical and economical.

## HPV test in primary screening: possible strategies

- Adjunctive Test = cytology + HPV for all women
- Standalone Test = HPV for all women and cytology for HPV + ve women

  *OR*

  Cytology for all women and HPV on cytology +ve women

- Cessation of routine screening after the menopause if a woman has been regularly screened and always cytologically or HPV-negative
- Primary screening with HPV together with cytology ('DNA PAP') for women over 30 years and extend the screening interval for women who are both cytology and HPV-negative
- For practical purposes cytology laboratories may be asked to adopt one of the following scenarios:
  - Current policy of LBC or conventional cytology screening only
  - Cytology and HPV in all women
  - HPV primary screening with LBC sampler and LBC cytology from same vial for HPV +ve women
  - HPV primary screening with HPV sampler/second LBC or conventional cytology sample for HPV +ve women
  - LBC cytology with HPV triage for ASCUS (borderline) and LSIL (mild dyskaryosis) or only for ASCUS.

## Implications of introducing HPV test in an organised screening programme

### Practical issues

There are several HPV tests on the market and new ones are emerging. There are two LBC systems from which residual material has been tried by some of the HPV companies but *not* by all and new LBC tests are emerging. Even with the much tested Hybrid Capture2® (HC2), in the NHSCSP, various trials have used different relative light units (RLU) for the cut-off point and the ARTISTIC trial results are only on ThinPrep samples. The world of HPV testing is not straightforward and laboratories will have to take into consideration the following points which are only the initial list from the lessons learnt by the author (M.D.) from participation in the ARTISTIC and MAVARIC trials and the HPV triage and test of cure sentinel site project.

- Follow-up protocol: acceptability to five parties – cytologists, virologists, colposcopists, primary care staff and women – is a mammoth task
- Which LBC test and which HPV test?
- Which LBC system is FDA approved for which HPV test?
- Who will do the HPV testing. HC2 can be performed in a cytology setting, but virology or molecular biology laboratories may be more appropriate in some areas
- Issues related to transport of vial to a different laboratory for testing

- Need for space and training of staff if the HPV test is performed in cytology laboratories
- Specific issues with virology test, e.g. which cut-off point for HC2 test?
- Management of patients with inadequate virology result
- Patient information and consent (taboo of sexually transmitted disease)
- Dealing with cytology −ve, HPV +ve result when the colposcopy or biopsy outcome is negative
- Patient's right to refuse the test
- Training of sample-taker
- Modification of cytology reports and result letters
- Modifications to laboratory IT systems in cytology and virology
- Changes in the national computer system to allow BNC and mild dyskaryosis results to go on routine recall if HPV −ve
- Changes in national and laboratory fail-safe system and letters to women
- Virology IQC and EQA scheme.

### Specific issues with ThinPrep and SurePath

- Lysis of blood in ThinPrep samples using acetic acid cannot be performed. This may increase cytology inadequacy rate
- For SurePath samples, residue from vials or tubes must be topped up with the manufacturer's preservative fluid otherwise there are more inadequate HPV results
- No need to store or transport SurePath samples at cold temperature (2–8°C) for HPV test with HC2 or Roch Amplicor method, ignoring the manufacturer's recommendation which is impractical[39]
- For the SurePath system, the HPV test should be performed no more than 4 weeks after taking the sample, therefore more than 2 weeks backlog of reporting is unworkable
- May not be able to make extra slides for teaching
- Transport:
  – SurePath samples: important to use correct residual material (original vial/cell-enriched tube)
  – ThinPrep samples: blood-stained samples treated with acetic acid cannot be tested for HPV.

## HPV test: emerging technologies

There are a number of commercial technologies under development, details of which are beyond the scope of this chapter.

## HPV test unanswered questions

- Which LBC? ARTISTIC used ThinPrep with no problem for the HC2 test and different genotyping tests. Will SurePath show similar results?
- Which cut-off point for HPV test? ARTISTIC used: (1) RLU/Sentinel sites, (2) RLU/MAVARIC automation trial, (3) RLU
  – More RLU = less +ve /better specificity, but at what cost?
- Where HPV test will be carried out? Cytology or virology laboratory?
- How will virology EQA be organised?

- Revision of performance indicators for cytology. Only a few abnormal samples in the future
- Focal point algorithm is based on cross-sectional population samples. Will this be suitable for small numbers of triage cytology samples if primary screening is performed by HPV?
- Will HPV test pick-up adenocarcinoma?

## HPV testing in the developing world

A recent large randomised study of HPV screening for cervical cancer in rural India[40] on 131 746 healthy women from 52 villages concluded that a single HPV test significantly reduced the incidence of advanced cervical cancer and cervical cancer mortality within 8 years – far more than one conventional cytology test or VIA *and no cancer death was recorded in HPV negative women*. HPV testing with a self-sampler has brought renewed hopes for the prevention of cervical cancer in the developing world. The START project (Screening Technologies to Advance Rapid Testing) coordinated by PATH (Seattle, WA, USA) in collaboration with China, India, the International Agency for Research on Cancer (IARC) and industrial partners, is funded by the Bill and Melinda Gates Foundation. This project has developed a rapid, simple and low-cost HPV test based on Hybrid capture technology called Care HPV. Its efficacy and cost-effectiveness are being investigated in randomised controlled trials.[41]

## Molecular markers

HPV screening has a higher sensitivity but lower specificity than cytology screening for the detection of cervical precancer and cancer. This will require an additional test in cytology −ve/HPV +ve women to assure the woman that she is at a higher risk of developing high-grade disease and colposcopy is advisable to detect and treat the lesion.

There are a number of tests that identify either persistence of oncogenic HPV types 16/18 or molecular markers of abnormal cellular proliferation (see Ch. 34). Two of these molecular markers have been widely investigated. They are MCM and P16.[42,43] They may have a role in the triage of HPV +ve/cytology −ve group of women. This will need further investigation in the NHSCSP setting.

## HPV vaccine

The advent of the HPV vaccine has raised hopes for cervical cancer prevention in the developed and developing world. Several countries of the developed world have already started population vaccination programmes.

In the UK, a new HPV vaccination programme started in September 2008. After a rigorous adjudication process, Cevarix® vaccine was selected for the national programme.[44] This commenced with vaccination of 12–13-year-old girls through a schools-based programme and within 1 year, 70% uptake has been achieved. This is in line with experience in other countries, including Australia. A catch-up programme will offer vaccination to all girls up to the age of 18 over the next 3 years. Vaccination with Cevarix® will offer immunity against type 16 and 18 oncogenic types but will not prevent pre-cancer and cancer related to other oncogenic types. It is possible that this vaccine will give cross-protection with these other oncogenic types but this will require more data. The unknown level of cross-protection, uncertainty about the exact distribution of HPV subtypes and acceptance that full uptake of vaccination cannot be achieved form the rationale for the recommendation to continue cervical cytology screening.

In the developing world, research on vaccines is concentrated on low-cost alternatives, including production of a one-dose oral vaccine, which can be started at a younger age and incorporated into other vaccination programmes.

## Impact of HPV vaccination programme on cytology laboratories

Screening will still be required in a vaccinated population due to incomplete coverage and causation by non-16/18 strains. Vaccination may strengthen the argument for HPV testing in primary screening followed by cytology triage in HPV positive cases. However, if this policy is implemented, then cytology activity will be at no more than 20% of the current level.

The alternative, primary cytology screening, will bring challenges related to maintaining expertise in cytology when fewer abnormalities are present, although this could be offset by automation. In either case, configuration and staffing of laboratories will clearly need to change.

## The future

Cervical screening programmes are entering a new era of molecular technologies and automation in the developed world. New technologies are being marketed each year but at present, regular cervical screening is still the basis for the prevention of cervical cancer in most countries. However, the gap between healthcare in the developing and developed world is expanding. In this context, it is becoming clear that HPV vaccination offers the best hope of bringing down the incidence and mortality of cervical carcinoma, thereby reducing this unacceptable inequality globally.

## REFERENCES

1. Raffle A, Gray M. Screening Evidence and Practice. Oxford: Oxford University Press; 2008.

2. Papanicolaou GN. New cancer diagnosis. Proceedings of the Third Race Betterment Conference, January 1928. Race Betterment Foundation, Battle Creek, Michigan; 1928:528–34.

3. Macgregor JE, Campbell MK, Mann EM, et al. Screening for cervical intraepithelial neoplasia in north east Scotland shows fall in incidence and mortality from invasive cancer with concomitant rise in preinvasive disease. BMJ 1994;308:1407–11.

4. Wells W. Review of Cervical Screening Services in Kent and Canterbury Hospitals NHS Trust. South Thames, London: NHS Executive; October 1997.

5. Peto J, Gilham C, Fletcher O, et al. The cervical cancer epidemic that screening has prevented in the UK. Lancet 2004;364:249–56.

6. Quinn M, Babb P, Jones J, et al. Effect of screening on incidence of and mortality from cancer of cervix in England: evaluation based on routinely collected statistics. BMJ 1999;318:904–8.

7. Sasieni P, Cusick J, Farmery E. Accelerated decline in cervical cancer mortality in England and Wales. Lancet 1995;346:1566–67.

8. NHS Statistics. Online. Available at: www.ic.nhs.uk/statistics-and-data-collections/screening/cervical-cancer/cervical-screening-programme-2007–uk/statistics-and-data-collections/screening/cervical-cancer/cervical-screening-pro08-%5Bns%5D.

9. NHS Cervical Screening Programme Publications. Online. Available at: www.cancerscreening.nhs.uk

10. Bolick DR. A critical look at Pap adequacy: are our criteria satisfactory? Cytopathology 2006;17(suppl 1):1–1.

11. Jordan J, Arbyn M, Martin-Hirsch P, et al. European guidelines for quality assurance in cervical cancer screening: recommendations for clinical management of abnormal cervical cytology. Cytopathology 2008;19:342–54. Part 1.

12. Jordan J, Martin-Hirsch P, Arbyn M, et al. European guidelines for clinical management of abnormal cervical cytology. Cytopathology 2009;20:5–16. Part 2.

13. Denton K, Herbert AJ, Turnbull LS, et al. The proposed BSCC terminology for abnormal cervical cytology. Cytopathology 2008;19:398–99.

14. IARC Working Group on the Evaluation of Cancer Prevention Strategies. IARC Handbooks of Cancer Prevention, Vol. 10. Cervix cancer screening. Lyon: IARC Press; 2005.

15. Anttila A, Pukkala E, Soderman B, et al. Effect of organized screening on cervical cancer incidence and mortality in Finland, 1963–1995: recent increase in cervical cancer incidence. Int J Cancer 1999;83:59–65.

16. McGoogan E, Reith A. Would monolayers provide more representative samples and improved preparations for cervical screening? Overview and evaluation of systems available. Acta Cytol 1996;40:107–19.

17. Fahey MT, Irwig L, Macaskill P. Meta-analysis of Pap test accuracy. Am J Epidemiol 1995;141:680–89.

18. Cuzick J, Clavel C, Petry K, et al. Overview of the European and North American studies on HPV testing in primary cervical cancer screening. Int J Cancer 2006;119:1095–101.

19. Cuzick J, Szarewski A, Cubie H, et al. Management of women who test positive for high-risk types of human papillomavirus: the HART study. Lancet 2003;362:1871–76.

20. Koss LG. Diagnostic Cytology and its Histopathologic Basis. 4th ed. Philadelphia: Lippincott; 1992. 399–414.

21. NICE. Online. Available at: www.nice.org.uk/guidance/TA5

22. Arbyn M, Bergeron C, Klinkhamer P, et al. Liquid compared with conventional cervical cytology: a systematic review and meta-analysis. Obstet Gynecol 2008;111:167–77.

23. NIHR Health Technology Assessment Programme. A comparison of automated technology and manual cervical screening (MAVARIC). Online. Available at: www.hta.ac.uk/1462

24. Desai M. Role of automation in cervical cytology. Diagn Histopatholy 2009;15:323–29.

25. NHS cervical screening programme. Achieving a 14 day turnaround time for results by 2010. Advice to the NHS. London: Department of Health; April 2008.

26. Sankaranarayanan R, Rajkumar R, Theresa R, et al. Initial results from a randomized trial of cervical visual screening in rural south India. Int J Cancer 2004;109:461–77.

27. Park SY, Follen M, Milbourne A, et al. Automated image analysis of digital colposcopy for the detection of cervical neoplasia. J Biomed Opt 2008;13:1–10.

28. Bosch FX, Lorincz A, Munoz N, et al. The causal relation between human papillomavirus and cervical cancer. J Clin Pathol 2002;55:244–65.

29. Munoz N, Bosch FX, de Sanjose S, et al. International Agency for Research on Cancer Multicenter Cervical Cancer Study Group. Epidemiologic classification of human papillomavirus types associated with cervical cancer. N Engl J Med 2003;348:518–27.

30. Naucler P, Ryd W, Tornberg S, et al. Human papillomavirus and Papanicolaou tests to screen for cervical cancer. N Engl J Med 2007;357:1589–97.

31. Bulkmans R, Berkhof J, Rozendaal F, et al. Human papillomavirus DNA testing for the detection of cervical intraepithelial neoplasia grade 3 and cancer: 5-year follow-up of a randomised controlled implementation trial. Lancet 2006;370:1764–72.

32. Naucler P, Ryd W, Törnberg S, et al. Human papillomavirus and Papanicolaou tests to screen for cervical cancer. N Engl J Med 2007;357:1589–97.

33. Kitchener HC, Almonte M, Thomson C, et al. HPV testing in combination with

liquid-based cytology in primary cervical screening (ARTISTIC): a randomised controlled trial. Lancet Oncol 2009;10:672–82.

34. Ronco G, Cuzick J, Pierotti P, et al. Accuracy of liquid-based versus conventional cytology: overall results of the new technologies for cervical cancer screening randomised controlled trial. BMJ 2007;335:28–31.

35. Williams A. Liquid-based cytology and conventional smears compared over two 12-month periods. Cytopathology 2006;17:82–85.

36. Meijer CJ, Snijders PJ, Castle PE. Clinical utility of HPV genotyping. Gynecol Oncol 2006;103:12–17.

37. Solomon D, Schiffman M, Tarone R. Comparison of three management strategies for patients with atypical squamous cells of undetermined significance: baseline results

from a randomized trial. J Natl Cancer Inst 2001;93:293–99.

38. Arbyn M, Buntinx F, Van Ranst M, et al. Virologic versus cytologic triage of women with equivocal Pap smears: a meta-analysis of the accuracy to detect high-grade intraepithelial neoplasia. J Natl Cancer Inst 2004;96:280–93.

39. Cubie HA, Moore C, Waller M, Moss S. National Cervical Screening Committee LBC/HPV Pilot Steering Group. The development of a quality assurance programme for HPV testing within the UK NHS cervical screening LBC/HPV studies. J Clin Virol 2005;33:287–92.

40. Sankaranarayanan R, Nene BM, Surendra SS, et al. HPV Screening for cervical cancer in rural India. N Engl J Med 2009;360:1385–94.

41. Qiao YL, Sellors JW, Eder PS, et al. A new HPV-DNA test for cervical-cancer screening in

developing regions: a cross-sectional study of clinical accuracy in rural China. Lancet Oncol 2008;9:929–36.

42. Murphy N, Ring M, Killalea AG, et al. p16INK4A as a marker for cervical dyskaryosis: CIN and cGIN in cervical biopsies and ThinPrep smears. J Clin Pathol 2003; 56:56–63.

43. Murphy N, Ring M, Heffron CC, et al. p16INK4A, CDC6, and MCM5: predictive biomarkers in cervical preinvasive neoplasia and cervical cancer. J Clin Pathol 2005;58:525–34.

44. Salisbury DM. (Not) warts and all: Government fully considered HPV vaccine. BMJ 2008;337:a2552.

# Cervical intraepithelial neoplasia and squamous cell carcinoma of the cervix

Peter A. Smith and Winifred Gray

## Chapter contents

**Table 23.1** Geographical variation in age standardised incidence rates for cancer of the cervix per 100 000 population

| | |
|---|---|
| Colombia, Cali | 27.9 |
| Brazil, Brasilia | 37.7 |
| Peru, Trujillo | 43.9 |
| India, Bombay (Mumbai) | 14.5 |
| India, Madras | 28.1 |
| Israel, Jews | 5.8 |
| Japan, Osaka | 5.6 |
| USA, Atlanta, Black | 8.7 |
| USA, Atlanta, White | 6.1 |
| Australia, NSW | 6.1 |
| UK, West Midlands | 8.1 |
| UK, Thames | 5.6 |

(Data from Curado MP, Edwards B, Shin HR, et al. (eds) Cancer Incidence in Five Continents, Vol IX. Lyon: IARC Scientific Publications; 2007.)[2]

## Introduction

It is estimated that in 2002, worldwide, there were 493 000 cases of, and 274 000 deaths from, carcinoma of the cervix. Overall, it is the second most commonly occurring visceral cancer in women, and the third most common cancer causing death in women (after cancers of the breast and lung), but in some parts of the developing world it is the commonest. About 83% of the mortality from this disease occurs in developing countries.[1] The epidemiology of cervical cancer shows wide geographical variation in its occurrence, and varies within local populations (Table 23.1).[2] These differences are related to social and economic conditions, as well as to religion, and the influence of these factors on sexual practices. Age standardised incidence rates of less than 14.5 per 100 000 are generally found in developed countries, and are usually associated with the implementation of successful population screening programmes; before the implementation of such programmes, rates were generally similar to those found in the developing world.[1]

The principal predisposing factors to the development of cancer of the cervix have long been known to be sexual intercourse and the commencement of it at an early age. The next most important epidemiological factor to early age of onset of sexual activity is the number of sexual partners, which is illustrated by the high risk of the disease in prostitutes in all parts of the world. Populations such as that of Cali, Columbia, where women are traditionally carefully shielded from sexual relations before marriage, but men customarily consort with prostitutes, have a high incidence of cervical cancer. Other factors involved include cigarette smoking, the use of the oral contraceptive pill and immunosuppression (see below).

Squamous cell carcinoma is the commonest histological type of cervical cancer. Traditionally, adenocarcinoma of the cervix has been said to account for about 10–15% of the total of invasive carcinomas, but this figure increases if staining for mucin is routinely applied to histopathological material. It has been suggested that pure squamous cell carcinomas account for only about 70% of the total, and the balance is accounted for by mixed adenosquamous carcinomas or poorly differentiated adenocarcinomas. Both relative and absolute increases in the incidence of adenocarcinoma of the cervix have been reported, possibly partly as a consequence of the prevention of squamous cell carcinoma by screening programmes, but the changes vary considerably between different countries.[3] Adenocarcinoma of the cervix is discussed further in Chapter 24.

*The authors acknowledge the contribution of Dr E. A. Hudson to this chapter in the first edition of Diagnostic Cytopathology and wish to dedicate our chapter to her and to Dr O. A. N. Husain, to thank them for all they taught us.*

## Clinical features of invasive carcinoma of the cervix

### Presentation

Clinical invasive carcinoma of the cervix usually presents with symptoms of abnormal vaginal bleeding, particularly post-coital bleeding, and vaginal discharge. After the menopause, postmenopausal bleeding may be the main presenting symptom. Advanced disease is associated with general symptoms such as weight loss and debility, and pelvic or abdominal pain. Inspection of the cervix may reveal an exophytic growth, or the cervix may be infiltrated by an endophytic or diffuse growth, in which case the condition may not be apparent to naked eye examination until necrosis causes ulceration. Some cancers remain in the endocervical canal and are not seen. Colposcopic examination of early invasive carcinoma may show characteristic features even when there is no exophytic growth.

### Spread of carcinoma of the cervix

Squamous cell carcinoma of the cervix spreads principally by local extension to the vagina, parametrium and adjacent structures, including the ureters, bladder and rectum, but also to the pelvic lymph nodes. Involvement of lymphatics or blood vessels carries a poor prognosis. Distant metastases are less common clinically, although they are frequently present at autopsy in patients who die of the disease. Local spread of the carcinoma is responsible for most of the serious effects, and infiltration or compression of the ureters is present in two-thirds of fatal cases. The clinical staging of carcinoma of the cervix of the International Federation of Gynecology and Obstetrics[4] is summarised in Table 23.2.

### Diagnosis

Diagnosis and staging are carried out by a sequence usually involving cytology, colposcopy, histology and clinical and imaging assessment. Cervical cytology samples taken in the presence of invasive carcinoma will usually show severe dyskaryosis and may show features suggestive of the presence of invasive carcinoma (see below). The cervical cytology test is, however, less sensitive for the detection of invasive carcinoma than for preinvasive disease, termed cervical intraepithelial neoplasia (CIN). Cytology preparations taken from invasive carcinomas of the cervix are frequently dominated by blood cells and purulent exudate to the exclusion of neoplastic cells. Further, the cells from invasive carcinoma are sometimes more difficult to interpret than those of CIN. Signs and symptoms that raise suspicion of invasive carcinoma are therefore an indication for referral to a specialist for colposcopic examination and histological biopsy, even if the cytology test is negative.

Examination of the cervix by colposcopy is a key step in the assessment of premalignant and early invasive carcinoma of the cervix. At colposcopy, the cervix is examined under low power magnification. CIN temporarily stains white ('aceto-white') when dilute acetic acid is applied to the cervix, and fails to stain if Lugol's iodine is applied. The reactions to this staining, combined with changes in the vascular pattern of the cervical

**Table 23.2** FIGO clinical staging of carcinoma of the cervix

| Stage | |
|---|---|
| 0 | Carcinoma *in situ* (pre-invasive carcinoma) |
| I | Carcinoma confined to cervix (extension to corpus should be disregarded) |
| IA | Invasive carcinoma diagnosed only by microscopy. All macroscopically visible lesions – even with superficial invasion – are Stage 1B |
| IA1 | Stromal invasion no greater than 3 mm in depth and 7 mm or less in horizontal spread |
| IA2 | Stromal invasion more than 3 mm and not more than 5 mm with a horizontal spread 7 mm or less[a] |
| IB | Clinically visible lesion confined to the cervix or microscopic lesion greater than IA2 |
| IB1 | Clinically visible lesion 4 cm or less in greatest dimension |
| IB2 | Clinically visible lesion more than 4 cm in greatest dimension |
| II | Tumour invades beyond the uterus but not to pelvic wall or to lower third of the vagina |
| IIA | Without parametrial invasion |
| IIB | With parametrial invasion |
| III | Tumour extends to pelvic wall and/or involves lower third of vagina and/or causes hydronephrosis or non-functioning kidney |
| IIIA | Tumour involves lower third of vagina, no extension to pelvic wall |
| IIIB | Tumour extends to pelvic wall and/or causes hydronephrosis or non-functioning kidney |
| IVA | Tumour invades mucosa of bladder or rectum and/or extends beyond true pelvis[b] |
| IVB | Distant metastasis |

(From: Hacker NF, Ngan HYS, Benedet JL. Staging, Classification and Clinical Practice Guidelines for Gynecologic Cancers. FIGO Committee on Gynecologic Oncology, 2nd edn. Int J Gynecol Obstet 2000; 70:207–312.)[4]

[a]The depth of invasion should not be more than 5 mm taken from the base of the epithelium, either surface or glandular, from which it originates. The depth of invasion is defined as the measurement of the tumour from the epithelial-stromal junction of the adjacent most superficial epithelial papilla to the deepest point of invasion. Vascular space involvement, venous or lymphatic, does not affect classification.

[b]The presence of bullous oedema is not sufficient to classify a tumour as T4.

mucous membrane enable the presence, degree and extent of CIN to be assessed and the appropriate site(s) for biopsy to be determined. It should be noted that the appearances of CIN lesions at colposcopy do not always conform with the standard descriptions. Furthermore, just as cytological and histological assessments of cell and tissue preparations from CIN are examples of 'continuous' morphological diagnosis, and as such are subject to observer variation, so are colposcopic assessments of the cervical epithelium. Lesions affecting the vaginal vault rather than the cervix are sometimes overlooked. Apparently significant discrepancies between cytological, colposcopic and histological findings in an individual case should be considered carefully by practitioners in all three disciplines. In current UK practice, this should be in the setting of a clinical multidisciplinary-team meeting.

## Histological classification

Cytological appearances reflect the histological types of invasive squamous cell carcinoma defined by the World Health Organization as follows:

### Invasive squamous cell carcinoma of the cervix

- Keratinising carcinoma
- Large cell non-keratinising carcinoma
- Small cell non-keratinising carcinoma.

This classification equates broadly with a grading system of well, moderately and poorly differentiated carcinoma. Mixed histological patterns of squamous cell carcinoma are commonplace but they may not be apparent cytologically; because of the limitations of sampling, the cells are restricted to those accessible to the sampling implement on the exposed surface of the carcinoma.

## Aetiology and pathogenesis of carcinoma of the cervix

### Human papillomavirus infection

The established relationship between patterns of sexual activity and carcinoma of the cervix is now clearly explained by recognition that certain strains of human papillomavirus (HPV) are causally related to virtually all carcinomas of the cervix.[5] Papillomaviruses have been widely implicated in the development of cancer in higher animals and man, and in excess of 130 HPV types have now been identified. Generally, papillomaviruses cause local epithelial infections, and are highly species specific. In man, HPV infections are fairly site specific. Infection with papillomaviruses is extremely common, and it has been suggested that there is a 70% lifetime risk of genital HPV infection in women in the UK. Genital HPV infection is usually, but not invariably,[6] sexually transmitted. Most infections are transient and typically resolve within 12–24 months. Infections may cause local cell proliferation resulting in such lesions as genital warts and cervical intraepithelial neoplasia (CIN). High-grade CIN and invasive carcinoma of the cervix are associated with persistent HPV infection. Carcinoma of the cervix is recognised as a rare outcome of a common sexually transmitted infection.[7]

Recognised 'low risk' genital HPV types are 6, 11, 42, 43 and 44 are they associated with clinical genital warts and low-grade intraepithelial neoplastic lesions (see below); they have a low risk of progression to high-grade intraepithelial lesions and invasive carcinoma. 'High risk' types include 16, 18, 31, 33, 35, 39, 45, 51, 52, 56, 58, 59 and 68; these are associated with a high risk of progression to high-grade intraepithelial lesions and invasive squamous cell carcinoma. The most commonly detected types of high risk HPV types in the UK are 16, 18, 31 and 45, in descending order. Intraepithelial pre-malignant glandular lesions and invasive adenocarcinoma of the cervix are closely associated with HPV type 18.

The E6 and E7 genes of HPV types 16 and 18 have been shown to be powerful oncogenes in experimental models. Papillomaviruses appear to infect the basal cells of stratified epithelium and low copy numbers of viral genomes are retained in circular (or episomal) form in the basal cells, while the virus reproduces in the maturing differentiated cells. Expression of E6 and E7 is controlled at low levels in the basal cells. In 'productive' infection the transcription of viral DNA results in the production of viral genomes and capsid proteins in the cytoplasm of the host cell. High levels of E6 and E7 expression only occur in differentiated cells which are lost from the surface of the epithelium continually as it is renewed, allowing these cells to pose no carcinogenic threat. Deregulation of this process in some high risk HPV infections allows high levels of oncogene expression in all the epithelial cells, and in particular the basal cells which, as the epithelial progenitor cells, are long lived and susceptible to carcinogenic events. CIN and the development of invasive carcinoma are sequelae of this process. It is apparent that high risk HPV infection is an essential, but not in itself a sufficient cause of carcinoma of the cervix, and other genetic or molecular changes are also required.[8] The integration of HPV DNA into host cell genomes is observed in a very high proportion of invasive carcinomas, and appears to be a key event, but the true significance of integration in relation to the temporal sequence of oncogenesis is uncertain, and the subject of continuing research.[9] Currently, it remains impossible to predict which HPV-related lesions, if untreated, will progress to invasive carcinoma.

Established HPV infections are cleared by cell mediated immune mechanisms. While humoral antibodies are also produced, they appear to be effective only against re-infection. The immunity resulting from immunisation (which uses vaccines prepared with artificial 'virus-like particles') appears to be much stronger and longer lasting than natural immunity.

The establishment of high risk strains of HPV as causal in cervical cancer opens new possibilities for screening, and primary prevention by vaccination. Testing for HPV DNA has potential roles in primary screening (for which it is more sensitive but less specific than cytology), triage of low-grade cytological abnormalities to assist clinical management, test of cure after treatment and potential lengthening of the routine cytology screening interval. These are discussed further in Chapter 22.

### Cigarette smoking

Cigarette smoking has been shown to increase the risk of developing high-grade intraepithelial lesions and invasive carcinoma,[10] with odds ratios of 2–5 for HPV-positive women who have ever smoked.[7] Both direct carcinogenic effects of absorbed products of tobacco smoke, including high levels of cotinine which is preferentially excreted into cervical mucus, and local effects on the immune system, have been suggested as mechanisms. Smoking has been shown to reduce the number of Langerhans cells in cervical epithelium which may interfere with local immunological mechanisms.

### Immunosuppression

In view of the mechanisms responsible for the normal elimination of HPV infection it is unsurprising that immunosuppressed individuals are abnormally susceptible to HPV infections and the development of carcinoma of the cervix. Carcinoma of the cervix is recognised as an acquired immune deficiency syndrome (AIDS)-defining disease in human immunodeficiency virus (HIV)-positive individuals.[11] Immunosuppressed individuals may be a special group who warrant more frequent cervical screening than the general population in view of their increased risk of rapidly progressive HPV-related lesions and cervical cancer.

## Other sexually transmitted infections

Infection with *Chlamydia trachomatis* and with Herpes simplex type 2 have been shown to be associated with an increased risk of invasive carcinoma of the cervix.[7]

## Oral contraceptive pill

Oral contraceptive use for 5 years or more is associated with an increased risk of both CIN and invasive carcinoma which appears to be directly related to the length of time of use, but the effect is mostly observed in countries without a properly organised screening programme.[7,12]

## Parity

More than five full-term pregnancies are associated with an increased risk of invasive carcinoma of the cervix.[7]

## The relationship between CIN and cervical cancer

With the increase in knowledge of cancer pathology, it is now apparent that most cancers, particularly those of epithelial cells, have a prolonged pre-invasive phase. These are recognisable histologically and cytologically, and tend to progress in severity and extent with time, until they become invasive carcinomas. These morphological changes are consistent with the multi-step theory of neoplasia. The association of HPV infection with cervical carcinogenesis, in the light of the natural history of HPV infection, helps explain the pre-invasive changes recognised histologically and cytologically, and the progression and regression of these lesions.

Invasive squamous cell carcinoma of the cervix is preceded by precancerous changes in the cervical epithelium of the transformation zone, which can be identified histologically; the preinvasive (precancerous or premalignant) changes are now usually described as cervical intraepithelial neoplasia (CIN).

## Evidence that CIN is a precursor for invasive squamous cell carcinoma

- Studies of patients with CIN who did not receive treatment
- Temporal relationship between CIN, microinvasive carcinoma and invasive carcinoma
- CIN is found at the periphery of invasive carcinoma in histological sections
- Cells from CIN show morphological and cytogenetic similarities to those from invasive carcinoma
- Successful screening programmes are based on the detection and elimination of CIN.

The preinvasive changes represent a continuous spectrum of morphology, which has been divided into three stages, CIN 1, CIN 2 and CIN 3. These are equivalent to the older conventional terminology respectively to mild dysplasia, moderate dysplasia and severe dysplasia/carcinoma *in situ*. Estimation of the duration of the pre-invasive changes is based on the mean age at diagnosis of CIN 3 and the mean age of development of invasive cancer, some 10–15 years later. Similarly, the mean age for diagnosis of the grades of CIN is consistent with the progression from CIN 1 (mild dysplasia) through CIN 2 (moderate dysplasia) to CIN 3 (severe dysplasia and carcinoma in situ) over a further period of around 10 years. CIN lesions may regress as well as progress and regression may occur spontaneously or be induced by such limited interventions as diagnostic punch biopsy. Regression is more likely at the mild end of the spectrum of change, which is represented in Figure 23.1. It is important to recognise the limitations of a negative cervical cytology test as a test of cure, largely because of sampling problems, and patients with abnormal cytology need follow-up for prolonged periods before regression can be confirmed.

## Progression of CIN 3 to invasive carcinoma

Appropriately designed prospective trials to determine the probability of progression of CIN 3 to invasive carcinoma have never been carried out, and it would now be unethical to perform such trials, because of the known significant risk of progression, and the lack of markers to indicate which particular cases of CIN 3 might progress. A conversion rate of about 30% of cases of CIN 3 to invasive carcinoma over a 30-year period has generally been assumed from the available historical evidence on conversion rates. An extended study has recently been published on a group of women from whom treatment for CIN 3 was withheld, in an unethical clinical trial in New Zealand, between 1965 and 1974. In 143 women managed only by punch or wedge biopsy, the cumulative incidence of invasive carcinoma of the cervix or vaginal vault was 31.3% at 30 years, and 50.3% in a subset of 92 such women who had evidence of persistent CIN within 24 months. In contrast, the cancer risk at 30 years was only 0.7% in 593 women whose treatment was

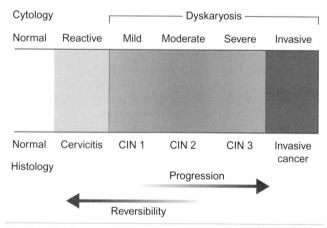

**Fig. 23.1** The diagram represents the spectrum of changes in the cervical epithelium between normal, through intraepithelial neoplasia to invasive squamous cell carcinoma with arrows depicting potential for progression and reversibility.

reviewed as adequate or probably adequate in retrospect.[13] It should be borne in mind that these lesions were in a group of women of a median age of 38 years with extensive lesions, and that CIN 3 lesions in younger women, detected by screening, are generally much smaller in extent, and may not behave in the same way; rates of progression and regression of small CIN 3 lesions in younger women are unknown.[13,14]

If a normal distribution of progression rate is assumed, some cases will develop rapidly and may outstrip the most assiduous preventive screening (resulting in a true 'interval cancer'), whereas cases at the other end of the distribution will not progress to invasive carcinoma within the woman's lifetime. When screening of a population starts the ratio of cases of CIN 3 to invasive carcinoma is of the order of 4:1, which correlates reasonably with the known risk of progression to invasive carcinoma. When data are available from a screened population, very many more cases of CIN 3 are detected than clinical cancers, and a ratio of 10:1 has been reported.[15]

## Area of cervical epithelium with CIN

The proportion of the transformation zone affected by CIN, including crypt involvement, appears to be related to the risk of progression. The cervical cytology test does not detect all CIN, particularly low-grade CIN and/or CIN involving small areas of the transformation zone. The probability of detection by the cervical cytology test rises with an increase in the grade of CIN and an increase in the area of affected epithelium. In earlier successful screening programmes, such as that in North-east Scotland, treatment by cone biopsy or hysterectomy was only given to women whose smears indicated severe dysplasia or carcinoma *in situ* (CIN 3), from which it is deduced that some women with very small areas of CIN 3 had cytology tests reported as only mildly abnormal, and were followed-up by cytology alone; some may even have had normal tests. Progression of these under-graded abnormalities to involve larger areas of the cervix, and increase in cytological abnormality at a subsequent screening, would prevent progression to invasive carcinoma in most cases.

## Screening for prevention of carcinoma of the cervix

The observations of George Papanicolaou of abnormal cells exfoliated from the cervix gave rise to the use of the cervical smear test for the detection of preinvasive cancer. The long natural history of CIN and progression to invasive carcinoma of the cervix, and the probability of successful treatment of CIN approaching 100%, make the disease process an ideal target for population screening. Organised screening programmes are considered in Chapter 22.

## The conventional cervical smear test

The aim of the smear taker is to obtain a representative sample of cells from the transformation zone (see Ch. 21). The material must be spread evenly on the microscope slide and suitably preserved with fixative, so that abnormal cells can be identified by the microscopist. The smear is usually taken using a wooden or plastic spatula. Since the original Ayre spatula, a range of spatulae and brushes have been developed with the aim of improving transformation zone and/or endocervical sampling. Opinion is divided between those who recommend that a brush sample as well as a spatula sample is essential for every cervical screening test, and others who take a brush sample only when the external os is too narrow to admit the tip of a spatula, or if an endocervical glandular abnormality is being investigated or followed up. Stenosis of the os occurs principally with postmenopausal atrophy or after treatment of CIN. Submission of two slides for each sample doubles screening time, with profound resource implications for laboratories, particularly in organised screening programmes. Submission of a combined spatula and brush smear on one slide is a compromise but one or both components of such a smear are likely to show airdrying artifact. An advantage of liquid-based cytology (LBC) is that material from two sampling techniques may be combined in a single preparation yielding one slide for examination with no adverse effects on technical quality. The importance of sampling technique and sample quality for effective screening have been recognised and comprehensive guidance is available to smear takers, most of whom operate in a primary care setting.[16,17]

## LBC

The conventional cervical smear test ('PAP smear') has been described as the most successful cancer screening test ever devised and has served screening programmes well for over half a century, but has now been superseded by LBC in some parts of the developed world. LBC preparation systems were devised primarily with automated or semi automated smear reading in view; in conventional smears cell clumping and overlap, and the inhomogeneous nature of the samples are likely to be problematic for automated cytology reading systems. They also have other potential advantages, which may justify their introduction for conventional microscopic screening. The whole of the UK NHS Cervical Screening Programme (NHSCSP) has now converted to LBC (see Ch. 22).

When a conventional cervical smear is made, significant quantities of cellular material may be discarded with the sampler. The technical preparation is then largely dependent on the smear taker, with individual variation in technique, and inevitably resulting in a cellular preparation of uneven thickness. In liquid-based techniques, the sampler is rinsed or placed in a vial of proprietary fixative and transported to the laboratory for further preparation, thus removing responsibility of the smear-taker for the technical preparation of the smear. Cell preparation systems are designed to produce a thin cell layer of a representative sample of the cells present in the vial, and remove red blood cells and inflammatory cells, although not necessarily completely.

Many papers have indicated that the advantages of LBC include improved sensitivity and specificity for detection of abnormalities, and reduction of the inadequate sample rate, but many of the studies from which these conclusions were drawn have been criticised as having methodological deficiencies.[18,19]

The effect of retraining has also not been taken into account. It is recognised that retraining of laboratory staff is an essential part of the adoption of LBC, and a 'learning curve' is acknowledged.[20] It is questionable to what extent retraining of staff might have improved the sensitivity of conventional smears, especially when problems in the detection and interpretation of some patterns of abnormality have previously been described.[21,22] A further important advantage of LBC is that an aliquot of the sample remains available for ancillary tests such as for HPV DNA, eliminating the need for a further clinic visit for this purpose.

Implementation of LBC in England followed from pilot studies which suggested that the adoption of LBC would significantly improve the programme and that the increased costs associated with LBC (training, equipment capital/leasing costs, consumables) would be offset by savings associated with reduced numbers of tests because of the anticipated fall in inadequate rate and resulting repeat tests.[23] In the pilot studies the inadequate rate fell by 82.7%. Subsequently, guidance was issued by the National Institute for Clinical Excellence (NICE) directing the implementation of LBC in England using either of the systems used in the pilot studies, SurePath® (formerly TriPath Imaging® Inc., now BD-TriPath, Burlington, NC, USA) and ThinPrep® (formerly Cytyc® Corporation, now Hologic Inc. Bedford, MA, USA).[24]

Assessment of sample adequacy has always been controversial, and that for LBC has to date proved no less so than for conventional cervical smears.

Comparison of adequacy rates between conventional smears and LBC samples may be fallacious in the absence of comparable criteria for the two types of test. In conventional smears the criteria have been, at best, subjective and semi-quantitative. The claimed homogeneity of LBC samples makes quantitative assessment of cell numbers possible. In the Bethesda System terminology (TBS), an adequate LBC sample is one with 5000 or greater squamous epithelial cells. In the UK NHS Cervical Screening Programme, with its 3–5 yearly routine screening interval, more stringent criteria are considered appropriate than those adopted by TBS, but none have yet been agreed nationally, and sample adequacy is the subject of a Health Technology Assessments (HTA) study which has yet to report. At the Royal Liverpool University Hospital a criterion for adequacy of 15 000 squamous cells in an LBC preparation has been used, counts being made on a small number of sample fields according to a standard protocol. Previously, reporting of inadequate conventional samples was by the then current NHSCSP guidelines.[25] The Royal Liverpool University Hospital converted to LBC (using both SurePath® and ThinPrep® systems) in December 2004 and the inadequate sample rate fell from 14.5% in the calendar year 2004 to 3.9% in the second half of 2005, when LBC conversion was complete.

## Automated and semi-automated screening systems

The automation or semi-automation of reading cervical cytology has now been achieved, and offers the potential of greater laboratory productivity and accuracy than with conventional human reading (see Ch. 22). In particular, it may enable false negative test results associated with the limitations of human observation[26–29] to be reduced. In 2003, the ThinPrep® Imager (Cytyc® Corporation, now Hologic Inc.), which uses ThinPrep slides was approved for use as a primary screening device in the USA by the Food and Drugs Administration (FDA)[30] and by the end of 2004 over 140 devices were in routine laboratory use. Several studies in the USA, Europe and Australia have reported at least equivalent, and sometimes improved, sensitivity and specificity,

and considerable improvements in productivity with the Imager compared with manual screening.[31–36] The Focal Point Slide Profiler™ (TriPath Imaging® Inc., now BD-TriPath) which can scan SurePath (or conventional) slides and rank them in order of those most likely to be abnormal is also approved for use in the USA by the FDA, and the 25% of slides ranked lowest may be reported as negative without the need for human review. The Slide Profiler also identifies the 15% of slides most likely to be abnormal and has been shown to be superior to human screening in the detection of high-grade intraepithelial abnormalities. The BD Focal Point™ GS Imaging System additionally identifies 15 fields of view requiring further review. In 2002, Wilbur et al. concluded that the Focal Point GS system was more accurate and productive than human screening.[37] The BD Focal Point™ Imaging System received pre-market approval from the FDA in December 2008.[38]

The potential application of both of these systems in the UK is being investigated. A trial funded by the UK HTA is in progress in Manchester. This is known as the MAVARIC trial (MAnual Versus Automated Reading In Cytology) and is designed to compare human screening with both the ThinPrep Imager and Focal Point GS systems in a randomised trial of 100 000 samples. The trial is due to report at the end of 2009.

## Cytological terminology of cervical pre-cancer

## Introduction

Developments in the practice of cervical and vaginal cytology have led to changes in the terminology used. The tendency of early practitioners of cytology to work independently of histopathologists, and possibly promote cytological diagnosis as equivalent to histological diagnosis, has influenced the use of terminology in gynaecological cytology.

## The Papanicolaou classification

Papanicolaou's classification (Table 23.3) was used for many years and his classes I–V have been adhered to until relatively recently by some cytologists and gynaecologists. In 1953, Reagan et al. proposed the term dysplasia to replace atypical metaplasia and atypical hyperplasia and this suggestion was approved by the First International Congress of Exfoliative Cytology in Vienna.

**Table 23.3** Papanicolaou classification of cytology smear reports

| Class I | Negative | Absence of atypical or abnormal cells |
|---------|----------|----------------------------------------|
| Class II | Negative | Atypical cells present but without abnormal features |
| Class III | Suspicious | Cells with abnormal features suggestive but not conclusive for malignancy |
| Class IV | Positive | Cells and cell clusters fairly conclusive for malignancy |
| Class V | Positive | Cells and cell clusters conclusive for malignancy |

## World Health Organization classification

Ritton and Christopherson defined the normal and abnormal cells of cervical and vaginal smears in the World Health Organization (WHO) International Classification in 1973. The abnormal cells were described in terms of the histological condition with which they correlated. The conventional histological terminology of mild, moderate and severe dysplasia and carcinoma *in situ* was used as well as atypical metaplasia. The WHO publication was widely distributed and the concise text and clear illustrations have contributed to international agreement on the application of these definitions. Grades of dysplasia, carcinoma *in situ* and invasive carcinoma were used by a generation of cytologists to describe cervical cytology.

## Dissatisfaction with older terminologies

Dissatisfaction with the Papanicolaou classification led to the introduction of subdivisions, particularly of Class III, but variation in the use of the classification between centres, and idiosyncratic applications resulted in deterioration of its reproducibility. Although some cytologists prefer to describe cells in terms of expected histology, there is also reluctance by others, particularly in the UK, to use histological terms to describe cell preparations. The disadvantage of using histological terms for reporting cervical cytology is the potential for misunderstanding of the report by the recipient who, untrained in pathology, may be misled into believing that the cervical smear test is as definitive as the histological biopsy. It is well established in the literature that, largely because of sampling error, cervical cytology underestimates the abnormality actually present in a significant minority of cases. This is the main reason why women with persistent mild or low-grade cytological abnormalities should be referred for colposcopy. In a screening sense the abnormal cervical cytology report should be taken as indicating the least abnormality that is likely to be found on the cervix when the patient is investigated.

## British Society for Clinical Cytology (BSCC) terminology

The BSCC held a first working party which reported in 1978 and recommended use of the term dyskaryosis, originally coined by Papanicolaou, and translated from the Greek meaning abnormal nucleus, to describe cells from preinvasive and invasive cancer. The first working party classified dyskaryosis as superficial cell dyskaryosis, intermediate cell dyskaryosis and parabasal cell dyskaryosis, according to the cytoplasmic differentiation of the dyskaryotic cell and its expected correlation with mild, moderate and severe dysplasia and carcinoma *in situ*. Dyskaryosis and dyskaryotic proved an acceptable concept for description of abnormal cells in cervical smears but classification according to cytoplasmic differentiation using the same words used to describe normal squamous epithelial cells revealed inconsistencies. For example, parabasal cell dyskaryosis is an appropriate description of the classical or oval dyskaryotic cells with a narrow rim of dense cytoplasm from CIN 3, but it is not a suitable description for some of the variations in appearance of cells from CIN 3 and invasive squamous cell carcinoma.

**Table 23.4** Terminology for reporting squamous epithelial cell abnormalities in cervical smears

| Cytology | Expected histology |
|---|---|
| Mild dyskaryosis | CIN 1 (mild dysplasia) |
| Moderate dyskaryosis | CIN 2 (moderate dysplasia) |
| Severe dyskaryosis | CIN 3 (severe dysplasia/carcinoma *in situ*) |
| | Invasive cancer |

(Evans DMD, Hudson EA, Brown CL et al. Terminology in gynaecological cytopathology: report of the Working Party of the British Society for Clinical Cytology. J Clin Pathol 1986; 39:933–944).[39]

The BSCC Working Party produced a further review in 1986[39] in which dyskaryosis remained the recommended term but it was graded into mild, moderate and severe (Table 23.4). This terminology replaced dysplasia and carcinoma *in situ* in the UK NHSCSP. Broadly, the 1986 terminology worked well and has been in use since that date, but from the late 1990s onwards there has been pressure to modify it for a number of reasons:

- Clinical management of women with CIN falls clearly into two groups depending on the degree of abnormality, rather than three
- It is increasingly important to be able to translate findings into different terminologies for purposes of epidemiology and comparative research, and particularly with the Bethesda System (see below)
- Concerns about the reproducibility of moderate dyskaryosis as a grade
- The 1986 BSCC area criteria for grading dyskaryosis have been show to be incorrect (see below)
- Concerns that LBC preparations would change the grading criteria
- Understanding of the role of HPV infection modifies the likely clinical management of mild dyskaryosis and 'borderline' changes.

Following a conference in 2002, broad consensus was reached, although the proposed changes were not published until 2008.[40] The modified terminology has not at the time of writing been accepted by the NHSCSP. There has been considerable resistance to change, largely because of the changes required to national computer systems. The 1986 terminology, problems in its application, and 2008 modifications will be described in detail below. It was felt inappropriate to adopt the Bethesda System in the UK, as TBS does not include management and was designed for a different clinical environment from the UK. However, the new BSCC terminology and TBS can now be correlated very closely.

## Cervical intraepithelial neoplasia (CIN) terminology

The disciplines of cytology and histology have converged and both cytologists and histologists have a clearer understanding of the role of cervical cytology for screening and reporting normal cells/samples and for making a preliminary diagnosis when abnormal cells are present. Richart recommended the use of the term cervical intraepithelial neoplasia (CIN) to replace dysplasia and carcinoma *in situ* for histological diagnosis. CIN is classified into grades 1, 2 and 3 in which the artificial distinction between severe dysplasia and carcinoma *in situ* is avoided by including them both in CIN 3.[41] The term has been widely adopted for histological diagnosis.

## The Bethesda System (TBS)

The 1988 *Bethesda System for Reporting Cervical/Vaginal Cytologic Diagnoses* was published by a Workshop of North American experts convened by the Division of Cancer Prevention and Control of the USA National Cancer Institute to review existing terminology and recommend effective methods of reporting. The Workshop agreed that the Papanicolaou classification was no longer appropriate and proposed the Bethesda System. TBS included a new term, squamous intraepithelial lesion (SIL) which is divided into two grades: low-grade SIL, to include cells from HPV and CIN 1 and high-grade SIL for cells from CIN 2 and CIN 3.

The division by the Bethesda Workshop of cells from precancerous lesions of the squamous epithelium into two grades instead of three was intended to improve reproducibility of reports of abnormal cervical cytology and to relate classification to the management of the patient. High-grade SIL is an indication for excision or ablation of the abnormal tissue whereas low-grade SIL may be followed-up initially by cytology alone. Minor amendments were made in 1991 and in 2001, a further Bethesda Workshop was held resulting in further modifications.[42] The Bethesda 2001 Terminology is summarised in Box 23.1. The BSCC 1986, BSCC 2008, Bethesda 2001, ECTP and AMBS 2004 terminologies are compared in Table 23.5.

## The cytology of CIN and invasive squamous cell carcinoma

A continuous range of abnormal nuclear morphology is seen in epithelial cells in cervical cytology samples. The morphology reflects those abnormalities of the cervical epithelium which involve the cells on the surface. Hence, a simple basal cell hyperplasia does not produce changes at the surface of the epithelium or in the cervical cytology sample. Lesser changes in the sampled cells are normally associated with inflammatory or reactive conditions which are benign. The more striking changes described as dyskaryotic, as recommended and defined in the BSCC 1986 terminology, are associated with cervical intraepithelial neoplasia (CIN). The continued use of the term dyskaryosis was endorsed in the BSCC 2008 terminology. If a cervical cytology sample is correctly taken and represents the whole of the transformation zone, an accurate correlation may be expected between the cytological abnormality and the subsequent histological findings when CIN is present. Factors influencing the accuracy of cervical cytology for the detection of CIN are described below.

## Features of dyskaryosis

The term dyskaryosis means literally 'abnormal nucleus'. It was used by Papanicolaou and subsequently with slightly different

---

### Box 23.1  The 2001 Bethesda System (abridged)

**Specimen adequacy**

Satisfactory for evaluation (note presence/absence of endocervical/transformation zone component)
Unsatisfactory for evaluation (specify reason)
Specimen rejected/not processed (specify reason)
Specimen processed and examined, but unsatisfactory for evaluation of epithelial abnormality because of (*specify reason*)

**General categorisation (*optional*)**

Negative for intraepithelial lesion or malignancy
Epithelial cell abnormality
Other

**Interpretation/result**

***Negative for intraepithelial lesion or malignancy***

*Organisms*

- *Trichomonas vaginalis*
- Fungal organisms morphologically consistent with *Candida* species
- Shift in flora suggestive of bacterial vaginosis
- Bacteria morphologically consistent with *Actinomyces* species
- Cellular changes consistent with herpes simplex virus

*Other non-neoplastic findings (optional to report; list not comprehensive)*

- Reactive cellular changes associated with inflammation (includes typical repair)
- Radiation
- Intrauterine contraceptive device

*Glandular cells post-hysterectomy*

*Atrophy*

**Epithelial cell abnormalities**

*Squamous cell*

- Atypical squamous cells (ASC)
  - Of undetermined significance (ASC-US)
  - Cannot exclude HSIL (ASC-H)
- Low-grade squamous intraepithelial lesion (LSIL)
  - Encompassing: human papillomavirus/mild dysplasia/cervical intraepithelial neoplasia (CIN)1
- High-grade squamous intraepithelial lesion (HSIL)
  - Encompassing: moderate and severe dysplasia, carcinoma *in situ*; CIN 2 and CIN 3
- Squamous cell carcinoma

*Glandular cell*

- Atypical glandular cells (AGC) (specify endocervical, endometrial or not otherwise specified)
- Atypical glandular cells, favour neoplastic (*specify endocervical or not otherwise specified*)
- Endocervical adenocarcinoma *in situ* (AIS)
- Adenocarcinoma

*Other (list not comprehensive)*

- Endometrial cells in a woman ≥40 years of age

**Automated review and ancillary testing (*include as appropriate*)**

**Educational notes and suggestions (*optional*)**

**Table 23.5** Comparison of different terminology systems

| BSCC 1986 and NHSCSP | BSCC proposed new terminology | The Bethesda System 2001 | ECTP terminology | AMBS 2004 |
|---|---|---|---|---|
| Negative | Negative | Negative for intraepithelial lesion or malignancy | Within normal limits | Negative |
| Inadequate | Inadequate | Unsatisfactory for evaluation | Unsatisfactory due to… | Unsatisfactory |
| Borderline nuclear change | Borderline change, sqamous, but not otherwise specified | Atypical sqamous cells of (ASC-US) undetermined significance | Koilocytes (without changes suggestive of intraepithelial neoplasia) | Possible low-grade squamous intraepithelial lesion |
| | | | Sqamous cell changes (not definitely neoplastic but merit early repeat) | |
| | Borderline change, high-grade dyskaryosis not excluded | ASC-H (cannot exclude HSIL) | | Possible high-grade sqamous intraepithelial lesion |
| | Borderline change in endocervical cells | Atypical endocervical, endometrial or glandular (NOS or specify in comments) | Atypical glandular cells (quality) | Atypical endocervical cells of undetermined significance |
| | | Atypical endocervical or glandular cells, favour neoplastic | | Atypical glandular cells of undetermined significance |
| Mild dyskaryosis | Low-grade dyskaryosis (includes all cases of koilocytosis provided that no high-grade dyskaryosis is present) | Low-grade sqamous intra-epithelial lesion (LSIL) | Mild dysplasia (CIN1) | Low-grade sqamous intraepithelial lesion |
| Moderate dyskaryosis | High-grade dyskaryosis | High-grade squamous intra-epithelial lesion (HSIL) | Moderate dysplasia (CIN2) | High-grade squamous intraepithelial lesion |
| Severe dyskaryosis | | HSIL | 1. Severe dysplasia (CIN3) | |
| | | | 2. Carcinoma *in situ* (CIN3) | |
| Severe dyskaryosis? invasive | High-grade dyskaryosis? Invasive | Squamous cell carcinoma | 1. Severe dysplasia? invasive | Squamous cell carcinoma |
| | | | 2. Invasive squamous cell carcinoma | |
| ? Glandular neoplasia | ? Glandular neoplasia | 1. Endocervical carcinoma *in situ* | Adenocarcinoma | Endocervical adenocarcinoma |
| | Endocervical | 2. Adenocarcinoma | AIS | *in situ* |
| | Non-cervical | Endocervical | Endocervical | Adenocarcinoma |
| | | Endometrial | Endometrial | |
| | | Extrauterine | Extrauterine | |
| | | NOS | NOS | |

BSCC, British Society for Clinical Cytology; ECTP, European Commission Training Programme; AMBS, Australian Modified Bethesda System. (Table reproduced with permission of Wiley-Blackwell, from Denton KJ, Herbert A, Turnbull LS, et al. The revised BSCC terminology for abnormal cervical cytology. Cytopathology 2008; 19:137–57.[40])

meanings by some to describe cells from CIN 1 and CIN 2 only, and by others for cells from CIN 3 only. Redefined in the BSCC 1986 terminology, dyskaryosis or dyskaryotic describes all abnormal cells with appearances that suggest derivation from CIN or invasive carcinoma of the cervix.

The morphological abnormalities seen in the nucleus in epithelial cells in cervical cytology preparations include a combination of any number of the following:

- Disproportionate nuclear enlargement
- Hyperchromasia

- Bi- and multinucleation
- Irregularity in form and outline
- Abnormal chromatin pattern, appearing as coarsening, stippling, formation of clumps or strands, and sometimes as condensation beneath the nuclear membrane producing apparent irregularities in its thickness
- Abnormalities of number, size and form of nucleoli.

The nuclear abnormalities produced by inflammation alone are usually limited to a mild degree of nuclear enlargement and hyperchromasia. A dyskaryotic cell may show no more than a marked degree of nuclear enlargement and hyperchromasia, but the most significant and definitive feature of dyskaryosis is abnormality of the chromatin pattern (Figs 23.2–23.4). Irregularity of the nuclear membrane may appear either as an irregular outline of the nucleus or irregular lines or folds across its surface. This must be distinguished from the wrinkling of the nuclear membrane in a degenerate cell as a result of inflammation. Hyperchromasia is a very common feature of dyskaryosis (Figs 23.5, 23.6) and easy to detect on screening examination of cervical cytology preparations, but it is not invariably present. Haematoxylin is not a stoichiometric stain for DNA and the intensity of staining of dyskaryotic nuclei is very variable. Some dyskaryotic nuclei are normochromatic or hypochromatic (in comparison with normal nuclei) (Figs 23.4, 23.7) and it is important that these less common presentations of dyskaryosis are not overlooked. Experience at least in the UK suggests that in the past the occurrence of 'pale' dyskaryosis has not received sufficient emphasis in the training of cytology medical and technical staff.[21,22] Dyskaryotic cells of these appearances are described as a significant factor leading to false negative reporting in

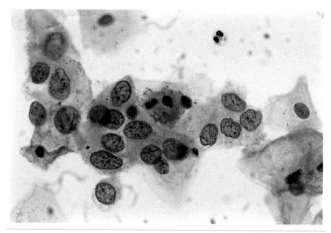

**Fig. 23.4** Low-grade and high-grade (mild and moderate) dyskaryosis. Compare the nuclei and nuclear/cytoplasmic ratios of the dyskaryotic cells with that of the normal intermediate squamous cell on the extreme right of the field. The four dyskaryotic nuclei on its immediate left are an example of 'pale' dyskaryosis (PAP; ThinPrep®).

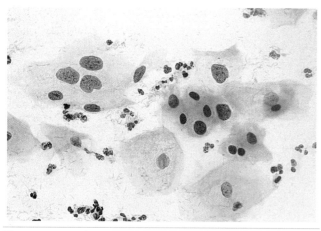

**Fig. 23.2** Low-grade (mild) dyskaryosis. Abnormal chromatin pattern and irregularity of nuclear outline are seen in the upper part of the field as well as nuclear enlargement and hyperchromasia. The dyskaryotic cells have plentiful cytoplasm. Normal intermediate cells are present in the lower part of the field (PAP).

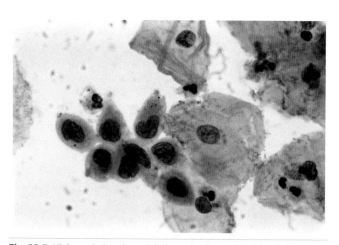

**Fig. 23.5** High-grade (moderate) dyskaryosis. The nuclei of the dyskaryotic cells are hyperchromatic, have irregular outlines and show complex folding (PAP; ThinPrep®).

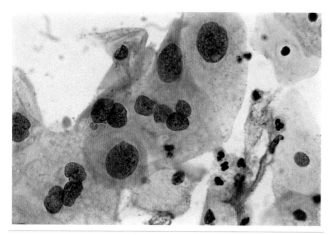

**Fig. 23.3** Low-grade (mild) dyskaryosis. The dyskaryotic cells show varying nuclear enlargement, abnormal chromatin pattern, mild irregularities of outline and multinucleation. Normal superficial and intermediate squamous cells are seen on the right of the field (PAP; ThinPrep®).

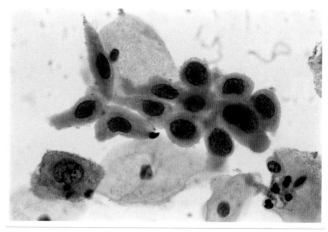

**Fig. 23.6** Low- and high-grade (mild and moderate) dyskaryosis. The dyskaryotic nuclei show varying hyperchromasia, abnormal chromatin pattern and sometimes irregularities of nuclear outline. Compare with the adjacent normal superficial and intermediate squamous cell nuclei (PAP; ThinPrep®).

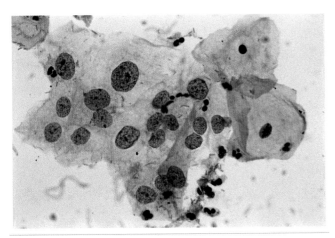

**Fig. 23.7** Low-grade (mild) dyskaryosis. The abnormal nuclei are not hyperchromatic and are an example of 'pale' dyskaryosis (PAP; ThinPrep®).

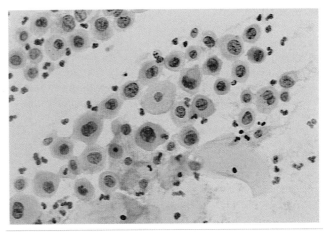

**Fig. 23.8** High-grade (severe) dyskaryosis from a case of CIN 3. Some of the cells have nuclear/cytoplasmic ratios more appropriate to low-grade dyskaryosis. Conceptually it is difficult to regard small dyskaryotic parabasal cells with dense cytoplasm as having arisen other than from CIN 3 (PAP).

cervical cytology.[21,27] Three-dimensional cell groups, or 'hyper-chromatic crowded groups'[43] are another recognised problem area in the detection of dyskaryosis, as is 'bland dyskaryosis' in LBC preparations.[44] Nucleoli are not usually a conspicuous feature of dyskaryotic cells from CIN. The presence of prominent nucleoli in dyskaryotic squamous cells from the cervix suggests either extensive CIN 3 or invasive disease.

The difficulty in defining objective criteria for the diagnosis of dyskaryosis, the merging at the mild end of the spectrum of change with reactive or inflammatory change, and the fact that some cells from dyskaryotic populations are not always recognisable as such on an individual basis from first principles,[22] are the main reasons for the necessity to use an indeterminate reporting category in practice. These changes are described as borderline nuclear changes in the BSCC terminology and will be discussed later.

## Grading of dyskaryosis

Squamous cell dyskaryosis is subdivided to give a more precise indication of the severity of the abnormality. The grading depends on the nuclear/cytoplasmic (N:C) ratio of the cell, the cytoplasmic shape and staining quality, and sometimes the degree and diversity of the nuclear abnormalities listed above.

No quantitative or objective criteria for assessing severity of abnormal nuclear morphology have been laid down, but in general the abnormalities listed may be said to tend to increase with grade of dyskaryosis. It is, however, important to note that high-grade dyskaryotic cells may show only subtle abnormalities of chromatin pattern in round or oval nuclei of normo- or hypochromatic staining reaction. In contrast to the emphasis on nuclear abnormalities of the 1986 BSCC terminology,[39] the 2008 document states 'Chromatin pattern and hyperchromasia do not influence grading of dyskaryosis'.[40] Nevertheless, it is important that grading of dyskaryosis does not depend on the quantity and maturation of the cytoplasm alone, because allowance must be made for dyskaryotic cells with mature, sometimes even keratinised cytoplasm which can be seen in CIN 3 and invasive squamous cell carcinoma. In these circumstances the nuclear features are likely to be more pronounced

in degree and diversity than those usually associated with CIN 1, and the nuclear changes outweigh any apparent cytoplasmic maturation. (It is notable that in TBS, 'keratinising dysplasia' is, by definition, considered a 'high-grade' lesion.) The situation perhaps may best be summarised by saying that if the nuclear morphological abnormalities observed are greater than those usually associated with mild or low-grade dyskaryosis, the use of N:C ratio as a sole grading criterion may lead to underestimation of the abnormality. Cells with a diameter N:C ratio of greater than 50% must not be downgraded to low-grade dyskaryosis because they only show subtle features of dyskaryosis, but dyskaryotic cells with a diameter N:C ratio of less than 50% may need to be upgraded to high-grade dyskaryosis on the basis of severely abnormal nuclear morphological features. Another situation where N:C ratio may mislead is in small dyskaryotic parabasal cells. These sometimes have ratios more commonly associated with mild or moderate dyskaryosis (1986 BSCC terminology) but conceptually it is difficult to regard them as having arisen other than from CIN 3 (Fig. 23.8).[22] Some normal cells seen in cervical cytology preparations have very high N:C ratios, making it essential to recognise the cell type and to confirm that, if epithelial, they are indeed dyskaryotic, before assessing them as high-grade dyskaryotic squamous cells on the basis of N:C ratio.

Definitions of the grades of dyskaryosis are made, but the changes are part of a continuous progression or spectrum of abnormality and absolute distinction between grades is not always possible. Grading follows careful scrutiny of the available material and rarely depends on the appearance of a single cell, which may be on the borderline between accepted definitions. Normal cells usually outnumber abnormal cells but the number of such cells is very variable. Dyskaryotic squamous cells of all grades may be seen dispersed singly or in cohesive clusters. Cell clusters, especially if large and three dimensional, may be very difficult to interpret. Cell boundaries may not be visible, in which case assessment of N:C ratios may be impossible. Even in predominantly clustered dyskaryotic cell populations, small numbers of dispersed dyskaryotic cells are usually present. Samples with clustered dyskaryotic squamous cells with no accompanying single dyskaryotic cells occur rarely.

For assessing N:C ratios in grading dyskaryosis, the BSCC 1986 terminology used area ratios. Thus mildly dyskaryotic cells had nuclei occupying less than half the total area of the cytoplasm, moderately dyskaryotic cells had nuclei half to two-thirds of the total area of the cytoplasm and severely dyskaryotic cells had nuclei occupying more than two-thirds of the total area of the cytoplasm. Slater et al.[45] made a quantitative investigation of these definitions on the images used in the BSCC 1986 terminology, external quality assurance and training school slide sets, and showed that these definitions were wrong. Their results indicate that diameter, rather than area, ratios are appropriate in the grading of dyskaryosis, and the authors commented 'The closeness of the diameter results to the BSCC N:C ratio figures of 50% and 66%, if they had been expressed as diameter rather than area, can only be regarded as remarkable'. Slater et al. also noted that mild, moderate and severe dyskaryosis existed as statistically different populations but that the usefulness of moderate dyskaryosis was limited by overlap with the other two grades. There was no overlap between mild and severe dyskaryosis. They also reported that, except for moderate dyskaryosis, there were no significant differences between conventional smears, ThinPrep® and SurePath™ LBC preparations with regard to diameter N:C ratios. By contrast, if area ratios were used there were significant differences between these two commercial methodologies. This is of relevance to some area definitions used in TBS, and the subject of a parallel study by Slater et al.[46] indicating that some of the Bethesda area definitions area also incorrect. The need to take qualitative morphological details into account in the grading of dyskaryosis, especially that of chromatin pattern, as well as assessment of N:C ratio, was re-emphasised.

## Differences between conventional and LBC cytology preparations

The similarities between conventional and LBC cervical cytology preparations are considerable, and far greater than the differences, but it is acknowledged that specific training in screening and reporting LBC samples is necessary.

In LBC preparations, by various processes which differ in the different commercial systems, the cells are dispersed, separated from blood and inflammatory cells and a representative sample of the epithelial cells deposited as a layer on a slide. The cells are distributed in thin layers, not monolayers, and are thicker than parts of some conventional smears. The need to focus through the full thickness of the layer of cells while screening is important, particularly in SurePath™ samples. Because of the nature of the processing of the specimen, it should be remembered that the cellularity of the slide does not necessarily reflect the cellularity of the original specimen (see discussion on specimen adequacy, above).

The cells tend to be more dispersed and, although clusters of cells are still common, they tend to be smaller. Some architectural features in cell groups are more subtle (particularly in CGIN, see Chapter 24). Dispersion of cells results in the disruption of some cell groupings into single dissociated cells which are unrelated to each other in LBC preparations The broom-like device used for sampling the cervix (Cervex-Brush®, Rovers Medical Devices BV, the Netherlands) includes central bristles designed to enter the endocervical canal and sampling of 'glandular' material including tubal or tuboendometrial metaplasia or directly sampled lower uterine segment endometrium is common in LBC samples.

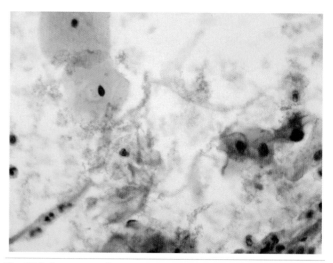

**Fig. 23.9** Squamous cell carcinoma. Malignant diathesis. Normal and dyskaryotic squamous cells, and anucleate keratinised and non-keratinised cytoplasmic fragments are present in a background of particulate material, red cell fragments and leucocytes (PAP; ThinPrep®).

Endocervical epithelium is more commonly seen in post menopausal women with LBC.

The cell sample is much smaller, and quicker and easier to screen than that of a conventional smear. Conversely, because only a representative sample of cells is present, dyskaryotic cell populations may be represented by many fewer cells in an LBC preparation. All small single cells with high N:C ratios need to be examined carefully at high power to ensure that scanty high-grade dyskaryotic cells are not overlooked. Likewise, all cell clusters should be examined closely.

SurePath™ specimens have a very high cell density and in atrophic smears in particular it may be preferable to use an X20 rather than X10 objective lens for screening.

Because of the rapid fixation, cellular details tend to be better preserved than in conventional preparations. Irregularities of nuclear outline tend to be greater resulting in dyskaryotic cells often having complexly folded, three-dimensional nuclei described as walnut-like. Minor irregularities in nuclear outline are commoner in LBC and should be disregarded in the absence of an abnormal chromatin pattern. Chromatin is better preserved than in conventional smears and it is important not to misinterpret the granular chromatin of normal metaplastic and endocervical cells in particular as representing dyskaryosis, especially in ThinPrep®.

The staining process used with SurePath™ is an incomplete Papanicolaou stain and the dense orange colour usually associated with keratinisation is not seen. Dyskeratotic cells and cell groups such as pearls, spikes and rafts have green or pink cytoplasm.

Malignant diathesis associated with invasive carcinoma can still be recognised, but it is very different from that seen in conventional smears. It is seen as proteinaceous material containing fragments of red cells and leucocytes. In ThinPrep® specimens (Fig. 23.9), it tends to be present mainly at the periphery of the deposit. In SurePath™ (Fig. 23.10), the material tends to be adherent to malignant cells and has been referred to as 'clinging' diathesis.

In LBC, the cytoplasm is often folded at the edges (especially in SurePath™, which uses a cell sedimentation technique) simulating the appearance of koilocytosis and it is important not to over-interpret this finding. Confirmation of an accompanying

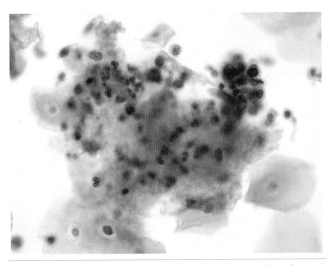

**Fig. 23.10** Squamous cell carcinoma. Malignant diathesis. High-grade (severely) dyskaryotic squamous cells are clumped with exudate, red cells and leucocytes (PAP; SurePath™).

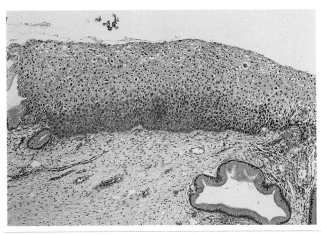

**Fig. 23.11** Section of cervical squamous mucosa showing CIN 1. There is crowding of the cells in the basal third of the epithelium, so that the basal layer is no longer distinct. Nuclei in this area are enlarged and hyperchromatic and show some loss of polarity. The middle and upper layers show persistence of nuclear enlargement, but the changes are less marked and the epithelium matures normally. Koilocytes are visible towards the surface (H&E).

nuclear abnormality will avoid this pitfall. Koilocytes and 'pseudokoilocytes' may co-exist in the same sample.

## Current recommendations of the 2008 BSCC terminology[40]

For squamous cell abnormalities, the following major recommendations are made:

- *Dyskaryosis* should be retained as a term for describing the nuclear abnormalities associated with CIN and invasive carcinoma
- The existing grades of moderate and severe dyskaryosis should be merged into a single category, *high-grade dyskaryosis*
- Mild dyskaryosis will be replaced by *low-grade dyskaryosis*. Koilocytosis will also be included in this group even if the nuclear abnormality corresponds with change hitherto described as borderline
- For grading purposes, N/C diameter and not area ratios should be used. High-grade dyskaryotic cells have a nuclear diameter of greater than 50% of the cell diameter and low-grade dyskaryotic cells a nuclear diameter of less than 50%
- Borderline nuclear changes should be subdivided into three groups: borderline change, high-grade dyskaryosis not excluded, borderline change, squamous, not otherwise specified (NOS) and borderline changes in endocervical cells.

## Low-grade (formerly mild) dyskaryosis, including koilocytosis: CIN 1

### Histology of CIN 1 (Fig. 23.11)

Despite controversy over the optimal histological classification of pre-invasive lesions of the cervix there are, nevertheless, clear definitions of cervical intraepithelial neoplasia and its three tier grading system. The CIN terminology continues to be widely used and is the recommended system in guidelines issued by the Royal College of Pathologists and NHSCSP.[47] CIN 1 is recognised in histological sections by increased cellularity and loss of polarity of the cells of the basal third of the epithelium due to replacement of the basal and parabasal layers by abnormal immature cells. Maturation appears to proceed more normally in the middle and upper thirds.

The immature cells are neoplastic and have nuclear abnormalities that relate closely to the cytological findings of dyskaryosis. They include enlargement and pleomorphism of nuclei, leading to a raised N:C ratio, which is in part responsible for the appearance of cell crowding. There are also some alterations in chromatin, usually with mild hyperchromasia and stippling of the chromatin pattern. Mitoses are not infrequent, and normal and abnormal mitotic figures can be seen in the basal third of the mucosa in up to 50% of cases in CIN 1.

Other changes frequently seen in the upper layers include dyskeratosis due to premature keratinisation of individual squamous cells, bi- and multinucleation, pyknotic nuclei and koilocytosis, suggesting concomitant HPV infection. It is important to note that the nuclear changes of CIN 1 persist in the mature superficial and intermediate squamous cells overlying the abnormal cells in the basal third of the epithelium. This enables recognition of lesser grades of CIN in cervical cytology preparations and allows prediction of the grade of lesion based on a combination of cell maturation and degree of nuclear abnormality.

### Cytological findings: low-grade dyskaryosis

The morphological features of low-grade (formerly mild) dyskaryosis (Figs 23.2, 23.3, 23.7, 23.12–23.15) include a combination of any of the following:

- Disproportionate nuclear enlargement, with the diameter of the nucleus less than one-half the diameter of the cell
- Nuclear hyperchromasia
- Abnormal chromatin pattern
- Irregularity of the nuclear membrane
- Multiple abnormal nuclei
- Cytoplasm reduced and relatively thin
- Cell borders usually angular.

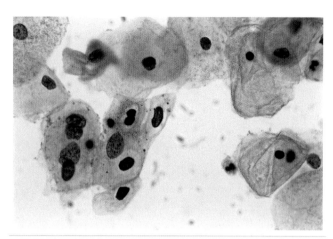

**Fig. 23.12** Low-grade (mild) dyskaryosis. Nuclear enlargement and hyperchromasia are seen in the enlarged nuclei on the left of the field. The small abnormal pyknotic nuclei have no visible chromatin structure and amount to borderline nuclear change. The binucleated cells and cytoplasmic clearing may indicate HPV infection but do not amount to classical koilocytosis (PAP; ThinPrep®).

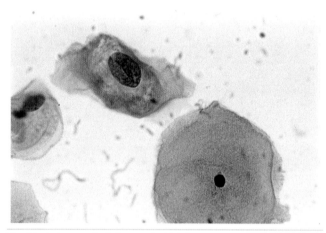

**Fig. 23.13** Low-grade dyskaryosis (mild dyskaryosis and koilocytosis). The cell in the upper part of the field is a koilocyte with a broad cytoplasmic perinuclear halo and condensed cytoplasm at its margin. The nucleus has a simple fold and slight coarsening of the chromatin, but is grossly enlarged, amounting to dyskaryosis (PAP; ThinPrep®).

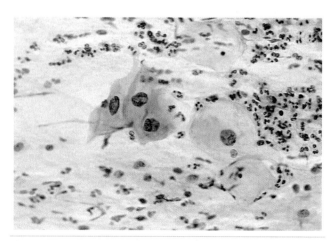

**Fig. 23.14** Low-grade (mild) dyskaryosis. The abnormal chromatin pattern clearly distinguishes the low-grade dyskaryosis from inflammatory nuclear change (PAP).

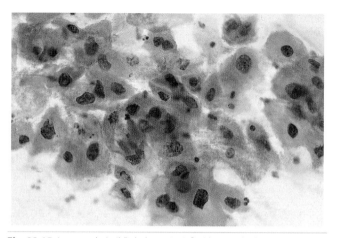

**Fig. 23.15** Low-grade (mild) dyskaryosis. A florid example showing some binucleation and orangeophilia of keratin associated in this case with HPV infection (PAP).

Cells sampled from an area of CIN 1 will show low-grade dyskaryosis. Low-grade dyskaryotic cells have additional and more striking nuclear abnormalities compared with those seen in inflammatory change. The cytoplasm is usually thin, transparent and plentiful, with angular borders as seen in normal superficial and intermediate squamous cells; keratinisation is sometimes seen in single cells or sheets of cells.

The nucleus is enlarged but generally occupies less than half the diameter of the cell. Nuclear hyperchromasia, abnormally shaped nuclei and multiple nuclei are striking features if present, but low-grade dyskaryosis may be represented by the more subtle changes of disproportionate nuclear enlargement and abnormal chromatin pattern. Nucleoli, if discernible, are indistinct. The abnormal nuclei associated with 'productive' HPV infections cannot be distinguished reliably from dyskaryosis by light microscopy and should be evaluated according to the same criteria as dyskaryosis.

## Cytological findings: HPV infection

The morphological changes due to HPV infection are summarised below. They are described more fully with infection of the female genital tract (see Ch. 21) but they must be considered further in relation to CIN.

- Koilocytosis
- Enlarged hyperchromatic nuclei
- Bi- and multinucleation
- Cytoplasmic keratinisation.

HPV infection may occur with or without concomitant CIN or in the same cervix as CIN but at a different site. These distinctions may be made from a histological section of a biopsy of the cervix, but cannot be made from a cervical cytology preparation. The four features of HPV are koilocytosis, abnormal nuclei, bi- and multinucleation and keratinisation, but not all of these characteristics are necessarily seen together. Koilocytes have a broad, clear perinuclear cytoplasmic vacuole with a condensed cytoplasmic rim. Their presence in a cervical cytology preparation is generally considered pathognomonic of HPV infection, but the other changes are less specific. The abnormal nuclei of HPV infection are enlarged and usually hyperchromatic and typically have a wrinkled or collapsed nuclear membrane. Nevertheless, the exclusion of CIN cannot be relied upon from the morphological changes and for many years it has been widely established convention that such patients should be managed according to the degree of nuclear abnormality.

In view of the increasing clinical role of HPV DNA testing, especially in the triage of low-grade cytological abnormalities (see below), it is probably appropriate to refer to the morphological changes suggesting viral infection, seen in cervical cytology preparations, in descriptive terms. The assumption that the morphological changes are necessarily related to HPV may be confusing to the clinician receiving the result, since HPV positive DNA test results are more definitive than cytology and are likely only to refer to tests positive for high risk HPV types. The morphological changes of HPV infection may result from high risk or low risk types. Thus koilocytosis, defined as a broad, clear perinuclear cytoplasmic halo with a condensed cytoplasmic rim, and almost always associated with nuclear abnormality of some degree, is included with low-grade dyskaryosis (unless high-grade dyskaryosis is also present). There is evidence that the majority of women with koilocytosis and nuclear changes hitherto reported as borderline do have high risk HPV infections, justifying this inclusion.[48]

Less specific changes of bi- and multinucleation and keratinisation should not be reported as indicating HPV infection and if the cervical cytology test is considered abnormal it should be managed according to the degree of nuclear abnormality present. Squamous cells infected with HPV sometimes appear larger than the normal equivalent squamous cells of equivalent maturation. When such cells are present the diameter N:C ratio should be taken into account as there may be a tendency to overestimate the degree of dyskaryosis present when very large nuclei are seen.

From the above definition of koilocytosis and considering the N:C ratios of the cells in question, it should be apparent that koilocytosis will usually be associated with low-grade dyskaryosis; it may be associated with high-grade (formerly moderate) dyskaryosis but is unlikely to be identifiable in high-grade (formerly severely) dyskaryotic cells.

### Diagnostic pitfalls: low-grade dyskaryosis

Low-grade dyskaryosis should be distinguished from the following:

- Reactive/inflammatory change
- Navicular cells
- Atrophic change
- Keratinising or verrucous carcinoma.

Inflammatory and reactive changes involve nuclear degeneration as well as reparative and regenerative changes (see Ch. 21). Nuclear hyperchromasia and disproportionate nuclear enlargement are the principal features which are also present in low-grade dyskaryosis but the abnormal chromatin pattern is the most distinctive characteristic (Figs 23.2, 23.3, 23.12–23.14). The spectrum of nuclear change is described as commencing with inflammation and continuing through the grades of dyskaryosis, but this important diagnostic sign of abnormal chromatin pattern distinguishes mild dyskaryosis from simple reactive or inflammatory change. Severe inflammatory changes tend to affect all the cells in a sample to some extent or are at least widespread (see Fig. 23.21); it may not to be

easy to pick out particularly worrying examples because many similar cells are seen throughout the preparation. Low-grade dyskaryosis, by contrast, will be seen in a population which is distinct from the normal and reactive squamous epithelial cells.

Nuclear degeneration leads to pyknosis and the process often includes wrinkling of the nuclear membrane at some stage. Pyknosis involves complete loss of the visible chromatin structure and it is unwise to make a diagnosis of dyskaryosis unless the diagnostic abnormal chromatin pattern is seen in some of the abnormal cells. An irregular nuclear membrane resulting from degenerative change is a sign of shrinkage of the nucleus, in contrast to the folding and bulging of the nuclear membrane seen in a viable dyskaryotic cell.

Navicular cells (see Fig. 23.21) are boat-shaped cells found in the presence of prolonged progesterone stimulation. They have eccentric nuclei and are filled with glycogen. A navicular cell may simulate a koilocyte if it has a central nucleus surrounded by a pale area in which the granular glycogen is lightly stained. Navicular cells may have hyperchromatic nuclei but they are not enlarged or multiple. If present in a cervical cytology sample the cells are usually numerous and the identity of a problem cell can easily be determined by comparison with neighbouring cells of similar appearance.

An atrophic cervical or vaginal cytology sample commonly shows inflammatory changes with all its nuclear manifestations (see Fig. 23.21). High magnifications reveal coarser chromatin aggregation than is normal in mature squamous epithelial cells and there is often considerable nuclear enlargement. Comparison is made with the normal appearance of the nucleus in parabasal squamous cells and a distinct population of dyskaryotic squamous cells should be identified before a definite diagnosis of dyskaryosis is made. If doubt persists, another test taken immediately after completion of a 7–10 day course of topical application of a suitable oestrogen cream, in order to mature the epithelium, will usually resolve the difficulty.

Because of the N:C ratios of many keratinised cells, cells from a keratinising, that is, well-differentiated squamous cell carcinoma may be mistaken for low-grade dyskaryosis if N:C ratio alone is relied upon for assessment of dyskaryosis. With these lesions, assessment of nuclear detail in terms of grading may be difficult and the assessment of other features such as a 'malignant diathesis' may be very important. Verrucous carcinoma (Fig. 23.16) is a rare, but important, differential diagnosis from low-grade dyskaryosis of CIN. Typically, the cervical cytology preparation contains a large quantity of anucleate fragments of thick keratinised cytoplasm. Nucleated cells tend to contain small, hyperchromatic but pyknotic nuclei. The distinction from benign reactive hyperkeratosis of HPV infection is difficult without a description of the patient's clinical symptoms and signs.

### High-grade dyskaryosis (incorporating moderate and severe dyskaryosis): CIN 2 and CIN 3

### Histology of CIN 2 and CIN 3 (Figs 23.17, 23.18)

Histological sections from CIN 2 show replacement of normal squamous epithelium by abnormal immature cells extending into the middle-third of the epithelium, but by definition, not

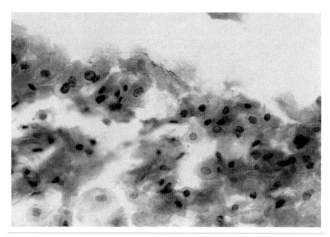

**Fig. 23.16** Verrucous squamous cell carcinoma. Hyperkeratotic and keratinised cells with small degenerate nuclei dominate the cytology. Nuclear features of only low-grade (mild) dyskaryosis may misrepresent the malignant nature of the tumour. Awareness of the clinical appearance of the cervix should lead to early referral of the patient for biopsy (PAP).

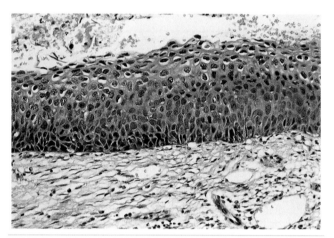

**Fig. 23.17** Section of cervical squamous mucosa showing CIN 2. The squamous cells show nuclear crowding, enlargement, hyperchromasia and disorganisation extending into the middle third. Above this the cells are maturing but abnormality persists to the surface (H&E).

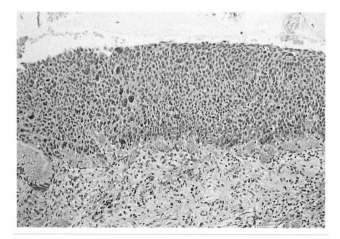

**Fig. 23.18** Section of cervical squamous mucosa showing CIN 3. There is complete replacement of normal squamous cells by crowded abnormal cells with marked nuclear pleomorphism, hyperchromasia and loss of polarity. No evidence of cell maturation can be seen. Note that the basement membrane is intact. The underlying stroma shows non-specific inflammation and marked vascular engorgement (H&E).

into the uppermost third. This change imparts a crowded, disorganised appearance concentrated in the deeper layers of the epithelium, although, as with CIN 1, abnormal nuclei persist in maturing cells up to the surface. Not only do the immature cells replace more of the epithelium, but in addition they usually show greater nuclear abnormality than is seen in CIN 1. Usually, pleomorphism is marked, the chromatin pattern is coarser and irregular, and hyperchromasia is more obvious. Abnormal mitotic figures may be quite frequent and may occur throughout the lower two-thirds of the epithelium. Nucleoli remain inconspicuous. The basement membrane of the squamous mucosa remains intact. HPV changes including koilocytosis can often be seen in the upper layers of the epithelium, affecting cells with dyskaryotic nuclei as well as less abnormal cells. The mucosa adjacent to CIN 2 frequently shows CIN 1 or HPV infection.

In cases of CIN 3, the cervical squamous epithelium is replaced by immature neoplastic cells, which extend into its uppermost third and often completely replace the entire thickness. Thus the category of CIN 3 includes both severe dysplasia and carcinoma *in situ* of previous terminology. There is much more obvious cellular and nuclear abnormality than in lesser grades of CIN, with greater loss of polarity and crowding of cells and a tendency to vertical orientation of nuclei. The cells and their enlarged nuclei may present a monotonous appearance or can exhibit marked nuclear pleomorphism with greater cytoplasmic maturation. This has led to subtyping of CIN 3 into small and large cell non-keratinising types, respectively. Less commonly, the epithelium is replaced by large, pleomorphic squamous cells with bizarre shapes and individual cell keratinisation, giving the third subtype, keratinising CIN 3. Combinations of the three different subtypes may be seen.

Nuclear changes usually include hyperchromasia, coarse granularity or irregularity of chromatin pattern, irregularities of nuclear contour and mitoses. Mitoses may include obviously abnormal forms and may extend into the upper one-third of the epithelium. By definition, the basement membrane is intact in CIN 3. The abnormal epithelium extends progressively over the ectocervix and/or along the endocervical canal, and also into endocervical crypts. There may be a pronounced chronic inflammatory cell infiltrate in the underlying cervical stroma, representing a host response to the epithelial abnormality. There is evidence that very extensive CIN 3 lesions are associated with a greater likelihood of invasion. Lesser grades of CIN and HPV changes are usually, but not invariably, present adjacent to areas of CIN 3.

### Cytological findings: high-grade dyskaryosis

Cells exhibiting high-grade dyskaryosis (Figs 23.19–23.39, and see Figs 23.4–23.6, 23.8) are expected to correlate with cells from the surface of CIN 2, CIN 3 or invasive squamous cell carcinoma.

The cytological findings may include any number of the following:

- Disproportionate nuclear enlargement, with the nucleus occupying more than 50% of the diameter of the cell
- Abnormal chromatin pattern, often (but not necessarily) more abnormal than that associated with low-grade dyskaryosis
- Irregular nuclear membrane

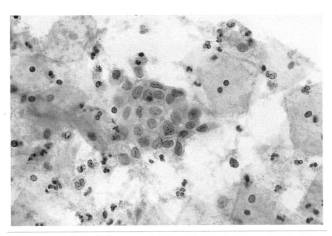

**Fig. 23.19** High-grade (moderate) dyskaryosis. Another example of 'pale' dyskaryosis. Irregular nuclear outlines and abnormal chromatin pattern are seen (PAP).

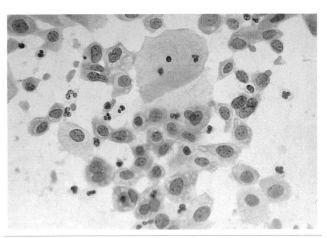

**Fig. 23.22** Dyskaryotic cells of all grades are seen in this case of CIN 3. Examples of nuclei with abnormal chromatin clumping, irregular nuclear outlines and of multinucleation of dyskaryotic cells are seen. The cytoplasm of the dyskaryotic cells is of variable density (PAP).

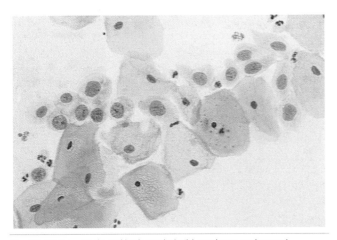

**Fig. 23.20** Low-grade and high-grade (mild, moderate and severe) dyskaryosis (PAP).

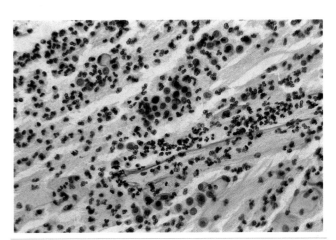

**Fig. 23.23** High-grade (severe) dyskaryosis in a case of small cell CIN 3. Streaks of high-grade dyskaryotic cells are mixed with polymorphs and may be difficult to identify (PAP).

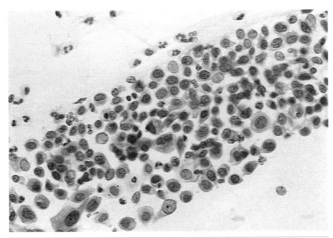

**Fig. 23.21** High-grade (severe) dyskaryosis. This streak of cells from a case of CIN 3 includes hypochromatic nuclei and 'bare' nuclei. Both of these may give rise to diagnostic difficulty if seen on their own (PAP).

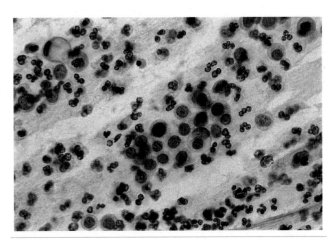

**Fig. 23.24** High-grade (severe) dyskaryosis in a case of small cell CIN 3, same field as Figure 23.23. There is marked hyperchromasia of a nucleus in the centre, but the abnormalities of the other nuclei are more subtle (PAP).

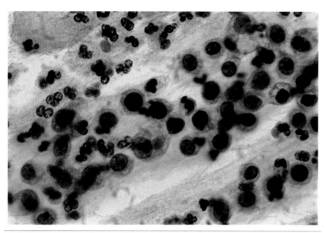

**Fig. 23.25** High-grade (severe) dyskaryosis in a case of small cell CIN 3, same case as Figures 23.23 and 23.24. Five nuclei in the centre of the field show obvious hyperchromasia and abnormal chromatin, but other dyskaryotic nuclei in the field are much more difficult to identify as such (PAP).

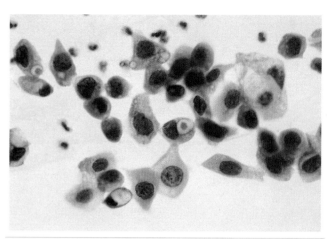

**Fig. 23.28** High-grade (severe) dyskaryosis. The cell pattern shows some features of immature squamous metaplasia but the nuclear chromatin, variation in nuclear size and shape and diminished cytoplasm indicate high-grade dyskaryosis, in this case of CIN 3 (PAP).

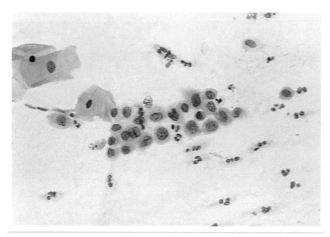

**Fig. 23.26** High-grade (severe) dyskaryosis. Small polychromatic cells of similar size and shape. The nuclear hyperchromasia, abnormal chromatin pattern and narrow band of cytoplasm indicate high-grade dyskaryosis in this case of CIN 3 (PAP).

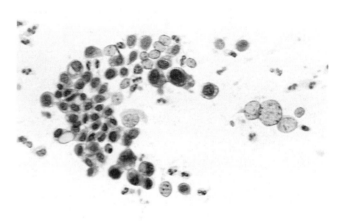

**Fig. 23.29** High-grade (severe) dyskaryosis. Bare, hypochromatic nuclei are associated with smaller high-grade dyskaryotic cells from a case of CIN 3. Bare nuclei of this type should not be mistaken for endocervical cell nuclei (PAP).

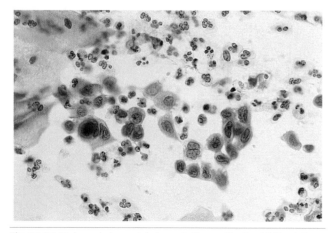

**Fig. 23.27** High-grade (severe) dyskaryosis. The small cells exhibit variation of size and shape as well as abnormal chromatin pattern and scanty cytoplasm. Engulfment of one cell by another is seen on the left of this field from a case of CIN 3 (PAP).

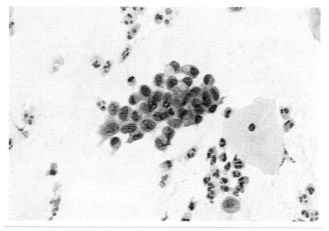

**Fig. 23.30** High-grade (severe) dyskaryosis. A cluster of cells from a case of CIN 3. Cytoplasmic vacuolation, as seen here, may be a feature of high-grade dyskaryotic cells in CIN 3 and invasive squamous cell carcinoma (PAP).

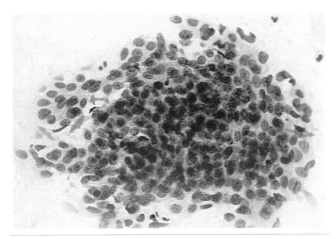

**Fig. 23.31** High-grade (severe) dyskaryosis. A sheet of crowded, overlapped dyskaryotic cells from a case of small cell non-keratinising CIN 3. Sheets and clusters of abnormal cells may be more difficult to identify than dispersed dyskaryotic cells (PAP).

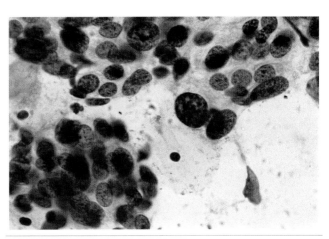

**Fig. 23.34** High-grade (severe) dyskaryosis, same case as Figure 23.33. Abnormal chromatin clumping is confirmed and is obvious in the large nucleus near the centre of the field (PAP).

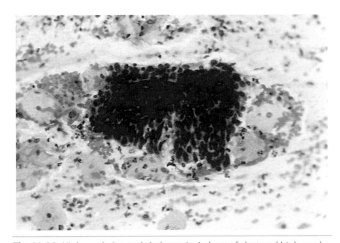

**Fig. 23.32** High-grade (severe) dyskaryosis. A sheet of clustered high-grade dyskaryotic cells from a case of CIN 3. Dispersed dyskaryotic cells are usually present, but if they are scanty, or in occasional cases even entirely absent, correct identification of clustered dyskaryotic cells may be very difficult (PAP).

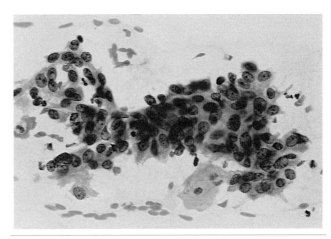

**Fig. 23.35** High-grade (severe) dyskaryosis. A sheet of cells of a case from widespread CIN 3. Punctate nucleoli, as seen in some of the nuclei, are not usually a feature of CIN 3 unless it occupies a large proportion of the transformation zone (PAP).

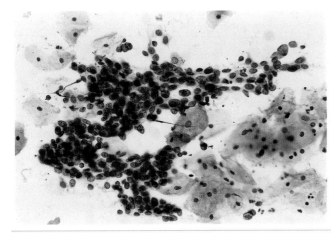

**Fig. 23.33** High-grade (severe) dyskaryosis. Clumped high-grade dyskaryosis from a case of CIN 3. Compare with the endometrial cells in Figure 23.44. Careful examination of individual nuclei at high power may be necessary to make the diagnosis (PAP).

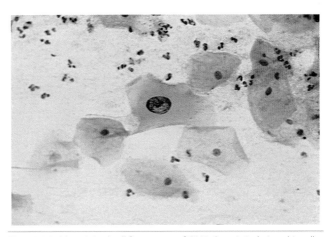

**Fig. 23.36** A keratinised cell from a case of CIN 3. Seen in isolation, this cell might be interpreted as showing only low-grade dyskaryosis (PAP).

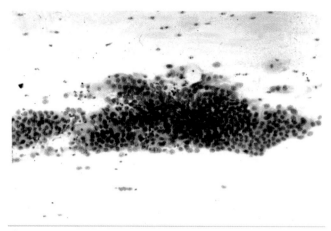

**Fig. 23.37** High-grade (severe) dyskaryosis of large cell non-keratinising type. Groups of this appearance may be mistaken for endocervical cells at screening power (PAP).

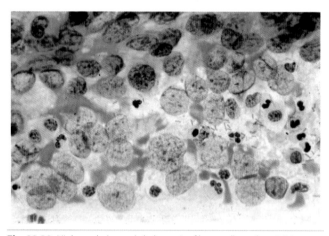

**Fig. 23.38** High-grade (severe) dyskaryosis of large cell non-keratinising type. Same area of same case as Figure 23.37. The abnormal chromatin pattern may be subtle and varies between nuclei, but is clearly apparent on high power examination. Where the nuclei are not overlapped the nuclear staining is markedly hypochromatic (PAP).

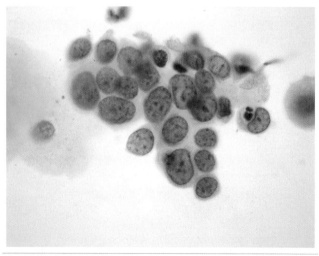

**Fig. 23.39** High-grade (severe) dyskaryosis of large cell non-keratinising type. A similar case to Figures 23.37 and 23.38 in a liquid-based preparation (PAP; ThinPrep®).

- Nuclear hyperchromasia
- Multiple abnormal nuclei
- Cytoplasm reduced
- Abnormal cytoplasmic maturation. It may be thin, dense or keratinised
- Cell borders may be angular or rounded. Bizarrely shaped cells may be seen, especially associated with CIN 3
- Prominent nucleoli may be seen, usually associated with extensive CIN 3 lesions.

In view of the evidence presented by Slater et al.,[45] if the terms moderate and severe dyskaryosis are retained for descriptive purposes, then the N:C ratios should be estimated according to the criteria of up to 50% (low-grade or mild), 50–66% (moderate) and greater than 66% (severe) but using diameter, and not area, ratios.

It is clear from the descriptions of the histological findings in CIN 2 and 3 that the appearances may be very variable. Similarly, the cytological findings will reflect this, and may be relatively uniform in an individual case. Failure to obtain a representative sample of the whole lesion (which may well be unavoidable, and not restricted to cytology preparations) may also limit the range of abnormal cellular material available for assessment and correlation.

High-grade dyskaryotic cells usually have nuclear morphology more abnormal than that associated with low-grade dyskaryosis and CIN 1, but have plentiful and sometimes keratinised cytoplasm. The diagnosis of high-grade dyskaryosis may frequently be confirmed by the presence of cells elsewhere in the cytology preparation with N:C ratios more commonly associated with high-grade dyskaryosis.

Abnormal chromatin pattern is usually the most significant nuclear abnormality associated with high-grade dyskaryosis. This may be accompanied by hyperchromasia, abnormal nuclear outline and multinucleation, or a combination of any number of these features. However, in some cervical cytology preparations with high-grade dyskaryosis the cytological abnormality is confined to an abnormal chromatin pattern in a round to oval nucleus in a cell in which the nuclear diameter exceeds 50% of the diameter of the cell. This appearance has recently been emphasised as a particular diagnostic pitfall in LBC preparations.[44] Nucleoli are not usually prominent in high-grade dyskaryosis but are sometimes seen, usually in association with extensive CIN 3 lesions on the cervix. Mitotic figures are infrequently observed in dispersed dyskaryotic cell populations but may sometimes be easily seen in large cohesive clusters or 'microbiopsy' fragments of dyskaryotic cells.

Although, as noted above, three cytological and histological types of high-grade dyskaryosis and CIN 3 are recognised, they are not usually reported in routine practice. Reporting of sub-types may, however, sometimes be useful for the purposes of clinico-pathological correlations in apparently discrepant cases. For example, small cell non-keratinising severe dyskaryosis and the corresponding CIN 3 lesion are likely to occur within the endocervical canal. This may explain the occasional failure of the colposcopist to visualise and biopsy a lesion diagnosed cytologically, thereby expediting appropriate management of the patient. Similarly, the histological diagnosis of keratinising CIN 3 may adequately explain bizarre keratinised squamous cells in a cytology preparation reported as possibly from an invasive squamous cell carcinoma.

## Diagnostic pitfalls: high-grade dyskaryosis

High-grade squamous dyskaryosis should be distinguished from the following:

- Immature squamous metaplasia
- Endocervical cells
- Histiocytes
- Follicular cervicitis
- Endometrial cells
- Endometrial exfoliation due to an IUCD
- Other 'glandular' cell groups
- HPV infection
- Intraepithelial and invasive adenocarcinoma.

*Immature squamous metaplasia* (see Ch. 21) may exhibit features of both squamous and endocervical glandular epithelium. The nuclei are relatively larger than those of mature squamous cells, with high nuclear cytoplasmic ratios, and frequently hyperchromasia, which may lead to misinterpretation as high-grade dyskaryosis if the architectural pattern of squamous metaplasia, uniformity of the cells and absence of a chromatin abnormality is not recognised (Fig. 23.40). Caution is necessary, however, because dyskaryosis may be present in what appear to be metaplastic cells (see Fig. 23.28). Atypical metaplasia is a term that has been applied to these appearances but to avoid misunderstanding they should be described as dyskaryotic and managed accordingly.

*Endocervical cells* (Fig. 23.41) are less likely to be confused with squamous cell dyskaryosis unless they show degenerative changes and marked hyperchromasia, in which case the nuclei tend to be pyknotic and lack a chromatin structure. Endocervical cell cytoplasm is delicate and in conventional cervical smears, loss of endocervical cytoplasm resulting in the presence of bare endocervical cell nuclei is common. A similar effect occurs in tubal type epithelial cells which are another common component of cervical cytology samples. Bare nuclei may also originate from CIN lesions and may cause concern, but the nuclei should be assessed by comparison with those of neighbouring well-preserved cells. If the bare nuclei can be assigned to a non-neoplastic cell population the problem

may be resolved (Fig. 23.42). In conventional smears, because degenerative changes are frequently present, dyskaryosis should not be diagnosed from the appearances of bare nuclei alone in the absence of dyskaryotic cells. In LBC preparations, loss of cytoplasm by endocervical cells appears to be much less of a problem because of the very rapid fixation of the samples. Conversely, the occurrence of bare nuclei is more difficult to interpret because of dispersion of the cells and disruption of the relationships seen in a conventional smear. In SurePath™ LBC preparations in particular, the presence of bare nuclei appears very closely linked with the presence of high-grade squamous dyskaryosis.

It should be remembered that postmenopausal atrophy of the cervix affects the endocervical as well as the ectocervical epithelium. *Atrophic endocervical cell* groups may be misinterpreted as high-grade dyskaryosis. Careful observation of the cell detail and comparison with neighbouring cells will usually enable the correct interpretation to be made.

*Large cells, often with hypochromatic nuclei* with uneven chromatin distribution and anisonucleosis, and a tendency to lose their cytoplasm and become bare nuclei, and which

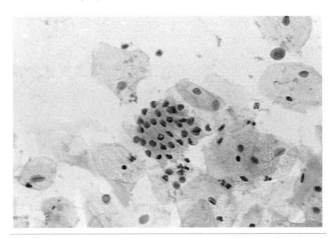

**Fig. 23.41** Degenerate endocervical cells: differential diagnosis from dyskaryosis. The uniform size and distribution of the pyknotic nuclei, distinct cell borders and weak haematoxylin staining of cytoplasmic mucin identifies the central group as endocervical cells (PAP).

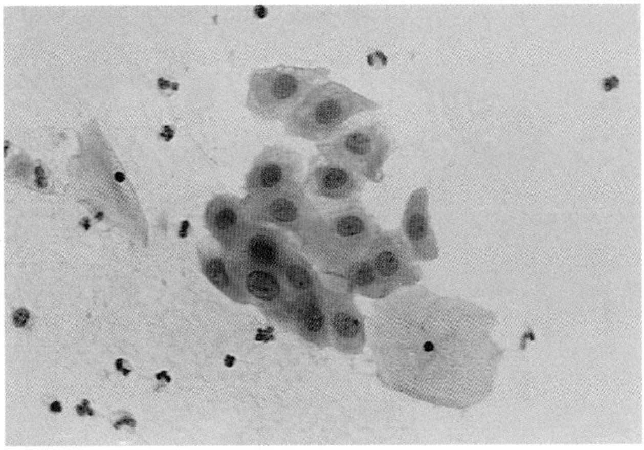

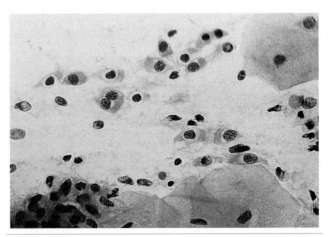

**Fig. 23.42** Stripped or bare nuclei and ciliated columnar cells: differential diagnosis of dyskaryosis. The hyperchromatic nuclei with coarse but uniformly distributed chromatin may be identified within the intact columnar cells, which have terminal bars and cilia. If the bare nuclei are seen alone they may be misinterpreted as dyskaryotic (PAP).

**Fig. 23.40** Immature squamous metaplasia: to be distinguished from high-grade (moderate) dyskaryosis. The uniformity of nuclear size and texture, the abundant cytoplasm and pattern of metaplastic cells is characteristic of these normal cells (PAP).

may resemble reactive endocervical cells, at least at screening magnification, are sometimes seen (Figs 23.37–23.39). Although they have in the past been described as atypical reserve cells, the authors consider that these cells are a (sometimes very subtle) presentation of high-grade squamous dyskaryosis from large cell non-keratinising CIN 3.

*Histiocytes* (Figs 23.43, 23.44) classically appear as dispersed single cells but they may sometimes be seen in clusters especially if they are numerous, as in the late menstrual 'exodus'. Although usually small, they may vary in size. Both nucleus and cytoplasm may show degenerative changes, which occasionally may mimic small keratinised or non-keratinised squamous cells very closely. If the characteristic reniform nuclei and foamy cytoplasm are not observed, distinction from a high-grade dyskaryotic squamous cell may usually be made by comparison with other neighbouring or similar cells showing more distinctive features. Engulfed material may sometimes be present in the cytoplasm.

*Follicular (lymphocytic) cervicitis* (Fig. 23.45) may result in streaks of follicular cells in a conventional smear, usually very focally but sometimes dominating large areas or even the whole of a smear. The cells characteristically are dispersed and include small lymphocytes and mature plasma cells, with coarse chromatin, larger less mature follicle centre cells which may show mitotic figures, and histiocytes containing tingible bodies (see Ch. 21). Paradoxically, in LBC preparations these cells often remain in aggregates,[49] particularly in ThinPrep® (Fig. 23.46), which may make the appearances of follicular cervicitis less likely to be confused with high-grade dyskaryosis.

*Endometrial cells* (Fig. 23.47) have small hyperchromatic nuclei and scanty cytoplasm and are usually present in clusters (see Chs 21, 26). They are not usually difficult to distinguish from cells of CIN or invasive carcinoma but it is necessary to be aware that clustered, and sometimes single cells from small cell non-keratinising CIN 3 or invasive carcinoma can sometimes look very similar to endometrial cells (Fig. 23.33). The presence of characteristic biphasic endometrial cell groups is helpful to confirm endometrial exfoliation, but if there is a possibility of co-existent CIN or carcinoma, further investigation may be necessary.

*Intrauterine contraceptive devices* (IUCD) cause reactive changes in the endometrial epithelium at points of contact, sometimes

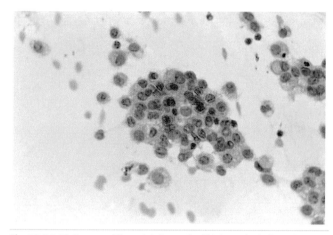

**Fig. 23.44** Histiocytes: differential diagnosis of high-grade dyskaryosis. Reniform nuclei, nucleoli, vacuolated cytoplasm and size are features which aid in the identification of histiocytes. These features are seen more clearly in the single cells surrounding the cluster (PAP).

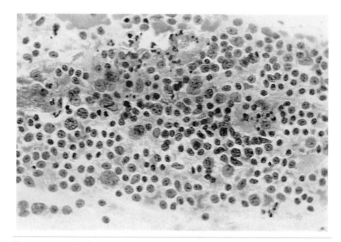

**Fig. 23.45** Follicular (lymphocytic cervicitis): differential diagnosis of high-grade dyskaryosis. The very coarse chromatin pattern of small lymphocytes and the presence of tingible body macrophages are important features in the identification of these cells (PAP).

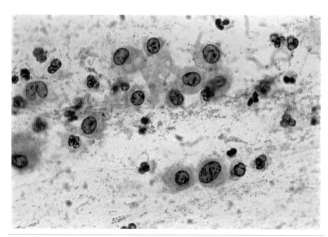

**Fig. 23.43** Histiocytes. Note the coarseness of clumping of the chromatin in the nuclei of these normal cells. Failure to identify such cells as histiocytes may lead to an erroneous diagnosis of high-grade dyskaryosis in squamous cells (PAP).

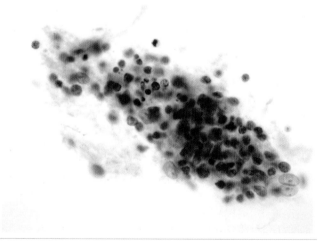

**Fig. 23.46** Clustered cells in follicular cervicitis in a liquid-based preparation. Note the tingible body macrophages above the centre of the field (PAP; Thin Prep®).

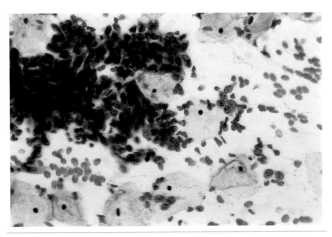

**Fig. 23.47** Endometrial cells: differential diagnosis of severe dyskaryosis. Exfoliated endometrial cells tend to form three-dimensional clusters. Distinction of such clusters from fragments of small cell CIN 3 or invasive carcinoma may require careful scrutiny of the whole sample for additional diagnostic features. Compare with Figure 23.33 (PAP).

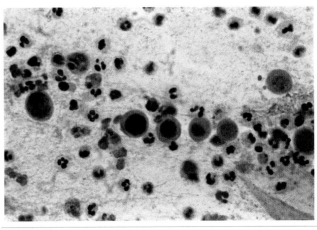

**Fig. 23.49** Endometrial cells in the smear of an IUCD user, same smear as Figure 23.48. The single cells with high nuclear/cytoplasmic ratios and hyperchromatic nuclei were felt probably to be degenerate endometrial cells, but that exclusion of high-grade squamous dyskaryosis was not possible. The patient subsequently underwent a cone biopsy and diagnostic uterine curettage. No neoplastic pathology was demonstrated in either specimen (PAP).

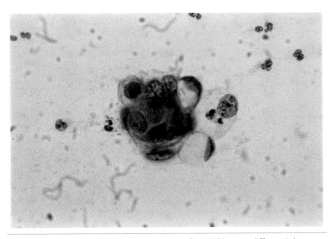

**Fig. 23.48** Endometrial cells in the smear of an IUCD user: differential diagnosis of high-grade dyskaryosis. This small three-dimensional group of endometrial cells with characteristic cytoplasmic vacuolation is easily identified, but see Figure 23.49 (PAP).

resulting in the exfoliation of abnormal endometrial cells which appear in cervical cytology samples (see Ch. 21) The abnormal endometrial cells are round but enlarged, sometimes multinucleated and sometimes have visible nucleoli. The cytoplasm may be vacuolated but often forms a dense narrow rim around the nucleus, closely mimicking high-grade dyskaryosis. The presence of tell-tale degenerate leucocytes, debris and endometrial material in streaks of mucus, and the known presence of an IUCD, are helpful in arriving at the correct interpretation (Figs 23.48, 23.49). The dissociation of the cellular components in an LBC preparation may make such distinction more difficult than in a conventional smear.

*Other clusters of 'glandular' material* may occasionally cause confusion with high-grade dyskaryosis, especially of small cell non-keratinising type.

Sampling of the lower uterine segment (LUS) (isthmic or directly sampled endometrium), endometriosis and tubal (or tuboendometrioid) metaplasia, all of which occur more frequently after cone biopsy or diathermy loop

excision procedures, may on occasion cause difficulties of interpretation. The recognition of a glandular epithelial cell component, and usually a 'biphasic' glandular epithelial and stromal population in LUS and endometriosis, are valuable guides to the correct interpretation.

*Cervical adenocarcinoma*, either intraepithelial or invasive, if not well differentiated may be indistinguishable from CIN 3 or non-keratinising carcinoma in a cervical cytology preparation. The characteristic features of rosettes, nuclear pseudostratification or palisading and feathered edges of sheets of dyskaryotic cells suggest cervical glandular intraepithelial neoplasia (CGIN) or invasive adenocarcinoma (see Ch. 24) but in the absence of these or distinctive features of squamous differentiation, the presence of adenocarcinoma or a mixed adenosquamous carcinoma may be difficult to determine. Prominent, sometimes multiple and irregular nucleoli may be present in squamous cell carcinoma or adenocarcinoma. It should also be borne in mind that a significant proportion of CGIN lesions and invasive adenocarcinomas are associated with concomitant CIN 3, an unsurprising finding in view of the now known common association with HPV type 18 in particular.

*Adenocarcinoma cells from carcinomas of the endometrium* or, less commonly, adenocarcinomas of the ovary or fallopian tube, can usually be distinguished from severe squamous dyskaryosis because of the tendency to form three-dimensional cell clusters, as well as by the presence of prominent nucleoli and cytoplasmic vacuolation (see Chs 26, 27). Poorly differentiated carcinoma cells from these sites may be more problematic to interpret but in general the cells are likely to be much less numerous than high-grade dyskaryotic cells originating from the cervix.

*Adenosquamous carcinoma* of the endometrium is occasionally represented in a cervical cytology preparation (see Ch. 26). A keratinising squamous component can mislead the cytologist towards a diagnosis of cervical squamous cell carcinoma, unless the adenocarcinomatous cells are represented and identified in the rounded clusters typical of endometrial origin. The dyskaryotic cells will usually be fewer than might be expected from a cervical carcinoma.

## Invasive squamous cell carcinoma

### Histology of microinvasive and invasive squamous cell carcinoma

Invasive carcinoma is recognised histologically by the presence of neoplastic squamous cells (Figs 23.50–23.53) which are no longer confined to the surface of the cervix or endocervical crypts by intact basement membrane, but have extended into the underlying stroma. The extent of invasion determines whether the lesion is regarded as microinvasive or frankly invasive carcinoma. The distinction is made because very early invasive (or microinvasive) carcinoma is amenable to conservative treatment, namely cone biopsy, rather than radical hysterectomy, trachelectomy or radiotherapy, as the risk of spread of carcinoma beyond the cervix is extremely low. Definitions of microinvasive carcinoma continue to evolve and in recent versions of the FIGO staging[4] the term microinvasive is itself no longer used (see Table 23.2). FIGO stage IA1 disease, i.e. with measured stromal invasion to a maximum depth of 3 mm and to a maximum width of 7 mm is generally considered that for which cone biopsy is considered adequate treatment.

In histological sections, early stage invasive carcinoma (Fig. 23.50) usually displays extensive CIN 3 as already described, from which tongues and islands of neoplastic cells extend through the basement membrane in a spray-like pattern or later as confluent invasion. The invading neoplastic cells frequently show greater maturation, with more cytoplasmic development than the cells of the CIN 3 from which they have arisen, a feature which may, importantly, be reflected in the cytology (see below) (Fig. 23.50). As growth proceeds beyond the stage of microinvasion, the islands of neoplastic cells become larger and a surrounding desmoplastic infiltrate may be seen, together with a variable inflammatory cell infiltrate. Lymphatic or vascular permeation by malignant cells is increasingly likely to be found. Ultimately there is a tumour mass, frequently ulcerated and recognisable clinically as an invasive carcinoma. Carcinomas are generally divided into

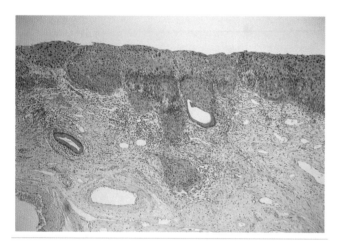

**Fig. 23.50** Microinvasive carcinoma of cervix. CIN 3 is present, extending into some of the endocervical glands. Deep to this, irregular groups of squamous cells extend into the stroma to a depth of less than 3 mm (H&E). A tiny focus of microinvasion FIGO Stage Ia1 is seen extending from the basement membrane into the inflamed stroma. The invasive component shows increased cytoplasm and nesting [redifferentiation] (H&E).

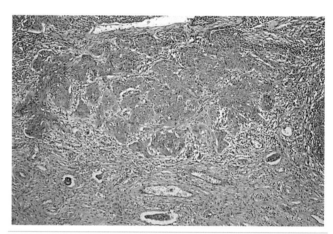

**Fig. 23.52** Section of cervix with moderately differentiated invasive squamous cell carcinoma. Multiple islands of carcinoma cells infiltrate the cervical stroma and lymphatic channels deep to the tumour contain small groups of malignant cells (H&E).

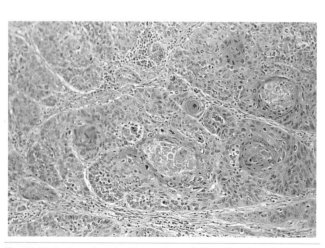

**Fig. 23.51** Section of cervix with invasive welldifferentiated keratinising squamous cell carcinoma. Nests of large eosinophilic tumour cells forming keratin pearls are present (H&E).

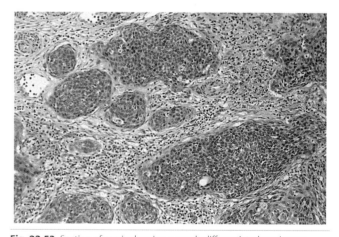

**Fig. 23.53** Section of cervix showing a poorly differentiated carcinoma composed of irregular groups of crowded abnormal epithelial cells with hyperchromatic nuclei and scattered mitoses. No differentiation can be seen but the pattern of infiltration, an origin from CIN 3 at the surface, and negative stains for mucin production indicate that this is a poorly differentiated squamous cell carcinoma (H&E).

well-, moderately or poorly differentiated grades relating to the pattern of invasion and to the cytoplasmic development of the neoplastic cells. Grading correlates broadly with prognosis for the patient and has a bearing on the cytological findings.

Features indicating a well-differentiated squamous cell carcinoma (Fig. 23.51) include the presence of large islands of infiltrating neoplastic cells with intercellular bridges, epithelial pearl formation and obvious keratinisation of the cell cytoplasm. Moderately differentiated carcinomas (Fig. 23.52) show some evidence of squamous differentiation, consisting of solid islands and smaller groups of polygonal pleomorphic cells, but keratinisation and intercellular bridges are less obvious and pearl formation is not seen. Approximately 60% of squamous cell carcinomas are moderately-differentiated. Poorly differentiated squamous cell carcinomas (Fig. 23.53) invade as sheets, islands and single cells, often invoking a pronounced inflammatory reaction. No definite squamous features are seen and their origin may only be established with the help of special stains to exclude mucin production, or immunocytochemistry to exclude other poorly differentiated neoplastic cell types. Identification of the pattern of keratin expression in carcinoma of the cervix by the use of poly- and monoclonal antibodies has proved useful in confirming the squamous nature of some poorly differentiated cervical neoplasms.

The World Health Organization has adopted a different grading system in which neoplasms are graded as keratinising, large cell non-keratinising and small cell non-keratinising squamous cell carcinomas. These groups correlate broadly with the three grades used above, but the last group includes a number of cases that have small cell neuroendocrine features similar to those of small cell carcinoma of the bronchus (see below). Glandular differentiation with mucin production may be noted in isolated cells within the tumour, but this does not denote an adenosquamous carcinoma unless mucin secreting cells form more than one-third of the neoplastic cell population.

## Cytological findings: invasive squamous cell carcinoma (Figs 23.54–23.70)

Microinvasive and invasive squamous cell carcinoma cannot be diagnosed reliably by cervical cytology because the high-grade dyskaryosis of CIN 3 may be morphologically indistinguishable from the high-grade dyskaryosis of invasive carcinoma. However, there are cytological features which imply the presence of an invasive carcinoma:

- Very large numbers of dyskaryotic cells reflecting the widespread CIN 3 generally present with early invasive lesions
- Variation in size and shape of the dyskaryotic cell nuclei more than that associated with CIN 3 and often including very small cells
- Abnormal chromatin clumping with such coarse aggregation that areas of lucency appear between the aggregates ('windowing')
- Tissue fragments or 'microbiopsies' of high-grade dyskaryotic cells
- Large and sometimes irregular macronucleoli especially in large cell non-keratinising carcinoma
- Cytoplasmic keratinisation including thick anucleate fragments in keratinising squamous cell carcinoma
- Bizarrely shaped dyskaryotic squamous cells including 'fibre cells' and 'tadpole' cells

- Smear background including fibrin, debris, leukocytes and blood described as a 'tumour' or 'malignant diathesis'. This is not sufficiently specific for diagnosis but may be a very important sign drawing attention to other features.

It is useful to report these features seen with high-grade dyskaryosis in order to convey the need for urgent investigation of the patient.

It is noteworthy that the BSCC 1986 classification concentrated on the presence of 'malignant diathesis' and the presence of abnormal keratinisation as features suggestive of invasive squamous cell carcinoma. Consequent on the success of screening programmes, invasive cervical carcinoma tends to be diagnosed at an earlier point in the natural history (lower FIGO clinical staging) than formerly. A substantial proportion of invasive disease is now diagnosed at clinical stage IA when ulceration and necrosis (from which the appearance of 'malignant diathesis' results) are unlikely to have occurred. Furthermore, the classical keratinising invasive lesions are less

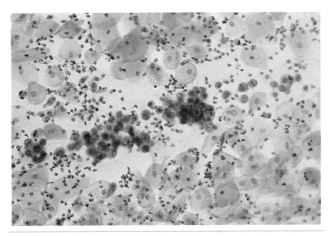

**Fig. 23.54** High-grade (severe) dyskaryosis from a case of early invasive squamous cell carcinoma. The smear contains many groups of high-grade dyskaryotic cells as well as small single keratinised cells which are seen in the background. These two features should alert the pathologist to the possibility of early invasion (PAP).

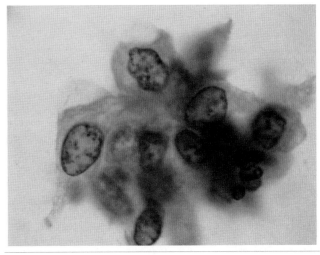

**Fig. 23.55** High-grade (severe) squamous dyskaryosis from an invasive squamous cell carcinoma. The chromatin is abnormally clumped with areas of lucency or 'windowing' (PAP; ThinPrep®).

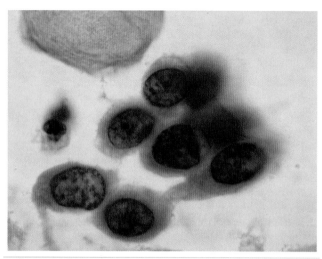

**Fig. 23.56** High-grade (severe) squamous dyskaryosis from an invasive squamous cell carcinoma. The chromatin is abnormally clumped with areas of lucency or 'windowing' (PAP; SurePath™).

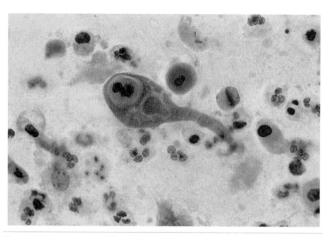

**Fig. 23.59** Squamous cell carcinoma. In the centre is a bizarrely shaped keratinised dyskaryotic cell, often described as a tadpole cell (PAP).

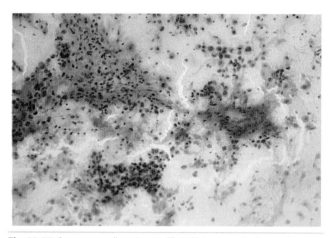

**Fig. 23.57** Squamous cell carcinoma. The whole picture is abnormal. Keratinisation of cytoplasm is a striking feature and high-grade (severe) dyskaryosis is clearly seen in the small cells, even at this magnification (PAP).

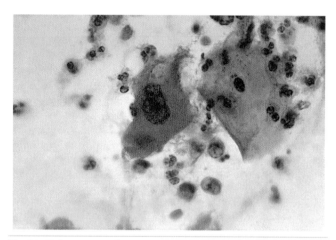

**Fig. 23.60** Squamous cell carcinoma. A high-grade (severely) dyskaryotic squamous cell with abundant keratinised cytoplasm lies next to a normal squamous cell (PAP).

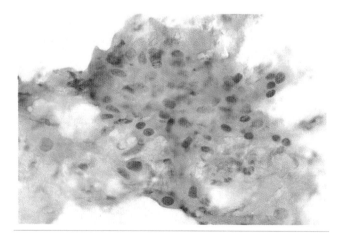

**Fig. 23.58** Squamous cell carcinoma; keratinising, well-differentiated type. Abnormal nuclear morphology is present but is less well defined in the degenerate cells (PAP).

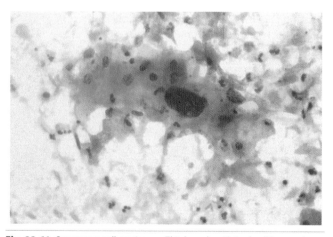

**Fig. 23.61** Squamous cell carcinoma. This large keratinised cell has nuclear features amounting to high-grade (severe) dyskaryosis (PAP).

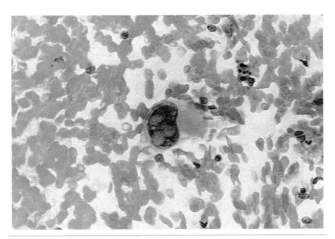

**Fig. 23.62** Squamous cell carcinoma. A high-grade (severely) dyskaryotic cell with a degenerate nucleus (PAP).

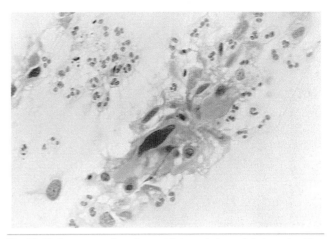

**Fig. 23.65** Squamous cell carcinoma. High-grade (severe) dyskaryosis with elongated nuclei. Eosinophilic and cyanophilic fragments of cytoplasm and neutrophil polymorphs in the background suggest an invasive carcinoma (PAP).

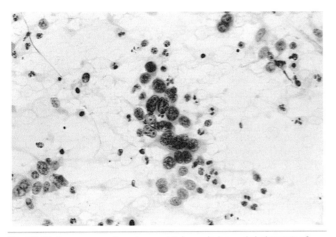

**Fig. 23.63** Squamous cell carcinoma. High-grade (severe) dyskaryosis of small cell type in a background of streaked exudate, debris and leukocytes (PAP).

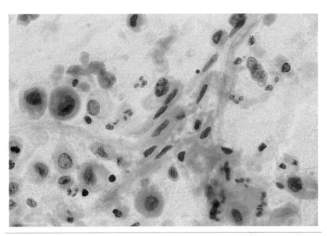

**Fig. 23.66** Squamous cell carcinoma. High-grade (severe) dyskaryosis with variation in size and shape of cells including elongated forms described as fibre cells (PAP).

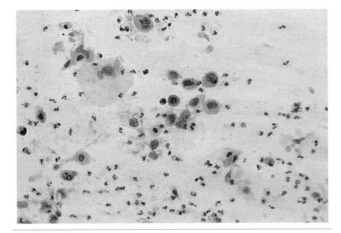

**Fig. 23.64** Squamous cell carcinoma. Small high-grade (severely) dyskaryotic cells with scanty cytoplasm with keratinisation in a few cells. The background 'diathesis' of leukocytes and cell debris suggests an invasive carcinoma (PAP).

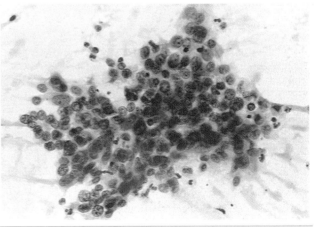

**Fig. 23.67** Squamous cell carcinoma. A fragment of small cell non-keratinising carcinoma (PAP).

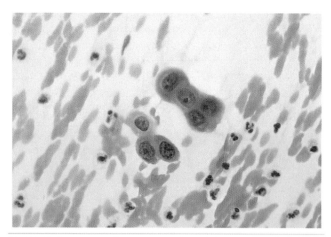

**Fig. 23.68** Squamous cell carcinoma. High-grade (severe) dyskaryosis from a non-keratinising squamous cell carcinoma in which the tumour cells have prominent nucleoli and a variable amount of dense cytoplasm. Cells of these appearances need to be distinguished from non-neoplastic cells seen in metaplasia or 'repair' change (PAP).

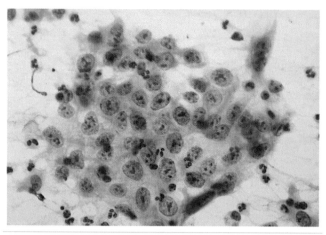

**Fig. 23.70** Squamous cell carcinoma. High-grade (severe) dyskaryosis from a non-keratinising squamous cell carcinoma in which the cells have large, multiple and irregular nucleoli (PAP).

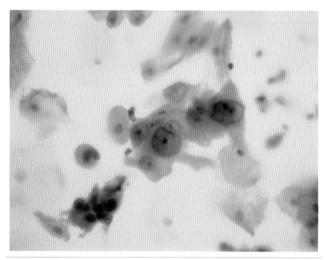

**Fig. 23.69** Squamous cell carcinoma. High-grade squamous dyskaryosis. The cells at the centre of the field have non-keratinised cytoplasm but some are of irregular shape. There is focal condensation of chromatin on the nuclear membranes and the nuclei have prominent nucleoli. Such cells should be distinguished from non-neoplastic cells seen in metaplasia or 'repair' change (PAP; SurePath™).

failure to appreciate the significance of a poor or inadequate sample. In slide reviews for audit of invasive carcinoma or medicolegal cases, one of the authors (PAS) has seen non-keratinising high-grade dyskaryotic squamous cells with prominent nucleoli, fairly dense, often grey staining cytoplasm, and sometimes diameter nuclear/cytoplasmic ratios of less than 50%, overlooked on a number of occasions. These appear to have been mistaken for normal immature metaplastic cells, when careful observation of the nuclear features should have led to the correct diagnosis of high-grade dyskaryosis (Figs 23.68, 23.69). The well-established histological observation, noted above, that the cells of invasive squamous cell carcinoma tend to appear better-differentiated than those of the CIN 3 lesion from which they arise, appears to have been inadequately translated into the corresponding cytological findings.

## Verrucous carcinoma (Fig. 23.71 and see Fig. 23.16)

This uncommon variant of squamous cell carcinoma affects the cervix rarely. It is a slowly growing exophytic tumour with a histologically well-defined deep margin which extends by pushing into the neighbouring tissue. It rarely metastasises. The cytology can be misleading because of the absence of nuclear characteristics of malignancy. Cervical cytology samples are dominated by cells with thick, keratinised cytoplasm and small pyknotic nuclei. Ulceration of the tumour and purulent discharge may be reflected by blood and leukocytes in the cytology preparation.

The distinction from condyloma acuminatum is important, and it may be the persistence or recurrence of the clinical abnormality which eventually leads to a sufficiently large biopsy being taken to establish the correct diagnosis. Human papillomavirus has been identified in the tumour cells.

## Borderline nuclear changes

Borderline nuclear changes is the term used in the BSCC terminology to categorise changes where there is genuine doubt as

frequently seen. The cytological suspicion of possible invasion is now likely to be much more dependent on the observation on marked abnormalities of cell size and shape and of striking chromatin abnormalities such as coarse clumping and 'windowing', as described above.

### Diagnostic pitfalls: invasive squamous cell carcinoma

The recognition of malignant diathesis is important, because it should draw the attention of the observer to the need to search for, and carefully assess the detail of, any abnormal cells present. This is a problem as its occurrence in screening samples is becoming much less frequent, and so for individual screeners, the opportunity to observe a malignant diathesis in their own primary screening activity has become a rare event. Failure to recognise diathesis and appreciate its significance may result in the under-grading of keratinised cells as discussed above, or

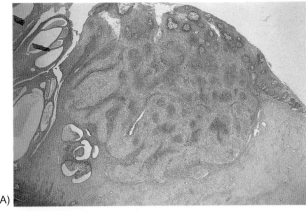

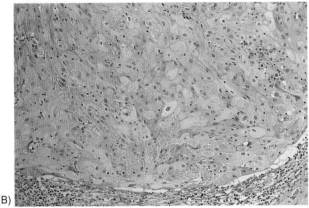

**Fig. 23.71** (A,B) Verrucous squamous cell carcinoma. Histology shows a raised exophytic tumour mass composed of pale squamous cells with ample cytoplasm and bland nuclei. The lower border of the tumour has a pushing margin but islands of invasive carcinoma cells can be seen in the stroma (H&E).

to whether or not they represent neoplasia. The use of a borderline or atypical category (atypical squamous cells and atypical glandular cells in TBS) is necessary in the practice of cervical cytology because some samples cannot confidently be classified as either normal or dyskaryotic. This relates to the lack of robust and objective criteria for clear distinction between reactive or inflammatory change and dyskaryosis, which form a continuum of cytological change; the difficulty in assessing the significance of minor changes associated with HPV infection; and the difficulty of confident diagnosis of the more subtle presentations of dyskaryosis, especially if the suspect cell population is scanty.

In screening terms, the significance of the borderline category is that a proportion of women with persistent borderline changes will be found to have CIN when they are investigated by colposcopy. For example, Parham et al.[50] found that there was a 23% excess of dyskaryosis in the repeat smear of patients after a report of borderline nuclear change compared with controls, and of those who attended for colposcopy 11% had biopsy confirmed CIN. In the USA estimates have suggested that 10–20% of women with atypical squamous cells have underlying CIN 2 or 3 and that 1 in 1000 may even have invasive cancer.[51] The possibility that tests from occasional women harbouring an invasive carcinoma will have cytological changes reported only as borderline is also acknowledged in UK practice.[25]

Nevertheless, the vast majority of these women do not have CIN, and the consequence is that large numbers of women who have no risk of developing invasive carcinoma in the next screening interval are investigated by colposcopy. This adds substantially to the costs of screening and is a significant cause of psychosexual morbidity. This need for investigation seriously impairs the effective specificity of the cervical cytology test, and probably the most valid criticism of cervical screening based on cytology is the overall lack of specificity of the test. The advent of testing for HPV-DNA as a routine and relatively inexpensive test offers an improvement in the management of these women, and the use of HPV testing in the management of women with borderline nuclear changes and low-grade dyskaryosis will be discussed further below.

The reporting of borderline nuclear change may be regarded as an unsatisfactory outcome of the test and, within the limits of safe reporting practice, its use should be minimised.

The 1986 BSCC terminology stressed that the borderline categorisation should only be made after scrutiny of all the material on the slide, as this may reveal unequivocal abnormalities in other cells. In practice, its use is difficult to monitor. Cervical cytology is less sensitive for minor abnormalities, the area from which the cells are sampled may be small and difficult to sample reliably, the lesion is likely to progress or regress in a short timescale, and there is no definite histological equivalent. The use of the borderline (or atypical) cervical cytology report tends to vary widely between centres and individual cytologists. In the early 1990s in the UK the problem of high and very variable reporting rates of borderline nuclear change was causing concern. A working party was convened to address the problem and attempt to refine the use of the term borderline nuclear change.[52] A formal subdivision into borderline nuclear changes not otherwise specified (NOS), borderline nuclear change, high-grade dyskaryosis not excluded, and borderline nuclear change in endocervical cells was proposed in the BSCC 2008 terminology, and further guidelines on reporting were given.[40]

Performance indicators are used in the UK NHS Cervical Screening Programme to assess abnormal reporting rates.[25] The target ranges used are evidence based and are quoted as 10–90 percentile ranges for all laboratories reporting more than 15 000 tests per year (England). The groups for mild dyskaryosis and borderline nuclear abnormalities are combined into one group, and the range was 3.4–6.8% for the financial year 2006/7 [53] (the need to combine the two categories is itself an indication of the difficulty in consistent classification of the two groups). An appropriate target range will vary with the population being screened and the reporting system in use, but the establishment of a range for a particular screening programme may be a valuable quality assurance tool. The Bethesda System suggests as a general guide that the rate of reporting ASC should not exceed 5% of all reports with ASC:SIL ratios of 2:2–3:1 in a general screening practice.[54]

## Cytomorphology of borderline nuclear changes

The cytological appearances associated with HPV infection have been described above and in Chapter 21. Cells showing koilocytosis are now to be classified with low-grade dyskaryosis (unless high-grade dyskaryosis is also present), but in isolation the less specific changes of bi- and multinucleation and keratinisation are not. Nuclear abnormality is often apparent with these changes, but falling short of dyskaryosis. The changes may include nuclear enlargement, minimal irregularities of outline, pyknosis or coarsening of the chromatin pattern (Figs 23.72–23.76). Abnormal keratinisation or dyskeratosis frequently accompanies HPV infection but is not specific for it. If anucleate or dyskeratotic cells are present in cervical cytology samples they should be examined carefully but if the nuclei are normal and no koilocytes are present, in the absence of other significant abnormality, they may be reported as negative. Dyskeratotic cells with nuclear enlargement and chromatin condensation (Fig. 23.74) not amounting to mild dyskaryosis should be reported as borderline nuclear change.

## Changes associated with inflammation

Mild nuclear hyperchromasia and nuclear enlargement are commonly associated with inflammatory and reactive changes, but if coarsening of the chromatin is present or there are degenerative changes or minor irregularities of outline, confident distinction from dyskaryosis may not be possible. Immature

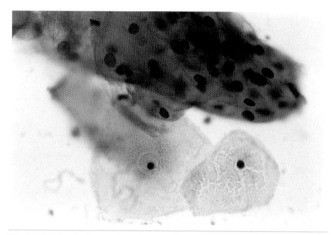

**Fig. 23.74** Borderline nuclear change. This dyskeratotic cell group shows mild nuclear enlargement and anisonucleosis. Peripheral condensation of chromatin can be seen in some of the nuclei. Compare with the adjacent superficial cell nuclei (PAP; ThinPrep®).

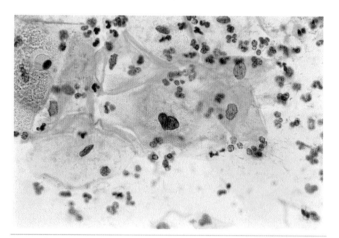

**Fig. 23.72** Borderline nuclear change. In the centre is a binucleated cell with slight nuclear enlargement and hyperchromasia, but no abnormality of chromatin pattern. Compare with the adjacent normal nuclei. The change may be HPV-related (PAP).

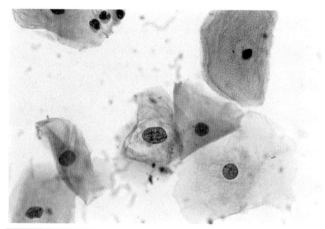

**Fig. 23.75** HPV-related changes. The cell in the centre is a koilocyte with nuclear enlargement, longitudinal nuclear folding and slight coarsening of the chromatin pattern. The nuclear appearances may be regarded as 'borderline,' but because of the presence of koilocytosis this cell would be graded as low-grade dyskaryosis in the BSCC 2008 terminology (PAP; ThinPrep®).

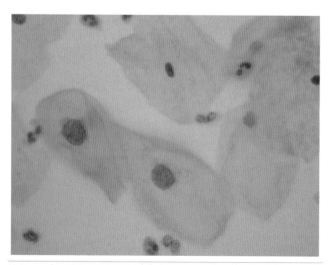

**Fig. 23.73** Borderline nuclear change. Two intermediate squamous cell nuclei show nuclear enlargement and slight coarsening of the chromatin falling short of dyskaryosis (PAP; SurePath™).

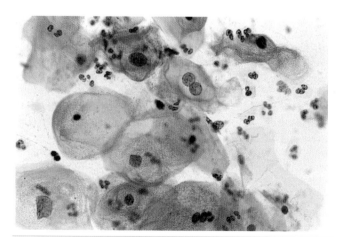

**Fig. 23.76** HPV-related changes. The nuclear features of binucleation, nuclear enlargement and slight coarsening of the chromatin may be regarded as 'borderline' but in the presence of koilocytosis these cells would be graded as low-grade dyskaryosis in the BSCC 2008 terminology (PAP).

metaplastic cells may present particular problems as a wider range of morphological features is acceptable as normal, than in mature squamous cells. Small metaplastic squamous cells in particular may have high N:C ratios. Simple nuclear folds are not uncommon and degenerative changes may occur. Some metaplastic cells have cytoplasmic vacuoles which indent the nucleus leading to apparent irregularities of nuclear outline which may be deceptive, especially at screening magnification. There may be bi- or multinucleation. The usual problems leading to categorisation of such cells as borderline are: hyperchromasia beyond that acceptable as reactive change; coarsening of the chromatin pattern in the absence of overt dyskaryosis; difficulty in distinguishing between simple nuclear folding, degenerative change and the irregular folding associated with dyskaryosis; minor variations in nuclear shape but with smooth outlines.

Interpretation of such details may be exceptionally difficult especially in scanty preparations, or (mainly in conventional smears) if the cells are partly obscured by polymorphs or other smear components. When a confident decision cannot be made the borderline category may have to be used.

### Repair and regeneration

Usually it is recognisable as an entity and may be dismissed as an insignificant finding (see Ch. 21). Although the cells may have large nuclei with prominent, sometimes multiple nucleoli and coarsening of the chromatin pattern, the chromatin remains evenly distributed. Repair cells often occur in more or less monolayered sheets, especially in conventional cervical smears, and consist of cells usually with low N:C ratios. If the cells are not monolayered, and particularly if they occur in three-dimensional groups, the nuclear detail may be difficult to observe and dismiss as insignificant. In these circumstances, the borderline nuclear change category may need to be used. Care should be taken in the assessment of apparent repair change, especially when the cells form three-dimensional clusters. Occasionally high-grade dyskaryosis mimics repair change, and it is important not to overlook this especially when large nucleoli are present in high-grade dyskaryosis, a feature likely to be associated with invasive squamous cell carcinoma. Squamous dyskaryosis of more usual appearance can usually be found in the sample when this occurs.

### Borderline nuclear changes; high-grade dyskaryosis not excluded

In most cases when borderline nuclear changes are reported, the cytological differential diagnosis is between normal, reactive or inflammatory conditions on the one hand and low-grade dyskaryosis on the other. In a small minority of cases, generally because the cells have diameter N:C ratios of greater than 50%, and there are doubts about the correct interpretation of the chromatin of the cells in question, the differential diagnosis lies between normal reactive or inflammatory conditions, and high-grade squamous dyskaryosis. This situation was acknowledged in the 1986 BSCC terminology[39] and by Buckley et al.,[52] but has now been made a specific sub-category of borderline nuclear change in the BSCC 2008 terminology.[40] The need to use this categorisation is particularly likely to arise when dealing with equivocal nuclear changes in immature metaplastic squamous cells, or in three-dimensional cell groups

(see below). This reporting category should be used very carefully and sparingly. It warrants immediate referral of the patient for colposcopy for the exclusion of the presence of high-grade disease. Women who have negative colposcopic and biopsy findings after such a cytology report may be difficult to manage, although the use of testing for high risk HPV types may be used to justify conservative management of these women when they test HPV-negative (see below).

### Three-dimensional cell clusters

Three-dimensional cell clusters frequently pose problems in interpretation of cervical cytology preparations. DeMay[43] has emphasised that 'hyperchromatic crowded cell groups' frequently consist of normal, benign cells, but when they are abnormal, tend to be from high-grade pre-malignant disease or invasive carcinoma. Careful examination of the architecture of the group in question may readily reveal the cell type as squamous, endocervical or endometrial. Lower uterine segment (LUS) or directly sampled endometrium have very characteristic appearances[55] in both conventional and liquid-based samples and similar findings may be seen in endometriosis of the cervix (see Ch. 25). Abnormal cell clusters frequently have 'steep' or thick edges and disorderly cell arrangements. Especially when the cluster is crowded, it may be very difficult to discern individual nuclear detail. There may be doubt about the type of cell within the group leading to, for example, a differential diagnosis of high-grade small cell squamous dyskaryosis *versus* endometrial cells. Alternatively, the cell type may be in no doubt, but there is difficulty in deciding whether the nuclei are dyskaryotic or not. Careful attention to cytological detail where the cells can clearly be seen is necessary, and sometimes this is only possible if cells are breaking away at the edges of such groups. While disorderly nuclei showing loss of polarity are an important feature in most abnormal cell groups, it should be noted that in some case of CIN 3 the cells in three-dimensional groups may appear deceptively orderly. Occasionally, cytomorphologically normal endocervical cells merge with high-grade squamous dyskaryosis. Mitotic figures may be seen in both benign and neoplastic cell groups and unless numerous or recognisably abnormal, their recognition may not be helpful in reaching a diagnosis. In abnormal three-dimensional cell clusters nuclear crowding and overlap, and difficulty in defining cell boundaries may lead to difficulty in assessing the grade of dyskaryosis present. In assessing three-dimensional cell groups, a particular pitfall is to assume that only one type of three-dimensional group is present in a sample, when there are both normal and abnormal cell groups. Every three-dimensional group of cells warrants individual attention when assessing a cervical cytology sample.

If a diagnostic decision cannot be made it will be necessary to use the borderline reporting category and this will frequently be 'borderline; high-grade dyskaryosis not excluded'. The nature of the cytological problem should be transmitted in the report.

### Borderline nuclear changes in endocervical cells (Figs 23.77, 23.78)

The range of inflammatory or reactive change seen in endocervical cells is considerable. At least in conventional cervical smears, there is overlap in the range of nuclear features which may be seen in extreme inflammatory change and those which may be seen in at least some examples of cervical glandular

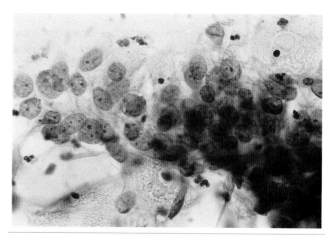

**Fig. 23.77** Borderline nuclear change in endocervical cells. This cell group is three-dimensional with nuclear crowding. Where individual nuclei can be seen there is anisonucleosis and mild coarsening of the chromatin (PAP).

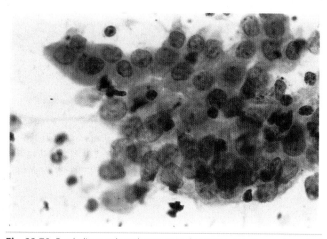

**Fig. 23.78** Borderline nuclear change in endocervical cells. The endocervical cells in the upper part of the field appear normal but they merge with cells showing disorderly, crowded and enlarged nuclei with coarsening of the chromatin pattern (PAP).

intraepithelial neoplasia (CGIN) (see Ch. 24). Recognition of the characteristic architectural features of CGIN is very important; in the absence of unequivocal and obvious endocervical cell dyskaryosis the cytological diagnosis of CGIN should not be made in the absence of those architectural features. In the absence of overt dyskaryosis, the likely circumstances when the use of the borderline category may be used in relation to endocervical abnormalities include:

- Three-dimensional cell groups with disorderly cell arrangements
- Coarse grainy chromatin
- Scanty suspect endocervical material.

It should be noted that none of the characteristic architectural abnormalities is absolutely specific for CGIN and if CGIN is present repeated examples of those abnormalities will usually be present in the cell population in question. If the suspect cellular material is scanty, a confident diagnosis of CGIN may not be possible, justifying the use of the borderline category. In LBC preparations, possibly because of better chromatin preservation and smaller cell groups, distinction between benign endocervical cell changes and CGIN is easier.[42]

## Management of borderline nuclear changes

Hitherto, the management of borderline nuclear changes has generally been by repeat cytology with referral for colposcopy for persistent abnormalities, practice tending to vary in detail locally. Within the NHSCSP, a maximum of three borderline reports within a 10-year period is allowed before referral, but most patients with persistent borderline changes will be referred within 18 months of their first test showing borderline nuclear changes. Of the subcategories, women with 'borderline nuclear change, high-grade dyskaryosis not excluded' should be referred immediately for colposcopy.[40] While in the past it was recommended that women with tests showing borderline nuclear changes in endocervical cells should have a repeat test including endocervical brushings in not more than 6 months,[52] immediate referral for colposcopy in now recommended in the NHSCSP.[56] This is based on the high incidence of invasive and high-grade disease found in these women. Some series of borderline nuclear change in endocervical cells show an excess of high-grade squamous lesions which may relate to difficulties in the recognition, definition and distinction of endocervical cells in comparison with small or immature metaplastic squamous cells.[57–61]

The fact that virtually all invasive squamous cell carcinomas of the cervix are related to high risk HPV infection offers the possibility of improvement of the management of women with borderline nuclear changes and low-grade dyskaryosis. In screening terms, women with borderline nuclear changes and low-grade dyskaryosis who test negative for high risk HPV infection have a negligible risk of development of invasive carcinoma in the next screening interval, and their clinical management may be modified accordingly. Information from the ALTS study in the USA,[62] and from the UK NHSCSP LBC/HPV pilot studies[48,63] shows that such 'triage' of low-grade abnormalities is effective, and cost effective, in practice. Following the UK studies, a small number of 'Sentinel Sites' have been funded in the UK from 2008 to implement triage of low-grade abnormalities by HPV testing to provide further information before national implementation of HPV testing. All women with a first cytology report of borderline nuclear changes or low-grade dyskaryosis will have 'reflex' testing for high risk HPV types using the Hybrid Capture™ 2 test (Qiagen). (The borderline nuclear change cases included in the protocol will include the categories of borderline, high-grade dyskaryosis not excluded and borderline nuclear change in endocervical cells.) Women testing negative for high risk HPV will be returned to routine screening (3- or 5-yearly depending on age). Women testing positive will be referred for colposcopy. Following satisfactory colposcopy, women with high-grade lesions will be treated. Those with changes of less than CIN 1 on biopsy will not undergo treatment and will be referred back for routine 3 or 5-yearly screening appropriate to their age. Those who have CIN 1 on biopsy will be followed up by cytology 1 year later (with or without colposcopy). If cytology only is used at this stage, follow-up will continue according to existing national protocols.

## The cervical cytology test in pregnancy

Dyskaryosis is seen in pregnant women, and the cytological appearances and their origin from CIN are the same as in non-pregnant women. Contrary to the opinion expressed in some early papers, there is no evidence that pregnancy has an adverse effect on the prognosis of invasive carcinoma of the cervix.[64]

Because of the complications of management of pregnant women with dyskaryosis, in the NHSCSP it is recommended that in adequately screened women routine tests should be deferred during pregnancy. If a woman who is pregnant has abnormal cytology, she should be referred for colposcopy by the usual criteria. A woman who has had a previous abnormal test requiring repeating may have such a repeat test in the mid-trimester, unless there is a clinical contraindication.[56] During pregnancy, the primary aim of colposcopy is to exclude the presence of invasive carcinoma, as it has been shown that delaying the treatment of CIN in pregnant women is safe,[65,66] and the incidence of invasive carcinoma of the cervix in pregnancy is low. If invasive disease is suspected clinically or colposcopically, a large enough biopsy to make the diagnosis is essential, be it a wedge, diathermy loop or cone biopsy; all of these procedures are associated with the risk of haemorrhage.[67]

Postpartum assessment and follow-up of all women with cytological abnormalities or biopsy proven CIN during pregnancy is essential. In the past it has been recorded that some CIN lesions are found to have regressed postpartum; it has been suggested that this was due to the trauma of delivery, and even the one-time routine application of diathermy to the cervix postpartum. Nevertheless, recent studies indicate that regression rates of CIN 2 and CIN 3 during pregnancy are low following delivery, and not related to its mode.[68] A high rate of disease persistence has been reported for high-grade CIN and early invasive carcinoma treated by cone biopsy during pregnancy. Excisional procedures carried out during pregnancy cannot be considered therapeutic, and colposcopic reassessment postpartum is essential.[56]

## Accuracy of cervical cytology

The preceding descriptions of dyskaryotic cells are comparable with the surface cells of histological sections of the cervix with CIN. It is this close relationship which gives the cervical cytology test its remarkable value as an indication of the whole thickness of the epithelium. In practice, however, the relationship is not perfect and merits further scrutiny.

## Positive predictive value of the test

Since 1995, the positive predictive value of the cervical cytology test has been used as a performance indicator in NHSCSP laboratories in the UK.[69] The figure is calculated as the percentage of tests showing moderate dyskaryosis or worse which have a biopsy showing CIN 2 or worse. Standard ranges were initially calculated from data from 1992/3 and 1993/4 from 12 laboratories all involved in cervical cytology training and/or external quality assurance, and which purported to follow BSCC reporting guidelines. Subsequently, the figures have been calculated as above from actual annual laboratory returns and the range is based on the 10th–90th centiles of values from all laboratories in England with a workload greater than 15 000 tests per year. The figures are thus now more firmly evidence-based, but there was remarkable consistency between the figures calculated initially from limited laboratory data and the subsequent comprehensive data. In 1995 the target range (calculated from the

above 1992/3 and 1993/4 data) was 65–85% and for 2006/7 it was 70.5–86.4%. For all laboratories in England in 2006/7 the overall outcome for tests showing CIN 2 or worse was: invasive cervical carcinoma 2.3%, CIN 3 or CGIN 51.8%, CIN 2 22.9%, CIN 1 10% and non-cervical carcinoma 0.7%.[53]

## Sensitivity of the cervical cytology test

The accuracy of a normal (or negative) cervical cytology test result, if the specimen is properly taken and reliably screened and interpreted, gives good protection against the development of cervical cancer within the next 3–5 years, but it does not exclude the possibility of small areas of usually low-grade CIN. The exact sensitivity of the cervical cytology is difficult or impossible to determine, partly because of the long natural history of the disease and the long time lapse before false negative tests are identified, if indeed they ever are. Colposcopic examination and cervicography are more sensitive tests for CIN, but they are not practical screening procedures, because they are too sensitive and would involve too many women in largely unnecessary investigations and treatment for small, mostly low-grade CIN lesions and HPV infection.

Estimating the sensitivity of the smear test has been made easier by the availability of colposcopy. In a study comparing the sensitivity of colposcopy and cervicography with the cervical cytology test, Campion et al. reported the sensitivity of cytology for the detection of CIN 2 and CIN 3 of 78% and an overall sensitivity of 68%.[70] Failure to detect all CIN 3 is largely due to the sampling method. A small area of epithelium may not be abraded by the sampling implement if pressure is too light or if the whole of the transformation zone is not scraped. Cells from a relatively large area of CIN 1, for example, may be present in the sample, but smaller areas of CIN 2 or CIN 3 may not be represented. A significant proportion of the cellular material sampled by a wooden spatula remains adherent to the spatula and is not transferred to the glass slide. Some areas of the traditionally prepared smear may be too thick for accurate microscopy. Thus, even when abnormal cells are scraped from the cervix they may not be transferred to, or be visible on the slide. LBC offers a solution to these last two factors. Unfortunately, laboratory errors also occur, resulting in false negative test results. Some laboratory errors are difficult to explain, but scanty abnormal cells are difficult to detect. There is now strong evidence suggesting that small numbers of dyskaryotic cells, especially if dispersed singly, confined to only part of a smear, and not showing marked nuclear hyperchromasia, are likely to be missed by a human screener.[27–29] This evidence relates to conventional smears and the equivalent figures for LBC preparations have yet to be defined. Computerised semi-automated or automated screening may offer at least a partial solution to this problem.

The sensitivity of primary screening is used as a performance indicator in the NHS Cervical Screening Programme.[25] The main method of internal quality control used is that of 'rapid review' in which all tests primary screened as negative or inadequate are subject to rescreening at normal screening magnification but for a restricted time, usually 75–90 seconds. Exact methods vary, and the use of rapid preview, in which all tests are examined before the main primary screening examination, is recommended by some as a superior method.[71] Sensitivity of primary screening based on rapid review assumes that primary screening plus rapid review detects 100% of all abnormalities, which is not the case in reality, as any cases actually reported falsely negative are, by definition, excluded from the calculation. Nevertheless, sensitivity of primary screening assessed in this way is a useful performance indicator, but it must be appreciated that it is critically dependent on the quality of rapid review examination. Monitoring the pick up rates of abnormal smears by primary screeners has been advocated as an alternative performance indicator, and it is independent of the quality of rapid review.[72]

Nevertheless, despite the above imperfections, the cervical smear is a sufficiently accurate test for a screening programme for prevention of cervical cancer, as indicated by the successful screening programmes described in Chapter 22.

## Management of the patient with abnormal cytology

It is widely agreed that the risk of progression to invasive cancer is an indication for further investigation and treatment of women who have cervical smears showing high-grade (moderate or severe) dyskaryosis (high-grade SIL in the Bethesda System). The management of the much more common cytological diagnosis of mild dyskaryosis (low-grade SIL in the Bethesda System) and changes due to HPV is less well defined. Until there is a means of distinguishing premalignant mild dyskaryosis from the mild dyskaryosis that will regress, many more women will be treated for CIN than would develop cancer if they were not treated.

As described above, the use of high risk HPV testing offers a significant refinement in the management of women with low-grade dyskaryosis. Referral for colposcopy at the first occurrence of mild dyskaryosis became the favoured management for mild dyskaryosis in the UK in 2004.[56]

## Treatment of CIN

Treatment of CIN may be carried out by a number of local destructive methods including cryotherapy, diathermy, laser ablation and 'cold' coagulation, the last two being the local destructive treatment methods of choice in recent times in the UK. Local destructive therapy, which must be preceded by incisional biopsy confirmation of the presence and grade of CIN present, has been shown to be just as effective in treating CIN as excisional treatments. Currently, excisional treatments are generally preferred, where possible diathermy large loop excision of the transformation zone (LLETZ, also known as loop electro-excision procedure, LEEP), rather than a cone biopsy. The advantage of excisional treatment is that the whole of the area of CIN removed may be examined histologically, and therefore there is a much smaller likelihood of an early invasive squamous cell carcinoma being overlooked. With local destructive therapy, failure to recognise or biopsy an area of early invasive disease is a possibility. The complications of LLETZ for childbearing were generally considered less significant than those of cone biopsy (e.g. cervical stenosis and incompetence) but a recent meta-analysis concluded that all excisional treatments for CIN show a similar pregnancy-related morbidity including preterm delivery and low birth weight.[73]

As noted above, early referral for colposcopy is now favoured in the UK for the management of women with cervical cytology tests showing mild dyskaryosis. Once they have been assessed at colposcopy, there is an increasing trend to manage low-grade CIN lesions conservatively, in the expectation that a proportion of such lesions will resolve spontaneously and not require any form of treatment.

## Follow-up after treatment and HPV testing as a test of cure

Women retain an increased risk of recurrent CIN and invasive squamous cell carcinoma after treatment for CIN and follow-up is essential. It is usual practice to follow treated women by a combination of colposcopy and cytology. Within the NHS Cervical Screening Programme, standard follow-up schedules are recommended. Women treated for CIN 2 and worse should have negative follow-up cytology at 6 and 12 months after treatment and then annually for at least a further 9 years, before being returned to the routine screening interval. Women treated for low-grade disease should have follow-up cytology at 6, 12 and 24 months and may then be returned to the routine screening interval if all are negative.

Following treatment of the cervix, residual or recurrent CIN may be more difficult to sample and detect by cytology because of alteration of the cervix (e.g. cervical stenosis) or because of 'buried' residual disease. Testing for HPV-DNA is a potentially valuable test in this setting.[74] It is more sensitive than cytology and a negative test for high risk HPV-DNA has a high negative predictive value for the presence of CIN.

The use of HPV testing as a test of cure for CIN is being introduced at the UK HPV testing 'Sentinel Sites' described under the management of borderline nuclear changes described above. After treatment for CIN (all grades) women will have a cytology test at 6 months. If it is abnormal they will be referred back for colposcopy and if that is normal they will have an HPV test. If the HPV test is positive they will be referred back for colposcopy. If it is negative they will have a further cytology test 3 years later and if that is negative be returned to the routine screening interval. The model follow-up schedules for high-grade disease involve some 10 fewer follow-up smears in negative women with a significant saving in costs.[75,76]

After conservative treatment for early invasive disease (cone biopsy or radical trachelectomy), follow-up cytology may be made difficult to interpret by the presence of directly sampled endometrium, endometriosis or tubo-endometrioid (tubal) metaplasia. After more radical treatment, which may include radical hysterectomy and usually radiotherapy and/or chemotherapy, iatrogenic cytological changes are likely to cause extreme difficulty in interpretation and cytological follow-up of these patients is not recommended.

## Vaginal intraepithelial neoplasia (VaIN)

Some women with CIN have disease which extends into the vaginal vault and following hysterectomy there is a risk of the occurrence of vaginal intraepithelial neoplasia (VaIN) and subsequently invasive carcinoma of the vagina, although the latter risk appears to be low (see Ch. 25). VaIN may be difficult to identify by colposcopic examination of the vault. Within the NHS cervical screening programme, the following recommendations are made for follow-up of the vaginal vault after hysterectomy[56]:

- For women on routine screening recall for at least 10 years prior to hysterectomy and no CIN in the hysterectomy specimen, no vault cytology is required
- For women with less than 10 years' routine screening recall and no CIN at hysterectomy, a sample should be taken

from the vault 6 months after surgery and there should be no further cytology follow-up if it is negative

- For women with completely excised CIN at hysterectomy, vault smears should be taken at 6 and 18 months following surgery and there should be no further cytology follow-up if both are negative
- For women with incomplete or uncertain excision of CIN, follow-up should continue as if the cervix were still present.

## REFERENCES

1. Parkin DM, Bray F, Ferlay J, et al. Global Cancer Statistics, 2002. CA Cancer J Clin 2005;55:74–108.

2. Curado MP, Edwards B, Shin HR, et al. editors. Cancer incidence in five continents, Vol. IX. Lyon: IARC Scientific Publications; 2007.

3. Vizcaino AP, Moreno V, Bosch FX, et al. International trends in the incidence of cervical cancer: 1 adenocarcinoma and adenosquamous cell carcinomas. Int J Cancer 1998;75:536–45.

4. Hacker NF, Ngan HYS, Benedet JL. Staging, classification and clinical practice guidelines for gynaecologic cancers. FIGO committee on gynecologic oncology. Int J Gynecol Obstet 2000;70:207–312.

5. Walboomers J, Jacobs MV, Manos MM, et al. Human papillomavirus is a necessary cause of invasive cervical cancer worldwide. J Pathol 1999;189:12–19.

6. Mant C, Cason J, Rice P, et al. Non-sexual transmission of cervical cancer-associated papillomaviruses: an update. Papill Report 2000;11:1–5.

7. Bosch FX, Iftner T. The aetiology of cervical cancer NHSCSP Publication No 22. Sheffield: NHS Cancer Screening Programmes; 2005.

8. Subramanya D, Grivas PD. HPV and cervical cancer: updates on an established relationship. Postgrad Med 2008;120:7–13.

9. Pett M, Coleman N. Review article. Integration of high-risk human papillomavirus: a key event in cervical carcinogenesis? J Pathol 2007;212:356–67.

10. Appleby P, Beral V, Berrington de Gonzalez A, et al. International collaboration of epidemiological studies of cervical cancer. Carcinoma of the cervix and tobacco smoking: collaborative reanalysis of individual data for 13,541 women with cervical cancer and 20,017 women without cervical cancer from 23 epidemiological studies. Int J Cancer 2006;118:1481–95.

11. Stein L, Urban MI, O'Connell D, et al. The spectrum of human immunodeficiency virus-associated cancers in a South African black population: results from a case-control study, 1995–2004. Int J Cancer 2008;122:2260–65.

12. Appleby P, Beral V, Berrington de Gonzalez A, et al. International collaboration of epidemiological studies of cervical cancer. Cervical cancer and hormonal contraceptives: collaborative reanalysis of individual data for 16,573 women with cervical cancer and 35,509 women without cervical cancer from 24 epidemiological studies. Lancet 2007;370:1609–21.

13. McCredie RE, Sharples KJ, Paul C, et al. Natural history of cervical neoplasia and risk of invasive cancer in women with cervical intraepithelial neoplasia 3: a retrospective cohort study. Lancet Oncol 2008;9:425–34.

14. Schiffman M, Rodriguez AC. Heterogeneity in CIN 3 diagnosis. Lancet Oncol 2008;9:404–6.

15. Herbert A, Smith JAE. Cervical intraepithelial neoplasia grade III (CIN III) and invasive cervical carcinoma: the yawning gap revisited and the treatment if risk. Cytopathology 1999;10:161–70.

16. NHSCSP. Resource pack for training smear takers NHSCSP Publication No. 9. Sheffield: NHS Cervical Screening Programme; 1998.

17. British Society for Clinical Cytology. How to take a cervical smear. Video and Booklet 'Taking Cervical Smears', 3rd edn. Revised by Craddock P, London; 2004. BSCC/Creation Video.

18. Moseley RP, Paget S. Liquid-based cytology: is this the way forward for cervical screening? Cytopathology 2002;13:71–82.

19. Davey E, Barratt A, Irwig L, et al. Effect of study design and quality on unsatisfactory rates, cytology classifications and accuracy in liquid-based versus conventional cytology: a systematic review. Lancet 2006;367:122–32.

20. Denton K. Liquid-based cytology: applying international experience to the United Kingdom. Cytopathology 2004;15:129–30.

21. Stanbridge CM, Suleman BA, Persad RV, et al. A cervical smear review in women developing carcinoma with particular respect to age, false negative cervical cytology, and the histologic type of the invasive carcinoma. Int J Gynecol Cancer 1992;2:92–100.

22. Smith PA, Turnbull LS. Small cell and 'pale' dyskaryosis. Cytopathology 1997;8:3–8.

23. Moss SM, Gray A, Legood R, et al. First Report to the Department of Health on evaluation of LBC. Unpublished report, December 2002.

24. National Institute for Health and Clinical Excellence. Guidance on the use of liquid-based cytology for cervical screening Technology Appraisal Guidance No. 5. London: NICE; 2002.

25. Johnson J, Patnick J, editors. Achievable standards, benchmarks for reporting and criteria for evaluating cervical cytopathology. NHSCSP Publication No 1, 2nd edn. Sheffield: NHS Cervical Screening Programme; 2000.

26. Bosch MMC, Rietveld-Scheffers PEM, Boon ME. Characteristics of false-negative smears tested in the normal screening situation. Acta Cytol 1992;36:711–16.

27. Mitchell H, Medley G. Differences between cervical smears with correct and incorrect diagnoses. Cytopathology 1995;6:368–75.

28. O'Sullivan JP, A'Hern RP, Chapman PA, et al. A case control study of true-positive versus false-negative cervical smears in women with cervical intra-epithelial neoplasia (CIN) III. Cytopathology 1998;9:155–61.

29. Baker RW, O'Sullivan JP, Hanley J, et al. The characteristics of false negative cervical smears: implications for the UK cervical

screening programme. J Clin Pathol 1999;52:358–62.

30. Summary of Safety and Effectiveness Data (ThinPrep Imaging System). Online. Available at: http://www.fda.gov/cdrh/pdf2/P020002b.pdf (accessed 1 June 2008).

31. Dawson AE. The changing face of cervical screening. Challenges for the future. Diagn Cytopathol 2005;33:63–64.

32. Biscotti CV, Dawson AE, Dziura B, et al. Assisted primary screening using the automated ThinPrep imaging system. Am J Clin Pathol 2005;123:281–87.

33. Underwood D, Dawson AE. Implementation of the ThinPrep imaging system: impact on cytology laboratory workload, turnaround time, and quality parameters. Acta Cytol 2004;48:662.

34. Weintraub J, Wenger D, Berger SD. Detection of abnormal cervicovaginal cytology specimens: a comparison between location guided (ThinPrep imaging system TIS) and manual screening of ThinPrep samples (TP). Acta Cytol 2004;48:662–63.

35. Qureshi MN, Ringer PJ. Validation of the accuracy of the ThinPrep imaging system to identify abnormalities. Acta Cytol 2004;48:663.

36. Lindfield KC, Chenette NL, Boersch C, et al. Validation of the ThinPrep imaging system: a multi-center European study. Acta Cytol 2004;48:702.

37. Wilbur DC, Parker EM, Foti JA. Location guided screening of liquid-based cytology specimens. Am J Clin Pathol 2002;118:399–407.

38. Summary of Safety and Effectiveness Data (BD Focal Point Imaging System). Online. Available at: http://www.fda.gov/cdrh/pdf/P9500095008b.pdf (accessed 18 February 2009).

39. Evans DMD, Hudson EA, Brown CL, et al. Terminology in gynaecological cytopathology: report of the Working Party of the British Society for Clinical Cytology. J Clin Pathol 1986;39:933–44.

40. Denton KJ, Herbert A, Turnbull LS, et al. The revised BSCC terminology for abnormal cervical cytology. Cytopathology 2008;19:137–57.

41. Richart RM. A modified terminology for cervical intraepithelial neoplasia. Obstet Gynecol 1990;75:131–33.

42. Solomon D, Davey D, Kurman R, et al. The 2001 bethesda system. Terminology for reporting results of cervical cytology. JAMA 2002;287:2114–19.

43. DeMay RM. Hyperchromatic crowded groups. Pitfalls in Pap smear diagnosis. Am J Clin Path 2000;114(Suppl 1):S36–43.

44. Denton K, Rana D, Lynch MA, et al. Bland dyskaryosis: a new pitfall in liquid-based cytology. Cytopathology 2008;19:162–66.

45. Slater DN, Rice S, Stewart R, et al. Proposed Sheffield quantitative criteria in cervical cytology to assist the grading of squamous cell dyskaryosis, as the British society for clinical cytology definitions require amendment. Cytopathology 2005;16:179–92.

46. Slater DN, Rice S, Stewart R, et al. Proposed Sheffield quantitative criteria in cervical cytology to assist the diagnosis and grading of squamous intra-epithelial lesions, as some Bethesda system definitions require amendment. Cytopathology 2005;16:168–78.

47. Working Party of the Royal College of Pathologists and NHS Cervical Screening Programme. Histopathology reporting in cervical screening NHSCSP Publication No. 10. Sheffield: NHS Cervical Screening Programme; 1999.

48. Moss S, Gray A, Legood R, et al. Effect of testing for human papillomavirus as a triage during screening for cervical cancer: observational before and after study. BMJ 2006;332:83–85.

49. Halford JA. Cytological features of chronic follicular cervicitis in liquid-based specimens: a potential diagnostic pitfall. Cytopathology 2002;13:364–70.

50. Parham DM, Wiredu EK, Hussein KA. Significance of borderline nuclear abnormality in cervical smears. Cytopathology 1992;3:85–91.

51. Solomon D, Schiffman M, Tarone R. for the ALTS Group. Comparison of three management strategies for patients with atypical squamous cells of undetermined significance: baseline results from a randomized trial. J Natl Cancer Inst 2001;93:293–99.

52. Buckley H, Herbert A, McKenzie EFD, et al. Borderline nuclear changes in cervical smears: guidelines on their recognition and management. J Clin Pathol 1994;47:481–92.

53. The Information Centre. Cervical Screening Programme, England 2006/6. National Statistics, 2007. London: National Health Service.

54. The Bethesda System. Online. Available at: http://bethesda2001.cancer.gov/postwrkshp_recs.html (accessed 21 July 2008).

55. de Paralta-Venturino MN, Purslow MJ, Kini SR. Endometrial cells of the 'lower uterine segment' (LUS) in cervical smears obtained by endocervical brushings: a source of potential diagnostic pitfall. Diagn Cytopathol 1995;12:263–68.

56. Luesley D, Leeson S, editors. Colposcopy and programme management. NHSCSP Publication No. 20. Sheffield: NHS Cervical Screening Programme; 2004.

57. Cullimore J, Scurr J. The abnormal glandular smear: cytologic prediction, colposcopic correlation and clinical management. J Obstet Gynaecol 2000;20:403–7.

58. Mohammed DKA, Lavie O, Lopes AdeB, et al. A clinical review of borderline glandular cells on cervical cytology. Br J Obstet Gynaecol 2000;107:605–9.

59. Zweizig S, Noller K, Reale F, et al. Neoplasia associated with atypical glandular cells of undetermined significance of undetermined significance on cervical cytology. Gynecol Oncol 1997;65:314–18.

60. Kennedy AW, Salmieri SS, Wirth SL, et al. Results of the clinical evaluation of atypical glandular cells of undetermined significance (AGCUS) detected on cervical cytology screening. Gynecol Oncol 1996;63:14–18.

61. Mathers ME, Johnson SJ, Wadehra V. How predictive is a cervical smear suggesting glandular neoplasia? Cytopathology 2002;13:83–91.

62. Kulasingam SI, Kim JJ, Lawrence WF, et al. Cost effectiveness analysis based on the atypical squamous cells of undetermined significance/low-grade squamous intraepithelial lesion triage study (ALTS). J Nat Cancer Inst 2006;98:82–93.

63. Legood R, Gray A, Wolstenholme J, et al. Lifetime effects, costs and cost effectiveness of testing for human papillomavirus to manage low-grade cytological abnormalities: results of the NHS pilot studies. BMJ 2006;332:79–82.

64. Nevin J, Soeters S, Dehaeck CM, et al. Cervical carcinoma associated with pregnancy. Obstet Gynecol Survey 1995;50:228–39.

65. Coppola A, Sorossky T, Casper R, et al. The clinical course of carcinoma in situ diagnosed during pregnancy. Gynecol Oncol 1997;67:162–65.

66. Woodrow N, Permezel M, Butterfield I, et al. Abnormal cytology in pregnancy. ANZ J Obst Gynaecol 1998;38:161–65.

67. Robinson WR, Webb S, Tirpack J, et al. Management of cervical intraepithelial neoplasia during pregnancy with loop excision. Gynecol Oncol 1997;64:153–55.

68. Yost NP, Santosa IT, McIntire DD, et al. Postpartum regression rates of antepartum cervical intraepithelial neoplasia II and III lesions. Obstet Gynaecol 1999;93:359–62.

69. NHSCSP. Achievable Standards, Benchmarks for Reporting and Criteria for Evaluating Cervical Cytopathology. Report of a Working Party set up by the RCPath, BSCC and NHSCSP. NHSCSP Publication No. 1, 1st edn. Sheffield: NHS Cervical Screening Programme; 1995.

70. Campion MJ, di Paola FM, Vellios F. The value of cervicography in population screening. J Exp Clin Cancer Res 1990(Suppl):FC/107.

71. Cross P. Editorial. Rapid screening in cervical cytology – a simple method with a big impact. Cytopathology 2004;15:71–73.

72. Houliston DC, Boyd CM, Nicholas DS, et al. Personal performance profiles: a useful adjunct to quality assurance in cervical cytology. Cytopathology 1998;9:162–70.

73. Kyrgiou M, Koliopoulos G, Martin-Hirsch P, et al. Obstetric outcomes after conservative treatment for intraepithelial or early invasive cervical lesions: systematic review and meta-analysis. Lancet 2006;376:489–98.

74. Arbyn M, Paraskevaidis E, Martin-Hirsch P, et al. Clinical utility of HPV-DNA detection: triage of minor cervical lesions; follow-up of women treated for high-grade CIN: an update of pooled evidence. Gynecol Oncol 2005;99:S7–S11.

75. Coleman D, Day N, Douglas G, et al. European guidelines for quality assurance in cervical cancer screening. Europe against cancer programme. Eur J Cancer 1993;29A(Suppl. 4): S1–S38.

76. National Health and Medical Research Council. Screening to prevent cervical cancer: Guidelines for the management of women with screen detected abnormalities. Sydney: Australian Government; 2006.

# Glandular neoplasms of the cervix

Christine Waddell and Ashish Chandra

## Chapter contents

## Introduction

Glandular tumours of the cervix present diagnostic and management difficulties affecting both pathologist and clinician. This chapter examines the current classification, terminology, diagnostic cytological features and pitfalls in the diagnosis of preinvasive and invasive neoplasia of endocervical cell origin, including the less common cell variants that reflect the müllerian derivation of the lining of the endocervical canal. Modern diagnostic techniques are reviewed and, in conclusion, the clinical management of cytological glandular abnormalities of the cervix in relation to the role of the cytopathologist is discussed.

## Epidemiology

### Incidence

Evidence is accumulating which shows that the incidence of adenocarcinoma of the cervix is rising[1-5] but following analysis of data from 60 population-based cancer registries, it appears that the trends are complex.[6] While an increase in incidence of adenocarcinoma and adenosquamous carcinoma has been shown in young women in many countries, including America, Australia and the UK, in other developed countries, including the Netherlands, Germany and New Zealand, there has been no significant change. A study from Southampton showed no rise or fall in the incidence of adenocarcinoma over a 12–year period in that region.[7] In Finland, France and Italy there have been falls in incidence. The increase, where present, is seen particularly in women born from 1935 onwards, with women born around 1955 having a three times greater risk than those born in 1935.

Recent data from Sweden[8] showed no clear benefit in the detection of glandular compared with squamous carcinoma through screening. In Denmark,[9] a reduction in the incidence of adenocarcinoma has been reported in women over 40 years of age but an increased incidence in 20–29 year old women in spite of improved coverage over a 15-year period. Some[10] have suggested that it takes 10–15 years to develop expertise in accurately identifying glandular lesions and others[11] predict a decrease in the cumulative incidence of cervical adenocarcinoma in the current decade.

### Risk factors

Epidemiological factors for cervical adenocarcinoma are less well-defined than for squamous carcinoma. As with squamous carcinoma, the increase in cervical adenocarcinoma is related to the number of sexual partners and intercourse at an early age.[12] In a meta-analysis by Berrington de González[13] high parity and long duration of oral contraceptive usage were associated with both histological types; however, adenocarcinoma showed a significantly lower association with current smoking than squamous carcinoma. Other factors affecting recorded incidence include changes in reporting practice, with increasing awareness of glandular lesions,[14] changes in choice of sampling devices leading to better sampling of the endocervical canal[15] and the effects of organised screening programmes leading to a relative decrease in squamous lesions.[6]

There is strong evidence that up to 50% of endocervical adenocarcinomas are associated with cervical intraepithelial neoplasia (CIN). It is tempting to speculate that both lesions share a common pathogenesis, namely an aberrant proliferation of reserve cells, which may result in the formation of either a glandular or a squamous neoplasm. Human papillomavirus (HPV) types 16 and 18 have been demonstrated in invasive and intraepithelial endocervical neoplasia, supporting the concept of a common pathogenesis for at least some lesions.[16-20] HPV testing is likely to prove useful in the investigation of borderline glandular lesions,[21] although on histology many of these will reveal high grade CIN.[22]

Finnish[16] and Dutch studies[23] demonstrated that adenocarcinoma is more likely to be associated with HPV 18 than with HPV 16. Adenocarcinoma and squamous carcinoma also differ in intratypic variants of HPV strains.[24] It has also been shown that HPV-negative cervical carcinoma is more likely to be adenocarcinoma.[25]

## Endocervical adenocarcinoma precursor lesions

The endocervical canal is lined by columnar epithelium, which forms a single layer over the stromal ridges, villi and crypts.

*The authors gratefully acknowledge their debt to the late Pauline Cooper whose contribution to the first edition of this chapter forms the basis for this revised edition.*

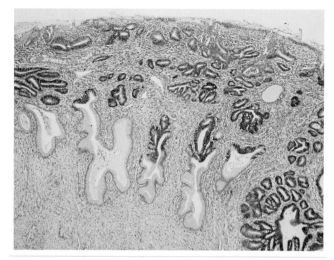

**Fig. 24.1** Cervical biopsy. HG-CGIN showing abrupt change from benign to neoplastic epithelium within gland crypts (H&E).

With the onset of neoplasia, the single layering is disturbed, initially by the development of pseudostratification. Cytologically this appears as overlapping and crowding of nuclei in sheets of epithelial cells. Most endocervical adenocarcinomas are of an endocervical type, but müllerian epithelium has the capacity to differentiate along several pathways, with the result that some tumours have histological features that closely resemble those usually arising in the endometrium or ovary. Müllerian epithelium also readily undergoes metaplastic change and so, for example, an adenocarcinoma of enteric type may be seen.[26] This diversity of histological pattern is reflected in the classification of endocervical tumours.[27]

## Cervical glandular intraepithelial neoplasia (CGIN): adenocarcinoma *in situ* (AIS)

This lesion was first described histologically in 1953, by Friedell and McKay.[28] They noted that the average age of patients with CGIN was several years less than that of patients with invasive disease, suggesting that the *in situ* form precedes the development of invasive cancer. This concept has been supported by other studies.[29–31]

On histology CGIN retains the architectural pattern of normal endocervical crypts. Usually the surface epithelium and both superficial and deep crypts are involved at or near the squamocolumnar junction. Partial crypt involvement is a frequent finding, with an abrupt transition from normal to neoplastic epithelium (Fig. 24.1).[32] High-grade (HG-) CGIN is usually a single lesion, less often multifocal and frequently extends into the endocervical canal.[33]

In the affected area, the glandular epithelium is composed of columnar cells which show an increase in nuclear size, nuclear pleomorphism, normal and abnormal mitotic activity, apoptosis and nuclear stratification. In preinvasive lesions and tumours of endocervical type, which are the commonest type, the cells may show abundant mucin production, but often cytoplasmic mucin is diminished.

Cases with an endometrioid or intestinal pattern (Fig. 24.2)[29] may be seen together with other histological variants, usually as focal areas within a lesion which is predominantly of

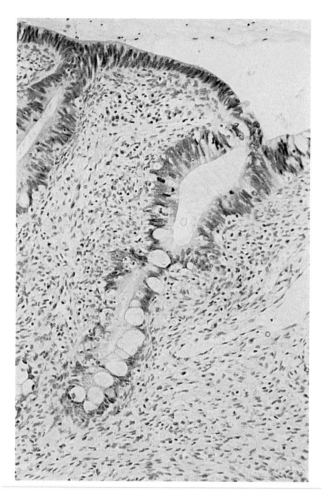

**Fig. 24.2** Cervical biopsy. HG-CGIN (intestinal type). Cells in the upper part of the crypt show mucous secretion. Goblet cells are conspicuous in the deeper portion of the crypt (H&E).

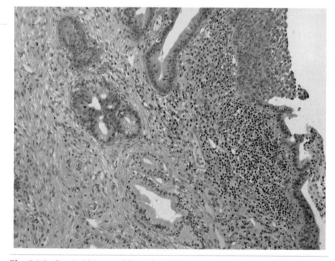

**Fig. 24.3** Cervical biopsy. CGIN adjacent to an area of CIN3. Note also adjacent normal gland crypts below the area of CGIN (H&E).

endocervical type.[33] When high-grade CGIN is associated with an *in situ* or invasive squamous carcinoma, the two cell types may be seen as adjacent areas of abnormality (Fig. 24.3). This almost certainly leads to underdiagnosis of the glandular component in lesions of mixed squamous and glandular types.[34]

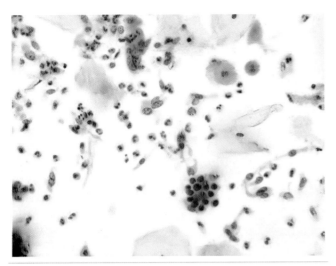

**Fig. 24.4** Cervical cytology. Atypical cells both single and in small clusters from a case of well-differentiated endocervical adenocarcinoma (SurePath).

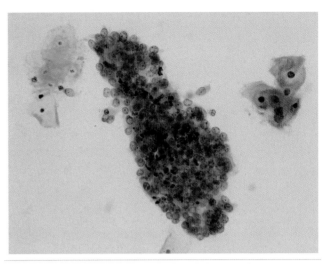

**Fig. 24.5** Cervical cytology. HG-CGIN and CIN1. Subtle disturbance in honeycomb, nuclear crowding, almost absent cytoplasm at periphery, even nuclear size and chromasia, several mitotic figures, small nuclear size – compare with adjacent squamous cells which show minor cytological atypia (ThinPrep).

While features of high-grade CGIN are relatively well described, low-grade CGIN remains a poorly reproducible entity. Histological criteria for low-grade CGIN have been proposed[32] and cytological criteria have also been published, but these are controversial.[35–37] There is currently no proof that low-grade glandular atypia is a precursor to adenocarcinoma.[38] Atypia in glandular cells often relates to non-neoplastic conditions[39] that mimic high-grade CGIN rather than represent low-grade CGIN. Nowadays, this dilemma can be investigated by HPV testing and the use of molecular markers.[31]

## Cytological findings: CGIN/AIS

Cytological manifestations of CGIN were first published by Barter and Waters in 1970.[40] Since then, evidence has accrued on which to base a prediction of glandular neoplasia.[41–45] In conventional cytology, prediction is usually made on the presentation of cells in sheets and clusters and rarely on abnormality in individual cells alone. Raab et al. identified in conventional cytology the three most useful individual cellular criteria on which to discriminate between benign and neoplastic changes in endocervical cells. These are irregularity of nuclear membrane thickness, raised nuclear/cytoplasmic (N/C) ratio and presence of atypical single cells (Fig. 24.4).[44,46,47] Using liquid-based cytology (LBC) there are slight differences compared to conventional smears as the nuclear details are more pronounced and architectural features more subtle.[39,48–51] However, comparing conventional cytology and the two most commonly used LBC methods, SurePath (SP) and ThinPrep (TP), Belsley et al. concluded that differences between the three methods are minimal.[52]

### *Exfoliation pattern (Fig. 24.5)[41,53]*

- Cohesive sheets and tissue fragments of varying size (especially in SurePath)
  - Cell clusters smaller in LBC than in conventional smears
  - Subtle disturbance in 'honeycomb' pattern
  - Crypt openings may be seen
  - Cells crowded with overlapping nuclei
  - Papillary fragments in serous subtype
- Single abnormal glandular cells throughout the background

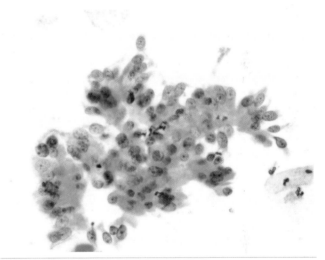

**Fig. 24.6** HG-CGIN. Disrupted rosette with peripheral palisading, pseudostratification and feathering. Note snake and egg pattern and delicate cytoplasmic tags at edge (ThinPrep).

- Common particularly in SurePath, less so in conventional cytology and uncommonly in ThinPrep[52]
  - Occasional apoptotic bodies in cell clusters[42]
- Feathering: at periphery of pseudostratified groups and rosettes: (Fig. 24.6)
  - Nuclei lie at different levels
  - Cytoplasm usually absent or partially lost
  - Protruding bare nuclei or nuclei tipped by wispy cytoplasmic tags.[54]

Whereas feathering is frequently the most useful criterion to distinguish between squamous lesions and glandular neoplasia in conventional cytology[45] with the rounding up of cell clusters in LBC, it is less common in TP and infrequent in SP.[52]

- Pseudostratification:[43]
  - In profile, nuclei seen at different levels in neighbouring cells (Fig. 24.7)
  - En face sheets appear as crowded with overlapping nuclei appearing at several levels of focus especially in SP (Fig. 24.8)

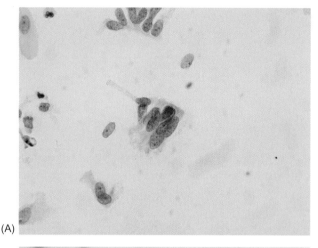

(A)

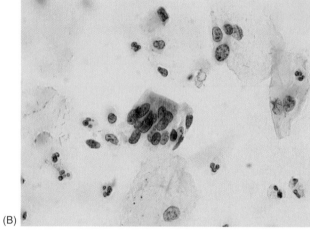

(B)

**Fig. 24.7** (A,B) Cervical cytology. HG-CGIN. Pseudostratified nuclei in strips of cells with common cytoplasmic borders. Note small nuclear size compared with adjacent intermediate cell nuclei (SurePath).

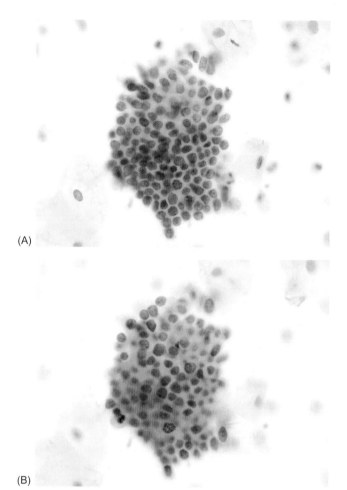

(A)

(B)

**Fig. 24.8** (A,B) Cervical cytology. HG-CGIN. Pseudostratification from above showing views of nuclei appearing in different planes of focus (SurePath).

- Polarity maintained giving a palisade effect in elongated forms
- In conventional and ThinPrep samples the pseudostratified strips are usually relatively straight sided
- In SurePath there is a tendency for the dyskaryotic nuclei to fan out
- Feathering, if present, is commonly seen in pseudostratified groups
- Rosettes:
  - Rounded group of cells with nuclear palisades at periphery and cytoplasm in the centre (Fig. 24.9)[55]
  - Rosettes in conventional smears and TP are similar
  - Peripheral polarisation of pseudostratified elongated nuclei
  - SurePath rosettes tend to be more three dimensional
  - Delicate frond-like cytoplasm with nuclei carried at the tips of the fronds giving an impression of clubbing (Figs 24.10, 24.11).[51]

### Nuclear features

- Size uniform within a cell sheet but may vary between sheets
- Size not always greater than in nuclei of benign epithelial cells. If nuclei are of normal size or smaller they may be misinterpreted as benign endometrial cells,[56,57] the diagnosis then depends on the recognition of the raised N/C ratio and the exfoliation pattern

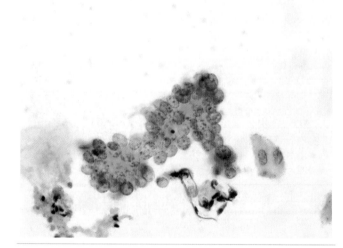

**Fig. 24.9** Cervical cytology. HG-CGIN. Rosette formation. Note palisading of peripheral nuclei, even nuclear size and chromasia and stippled chromatin pattern (ThinPrep).

- May be round but more frequently oval
- In LBC distortion of nuclear outline is noticeable especially in larger nuclei with flattening along the adjacent long axes of elongated nuclei in pseudostratified strips (Fig. 24.7)[53]

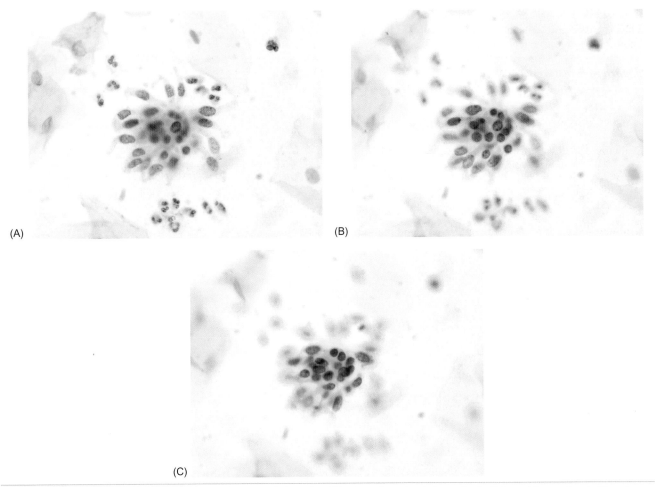

Fig. 24.10 (A,B,C) Cervical cytology. HG-CGIN. Rosette formation. Delicate frond-like three-dimensional cluster of cells. Note nuclei appearing at different planes of focus (SurePath).

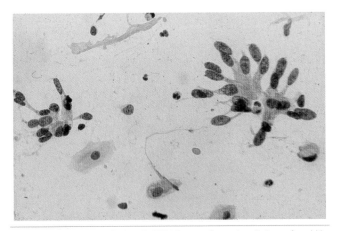

Fig. 24.11 Cervical cytology. HG-CGIN. Rosette formation. Delicate frond-like cluster of cells with almost bare nuclei (snake and egg effect) radiating from the centre and wispy cytoplasmic tags (conventional smear).

- Nuclear membrane is usually smooth in outline but may vary in thickness[46,47]
- Chromatin:[58] pattern variable, but evenly distributed. Fine to coarse granularity with moderate granularity the most common resulting in salt and pepper appearance
- Nucleoli are not a consistent feature of CGIN, but when present they are usually distinct and pink/red in colour[39,59]

- Frequency of mitoses varies and may appear greater in LBC[49] but can be a helpful feature especially in clusters of cells with banal looking nuclei of uniform size. Usually of normal morphology

### Cytoplasmic features

- Usually cyanophilic
- Delicate, finely vacuolated, fading towards the periphery of the cell
- Cytoplasmic tags[54] are often seen around the edges of cell groups and rosettes.

This feature helps in discrimination between the rosettes of CGIN and those of benign entities such as tuboendometrioid metaplasia. The absence or near absence of cytoplasm around the periphery of clusters of glandular cells acts as a trigger to alert the microscopist to the likelihood of glandular neoplasia. Particularly in SurePath, the absence of discernible cytoplasmic clothing of the nuclei frequently leads to a sharp, guttate (rain drop) appearance in clusters from CGIN (Fig. 24.12). In individual cells, and those involved in feathering, the stretching of the cytoplasm over the nucleus is sometimes termed the 'snake and egg' effect (Fig. 24.11). Occasionally, goblet cells characteristic of intestinal differentiation are seen (see pitfalls, below).

The classic architectural features of rosette formation, feathering and pseudostratification are manifestations mainly of endocervical-type differentiation of CGIN but co-existing subtypes may be present in up to two-thirds of glandular lesions, although they rarely occur alone.[43]

### Characteristic features of CGIN subtypes

- Intestinal CGIN: large single vacuoles (goblet cells) (Fig. 24.13)
- Serous CGIN: papillary clusters of abnormal glandular cells (Fig. 24.14)
- Endometrioid CGIN: small even-sized nuclei (Fig. 24.15).[57]

## Diagnostic accuracy of CGIN/AIS

Interobserver variability in interpretation of glandular entities is well documented.[60,61] In both conventional cytology and LBC, sensitivity in detection of endocervical glandular lesions is lower than for CIN.[62] The positive predictive value (PPV), which may be used as a surrogate marker for specificity, is also lower.[14,63–65] While the former may be the result of sampling failure changes in sensitivity and PPV may be manifestations of interpretation error[66] and is influenced over time by changes in awareness leading to alteration in cytological and histological recognition[6,67] Initially in the UK, pilot sites examining direct-to-vial screening population samples found lower sensitivity to glandular abnormalities[68] but post-pilot audits have demonstrated no change in sensitivity and increased accuracy in discrimination between glandular neoplasia and benign mimics.[69]

For LBC, use of residual material has been implicated as contributing to poorer sensitivity in split-sample studies[70,71] and, although lack of familiarity with the cellular presentation, in particular the absence of feathering, has been deemed likely to be a significant additional factor,[65,72] some workers have found little change in architectural features traditionally used for identification of glandular neoplasia and recognition of benign look-alikes.[45,39,59] In one centre, changeover from conventional smear preparation to LBC reduced the false negative rate for glandular neoplasia from 43.6% in conventional to 15.4% in thin-layer samples and reduced false positive reports associated with squamous look-alikes from 30.4% to 11.1%, thereby demonstrating both enhanced sensitivity and accuracy.[73]

Cell block preparations have been used from residual material from LBC vials as a further aid to interpretation.[74,75] Identification of glandular neoplasia based on examination of well-presented three-dimensional microbiopsies has been found to be more useful than reliance on feathering and other artefacts used in conventional preparations.

### Diagnostic pitfalls: CGIN/AIS

A comprehensive account of the interpretive difficulties in conventional cytology was published by Crum et al. in 1997.[76] These difficulties are reflected in the published positive predictive value (PPV) estimations for glandular prediction. PPV estimations vary from 77.4% for firm predictions to 25.9% for samples showing less definite features of glandular neoplasia.[63,77] With the advent of LBC techniques several authors have reported reduction in false positive reporting associated with mimics.[39,59,60,69,78,79] The following however, may cause some diagnostic confusion (Table 24.1).

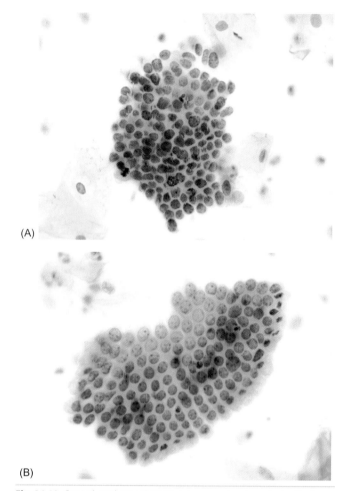

(A)

(B)

**Fig. 24.12** Cervical cytology. HG-CGIN versus normal endocervical epithelium. (A) Guttate appearance in crowded group from HG-CGIN showing disturbed honeycomb formation and bare periphery. (B) Normal neat honeycomb pattern of benign endocervical cells with well-defined cytoplasmic border (SurePath).

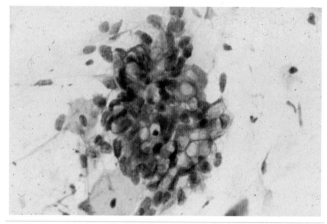

**Fig. 24.13** Cervical cytology. HG-CGIN Type II. Goblet cell like vacuoles in a cluster of disorganised glandular cells from CGIN with foci of intestinal differentiation. Note cellular dissociation at edge of cluster (conventional smear).

### Severely dyskaryotic squamous cells

Cells from gland crypts involved in CIN pose major diagnostic difficulties.[14,46,53,62,80,81] In conventional cytology, these are often associated with the use of the more pointed samplers such as the Aylesbury spatula and endocervical brushes. Selvaggi has described the cytological manifestations of CIN with crypt

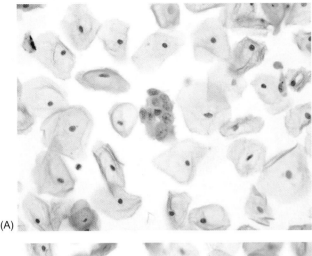

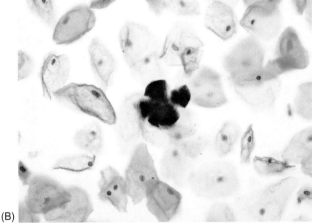

**Fig. 24.14** Cervical cytology. HG-CGIN Type II. (A) cluster of bland enlarged pale nuclei with modest anisonucleosis. Note the easy to overlook cytological atypia in this case of CGIN with serous differentiation. The presence of psammoma bodies (B) was the screening trigger for careful search for evidence of glandular neoplasia (SurePath).

**Table 24.1** Cytological prediction of CGIN: Diagnostic difficulties and look-alikes (see Ch. 25)

| Non-neoplastic | Neoplastic |
|---|---|
| Cervicitis | Gland crypt involvement in CIN |
| Endocervical polyps | Type II CGIN |
| Tubal metaplasia | Early invasive adenocarcinoma |
| | Endometrial hyperplasia and neoplasia |
| Endometriosis | Extrauterine carcinoma |
| Microglandular hyperplasia | |
| Arias-Stella reaction | |
| Isthmic (lower uterine segment) sampling | |

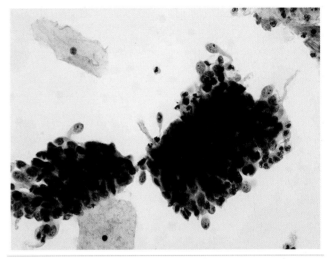

**Fig. 24.16** Cervical cytology. CIN3. Hyperchromatic crowded group from crypt involvement. Note crowded 'piled up' cells in centre of this brick-shaped microbiopsy with untidy frayed edges and some 'snake and egg'-like nuclei protruding. Group architecture and variation in nuclear shape size and chromasia would favour squamous rather than glandular origin of this group (ThinPrep).

involvement in both conventional and LBC preparations.[81,82] In hyperchromatic crowded groups the central areas show architectural anarchy with piling up of dyskaryotic nuclei. In LBC, mitotic figures and nucleoli are more readily seen. Nucleoli, if present in squamous lesions tend to be smaller than those seen in glandular neoplasia. These features are seen in both ThinPrep and SurePath preparations (Figs 24.16, 24.17).

Although cellular disorder is to be anticipated at the periphery of cell groups from CIN, occasionally architecture akin to CGIN is present with elongated nuclei protruding from cell clusters,[82] with peripheral palisading and discernible pseudostratification and even an impression of feathering (Fig. 24.18).[76] Features that help to identify squamous neoplasia include smooth chromatin texture in nuclei which have evenly distributed chromatin, or chromatin clumping and clearing in those with maldistribution of chromatin. The peripheral nuclei show variation in shape, size and chromasia. A relative denseness of cytoplasm with absence of peripheral cytoplasmic tags also favours squamous over endocervical neoplasia. Irregularity in thickness of nuclear membranes and the presence of nucleoli are more in keeping with glandular neoplasia.[44] The nuclear outline in squamous neoplasia is more likely to show sharp notches, not associated with nuclear folds (Table 24.2) (see Ch. 23).

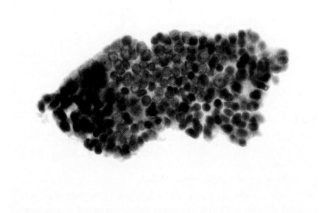

**Fig. 24.15** Cervical cytology. HG-CGIN Type II. Multilayered crowded cluster composed of small nuclei with acinar-like spaces. Histology predominantly endometrioid subtype (ThinPrep).

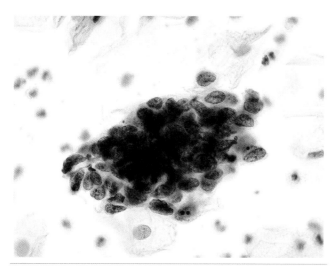

**Fig. 24.17** Cervical cytology. CIN3. Hyperchromatic crowded group from crypt involvement in CIN. Angular crowded cluster with crowded centre and variation in nuclear shape, size, chromasia and orientation at the periphery would favour squamous over glandular origin (SurePath).

**Table 24.2** Characteristics of cell clusters in crypt involvement in CIN versus HG-CGIN

|  | Crypt involvement | CGIN |
|---|---|---|
| Group contour | Thick steep-sided microbiopsies | Shallow clusters 2–3 cells deep |
| Group centre | Crowded disordered | Residual honeycomb pattern |
| Group periphery | Haphazard cell arrangement | Palisading or feathering |
| Nuclear morphology | Variable shape, size, chromasia | Relatively even shape, size, chromasia |
| Nuclear membrane | Irregular thickness | Irregular thickness |
| Nuclear outline | Irregular may be notched | Smooth round/oval |
| Chromatin | Usually fine granules | Coarse irregular sized granules |
|  | May be maldistributed | Commonly evenly distributed |
| Nucleoli | Small | Prominent, may be large |
| Cytoplasm | Dense smooth edged | Finely vacuolated, wispy edged |

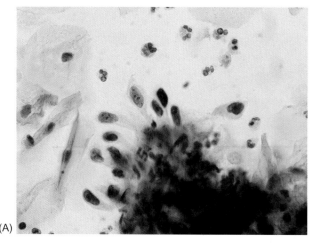

(A)

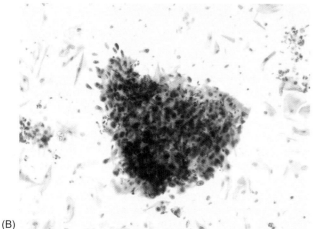

(B)

**Fig. 24.18** (A,B) Cervical cytology. CIN3. Hyperchromatic crowded group from crypt involvement in CIN. Note untidy crowded centre and frayed edge. Nuclei protruding from edge have 'snake and egg' appearance but nuclear variation in shape, size, chromasia and discernable cytoplasm clothing the nuclei favour squamous origin (SurePath).

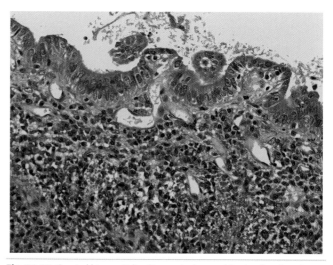

**Fig. 24.19** Cervical biopsy. Palisading and minor architectural and nuclear atypia at surface of endocervical polyp (H&E). (Courtesy of Dr G Spiegel, Guy's and St Thomas' NHS Foundation Trust.)

### Inflammatory change in endocervical cells

Normal endocervical cells are usually present singly or in small clusters and sheets with minimal nuclear overlapping. In inflammatory conditions, including polyps and cervicitis (Fig. 24.19),[44,78,83] they may present in moderately crowded groups but with discernible inter-nuclear spacing. Cytoplasm may be dense, cyanophilic or eosinophilic; terminal bars and occasionally cilia may be seen.[84] Where there is peripheral palisading, with crowding there may be a spurious impression of nuclear stratification. In LBC this is sometimes seen also in short strips of glandular cells with well-demarcated cytoplasm and angular borders (Fig. 24.20).[51,85] Mild anisonucleosis is common in otherwise unremarkable round or oval nuclei. Chromatin is usually vesicular but may be hyperchromatic and

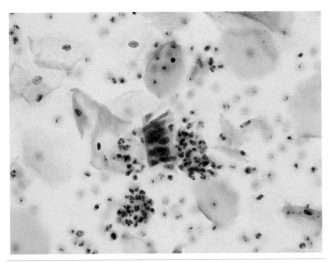

**Fig. 24.20** Cervical cytology. Short strip of glandular cells with sharp angular cytoplasmic borders on the long parallel sides and apparent nuclear stratification. Note dense relatively abundant well-demarcated cytoplasm and smudged chromatin pattern. Outcome at 3-year follow-up with normal cytology and colposcopy. Interpreted as reactive change (SurePath).

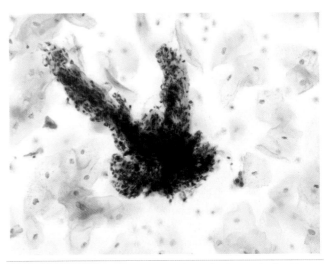

**Fig. 24.22** Cervical cytology. LUS. An untidy tangle of stromal cells with small bland nuclei and ill-defined cytoplasm in association with tube-like microbiopsies of cuboidal cells (Fig. 26.21) (SurePath).

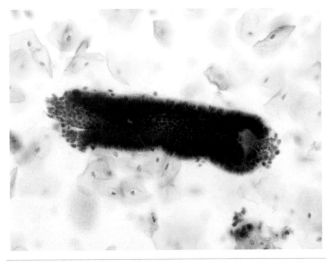

**Fig. 24.21** Cervical cytology. LUS. Three-dimensional tube of small uniform cuboidal cells with well-demarcated outline and peripheral palisading in association with stromal fragments (Fig. 26.22) (SurePath).

smudged.[86] Nucleoli, if present, may be conspicuous and round; very occasional mitoses are seen in regenerating epithelial cells.

### Endometrial cells and cervical endometriosis

The presence of endometrial cells in cervical samples can cause confusion. This is particularly so after loop/cone biopsy, trachelectomy or in endocervical brush samples.[87–89] The sampler may reach high into the endocervical canal and harvest cells from the lower uterine segment (LUS). These may present as blowzy poorly cohesive cuboidal cells lacking the exfoliative pattern required for a prediction of CGIN, and with delicate vesicular nuclei consistent with cells of endometrial origin. More striking are the large and sometimes branching fragments of crowded glandular tissue. Dense straight-sided tubular microbiopsies with peripheral palisading and associated tangles of delicate stromal cells are characteristic features particularly identifiable on low power inspection (Figs 24.21, 24.22). Capillaries may be observed running

through the stromal component and mitotic figures may be evident in samples taken during the first half of the menstrual cycle.[63,87,89,90] Adenomyomatous polyps in the lower uterine segment may present cytologically as bland stromal cells in loose frayed clusters. The epithelial content is variable from a few cells to tight packed clusters of crowded nuclei.[91]

Endometriosis is common in post-cone biopsy crevices but can also be seen in women with no history of previous surgery (Fig. 24.23).[92] Conflicting reports have been published of the cytological appearance of superficial cervical endometriosis which have been attributed to hormonal influences. Szyfelbein described similarities with endocervical neoplasia including feathering and Hanau et al. reported macronucleoli which may even lead to an erroneous prediction of adenocarcinoma.[93,94] Mulvaney and Surtees described changes similar to those attributed to direct LUS sampling or tubal metaplasia, with absence of feathering and pseudostratification.[95] Nevertheless, the endometrioid variant of CGIN should be considered if, in the absence of endometrial stroma, extreme crowding is a feature in samples with small well-preserved endometrial-type cells.[57]

### Tubal metaplasia

The upper-third of the endocervical canal and crypts may be lined by cuboidal epithelium composed of ciliated, secretory and small dark intercalated cells resembling the normal lining of the fallopian tube (Fig. 24.24).[88,96] Cytological features overlap those of CGIN and adenocarcinoma[97] with the appearance of crowding, sometimes the presence of pseudostratified strips and even rosettes. Apart from the smooth chromatin pattern of the nuclei, the most valuable feature for identification of tubal metaplasia is the presence of well-demarcated peripheral cytoplasm with blunted margins and sometimes cilia (Fig. 24.25). Diagnostic difficulties arise when cilia are not identified[86,98,99] or when numerous mitotic figures are seen.[100] Then the possibility of coexistence of tubal metaplasia and glandular neoplasia must be borne in mind. Such a case of ciliated adenocarcinoma of the cervix was reported by O'Connell and Cibas. This was initially interpreted and subsequently reviewed after diagnosis as entirely in keeping with tubal metaplasia.[101] Although the presence of cilia is generally accepted as a feature of the benign epithelial

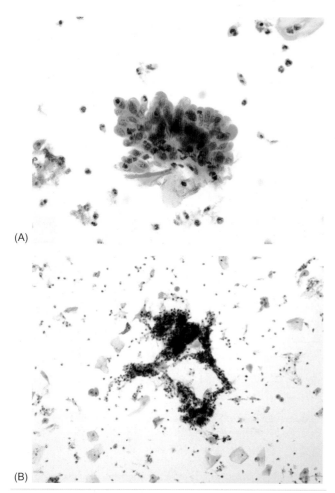

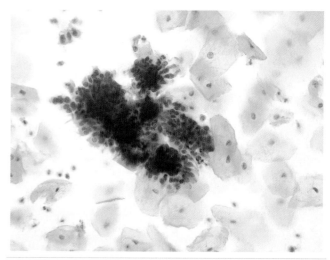

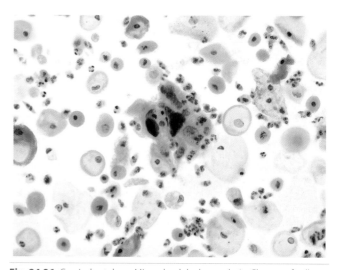

**Fig. 24.25** Cervical cytology. Tubal metaplasia. Crowded cluster of glandular cells with a well-defined rim of cytoplasm with focal cilia (SurePath).

**Fig. 24.23** Cervical cytology. Cervical endometriosis. (A) A cluster of blowzy cuboidal cells with well-demarcated cytoplasmic border. (B) A tangled cluster of stromal cells from the same sample, in a background of collections of altered blood and debris (SurePath).

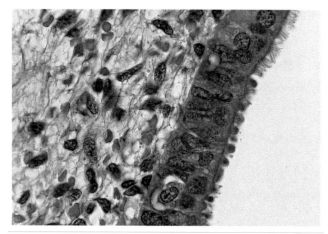

**Fig. 24.26** Cervical cytology. Microglandular hyperplasia. Clusters of cells with marked variation in nuclear size and chromasia, but bland chromatin pattern and abundant cytoplasm suggest benign change. Patient receiving tamoxifen (SurePath).

**Fig. 24.24** Cervical biopsy. Tubal metaplasia in an endocervical crypt. Although nuclei are enlarged and chromatin pattern vesicular, ciliated cells are numerous (H&E).

cell ciliated adenocarcinoma of the endometrium has also been reported in endocervical brush sampling.[102]

### Microglandular hyperplasia

Microglandular hyperplasia of the uterine cervix may occur during pregnancy and with oral contraceptive use, but has

been described in postmenopausal women.[103] The cytological features are non-specific with only the most florid papillary forms causing confusion with endocervical, endometrial or squamous neoplasia.[38,97,104,105] Alvarez-Santín et al. in 1999[106] proposed cytological identification based on the histological criteria.[103] These are the presence of two- and three-dimensional fenestrated sheets of a mixed population of cells consisting of cuboidal and columnar glandular cells with finely vacuolated cytoplasm, immature metaplastic cells with dense basaloid cytoplasm and reserve cells with little or no cytoplasm. Reactive changes resulting in anisonucleosis, nuclear enlargement and prominent nucleoli may lead to suspicion of either glandular or squamous neoplasia (Fig. 24.26).

### Radiation change

Early radiation change in endocervical cells may produce disorganised clusters of glandular cells with loss of the normal honeycomb pattern but with little overlapping of nuclei and ample cytoplasm, leading the cytologist to a non-neoplastic prediction. Nuclear enlargement with anisonucleosis

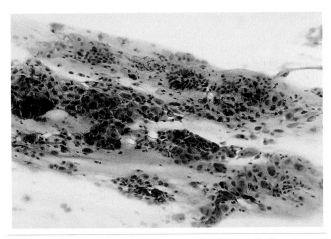

**Fig. 24.27** Cervical smear. Radiation change in endocervical cells. Disorganised clusters of cells with anisonucleosis, abundant cytoplasm and minimal overlapping of nuclei (conventional smear).

is common, together with nucleolar enlargement and multinucleation (Fig. 24.27). Unlike radiation change in squamous cells, bizarre nuclear shape is unusual.[107]

### Mesonephric duct remnants

The mesonephric (Wölffian) ducts in the male develop into the efferent ducts of the testis, epididymis, vasa deferentia, seminal vesicles and ejaculatory ducts. In the female the mesonephric ducts degenerate, but remnants may persist in the broad ligament and in the lateral wall of the uterine cervix and vagina. Because the remnants are situated within cervical stroma and rarely reach the surface, cytological presentation is uncommon. Stewart et al. reviewed cytology from a patient with mesonephric adenocarcinoma arising in an area of diffuse mesonephric hyperplasia.[108] They were both considered to show reactive changes only. Non-specific glandular atypia was similarly reported by Hejmadi et al. in three cases of proven mesonephric hyperplasia.[109]

### Arias-Stella reaction

This is a normal phenomenon in pregnancy and may affect glandular epithelium throughout the genital tract. These changes may take place within days of fertilisation.[110] However, the presence of large cells with ill-defined vacuolated cytoplasm, large nuclei with coarse chromatin and prominent nucleoli, accompanied by clusters of endometrial cells, is more likely to result in erroneous prediction of endometrial than endocervical neoplasia (Fig. 24.28). Moulded papillary fragments of placental tissue have also been described in post-partum and post-abortion smears which are open to misinterpretation as adenocarcinoma of the endocervix or of the ovary (Fig. 24.29).[111]

### Artefacts and other pitfalls

The cytologist needs to be mindful not only of the benign mimics of glandular neoplasia but also that benign and neoplastic entities may coexist. Masuda et al. have reported endometrioid adenocarcinoma arising in the lower uterine segment in a 27-year-old patient.[112] Sampling artefacts affecting the appearance of endocervical cells are also a potential pitfall. Endocervical brush samplers may produce a similar appearance to crypt involvement with no CIN confirmed histologically.[113] The cytological presentation of glandular

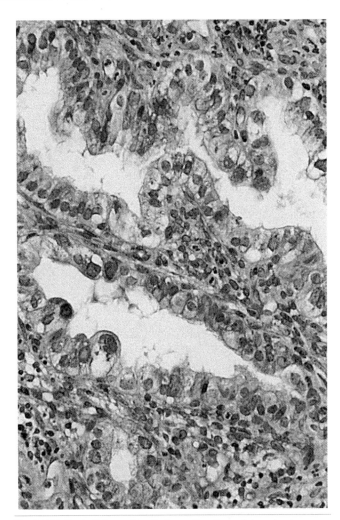

**Fig. 24.28** Cervical biopsy. Arias-Stella reaction. The cells have large pleomorphic nuclei which are surrounded by abundant cytoplasm. Mitoses are absent (H&E).

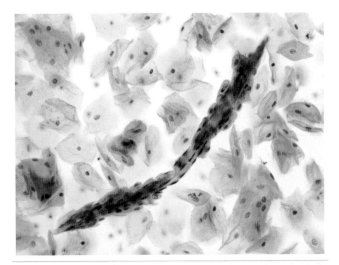

**Fig. 24.29** Cervical cytology. Decidual fragment. Moulded papillary fragment in sample taken 6 weeks post-partum (SurePath).

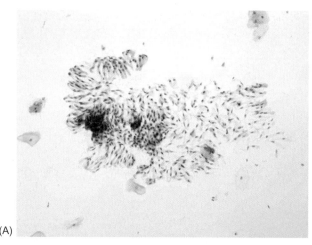

(A)

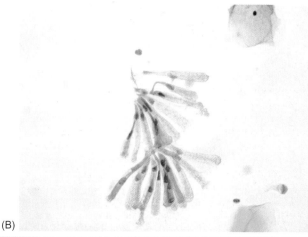

(B)

**Fig. 24.30** (A,B) Cervical sample. Acetic acid artefact. Grossly attenuated endocervical cells in sample taken at colposcopy (SurePath).

**Table 24.3** Comparison of cytological characteristics of CIN versus CGIN

| CGIN more likely | HG-CGIN unlikely |
| --- | --- |
| Rosettes | Disorganised crowded groups |
| Subtle disturbance in architecture | Central piling up of nuclei |
| Nuclear peripheral polarisation | Variation in nuclear shape/size/chromasia |
| Overlapping nuclei | Anisonucleosis |
| Dissociated abnormal nuclei | Multinucleation |
| Irregular nuclear membrane thickness | Chromatin clumping |
| Round/oval nuclei | Irregular nuclear outline |
| Stippled chromatin | Stromal and epithelial cells |
| Mitotic figures | Cilia |
| Delicate cytoplasm | Dense cytoplasm |

cells may be affected by the method both of cell collection and fixation. Cytobrush sampling frequently results in harvest of a surfeit of glandular cells in sheets and microbiopsies with associated difficulties in interpretation. Changeover to LBC has resulted in the 'rounding-up' of cell groups thus losing architectural features especially feathering.[38,51] Events

preceding cell collection also may also modify the appearance of glandular cells. Grossly attenuated endocervical cells may be observed in samples taken immediately after the application of acetic acid or Lugol's iodine used at colposcopic examination (Fig. 24.30).[114,115] Table 24.3 summarises useful features to take into account in the event of equivocal cytological findings.

## Invasive adenocarcinoma of the cervix

### Invasive endocervical adenocarcinoma

The term *microinvasive adenocarcinoma* is controversial: there is no agreed definition[32,116,117] and the term early invasive adenocarcinoma is preferred by some.[118] Cytological features of high-grade CGIN and early invasive adenocarcinoma overlap.[119] Mulvaney and Östör reported 30% sensitivity in prediction of invasion in women with abnormal glandular cells on cytology and with a histological diagnosis of high-grade CGIN and stromal invasion.[116]

### Cytological findings: invasive adenocarcinoma

**Sample background**

- Frequently inflammatory
- Less often there is a recognisable tumour diathesis especially in LBC
- Dissociated abnormal glandular cells.

**Exfoliation pattern**

- Very often indistinguishable from high-grade CGIN
- Crowded pseudosyncytial clusters of enlarged, pleomorphic nuclei
- Super-crowding in some groups with tiny cells packed in very tight sheets
- Papillary fragments.

**Nuclear features**

- Usually hyperchromatic
- Often round but variation in size and shape is common
- Nuclear membrane irregularity not consistent
- Chromatin pattern and distribution are unhelpful
- Nucleoli not consistently present, often small and single, but occasionally large and multiple.

The diversity in appearance in subtypes of cervical adenocarcinoma recognised histologically[32,118] is reflected in cytology. Cells from adenocarcinomas may present singly, in small acinar or papillary clusters, some as highly vacuolated groups and some in large complex microbiopsies.[51] Nuclear morphology ranges from relative uniformity of well-differentiated carcinomas to highly pleomorphic nuclei of high-grade undifferentiated tumours (Figs 24.31–24.33). Although nuclear crowding is an important feature in many invasive lesions, for adenocarcinomas this is unreliable, with mucinous, endometrioid and serous lesions often having moderate amounts of vacuolated cytoplasm and clear cell and glassy cell carcinomas having abundant cytoplasm.

As yet, there are few published accounts of the appearances of uncommon subtypes of cervical adenocarcinoma in LBC. For the common subtypes conventional and LBC samples are similar except for a relative absence of tumour diathesis and blood in

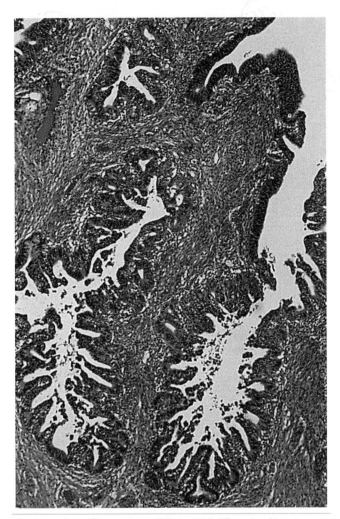

**Fig. 24.31** Cervical biopsy. Cervical biopsy. Well-differentiated invasive endocervical adenocarcinoma (Adeno CaCx).

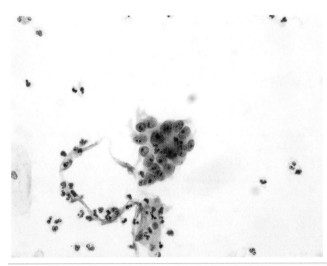

**Fig. 24.32** Cervical cytology. Well-differentiated endocervical type adenocarcinoma with deceptively bland chromatin but prominent nucleoli (ThinPrep).

the latter with a tendency for fewer false negative results.[120] In LBC there may be a spurious impression of increased cellular cohesion with rounding up of malignant cell clusters but, on careful inspection, dissociated single malignant cells are often

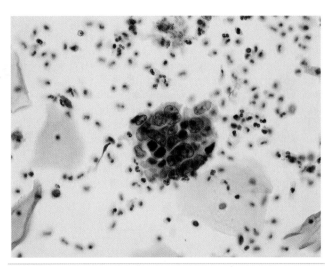

**Fig. 24.33** Cervical cytology. Moderately well-differentiated endocervical adenocarcinoma. A shallow three-dimensional cluster of cells with nuclear pleomorphism and ill-defined but discernible delicate cytoplasm (SurePath).

observed throughout the background of the sample. Although cell clusters may have a scalloped outline with nuclei pushed towards the periphery of the group, this is inconsistent and nuclear enlargement may be modest. Irregularity in nuclear outline, abnormal chromatin content and pattern, the presence of prominent and sometimes multiple nucleoli, variation in nuclear size and shape and mitotic figures are features in keeping with, but not diagnostic of, malignancy.[119]

## Endometrioid adenocarcinoma

Histological recognition of this subtype is contentious with wide variation between centres in reporting rates compared with the usual endocervical type.[118] While tumours of endocervical type are more likely to be cervical in origin, it is not possible on morphology alone to be certain of the site of origin of endometrioid, or indeed any other subtypes of adenocarcinoma.[119,121] Histologically and cytologically, these tumours are identical to those arising in the endometrium and may even contain areas of intraglandular squamous differentiation.[122]

### Cytological findings: endometrioid adenocarcinoma

- Small cuboidal or columnar cells
- Eccentric nuclei
- Small nucleoli
- Scanty dense cyanophilic coarsely granular cytoplasm.

It is important to be aware that following subtotal hysterectomy for pathology within the uterus, the continuing risk of an endometrioid adenocarcinoma arising in residual isthmic endometrial tissue must be considered when assessing cytology from the cervical stump.[123]

## Minimal deviation adenocarcinoma (MDA) – adenoma malignum

This rare tumour is the most differentiated form of endocervical adenocarcinoma. Histologically the tumour is characterised by increased complexity of crypt architecture, glands are usually lined by a single layer of columnar cells showing minimal cytological atypia with basal nuclei and abundant delicate cytoplasm. When nuclear pleomorphism is more pronounced, large nucleoli may be seen. On histology, discrimination between MDA and lobular endocervical glandular hyperplasia is difficult. Cytologically, the presence of intranuclear cytoplasmic inclusions has recently been described by Hashi et al. as predictive of this benign entity.[124]

Likewise, on cytology, MDA is difficult to recognise and in many cases this is retrospective.[54,125,126] An abundance of glandular material in the sample, excessive lacy cytoplasm and occasional mitotic figures in sheets of otherwise banal uniform looking cells, are particularly helpful diagnostic features (Figs 24.34, 24.35).

### Cytological findings: minimal deviation adenocarcinoma

- Flat honeycomb sheets with focal disorganisation
- Abundant, lacy or vacuolated cytoplasm
- Wispy cytoplasmic tails at the periphery of the groups

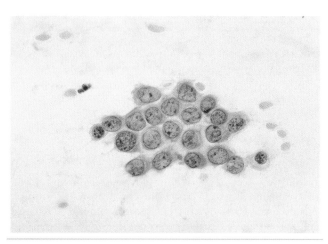

**Fig. 24.34** Cervical smear. Minimal deviation adenocarcinoma. Endocervical cells retain their 'honeycomb' arrangement, but show nuclear enlargement. The cytoplasm is delicate with some fine vacuolation (conventional smear).

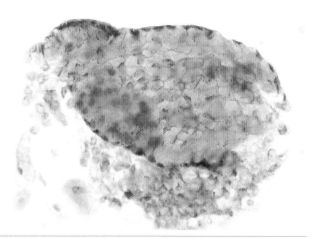

**Fig. 24.35** Cervical cytology. Minimal deviation adenocarcinoma. Flat sheet of cells with subtle disorganisation of the honeycomb pattern and striking yellow cytoplasmic stain (Conventional smear). (Courtesy of Buckinghamshire Hospitals NHS Trust.)

- Yellow-orange cytoplasmic mucin staining[127]
- Nuclei are round or oval
  - Up to twice normal size
  - Fine to coarsely granular chromatin
  - Occasional conspicuous nucleoli.

## Villoglandular adenocarcinoma

This is an uncommon tumour, mainly occurring in young women and with a relatively good prognosis. Histologically, the diagnosis is made on recognition of papillae with normal stromal cores covered by endocervical, endometrioid or intestinal-type cells exhibiting only minor degrees of atypia.[118] Because of the banal cellular features, cytological identification may be retrospective (Fig. 24.36).[128–132]

### Cytological findings: villoglandular adenocarcinoma

#### Exfoliation pattern

- Branching papillary fronds with smooth borders
- Occasional peripheral palisading or feathering
- Crowding and overlapping of cells
- Loss of honeycomb architecture.

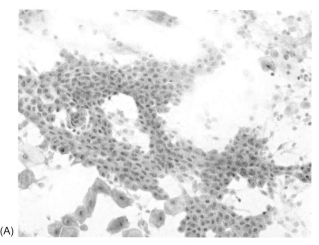

(A)

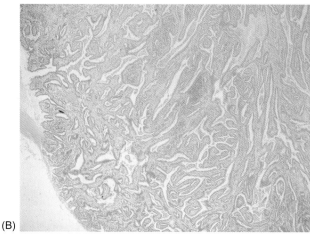

(B)

**Fig. 24.36** (A,B) Cystoscopy urine and cervical biopsy. Papillary fragment of bland cells from bladder involvement in cervical villoglandular carcinoma (A, PAP; B, H&E).

*Cell morphology*

- Nuclei:
  - Moderate hyperchromasia
  - Small uniform, up to twice the size of intermediate cell nuclei
  - Round/oval
  - Granular evenly dispersed chromatin
  - Nucleoli usually absent
  - Occasional mitotic figures and apoptosis
- Cytoplasm inconspicuous.

Caveat: papillary squamous and squamotransitional cell neoplasms and papillary CIN 3 are also recognised cytologically.[133] The identification of basaloid morphology in the cells at the papillary surfaces is a useful discriminator.

## Papillary serous adenocarcinoma

Histologically, this rare tumour differs from villoglandular adenocarcinoma in that the papillae are finer with delicate fibrous cores, psammoma bodies may be present and the epithelial covering shows marked cellular pleomorphism displaying unequivocal evidence of malignancy. Cytologically, they are identical to serous carcinoma of the ovary presenting as three-dimensional balls and papillary fragments made up of pleomorphic malignant cells (Fig. 24.37) (see Ch. 27).[130,134]

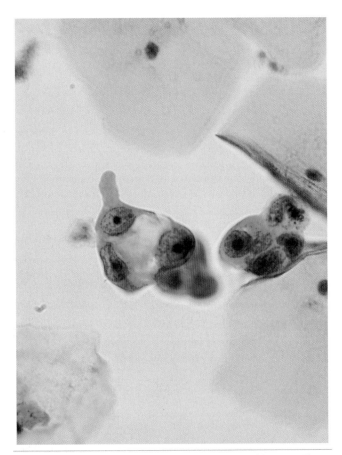

**Fig. 24.37** Cervical cytology. Papillary serous carcinoma of the cervix. Three-dimensional cluster of malignant cells showing nuclear pleomorphism and abundant fine and coarse cytoplasmic vacuolation (SurePath). (Courtesy of Manchester Cytology Training Centre.)

## Clear cell adenocarcinoma

This is an uncommon lesion in the cervix but may occur as *in situ* foci.[135] Although vaginal and cervical clear cell carcinoma in young women was previously associated with pre-natal diethylstilboestrol (DES) exposure, its use was discontinued in the UK in the early 1970s (see Chs 21, 23, 25). Cervical lesions do occur in non-exposed women but usually today, the malignant cells observed in cytology are of endometrial origin and are be more readily identifiable in LBC samples.[136] On histology, the tumours show a mixed papillary and tubular pattern, the lining cells having characteristic apical or 'hob nail' nuclei and prominent nucleoli (Fig. 24.38).[137]

### Cytological findings: clear cell adenocarcinoma

#### Exfoliation pattern

- Abnormal cells, single and in small clusters
- Anisonucleosis.

#### Cell morphology

- Nuclei:
  - Round/oval
  - Delicate nuclear border
  - Finely granular chromatin
  - Large eosinophilic nucleoli ± multiple
- Cytoplasm:
  - Delicate finely granular
  - Varying amounts from little or none to abundant.

## Enteric adenocarcinoma

These tumours are usually seen as part of a mixed pattern of differentiation; they rarely occur in pure form. The involved glands are lined by columnar cells with a prominent brush border and goblet cells are usually numerous. Occasionally, Paneth cells and argyrophil cells may be present.[26] The presence of

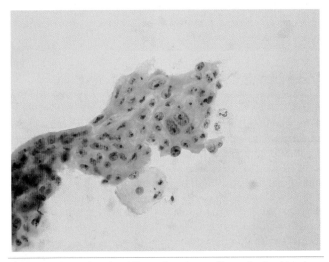

**Fig. 24.38** Cervical cytology. Clear cell carcinoma. Sheet of cells with pale vesicular nuclei showing anisonucleosis and prominent mainly off-centre nucleoli. Compare nuclear size with adjacent intermediate cell nucleus. Abundant cytoplasm could result in difficulty in discrimination between neoplasia and florid repair (ThinPrep). (Courtesy of University Hospitals of Leicester NHS Trust.)

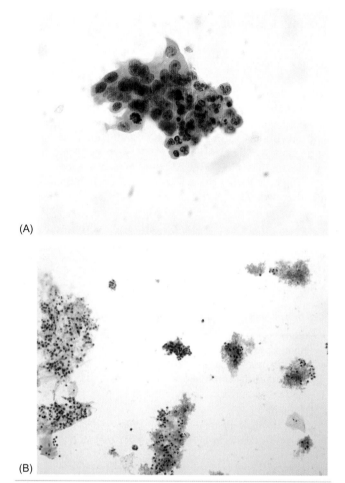

(A)

(B)

**Fig. 24.39** Cervical cytology. (A) Poorly differentiated adenosquamous carcinoma of the endocervix. A hyperchromatic crowded cluster of cells with nuclear pleomorphism and mitotic figures. Cytoplasm is relatively abundant and dense. Either squamous or glandular neoplasia could account for this appearance. (B) Blood and debris is in keeping with invasion (ThinPrep).

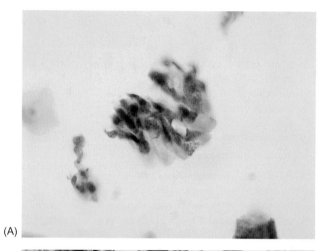

(A)

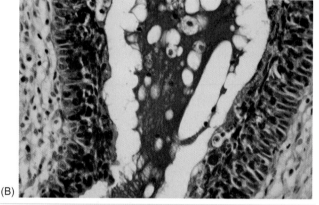

(B)

**Fig. 24.40** Cervical cytology and cervical biopsy. (A) Stratified mucin-producing intraepithelial lesion (SMILE). Disorganised cluster of cells with marked nuclear pleomorphism and dense but finely vacuolated cytoplasm. Non-specific abnormality, could be from either squamous or glandular neoplasia. (B) Biopsy shows intraepithelial mucin from SMILE. Histological outcome: HG-CGIN and SMILE (A, SurePath; B, PAS + diastase).

goblet cells on cytology should alert the microscopist to the presence of either a preinvasive or invasive lesion of enteric differentiation.

## Adenosquamous carcinoma including glassy cell carcinoma

Both squamous and glandular cervical tumours arise from undifferentiated reserve cells.[138] Consequently, it is not surprising that in some instances both patterns of differentiation are seen, either as discrete areas within a tumour (adenocarcinoma and squamous carcinoma) or with intermingling of the glandular and squamous cell components, adenosquamous carcinoma (Fig. 24.39) or its pre-invasive precursor – stratified mucin-producing intraepithelial lesion (SMILE). In the former there is a tendency for the glandular component to be overlooked in a background of dispersed dyskaryotic or malignant squamous cells frequently consisting of balls of cells and papillae covered with palisaded columnar cells and in SMILE, the cytological features are not specific for glandular differentiation and virtually impossible to tell apart from a pure squamous lesion (Fig. 24.40) (see Chs 23 and 25).[119,139]

Glassy cell carcinoma is an uncommon variant of poorly differentiated adenosquamous carcinoma which shows both glandular and squamous differentiation ultrastructurally. Histologically, it presents as sheets and nests of malignant cells with macronucleoli and marked mitotic activity. The findings on conventional cytology and LBC are similar.[140,141] It is most likely to be misinterpreted as large cell non-keratinising squamous carcinoma (Fig. 24.41).

### Cytological findings: adenosquamous carcinoma

#### Exfoliation pattern

- Syncytial aggregates of large malignant cells
- Dissociated malignant cells
- Admixed polymorphs, eosinophils and malignant cells (granuloepithelial complexes)
- Proteinaceous background/tumour diathesis.

#### Cell morphology

- Nuclei:
  - Round/oval
  - Delicate nuclear membrane
  - Chromatin evenly distributed finely granular
  - Large irregular single nucleoli

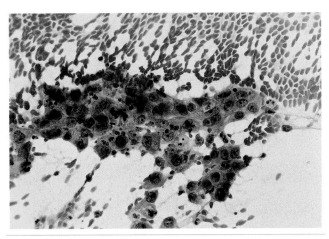

Fig. 24.41 Cervical smear. Glassy cell adenocarcinoma. Syncytial sheet of cells with round/oval nuclei and macronucleoli (conventional smear).

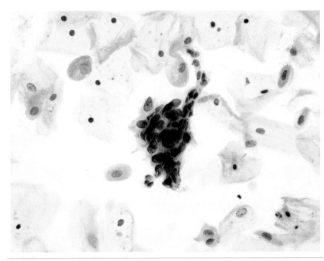

Fig. 24.43 Cervical cytology. Adenoid basal carcinoma. Hyperchromatic crowded group of cells with slight enlargement but minimal nuclear atypia. May be misinterpreted as of endometrial origin (SurePath). (Courtesy of Heart of England NHS Foundation Trust.)

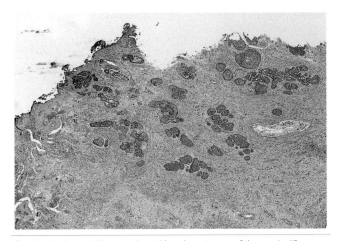

Fig. 24.42 Cervical biopsy. Adenoid basal carcinoma of the cervix. (Courtesy of Sandwell and West Birmingham Hospitals NHS Trust.)

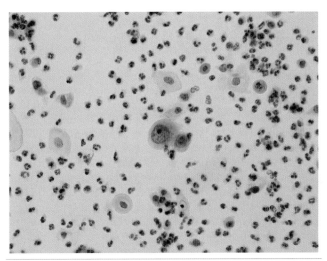

Fig. 24.44 Cervical cytology. Metastatic carcinoma of the stomach. Small cluster of malignant cells only slightly larger than accompanying parabasal cells but with nuclear enlargement, anisonucleosis and prominent nucleoli (SurePath).

- Cytoplasm:
  – Abundant, polygonal or elongated cells
  – Finely granular cyanophilic
  – Polymorph ingestion.

## Mesonephric, adenoid basal and adenoid cystic adenocarcinoma

These are very rare tumours in older women, usually inaccessible to cytological sampling, being either deep in the lateral wall of the cervix (mesonephric)[108] or beneath intact mucosa (adenoid basal and adenoid cystic) (Fig. 24.42). Cytologically, adenoid basal and adenoid cystic carcinomas appear as groups and sheets of small cells with a high N/C ratio, and uniform round or oval hyperchromatic nuclei with small nucleoli. They may be misinterpreted as of endometrial origin (Fig. 24.43). Differential diagnosis includes small cell neuroendocrine carcinoma and carcinoid tumours (see Ch. 25).[142–144]

## Non-cervical adenocarcinoma including metastatic carcinoma

Precise determination of site of origin of cytological glandular abnormalities may not be always possible, particularly in the absence of relevant clinical information (Figs 24.44, 24.45). Abnormal glandular cells presenting in cervical samples are neither site nor type specific and may be metastatic from a variety of distant sites (see Ch. 25).[145–147] In more than 25 years of glandular reporting, Sasagawa et al. found the site of disease was endometrial in 53% followed by 38% were of cervical origin, with ovary (8%) and tube (1%) represented rarely.[145] Metastatic tumour cells from extragenital sites presenting in smears were not included in this study. Similar proportions of endometrial versus endocervical carcinomas were reported by Hare et al.[121] and in LBC by Schorge et al.[120]

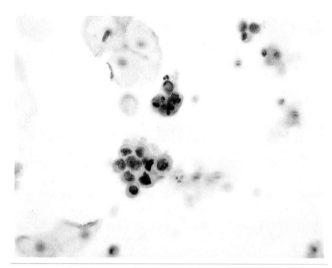

**Fig. 24.45** Cervical cytology. Metastatic lobular carcinoma of the breast. Clusters of small hyperchromatic cells with marked irregularity in nuclear contour and well- demarcated cytoplasm (SurePath).

**Table 24.4** Comparison of BSCC terminology and the Bethesda System for reporting glandular abnormalities (see pp. 615–617)

| BSCC terminology (proposed in 2008) | The Bethesda System (TBS) (2001) |
|---|---|
| **Negative** | **WNL** <br> Within normal limits <br> Benign atypia |
| **Borderline nuclear changes – endocervical** <br> (for endocervical prediction only) | **AGC NOS** (atypical glandular cells – not otherwise specified) <br> (for abnormality from all sites) |
| **?Glandular neoplasia** <br> Cervical glandular intraepithelial neoplasia (CGIN) and endocervical adenocarcinoma <br><br> Non-cervical adenocarcinoma from all non-cervical sites | **AGC favour neoplasia** (from all sites) |
| | **Adenocarcinoma in situ** (AIS) |
| | **Adenocarcinoma** (from all sites) |

BSCC: British Society for Clinical Cytology

## Immunochemical and molecular markers in glandular neoplasia

Ancillary techniques have been used on histological and cytological specimens of cervical glandular neoplasia with promising results. These are mostly based on the detection of HPV- associated cell proteins such as p16[INK,4a] similar to those well described in CIN.[148,149] Immunochemistry may be used to differentiate between endocervical and endometrial adenocarcinoma. Gene microarrays have revealed markers that may distinguish cervical adenocarcinoma from squamous carcinoma.

McCluggage and Jenkins demonstrated that primary endocervical adenocarcinoma was characterised by strong, diffuse positivity of 100% of cells with p16.[150] Others have also shown an excellent correlation between p16[INK4a] and high risk HPV DNA expression in cytological specimens.[151–153]

Murphy et al. showed that p16[INK4a] was the most reliable marker of cervical dysplasia and that combinations of biomarkers may be useful in diagnostically difficult cases.[154] MCM5 staining was independent of high risk HPV infection, highlighting its potential as a biomarker in both HPV-dependent and non-dependent cervical dysplasia. In addition, p16[INK4a] has been shown to be useful as a marker in investigating cytologically negative and equivocal cases.[155]

Alkushi et al.[155] described immunoprofiles that were specific for endocervical adenocarcinoma (negative for ER, vimentin and CK8/18, and positive for CEA) and endometrial adenocarcinoma (positive for ER, vimentin, CK8/18, and negative for CEA); however, most tumours showed an intermediate, non-specific immunophenotype.[156] McCluggage and Ansari-Lari showed the value of p16 in distinguishing between endocervical and endometrial adenocarcinoma.[150,156,157] Strong diffuse positivity is associated with the former, although endometrial adenocarcinoma may show focal staining, occasionally up to 50% of cells being positive.

Chao et al. analysed paired total RNA (cancer and normal tissues) with cDNA microarrays containing duplicate spots of 7334 sequence-verified human cDNA clones.[158] Genes including CEACAM5, TACSTD1, S100P and MSLN were upregulated in cervical adenocarcinoma. S100A9 and ANXA8, genes involved in the epidermal differentiation complex, were upregulated in squamous carcinoma. Baltazar et al. studied the differences in expression of COX-2 and EGFR in cervical adenocarcinoma, adenosquamous and squamous carcinoma.[159] COX-2 expression was stronger ($p = 0.003$) in adenocarcinoma compared with adenosquamous carcinoma. Expression of COX-2 and EGFR was significantly different when comparing squamous with adenocarcinoma ($p < 0.001$ and $p = 0.04$, respectively).

## Management of women with cytological prediction of glandular abnormality

The cytology report should indicate to the clinician the degree of risk of significant neoplasia based on cellular morphology. UK guidelines require urgent referral for investigation of all women for whom a ?'glandular neoplasia' report has been issued. This encompasses high-grade lesions from all sites including prediction of CGIN.[160] Where there is genuine doubt that the cytological features are truly neoplastic a 'borderline' report may be issued. Management of the 'borderline' category is subject of debate and either early repeat[51] or immediate referral[161] may be recommended depending on local practice. UK and American (TBS) terminologies are similar (Table 24.4).[47]

Besides its value in identifying glandular abnormalities in asymptomatic women taking part in population screening, cytology may provide additional information on women with signs and/or symptoms of cervical cancer. Colposcopic appearances are non-specific in those with preinvasive or very early invasive glandular lesions and even in women with established but occult adenocarcinoma. Also as lesions predicted on cervical samples may lie elsewhere within the genital tract or may rarely be extrauterine,[67,145,146,162] good communication between clinician and cytopathologist is of utmost importance to ensure optimal patient management.[163]

With 'borderline' category results, cytological surveillance may be justified[47,51,77,161] but because of the focal nature of glandular lesions within the endocervical canal and the inability of cytology to discriminate between CGIN and early invasive adenocarcinoma, small diagnostic biopsies cannot be relied upon to provide representative sampling.[164] Cone biopsy or large loop excision biopsy is regarded as the minimum on which to diagnose and treat CGIN.[165,166] Conservative surgery – trachelectomy – is also used in the treatment of early stage cervical cancer. This involves amputation of the cervix with conservation of the uterus and adnexae. Lack of endocervical sampling is to be anticipated on follow-up, not only because of stenosis at the isthmic-vaginal junction but also as a result of complete excision of all endocervical tissue. Difficulties may arise in interpretation of glandular cells from the isthmus mimicking glandular neoplasia.[89,167]

In the UK, there are no specific guidelines, separate from those for CIN, for follow-up management of CGIN other than that cervical samples must contain endocervical cells.[161] Johnston recommends 6-monthly smears to be undertaken indefinitely[168] and Hwang et al., finding late recurrences at 97

and 153 months, advocate at least 10 years of follow-up for women post-conservative treatment or hysterectomy.[169] Post-loop or cone biopsy cytology is particularly difficult to interpret especially after management of CGIN as there is the potential for the development of endometriosis, tuboendometrial metaplasia, and the likelihood of lower uterine segment sampling. Heightened awareness of the possibility of glandular neoplasia also introduces bias, with increased risk of false positive reporting of residual glandular abnormality in the presence of these benign look-alikes.[60,77] It is half a century since Friedell and McKay described adenocarcinoma *in situ* of the endocervix and still there remain problems for clinicians and pathologists alike in recognition of this lesion and in clinical management.[28]

The variable terminology used for glandular cells in cervical smears, their diverse outcomes in relation to histology and the emerging impact molecular techniques have been reviewed fully recently, with emphasis on the role of cytology combined with colposcopy in ensuring good patient management.[170-174]

## REFERENCES

1. Tasker JT, Collins JA. Adenocarcinoma of the uterine cervix. Am J Obstet Gynecol 1974;118:344–48.

2. Shorrock K, Johnson J, Johnson IR. Epidemiological changes in cervical carcinoma with particular reference to mucin-secreting subtypes. Histopathology 1990;17:53–57.

3. Sasieni P, Adams J. Changing rates of adenocarcinoma and adenosquamous carcinoma of the cervix in England. Lancet 2001;357:1490–93.

4. Bulk S, Visser O, Rozendaal L, et al. Cervical cancer in the Netherlands 1989–1998: decrease of squamous cell carcinoma in older women, increase in adenocarcinoma in younger women. Int J Cancer 2005;113:1005–9.

5. Smith HO, Tiffany MF, Qualls CR, et al. The rising incidence of adenocarcinoma relative to squamous cell carcinoma of the uterine cervix in the United States – a 24-year population-based study. Gynecol Oncol 2000;78:97–105.

6. Vizcaino AP, Moreno V, Bosch FX, et al. International trends in the incidence of cervical cancer: 1. Adenocarcinoma and adenosquamous cell carcinomas. Int J Cancer 1998;75:536–45.

7. Herbert A, Singh N, Smith JA. Adenocarcinoma of the uterine cervix compared with squamous cell carcinoma: a 12-year study in Southampton and south-west Hampshire. Cytopathology 2001;12:26–36.

8. Gunnell AS, Ylitalo N, Sandin S, et al. A longitudinal Swedish study on screening for squamous cell carcinoma and adenocarcinoma: evidence for effectiveness and overtreatment. Cancer Epidemiol Biomarkers Prev 2007;16:2641–48.

9. Kyndi M, Frederikson K, Krüger Kjaer S. Cervical cancer incidence in Denmark over six decades (1943–2002). Acta Obstet Gynaecol Scand 2006;85:106–11.

10. Schoolland M, Segal A, Allpress S, et al. Adenocarcinoma in situ of the cervix. Cancer 2002;96:330–37.

11. Mitchell H, Hocking J, Saville M. Improvement in protection against adenocarcinoma of the cervix resulting from participation in cervical screening. Cancer 2003;99:336–41.

12. International Collaboration of Epidemiological Studies for Cervical Cancer. Comparison of risk factors for invasive squamous cell carcinoma and adenocarcinoma of the cervix: collaborative reanalysis of individual data on 8,097 women with squamous cell carcinoma and 1,374 women with adenocarcinoma from 12 epidemiological studies. Int J Cancer 2007;120:885–91.

13. Berrington de Gonzáles A, Sweetland S, Green J. Comparison of risk factors for squamous cell and adenocarcinoma of the cervix: a meta-analysis. Br J Cancer 2004;90:1787–91.

14. Mathers ME, Johnson SJ, Wadehra V. How predictive is a cervical smear suggesting glandular neoplasia? Cytopathology 2002;13:83–91.

15. Howlett RI, Marrett LD, Innes MK, et al. Decreasing incidence of cervical adenocarcinoma in Ontario: is this related to improved endocervical Pap test sampling? Int J Cancer 2007;120:362–67.

16. Iwasawa A, Nieminen P, Lehtinen N, et al. Human Papillomavirus DNA in uterine cervix squamous cell carcinoma and adenocarcinoma detected by polymerase chain reaction. Cancer 1996;77:2275–79.

17. Moreira MA, Longato-Filho A, Taromaru E, et al. Investigation of human papillomavirus by hybrid capture II in cervical carcinomas including 113 adenocarcinomas and related lesions. Int J Gynecol Cancer 2006;16:586–90.

18. Castellsagué X, Diaz M, de Sanjosé S, et al. Worldwide human papillomavirus etiology of cervical adenocarcinoma and its cofactors: implications for screening and prevention. J Nat Cancer Inst 2006;98:303–15.

19. Brink AA, Zielinski GD, Steenbergen RD, et al. Clinical relevance of human papillomavirus testing in cytopathology. Cytopathology 2005;16:7–12.

20. Pirog EC, Kleter B, Olgac S, et al. Prevalence of human papillomavirus DNA in different histological subtypes of cervical adenocarcinoma. Am J Pathol 2000;157:1055–62.

21. Oliveira ERZM, Derchain SFM, Rabelo-Santos SH, et al. Papillomavirus (HPV) DNA by Hybrid Capture II in women referred due

to atypical glandular cells in the primary screening. Diagn Cytopathol 2004;31:19–22.

22. Saqi A, Gupta PK, Erroll M, et al. High-Risk Human Papillomavirus DNA testing: a marker for atypical glandular cells. Diagn Cytopathol 2006;34:235–39.

23. Bulk S, Berkhof J, Bulkmans NW, et al. Preferential risk of HPV16 for squamous cell carcinoma and of HPV18 for adenocarcinoma of the cervix compared to women with normal cytology in The Netherlands. Br J Cancer 2006;94:171–75.

24. Burk RD, Terai M, Gravitt PE, et al. Distribution of human papillomavirus types 16 and 18 variants in squamous cell carcinomas and adenocarcinomas of the cervix. Cancer Res 2003;63:7215–20.

25. Zielinski GD, Snijders PJ, Rozendaal L, et al. The presence of high-risk HPV combined with specific p53 and p16INK4a expression patterns points to high-risk HPV as the main causative agent for adenocarcinoma in situ and adenocarcinoma of the cervix. J Pathol 2003;201:535–43.

26. McCluggage WG, Shah R, Connolly LE, et al. Intestinal-type cervical adenocarcinoma in situ and adenocarcinoma exhibit a partial enteric immunophenotype with consistent expression of CDX2. Int J Gynecol Pathol 2008;27:92–100.

27. Wells M, Östör AG, Crum CP, et al. Tumours of the uterine cervix: epithelial tumours. In: Tavassoli FA, Devilee P, editors. World Health Organization Classification of Tumours Pathology and Genetics Tumours of the Breast and Female Genital Organs. Lyon: IARC Press; 2003. p. 272–73.

28. Friedell GH, McKay DG. Adenocarcinoma in situ of the endocervix. Cancer 1953;6:887–97.

29. Lee KR, Flynn CE. Early invasive adenocarcinoma of the cervix. Cancer 2000;89:1048–55.

30. Östör AG. Early invasive adenocarcinoma of the uterine cervix. Int J Gynecol Pathol 2000;19:29–38.

31. Lee KR, Rose PG. Glandular neoplasia of the cervixCh. 14. In: Crum CP, Lee KR, editors. Diagnostic Gynaecologic and Obstetric Pathology. London: Elsevier Saunders; 2006.

32. Fox H, Buckley CH. Working Party of the Royal College of Pathologists and the NHS Cervical Screening Programme. Histopathological reporting in cervical screening. Sheffield: NHS Cervical Screening Programme Publication; 1999 10:16–36.

33. Young RH, Clement PB. Endocervical adenocarcinoma and its variants: their morphology and differential diagnosis. Histopathology 2002;41:185–207.

34. Drijkoningen M, Meertens B, Lauweryns J. High-grade squamous intraepithelial lesion (CIN3) with extension into endocervical clefts. Difficulty of cytologic differentiation from adenocarcinoma in situ. Acta Cytol 1996;40:889–94.

35. Cenci M, Mancini R, Nofroni I, et al. Endocervical atypical cells of undetermined significance I: morphometric and cytologic characterization of cases that 'cannot rule out adenocarcinoma in situ'. Acta Cytol 2000;44:319–26.

36. Cenci M, Mancini R, Nofroni I, et al. Endocervical atypical cells of undetermined significance II: morphometric and cytologic analysis of nuclear features useful in characterizing differently correlated subgroups. Acta Cytol 2000;44:327–31.

37. Chhieng DC, Elgert PA, Cangiarella JF, et al. Clinical significance of atypical glandular cells of undetermined significance. A follow-up study from an academic medical center. Acta Cytol 2000;44:557–66.

38. Goldstein NS, Ahmad E, Hussain M. Endocervical glandular atypia: does a preneoplastic lesion of adenocarcinoma in situ exist? Am J Clin Pathol 1998;110:200–9.

39. Johnson JE, Rahemtulla A. Endocervical glandular neoplasia and its mimics in ThinPrep Pap tests. A descriptive study. Acta Cytol 1999;43:369–75.

40. Barter RA, Waters ED. Cyto- and histo-morphology of cervical adenocarcinoma in situ. Pathology 1970;2:33–40.

41. Bousfield L, Pacey F, Young Q, et al. Expanded cytologic criteria for the diagnosis of adenocarcinoma in situ of the cervix and related lesions. Acta Cytol 1980;24:283–96.

42. Biscotti CV, Gero MA, Toddy SM, et al. Endocervical adenocarcinoma in situ: an analysis of cellular features. Diagn Cytopathol 1997;17:326–32.

43. Van Aspert-Van Erp AJ, Smedts FM, Vooijs GP, et al. Severe cervical glandular cells lesions with coexisting squamous cells lesions. Cancer (Cancer Cytopathol) 2004;102:218–27.

44. Torres J, Derchain S, Gontijo R, et al. Atypical glandular cells: criteria to discriminate benign from neoplastic lesions and squamous from glandular neoplasia. Cytopathology 2005;16:295–302.

45. Rabelo-Santos S, Derchain S, do Amaral Westin M, et al. Endocervical glandular cell abnormalities in conventional cervical smears: evaluation of the performance of cytomorphological criteria and HPV testing in predicting neoplasia. Cytopathology 2008;19:34–43.

46. Raab SS, Isacson C, Layfield LJ, et al. Atypical glandular cells of undetermined significance: cytologic criteria to separate clinically significant from benign lesions. Am J Clin Pathol 1995; 104:574–582.

47. Solomon D, Frable W, Vooijs G, et al. ASCUS and AGUS criteria: IAC Task Force Summary. Acta Cytol 1998;42:16–24.

48. The American Society for Colposcopy and Cervical Pathology. Online. Available at: www.asccp.org/consensus.shtml.

49. Ozkan F, Ramzy I, Mody DR. Glandular lesions of the cervix on thin-layer Pap tests. Validity of cytologic criteria used in identifying significant lesions. Acta Cytol 2004;48:372–79.

50. National Health Cervical Screening Programme Cervical Cytopathology Atlas. Glandular abnormalities: 98–109 and Theme 7, Palisading and honeycombs: 124–125. Sheffield: NHS Cancer Screening Programmes; 2006.

51. Denton K, Herbert A, Turnbull L, et al. The revised BSCC terminology for abnormal cervical cytology. Cytopathology 2008;19:137–57.

52. Belsley NA, Tambouret RH, Misdraji J, et al. Cytologic features of endocervical glandular lesions: Comparison of SurePath, ThinPrep, and Conventional smear specimen preparations. Diagn Cytopathol 2008;36:232–37.

53. Johnson J. Atypical glandular cells NOS and Endocervical adenocarcinoma in situ. In: Werneke S & Brahm C. editors. ThinPrep Pap Test Morphology Reference Atlas Boxborough: Cytyc; 2003: 84–97.

54. Vogelsang PJ, Nguyen G-K, Honoré LH. Exfoliative cytology of adenoma malignum (minimal deviation adenocarcinoma) of the uterine cervix. Diagn Cytopathol 1995;13:146–50.

55. Siziopikou K, Wang H, Abu-Jawdeh G. Cytological features of neoplastic lesions in endocervical glands. Diagn Cytopathol 1997;17:1–7.

56. Lee KR, Manna EA, Jones MA. Comparative cytologic features of adenocarcinoma in situ of the uterine cervix. Acta Cytol 1991;35:117–26.

57. Lee KR. Adenocarcinoma in situ with a small cell (endometrioid) pattern in cervical smears: a test of the distinction from benign mimics using specific criteria. Cancer (Cancer Cytopathol) 1999;87:254–58.

58. Wantanabe S, Iwasaka T, Yokoama M, et al. Analysis of nuclear chromatin distribution in cervical glandular abnormalities. Acta Cytol 2004;48:505–13.

59. Bai H, Sung CJ, Steinhoff MM. ThinPrep Pap test promotes detection of glandular lesions of the endocervix. Diagn Cytopathol 2000;23:19–22.

60. Lee KR, Darragh TM, Joste NE, et al. Atypical glandular cells of undetermined significance (AGUS). Interobserver reproducibility in cervical smears and corresponding thin-layer preparations. Am J Clin Pathol 2002;117:96–102.

61. Simsir A, Hwang S, Cangiarella J, et al. Glandular atypia on Papanicolaou smears. Interobserver variability in the diagnosis and prediction of the cell of origin. Cancer (Cancer Cytopathol) 2003;99:323–30.

62. van Aspert-van Erp AJ, Smedts FM, Vooijis GP. Severe cervical glandular lesions and severe cervical combined lesions. Predictive value of the Papanicolaou smear. Cancer (Cancer Cytopathol) 2004;102:210–17.

63. Segal A, Frost F, Miranda A, et al. Predictive value of diagnoses of endocervical glandular abnormalities in cervical smears. Pathology 2003;35:198–203.

64. Kirwan J, Herrington C, Smith P, et al. A retrospective clinical audit of cervical smears reported as 'glandular neoplasia'. Cytopathology 2004;15:188–94.

65. Moreira A, Filho A, Castelo A, et al. How accurate is cytological diagnosis of cervical glandular lesions? Diagn Cytopathol 2008;36:270–74.

66. Ruba S, Schoolland M, Allpress S, et al. Adenocarcinoma in situ of the uterine cervix. Screening and diagnostic errors in Papanicolaou smears. Cancer Cytopathol 2004;102:280–97.

67. Jackson SR, Hollingworth TA, Anderson MC, et al. Glandular lesions of the cervix–cytological and histological correlation. Cytopathology 1996;7:10–16.

68. NICE. Online. Available at: http://guidance.nice.org.uk/TA69

69. Williams A. Liquid based cytology and conventional smears compared over two 12-month periods. Cytopathology 2006;17:86–93.

70. Roberts JM, Gurley AM, Thurloe JK, et al. Evaluation of the ThinPrep Pap test as an adjunct to the conventional Pap smear. Med J Aust 1997;167:466–69.

71. Corkill M, Knapp D, Martin J, et al. Specimen adequacy of ThinPrep sample preparations in a direct-to-vial study. Acta Cytol 1997;41:39–44.

72. Roberts JM, Thurloe JK, Bowditch RC, et al. Comparison of ThinPrep and Pap smear in relation to prediction of adenocarcinoma in situ. Acta Cytol 1999;43:74–80.

73. Ashfaq R, Gibbons D, Vela C, et al. ThinPrep Pap test. Accuracy for glandular disease. Acta Cytol 1999;43:81–85.

74. Yeoh GPS, Chan KW. Cell block preparation on residual ThinPrep sample. Diagn Cytopathol 1999;21:427–31.

75. Diaz-Rosario L, Kabawar S. Cell block preparations by inverted filter sedimentation is useful in differential diagnosis of atypical glandular cells of undetermined significance in ThinPrep specimens. Cancer Cytopathol 2000;90:265–72.

76. Crum CP, Cibas ES, Lee KR, editors. Glandular precursors, adenocarcinomas, and their mimics. In: Contemporary Issues in Surgical Pathology: Pathology of Early Cervical Neoplasia. New York: Churchill Livingstone; 1997:177–240.

77. Roberts JM, Thurloe JK, Bowditch RC, et al. Subdividing atypical glandular cells of undetermined significance according to the Australian modified Bethesda system: Analysis of outcomes. Cancer (Cancer Cytopathol) 2000;90:87–95.

78. Wood M, Horst J, Bibbo M. Weeding atypical glandular cell look-alikes from the true atypical lesions in liquid-based Pap tests: A review. Diagn Cytopathol 2007;35:12–17.

79. Ramsaroop R, Chu I. Accuracy of diagnosis of atypical glandular cells – conventional and ThinPrep. Diagn Cytopathol 2006;34:614–19.

80. Burja IT, Thompson SK, Sawyer WL, et al. Atypical glandular cells of undetermined significance on cervical smears. Acta Cytol 1999;43:351–56.

81. Selvaggi S. Cytologic features of high-grade squamous intraepithelial lesions involving endocervical glands on ThinPrep cytology. Diagn Cytopathol 2002;26:181–85.

82. Selvaggi SM. Cytologic features of squamous cell carcinoma in situ involving endocervical glands in endocervical cytobrush specimens. Acta Cytol 1994;38:687–92.

83. Ghorab Z, Mahmood S, Schinella R. Endocervical reactive atypia: a histo-cytologic study. Diagn Cytopathol 2000;22:342–46.

84. Di'Tomasso J, Ramzy I, Mody DR. Glandular lesions of the cervix. Validity of cytologic criteria used to differentiate reactive changes, glandular intraepithelial lesions and adenocarcinoma. Acta Cytol 1996;40:1127–35.

85. Waddell C. Glandular prediction: The liquid revolution. Scan 2007;18:5–11.

86. Lee K, Manna E. Atypical endocervical glandular cells: accuracy of cytologic diagnosis. Diagn Cytopathol 1995;13:202–8.

87. de Peralta-Venturino MN, Purslow MJ, Kini SR. Endometrial cells of the 'lower uterine segment' (LUS) in cervical smears obtained by endocervical brushings: a source of potential diagnostic pitfall. Diagn Cytopathol 1995;12:263–71.

88. Wilbur DC. Endocervical glandular atypia: A 'new' problem for the cytologist. Diagn Cytopathol 1995;13:463–69.

89. Feratovic R, Lewin SN, Sonoda Y, et al. Cytologic findings after fertility-sparing radical trachelectomy. Cancer (Cancer Cytopathol) 2008;114:1–6.

90. Lee KR, Genest DR, Minter LJ, et al. Adenocarcinoma in situ in cervical smears with small cell (endometrioid) pattern. Distinction from cells directly sampled from the upper endocervical canal or lower segment of the endometrium. Am J Clin Pathol 1998;109:738–42.

91. Chhieng DC, Elgert PA, Cangiarella JF, et al. Cytology of polypoid adenomyomas: a report of two cases. Diagn Cytopathol 2000;22:176–80.

92. Lundeen S, Horwitz C, Larson C, et al. Abnormal cervicovaginal smears due to endometriosis. Diagn Cytopathol 2002;26:35–40.

93. Hanau CA, Begley N, Bibbo M. Cervical endometriosis: a potential pitfall in the evaluation of glandular cells in cervical smears. Diagn Cytopathol 1997;16:274–80.

94. Szyfelbein WM, Baker PM, Bell DA. Superficial endometriosis of the cervix. A source of abnormal glandular cells in cervicovaginal smears. Diagn Cytopathol 2004;30:88–91.

95. Mulvaney NJ, Surtees V. Cervical/vaginal endometriosis with atypia: a cytohistopathologic study. Diagn Cytopathol 1999;21:188–93.

96. Ducatman BS, Wang HH, Jonasson JG, et al. Tubal metaplasia: a cytologic study with comparison to other neoplastic and non-neoplastic conditions of the endocervix. Diagn Cytopathol 1993;9:98–105.

97. Selvaggi SM, Haefner HK. Microglandular endocervical hyperplasia and tubal metaplasia: pitfalls in the diagnosis of adenocarcinoma on cervical smears. Diagn Cytopathol 1997;16:168–73.

98. Hirschowitz L, Eckford SD, Phillpotts B, et al. Cytological changes associated with tubo-endometrioid metaplasia of the uterine cervix. Cytopathology 1994;5:1–8.

99. Babkowski RC, Wilbur DC, Rutkowski MA, et al. The effects of endocervical canal topography, tubal metaplasia, and high canal sampling on cytologic presentation of nonneoplastic endocervical cells. Am J Clin Pathol 1996;105:403–10.

100. Ronnett B, Manos M, Ransley J, et al. Atypical glandular cells of undetermined significance (AGUS): cytopathologic feature, histopathologic results, and human papilloma DNA detection. Hum Pathol 1999;30:816–25.

101. O'Connell F, Cibas E. Cytologic features of ciliated adenocarcinoma of the cervix. Acta Cytol 2005;49:187–90.

102. Maksem JA. Ciliated cell adenocarcinoma of the endometrium diagnosed be endometrial brush cytology and confirmed by hysterectomy: a case report detailing a highly efficient cytology collection and processing technique. Diagn Cytopathol 1997;16:78–82.

103. Greeley C, Schroeder S, Silverberg S. Microglandular hyperplasia of the cervix: A true 'pill' lesion? Int J Gynecol Pathol 1995;14:50–54.

104. Valente PT, Schantz HD, Schultz M. Cytologic atypia associated with microglandular hyperplasia. Diagn Cytopathol 1994;10:326–31.

105. Cangiarella J. Atypical glandular cells – an update. Diagn Cytopathol 2003;29:271–79.

106. Alvarez-Santín C, Sica A, Rodríguez MC, et al. Microglandular hyperplasia of the uterine cervix. Cytologic diagnosis in cervical smears. Acta Cytol 1999;43:110–13.

107. Frierson HF, Covell JL, Andersen WA. Radiation changes in endocervical cells in brush specimens. Diagn Cytopathol 1990;6:243–47.

108. Stewart CJR, Taggart CR, Brett F, et al. Mesonephric adenocarcinoma of the uterine cervix with focal endocrine cell differentiation. Int J Gynecol Pathol 1993;12:264–69.

109. Hejmadi RK, Gearty JC, Waddell C, et al. Mesonephric hyperplasia can cause abnormal cervical smears: report of three cases with review of the literature. Cytopathology 2005;16:240–43.

110. Pisharodi L, Jovanoska S. Spectrum of cytologic changes in pregnancy. A review of 100 abnormal cervicovaginal smears with emphasis on diagnostic pitfalls. Acta Cytol 1995;39:05–908.

111. Quincey C, Persad RV, Stanbridge CM. Chorionic villi in post-partum cervical smears. Cytopathology 1995;6:149–55.

112. Masuda K, Yutani C, Akutagawa K, et al. Cytopathological observations in a 27 year old female patient with endometrioid adenocarcinoma arising in the lower uterine segment of the uterus. Diagn Cytopathol 1999;21:117–21.

113. van Hoeven KH, Hanau CA, Hudock JA. The detection of endocervical gland involvement by high-grade squamous intraepithelial lesions in smears prepared from endocervical brush specimens. Cytopathology 1996;7:310–15.

114. De May RM, editors. The Pap smear. In: The Art and Science of Cytopathology: exfoliative Cytology. Chicago: ASCP Press; 1996: 161.

115. Cronjé HS, Divall P, Bam RH, et al. Effects of dilute acetic acid on the cervical smear. Acta Cytol 1997;41:1091–94.

116. Mulvaney N, Östör A. Microinvasive adenocarcinoma of the cervix: a cytohistopathologic study of 40 cases. Diagn Cytopathol 1997;16:430–36.

117. Kurian K, Al-Nafussi A. Relation of cervical glandular intraepithelial neoplasia to microinvasive and invasive adenocarcinoma of the uterine cervix: a study of 121 cases. J Clin Pathol 1999;52:112–17.

118. McCluggage W. Endocervical glandular lesions: controversial aspects and ancillary techniques. J Clin Pathol 2002;56:164–73.

119. Hayes MM, Matisic JP, Chen C-J, et al. Cytological aspects of uterine cervical adenocarcinoma, adenosquamous carcinoma and combined adenocarcinoma-squamous carcinoma: appraisal of diagnostic criteria for in situ versus invasive lesions. Cytopathology 1997;8:397–408.

120. Schorge J, Saboorian M, Hynan L, et al. ThinPrep detection of cervical and endometrial adenocarcinoma: a retrospective cohort study. Cancer Cytopathol 2002;96:338–43.

121. Hare A, Duncan A, Sharp A. Cytology suggestive of glandular neoplasm: outcomes and suggested management. Cytopathology 2003;14:12–18.

122. Hirschowitz L, Sen C, Murdoch J. Primary endometrioid adenocarcinoma of the cervix with widespread squamous metaplasia – a potential diagnostic pitfall. Diagnostic Pathology 2007;2:40.

123. Goodman HM, Niloff JM, Buttlar CA, et al. Adenocarcinoma of the cervical stump. Gynecol Oncol 1989;35:188–92.

124. Hashi A, Yuminamochi T, Xu J-Y, et al. Intranuclear cytoplasmic inclusion is a significant diagnostic feature for the differentiation of lobular endocervical glandular hyperplasia from minimal deviation adenocarcinoma of the cervix. Diagn Cytopathol 2008;36:535–44.

125. Granter SR, Lee KR. Cytologic findings in minimal deviation adenocarcinoma (adenoma malignum) of the cervix. A report of seven cases. Am J Clin Pathol 1996;105:327–33.

126. Hirai Y, Takeshima N, Haga A, et al. A clinicocytopathologic study of adenoma malignum of the uterine cervix. Gynecol Oncol 1998;70:219–23.

127. Ishii K, Katsuyama T, Ota H, et al. Cytologic and cytochemical features of adenoma malignum of the uterine cervix. Cancer (Cancer Cytopathol) 1999;87:245–53.

128. Ballo MS, Silverberg SG, Sidawy M. Cytologic features of well-differentiated villoglandular adenocarcinoma of the cervix. Acta Cytol 1996;40:536–40.

129. Novotny DB, Ferlisi P. Villoglandular adenocarcinoma of the cervix: cytologic presentation. Diagn Cytopathol 1997;17:383–87.

130. Chang WC, Matisic JP, Zhou C, et al. Cytologic features of villoglandular adenocarcinoma of the uterine cervix: comparison with typical endocervical adenocarcinoma with a villoglandular component and papillary serous carcinoma. Cancer (Cancer Cytopathol) 1999;87:5–11.

131. Khunamornpong S, Siriaunkgul S, Suprasert P. Well-differentiated villoglandular adenocarcinoma of the uterine cervix: cytomorphologic observation of five cases. Diagn Cytopathol 2002;26:10–14.

132. Ajit D, Dighe S, Gujral S. Cytologic features of villoglandular adenocarcinoma of the cervix. Acta Cytol 2004;48:288–89.

133. Nguyen G-K, Daya D. Exfoliative cytology of papillary serous adenocarcinomas of the uterine cervix. Diagn Cytopathol 1997;16:548–50.

134. Ng W-K. Thin-layer (liquid-based) cytologic findings of papillary squamotransitional cell carcinoma of the cervix. Acta Cytol 2003;47:141–48.

135. Hasumi K, Ehrmann R. Clear cell carcinoma of the uterine endocervix with an in situ component. Cancer 1978;42:2435–38.

136. Guidos B, Selvaggi S. Detection of endometrial adenocarcinoma with the ThinPrep Pap test. Diagn Cytopathol 2000;23:260–65.

137. Young Q, Pacey NF. The cytologic diagnosis of clear cell adenocarcinoma of the cervix uteri. Acta Cytol 1978;22:3.

138. Fox H, Wells M, Harris M, et al. Enteric tumours of the lower female genital tract: a report of three cases. Histopathology 1988;12:167–76.

139. Ng W-K. Thin-layer cytology findings of papillary adenosquamous carcinoma of the cervix. Acta Cytol 2003;47:649–56.

140. Chung J, Lee S, Cho K. Glassy cell carcinoma of the uterine cervix: cytologic features and expression of progesterone receptors. Acta Cytol 2000;44:552–56.

141. Ng W-K, Cheung L, Albert S. Liquid-based cytology findings of glassy cell carcinoma of the cervix. Acta Cytol 2004;48:99–106.

142. Powers C, Stastny J, Frable W. Adenoid basal carcinoma of the cervix: a potential pitfall in cervicovaginal cytology. Diagn Cytopathol 1996;14:172–77.

143. Ravinsky E, Safneck J, Chantziantoniou N. Cytologic features of primary adenoid cystic carcinoma of the uterine cervix. Acta Cytol 1996;40:1304–8.

144. Vuong P, Neveux Y, Schoonaert M-F, et al. Adenoid cystic (cylindromatous) carcinoma associated with squamous cell carcinoma of the cervix uteri. Acta Cytol 1996;40:289–94.

145. Sasagawa M, Nishino K, Honma S, et al. Origin of adenocarcinoma cells observed on cervical cytology. Acta Cytol 2003;47:410–14.

146. Fiorella RM, Beckwith LG, Miller LK, et al. Metastatic signet ring carcinoma of the breast as a source of positive cervicovaginal cytology. A case report. Acta Cytol 1993;37:948–52.

147. Matsuura Y, Saito R, Kawagoe T, et al. Cytologic analysis of primary stomach adenocarcinoma metastatic to the uterine cervix. Acta Cytol 1997;41:291–94.

148. Baak JPA, Kruse AJ, Robboy SJ, et al. Dynamic behavioural interpretation of cervical intraepithelial neoplasia with molecular biomarkers. J Clin Path 2006;59:1017–28.

149. Guimarães MCM, Gonçalves MAG, Soares CP, et al. Immunohistochemical Expression of p16INK4a and bcl-2 According to HPV Type and to the Progression of Cervical Squamous Intraepithelial Lesions. J Histochem Cytochem 2005;53:509–16.

150. McCluggage WG, Jenkins D. p16 immunoreactivity may assist in the distinction between endometrial and endocervical adenocarcinoma. Int J Gynae Pathol 2003;22:231–35.

151. Mitsuya I, Takuma F, Nobuo M, et al. Correlation of p16INK4A overexpression with human papillomavirus infection in cervical adenocarcinomas. Int J Gynecol Pathol 2003;22:378–85.

152. Negri G, Egarter-Vigl E, Kasal A, et al. p16INK4a is a useful marker for the diagnosis of adenocarcinoma of the cervix uteri and its precursors: an immunohistochemical study with immunocytochemical correlations. Am J Surg Pathol 2003;27:187–93.

153. Saqi A, Pasha TL, McGrath CM, et al. Overexpression of p16INK4A in liquid-based specimens (SurePathTM) as marker of cervical dysplasia and neoplasia. Diagn Cytopathol 2002;27:365–70.

154. Murphy N, Ring M, Heffron CCBB, et al. P16INK4a, CDC6 and MCM5: predictive

biomarkers in cervical preinvasive neoplasia and cervical cancer. J Clin Pathol 2005;58:525–34.

155. Alkushi A, Irving F, Hsu F, et al. Immunoprofile of cervical and endometrial adenocarcinomas using a tissue microarray. Virchows Archiv 2004;442:271–77.

156. Ansari-Lari MA, Staebler A, et al. Distinction of endocervical and endometrial adenocarcinomas: immunohistochemical p16 expression correlated with human papillomavirus (HPV) DNA detection. Am J Surg Pathol 2004;28:160–67.

157. Filho AL, Utagawa ML, Shirata NK, et al. Cytochemical expression of p16INK4A and Ki-67 in cytologically negative and equivocal Pap smears positive for oncogenic human papillomavirus. Int J Gyn Pathol 2005;24:118–24.

158. Chao A, Wang T, Lee Y, et al. Molecular characterisation of adenocarcinoma and squamous carcinoma of the uterine cervix using microarray analysis of gene expression. Int J Cancer 2006;19:91–98.

159. Baltazar F, Filho AL, Pinheiro C, et al. Cyclooxygenase-2 and epidermal growth factor receptor expressions in different histological subtypes of cervical carcinomas. Int J Gyn Pathol 2007;76:235–41.

160. Johnson J, Patnick J, editors. Achievable standards, benchmarks for reporting, criteria for evaluating cervical pathology. 2nd edn. Sheffield: NHSCSP; 2000. Publication No. 1.

161. Luesley D, Leeson S. Colposcopy and programme management: guidelines for the NHS Cervical Screening Programme. Sheffield: NHSCSP; 2004 Publication No. 20: 50–54.

162. Cullimore J, Scurr J. The abnormal glandular smear: cytologic prediction, colposcopic correlation and clinical management. J Obstet Gynaecol 2000;20:403–7.

163. Leeson SC, Inglis TCM, Salman WD. A study to determine the underlying reason for abnormal glandular cytology and the formulation of a management protocol. Cytopathol 1997;8:20–26.

164. Cullimore JE, Luesley DM, Rollason TP, et al. A management of cervical intraepithelial

glandular neoplasia (CIGN): a preliminary report. Br J Obstet Gynaecol 1992;99:314.

165. Soutter W, Haidopoulos D, Gornall R, et al. Is conservative treatment for adenocarcinoma in situ of the cervix safe? Br J Obstet Gynaecol 2001;108:1184–89.

166. Wright T, Massad S, Dunton C, et al. 2006 consensus guidelines for the management of women with cervical intraepithelial neoplasia or adenocarcinoma in situ. Am J Obstet Gynecol 2007:340–45.

167. Singh N, Titmuss E, Aleong J, et al. A review of post-trachelectomy isthmic and vaginal smear cytology. Cytopathology 2004;15:97–103.

168. Johnston C. Cervical adenocarcinoma in situ: a persistent clinical dilemma. Lancet 1997;350:1337.

169. Hwang D, Lickrish G, Chapman W, Colgan T. Long-term surveillance is required for all women treated fro cervical adenocarcinoma in situ. J Lower Genital Tract Disease 2004;8:125–31.

170. Negri G. Atypical glandular cells in cervical cytology: what are we talking about? Terminology and the impact of molecular techniques. Cytopathology 2009;20: 347–50.

171. Kumar N, Bongiovanni M, Molliet M-J, et al. Diverse glandular pathologies coexist with high-grade squamous intraepithelial lesion in cyto-histological review of atypical glandular cells on ThinPrep specimens. Cytopathology 2009;20:351–58.

172. Ullal A, Roberts M, Bulmer JN, et al. The role of cervical cytology and colposcopy in detecting cervical glandular neoplasia. Cytopathology 2009;20:359–66.

173. Finall Al, Olafsdottir R. Outcomes of cervical liquid-based cytology suggesting a glandular abnormality. Cytopathology 2009;20:367–74.

174. Adhya AK, Mahesha V, Srinivasan R, et al. Atypical glandular cells in cervical smears: histological correlation and a suggested plan of management based on age of the patient in a low resource setting. Cytopathology 2009;20:375–79.

# Other tumours and lesions of cervix, vulva and vagina

John H. F. Smith

## Chapter contents

## Introduction

The preceding chapters have covered the cytopathology of the commonest types of neoplasms arising in the cervix. This chapter will concentrate on the cytology of non-neoplastic conditions of the cervix that may present as a tumour clinically or microscopically; the cytological findings in some less common tumours and tumour variants; and the cytology of tumours and tumour-like conditions of the vagina and vulva.

## Tumour-like conditions of the cervix

### Cervical polyps

The term polyp simply refers to a protuberant mass of tissue. The tissue may be regenerative, inflammatory or neoplastic in origin; less often, it may be congenital or hamartomatous. In gynaecological practice, a cervical polyp is usually a benign polypoid overgrowth of the endocervical tissues possibly due to chronic inflammation, although other types of polypoid lesion are also encountered.

Cervical polyps of endocervical origin are common, occurring in approximately 5–8% of women, most of whom are multiparous and over the age of 40 years. The polyps are usually solitary, less than 3 cm across, asymptomatic, and often an incidental finding at the time of routine cervical cytology sampling. They may, however, cause vaginal discharge or bleeding. The presence of a polyp may also compromise cervical cytology sampling if overlying part of the transformation zone.

Histologically, they are composed of endocervical tissue covered by columnar, squamous or immature metaplastic epithelium and are often inflamed (Fig. 25.1). Microglandular endocervical hyperplasia may be present focally.

Although cervical intraepithelial neoplasia (CIN) is no more likely to be found in an endocervical polyp than in the native cervix and the incidence of adenocarcinoma or squamous carcinoma

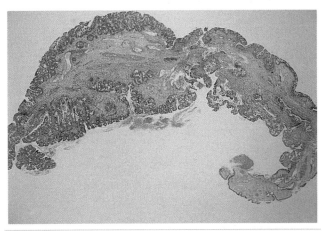

**Fig. 25.1** Section of a benign endocervical polyp covered by endocervical and metaplastic epithelium. The stroma shows a light non-specific inflammatory cell infiltrate (H&E).

arising in a polyp is low (0.2–0.4%),[1] removal of cervical polyps, accompanied by curettage to exclude coexisting endometrial pathology, is generally advisable, particularly in symptomatic women.[2] Histological examination is imperative and may reveal that the polyp is in fact an unsuspected condyloma or a neoplasm.

### Cytological findings: cervical polyps

- Cytology samples are usually entirely normal
- Endocervical cells may show reactive features.

### Diagnostic pitfalls: cervical polyps

The cytology sample may be of poor quality if the polyp has significantly interfered with sample taking, caused bleeding or is associated with cervicitis. Sometimes, endocervical cells from the polyp show reactive changes including marked nuclear enlargement with pleomorphism, hyperchromasia and prominent nucleoli (Fig. 25.2). Occasionally, polypoidal tissue fragments from the polyp appear in cervical cytology samples, comprising an inner core of numerous small dark stromal cells, covered by a layer of columnar cells with basal nuclei.[3] If there are interpretative problems, the investigation should be repeated after removal of the polyp.

Microglandular hyperplasia, as described in the previous chapter, is sometimes seen in cytology samples from a polyp. Human papillomavirus associated changes, squamous or glandular precancer or invasive neoplasia within a polyp, if appropriately sampled, yields the same cytological findings as described in the preceding chapters.

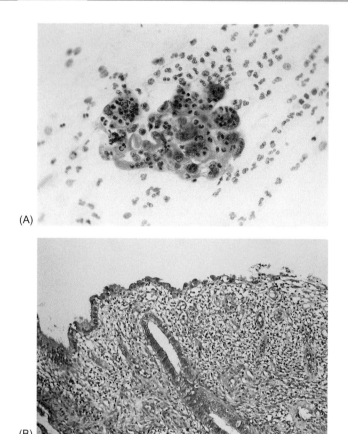

(A)

(B)

**Fig. 25.2** (A) Endocervical cell cluster with reactive changes in cervical smear with a heavy inflammatory exudate. A cervical polyp was recorded in the clinical details. The smear was repeated after polypectomy and was found to be normal. The polyp showed non-specific inflammation (PAP). (B) Polypectomy specimen showed similar changes at the surface of the polyp (H&E).

## Lower uterine segment polyps

This term is used to describe polyps arising at or just above the junction of endocervix with endometrium. They typically have a low gland to stroma ratio. The cytological features of two such polyps presenting in cervical smears have been described.[3] Both smears contained tissue fragments comprising small vessels running in various directions, connected by thin sheets of small ovoid cells with indistinct cytoplasm.

## Decidual polyps

During pregnancy the cervical stroma frequently undergoes focal decidual change and this reaction may be so extensive as to form a polypoid protrusion of the cervical stroma known as a decidual polyp. The decidual change is typically subepithelial in location, often disrupting the overlying epithelium. The histological appearance may be misinterpreted as carcinoma since decidualised stromal cells have large nuclei, prominent nucleoli and abundant cytoplasm, imparting an epithelioid appearance (Fig. 25.3A).[4]

### Cytological findings: decidual polyps

- Loose sheets of polygonal cells
- Abundant pale cytoplasm
- Large nuclei, prominent nucleoli.

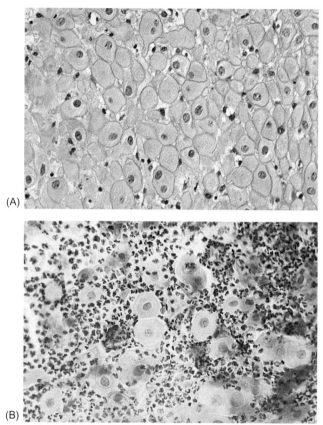

(A)

(B)

**Fig. 25.3** (A) Decidual reaction in cervical stroma of a young woman at 10 weeks of pregnancy. The cervix had a clinically suspicious appearance and was biopsied to exclude a tumour. The stroma shows swollen pale cells with abundant cytoplasm, well-defined cell membranes and regular nuclei (H&E). (B) Decidual cells in a cervical smear taken from the same patient. The cells are similar to those in the biopsy, appearing swollen and pale against the background of neutrophil polymorphs (PAP). (Courtesy of Professor B. Naylor, Michigan, USA.)

Decidual cells have been found in 34% of conventional smears from women with histologically confirmed decidual change in the cervix.[4] The number of decidual cells per smear varied from 11 to 208 with a mean of 105 and they tend to be arranged in loose sheets accompanied by neutrophil polymorphs. The cells are usually polygonal, more rarely having a spindled shape. Nuclei are large and usually have finely granular chromatin with prominent eosinophilic nucleoli. The cytoplasm is plentiful, transparent and basophilic or amphophilic (Fig. 25.3B).

A history of pregnancy is helpful in avoiding confusion of decidual cells with repair cells and neoplastic glandular or squamous cells.

## Arias–Stella change

Interpretive problems may arise during pregnancy if the endocervical glandular epithelium undergoes the type of extreme hypersecretory activity known as Arias–Stella change. This has been observed in 9% of cervices from hysterectomy specimens obtained during pregnancy[5] and is due to the action of human chorionic gonadotrophin. It can also occur in other hyperprogestational states such as gestational trophoblastic disease and with high-dose progestogen or ovulation-inducing therapy.[6] Histologically, the cervix shows an exaggerated secretory pattern in the glands, associated with papillary infoldings of the epithelium, mirroring the findings in endometrium (see Ch. 26). The nuclei may be pleomorphic and hyperchromatic and the cytoplasm is vacuolated, producing a hobnail appearance at the cell surface. When superficial endocervical glands show Arias–Stella change it is possible for cells from these glands to be seen in a cervical smear.

## Cytological findings: Arias–Stella change

- Atypical glandular cells in the presence of pregnancy or other hyperprogestational state
- Large pleomorphic eccentric nuclei, vacuolated cytoplasm.

The cytological features have been described in single case reports,[7,8] and in one of these, the cervical Arias–Stella reaction was associated with a cervical pregnancy. Atypical glandular cells occur singly, in syncytial clusters and cohesive sheets. They have large, hyperchromatic, pleomorphic nuclei with finely granular or smudged chromatin and one or two small nucleoli. The nuclear cytoplasmic ratio is low and the cells have abundant, frequently microvacuolated cytoplasm. A few intranuclear cytoplasmic inclusions and large, bare, hyperchromatic nuclei may also be present. Arias–Stella cells could be misinterpreted as malignant glandular cells if the history of pregnancy is not known.[9]

## Endometriosis

Endometriosis refers to the presence of endometrial glands and stroma outside the body of the uterus. Cervical endometriosis is uncommon unless there has been a previous operative procedure, superficial endometriosis then resulting from direct implantation, as a response to injury, or as a metaplastic or neoplastic process (Fig. 25.4). In a study of 42 cervices from hysterectomies following conisation, Ismail reported the presence of endometriosis in 43% of cases.[10] This ectopic tissue is hormonally responsive and friable and the patient may therefore present with irregular contact bleeding.

## Cytological findings: endometriosis

- Bloodstained conventional smears due to contact bleeding
- Strips and sheets of endometrial epithelial cells
- Endometrial stromal cells in loose groups or admixed with epithelial cells
- Mitoses and mild nuclear atypia may be present
- Aspirated specimens may include degenerate red blood cells and haemosiderin-laden macrophages.

In cervical cytology samples, endometrial cells from the cervix are well preserved and are arranged in large sheets or strips showing gland openings and nuclear stratification respectively (Fig. 25.4B). The smears are often heavily blood-stained.

Endometrial cells have a high nuclear/cytoplasmic ratio, relatively hyperchromatic nuclei with irregular contours and coarse chromatin; they may have prominent nucleoli and mitoses may be found. These features, together with the exfoliation pattern described, carry the risk that the cells may be mistaken for dyskaryotic endocervical cells. The latter cells, however, typically show flat sheets of monotonous cells with crowded overlapping nuclei and the sheets have more striking architectural abnormalities (see Ch. 24). Nevertheless,

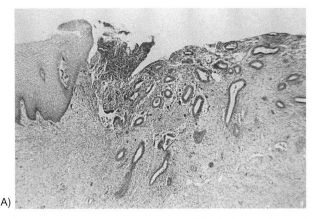

(A)

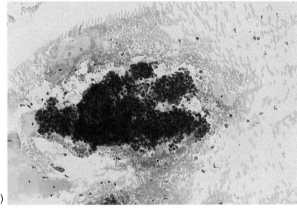

(B)

**Fig. 25.4** (A) Endometriosis of cervix. The biopsy was taken from a haemorrhagic friable area at the external os in a middle-aged woman presenting with contact bleeding 9 months after diathermy to a prominent nabothian follicle. Note the cellular endometrial stroma surrounding irregular glands lined by darkly stained epithelium of endometrial type (H&E). (B) Endometrial cell group composed of crowded cells with hyperchromatic nuclei in a haemorrhagic background. Cervical smear is from the patient whose biopsy is shown in (A) (PAP).

diagnostic problems may arise, especially if endometriosis has developed following treatment for cervical glandular neoplasia.

Endometrial stromal cells may also be present, either in loose groups with ragged edges or admixed with the epithelial cells. Stromal cells are oval or round with rounded or reniform nuclei and scanty ill-defined cytoplasm, which is more abundant during the secretory phase of the cycle. Their presence enables the diagnosis of endometriosis to be made.[11,12]

The possibility of endometriosis should also be considered when reporting fine needle aspirates from the cervix or other sites. Aspirated specimens contain endometrial epithelial and stromal cells arranged in biphasic clusters or in separate groups of one cell type. Haemosiderin-laden macrophages and degenerate red blood cells are also usually present. The problem of misinterpreting mildly atypical glandular cells as adenocarcinoma in an aspirate from a caecal endometriotic mass has been reported.[13]

## Nabothian follicles

Nabothian follicles or mucus retention cysts are cystically dilated endocervical crypts, which develop because the opening of the gland becomes occluded by inspissated mucus or

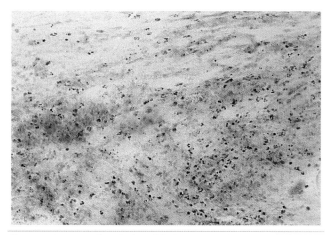

**Fig. 25.5** Contents of a nabothian follicle in a cervical smear showing granular inflammatory debris mixed with thick mucoid material (PAP).

metaplastic epithelium at the orifice of the crypt. If a follicle is ruptured while taking a conventional smear, streaks of mucoid inflammatory debris may be obtained (Fig. 25.5), associated with multinucleate cells having abundant foamy cytoplasm. While some of these cells are clearly histiocytes, others are endocervical in origin. Degenerate forms with pyknotic nuclei may be confused with dyskaryotic cells.

## Microglandular endocervical hyperplasia

The term microglandular hyperplasia is applied to an alteration in endocervical glandular tissue frequently seen in pregnancy or during oral contraception and other hormone therapy. It is thought to be due to progestogen stimulation and does not appear to have any premalignant potential. Typically, there are one or more small polypoid areas arising from the endocervical canal but more extensive involvement of the endocervical epithelium also occurs. The microscopic features have been fully described in Chapter 24.

## Malakoplakia

Malakoplakia is an uncommon chronic inflammatory condition usually involving the urinary tract but which can affect many other organs. It is thought to result from an acquired defect in macrophage function resulting in an inability to degrade ingested bacteria, particularly *E. coli*. It is often associated with primary or acquired immunodeficiency.

Malakoplakia of the female genital tract is rare, occurring most often in the vagina.[14] The patient is typically elderly and presents with postmenopausal bleeding. Polypoid friable lesions may be seen in the vagina and on the cervix, simulating malignancy. Histologically, there is an infiltrate of histiocytes with abundant granular eosinophilic cytoplasm. Some of these cells contain the pathognomonic intracytoplasmic calcified laminated spherules known as Michaelis–Gutmann bodies and microorganisms may sometimes be demonstrated.

### Cytological findings: malakoplakia

- Numerous plump histiocytes with large vesicular nuclei
- Endothelial-lined capillaries associated with histiocytes

- Background of mixed inflammatory cells
- Intracytoplasmic bacilli and Michaelis–Gutmann bodies may be seen.

The cytological features have been described in cervical smears[15] and in fine needle aspiration (FNA) material from a vaginal mass.[16] Both types of specimen tend to be highly cellular, the majority of cells being single histiocytes with a background of other inflammatory cells, usually neutrophil polymorphs, lymphocytes and plasma cells. The histiocytes have large vesicular nuclei with abundant granular or finely vacuolated cytoplasm.

The number of Gram-negative bacilli and Michaelis–Gutmann bodies recognised within the histiocytes varies widely from case to case. Stewart and Thomas describe the presence of prominent endothelium-lined capillaries associated with many of the histiocytes.[15]

## Epithelial changes simulating neoplasia

## Reserve cell hyperplasia

Single reserve cells, as described in Chapter 23, lie between the columnar endocervical cells and the basement membrane, predominantly in the proximal part of the endocervical canal. When they proliferate without maturing this is described as reserve cell hyperplasia. It is often seen in pregnant or postmenopausal women and in women using oral contraceptives, representing the earliest stage in the evolution of immature squamous metaplasia. It may also result from tamoxifen therapy.[17]

Histologically, there are several layers of small primitive cells beneath the columnar endocervical epithelium (Fig. 25.6A). The cells have round or oval nuclei, finely granular chromatin and ill-defined cell boundaries. Atypical reserve cell hyperplasia is thought to be capable of progressing to either CIN 3 or endocervical neoplasia, thus reflecting the bipotential role of the reserve cell.

### Cytological findings: reserve cell hyperplasia

- Cells in sheets, clumps and pairs, and that are dissociated
- Little or no cytoplasm
- Nuclei are pale or normochromatic
- Columnar cells may be attached
- Anisocytosis, nucleoli and mitoses are found in atypical hyperplasia.

Hyperplastic reserve cells are typically shed in sheets and are also seen in rows with ramifications, in clumps, paired and single. Columnar endocervical cells may be attached to these cells, arranged in a single layer (Fig. 25.6B).

The reserve cells have oval, round or bean-shaped nuclei, slightly smaller than those of endocervical cells. One end of the nucleus may be pointed and there may be a longitudinal groove. Nuclear moulding is also a recognised feature. The chromatin is finely granular and a small nucleolus may be apparent. Most nuclei are naked when the cells are dissociated, although a small amount of poorly defined cytoplasm is occasionally present (Fig. 25.6B). Sheets of reserve cells typically have a syncytial appearance because cell borders are poorly defined.

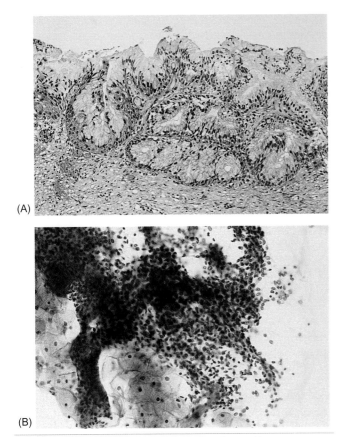

(A)

(B)

**Fig. 25.6** (A) Reserve cell hyperplasia in section of cervix. There is a multilayered row of immature cells beneath the tall columnar epithelium of the endocervical canal, showing no evidence of squamous metaplasia (H&E). (B) Reserve cell hyperplasia in cervical smear. This large cellular group of endocervical origin is more crowded than normal and shows many dissociated bare nuclei at the margins. The degree of crowding was thought suggestive of endocervical dyskaryosis, but biopsy showed reserve cell hyperplasia only (PAP).

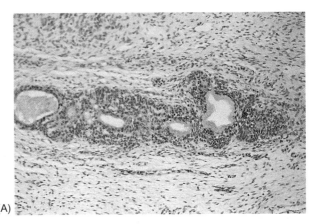

(A)

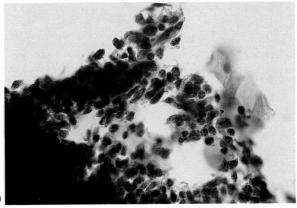

(B)

**Fig. 25.7** (A) Atypical reserve cell hyperplasia in cervical cone biopsy. There is a zone of multilayered reserve cells forming a cuff around most of the glands. The cells are crowded and disorganised in contrast to Figure 25.6A, but no mitoses are seen (H&E). (B) Atypical reserve cell hyperplasia in the cervical smear from the patient whose histology is illustrated in (A). Fragments of crowded small cells with hyperchromatic nuclei are seen, and were interpreted as severe glandular dyskaryosis. The cone biopsy showed CIN 1 in addition to the atypical reserve cell hyperplasia but no evidence of glandular intraepithelial neoplasia was found (PAP).

### Diagnostic pitfalls: reserve cell hyperplasia

In atypical reserve cell hyperplasia the cells show the same exfoliation pattern, but the nuclei show anisokaryosis which may be marked. The nuclear border is prominent and the chromatin is slightly granular but evenly dispersed (Fig. 25.7). The nuclei are normo- or hypochromatic rather than hyperchromatic. Nucleoli may be visible and mitoses can be seen. Atypical reserve cells are rarely seen in negative samples, tending to be present when dyskaryotic squamous or glandular cells are also present. The higher the grade of dyskaryosis the more likely is the finding of atypical reserve cells. They can usually be distinguished from dyskaryotic cells, which have denser cytoplasm and hyperchromatic nuclei.[18,19]

## Tubal metaplasia

Tubal metaplasia refers to replacement of epithelium at müllerian-derived sites, such as the endometrial cavity or endocervix, by benign epithelium resembling that of the fallopian tube. It has been found in between 31% and 100% of adequately sampled cervices removed for both neoplastic and non-neoplastic reasons.[20–22] Tubal metaplasia frequently includes cells of endometrial type, so-called tuboendometrioid

metaplasia (Fig. 25.8). Ismail has also reported finding tubal or tuboendometrioid metaplasia in 26% of cervices removed after cone biopsy.[10]

The changes tend to be multifocal and involve upper endocervical crypts more commonly than the lower endocervix and surface epithelium: the findings are more likely to be encountered in cervical cytology specimens following the use of brush devices for LBC sampling.[22,23] Endometriosis may also occur in the same group of patients, as already described, although it is a less frequent event.

Although not thought to be preneoplastic, it is important that the cytological appearances are recognised and not misinterpreted as indicating endocervical glandular dysplasia. In a study by Novotny and co-workers[24] tubal metaplasia accounted for the smear appearances in 76% of cases in which endocervical glandular dysplasia had been suggested.

### Cytological findings: tubal metaplasia (Fig. 25.9)

- Numerous columnar cells, some ciliated and non-ciliated
- Large- to medium-sized sheets and clusters, and single cell arrangements
- Nuclei larger and darker than endocervical cells
- Intercalary cells may be recognised.

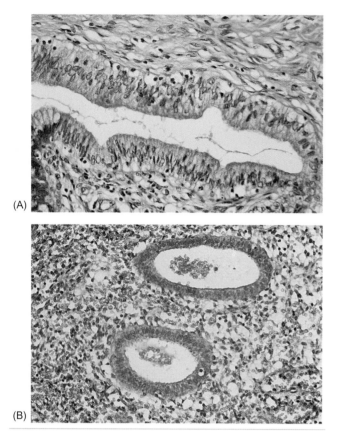

(A)

(B)

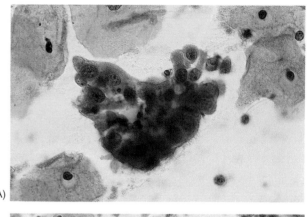

(A)

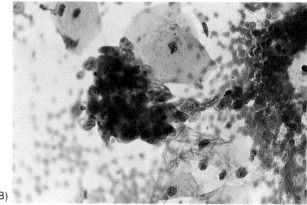

(B)

**Fig. 25.8** (A) Tubal metaplasia in histological section of cervix. The endocervical gland lining consists of ciliated cells with slight multilayering imparting a more disorganised appearance than is usually seen in endocervical mucosa or glands (H&E). (B) Tuboendometrioid metaplasia of cervix showing two glands lined by cells with tubal and endometrial features, set in inflamed stroma (H&E).

**Fig. 25.9** (A) Tubal metaplasia in a group of glandular cells in a cervical smear taken as follow-up of treated CIN. There is a columnar border showing ciliated cells along the lower edge of the group. Intercalary cells cannot be identified (PAP). (B) Tuboendometrioid metaplasia in the same smear as shown (A). This group shows degenerative features with nuclear irregularities and crowding as seen in endometrial cells, although without the characteristic central core of stroma (PAP).

The changes in both conventional smears and liquid-based preparations have been described in detail.[23–28] The three cell types seen in fallopian tube epithelium should be present, namely ciliated cells, secretory non-ciliated cells and intercalary cells. Their proportion in a sample varies greatly, but ciliated columnar cells with apical terminal bars are necessary for diagnosis.

The cells are arranged in flat sheets, three-dimensional clusters, small poorly cohesive groups or they may occur singly. Cells are smaller than endocervical cells but nuclei tend to be larger and evenly spaced, although there may be overlapping of nuclei in the three-dimensional groups.

They are oval, round or elongated and are usually basal in position. The chromatin is finely granular and typically slightly darker than that of endocervical cell nuclei. Nucleoli are more often visible in LBC preparations and are small and single.

Intercalary cells, exclusive to tubal metaplasia yet not readily seen in cytology samples, have triangular dark staining nuclei and little cytoplasm, in contrast to the other cells which have varying amounts of granular or vacuolated cytoplasm. Mitoses are rare.

### Diagnostic pitfalls: tubal metaplasia

The presence of aligned ciliated cells is one of the most helpful features in distinguishing tubal metaplasia from endocervical glandular dysplasia, although cilia are not often preserved

in all groups in a sample. Rosettes, palisades of cells and the feathered appearance at the edge of sheets of cells typically seen in adenocarcinoma *in situ* (AIS) are rarely seen in tubal metaplasia. The nuclei are also different in AIS, since they tend to be elongated and hyperchromatic with coarsely granular chromatin and prominent nucleoli. They are invariably crowded and stratified and mitotic figures are usually present.

Other differential diagnoses include cervical endometriosis, endometrial cells from the lower uterine segment, microglandular and reserve cell hyperplasia, 'reactive' endocervical cells and dyskaryotic cells from CIN 3 involving endocervical glands.

## Transitional cell metaplasia

Occasionally, metaplasia on the ectocervix to a transitional type of epithelium has been identified in histological sections of the cervix, particularly in older postmenopausal women. This change causes no symptoms and its importance lies principally in the potential for a mistaken diagnosis of high-grade CIN in hysterectomy specimens because of the lack of maturation of cells in crowded epithelium.[29] However, careful examination of tissue sections reveals uniformity of nuclei, an even chromatin pattern and lack of mitotic activity, thereby excluding the possibility of neoplasia. No direct relationship to cervical pre-cancer or invasive disease has been established but a recent study has suggested that transitional cell metaplasia may be related to human papillomavirus infection.[30]

Descriptions of the cytological findings when cells from this type of mucosa are sampled have been published. The finding of cohesive groups of cells containing streaming spindled nuclei with haloes, grooves, tapered ends and wrinkled contours permits distinction from squamous dyskaryosis.[30,31]

## Leukoplakia

Leukoplakia is a clinical concept describing the presence of white patches on the mucosa of the ectocervix or other areas of genital tract squamous epithelium. Typically, at the cervix, lesions are due to hyperkeratosis or parakeratosis of the ectocervical epithelium. The squamous mucosa may be atrophic or normal but is often hyperplastic and is covered by a thick layer of anucleate keratin (hyperkeratosis) or keratin in which pyknotic nuclei persist (parakeratosis). There is usually a well-defined granular layer beneath the layer of keratin.

These changes are often due to chronic irritation of the epithelium, for example, when there is uterine prolapse (Fig. 25.10A), if a pessary is in place or with severe chronic inflammation. Sometimes, however, the underlying epithelium is abnormal, showing evidence of HPV infection, CIN or invasive squamous carcinoma. Colposcopic examination is therefore appropriate if leukoplakia is present, even in the absence of dyskaryotic squamous cells in the cytology sample, to rule out serious underlying pathology.

### Cytological findings: leukoplakia

- Sheets of and single anucleate mature squamous cells
- Keratohyaline granules in squamous cell cytoplasm
- Small irregular pyknotic nuclei within keratotic squames in parakeratosis.

Anucleate squamous cells are present singly or in sheets or plaques. They are of intermediate or superficial cell size and stain bright orange or yellow with the Papanicolaou stain (Fig. 25.10B) in conventional smears. Some may contain pink or basophilic intracytoplasmic granules of keratohyaline. Parakeratotic cells are seen as smaller keratinised cells lying singly or in sheets with small slightly irregular pyknotic nuclei. Abnormal cells derived from underlying pathology may also be present.

## Repair and regeneration

When cervical mucosa is ulcerated or damaged re-epithelialisation of denuded stroma occurs, initially by immature metaplastic epithelium, to be replaced later by mature squamous epithelium. Changes due to repair and regeneration may be seen in cases of severe cervicitis and cytology samples taken after cervical biopsy, ablative therapy, or irradiation.[32–34] The cells obtained can be confused with dyskaryotic squamous and glandular cells. It is therefore advisable to delay follow-up smears for at least 4 months and preferably for 6 months after treatment.

Features seen histologically include thickening of the squamous epithelium, basal cell hyperplasia and immature squamous metaplasia. The nuclei may be hyperchromatic and have prominent nucleoli but there is no nuclear crowding or overlapping

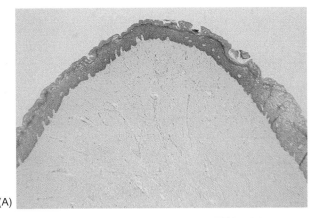

(A)

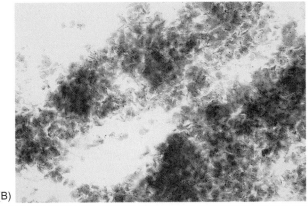

(B)

**Fig. 25.10** (A) Section of cervix from a case of uterine prolapse. The squamous mucosa is thickened and covered by a dense layer of keratin (H&E). (B) Hyperkeratosis in a cervical smear from a patient with procidentia. Much of the smear consisted of deeply stained anucleate squames from the keratinised surface of the cervix (PAP).

and normal maturation of cells in the upper layers of the mucosa. Endocervical epithelium may also display similar reactive features with nuclear enlargement and hyperchromasia, loss of cytoplasmic mucus and mitotic figures. Both mucosa and underlying stroma are inflamed and there may be granulation tissue formation.

### Cytological findings: repair and regeneration[32–36]

- Immature population of parabasal, metaplastic and reserve cells
- Repair cells, fibroblasts and inflammatory cells.

Repair cells are thought to originate from both epithelial and stromal cells,[30] the former showing varying degrees of differentiation towards squamous and columnar epithelium. Epithelial cells tend to occur in flat syncytial sheets in which uniform polarity is maintained, often resulting in a streaming appearance. They have enlarged oval pleomorphic nuclei containing one or more eosinophilic large nucleoli (Fig. 25.11), which indicate active protein synthesis in fast growing cells, and multinucleation is often present. The chromatin pattern is usually fine and regular but may be slightly coarse and hyperchromatic. The cytoplasm is abundant and has ragged margins; there is often evidence of leucophagocytosis. Mitotic figures may be seen.

Cells thought to be fibroblasts or stromal cells tend to occur in aggregates with oval nuclei and ribbon-like extensions of poorly defined cytoplasm (Fig. 25.12). The chromatin is

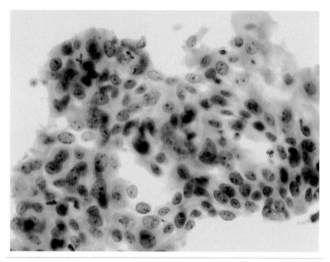

**Fig. 25.11** Repair changes in metaplastic squamous cells. The cells form a flat syncytial sheet and have enlarged nuclei with prominent nucleoli and sharply defined uniform nuclear borders. Note also the intercellular 'windows' and associated acute inflammatory cells (PAP).

uniformly finely granular. Single or multiple macronucleoli are present and are occasionally irregular. Other cell types to be found include parabasal cells, metaplastic squamous cells, reserve cells which may be atypical, neutrophil polymorphs, red blood cells and cellular debris.

### Diagnostic pitfalls: repair and regeneration

Although the repair process shares some features with adenocarcinoma and large cell non-keratinising squamous carcinoma, repair cells tend to display uniformity in numbers of chromocentres and nucleoli, an even distribution of chromatin and round smooth nuclear outlines with thin nuclear membranes, and uniform polarity; these features are not seen in malignant cells. Malignant cells occur singly as well as in groups, whereas repair cells are almost invariably grouped. A tumour diathesis may accompany carcinoma cells, while repair cells are frequently associated with neutrophil polymorphs.

When the chromatin of repair cells is coarse and hyperchromatic and the macronucleoli are pleomorphic and very prominent, they are said to be atypical and are difficult to distinguish from malignant cells. While the clinical significance of atypical repair is controversial, a repeat sample for borderline nuclear abnormality (atypical squamous cells of undetermined significance), as discussed in previous chapters, may be necessary, or a biopsy if there is a clinical suspicion of malignancy.[36–39] A recent study has suggested that reflex molecular analysis for HPV performed on LBC samples is helpful in predicting the possible association with underlying CIN.[40]

## Uncommon tumours of the cervix

## Special types of carcinoma

### Adenosquamous carcinoma

Adenosquamous carcinoma, defined as a tumour containing variable proportions of malignant squamous and glandular elements clearly recognisable without the use of special stains, comprises 3.6% of cervical carcinoma and presents in slightly

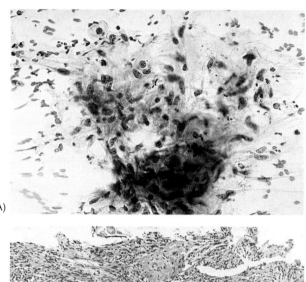

(A)

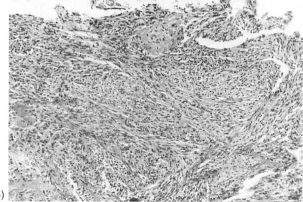

(B)

**Fig. 25.12** (A) Repair changes in stromal cells in a cervical smear from a 78-year-old-woman. The cells are elongated, with ill-defined cytoplasm and have prominent nucleoli (PAP). (B) Granulation tissue found on biopsy of cervix of patient whose smear is illustrated in (A). The fibroblasts within the newly formed tissue are similar to the stromal cells found in the smear (H&E). (Courtesy of Professor B. Naylor, Michigan, USA.)

younger women than squamous cell carcinoma (Fig. 25.13).[41,42] It is disputed whether adenosquamous carcinoma has a similar prognosis to adenocarcinoma and squamous cell carcinoma of the cervix.[41,43,44] Uncommitted subcolumnar reserve cells are probably the cell type from which this neoplasm arises.

### Cytological findings: adenosquamous carcinoma (see Fig. 24.39)

- Severely dyskaryotic squamous and glandular cells
- Tumour diathesis.

Carcinoma cells are present and may consist of an obvious mixture of squamous and glandular cells, or only one type of differentiation may be apparent.

## Glassy cell carcinoma

Glassy cell carcinoma is considered to be a variant of adeno-squamous carcinoma since ultrastructurally, there is evidence of both glandular and squamous differentiation.[45] The prognosis is generally poor. Histologically, the tumour has an undifferentiated appearance, being composed of sheets of malignant cells with abundant finely granular eosinophilic cytoplasm and sharply defined cytoplasmic borders, large vesicular nuclei and prominent nucleoli (Fig. 25.14A). Mitoses tend to be numerous and the stroma is often infiltrated by lymphocytes, plasma cells and eosinophils.

Evidence of glandular and squamous differentiation may be present as focal acinar formation, demonstrable intra-cytoplasmic mucin, dyskeratotic cells and an occasional keratin pearl.

### Cytological findings: glassy cell carcinoma

- Numerous large malignant cells in syncytial groups

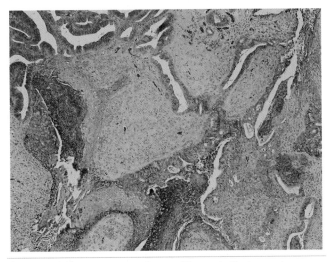

**Fig. 25.13** Adenosquamous carcinoma of the cervix. The tumour is composed of an intimate admixture of malignant squamous and glandular epithelium (H&E).

- Large hyperchromatic nuclei, finely granular cytoplasm
- Prominent nucleoli
- Tumour diathesis.

The cytological features in both conventional smears and liquid-based preparations have been described.[46,47] The tumour cells tend to be numerous and arranged in groups with a syncytial appearance or in sheets and clusters. A few single tumour cells may also be present. They are larger than severely dyskaryotic squamous cells and show marked anisokaryosis. The nuclei are large and hyperchromatic, the chromatin having a finely granular appearance. Large irregular nucleoli are often present.

A moderate amount of cytoplasm is present which may have a finely granular appearance (Fig. 25.14B, C). Inflammatory cells, including eosinophils, may be conspicuous in the background and may be seen closely associated with tumour cells.

The cytological features can be confused with poorly differentiated large cell non-keratinising squamous carcinoma, the nuclei of which tend to have coarser chromatin and less nucleolar abnormality, and with atypical reparative cells which do not fulfil the nuclear criteria of malignancy. Misdiagnosis as a low-grade squamous abnormality can occur if the sheets of cells have bland nuclear features, leading to delay in diagnosis.[48]

### Adenoid cystic and adenoid basal carcinoma

These are both rare types of cervical carcinoma that have a number of features in common, namely cells with basaloid

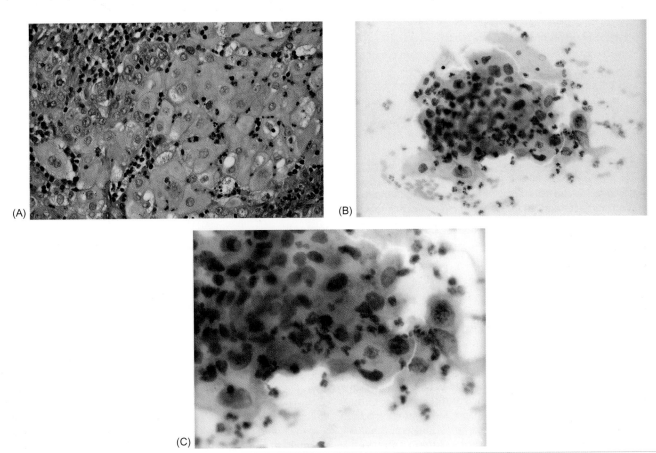

**Fig. 25.14** (A) Glassy cell carcinoma in histological section of cervix showing a compact arrangement of medium to large malignant cells with pale cytoplasm, pleomorphic nuclei, prominent nucleoli and frequent mitoses. Mucin stains showed occasional cells with mucin secretion but the majority resemble a non-keratinising squamous carcinoma. Medium (B) and high power (C) views of cells from a glassy cell carcinoma of cervix showing syncytial sheets with anisokaryosis (PAP).

morphology, an association with HPV infection, occurrence in postmenopausal women, an association with squamous neoplasia and similar cytological appearances in cervical cytology samples. In addition, they may occur together and be associated with carcinosarcoma.[49]

Adenoid cystic carcinoma usually presents as a symptomatic cervical mass. It has a similar histological appearance to adenoid cystic carcinoma more commonly seen in the salivary glands, consisting of cribriform sheets of crowded basaloid cells with nuclei containing dense chromatin and frequent mitoses. The glandular spaces contain clear hyaline or PAS-positive eosinophilic basement membrane-like material and there may also be a trabecular, solid or undifferentiated growth pattern surrounded by hyaline material. Vascular and perineural lymphatic space invasion is a characteristic finding responsible for the high incidence of recurrence and metastases and consequent poor prognosis.

Adenoid basal carcinoma is usually an incidental finding during investigation for a squamous lesion or non-neoplastic gynaecological disorder. It consists of rounded nests or islands of uniform basaloid cells with peripheral palisading that invade the cervical stroma with minimal or no desmoplastic reaction. There may be focal cystic change, columnar cell or squamous differentiation. The absence of basement membrane material, necrosis, vascular or lymphatic space invasion and low mitotic count allow distinction from adenoid cystic carcinoma. The prognosis is excellent: metastases and death from adenoid basal carcinoma have not been reported.

### Cytological findings: adenoid cystic and adenoid basal carcinoma

- Groups and sheets of small uniform cells
- Hyperchromatic nuclei, indistinct nucleoli and scant cytoplasm.

These tumours are rarely diagnosed in cervical cytology samples, either because no tumour cells are present, reflecting the fact that the overlying mucosa is usually intact, or because the tumour cells present are misinterpreted as benign or abnormal endometrial cells. The cells are small, tend to be arranged in irregularly shaped three-dimensional groups and sheets, and have small uniform hyperchromatic nuclei, occasional small nucleoli and scanty cytoplasm. They may also form cords and acini, some of which contain globules of hyaline material if derived from an adenoid cystic carcinoma.

The differential diagnosis includes endocervical adenocarcinoma, endometrial adenocarcinoma, small cell neuroendocrine carcinoma, in which nuclear moulding and frequent mitoses are seen, and severe squamous dyskaryosis, in which the cells tend to be larger and less uniform.

If the tumours occur in association with *in situ* or invasive squamous neoplasia both tumour cell types may be present in the same smear.[50–52]

## Neuroendocrine carcinoma

Neuroendocrine carcinoma of the cervix is rare. It is typically seen in young to middle-aged women and presents as a symptomatic cervical mass. Generally, it has a poorer prognosis than squamous or adenocarcinoma. The origin is uncertain but the observation that some neuroendocrine carcinomas are associated with areas of squamous, glandular or adenosquamous differentiation lends support to the theory that they are derived from pluripotential basal or reserve cells.

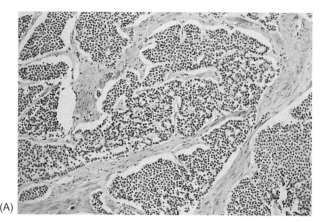

(A)

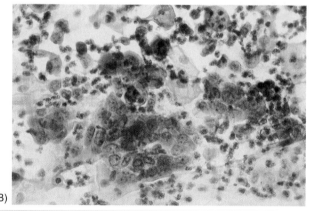

(B)

**Fig. 25.15** (A) Neuroendocrine tumour of cervix of carcinoid type, composed of nests, clumps and ribbons of small regular cells set in dense fibrous stroma (H&E). (B) Neuroendocrine carcinoma cells in cervical smear showing a cohesive group of crowded cells with hyperchromatic nuclei and well-defined nucleoli (PAP). (Courtesy of Dr C. Waddell and Dr M. Light, Birmingham, UK.)

The appearances range from a well-differentiated tumour (Fig. 25.15) with a trabecular or solid streaming pattern typical of a carcinoid tumour, to a small cell undifferentiated carcinoma resembling oat cell carcinoma of bronchus (Fig. 25.16).[53] The latter is the commonest type of cervical neuroendocrine carcinoma. The frequency with which argyrophilic neurosecretory granules are demonstrable in the cytoplasm varies between the types of cervical neuroendocrine carcinoma and definitive diagnosis is more reliable achieved, particularly in the undifferentiated carcinomas, by immunohistochemistry: most tumours stain positive for chromogranin, synaptophysin or both.

### Cytological findings: neuroendocrine carcinoma

- Small cells, scanty cytoplasm
- Round or oval nuclei with indistinct nucleoli
- Coarse chromatin and nuclear moulding in conventional smears if poorly differentiated
- Malignant squamous and glandular cells often also present
- Tumour diathesis usually seen.

If the tumour is well-differentiated the cells are usually in nests and have round to oval mildly pleomorphic nuclei containing small punctate reddish nucleoli and finely granular chromatin. Cytoplasm is scant and eosinophilic or basophilic, the cytoplasmic borders being ill-defined.[54]

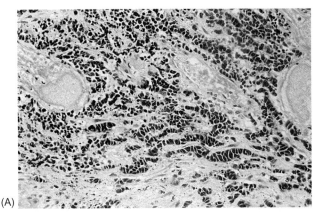

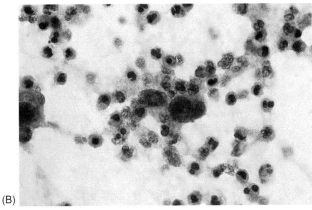

(A)

(B)

**Fig. 25.16** (A) Poorly differentiated neuroendocrine carcinoma of cervix in histological section. The tumour cells are similar to those seen in an oat cell carcinoma of bronchus, infiltrating in sheets and ribbons, with a high nuclear/cytoplasmic ratio and hyperchromatic nuclei. Nuclear moulding and pyknosis are also seen. Immunohistochemistry was in keeping with the diagnosis of neuroendocrine carcinoma (H&E). (B) Cervical smear from the same patient showed marked tumour diathesis and a few small clusters of malignant cells with little cytoplasm and coarsely granular hyperchromatic nuclei (PAP).

The cells of poorly differentiated tumours tend to be ovoid and to occur singly, although papillary clusters with associated psammoma bodies have been described.[55,56] Nuclear moulding is typically present in conventional cervical smears but may not be conspicuous in LBC preparations.[57] The nuclei are oval and hyperchromatic with coarse or smudged chromatin and show minimal anisokaryosis. Nucleoli are indistinct. There is a thin rim of cytoplasm (Figs 25.15, 25.16).

### Diagnostic pitfalls: neuroendocrine carcinoma

Neuroendocrine carcinoma cells can be confused with poorly differentiated squamous carcinoma, adenocarcinoma or lymphoma.[58] If the sample contains two cell populations, because a squamous or glandular component is present, confusion with an adenosquamous carcinoma can arise or the neuroendocrine component may be completely overlooked. The presence of nuclear moulding, indistinct nucleoli and scanty cytoplasm are helpful features in detecting neuroendocrine carcinoma. Metastatic pulmonary small cell carcinoma must be considered, although metastases to the cervix are usually within the stroma and covered by intact mucosa, at least in the early stages; an appropriate history of lung tumour should be sought.

## Lymphoepithelioma-like carcinoma

This variant of squamous carcinoma may have a more favourable prognosis than the usual squamous cell carcinoma. Although morphologically similar to nasopharyngeal lymphoepithelioma-like carcinoma (LEC), there is geographical variation in the association with Epstein–Barr virus, and it is unclear whether the tumour has the same high degree of radiosensitivity.

Histologically, the tumour comprises syncytial groups of anaplastic cells, intimately associated with a prominent lymphoid infiltrate.

### Cytological findings: lymphoepithelioma-like carcinoma

- Uniform large tumour cells with indistinct borders
- Round or oval hyperchromatic nuclei
- Finely granular to flocculent cytoplasm
- Lymphocytes are often closely associated with tumour cells
- Background of blood and inflammatory cells.

Reich et al.[59] and Proca et al.[60] have reported the cytological features in three cases of LEC. The tumour cells occur singly and in small clusters. They have a high nuclear cytoplasmic ratio. The nuclear chromatin has an irregular pattern and tends to show peripheral margination. One or more prominent nucleoli may be present. There is no evidence of dyskeratosis, keratinisation or koilocytosis and no glandular features are present. Proca et al.[60] emphasise that the tumour cells can easily be overlooked in a smear containing numerous red blood cells and inflammatory cells.

LEC may be confused cytologically with squamous cell carcinoma, glassy cell carcinoma and non-Hodgkin lymphoma, particularly of Lennert's type. The cells of a usual squamous cell carcinoma are more pleomorphic and hyperchromatic than those of a lymphoepithelioma-like carcinoma and have distinct cell borders, as do glassy cell carcinoma cells, which are also recognised by the ground-glass appearance of their cytoplasm.

## Carcinosarcoma (malignant mixed müllerian tumour)

This tumour is now generally accepted to be a metaplastic carcinoma.[61] In the majority of cases, carcinosarcoma of the cervix represents spread of tumour from the endometrium. In a series of 202 patients with cervical involvement by this tumour, only one case was shown to be a primary cervical neoplasm.[62] Most present at around the age of the menopause and the prognosis is generally poor. There is a well-established association with prior pelvic irradiation where these tumours occur at a younger age.[63]

The histological blend of carcinomatous and sarcomatous elements is variable but there is always a component of undifferentiated small cells and spindle cells. Heterologous elements of rhabdomyosarcomatous, chondrosarcomatous or other type are present in about 50% of cases.[64]

### Cytological findings: carcinosarcoma (Fig. 25.17)

- Carcinomatous cells, usually adenocarcinomatous
- Pleomorphic and spindle-shaped sarcomatous cells
- Small undifferentiated cells
- Tumour diathesis, blood-stained smears.

Most studies of smear findings are based largely on endometrial tumours, and abnormal cells are detected by cervical cytology

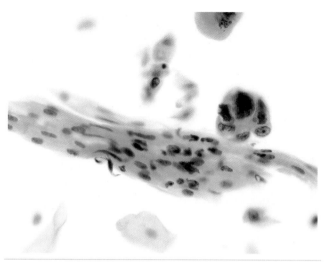

**Fig. 25.17** Cells from a carcinosarcoma (malignant mixed müllerian tumour) of the endometrium in a LBC cytology sample. Highly atypical malignant epithelial cells are associated with atypical spindle-shaped cells on a clean background (SurePath).

in only a low proportion of such cases.[65,66] Adenocarcinoma cells are the commonest epithelial abnormality to appear in cervicovaginal smears, often having a papillary arrangement.[67] Spindle-shaped malignant cells represent the sarcomatous component and these show pleomorphism and multinucleation. Heterologous elements are rare and are difficult to recognise with certainty in smears. The small undifferentiated cells of carcinosarcoma are usually present.

The related, but less common müllerian carcinofibroma has a better prognosis than carcinosarcoma and occurs principally in the uterine body, but can arise in the cervix. It comprises a mixture of malignant epithelium and a benign mesenchymal component, usually a fibroma. The adenocarcinoma cells in the case reported by Imai et al.[68] showed papillary and tubular arrangements. The spindle-shaped and ovoid cells were numerous and scattered throughout the smear. They had a thin nuclear membrane, fine chromatin and narrow, pale cytoplasm. They were larger than normal endometrial stromal cells and no mitotic activity or nuclear atypia were evident, but a tumour diathesis was present in the blood-stained smear.

## Mesenchymal tumours

### Benign mesenchymal tumours

Approximately 8% of uterine leiomyomas (fibroids) occur in the cervix, making these the commonest benign mesenchymal neoplasms at this site. They are usually solitary. If the overlying mucosa is ulcerated benign smooth muscle cells from the lesion may be present in cervical cytology samples, but their site of origin cannot be identified without appropriate clinical information. The cytological findings are described in Chapter 27.

Other benign mesenchymal tumours, namely haemangioma, neurilemmoma, lipoma, paraganglioma and adenofibroma are uncommon and the cytological findings have not so far been documented in cervical smears.

Adenomyomas and polypoid adenomyomas are rare. They comprise a mixture of benign endocervical glands and stroma composed predominantly of smooth muscle.

Atypical polypoid adenomyoma also rarely arises in the cervix. The glandular component in this entity is indistinguishable from endometrial intraepithelial neoplasia and there are usually conspicuous squamous morules.

The cytological features of both typical and atypical polypoid adenomyoma have recently been described. In both cases cervical smears contained spindle-shaped smooth muscle cells but whilst in the case of polypoid adenomyoma there were sheets and strips of reactive endocervical cells in an inflammatory background, in the case of atypical polypoid adenomyoma there were tightly packed, crowded clusters of atypical glandular cells suspicious of adenocarcinoma.[69]

### Malignant mesenchymal tumours

Malignant mesenchymal tumours arising as a primary neoplasm of the cervix are very rare. The most frequently encountered types are leiomyosarcoma and endometrial stromal sarcoma. They have similar clinical behaviour and microscopic features to their more common counterparts in the uterine corpus as described in Chapter 27. Sarcoma botryoides (embryonal rhabdomyosarcoma), an aggressive rare tumour of the vagina in young girls, may very occasionally develop as a primary neoplasm of the cervix.

### Endometrial stromal sarcoma

This tumour arises primarily in the body of the uterus and, although spread to the cervix can occur, cervical or vaginal smears do not usually contribute to diagnosis. The cytological findings are described in Chapter 27.

### Embryonal rhabdomyosarcoma (sarcoma botryoides)

The cervix is very rarely the primary site of this aggressive tumour. It typically presents in the reproductive years with vaginal discharge or a vaginal mass. The tumour develops beneath the surface epithelium and produces a polypoid mass. The cytological features of a case have been described by Matsuura et al.[70]

**Cytological findings: embryonal rhabdomyosarcoma**

- Loose clusters of short spindle-shaped cells
- Elongated, scanty cytoplasm, with indistinct cell borders
- Tumour diathesis.

The tumour nuclei are elongated or oval with a thin nuclear membrane, variable but usually fine chromatin and tend to have macronucleoli which are partly clear. The degree of cellular atypia ranges from mild to severe. Cross striations are rarely present. Without immunocytochemistry to confirm rhabdomyoblastic differentiation, distinction from a leiomyosarcoma is difficult.

## Malignant melanoma

Malignant melanoma of the cervix is very rare and is usually secondary to vaginal melanoma, presenting as an ulcerated or polypoid mass, which bleeds readily. The prognosis is poor and most patients die within 2 years of diagnosis. The histological features (Fig. 25.18A) are typical of melanoma at other sites, showing infiltration of tissues by epithelioid or spindle-shaped tumour cells with large pleomorphic nuclei and prominent nucleoli. Multinucleate forms are common and intracytoplasmic melanin is often present.[71]

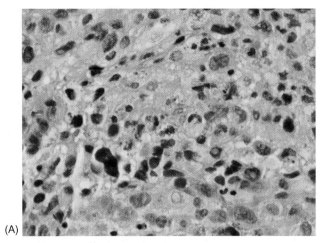

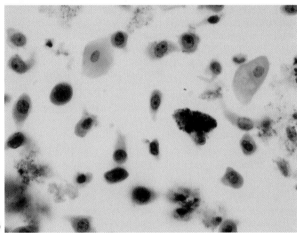

**Fig. 25.18** (A) Malignant melanoma forming a polypoid mass in the vagina that presented with post-menopausal bleeding. There was no evidence of melanoma elsewhere. Brown melanin pigment is visible in some of the pleomorphic tumour cells (H&E). (B) Liquid based cervical cytology sample from the patient whose histology is illustrated in (A) showing dissociated pleomorphic malignant cells, with prominent nucleoli and, in some, abundant intracytoplasmic brown melanin pigment (SurePath).

- Pleomorphic single cells or dissociating groups
- Eccentric nuclei and prominent nucleoli
- Intranuclear cytoplasmic inclusions
- Melanin may be visible
- Tumour diathesis.

The diagnosis of melanoma of the cervix may be suggested by exfoliative or FNA cytology.[72,73]

Although the cells can be arranged in loose groups and sheets, they typically occur singly. There is usually considerable cellular pleomorphism and the cells may be epithelioid or spindle shaped in appearance. The nuclei are pleomorphic and often eccentric. They can be hypo- or hyperchromatic, bi- or multinucleate and usually contain prominent nucleoli. The nuclear/cytoplasmic ratio is variable and nuclear moulding may be prominent. Cytoplasmic inclusions, appearing as rounded intranuclear vacuoles, are a feature of some melanomas. The cytoplasm may be abundant and contain melanin pigment. Cell borders tend to be ill-defined, having a lacy appearance.

**Diagnostic pitfalls: malignant melanoma**

Cellular pleomorphism is usually marked but melanoma cells can be small and uniform, blending with normal cervical cells on a smear, in which case they may be overlooked.

The differential diagnosis also includes squamous carcinoma, adenocarcinoma and sarcoma. Melanoma cells tend to be epithelioid but can be spindle shaped, in which case they may be misinterpreted as sarcomatous if the cells are exclusively of this type and no melanin is seen. A Masson–Fontana silver stain to detect melanin pigment may be helpful if pigment is not apparent on a Papanicolaou-stained smear. Immunocytochemistry, using antibodies to S100 protein or a more specific melanoma marker such as HMB 45, NKI C3 or Melan A, may be helpful if sufficient material is available.

## Lymphoma and leukaemia

Primary non-Hodgkin lymphoma of the cervix is a rare but well-documented event and is usually of diffuse large B cell type. Secondary involvement of the female genital tract by lymphoma or leukaemia is more commonly encountered, occurring in up to 40% of cases.[74] Advanced Hodgkin's disease also may involve the cervix.

Primary non-Hodgkin lymphoma of cervix usually presents in middle-aged or elderly patients with vaginal bleeding and a cervical tumour mass, which is then biopsied. Much less often, a cervical cytology sample reveals abnormal cells, which may be recognised as lymphoid.

**Cytological findings: lymphoma and leukaemia**

- Blood-stained specimen
- Dissociated abnormal lymphoid or plasma cells
- Tumour diathesis present.

The cytological features of lymphoma of the cervix have largely been limited to single case reports, although a few small series have been reported.[75,76] Smears are typically normal or only show non-specific inflammation if the neoplastic cells are covered by intact mucosa. Details of the diagnostic features of the different types of lymphoma are given in Chapter 13. Subtyping of lymphomas in conventional cervical smears is not reliable but liquid-based preparations offer the possibility of immunostaining the abnormal cells with a panel of antibodies for phenotyping and accurate classification.

Myeloma rarely affects the female genital tract. Atypical plasma cells have been described in the smear from a woman with postmenopausal bleeding in whom the diagnosis of myeloma had yet to be made.[77] Myeloma cells appeared as large single cells with scant or deeply basophilic cytoplasm, hyperchromatic eccentric nuclei, some of which were multinucleate and had prominent large irregular nucleoli.

Leukaemic deposits in cervical stroma may occasionally be sampled by cervical cytology. The appearance of the cells varies according to the type of leukaemia.[78]

**Diagnostic pitfalls: lymphoma and leukaemia**

Lymphomatous cells on a cervical cytology sample must be distinguished from chronic inflammatory cells, small cell carcinoma, small cell severe dyskaryosis, endometrial carcinoma, poorly differentiated adenocarcinoma, and sarcoma.

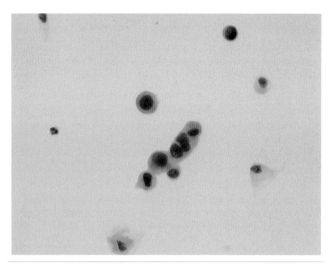

**Fig. 25.19** Metastatic carcinoma cells in a liquid based cervical cytology sample from a patient with known lobular carcinoma of the breast. The malignant epithelial cells form characteristic 'Indian files' similar to the appearance seen in histological sections. Breast is one of the commonest extragenital secondary tumours that involves the uterus (SurePath).

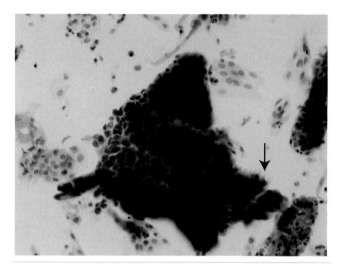

**Fig. 25.20** Metastatic adenocarcinoma in a liquid-based cervical cytology sample. Large complex folded sheets of malignant glandular cells are present. The palisaded border of tall columnar cells with intracytoplasmic mucin vacuoles (arrowed) is unlike the usual appearance of primary cervical adenocarcinoma. This patient had had a prior resection of a carcinoma of the rectum (PAP).

Reactive inflammatory cells will have a polymorphic appearance, being composed of a mixture of normal mature and immature lymphocytes, sometimes including plasma cells. A leukaemic infiltrate may be mistaken for follicular cervicitis if the appropriate history is not available. Small cell carcinoma cells tend to be irregularly shaped and pleomorphic with indistinct nucleoli. Characteristic nuclear moulding and clustering may be present. Cells of small cell severe dyskaryosis may present in sheets as well as singly and individual cells may show evidence of keratinisation.

Cells from a high-grade lymphoma may be mistaken for poorly differentiated adenocarcinoma. Features favouring the diagnosis of lymphoma include single dissociated cells with prominent nucleoli, nipple-like projections on the nuclei, chromatin clumping at the nuclear borders and scant cytoplasm.

## Metastatic tumours

Metastasis of carcinoma to the cervix is not uncommon and usually occurs in the presence of advanced disease. The cervical mucosa tends to remain intact so that tumour cells are not often seen in cytology preparations. The most common primary sites are elsewhere in the genital tract, the gastrointestinal tract and breast.[79] Tumour may also involve the cervix by direct invasion from the endometrium, bladder or rectum.

### Cytological findings: metastatic tumours

- Relative paucity of tumour cells
- Malignant nature of cells usually obvious
- Resemblance to known primary tumour.

The cytological findings are variable, depending on the nature of the original tumour, the presence or absence of ulceration and the extent of cervical involvement by the metastasis. In general there are fewer abnormal cells than in smears from primary tumours of cervix. The cells are readily recognised as malignant, but tumour typing may be difficult unless distinctive features are present (Fig. 25.19). Signet ring cell formation or large sheets of tall columnar vacuolated malignant cells palisaded along one edge may suggest an origin from the gastrointestinal tract (Fig. 25.20).

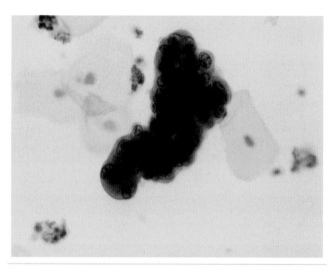

**Fig. 25.21** Papillary clustering of adenocarcinoma cells in a liquid based cervical cytology sample from a woman with ovarian serous carcinoma. The tumour had not spread to the cervix. The abnormal cells stand out on low power against a clean background (SurePath).

While strictly not true metastases, cells exfoliated from tumours of the fallopian tube, ovary or peritoneum may be found in cervical cytology specimens and often stand out from a clean background, with little or no tumour diathesis (Fig. 25.21) as discussed in Chapters 26 and 27. The cells may have a papillary pattern and psammoma bodies are sometimes noted. When psammoma bodies are identified, the likelihood of associated significant pathology is related to patient age, clinical symptoms and the presence of abnormal cells.[80]

In conclusion, awareness of the patient's history should alert one to the possibility of metastasis but it is important to remember that patients with one tumour are also more likely to develop further neoplasms. If abnormal cells are seen in a cervical cytology sample from a patient with a known carcinoma, the original tumour histology should be reviewed and compared with the cytological findings.

## Tumours of the vulva

## Introduction

Cytology specimens from the vulva are received in the laboratory far less frequently than those from the cervix. Vulval samples tend to be dry and, because many lesions have surface keratosis, they often consist mainly of anucleate squamous cells: as a result it has been difficult to establish a firm role for cytology in the diagnosis of vulval disease.

## Technical aspects

Smears taken from the vulva with a conventional spatula, unless from the introitus, will be dry. Improved cell preservation can be achieved by gently rubbing the area with a cotton wool swab dipped in saline and then squeezing and rolling the swab on to a glass slide to transfer the cells. Rapid fixation is essential, followed by Papanicolaou staining. When using these smears along with vulvoscopy in follow-up of vulval intraepithelial neoplasia, separate samples from the four vulval quadrants (right and left, anterior and posterior) can help to localise a recurrence. Recently, Levine et al. have described a brush and monolayer technique (cytospin) in the diagnosis and follow-up of vulval disease, allowing sampling from a wide area with minimum patient discomfort.[81] Touch preparations and brush samples may also be taken when lesions are ulcerated.

## Benign tumours of the vulva

The vulva is covered with skin and benign tumours seen elsewhere are also found at this site. Naevi, pyogenic granulomata, keratoacanthomas and seborrhoeic warts are among those most often diagnosed (see Ch. 30). Vulval skin includes numerous hair follicles and sebaceous, eccrine and apocrine glands but, despite this, skin adnexal tumours are unusual. Papillary hidradenoma is the most common.

### Papillary hidradenoma

This benign tumour of apocrine origin occurs almost exclusively in middle-aged white woman. It usually presents as a solitary, well circumscribed, mobile nodule less than 2 cm in diameter located in the interlabial sulcus. Although characteristically single, rare cases of women with multiple lesions have been reported.[82] Papillary hidradenoma may ulcerate and evert giving rise to a red, friable papillary mass. These tumours are most frequently diagnosed clinically, or on biopsy, but cases diagnosed by imprint or FNA cytology have been reported.[83,84]

Histologically, the lesions are composed of columnar eosinophilic glandular cells overlying a basal layer of smaller myoepithelial cells in a tubular and papillary growth pattern (Fig. 25.22).The cells seen on cytology are derived from the outer layer of cells and consist of clumps of slightly pleomorphic glandular cells with fine, evenly distributed chromatin and, in some cells, abundant rather granular looking cytoplasm.[84]

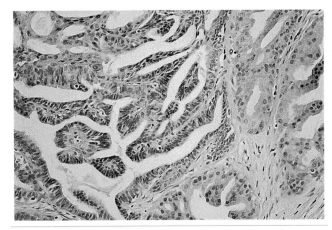

**Fig. 25.22** Vulval biopsy. A papillary hidradenoma. Note the papillary structure. The cells with granular cytoplasm have undergone 'apocrine metaplasia', similar to that seen in the breast. Nuclear pleomorphism and nucleoli can be seen (H&E).

## Malignant tumours of the vulva

Approximately 4% of malignant tumours in the female genital tract arise in the vulva and of these 90% are squamous cell carcinomas. The remainder include malignant melanoma, basal cell carcinoma and adenocarcinoma of Bartholin's gland.[85]

### Vulval intraepithelial neoplasia (VIN)

It is now well recognised that there are two types of VIN: undifferentiated VIN, associated with human papillomavirus (HPV) infection (especially type 16), and differentiated VIN, unrelated to HPV infection. Undifferentiated VIN occurs predominantly, but not exclusively, in younger women, tends to be multicentric and multifocal, is often associated with intraepithelial neoplasia elsewhere in the lower genital tract, and is of basaloid or Bowenoid histological type. By contrast, differentiated VIN is generally found in older women, is commonly unifocal and unicentric, associated with lichen sclerosus or squamous epithelial hyperplasia and shows evident squamous maturation. In addition, progression of undifferentiated VIN to invasive squamous cell carcinoma is relatively uncommon, whereas there is a strong association between differentiated VIN and invasive squamous carcinoma.[86]

Histologically, two patterns of undifferentiated VIN are seen; basaloid in which basal or parabasal type cells extend into the upper layers of the epidermis and Bowenoid or 'warty' in which premature cellular maturation, characterised by dyskeratosis, occurs in association with koilocytosis and multinucleation, (Fig. 25.23A, B). Both types of undifferentiated VIN may coexist in the same patient. In both types mitotic figures are found above the basal epithelial layer and are often of abnormal form. There is nuclear pleomorphism, a high nucleocytoplasmic ratio, irregular clumping of chromatin and parakeratosis or hyperkeratosis. Undifferentiated VIN is graded in the same way as CIN: nuclear abnormalities are present throughout the full epithelial thickness but when cellular abnormalities and lack of stratification and cytoplasmic differentiation are limited to the lower third the lesion is classed as VIN I. In VIN 2 abnormal cells extend into the middle third of the epithelium and in VIN 3 into the upper third.

In differentiated VIN the epithelium is thickened and parakeratotic with elongated anastomosing rete ridges. There is minimal atypia above the basal or parabasal layers where the cells are small

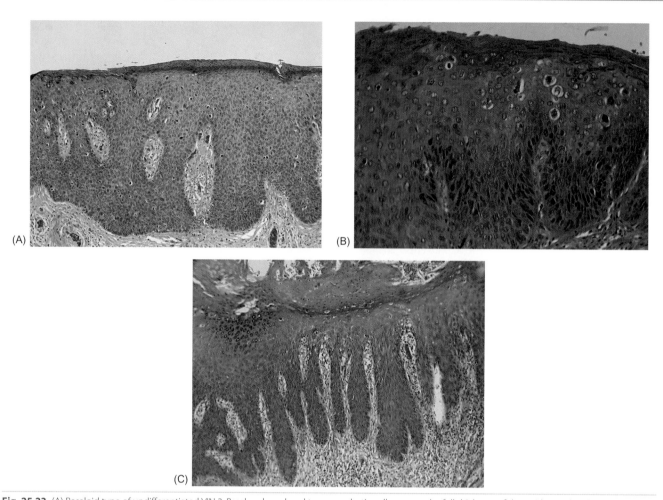

**Fig. 25.23** (A) Basaloid type of undifferentiated VIN 3. Basal and parabasal type neoplastic cells occupy the full thickness of the epidermis (H&E). (B) Bowenoid type of undifferentiated VIN 3. Note the characteristic dyskeratosis, koilocytosis and multinucleation of the neoplastic cells (H&E). (C) Differentiated VIN. Atypia is limited to the basal or parabasal layers and the more superficial layers are occupied by large eosinophilic keratinocytes with abnormal vesicular nuclei and prominent intercellular bridges (H&E).

and the nuclei have coarse chromatin and prominent nucleoli. The more superficial layers are occupied by large eosinophilic keratinocytes with abnormal vesicular nuclei and prominent intercellular bridges (Fig. 25.23C). Differentiated VIN is not graded.[86]

The most common presenting feature clinically is pruritus. On gross inspection, areas of VIN may be slightly raised and reddened, or keratotic. A colposcope may be used to help outline the areas of abnormal epithelium. It may be difficult clinically to distinguish VIN from viral warts and squamous carcinoma.[87]

### Cytological findings: vulval intraepithelial neoplasia

- Parakeratotic cells
- Dyskaryotic cells
- Anucleate squamous cells.

Descriptions of the cytological findings in VIN relate to undifferentiated VIN. Normal anucleate squamous cells are usually replaced by parakeratotic cells when significant degrees of VIN are present (Fig. 25.24). Parakeratosis alone should alert the observer to the possibility of VIN, although it may be seen in other dermatological conditions such as psoriasis. It is helpful for clinicians to know that if a lesion is clearly keratotic it is usually the cells beneath the white material, which rubs off, that are more likely to be diagnostic.

The cells may be single or in clumps. Dyskaryotic cells are identical to those seen in cervical cytology preparations.[81,87]

## Squamous cell carcinoma

By analogy to VIN, it is now recognised that there are two types of vulval squamous cell carcinoma. The more common, accounting for about two-thirds of cases, occurs in elderly women, is generally well-differentiated keratinising carcinoma, and associated with differentiated VIN, lichen sclerosus or squamous hyperplasia. The less common is seen in relatively young women, is usually moderately or poorly differentiated with basaloid or Bowenoid morphology and associated with undifferentiated VIN. It is disputed whether these two tumour types have a different prognosis.[86] The majority of tumours arise on the labia, especially the labia majora, and present as a mass, which is often ulcerated, or with pruritus, bleeding, discharge or pain.

### Cytological findings: squamous cell carcinoma

- Dyskaryotic squamous cells
- Bizarre cell types
- Tumour diathesis
- Parakeratotic groups
- Anucleate squamous cells.

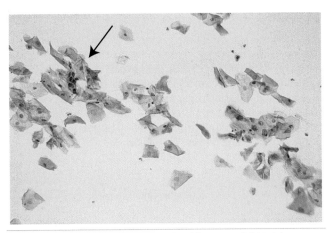

**Fig. 25.24** A swab smear from a case of undifferentiated VIN 3. A few parakeratotic cells are present in the centre of the field. Diagnostic severely dyskaryotic cells are in the group at the top (arrow) (PAP) × MP).

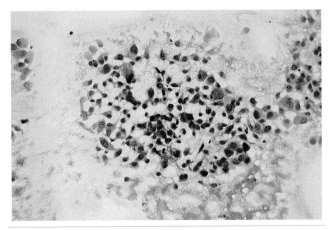

**Fig. 25.25** Malignant melanoma cells in a touch preparation. A loose cluster of cells with marked pleomorphism. Brown pigment can be seen in some of the cells (PAP).

The cytological features are identical to those seen in squamous carcinoma of the cervix and reflect the degree of differentiation of the tumour (see Ch. 26). Parakeratotic clusters and anucleate squamous cells derived from adjacent VIN may accompany the squamous carcinoma cells.

FNA cytology of inguinal lymph nodes may have a role in the management of vulval squamous carcinoma.[88]

## Basal cell carcinoma

This rare tumour usually involves the labia majora in postmenopausal women. The histological appearances are similar to those seen in basal cell carcinoma at other sites, including the characteristic peripheral palisading of cells (see Ch. 27).

## Malignant melanoma

This is a rare tumour of the vulva, but the second commonest malignant vulval tumour. The incidence progressively rises from teenage to peak in the sixth and seventh decade. The clitoris and labia majora are the principal sites and most patients present with a vulval mass, bleeding or itching. There is rarely evidence of a pre-existing naevus. The histological appearance is similar to that at extragenital sites and superficial spreading, nodular, mucosal lentiginous and neurotropic types have all been described in the vulva. As with other cutaneous melanomas, survival is principally related to the depth of invasion.[89,90]

---

**Cytological findings: malignant melanoma (Figs 25.25, 25.26)**

- Loose clusters of pleomorphic cells
- Nuclei of variable size and shape
- Pigment often present.

The cytological appearances are similar to those in extragenital sites and immunocytochemistry for S100 or more specific melanoma markers may be valuable, particularly in amelanotic lesions (see Ch. 26).

---

## Paget's disease of the vulva

This disease occurs most often in postmenopausal white women. The average age at diagnosis in most series is 65 years,

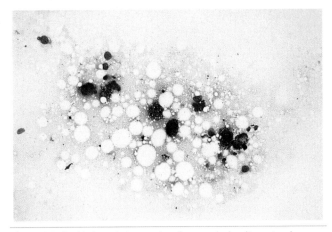

**Fig. 25.26** Air-dried touch preparations from a vulval malignant melanoma. The black pigment granules are more obvious (Giemsa).

and it is rarely diagnosed below 50 years of age. The lesions appear as intensely itchy, reddened, excoriated areas predominantly on the labia majora. There are only occasional multifocal lesions.[91]

Histologically, Paget's disease is a form of intraepithelial adenocarcinoma and is similar wherever it occurs (Fig. 25.27), but unlike Paget's disease of the nipple, where an underlying breast carcinoma is the usual finding, an underlying tumour is found in no more than 25% of cases of vulval Paget's disease.[92] When present, such tumours are usually adenocarcinoma in skin adnexae or Bartholin's gland, but less frequently there may be a transitional cell carcinoma of the urinary tract, cervical adenocarcinoma, adenocarcinoma of the lower gastrointestinal tract or squamous carcinoma.[86,93] Vulval Paget's disease may also occur in association with carcinoma of the breast, with or without evidence of Paget's disease of the nipple: such associations are unexplained.[94]

If left untreated, Paget's disease of the vulva spreads into adjacent perianal skin and the top of the thigh, and rarely into the vagina and on to the cervix.[95] The clinically visible extent usually underestimates the area of histological involvement and may lead to incomplete surgical excision unless accompanied by a wide apparently disease-free margin.

### Cytological findings: Paget's disease of the vulva[96]

- Single and clustered adenocarcinoma (Paget's) cells
- Pale indistinct cytoplasm
- Abnormal chromatin distribution
- Enlarged nuclei and nucleoli.

In scrapes from clinically involved areas, Paget's cells may be seen singly or in clusters. The cytoplasm is pale staining and has an indistinct outline. The nuclei are large and nucleoli are visible (Fig. 27.28). Occasionally, signet ring forms are present. The cells are indistinguishable from Paget's cells in the nipple and from cells in aspirates from breast ductal carcinoma (see Ch. 6).[94] If the disease extends to the vagina or cervix, diagnostic cells may be found in conventional cervical smears.[97]

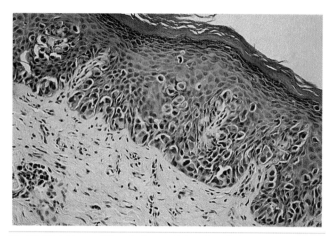

**Fig. 25.27** A biopsy of Paget's disease of the vulva. The large Paget's cells are present singly and in clusters in the epidermis (H&E).

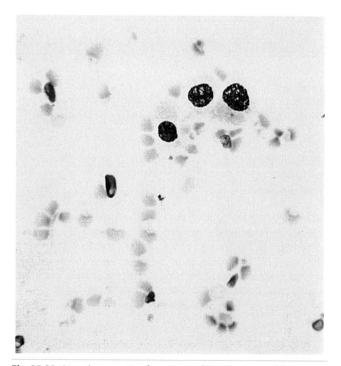

**Fig. 25.28** A touch preparation from a case of Paget's disease of the vulva. Note the very scanty Paget's cells here in a small cluster. They are clearly adenocarcinoma cells with very abnormal chromatin distribution. The cytoplasm is pale staining and has an indistinct cell boundary (MGG).

## Adenocarcinoma of Bartholin's gland

These lesions are exceedingly rare. They are usually mucin-producing and have a variety of growth patterns including papillary and mucoepidermoid. If they invade to the skin surface, they can be diagnosed on cytology.[98] They are distinguished from sweat gland carcinoma by their site. Squamous cell, neuroendocrine and adenoid cystic carcinomas may also arise within Bartholin's glands: the cytological appearances are similar to corresponding tumours of the cervix.

## Tumours of the vagina

Most vaginal samples are performed for follow-up of women with previously treated cervical or vaginal disease. The most common cytology specimens received are vault smears for follow-up of cervical neoplasia treated by hysterectomy. Current NHSCSP guidance is that two vault samples should be taken, 6 and 18 months post surgery, when there is evidence of completely excised CIN in the hysterectomy specimen, and if both are negative, further samples are not necessary. If the CIN is incompletely excised at the vaginal margin or adequacy of excision is uncertain, follow-up should be as if the cervix was still *in situ*. For CIN 1 this is vault cytology at 6, 12 and 24 and for CIN 2 or 3, vault cytology at 6 and 12 months followed by nine annual vault samples.[99] In some units, vault smears are also used for follow-up after hysterectomy for cervical cancer. However, the value of vault cytology in both these settings is uncertain and further research is warranted.[100]

The main problem areas in interpretation of vault samples are atrophy, changes induced by radiotherapy,[34] and the finding of glandular cells. The latter may be due to a variety of causes as shown in Table 25.1.[101–103]

## Benign tumours of the vagina

### Fibroepithelial stromal polyp

These lesions are benign, connective tissue tumours with stroma similar to that of the subepithelial layer of the normal vagina. They may represent a reactive hyperplasia of the vaginal wall rather than a true tumour. There are frequently giant fibroblasts scattered within the stroma and there may be a subepithelial condensation of fibroblasts.[104] Pedunculated leiomyomata and rhabdomyomas are also found. All these polypoid tumours are covered by benign vaginal squamous epithelium and cytology

**Table 25.1** Potential explanations for the finding of glandular cells in vaginal vault cytology samples

| | |
|---|---|
| Sub-total hysterectomy | Adenocarcinoma: recurrent, metastatic or primary |
| Vaginal endometriosis | Cytologic effects of 5-fluorouracil or previous $CO_2$ laser ablation |
| Vaginal adenosis | Rectovaginal fistula |
| Mesonephric duct remnants | Reparative fibroblasts in ulcers and granulation tissue |
| Fallopian tube prolapse | Reparative squamous parabasal and basal cells resembling columnar or goblet cells |

samples from the surface contain normal squamous cells. If the polyp has prolapsed through the introitus, however, the exposed squamous epithelium may become keratinised and anucleate squamous cells can be a predominant feature.

## Malignant tumours of the vagina

In the female genital tract, only carcinoma of the fallopian tube is diagnosed less frequently than primary carcinoma of the vagina, which accounts for 1–2% of gynaecological malignancies. The majority of neoplasms in the vagina are metastases, as a result of direct extension, implantation, lymphatic or vascular embolisation.[105] The commonest primary sites are endometrium and cervix and the cytological appearance is that of the primary tumour.[79]

### Vaginal intraepithelial neoplasia (VAIN)

Although most often seen in association with cervical intraepithelial neoplasia (CIN) and sharing the same risk factors, VAIN is much less common than CIN and occurs at a later age.[106] It may be multifocal and present in women with intraepithelial neoplasia elsewhere in the lower genital tract.[107] The diagnosis of VAIN is usually made on cytology with confirmatory colposcopy and biopsy. It has been reported that in post hysterectomy vault smears when VAIN is present, abnormal cells can be identified in 97% of conventional cervical smears with 83% sensitivity. False negatives were ascribed to obscuring inflammatory cells.[108]

Histologically, intraepithelial neoplasia of the vagina is similar to CIN, and the cytological patterns seen in cells from VAIN are those seen in CIN with all the same variants (see Ch. 26).

### Squamous cell carcinoma

The majority of vaginal squamous carcinomas occur in the sixth to eight decade, approximately 20 years older than the mean age for cervical squamous carcinoma, suggesting that factors in addition to HPV infection are implicated in the pathogenesis of these tumours.[109] Most tumours are of the large cell non-keratinising type, but all types of squamous cell carcinoma seen in the cervix also present in the vagina. The cytological appearances are identical to the corresponding cervical tumours as described in Chapter 26.

### Adenocarcinoma

In the early 1970s vaginal adenosis, the presence of endocervical or endometrial type glands in the vaginal lamina propria, and clear cell adenocarcinoma of the vagina and cervix were described in young women in the USA who had been exposed *in utero* to diethylstilboestrol (DES).[110] DES is a synthetic oestrogen that was prescribed to pregnant women in the UK between 1950 and 1975, to prevent miscarriage and other pregnancy complications. In 1974 it was estimated that approximately 7500 women in the UK had been prescribed DES during pregnancy. Approximately one in three 'DES daughters' are found to have vaginal adenosis and 1 in 1000 develop clear cell adenocarcinoma (see Ch. 26).[111,112] They also have a higher than expected risk of development of cervical and vaginal squamous neoplasia.[113] In women not exposed to DES, vaginal adenosis is very rare and clear cell adenocarcinoma occurs much later in life, in the sixth to ninth decade. While the clear cell adenocarcinoma cells may be readily identified in vaginal smears,[114] they are indistinguishable from those arising from clear cell adenocarcinoma elsewhere in the genital tract, and it should be remembered that a metastatic deposit from such a tumour would present far more commonly than DES associated clear cell carcinoma, even in a young woman.

Cells from other types of adenocarcinoma may also be found in vaginal smears, derived from either adjacent pelvic or distant primary tumours. The cytological appearances reflect that of the primary tumour.

### Malignant melanoma

This is a very rare primary tumour of the vagina.[115] The cytological features are the same as those seen in melanoma of the vulva.

### Malignant connective tissue and other tumours

There are no cytological descriptions of the rare germ cell and malignant mesenchymal tumours that may occur in the vagina in children and adults such as yolk sac tumour, leiomyosarcoma and angiosarcoma. The cytological appearances of vaginal embryonal rhabdomyosarcoma are as previously described for the cervix.[70]

## The role of the cytopathologist in clinical management

This chapter has described the cytology of relatively rare tumours and the more common tumour-like conditions of the lower female genital tract and the diagnostic pitfalls that may occur, especially if there is inadequate clinicopathological correlation. This highlights the absolute necessity for cytopathologists to participate in multidisciplinary-team meetings and regularly interact with colleagues in the other diagnostic specialties.

## REFERENCES

1. Craig P, Lowe D. Non-neoplastic conditions of the cervix. In: Fox H, Wells M, editors. Haines and Taylor Gynaecological and Obstetric Pathology. Edinburgh: Churchill Livingstone; 2003:290.

2. Golan A, Ber A, Wolman I, et al. Cervical polyp: evaluation of current treatment. Gynecol Obstet Invest 1994;37:56–58.

3. Ngadiman S, Yang GCH. Adenomyomatous, lower uterine segment and endocervical polyps in cervicovaginal smears. Acta Cytol 1995;39:643–47.

4. Schneider V, Barnes LA. Ectopic decidual reaction of the uterine cervix: frequency and cytologic presentation. Acta Cytol 1981;25:616–22.

5. Schneider V. Arias-Stella reaction of the endocervix: frequency and location. Acta Cytol 1981;25:224–28.

6. Lui M, Boerner S. Arias–Stella reaction in a cervicovaginal smear of a woman undergoing infertility treatment: a case report. Diagn Cytopathol 2005;32:94–96.

7. Mulvany NJ, Khan A, Ostor A. Arias–Stella reaction associated with cervical pregnancy. Report of a case with a cytologic presentation. Acta Cytol 1994;38:218–22.

8. Yates WA, Persad RV, Stanbridge CM. The Arias–Stella reaction in the cervix: a case report with cervical cytology. Cytopathology 1997;8:40–44.

9. Pisharodi LR, Jovanoska S. Spectrum of cytologic changes in pregnancy. A review of 100 abnormal cervicovaginal smears, with emphasis on diagnostic pitfalls. Acta Cytol 1995;39:905–8.

10. Ismail SM. Cone biopsy causes cervical endometriosis and tubo-endometrioid metaplasia. Histopathology 1991;18:107–14.

11. Szyfelbein WM, Baker PM, Bell DA. Superficial endometriosis of the cervix: a source of abnormal glandular cells on cervicovaginal smears. Diagn Cytopathol 2004;30:88–91.

12. Wood MD, Horst JA, Bibbo M. Weeding atypical glandular cell look-alikes from the true atypical lesions in liquid-based Pap tests: a review. Diagn Cytopathol 2007;35:12–17.

13. Srinivasan R, Nijhawan R, Das A, et al. Fine needle aspiration cytodiagnosis of endometriosis arising in scar tissue and in the caecum – case reports. Cytopathol 1993;4:357–60.

14. Chen KTK, Hendricks EJ. Malakoplakia of the female genital tract. Obstet Gynecol 1985;65:S84–7.

15. Stewart CJR, Thomas MA. Malakoplakia of the uterine cervix and endometrium. Cytopathology 1991;2:271–75.

16. Saad AJ, Donovan TM, Truong LD. Malakoplakia of the vagina diagnosed by fine-needle aspiration cytology. Diagn Cytopathol 1993;9:559–61.

17. Yang YJ, Trap kin LK, Demo ski RK, et al. The small blue cell dilemma associated with tamoxifen therapy. Arch Pathol Lab Med 2001;125:1047–50.

18. Beyer-Boon ME, Verdonk GW. The identification of atypical reserve cells in smears of patients with premalignant and malignant changes in the squamous and glandular epithelium of the uterine cervix. Acta Cytol 1978;22:305–11.

19. Boon ME, van Dunne FM, Vardaxis NJ. Recognition of atypical reserve cell hyperplasia in cervical smears and its diagnostic significance. Mod Pathol 1995;8:786–94.

20. Jonasson JG, Wang HH, Antonioli DA, et al. Tubal metaplasia of the uterine cervix: a prevalence study in women with gynecologic pathology. Int J Gynecol Pathol 1992;11:89–95.

21. Al-Nafussi A, Rahilly M. The prevalence of tubo-endometrial metaplasia and adenomatoid proliferation. Histopathology 1993;22:177–79.

22. Babkowski RC, Wilbur DC, Rutkowski MA, et al. The effects of endocervical canal topography, tubal metaplasia, and high canal sampling on the cytologic presentation of nonneoplastic endocervical cells. Am J Clin Pathol 1996;105:403–10.

23. Selvaggi SM, Haefner HK. Microglandular endocervical hyperplasia and tubal metaplasia: pitfalls in the diagnosis of adenocarcinoma on cervical smears. Diagn Cytopathol 1997;16:168–73.

24. Novotny DB, Maygarden SJ, Johnson DE, et al. Tubal metaplasia. A frequent potential pitfall in the cytologic diagnosis of endocervical glandular dysplasia on cervical smears. Acta Cytol 1992;36:1–10.

25. Ducatman BS, Wang HH, Jonasson JG, et al. Tubal metaplasia: a cytologic study with comparison to other neoplastic and non-neoplastic conditions of the endocervix. Diagn Cytopathol 1993;9:98–105.

26. Hirschowitz L, Eckford SD, Phillpotts B, et al. Cytological changes associated with tubo-endometrioid metaplasia of the uterine cervix. Cytopathology 1994;5:1–8.

27. Demay RM. Hyperchromatic crowded groups: pitfalls in pap smear diagnosis. Am J Clin Pathol 2000;114(Suppl):S36–43.

28. Johnson JE, Rahemtulla A. Endocervical glandular neoplasia and its mimics in ThinPrep Pap tests. A descriptive study. Acta Cytol 1999;43:369–75.

29. Weir MM, Bell DA, Young RH. Transitional cell metaplasia of the uterine cervix and vagina: an underrecognized lesion that may be confused with high-grade dysplasia. A report of 59 cases. Am J Surg Pathol 1997;21:510–17.

30. Ng WK, Cheung LK, Li AS, et al. Transitional cell metaplasia of the uterine cervix is related to human papillomavirus: molecular analysis in seven patients with cytohistologic correlation. Cancer 2002;96:250–58.

31. Weir MM, Bell DA. Transitional cell metaplasia of the cervix: a newly described entity in cervicovaginal smears. Diagn Cytopathol 1998;18:222–26.

32. Gondos B, Smith LR, Townsend DE. Cytologic changes in cervical epithelium following cryosurgery. Acta Cytol 1970;14:386–89.

33. Gonzalez-Merlo J, Ausin J, Lejarcegui JA, et al. Regeneration of the ectocervical epithelium after its destruction by electrocauterization. Acta Cytol 1973;17:366–71.

34. Shield PW, Daunter B, Wright RG. Post-irradiation cytology of cervical cancer patients. Cytopathology 1992;3:167–82.

35. Ueki M, Ueda M, Kurokawa A, et al. Cytologic study of the tissue repair cells of the uterine cervix with special reference to their origin. Acta Cytol 1992;36:310–18.

36. Rimm DL, Gmitro S, Frable WJ. Atypical reparative change on cervical/vaginal smears may be associated with dysplasia. Diagn Cytopathol 1996;14:374–79.

37. Sherman ME, Tabbara SO, Scott DR, et al. 'ASCUS, rule out HSIL': cytologic features, histologic correlates, and human papillomavirus detection. Mod Pathol 1999;12:335–42.

38. Snyder TM, Renshaw AA, Styer PE, et al. Altered recognition of reparative changes in ThinPrep specimens in the College of American Pathologists Gynecologic Cytology Program. Arch Pathol Lab Med 2005;129:861–65.

39. Levine PH, Elgert PA, Sun P, et al. Atypical repair on Pap smears: clinicopathologic correlates in 647 cases. Diagn Cytopathol 2005;33:214–17.

40. Ng WK, Li AS, Cheung LK. Significance of atypical repair in liquid-based gynecologic cytology: a follow-up study with molecular analysis for human papillomavirus. Cancer 2003;99:141–48.

41. Shingleton HM, Bell MC, Fremgen A, et al. Is there really a difference in survival of women with squamous cell carcinoma, adenocarcinoma, and adenosquamous cell carcinoma of the cervix? Cancer 1995;76:1948–55.

42. Young RH, Clement PB. Endocervical adenocarcinoma and its variants: their morphology and differential diagnosis. Histopathology 2002;41:185–207.

43. Look KY, Brunetto VL, Clarke-Pearson DL, et al. An analysis of cell type in patients with surgically staged stage IB carcinoma of the cervix: a Gynecologic Oncology Group study. Gynecol Oncol 1996;63:304–11.

44. Alfsen GC, Kristensen GB, Skovlund E, et al. Histologic subtype has minor importance for overall survival in patients with adenocarcinoma of the uterine cervix: a population-based study of prognostic factors in 505 patients with nonsquamous cell carcinomas of the cervix. Cancer 2001;92:2471–83.

45. Ulbright TM, Gersell DJ. Glassy cell carcinoma of the uterine cervix. A light and electron microscopic study of five cases. Cancer 1983;51:2255–63.

46. Chung J-H, Koh J-S, Lee S-S, et al. Glassy cell carcinoma of the uterine cervix. Cytologic features and expression of estrogen and progesterone receptors. Acta Cytol 2000;44:551–56.

47. Ng WK, Cheung LK, Li AS. Liquid-based cytology findings of glassy cell carcinoma of the cervix. Report of a case with histologic correlation and molecular analysis. Acta Cytol 2004;48:99–106.

48. Smith JHF. Cervical cytology through the looking glass. Cytopathology 2000;11:54–56.

49. Lee KR, Rose PG. Glandular neoplasia of the cervix. In: Crum CP, Lee KR, editors. Diagnostic Gynecologic and Obstetric Pathology. Philadelphia: Elsevier Saunders; 2006:389.

50. Vuong PN, Neveux Y, Schoonaert M-F, et al. Adenoid cystic (cylindromatous) carcinoma associated with squamous cell carcinoma of the cervix uteri. Cytologic presentation of a case with histologic and ultrastructural correlations. Acta Cytol 1996;40:289–94.

51. Powers CN, Stastny JF, Frable WJ. Adenoid basal carcinoma of the cervix: a potential pitfall in cervicovaginal cytology. Diagn Cytopathol 1996;14:172–77.

52. Khoury T, Lele S, Tan D. Pathologic quiz case: an asymptomatic 79-year-old woman with an abnormal Papanicolaou test. Arch Pathol Lab Med 2004;128:485–86.

53. Albores-Saavedra J, Gersell DJ, Gilks CB, et al. Terminology of endocrine tumours of the uterine cervix: results of a workshop sponsored by the College of American Pathologists and the National Cancer Institute. Arch Pathol Lab Med 1997;121:34–39.

54. Hirahatake K, Hareyama H, Kure R, et al. Cytologic and hormonal findings in a carcinoid tumour of the uterine cervix. Acta Cytol 1990;34:119–24.

55. Lee WY. Exfoliative cytology of large cell neuroendocrine carcinoma of the uterine cervix. Acta Cytol 2002;46:1176–79.

56. Russin V, Valente PT, Hanjani P. Psammoma bodies in neuroendocrine carcinoma of the uterine cervix. Acta Cytol 1987;31:791–95.

57. Hoerl HD, Schink J, Hartenbach E, et al. Exfoliative cytology of primary poorly differentiated (small-cell) neuroendocrine carcinoma of the uterine cervix in ThinPrep material: a case report. Diagn Cytopathol 2000;23:14–18.

58. Ciesla MC, Guidos BJ, Selvaggi SM. Cytomorphology of small-cell (neuroendocrine) carcinoma on ThinPrep cytology as compared to conventional smears. Diagn Cytopathol 2001;24:46–52.

59. Reich O, Pickel H, Purstner P. Exfoliative cytology of a lymphoepithelioma like carcinoma in a cervical smear. A case report. Acta Cytol 1999;43:285–88.

60. Proca DM, Hitchcock CL, Keyhani-Rofagha S. Exfoliative cytology of lymphoepithelioma like carcinoma of the uterine cervix. A report of two cases. Acta Cytol 2000;44:410–14.

61. McCluggage WG. Malignant biphasic uterine tumours: carcinosarcomas or metaplastic carcinomas? J Clin Pathol 2002;55:321–25.

62. Silverberg SG, Major FJ, Blessing JA, et al. Carcinosarcoma (malignant mixed mesodermal tumor) of the uterus. A gynecologic oncology group pathologic study of 203 cases. Int J Gynecol Pathol 1990;9:1–19.

63. Valera-Duran J, Nochomovitz LE, Prem KA, et al. Postirradiation mixed Müllerian tumours of the uterus. A comparative clinicopathologic study. Cancer 1980;45:1625–31.

64. Kurman RJ, Norris HJ, Wilkinson E. Tumours of the cervix, vagina, and vulva. In: Atlas of Tumour Pathology. Washington: Armed Forces Institute of Pathology; 1992:112.

65. Barwick KW, LiVolsi VA. Malignant mixed Müllerian tumors of the uterus. A clinicopathologic assessment of 34 cases. Am J Surg Pathol 1979;3:125–35.

66. Massoni EA, Hadju SI. Cytology of primary and metastatic uterine sarcomas. Acta Cytol 1984;28:93–100.

67. An-Foraker SH, Kawada CY. Cytodiagnosis of endometrial mixed mesodermal tumor. Acta Cytol 1985;29:137–41.

68. Imai H, Kitamura H, Nananura T, et al. Müllerian carcinofibroma of the uterus. A case report. Acta Cytol 1999;43:667–74.

69. Chieng DC, Elgert PA, Cangiarella JF, et al. Cytology of polypoid adenomyomas: a report of two cases. Diagn Cytopathol 2000;22:176–80.

70. Matsuura Y, Kashimura M, Hatanaka K, et al. Sarcoma botryoides of the cervix. Report of a case with cytopathologic findings. Acta Cytol 1999;43:475–80.

71. Clark KC, Butz WR, Hapke MR. Primary malignant melanoma of the uterine cervix: case report with world literature review. Int J Gynecol Path 1999;18:265–73.

72. Deshpande AH, Munshi MM. Primary malignant melanoma of the uterine cervix: report of a case diagnosed by cervical scrape cytology and review of the literature. Diagn Cytopathol 2001;25:108–11.

73. Gupta S, Sodhani P, Jain S. Primary malignant melanoma of uterine cervix: a rare entity diagnosed on fine needle aspiration cytology – report of a case. Cytopathol 2003;14:153–56.

74. Vang R, Mederios LJ, Ha CS, et al. Non-Hodgkin's lymphomas involving the uterus: a clinicopathologic analysis of 26 cases. Mod Pathol 2000;13:19–28.

75. al Talib RK, Sworn MJ, Ramsay AD, et al. Primary cervical lymphoma: the role of cervical cytology. Cytopathology 1996;7:173–77.

76. Chan JK, Loizzi V, Magistris A, et al. Clinicopathologic features of six cases of primary cervical lymphoma. Am J Obstet Gynecol 2005;193:866–72.

77. Figueroa JM, Huffaker AK, Diehl EJ. Malignant plasma cells in cervical smear. Acta Cytol 1978;22:43–45.

78. Ikuta A, Saito J, Mizokami T, et al. Primary relapse of acute lymphoblastic leukemia in a cervical smear: a case report. Diagn Cytopathol 2006;34:499–502.

79. Gupta D, Balsara G. Extrauterine malignancies. Role of Pap smears in diagnosis and management. Acta Cytol 1999;43:806–13.

80. Smith JHF. Psammoma bodies in cervical smears: sifting the grains of sand. Cytopathology 2007;18:140–42.

81. Levine TS, Rolfe KJ, Crow J, et al. The use of cytospin monolayer technique in the cytological diagnosis of vulval and anal disease. Cytopathology 2001;12:297–305.

82. Woodworth H Jr, Dockerty MB, Wilson RB, et al. Papillary hidradenoma of the vulva: a clinicopathologic study of 69 cases. Am J Obstet Gynecol 1971;110:501–8.

83. Hustin J, Donnay M, Hamels J. Identification of papillary hidradenoma of the vulva by imprint cytology. Acta Cytol 1980;24:466–67.

84. Rollins SD. Fine-needle aspiration diagnosis of a vulvar papillary hidradenoma: a case report. Diagn Cytopathol 1994;10:60–61.

85. Fox H, Buckley CH. Neoplastic disease of the vulva and associated structures. In: Fox H, Wells M, editors. Haines and Taylor Gynaecological and Obstetric Pathology. Edinburgh: Churchill Livingstone; 2003:114.

86. Fox H, Wells M. Recent advances in pathology of the vulva. Histopathology 2003;42:209–16.

87. Maclean AB. Vulval cancer: prevention and screening. Best Pract Res Clin Obstet Gynaecol 2006;20:379–95.

88. Hall TB, Barton DP, Trott PA, et al. The role of ultrasound-guided cytology of groin lymph nodes in the management of squamous cell carcinoma of the vulva: 5-year experience in 44 patients. Clin Radiol 2003;58:367–71.

89. Ragnarsson-Olding BK, Nilsson BR, Kanter-Lewensohn LR, et al. Malignant melanoma of the vulva in a nationwide, 25-year study of 219 Swedish females: clinical observations and histopathologic features. Cancer 1999;86:1274–84.

90. Verschraegen CF, Benjapibal M, Supakarapongkul W, et al. Vulvar melanoma at the M. D. Anderson Cancer Center: 25 years later. Int J Gynecol Cancer 2001;11:359–64.

91. Lee SC, Roth LM, Ehrlich C, et al. Extramammary Paget's disease of the vulva. A clinicopathologic study of 13 cases. Cancer 1977;39:2540–49.

92. Regauer S. Extramammary Paget's disease – a proliferation of adnexal origin? Histopathology 2006;48:723–29.

93. Taylor PT, Stenwig JT, Klausen H. Paget's disease of the vulva. A report of 18 cases. Gynecol Oncol 1975;3:46–60.

94. Russell Jones R, Spaull J, Gusterson B. The histogenesis of mammary and extramammary Paget's disease. Histopathology 1989;14:409–16.

95. Lloyd J, Evans DJ, Flanagan AM. Extension of extramammary Paget disease of the vulva to the cervix. J Clin Pathol 1999;52:538–40.

96. Castellano Megias V, Ibarrola de Andres., Martinez Parra D, et al. Cytology of extramammary Paget's disease of the vulva. A case report. Acta Cytol 2002;46:1153–57.

97. Gu M, Ghafari S, Lin F. Pap smears of patients with extramammary Paget's disease of the vulva. Diagn Cytopathol 2005;32:353–57.

98. Imachi M, Tsukamoto N, Shigematsu T, et al. Cytologic diagnosis of primary adenocarcinoma of Bartholin's gland. A case report. Acta Cytol 1992;36:167–70.

99. Luesley D, Leeson S, editors. Colposcopy and Programme Management, NHSCSP Publication 20. Sheffield: NHSCSP; 2004: 37–38.

100. Stokes-Lampard HJ, Macleod J, Wilson S. Variation in NHS utilisation of vault smear tests in women post-hysterectomy: a study, using routinely collected datasets. BMC Womens Health 2008;8:6.

101. Sodhani P, Gupta S, Prakash S, et al. Columnar and metaplastic cells in vault smears: cytologic and colposcopic study. Cytopathology 1999;10:122–26.

102. Ganesan R, Ferryman SR, Waddell C. Vaginal adenosis in a woman on Tamoxifen therapy: a case report. Cytopathology 1999;10:127–30.

103. Yavuz E, Ozluk Y, Kucucuk S, et al. Radiation-induced benign glandular cells in posthysterectomy smears: a cytomorphologic and clinical analysis. Int J Gynecol Cancer 2006;16:670–74.

104. McCluggage WG. A review and update of morphologically bland vulvovaginal mesenchymal lesions. In J Gynecol Pathol 2005;24:26–38.

105. Schmidt WA. Pathology of the vagina. In: Fox H, Wells M, editors. Haines and Taylor Gynaecological and Obstetric Pathology. Edinburgh: Churchill Livingstone; 2003. p. 216–19.

106. Micheletti L, Zanotto Valentino MC, Barbero M, et al. Current knowledge about the natural history of intraepithelial neoplasms of the vagina. Minerva Ginecol 1994;46:195–204.

107. Scholefield JH, Hickson WG, Smith JH, et al. Anal intraepithelial neoplasia: part of a multifocal disease process. Lancet 1992;340:1270–73.

108. Davila RM, Miranda MC. Vaginal intraepithelial neoplasia and the Pap smear. Acta Cytol 2000;44:137–40.

109. Hellman K, Silfversward C, Nilsson B, et al. Primary carcinoma of the vagina: factors influencing the age at diagnosis. The Radiumhemmet series 1956–96. Int J Gynaecol Cancer 2004;14:491–501.

110. Herbst AL, Ulfelder H, Poskanzer DC. Adenocarcinoma of the vagina. Association of maternal stilbestrol therapy with tumor appearance in young women. N Engl J Med 1971;284:878–81.

111. Herbst AL. Behaviour of estrogen-associated female genital tract cancer and its relation to neoplasia following intrauterine exposure to diethylstilboestrol (DES). Gynecol Oncol 2000;76:147–56.

112. Trimble EL. Guest editorial: update on diethylstilboestrol. Obstet Gynecol Surv 2001;56:187–89.

113. Bornstein J, Adam E, Adler-Storthz K, et al. Development of cervical and vaginal squamous cell neoplasia as a late consequence of in utero exposure to diethylstilboestrol. Obstet Gynecol Surv 1988;43:15–21.

114. Hanselaar AG, Boss EA, Massuger LF, et al. Cytologic examination to detect clear cell adenocarcinoma of the vagina or cervix. Gynecol Oncol 1999;75:338–44.

115. Chung AF, Murray JC, Flannery JT, et al. Malignant melanoma of the vagina – report of 19 cases. Obstet Gynecol 1980;55:720–27.

# Cytology of the body of the uterus

Tadao K. Kobayashi, Yoshiaki Norimatsu and Anna Maria Buccoliero

## Chapter contents

## Introduction

The uptake of endometrial cytology as a diagnostic procedure has been hampered in the past by the difficulties that arise in interpreting the cytological findings due to a number of factors that are intrinsic to this branch of cytology. These include the presence of excess blood in many samples, leading to poor display of the material, the tendency to overlapping of cells and problems with cell groups. There is also the complex physiology of the endometrium to be taken into account when assessing a specimen. Recently, the use of liquid-based cytology (LBC), with its ability to remove blood and mucus and to distribute cells uniformly in a thin layer on the slide has provided an opportunity to re-evaluate the role of endometrial cytology in cytodiagnosis.[1–6]

## Endometrial sampling and processing

Endometrial pathology may be detected cytologically in exfoliated cells in a cervical smear or by direct sampling methods from within the body of the uterus (see Chs 21, 24, 25).

## Endometrial sampling by cervical cytology

During the reproductive years, endometrial cells are normally detectable in the menstrual and early proliferative phases of the cycle. Beyond day 10–12 of the cycle the finding is considered abnormal, and should be evaluated in the light of clinical details such as the presence of an intrauterine contraceptive device, a recent pregnancy, contraceptive hormone use with break-through bleeding, recent uterine instrumentation or known endometrial pathology. In postmenopausal patients, any shedding of endometrial cells seen in cervico-vaginal cytological samples should be considered abnormal, since it is a potential indicator of endometrial pathology.

Possible endometrial conditions that may cause abnormal endometrial shedding include endometritis, endometrial polyps, submucosal leiomyomas, endometrial hyperplasia and endometrial carcinoma. However, the sensitivity of cervico-vaginal sampling for endometrial pathology is low since significant exfoliation does not occur even in cases of endometrial carcinoma.[7] Moreover the likelihood of degenerative changes in spontaneously exfoliated endometrial cells makes their interpretation difficult.

Direct abrasive sampling of endometrial tissue at cervical smear taking may be seen in cases of previous cone biopsy, high sampling with an endocervical brush or cervical endometriosis.

## Direct endometrial sampling

Direct endometrial sampling is significantly more reliable than cervico-vaginal sampling. Several procedures have been used to obtain direct samples of endometrium including:

1. Aspiration
2. Washing
3. Brushing.

The technique of direct aspiration of the uterine cavity by a rigid cannula was first introduced by Papanicolaou and Cary in 1943 and since then, a number of flexible devices have been used. Endometrial washings may be obtained under positive or negative pressure. However, the use of both endometrial aspiration and washing techniques has long been discontinued, mainly due to the potential risk of spreading malignant cells, particularly in the case of endometrial washings. Additional disadvantages are the lack of simplicity in these procedures and their high cost.

Today, the endometrial brushing method is the technique most frequently used for cytological endometrial sampling. The specimens may be obtained by means of several devices. The majority consist of an outer tube that reduces cervical and vaginal cell contamination and an inner stick which has a sampling tip on the end (Fig. 26.1). Before the introduction of the device into the uterus, the sampling tip is held inside the outer tube. Once inside the uterine cavity, the sampling tip is released

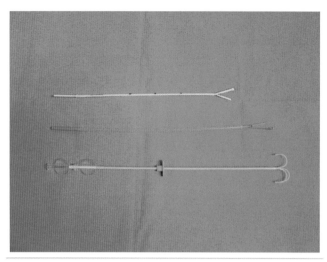

**Fig. 26.1** Endometrial brushing: three devices with different sampling tips.

and rotated clockwise and anticlockwise several times. After the collection of endometrial material the tip is retracted inside the outer tube and the device removed. Outside of the uterus, the device is cleaned with gauze to remove the cervical and vaginal cells and then the sampling tip is exposed.

The collected cells may be processed in several ways: conventionally by the 'flicked method' or by liquid-based processing.

## Conventional processing

In conventional endometrial cytology, the brush is rolled on to a glass slide, immediately fixed and subsequently stained by the Papanicolaou method.

## Direct endometrial sampling by the 'flicked method'

In 1968, Johnsson and Stormby[8] reported the use of a cytological brushing technique to obtain cells from endometrial lesions. However, the sensitivity of endometrial sampling depends in part on whether tissue fragments are obtained so that cytoarchitectural criteria can be used in direct endometrial sampling, especially for the diagnosis of endometrial hyperplasia and well-differentiated adenocarcinoma. We currently use the Uterobrush (Cooper Surgical, Trumbull, CT: ASKA Pharmaceutical, Tokyo, Japan) because insertion to the uterine cavity is easy and painless.[9,10]

The Uterobrush is pre-sterilised and consists of a sheath of polypropylene 175 mm in length with a thin wire 0.4 mm in diameter attached to a handle. The tip of the wire has a collecting brush 6 mm in length, composed of nylon bristles with an overall width of 20 mm. Graduation marks along the length of the Uterobrush provide guidance to the operator when introducing the instrument into the endometrial cavity. The tip of the instrument has a bulbous end to minimise the risk of perforation of the uterus.

To collect samples, the sheathed brush is inserted to the level of the uterine fundus and the sheath is slid down toward the

handle to expose the brush. Endometrial cells are collected by rotating the handle a few times then the sheath is replaced over the brush in order to entrap the sample as described above.

For specimen preparation, the procedure is improved by using the so-called 'flicked' method as follows (Fig. 26.2):

1. The stem of the brush is held in one hand, and forceps (or a thin stick) in the other.
2. The tip of the brush is placed on a glass slide and sharply flicked by forceps or stick.
3. The brush is moved little by little along the length of the slide, repeating step (2) several times.

Uterobrush samples prepared by the 'flicked' method have a much greater quantity of cell clumps than those using the earlier Endocyte sampler,[11] although the size of the cell clumps is the same as with the Endocyte brush. The same criteria are applicable to both types of sample. Besides improving the cytodiagnosis of endometrial lesions, the findings are helpful in the standardisation of criteria in direct intrauterine cell samples,[11] for example by allowing observation of cell clumps with either a tubular or sheet-like pattern, tube-shaped glands being symmetrical with nearby cohesive endometrial stromal cells but disrupted tube-shaped glands yield a sheet-like configuration (Fig. 26.3).

## Liquid-based processing

In liquid-based cytology, the brush head of the device is immersed in a vial of fixative solution where it is vigorously rotated several times to ensure release of the cells collected (Fig. 26.4). The device is then removed from the vial. The sample is ready for processing after about 30 minutes in fixative solution and is stable for several weeks thereafter. Excess blood and mucus are eliminated by means of washing through a succession of centrifugation and resuspension of the sample in mucolytic and haemolytic agents. The cells are then placed onto the slide by special automated or semi-automated processor machines which transfer a representative fraction of the collected cells for staining. Subsequently, further slides may be obtained from the remaining sample and these may be stained routinely or used for immunohistochemical or molecular investigations.

When endometrial brushings are suspension-fixed, cell aggregates maintain their three-dimensional pattern comprising, in essence, microbiopsies. Three-dimensional structures such as glands may be observed in cytology preparations and this allows direct correlation between histological and cytological features.[12]

## Cells present in endometrial samples

Cytological endometrial samples contain a heterogeneous mixture of cells including endometrial, cervical, ciliated and inflammatory cells.

## Endometrial cells

- Epithelial cell aggregates in tubular or sheet-like arrangements
- Small cells with scanty cytoplasm

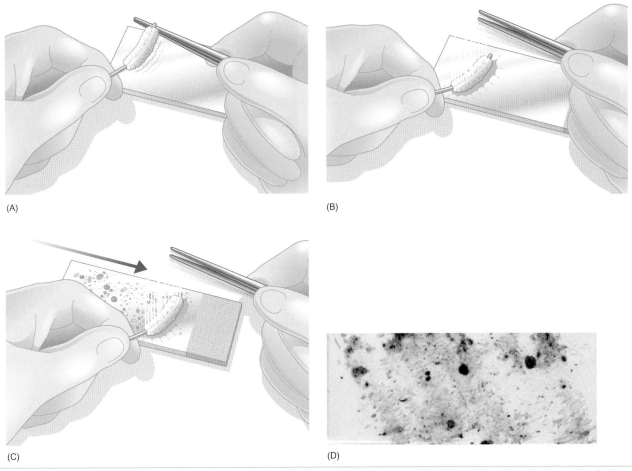

**Fig. 26.2** The manipulation procedure of the Uterobrush 'flicked' method. (A) The stem of a brush is held in one hand, and forceps (or a thin stick) is held in the other. (B) The tip of the brush is placed on a glass slide and is sharply flicked by forceps or stick. (C) The brush is moved little by little along the slide repeating step B several times. (D) Papanicolaou stained slide. (From Fujihara et al. 2006.[11])

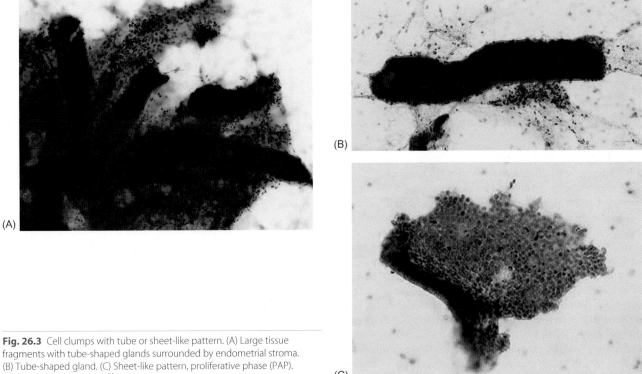

**Fig. 26.3** Cell clumps with tube or sheet-like pattern. (A) Large tissue fragments with tube-shaped glands surrounded by endometrial stroma. (B) Tube-shaped gland. (C) Sheet-like pattern, proliferative phase (PAP). (From Fujihara et al. 2006.[11])

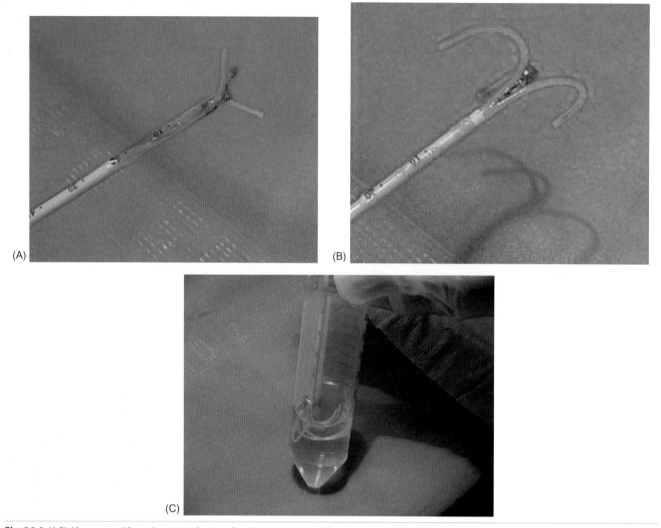

**Fig. 26.4** (A,B) After removal from the uterus the sampling tip is exposed and then immersed in a vial containing a fixative solution where it is vigorously rotated several times to ensure release of the endometrial cells (C). (Endoflower device; RI-MOS, Mirandola, Modena, Italy.)

- Uniform small round nuclei
- Fine granular chromatin with chromocentres
- Single or overlapping stromal cell groups or single spindle-shaped cells
- Epithelial and stromal cells are influenced by hormonal changes.

Endometrial cells, both epithelial and stromal, show several different cytoarchitectural features depending on the woman's age, the menstrual phase and any administration of hormonal therapy. Epithelial cells may be aggregated in three-dimensional cylindrical clusters or in two-dimensional sheets. They are small, only slightly larger than mature lymphocytes. The cytoplasm, apart from during the secretory phase, is scant. Nuclei are small, round and uniform in size and shape. The chromatin is finely granular and small chromocentres may be present (Fig. 26.5).

Stromal cells are present as single elements or as cell groupings. Stromal clusters may show cellular overlapping and irregularity in their outline with protruding bare nuclei. Individual cells may be spindle-shaped with scant cytoplasm or, when modified by decidual change, may be larger and polygonal with obvious cytoplasm. Under the influence of progesterone there is an increase in cytoplasmic volume due to glycogen accumulation. Nuclei are isomorphic and have finely granular chromatin. Nucleoli are generally small or absent, although with progesterone they may be prominent. The distinction between stromal and epithelial endometrial cells might sometimes be difficult to ascertain. In such cases, the immunocytochemistry, which is easily performed on liquid-based specimens, may help in this distinction. Indeed, endometrial stromal cells are CD10 (human membrane-associated neutral peptidase) positive while endometrial epithelial cells are not (Fig. 26.6).[13] Blood vessels may also be identified in liquid-based samples, as described below.

## Cervical cells

- Squamous, metaplastic and endocervical cells may be present
- Cytologically similar to appearances in cervical smears.

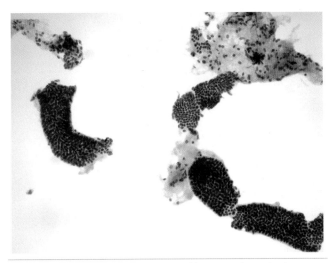

**Fig. 26.5** Tubular endometrial clusters (proliferative endometrium): endometrial cells show scant cytoplasm and small nuclei. LBC direct endometrial sampling.

Cervical cells, either columnar, squamous, intermediate and metaplastic, may variably contaminate the cytological endometrial specimens. Columnar mucin-secreting cells may be identified as single cells or they may occur as strips or sheets showing a honeycomb pattern. Nuclei are round or oval and, depending on their orientation on the slide, basally or centrally located. Chromatin is finely granular. Nucleoli are generally inconspicuous. Cytoplasm is abundant and clear. Superficial squamous cells are polygonal with eosinophilic or cyanophilic cytoplasm and small pyknotic nuclei. Intermediate cells have more vesicular, larger nuclei than superficial squamous cells. Cervical metaplastic cells are smaller than either of these. They are identified by their cytoplasmic prolongations and also may show prominent chromocentres. Metaplastic cells usually appear as cell clusters or as flat sheets.

Cylindrical ciliated cells, deriving from the isthmus, from endometrioid metaplasia or from the fallopian tube, are also sometimes visible in cytological endometrial samples. Such cells have thin wavy cilia extending from the luminal pole of the cell with its thick eosinophilic terminal bar (Fig. 26.7).

## Inflammatory cells

- Mononuclear and polymorphonuclear cells are common
- Relate to menstrual cycle and menopausal status
- Multinucleated histiocytes seen in menopausal samples.

Occasional inflammatory cells, either mono- or polymorphonuclear may be found in non-pathological endometrial samples. The number of polymorphs found in samples from women having menstrual cycles is greatly dependent on the phase of the cycle. Indeed, as with cervico-vaginal samples, endometrial samples obtained in the late secretory phase may be accompanied by a large number of granulocyte or 'K' cells. Multinucleated histiocytes are frequently found during the menopause, having no association with any endometrial pathology. They are oval to round in shape and may be huge. The cytoplasm is voluminous, the nuclei, often in dozens, are oval with slight variation in size and finely granular chromatin (Fig. 26.8).[14]

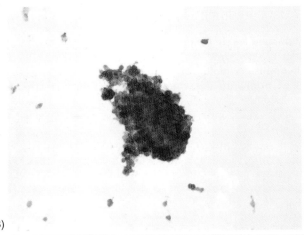

(A)

(B)

**Fig. 26.6** (A) Stromal cluster on progesterone: obvious cytoplasm and isomorphic nuclei showing finely granular chromatin and small chromocentres. (B) CD10 positive immunostaining. LBC direct endometrial sampling.

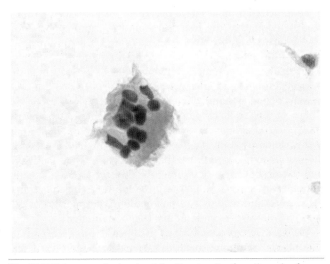

**Fig. 26.7** Columnar cells showing thin cilia extending from the pole of the cells where a thick terminal bar is clearly visible. LBC direct endometrial sampling.

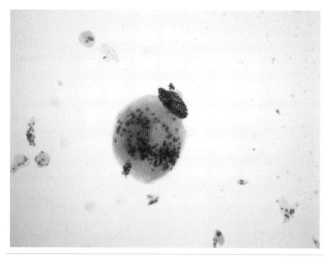

**Fig. 26.8** Multinucleated histiocyte close to atrophic endometrial gland. LBC direct endometrial sampling.

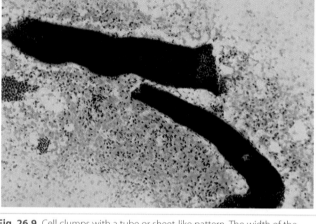

**Fig. 26.9** Cell clumps with a tube or sheet-like pattern. The width of the tube-shaped gland is approximately uniform, and shows adhesion of the endometrial stromal cells to the margins of the gland (PAP). (From Norimatsu et al. 2006.[28])

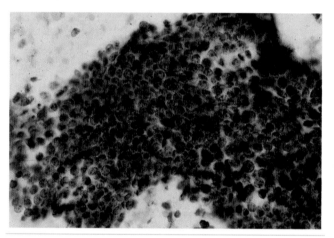

**Fig. 26.10** When a tube-shaped gland is disrupted and opened out, it shows a sheet-like form (PAP). (From Norimatsu et al. 2006.[28])

## Clinical correlation

As can be seen from the discussion so far, it is apparent that if optimal benefit is to be obtained in the detection of the endometrial pathology by the cellular approach, the provision of pertinent clinical informations is important. The age, the day of menstrual cycle, or menopausal status of the patient should be provided. Other important information such as any presenting symptoms, the use of exogenous hormones and details of any recent intrauterine instrumentation should be included.

## Cytological findings in direct preparations using cytoarchitectural features

It is well recognised that detection of pathological lesions ranging from endometrial hyperplasia to endometrial carcinoma is crucial for appropriate patient management. However, there is controversy over the value of cytology in diagnosing these conditions. Although the cellular features of endometrial hyperplasia in endometrial aspirates have been described by Morse,[21] other groups report that the lesions are under-diagnosed by cytology.[22,23] This is probably because routine cytology can never provide the architectural detail needed for an accurate diagnosis of this particular range of abnormalities. Consequently, the interpretation of endometrial smears requires special expertise as well as general training in histopathology.[24]

Recent diagnostic criteria have emerged that are reported to solve these problems[25,26] with the recognition of tissue fragments demonstrating papillary formation in malignant conditions. Byren[27] found that papillary, pseudo-papillary and fimbriated structures were present within the tissue fragments of malignant smears, similar to those found in the characteristic irregular protrusions and papillotubular formations of cell clumps from cases of endometrial adenocarcinoma.[28]

We have recently established cytological criteria for direct endometrial sampling methods[28] using cytoarchitectural features classified into four types:

1. Tubular or sheet-like pattern
2. Dilated or branched pattern
3. Irregular protrusion pattern
4. Papillotubular patten.

## Normal endometrial cell clumps (tissue fragments)

Endometrial cell clumps of various sizes are usually abundant in cytological material collected using the Endocyte or Uterobrush sampler. The cytological characteristics of fragments from normal uterine endometrium are illustrated below.

Endometrial glands appear as virtually straight and tube-shaped (Fig. 26.9). The width of the tube-shaped gland is approximately uniform, and cohesion of the endometrial stromal cells to the margins of the gland are noted. When the tube-shaped gland is disrupted and opened out, it has a sheet-like shape and adhesion of the stromal cells is observed. The surface covering of endometrial cells also appears as a sheet (Figs. 26.10, 26.11).

### Cytological findings: normal endometrial cell clumps (tissue fragments)

- Cell clumps of normal endometrium
- Gland width is approximately uniform (tubular form)

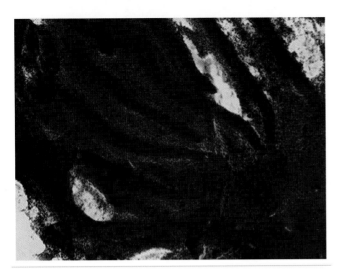

**Fig. 26.11** Frequent large tissue fragments with tube-shaped glands surrounded by endometrial stroma are seen (proliferative phase) (PAP). (From Norimatsu et al. 2006.[28])

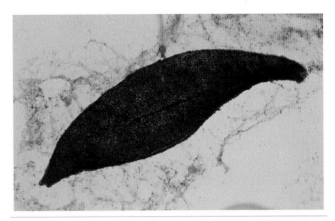

**Fig. 26.12** Cell clump with dilated pattern. Simple endometrial hyperplasia (PAP). (From Norimatsu et al. 2006.[28])

- Cohesion of the endometrial stromal cells to the margins of the gland
- Disrupted tubular glands open out and lie in a sheet-like pattern.

## Cytology of endometrial hyperplasia and neoplasia

In these conditions, the endometrial glands and their lining cells undergo a number of changes. The cytoarchitectural characteristics of the resulting abnormal endometrial and stromal cell clumps include the following.

### Dilated or branched patterns

In these examples, irregular dilation and branching were noted in tubular glands. The maximum width of a gland is more than twice that of its minimum width and shows adhesion of the endometrial stromal cells to the margins of the gland (Figs 26.12–26.15).

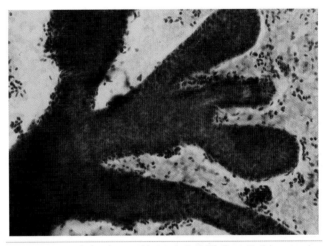

**Fig. 26.13** Complex endometrial hyperplasia (PAP). (From Norimatsu et al. 2006.[28])

#### Cytological findings: dilated or branched patterns

- Cell clumps of abnormal endometrium
- Tube-shaped gland have irregularly dilated or branched patterns
- The maximum width of a gland is greater than twice that of the minimum width
- Stromal cells adhere to the margins of the gland.

### Irregular protrusions patterns

Some irregular small projections were noted at the edges of cell clumps (Fig. 26.16). The margin of the cytoplasm of those small projections is clearly observed.

### Papillotubular patterns

The endometrial gland shows a papillary growth pattern with irregular branching and projections as described above (Figs. 26.17, 26.18). Cohesion of the endometrial stromal cells is not

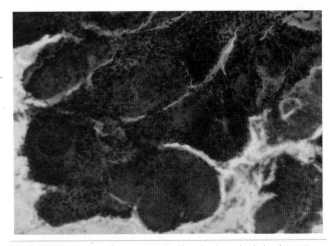

**Fig. 26.14** Large tissue fragments with dilated or branched glands are seen in, complex endometrial hyperplasia (PAP). (From Norimatsu et al. 2006.[28])

noted at the margins of the gland. When the papillary structure is complex and confluent, much glandular space is formed, and back-to-back structures with a cribriform pattern are also recognised (Figs 26.19–26.21). Occasionally, a fibrovascular core may be observed in the epithelial papillae.

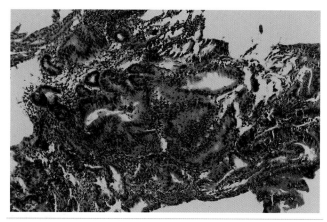

**Fig. 26.15** A cell block specimen from the case shown in Figure 26.14. The crowded glands show irregular dilatation with out-pouching into the endometrial stroma and branching (H&E). (From Norimatsu et al. 2006.[28])

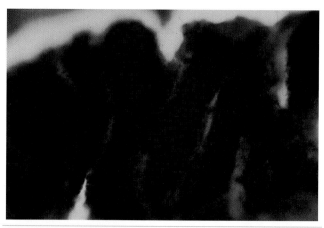

**Fig. 26.18** Large tissue fragment with a papillotubular pattern. A papillary growth pattern was observed in this Grade 1 adenocarcinoma (PAP). (From Norimatsu et al. 2006.[28])

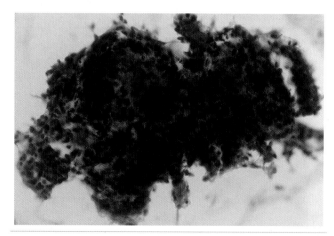

**Fig. 26.16** Cell clump with irregular protrusions. Some irregular small projections are observed from the margins of the cell clumps (PAP). (From Norimatsu et al. 2006.[28])

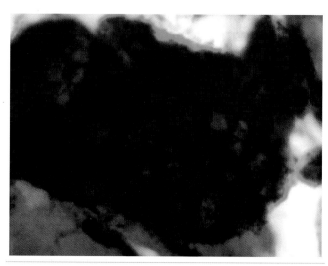

**Fig. 26.19** Large tissue fragment with a papillotubular pattern. A cribriform structure is recognised (Grade 1 adenocarcinoma) (PAP). (From Norimatsu et al. 2006.[28])

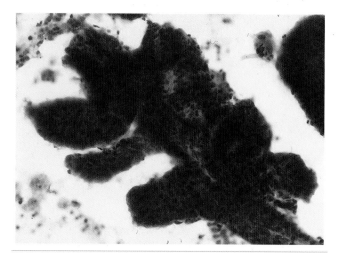

**Fig. 26.17** Cell clumps with a papillotubular pattern The gland shows a papillary growth pattern and irregular branching (PAP). (From Norimatsu et al. 2006.[28])

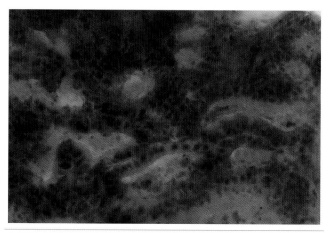

**Fig. 26.20** Large tissue fragment with a papillotubular pattern. The back-to-back structure is obvious (Grade 1 adenocarcinoma). (From Norimatsu et al. 2006.[28])

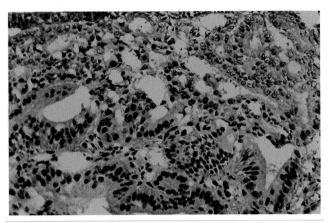

**Fig. 26.21** A cell block specimen from the case shown in Figure 26.20. The back-to-back pattern and cribriform structure are apparent (H&E). (From Norimatsu et al. 2006.[28])

### Cytological findings: papillotubular patterns

- Cell clumps of abnormal endometrium
- Papillary growth pattern and irregular branching with projections
- Back-to-back structures with a cribriform pattern
- Cohesion of the endometrial stromal cells at the gland margins is *not* seen.

## Cytological findings in LBC preparations using cytoarchitectural features: non-neoplastic endometrium

The adequacy of LBC for endometrial samples has already been described in the literature. Gracia et al.[29] noted that thin-layer endometrial cytology has good specificity and positive predictive value for the detection of endometrial abnormalities and has a lower rate of unsatisfactory diagnoses compared to biopsy. It has been reported[3] that examination of just one slide provides sufficient material for cytological evaluation of endometrial sampling. Therefore, although the preparation area of LBC is smaller than with conventional methods, nevertheless LBC preparations contain cells of adequate quantity and quality for a diagnosis to be possible (Tables 26.1A, 26.1B).[30]

### Normal endometrial cells

#### Proliferative endometrium (PE)

Proliferative endometrium shows uniform straight to curvilinear tubular or flat epithelial sheets with cohesion of the endometrial stromal cells (Fig. 26.22). The nuclei of epithelial cells are closely packed, oval to cigar-shaped with smooth contours, evenly dispersed chromatin, and small-sized nucleoli. Mitoses of normal configuration may be seen (Fig. 26.22).

#### Secretory endometrium (SE)

Early SE is similar to PE but with a lower nuclear/cytoplasmic ratio, smaller inconspicuous nucleoli, absent mitoses and

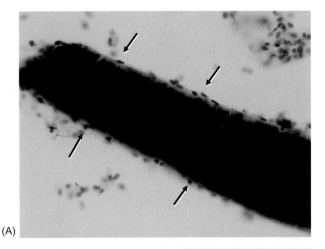

(A)

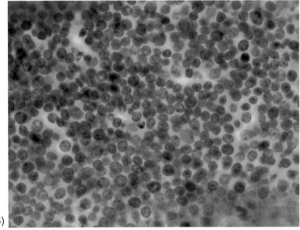

(B)

**Fig. 26.22** Proliferative endometrium shows uniform straight tubular (A) or flat epithelial sheets (B) with adhesion of the endometrial stromal cells (indicated by black arrow). (B) Epithelial cell nuclei are closely packed, oval to cigar-shaped with smooth contours, evenly dispersed chromatin, and small-sized nucleoli. (LBC, PAP). (From Norimatsu et al. 2006.[30])

greater spacing of nuclei (Fig. 26.23A). Mid-SE shows a honeycomb pattern with increased cytoplasm over that of early-SE, and accordion-pleated glands which are the three-dimensional equivalent of 'saw-toothed' glands (Fig. 26.23B). Nuclei are larger than those of PE, rounded and vesicular, and display a fine chromatin pattern (Fig. 26.23C).

### Atrophic endometrium

Atrophic endometrium is similar to PE but nuclear crowding and overlapping is not as striking as in PE. The uniform round nuclei are generally arranged in small monolayer sheets and present distinct cytoplasmic boundaries, with decreased or absent mitoses (Fig. 26.24).

### Blood vessels in LBC

These are identified by an elongated bundle of spindle-shaped cells including endothelial cells and/or perivascular smooth cells (Fig. 26.25). Vascular identification is easy, because the back ground is clean in LBC.

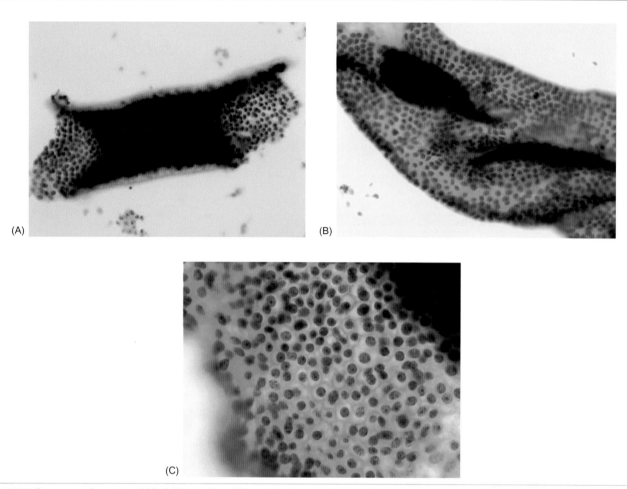

**Fig. 26.23** Secretory endometrium. (A) Early SE is similar to PE but with a lower nuclear/cytoplasmic ratio, smaller inconspicuous nucleoli, absent mitoses and greater spacing of inter-nuclear distance. (B) Mid-SE shows a honeycomb pattern with more cytoplasm than that of early SE, and accordion-pleated glands which are the three-dimensional equivalent of 'saw-toothed' glands. (C) The nuclei are larger than those of PE, rounded and vesicular and display a fine chromatin pattern. (LBC, PAP). (From Norimatsu et al. 2008.[30])

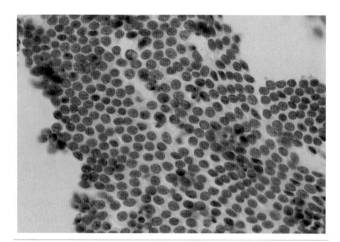

**Fig. 26.24** Atrophic endometrium is similar to PE but nuclear crowding and overlapping is not as striking as PE. The uniform round nuclei are generally arranged in small monolayer sheets and present distinct cytoplasmic boundaries with decreased or absent mitoses. (LBC, PAP). (From Norimatsu et al. 2008.[30])

### Cytological findings: blood vessels in LBC

- Proliferative endometrium shows uniform straight to curvilinear tubular structures or flat epithelial sheets

- Secretory endometrium shows a honeycomb pattern and accordion-pleated glands pattern
- Vascular identification is easy, because the back ground is clean in LBC.

### Hormone-dependent modifications

Hormonal administration, for birth control, for example, or for treatment of menopausal symptoms or dysfunctional uterine bleeding leads to morphological changes in the endometrium, depending on the type of hormone used, the dosage, the regime followed (combined or sequential oestrogen/progesterone administration) the duration of the administration and, in premenopausal women, the menstrual phase in which the hormone is administered. Moreover, every patient reacts uniquely, depending on the state of the endocrine system. The hormone-dependent endometrial modifications involve both the glands and the stroma. Exogenous and endogenous oestrogens when unopposed by progesterone induce proliferation of the endometrium leading to hyperplastic and even neoplastic changes. Secretion is suppressed.

By contrast, progestogens are responsible for proliferation arrest, glandular secretion and differentiation of stromal cells

**Table 26.1A** Comparison between the number of endometrial epithelial cell clumps obtained by CCP and LBC methods

|  | PE (*n* = 40) | SE (*n* = 42) | AE (*n* = 46) | EGBD (*n* = 30) |
|---|---|---|---|---|
| CCP | 37.3 (7-88) | 37.6 (9-111) | 46.2 (8-115) | 37.1 (9-114) |
| LBC | 21.2 (3-59) | 26.3 (6-106) | 19.1 (7-54) | 20 (2-56) |
| Significant difference | *p* < 0.0001 | *p* = 0.0149 | *p* < 0.0001 | *p* = 0.0006 |

CCP, conventional cytological preparation; LBC, liquid-based cytology; PE, proliferative endometrium; SE, secretory endometrium; AE, atrophic endometrium; EGBD, endometrial glandular and stromal breakdown. (From Norimatsu et al. 2008.[30])

**Table 26.1B** Presence of LBC > CCP cases on the number of endometrial epithelial cell clumps (%)

|  | PE (*n* = 40) | SE (*n* = 42) | AE (*n* = 46) | EGBD (*n* = 30) |
|---|---|---|---|---|
| Before correction | 8/40 (20.0) | 12/42 (28.6) | 6/46 (13.0) | 4/30 (13.3) |
| After correction | 40/40 (100) | 42/42 (100) | 46/46 (100) | 27/30 (90.0) |
| Significant difference | *p* < 0.0001 | *p* < 0.0001 | *p* < 0.0001 | *p* < 0.0001 |

*Preparation area of LBC is a circle of diameter 13 mm, and the area is about 133 mm². On the other hand, preparation area of CCP is a rectangle of 25 mm wide and 50 mm long, and the area is 1250 mm². The preparation area of CCP is about 9.4 times the area of LBC. Therefore, the number of cell clumps in LBC was multiplied by 9.4 to convert it into the same area as CCP. The number of cell clumps in LBC before and after correction was compared with CCP. (From Norimatsu et al. 2008.[30])

into decidual cells. Prolonged progesterone treatment induces progressive arrest of secretion and consequent atrophy of the glands with obvious decidualisation of the stroma.

By administering both oestrogens and progestogens, the oestrogen-related effects are commonly reduced. On the other hand, secretory changes are also reduced. In most cases, the administration of both hormones induces endometrial hypo-atrophy consisting in small glands in which only abortive secretory phenomena may be observed and progressive stromal decidual change (Fig. 26.26).

Cytological features in endometrial specimens reflect these hormone-induced modifications. Nowadays, the administration of oestrogens unopposed by progestogens is mainly avoided in view of the well-known neoplastic risk. Consequently, in the majority of the cases, cytological endometrial specimens display small tubular endometrial epithelial aggregates which may show clear cytoplasm as consequence of the weak secretory activity and decidualised stromal cells (Fig. 26.27).[15]

Tamoxifen is a synthetic drug which exhibits non-steroidal anti-oestrogenic activity in the breast. Since the early 1980s, it has been the standard adjuvant therapy in the management of women with endocrine-responsive breast cancer. Tamoxifen works by blocking the binding of oestrogens to the oestrogen receptors. Nevertheless, some metabolites of tamoxifen may show an oestrogenic effect particularly on the female genital tract. This oestrogenic activity, predominantly among long-term users who are aged 50 years or older, can promote uterine pathologies such as leiomyomas, endometrial polyps, hyper-plasias, and even neoplasms. Endometrial polyps are the most common endometrial lesion in patients receiving tamoxifen. The reported relative risk for uterine malignancies associated with tamoxifen therapy ranges from 0.6 to 15.2. Recently, liquid-based endometrial cytology has been proposed as an effective diagnostic method for endometrial surveillance in patients on tamoxifen.[16–20]

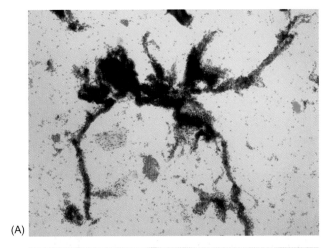

(A)

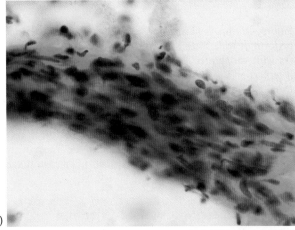

(B)

**Fig. 26.25** Presence of blood vessels in LBC. (A) Because the background is clean in LBC, vascular identification is easy. (B) The blood vessel has a run of bundled spindle-shaped cells including endothelial cells and/or perivascular smooth muscle cells (SE case) (LBC, PAP). (From Norimatsu et al. 2008.[30])

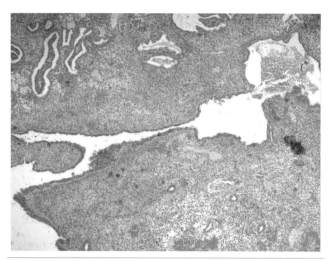

**Fig. 26.26** Endometrium on progesterone: obvious decidualisation of the stroma and secretory (up) and atrophic (down) endometrial glands.

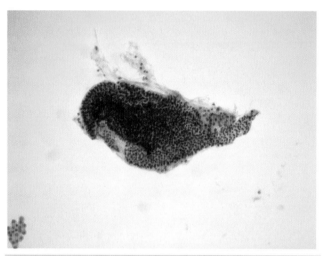

**Fig. 26.27** Endometrium on progesterone: endometrial gland showing secretory features (same case as Fig. 26.6A,B). Liquid based direct endometrial sampling.

## Endometrial hyperplasia

Endometrial hyperplasia appears in LBC cytological samples in the form of wide three-dimensional epithelial endometrial clusters with variable cellular crowding and architectural disorder. In typical endometrial hyperplasia the cytoplasm is commonly scant and the nuclei are isomorphic with finely granular chromatin and small or absent nucleoli. In atypical endometrial hyperplasia the cytoplasm becomes evident and the nuclei may show a moderate pleomorphism. Spindle-shaped stromal cells are abundant in typical hyperplasia, while they are scarce in atypical hyperplasia. The background may enclose inflammatory cells.

## Endometrial glandular and stromal breakdown (EGBD)

Anovulatory cycles may lead to dysfunctional uterine bleeding (DUB) with changes in the endometrium that are similar to

endometrial hyperplasia in cytological preparations. This type of bleeding occurs frequently and many patients are referred to the gynaecology out-patient clinics for evaluation Therefore, it is necessary that endometrial hyperplasia is correctly identified by cytology, with appropriate careful follow-up[31]; but recognition of the cytological findings in anovulatory cycle endometrium is also essential if endometrial hyperplasia is to be ruled out. The appearance of atypical glandular cells in cervicovaginal smears was described in 1975 by Ehrmann[32] in two cases with false positive cytology thought retrospectively to be associated with endometrial stromal breakdown. Since then, there has been no report of finding atypical cells in anovulatory cycle endometrium.

Uterine bleeding that occurs at irregular intervals, is prolonged, excessive, or scanty and prolonged, is regarded as DUB if there is no easily assignable cause. Anovulatory cycles are the most common cause of DUB in women of reproductive age.[33] There are various references to the histological features of DUB.[34,35] Sherman et al.[33] described the clinical and pathological changes in hormone-disordered endometrium associated with anovulatory cycles. These changes are characterised by extensive fragmentation of proliferative endometrium with anovulatory bleeding which is referred to as EGBD (Figs 26.28, 26.29).[36]

The EGBD cases in which histopathological diagnoses were obtained by endometrial curettage have been studied in order to improve the accuracy of cytodiagnosis. At the time of the menopause anovulatory cycles frequently cause changes in simple atrophic endometrium leading to abnormal bleeding in many cases. The endometrial changes may simulate endometrial hyperplasia, leading to difficulty in cytological interpretation. Anovulatory DUB due to raised oestrogen levels is most often associated histologically with persistent proliferative phase endometrium and hyperplasia. It is caused by prolonged endogenous hyperoestrogenism, unopposed by progesterone. Hence, the origin of breakthrough bleeding in persistent proliferative endometrium and hyperplasia can be traced to stromal breakdown, which is associated with pools of extravasated erythrocytes, platelet/fibrin thrombi in capillaries and repair-related changes.[37] Therefore, diagnosis of EGBD should be considered when the cytomorphological changes reveal fragmented clusters of endometrial glands (Fig. 26.30), and condensed clusters of stromal cells (Fig. 26.31). These cytological findings are significant and common and are the characteristic cellular changes of EGBD.

### Diagnostic pitfalls: endometrial glandular and stromal breakdown (EGBD)

- Abnormal bleeding due to other causes.
- Extensive fragmentation of normal proliferative endometrium
- Fragmented clusters of endometrial glands
- Condensed clusters of stromal cells
- Changes may be similar to endometrial hyperplasia.

## Papillary metaplastic change in endometrium

The problems of interpretation of endometrial cytology in anovulatory bleeding described above are compounded by various

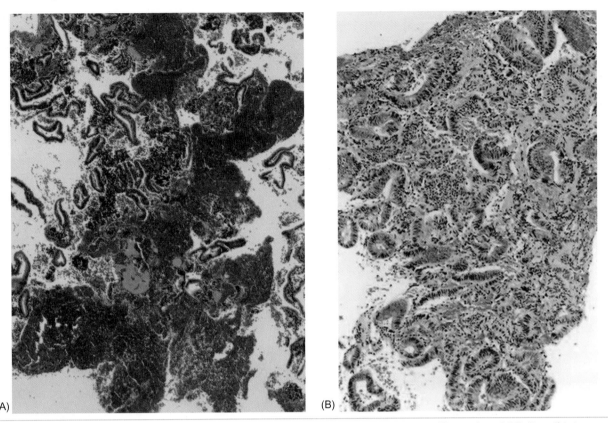

**Fig. 26.28** (A,B) Histological EGBD. Note the extensive fragmentation of proliferative glands, stromal necrosis and haemorrhage (H&E). (From Shimizu et al. 2006.[36])

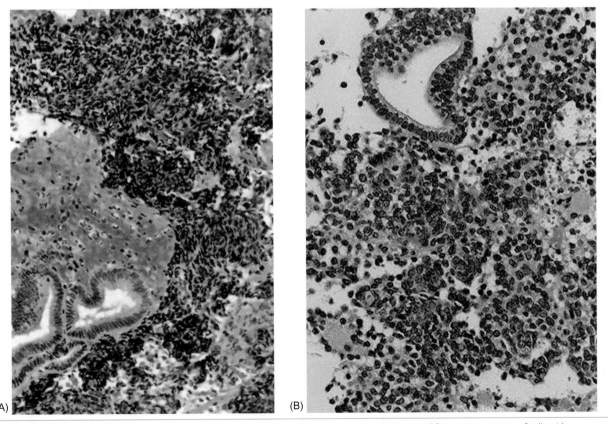

**Fig. 26.29** (A,B) Histological EGBD. As the ground substance undergoes dissolution, stromal cells condense and form compact nests of cells with hyperchromatic nuclei and little or no cytoplasm (H&E). (From Shimizu et al. 2006.[36])

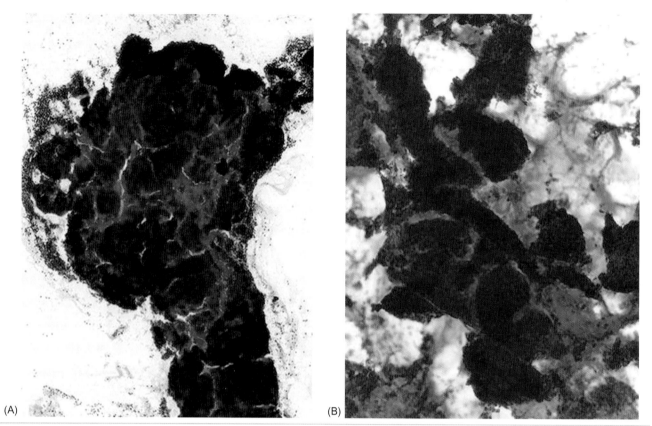

**Fig. 26.30** (A,B) Cytological EGBD showing fragmented clusters of endometrial glands. Cell clumps with associated endometrial stromal cells are produced by fragmentation of glands buried in blood and fibrin causing degenerate aggregation (PAP). (From Shimizu et al. 2006.[36])

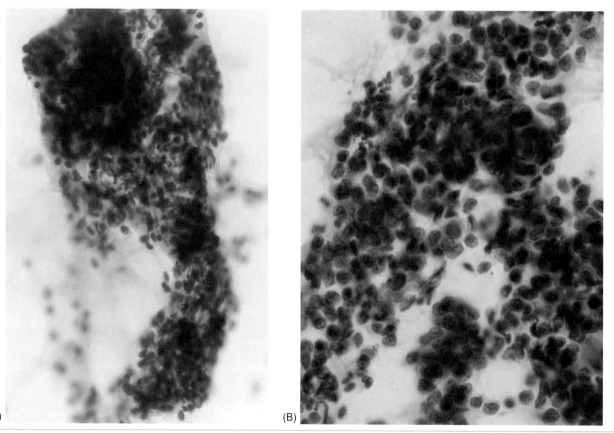

**Fig. 26.31** (A,B) Cytological EGBD showing a condensed cluster of stromal cells. These consist of condensed and compact nests with hyperchromatic nuclei and little or no cytoplasm (PAP). (From Shimizu et al. 2006.[36])

types of hormonally induced metaplastic changes in the endometrium as the histological changes progress from benign to malignancy.[38–42] Frequently, in the process of endometrial glandular and stromal breakdown metaplastic changes occur in the endometrial surface epithelium.[33,42,43] The cellular pattern of these metaplastic changes is similar to that of endometrial hyperplastic cells and, in many respects also to that of endometrial adenocarcinoma cells, creating diagnostic pitfalls in the cytomorphology.[32,44] Despite its frequent occurrence and potential for confusion with other endometrial pathology, very little has been written about the cellular manifestations of such lesions in endometrial samples.

Recently, we have found that the presence of metaplastic cells in cytological samples showing EGBD cases was significantly higher than in other endometrial lesions (Table 26.2). Both eosinophilic and ciliated metaplasia were recognised (Fig. 26.32).[45] Because metaplasias originate in high oestrogen levels, the finding is of relevance to endometrial hyperplasia.[33,37,40] Papillary metaplasia is situated on the endometrial surface epithelium,[33,38–40] therefore presenting as a structural atypia in cytological material. Distinction from endometrial hyperplasia can be particularly difficult as the metaplastic cells may be present in abnormal cell clumps in samples from women showing EGBD. The metaplastic cells show thick

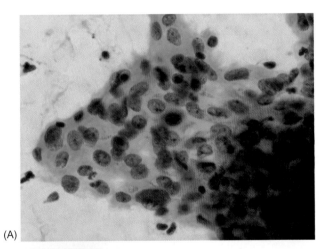

(A)

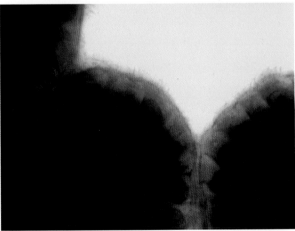

(B)

**Fig. 26.32** (A,B) Cytological EGBD. Typical cytomorphology (A) and ciliated cell metaplasia (B). (A) Cytologically bland cells have abundant eosinophilic cytoplasm and no nuclear pleomorphism. (B) These cells possess clearly visible luminal cilia (PAP). (From Norimatsu et al. 2006.[45])

**Table 26.2** Occurrence of metaplastic cells in each lesion

|  | NPE (n = 49) | EGBD (n = 32) | EH (n = 63) |
|---|---|---|---|
| Eosinophilic metaplasia | 10/49 (20.4%) | 11/32 (34.4%) | 12/63 (19.1%) |
| Ciliated cell metaplasia | 4/49 (8.2%) | 19/32 (59.4%) | 14/63 (22.2%) |
| Total | 14/49 (28.6%) | 30/32 (93.8%) | 26/63 (41.3%) |

NPE, normal proliferative endometrium; EGBD, endometrial glandular and stromal breakdown; EH, endometrial hyperplasia without atypia. (From Norimatsu et al. 2006.[45])

**Table 26.3** Occurrence of metaplastic clumps with irregular protrusions (MCIP) in each lesion

|  | NPE (n = 49) | EGBD (n = 32) | EH (n = 63) |
|---|---|---|---|
| Metaplastic clumps with irregular protrusion | 5/49 (10.2%) | 29/32 (90.6%) | 18/63 (28.6%) |

NPE, normal proliferative endometrium; EGBD, endometrial glandular and stromal breakdown; EH, endometrial hyperplasia without atypia. (From Norimatsu et al. 2006.[45])

eosinophilic cytoplasm and rounded slightly swollen nuclei; some irregular small projections can be seen from the edges of the cell clumps. We have defined these as metaplastic clumps with irregular protrusion (MCIP) (Fig. 26.33A,B). In EGBD cases, MCIP appears to be common, occurring in 90.6% of our cases, and they were rather characteristic in comparison with other lesions (Table 26.3).

Papillary metaplasia, also known as eosinophilic syncytial change, papillary syncytial change, and surface syncytial change, is seen with EGBD on the endometrial surface epithelium. Sherman et al.[33] demonstrated that papillary syncytial metaplasia is an epithelial alteration that is associated with stromal breakdown and these lesions typically involve the surface. Histopathological findings of acute endometrial breakdown, as shown previously by Zaman and Mazur[46] who reported such changes, were intimately admixed with foci of papillary syncytial change along surface epithelium. The papillary metaplasia in their cases was characterised by stratified eosinophilic cells often forming small papillary tufts that lacked connective tissue support; the degree of nuclear enlargement, pleomorphism, and irregularity is comparatively modest (Fig. 26.33C).[33,38,43] The MCIP which we have observed are considered to equate to this type of papillary metaplasia.

Sherman et al.[33] stated that the condensed stromal cell changes observed in the endometrium are associated with anovulatory cycles. There still remains the problem of understanding the cytomorphological alteration of these changes. Therefore, we classified three morphological variants of MCIP, and their tissue of origin is suggested.[45]

MCIP was present with condensed stromal clusters in 93.1% of EGBD cases, which was highly significant, compared with other lesions (Fig. 26.34A,B, Table 26.4). In histopathological samples of EGBD, papillary metaplasia was seen within

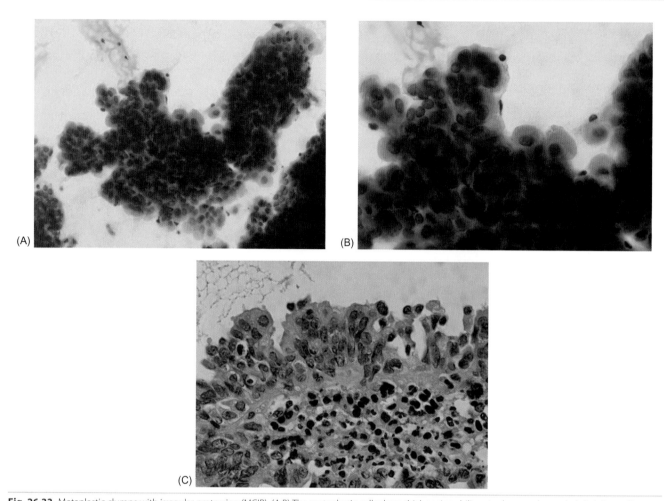

**Fig. 26.33** Metaplastic clumps with irregular protrusion (MCIP). (A,B) The metaplastic cells show thick eosinophilic cytoplasm and rounded slightly swollen nuclei. Some irregular small projections are seen at the edges of the cell clumps (EGBD case, PAP). (C) Papillary metaplasia on the endometrial surface epithelium. This type of metaplasia is characterised by stratified eosinophilic cells often forming small papillary tufts that lack connective tissue cores (EGBD case, H&E). (From Norimatsu et al. 2006.[45])

endometrial surface epithelium, and was both included in and attached to the condensed stromal clusters (Fig. 26.34C).[33,42,43,46] Papillary metaplastic tissue forms microscopic mounds on the endometrial surface overlying condensed stromal cells, as has been described by Sherman et al.[33] Zaman and Mazur[46] have shown that the dense clusters of endometrial stroma, often with a cap of epithelium, are the defining features of the process of acute endometrial breakdown. Lehman and Hart[43] found that the presence of rounded clumps of endometrial stromal cells associated with nuclear debris and neutrophils are a characteristic appearance. However, these lesions are not a pathological change nor even metaplastic, but are an expected reparative tissue response following endometrial breakdown bleeding. Therefore, the appearance of MCIP with condensed stromal clusters is thought to originate from papillary metaplasia. They occur on the endometrial surface epithelium, and the appearance of MCIP can be of great help in confirming the suggestion of EGBD endometrium.[45]

### Diagnostic pitfalls: papillary metaplastic change in endometrium

- Metaplastic changes are recognised as structural atypia in the cytological diagnosis

- Metaplastic clumps with irregular protrusion (MCIP)
- MCIP is similar to the cells of endometrial hyperplasia and endometrial adenocarcinoma
- MCIP with condensed stromal clusters is of high diagnostic value in EGBD.

**Table 26.4** Occurrence of MCIP with condensed stromal clusters (%)

|  | NPE (n = 5) | EGBD (n = 29) | EH (n = 18) |
|---|---|---|---|
| Type I MCIP | 1/5 (20.0%) | 15/29 (51.7%) | 1/18 (5.6%) |
| Type II MCIP | 0 | 6/29 (20.7%) | 2/18 (11.1%) |
| Types I + II MCIP | 0 | 6/29 (20.7%) | 0 |
| Total | 1/5 (20.0%) | 27/29 (93.1%) | 3/18 (16.7%) |

MCIP, metaplastic clumps with irregular protrusion; NPE, normal proliferative endometrium; EGBD, endometrial glandular and stromal breakdown; EH, endometrial hyperplasia without atypia. (From Norimatsu et al. 2006.[45])

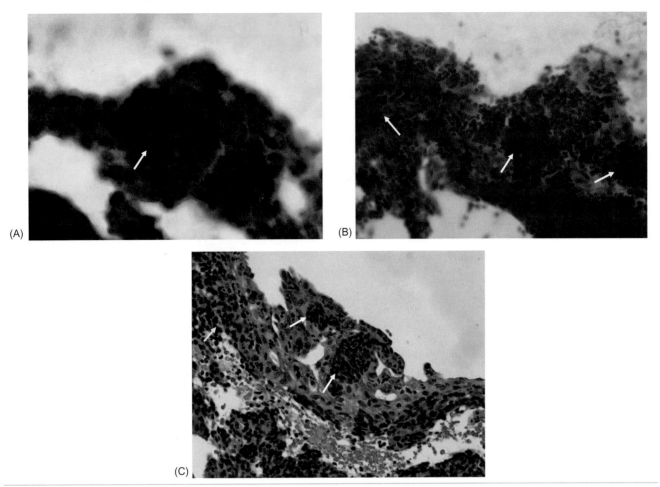

**Fig. 26.34** Cytomorphology of MCIP. (A) Type I MCIP arranged in condensed stromal clusters included within clumps. (B) Type II MCIP arranged in clumps partly attached condensed stromal clusters (EGBD case, PAP). (C) Papillary metaplasia on the endometrial surface epithelium. Histopathological appearance of EGBD with papillary metaplasia was seen within the endometrial surface epithelium. The metaplastic cells are included (see white arrow) and attached to condensed stromal clusters (indicated by yellow arrow) (EGBD case, H&E). (From Norimatsu et al. 2006.[45])

## Endometrial adenocarcinoma

### Epidemiology and classification

Endometrial carcinoma is the most common invasive malignancy of the female genital tract in developed countries. A significant increase in its frequency, both relative and absolute, has been documented during the last decades as a consequence of the effective screening to reduce the incidence of cervical cancer, of the extended life expectancy of women and of the increase in the incidence of risk factors such as obesity, diabetes mellitus, hypertension and low parity.

The majority of the cases are sporadic, whereas about 10% are hereditary. Most important among the latter, is the autosomal dominantly inherited hereditary non-polyposis colorectal cancer caused by mutation of DNA mismatch repair gene that determines constitutive microsatellite instability and Cowden syndrome in patients with germline PTEN inactivation.

Most women with endometrial cancer are diagnosed at an early stage as vaginal bleeding is a precocious, although non-specific, presenting symptom.

Two subtypes of endometrial carcinoma, named type I and type II, have been described on the basis of their different age at presentation, aetiology, pathogenesis, histopathological features and prognosis. *Type I carcinoma*, which accounts for most of cases (approximately 80%), occurs in perimenopausal women, is related to unopposed oestrogen stimulation, is more often well differentiated and of endometrioid histotype, frequently express oestrogen and progesterone receptors, and has a favourable prognosis with appropriate therapy. Conversely, the less frequent *type II carcinoma* mainly affects older post-menopausal women, is non-oestrogen dependent, displays a low frequency of expression of hormonal receptors, is predominantly of serous papillary or clear cell histotype, and has a worse prognosis with a high incidence of metastases. Type I adenocarcinoma develops from endometrial hyperplasia whereas type II is not related. Indeed, type II carcinoma derives from serous endometrial intraepithelial carcinoma (Fig. 26.35A) which arises on atrophic endometrium or within an endometrial polyp. However, endometrial intraepithelial carcinoma can show extrauterine spread. For this reason some authors have suggested that it should be considered a small uterine serous cancer rather than an intraepithelial precancer. In regard to this, recent studies identify endometrial glandular dysplasia as the precursor lesion of type II tumours, both serous intraepithelial carcinoma and serous carcinoma.

Type I carcinomas are associated with mutations in the *k-ras* proto-oncogene, and in the PTEN tumour suppressor gene, and often show microsatellite instability, but do not usually have

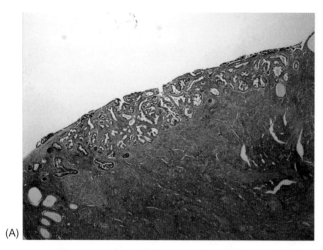

(A)

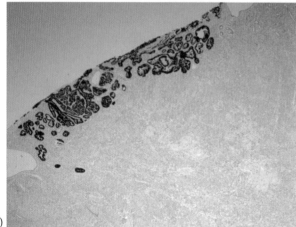

(B)

**Fig. 26.35** (A) Serous intraepithelial carcinoma arising in atrophic endometrium. (B) Positive p53 immunostaining.

mutations in the p53 tumour suppressor gene; by contrast, type II carcinomas show frequent p53 mutations (Fig. 26.35B), but rarely have microsatellite instability, and *k-ras* or PTEN mutations.[47–52]

## Histopathology of endometrial adenocarcinoma

The World Health Organization (WHO) classifies a number of endometrial adenocarcinomas (Box 26.1).[47]

### Endometrioid adenocarcinoma

Endometrioid adenocarcinoma forms the majority of the type I endometrial carcinomas. It replicates the histological features of the normal endometrium. The malignant glands have a back-to-back arrangement with scant or no intervening stroma and are lined by pseudostratified epithelium. Tumoral cells show an increased nuclear size and nuclear/cytoplasmic ratio (Fig. 26.36). Endometrioid adenocarcinoma may exhibit varied epithelial differentiation including squamous, secretory and ciliated and architectural patterns such as villous pattern. All these histological variants carry a prognosis similar to that of classic endometrioid adenocarcinoma. Endometrioid adenocarcinomas often disclose squamous differentiation in the form of keratinisation phenomena, intercellular bridges, and/or at least three of the following morphological features:

---

**Box 26.1  WHO histological classification of tumours of the uterine corpus**

**Epithelial tumours**

Endometrial carcinoma

- Endometrioid adenocarcinoma
  - Variant with squamous differentiation
  - Villoglandular variant
  - Secretory variant
  - Ciliated cell variant
- Mucinous adenocarcinoma
  - Microglandular adenocarcinoma
- Serous adenocarcinoma
- Clear cell adenocarcinoma
- Mixed cell adenocarcinoma
- Squamous cell adenocarcinoma
- Transitional adenocarcinoma
- Small cell carcinoma
- Undifferentiated adenocarcinoma
- Others

**Mesenchymal tumours**

Endometrial stromal and related tumours

- Endometrial stromal sarcoma, low grade
- Endometrial stromal nodule
- Undifferentiated endometrial sarcoma

Smooth muscle tumours

- Leiomyoma
- Leiomiosarcoma
- Smooth muscle tumour of uncertain malignant potential

**Mixed epithelial and mesenchymal tumours**

- Carcinosarcoma
- Adenosarcoma
- Carcinofibroma
- Adenofibroma
- Adenomyoma

**Gestational trophoblastic disease**

- Trophoblastic neoplasms
  - Choriocarcinoma
  - Placental site trophoblastic tumour
  - Epithelioid throphoblastic tumour
- Molar pregnancies
  - Hydatiform mole
  - Complete
  - Partial
  - Invasive
  - Metastatic

**Miscellaneous tumours**

**Lymphoid and haemopoietic tumours**

**Secondary tumours**

---

sheet-like growth without gland formation or palisading, sharp cell margins, eosinophilic and thick or glassy cytoplasm, and a decreased nuclear/cytoplasmic ratio (Fig. 26.37). The secretory variant shows sub-nuclear glycogen vacuoles analogous to

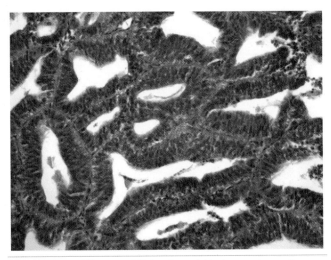

**Fig. 26.36** Well-differentiated (G1) endometrioid adenocarcinoma: the malignant glands have a back-to-back arrangement and are lined by pseudostratified epithelium; the stroma is scant.

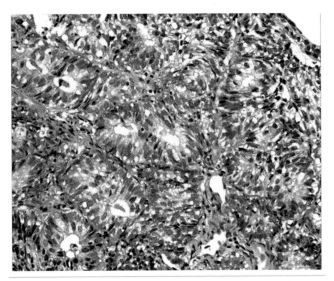

**Fig. 26.38** Endometrioid adenocarcinoma: secretory variant (note the sub-nuclear glycogen vacuoles).

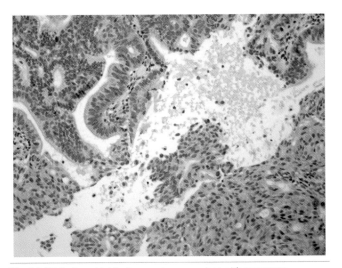

**Fig. 26.37** Endometrioid adenocarcinoma: variant with squamous differentiation.

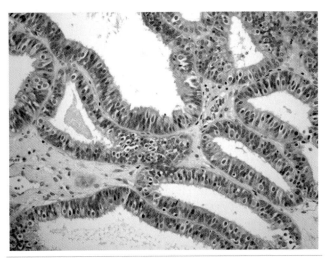

**Fig. 26.39** Endometrioid adenocarcinoma: ciliated cell variant.

those of early secretory endometrium (Fig. 26.38). In the ciliated cell variant, neoplastic cells are ciliated and resemble those of the tubal epithelium (Fig. 26.39). Villoglandular adenocarcinoma is a relatively common variant of endometrioid adenocarcinoma in which there are numerous villous fronds having a delicate central core lined by cells similar to those of the classic endometrioid adenocarcinoma (Fig. 26.40).

With respect to the grade of histological differentiation, endometrioid adenocarcinoma exists as high, intermediate, and low grade (G1, G2, G3) on the basis of nuclear atypia and architecture (Table 26.5). More highly differentiated endometrioid adenocarcinomas (G1) have a predominantly glandular architectural pattern with regular non-atypical columnar cells (Fig. 26.36). Less-differentiated tumours (G3) show a predominantly solid growth pattern and obvious atypia. Squamous components are excluded for grading (Fig. 26.41).

## Serous and clear cell carcinomas

Serous and clear cell carcinomas typify the type II endometrial carcinoma. Serous carcinoma is the most frequent among

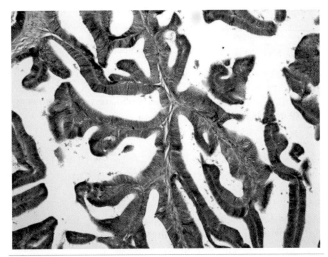

**Fig. 26.40** Endometrioid adenocarcinoma: villoglandular variant.

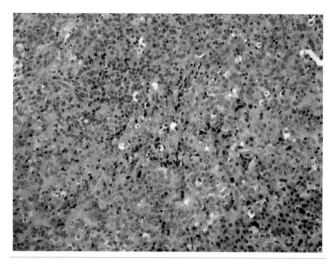

**Fig. 26.41** Grade 3 (G3) endometrioid adenocarcinoma with predominantly solid growth and obvious atypia.

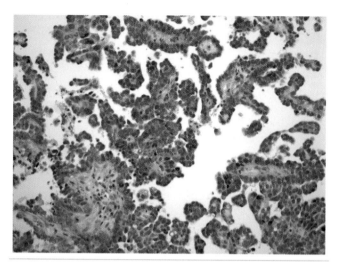

**Fig. 26.42** Serous carcinoma with prominent papillary architecture and marked cellular atypia.

**Table 26.5** Grading of type I endometrial adenocarcinoma

| Grade 1 (G1) | ≤5% solid growth pattern |
|---|---|
| Grade 2 (G2) | 6–50% solid growth pattern |
| Grade 3 (G3) | >50% solid growth pattern |

Squamous/morular components are excluded for grading; nuclear atypia should raise the grade by one (i.e. from 1 to 2 or from 2 to 3).

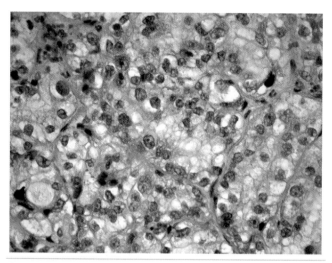

**Fig. 26.43** Clear cell carcinoma (solid pattern); neoplastic cells have clear glycogen-filled cytoplasm.

type II carcinomas. It resembles its most common and familial counterpart in the ovary and coexistent ovarian and endometrial serous carcinomas are not uncommon. The tumour may have a papillary (so-called serous papillary carcinoma), glandular or solid growth pattern (Fig. 26.42). Psammoma bodies are found in about 30% of the cases. Clear cell carcinoma is composed of clear, glycogen-filled, cells arranged in solid, tubulocystic or papillary pattern (Fig. 26.43).

In both serous and clear cell carcinomas cellular atypia is prominent. Large pleomorphic nuclei possessing prominent nucleoli are characteristically placed at the cellular apex giving rise to the so-called hob-nail appearance of the cells.

### Mucinous carcinoma

Mucinous carcinoma resembles endocervical adenocarcinoma. Its characteristic is the presence of intracytoplasmic mucin.

### Pure squamous, transitional and small cell carcinomas

Pure squamous, transitional and small cell carcinomas are infrequent histotypes.

### Cytological findings in LBC preparations using cytoarchitectural features: endometrial adenocarcinoma

In cases of malignancy, cytological endometrial specimens may show different features depending on the histotype and on the grade of differentiation of the tumour. Also, the cytological features of epithelial endometrial tumours will differ from those of mixed endometrial tumours, trophoblastic tumours and non-endometrial tumours such as cervical, tubal or ovarian carcinomas. Directly sampled specimens may also include non-pathological or hyperplastic endometrial cell aggregates.

### Main malignancy criteria

1. Architectural
   - Loss of polarity
   - Papillary cell clusters
   - Discohesive cells
2. Cellular
   - High nucleo/cytoplasmatic ratio
   - Anisonucleosis and poikilonucleosis
   - Coarse and/or marginated chromatin
   - Nucleolar prominence
   - Nuclear membrane indentations
   - Cell cannibalism
3. Background
   - Scarcity of stromal cells
   - Necrosis.

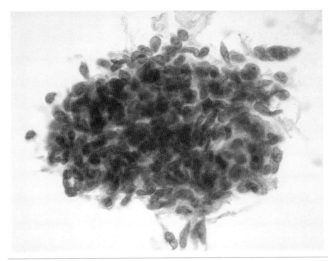

**Fig. 26.44** Neoplastic endometrial cellular group showing tumour cells protruding from the cluster silhouette. LBC direct endometrial sampling.

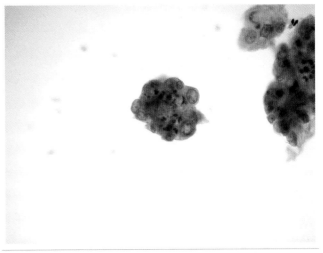

**Fig. 26.45** Papillary aggregate. LBC direct endometrial sampling.

Tumour cell groups usually lose their cell polarity. This feature is particularly obvious at the margin of the epithelial endometrial clusters where the typical palisade organisation of the cells disappears. Moreover, the presence of cells protruding from the cluster silhouette is suspicious for malignancy (Fig. 26.44). The degree of cellular crowding and the size of the tumoral clusters are variable. Papillary aggregates as well as rosettes, plum blossoms and cellular spheres are ominous for malignancy (Fig. 26.45). They are numerous in serous papillary carcinomas (see below).

The size and shape of the nuclei is variable. In general nuclei are enlarged with consequent high nuclear/cytoplasmic ratio. Nucleoli may be prominent and chromatin may appear coarse, condensed and sometimes marginated at the periphery of the nucleus giving a thickened appearance to the nuclear membrane. Indentations of the nuclear membrane may also be found. In well-differentiated (G1) endometrioid adenocarcinomas nuclear enlargement and nuclear atypia may be not evident. Mitoses may be prominent but this is not a reliable feature of malignancy as mitoses can be present in normal endometrium, particularly in the proliferative phase.

Stromal cells are generally scarce.[53] The background shows a variable amount, of tumour diathesis, from almost absent to intense, usually consisting of degenerate cells, nuclear debris, histiocytes and leucocytes.

Cell cannibalism, either epithelium-epithelium and epithelium-inflammatory cells, may be found (Fig. 26.46). Indeed, neutrophils are often present within neoplastic cells (neutrophilic emperipolesis) displacing the nucleus to the periphery of the cell.[28,54,55]

### Type I endometrioid endometrial carcinomas

In cases of well-differentiated endometrioid adenocarcinomas, endometrial epithelial clusters are commonly medium in size, usually smaller than those observed in hyperplastic samples, with prominent cellular overlapping (Fig. 26.47). The cellular polarity is, at least in part, lost and the tumour cells may protrude beyond the cluster (Fig. 26.44). Cytological atypia is inconspicuous. Indeed, the tumour cells are not very different

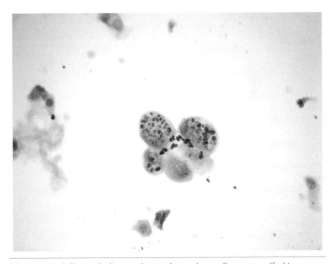

**Fig. 26.46** Cell cannibalism; polymorphonuclear cells are engulfed in the cytoplasm of the tumour cells (neutrophilic emperipolesis). LBC direct endometrial sampling.

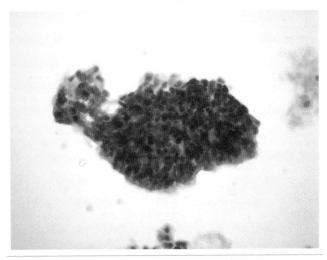

**Fig. 26.47** Well-differentiated endometrioid adenocarcinoma: medium-size three-dimensional group with cellular overlapping (crowding) and partial loss of cell polarity (that is, of the typical palisade organisation at the margin of the epithelial endometrial cluster). LBC direct endometrial sampling.

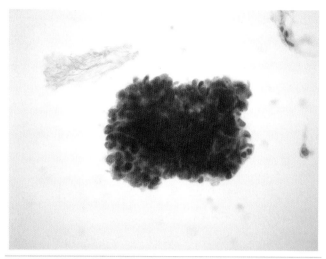

**Fig. 26.48** Well-differentiated endometrioid adenocarcinoma: medium-sized tumour cell cluster with cellular overlapping and complete loss of the cell polarity. LBC direct endometrial sampling.

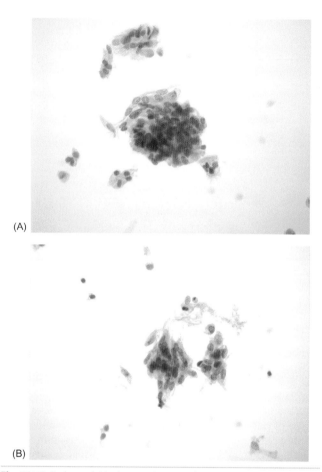

(A)

(B)

**Fig. 26.50** Endometrioid adenocarcinoma with squamous differentiation (A,B). Cytological features of the same case of the Figure 26.37. Note the spindle appearance of some of the neoplastic cells. LBC direct endometrial sampling.

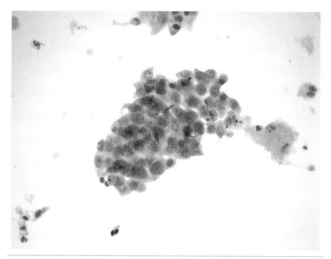

**Fig. 26.49** Poorly differentiated endometrioid adenocarcinoma: small and discohesive neoplastic sheet. LBC direct endometrial sampling.

from those of proliferative endometrium (Fig. 26.48). Tumour diathesis consisting of necrotic cellular debris and inflammatory cells is not constant.

Features suggesting the diagnosis of poorly differentiated endometrioid adenocarcinoma are the reduced size and crowding of the cell clumps which are a consequence of the reduced cellular cohesion, the crowding of the tumour cell clusters and the prominent cytological atypia (Fig. 26.49). Cell cannibalism is observed more often in low grade tumours compared with poorly differentiated tumours.

The endometrioid carcinoma variants may sometimes be identified on the basis of some typical cytological markers: endometrioid adenocarcinoma with squamous differentiation may exhibit squamous morules (Fig. 26.50); villoglandular adenocarcinoma shows more obvious papillary groups; secretory adenocarcinoma cells have abundant clear and vacuolated cytoplasm, while ciliated cell endometrioid adenocarcinoma has cilia. However, the recognition of these histological variants may be difficult as well as clinically irrelevant.

## Type II endometrial carcinomas

### Serous carcinoma

Cytological endometrial specimens from serous carcinomas show marked exfoliation of tumour cells either in the form of cellular clusters or as single cells or even single bare nuclei. Clusters are generally small and flat sheet-like or three-dimensional with inconspicuous cellular crowding. Papillae are present in many cases (Fig. 26.51). The tumour cells are larger and more atypical than those seen in endometrioid adenocarcinoma. Chromatin is commonly coarse and marginated and nucleoli are prominent. The nuclear contour is irregular. The cytoplasm is dense and well defined (Fig. 26.52). Psammoma bodies, naked or incorporated in a malignant cell group, can sometimes be seen (Fig. 26.53). The presence of numerous single cells and bare nuclei is the most striking diagnostic feature of serous carcinomas (Fig. 26.54, Table 26.6).[56,57]

Early lesions may show the hallmarks of serous papillary carcinoma as well as the cytological features of endometrial atrophy. Actually, the precursor of serous papillary carcinoma is serous intraepithelial tumour which is a focal lesion frequently arising on atrophic endometrium.

### Clear cell carcinoma

Clear cell and serous carcinoma closely overlap and at times are indistinguishable from one another. The malignant clear cells

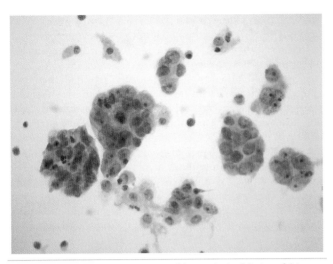

**Fig. 26.51** Serous carcinoma. Because of the marked exfoliation of this histotype, the cytological specimens are rich in neoplastic cells which frequently show a papillary architecture (serous papillary carcinoma. LBC direct endometrial sampling.

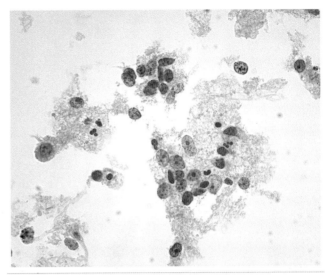

**Fig. 26.54** Serous carcinoma. Single cells and bare nuclei. LBC direct endometrial sampling.

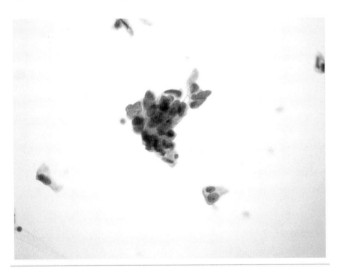

**Fig. 26.52** Serous carcinoma. A small cluster showing prominent atypia with irregular size and shape of the cells, coarse and marginated chromatin, prominent nucleoli, irregular nuclear contour. LBC direct endometrial sampling.

**Table 26.6** Cytological features of type I and type II endometrial carcinoma

| Cytological features | Endometrioid adenocarcinoma | Serous carcinoma |
|---|---|---|
| Tumour cells | | |
| Architecture | Middle- to small-sized neoplastic clusters depending on the grade of differentiation | Many single neoplastic cells |
| | | Small-sized neoplastic clusters |
| | | Papillae |
| Nuclei | Regular or variably pleomorphic | Pleomorphic |
| | Micronucleoli | Irregular nuclear membrane |
| | | Macronucleoli |
| | | Single bare nuclei |
| Psammoma bodies | Absent | Present in some cases |
| p53 | Negative | Positive |

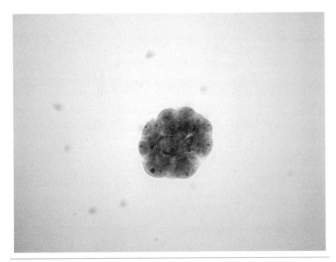

**Fig. 26.53** Serous carcinoma. Psammoma bodies incorporated in a papilla. LBC direct endometrial sampling.

are pleomorphic and characterised by abundant clear cytoplasm, large vesicular nuclei and prominent nucleoli (Fig. 26.55).

Peritoneal and pelvic washings in patients with type II endometrial carcinoma frequently contain malignant cells. Further support for the diagnosis comes from the overexpression of the p53 protein on immunohistochemistry which is typical of these tumours (Fig. 26.56).[58]

## Overlapping nuclei

Overlapping nuclei implies that there are at least more than two layers of cell nuclei in the sheets and this can clearly be

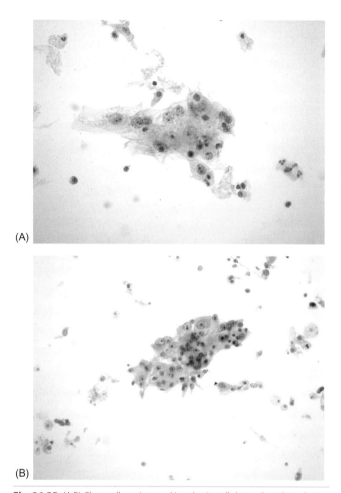

(A)

(B)

**Fig. 26.55** (A,B) Clear cell carcinoma. Neoplastic cells have abundant clear cytoplasm, large nuclei and prominent nucleoli. LBC direct endometrial sampling.

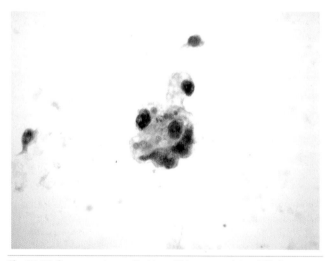

**Fig. 26.56** Serous carcinoma. Positive p53 immunostaining. LBC direct endometrial sampling.

seen under the microscope by moving the focus. While changing focus, the initial nucleus completely disappears, and if another nucleus then appears, the degree of overlapping nuclei is considered to be two layers. If the second nucleus disappears and another nucleus appears, it is considered to have three

layers of overlapping nuclei (Fig. 26.57).[59] However, when there is less overlapping the initial nucleus does not completely disappear. Furthermore, on changing focus, a stromal nucleus may appear as seen in Figure 26.58.

Meisels and Jolicoeur[60] and Morse[21] reported that overlapping nuclei are 'useful' as diagnostic criteria for endometrial lesions in conventional cytological preparations (CCP). Similarly, with LBC, Papaefthimiou et al.[3] reported that overlapping of two nuclei was observed in endometrial adenocarcinoma. However, the degree of overlapping between the nuclei in hyperplasia with or without atypia was slight. According to Norimatsu et al.,[59] comparison of the degree of overlapping of nuclei in endometrial carcinoma and normal endometrium showed that it decreased significantly from endometrial carcinoma to proliferative, secretory and atrophic endometrium in both conventional and LBC preparations (Table 26.7) so that defining the degree of overlapping is necessary to distinguish endometrial carcinoma from normal endometrium. However, while there is no significant difference in the extent of overlapping nuclei between CCP and LBC with regard to normal endometrial types, with endometrial carcinoma LBC reveals more overlapping ($p < 0.0001$) than CCP (Table 26.7). This evidence that the degree of overlapping nuclei in endometrial carcinoma is enhanced by LBC compared with CCP is a new finding, which is very useful in the diagnosis of endometrial carcinoma. It is assumed that the finding reflects a characteristic of the LBC (SurePath) method[61] whereby when the endometrial cells in clumps are collected into the vial the cellular architecture is preserved by the fixative. When making the smear, these clumps are absorbed onto the glass slide surface, being heavy cells of high specific gravity, both by cellular electric charge (glass slide surface is ' + ', cell is ' − ') and by cell gravity. Thus in LBC preparations it seems that the original architecture is retained in the preserved cell clumps.

**Table 26.7** Comparison of degree of overlapping nuclei in normal endometrium and carcinoma

|  | CCP | LBC | Significant difference[a] |
|---|---|---|---|
| EC (*n* = 30) | 2.07 ± 0.23[b,c,d] | 2.82 ± 0.38[b,c,d] | $p < 0.0001$ |
| PE (*n* = 30) | 1.48 ± 0.04[b,d] | 1.45 ± 0.07[b,d] | $p = 0.1501$ |
| SE (*n* = 30) | 1.16 ± 0.15[e] | 1.18 ± 0.14[f] | $p = 0.6768$ |
| AE (*n* = 30) | 1.07 ± 0.06 | 1.10 ± 0.14 | $p = 0.7379$ |

CCP, conventional cytological preparation; LBC, liquid-based cytology; EC, endometrial carcinoma; SE, secretory endometrium; PE, proliferative endometrium; AE, atrophic endometrium.

[a]Comparison of degree of overlapping nuclei between CCP and LBC, in EC and normal endometrium.

[b]Statistically significant difference between SE ($p < 0.001$).

[c]Statistically significant difference between PE ($p < 0.001$).

[d]Statistically significant difference between AE ($p < 0.001$).

[e]Statistically significant difference between AE ($p = 0.0219$).

[f]Statistically significant difference between AE ($p = 0.0168$).
(From Norimatsu et al. 2009.[59])

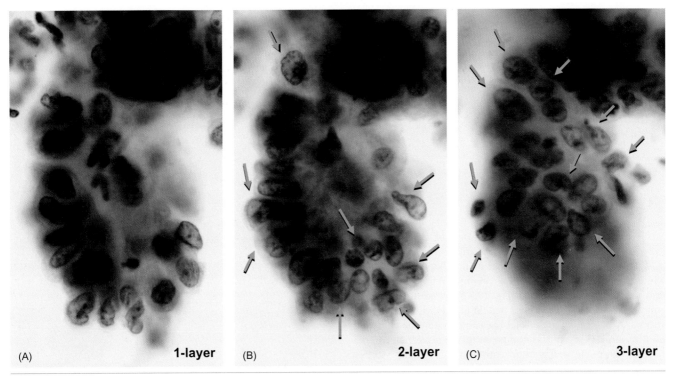

**Fig. 26.57** Overlapping nuclei in SurePath LBC. (A,B) On changing focus, the initial nucleus completely disappears. If another nucleus then appears (arrow), the degree of overlapping nuclei is considered to be two layers. (B,C) If the second nucleus disappears and another nucleus appears (arrow) it is considered to be three layers of overlapping (endometrioid adenocarcinoma Grade-2, PAP). (From Norimatsu et al. 2009.[59])

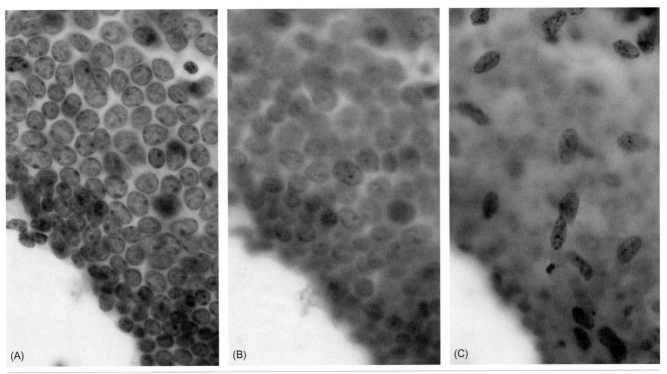

**Fig. 26.58** Overlapping nuclei in SurePath LBC. (A, B) On changing focus, the initial nucleus does not completely disappear. (B,C) With further changing of focus, a stromal nucleus appears. Therefore, no overlapping of nuclei was recognised (proliferative endometrium, PAP). (From Norimatsu et al. 2009.[59])

## Cytological findings: overlapping nuclei

- A significant difference in degree of overlapping nuclei is not recognised between CCP and LBC in normal endometrial types
- The degree of overlapping nuclei in endometrial carcinoma is enhanced in LBC preparations
- This new finding is very useful in the diagnosis of endometrial carcinoma.

## Malignant mixed müllerian tumour (carcinosarcoma)

Mixed müllerian tumours are composed of two phenotypically different cellular components: epithelial and mesenchymal. Both components are benign in papillary adenofibroma while they are both malignant in malignant mixed müllerian tumour (i.e. carcinosarcoma) (Fig. 26.59). When the tumour is composed of a combination of benign glands with a malignant stroma, it is termed adenosarcoma (Box 26.1). The commonest tumour of this group is malignant mixed müllerian tumour. It is a high-grade malignancy, commoner in elderly women. It frequently shows a polypoid appearance, even occasionally protruding through the cervical os (see Ch. 25).

Malignant mixed müllerian tumours express both malignant epithelial and mesenchymal differentiation. The epithelial component most commonly consists of conventional endometrioid adenocarcinoma. However, other forms of epithelial differentiation may be present either alone or in combination. The sarcomatous component is shed singly or in loose clusters and shows homologous (leiomyosarcoma or endometrial stromal sarcoma) or heterologous (e.g. rhabdomyosarcomatous or osteosarcomatous) differentiation.[47] In cytological endometrial specimens the dual phenotype is especially appreciable when the epithelial component has a striking glandular appearance and/or in cases with heterologous differentiation (Fig. 26.60).

## Trophoblastic tumours

Although, cytology has a marginal role in the routine diagnosis of trophoblastic tumours, their cytological features have been described. Malignant cytotrophoblasts appear singly or aggregated in small clusters. They are large and pleomorphic with abundant dispersed chromatin and prominent eosinophilic nucleoli and have dense cytoplasm which may be eosinophilic or cyanophilic (Fig. 26.61). Multinucleated trophoblastic cells may be also seen (Fig. 26.62). The background may be necrotic and contain inflammatory cells.[62]

## Non-endometrial tumours

Analogous to serous intraepithelial tumours, in cases of non-endometrial tumours there is a frank dichotomy comprising normal endometrial aggregates and neoplastic cellular groups. Non-endometrial neoplastic cells may result from contamination of the endometrial specimens by a cervical carcinoma

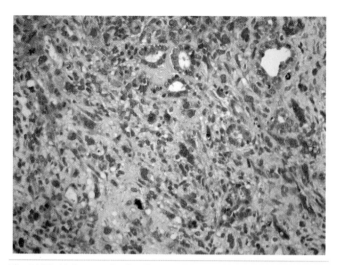

**Fig. 26.59** Malignant mixed müllerian tumour (carcinosarcoma): epithelial and mesenchymal components.

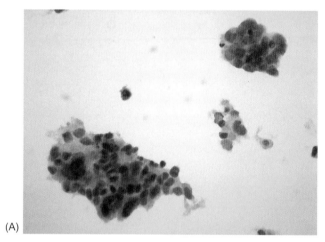

(A)

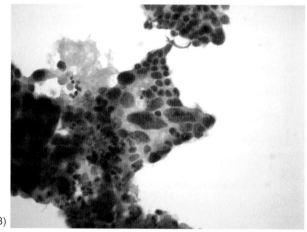

(B)

**Fig. 26.60** (A,B) Malignant mixed müllerian tumour (carcinosarcoma): epithelial components in (A) on the upper right field and mesenchymal elements in (A) on the lower left field, and also seen in (B). LBC direct endometrial sampling.

(Fig. 26.63), from metastatic spread of tumour to the endometrial cavity, or the malignant cells may enter the uterine cavity by traversing the lumen of the fallopian tube from an ovarian or extra-ovarian tumour (predominantly tumours arising in the pelvis and abdominal cavity).

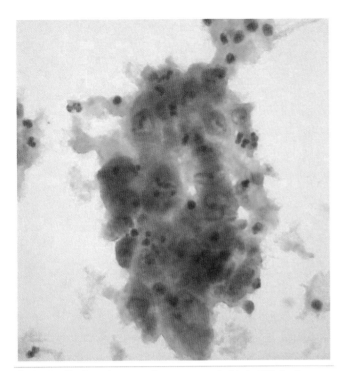

**Fig. 26.61** Choriocarcinoma: malignant cytotrophoblasts. LBC direct endometrial sampling.

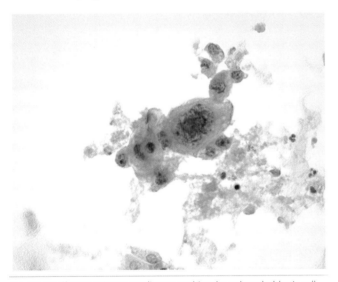

**Fig. 26.62** Choriocarcinoma: malignant multinucleated trophoblastic cell. LBC direct endometrial sampling. (Reproduced by permission of Carlos Bedroissian, Editor in Chief *Diagnostic Cytopathology*).

## Immunocytochemistry using LBC

Mutations of the PTEN, p53, and beta-catenin genes are the most frequent molecular defects in type I endometrial carcinomas. PTEN encodes a dual-specificity phosphatase with lipid phosphatase and protein tyrosine phosphatase activities that regulate both apoptosis and interactions with the extracellular matrix.[63] In a study of 38 cases of endometrial intraepithelial neoplasia (EIN), Norimatsu et al.[64] describe helpful histopathological findings using immunohistochemistry that immunohistochemical loss of PTEN and positive nuclear staining of beta-catenin were frequently seen in EIN but not in

**Table 26.8** Correlation between PTEN and nuclear beta-catenin immunoreactivity in EIN cases

| EIN (*n* = 38) | | Nuclear beta-catenin | |
| --- | --- | --- | --- |
| | | Positive (*n* = 10) | Negative (*n* = 28) |
| PTEN | Positive (*n* = 25) | 9 (23.7%) | 16 (42.1%) |
| | Negative (*n* = 13) | 1 (2.6%) | 12 (31.6%) |

EIN, endometrial intraepithelial neoplasia. PTEN, phosphatase and tensin homologue (see text). (From Norimatsu et al. 2007.[64])

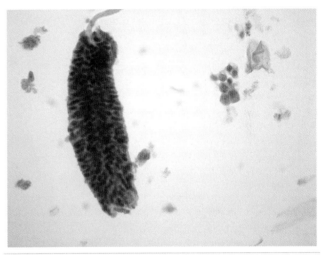

**Fig. 26.63** Cervical carcinoma: proliferative endometrial cluster (left) and neoplastic cervical squamous cells (right) with high nuclear/cytoplasmic ratio. LBC direct endometrial sampling.

normal proliferative endometrium cases. The combination of PTEN-negative/beta-catenin positive results may become a reliable marker for detecting EIN (Table 26.8).

## Immunocytochemical expression of PTEN, beta-catenin and p53 expression in benign endometrial samples

Recently, it has been reported[65] that PTEN expression of normal endometrial glandular epithelial cells changes with the hormonal status; cells from proliferative phase endometrium (PE) produce very high expression, from secretory endometrium (SE) shows attenuation or disappearance of PTEN expression, which in atrophic endometrium (AE) is diminished more in comparison with SE. PTEN expression in EGBD showed a tendency towards atten uation compared with PE and AE. As for the immunoreactivity of beta-catenin, in all phases (PE, SE, AE, and EGBD), activity was observed in the cytoplasm of glandular epithelial cells, with strong membranous staining, but there was no staining of nuclei. With p53 immunoreactivity, p53 positivity was not observed in the glandular epithelial cells in any

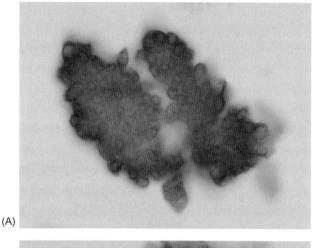

(A)

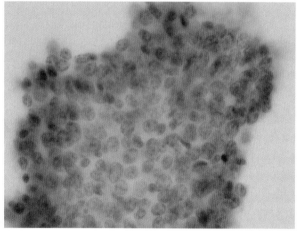

(B)

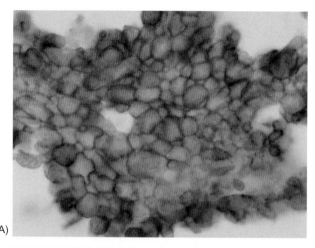

(A)

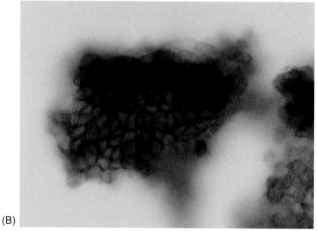

(B)

**Fig. 26.64** Immunoreactivity for PTEN in Grade 1 endometrioid adenocarcinoma. (A) The staining reaction of brown granules in cytoplasm and nuclei was considered positive, whereas (B) the lack of staining was considered negative (immunostain). (From Norimatsu et al. 2008.[67])

**Fig. 26.65** Immunoreactivity for beta-catenin. The staining reaction of brown granules in the cell was considered positive and was classified as membranous staining (A) and cytoplasmic staining (B). A and B show a Grade 1 endometrioid adenocarcinoma (immunostain). (From Norimatsu et al. 2008.[67])

of the phases (PE, SE, AE and EGBD) but was present in some metaplastic cells. The presence of weak p53 immunoreactivity in metaplastic cells was unexpected. In normal endometrium and EGBD, combining the immunocytochemical findings with the cytomorphological features might be useful for distinguishing these conditions from both precancer and carcinoma in endometrial cytology.

## Diagnostic utility of PTEN, beta-catenin and p53 for endometrial cancer

As already described above, endometrial carcinoma (EC) is currently divided into two types of malignant tumours; one associated with endometrial hyperplasia (type I) and the other without any associated endometrial hyperplasia (type II). The histological association between hyperplasia and type I carcinomas indicates oestrogen-dependency, whereas type II carcinomas appear to be a hormone-independent type of cancer.[58]

Today, the clinical and morphological differences between type I and type II carcinomas are firmly established by their differences in the alterations of type-specific genes. The most frequent molecular defects in type I carcinomas are mutations of the phosphatase and tensin homolog (PTEN), *k-ras*,

and beta-catenin genes and microsatellite instability; whereas type II carcinoma often exhibits mutations of the p53 tumour suppressor gene and loss of heterozygosity located on certain chromosomes.[58] In particular, in type II carcinoma, the cumulative effect of abnormalities of these genes is responsible for the transition from normal endometrial cells to pre-cancerous cells and to carcinoma.[66] Therefore, because the overexpression of gene products in types I and II carcinomas correlate with clinicopathological factors and prognosis, it is important to understand the expression of these gene products in normal endometrium, pre-cancerous endometrium and carcinoma.

Recently, the immunocytochemical expression of PTEN, beta-catenin and p53 in EC samples has been demonstrated using LBC.[67] With regard to PTEN immunoreactivity, a cut-off value of 50% of PTEN expression may be useful for the accurate diagnosis of EC in endometrial cytology (Fig. 26.64). For beta-catenin immunoreactivity, the cytoplasmic and nuclear beta-catenin expression and the loss of beta-catenin expression may be useful for more accurate diagnosis of EC in endometrial cytology and may aid in the stratification of tumour type (Figs 26.65, 26.66). For p53 immunoreactivity, the application of a cut-off score of >4 for nuclear p53 expression may be useful for evaluating type II EC in endometrial cytology (Fig. 26.67).

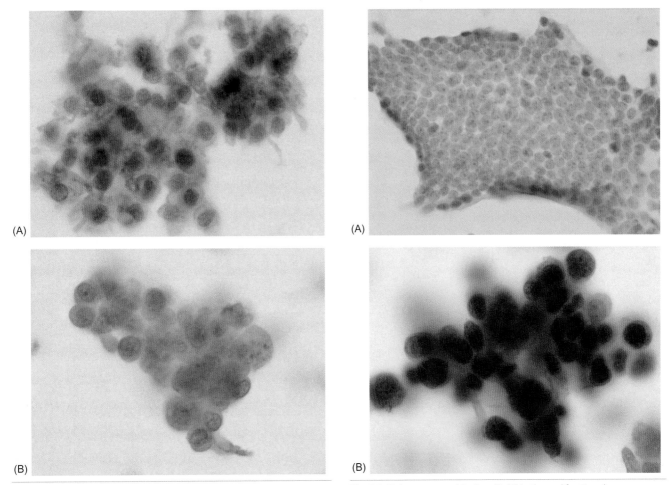

**Fig. 26.66** Immunoreactivity for beta-catenin. (A) The staining reaction of brown granules in the cell was considered positive and was classified as nuclear staining in a Grade 1 endometrioid adenocarcinoma. (B) Grade 3 endometrioid adenocarcinoma with no staining, indicating a negative reaction (immunostain). (From Norimatsu et al. 2008.[67])

**Fig. 26.67** Immunoreactivity for p53. (A) In the proliferative phase, the glandular epithelial cells show negative p53 immunoreactivity (immunostain). (Reproduced with permission from Norimatsu et al.[64]). (B) In papillary serous carcinoma the tumour cells show strong p53 positivity (immunostain). (From Norimatsu et al. 2008.[67])

Finally, it must be emphasised that the current immunocytochemical findings from the combination of PTEN, beta-catenin and p53, along with cytomorphological features, appears to be a valuable tool for the identification of EC using LBC.

## Reporting format for endometrial cytodiagnosis based on cytoarchitectural criteria

### Diagnostic criteria

Diagnostic criteria consist of two main elements (Box 26.2)[68]: the criteria that reflect the cytoarchitecture, and the conventional criteria (background, atypia of cells or cell clumps). Cell clumps are classified into two categories: normal and abnormal cell clumps. The normal category includes those cell groups with a tubular or sheet-like pattern. The abnormal category includes cell clumps with dilated or branched patterns, papillotubular patterns and irregular protrusions. Norimatsu et al.[28] have described all of these characteristics in detail. Cell clumps

composed of metaplastic cells and some irregular small projection figures, usually accompanied by condensed stromal cell clusters, were excluded from these four categories, since their diagnostic importance is not yet clear. Endometrial hyperplasia was suspected in specimens with a total of 10 or more cell clumps and an abnormal cell clump rate of 20–70%, provided there was no overlap with the over 70% group. Atypical endometrial hyperplasia or endometrial carcinoma was suspected in specimens with a total of 10 or more cell clumps and an abnormal cell clump rate of over 70%. The final cytological diagnosis was based on a combination of these results and the conventional criteria.

### The reporting of the endometrial cytological diagnosis

Once specimen adequacy has been described, the result can be categorised into four groups: negative, atypical endometrial cells of undetermined significance (AEC-US), atypical endometrial cells encompassing the spectrum of precursors

## Box 26.2  Diagnostic criteria for endometrial cytology

**Abnormal cell clumps rate[1]**

(B) + (C) + (D)/(A) + (B) + (C) + (D)

(A) tube or sheet-like pattern
(B) dilated or branched pattern
(C) papillotubular pattern
(D) irregular protrusions pattern

- Endometrial hyperplasia is suspected: frequency of abnormal cell clump ratio >20%
- Atypical endometrial hyperplasia or carcinoma is suspected: frequency of abnormal cell clump ratio >70%

**Background and cellular atypia**

- Small cell cluster[2] consisting of atypical cells
- Isolated atypical cells
- Necrotic background
- Metaplastic change (squamous (morule), eosinophilic, ciliated, mucinous, clear cell)

*Source*: Yanoh et al.[68]
[1]Exclusive of cell clumps consisting of metaplastic cells.
[2]Maximum diameter of the cell cluster <0.2mm.

## Box 26.3  A reporting system for endometrial cytology

**Specimen adequacy**

- Satisfactory for evaluation
- Less than optimal
- Unsatisfactory for evaluation

**Interpretation/result**

- Negative
  - Proliferative or secretory phase, or atrophic endometrium
- AEC-US (atypical endometrial cells of undetermined significance)
  - Suspicious for benign endometrial disease (bleeding due to ovarian dysfunction, iatrogenic changes, Infection), or simple endometrial hyperplasia (biopsy not recommended)
- AEC-PEMT (atypical endometrial cells encompassing the spectrum of precursors to endometrial malignant tumours)
  - Suspicious for complex endometrial hyperplasia, simple or complex atypical endometrial hyperplasia, adenocarcinoma *in situ* (biopsy recommended)
- Positive
  - Suspicious for malignant tumour

*Source*: Yanoh et al.[68]

---

to endometrial malignant tumour (AEC-PEMT), and positive. When normal endometrium with proliferative, secretory or menstrual phase changes or atrophy has been identified cytologically,[69] these cases can be reported as 'negative'. The term AEC-US is used for atypical findings in which clinically benign endometrial disease, such as endometrial bleeding due to ovarian dysfunction, iatrogenic changes or infection, is suspected.[69] In such cases, subsequent endometrial biopsy is usually not recommended unless the change persists on repeat cytology. The term AEC-PEMT applies to cases in which a premalignant lesion, such as atypical endometrial hyperplasia, is suspected, and a biopsy is recommended, as for 'positive' cases. All of these options should include additional information suggesting the histopathological diagnosis (Box 26.3).

## The importance of multidisciplinary team meetings for endometrial cytology reporting

In view of the complexity of the findings in normal endometrium and the range of pathological changes leading to endometrial carcinoma, the reporting of endometrial cytology, whether using conventional techniques or LBC, requires close contact between the reporting pathologist and the clinician responsible for the patient's care so as to ensure full understanding of the advantages and limitations of the cytological approach. This is best achieved by regular multidisciplinary meetings for discussion of the patient's care in the light of the reports. Such meetings have proved beneficial to the clinician and the cytopathologist, as well as ensuring appropriate patient management.

## REFERENCES

1. Buccoliero AM, Caldarella A, Noci I, et al. Thin layer method in endometrial cytology. Pathologica 2003;95:179–84.

2. Garcia F, Barker B, Davis J, et al. Thin-layer cytology and histopathology in the evaluation of abnormal uterine bleeding. J Reprod Med 2003;48:882–88.

3. Papaefthimiou M, Symiakaki H, Mentzelopoulou P, et al. Study on the morphology and reproducibility of the diagnosis of endometrial lesions utilizing liquid-based cytology. Cancer 2005;105:56–64.

4. Buccoliero AM, Gheri CF, Castiglione F, et al. Liquid-based endometrial cytology: cytohistological correlation in a population of 917 women. Cytopathology 2007;18:241–49.

5. Buccoliero AM, Gheri CF, Castiglione F, et al. Liquid-based endometrial cytology in the management of sonographically thickened endometrium. Diagn Cytopathol 2007;35:398–402.

6. Buccoliero AM, Castiglione F, Gheri CF, et al. Liquid-based endometrial cytology: its possible value in post-menopausal asymptomatic women. Int J Gynecol Cancer 2007;17:182–87.

7. Geldenhuys L, Murray ML. Sensitivity and specificity of the Pap smear for glandular lesion of the cervix and endometrium. Acta Cytol 2007;51:47–50.

8. Johnsson JE, Stormby NG. Cytological brush technique in malignant disease of the endometrium. Acta Obstet Gynecol Scand 1968;47:38–51.

9. Klemi PJ, Alanen KA, Salmi T. Detection of malignancy in endometrium by the brush sampling in 1042 symptomatic patients. Int J Gynecol Cancer 1995;5:222–25.

10. Sato S, Yaegashi N, Shikano K, et al. Endometrial diagnosis with the Uterobrush and endocyte. Acta Cytol 1996;40:907–10.

11. Fujihara A, Norimatsu Y, Kobayashi TK, et al. Direct intrauterine sampling with Uterobrush: cell preparation by the flicked method. Diagn Cytopathol 2006;34:486–90.

12. Maksem J, Sager F, Bender R. Endometrial collection and interpretation using the Tao brush and cytorich fixative system: a feasibility study. Diagn Cytopathol 1997;17:339–46.

13. Groisman GM, Meir A. CD10 is helpful in detecting occult or inconspicuous endometrial

stromal cells in cases of presumptive endometriosis. Arch Pathol Lab Med 2003;127:103–1006.

14. Nassar A, Fleisher SR, Nasuti JF. Value of histiocytes detection in pap smears for predicting endometrial pathology. An institutional experience. Acta Cytol 2003;47:762–67.

15. Feeley KM, Wells M. Hormone replacement therapy and the endometrium. J Clin Pathol 2001;54:435–40.

16. Mathelin C, Youssef C, Annane K, et al. Endometrial brush cytology in the surveillance of post-menopausal patients under tamoxifen: a prospective longitudinal study. Eur J Obstet Gynecol Reprod Biol 2007;132:126–28.

17. Buccoliero AM, Fambrini M, Gheri CF, et al. Surveillance for endometrial cancer in women on tamoxifen: the role of liquid-based endometrial cytology. Cytohistological correlation in a population of 168 women. Gynecol Obstet Invest 2008;65:240–46.

18. Savelli L, De Iaco P, Santini D, et al. Histopathologic features and risk factors for benignity, hyperplasia, and cancer in endometrial polyps. Am J Obstet Gynecol 2003;188:927–31.

19. Ben-Arie A, Goldchmit C, Laviv Y, et al. The malignant potential of endometrial polyps. Eur J Obstet Gynecol Reprod Biol 2004;115:206–10.

20. Fambrini M, Buccoliero AM, Bargelli G, et al. Clinical utility of liquid-based cytology for the characterisation and management of endometrial polyps in postmenopausal age. Int J Gynecol Cancer 2008;18:306–11.

21. Morse AR. The value of endometrial aspiration in gynecological practice. In: Koss LG, Coleman DV, editors. Advances in Clinical Cytology. London: Butterworth; 1981. p. 44–63.

22. Ginsberg NA, Padleckas R, Javaheri G. Diagnostic reliability of Mi-Mark helix technique in endometrial neoplasia. Obstet Gynecol 1983;62:225–30.

23. Crow J, Gordon H, Hudson E. An assessment of the Mi-Mark endometrial sampling technique. J Clin Pathol 1980;33:72–80.

24. Reagan JW. Can screening for endometrial cancer be justified?. Acta Cytol 1980;24:87–89.

25. Skaarland E. New concept in diagnostic endometrial cytology; diagnostic criteria based on composition and architecture of large tissue fragments in smears. J Clin Pathol 1986;39:36–43.

26. Ishii Y, Fujii M. Criteria for differential diagnosis of complex hyperplasia or beyond in endometrial cytology. Acta Cytol 1997;41:1095–102.

27. Byren AJ. Endocyte endometrial smears in the cytodiagnosis of endometrial carcinoma. Acta Cytol 1990;34:373–81.

28. Norimatsu Y, Shimizu K, Kobayashi TK, et al. Cellular features of endometrial hyperplasia and well differentiated adenocarcinoma using the endocyte sampler. Diagnostic criteria based on the cytoarchitecture of tissue fragments. Cancer 2006;108:77–85.

29. Gracia F, Barker B, Davis J, et al. Thin-layer cytology and histopathology in the evaluation of abnormal uterine bleeding. J Reprod Med 2003;48:882–88.

30. Norimatsu Y, Kouda H, Kobayashi TK, et al. Utility of thin-layer preparations in the endometrial cytology: evaluation of benign endometrial lesions. Ann Diagn Pathol 2008;12:103–11.

31. Kurman RJ, Kaminski PF, Norris HJ. The behavior endometrial hyperplasia a long-term study 'untreated' hyperplasia in 170 patients. Cancer 1985;56:403–12.

32. Ehrmann RL. Atypical endometrial cells and stromal breakdown tow case reports. Acta Cytol 1975;19:465–69.

33. Sherman ME, Mazur MT, Kurman RJ. Benign disease of the endometrium. In: Kurman RJ, editor. Blaustein's pathology of the female genital tract. 5th edn. New York: Springer-Verlag; 2001. p. 431–39.

34. Vakiani M, Vavilis D, Agorastos T, et al. Histopathological findings of the endometrium in patients with dysfunctional uterine bleeding. Clin Exp Obstet Gynecol 1996;23:236–39.

35. Livingstone M, Fraser IS. Mechanisms of abnormal uterine bleeding. Hum Reprod Update 2002;8:60–67.

36. Shimizu K, Norimatsu Y, Kobayashi TK, et al. Endometrial glandular and stromal breakdown, part 1: cytomorphological appearance. Diagn Cytopathol 2006;34:609–13.

37. Frenczy A. Pathophysiology of endometrial bleeding. Maturitas 2003;45:1–14.

38. Hendrickson MR, Kempson RL. Endometrial epithelial metaplasias:proliferations frequently misdiagnosed as adenocarcinoma. Report of 89 cases and proposed classification. Am J Surg Pathol 1980;4:525–42.

39. Andersen WA, Taylor PT, Fechner RE, et al. Endometrial metaplasia associated with endometrial adenocarcinoma. Am J Obstet Gynecol 1987;157:597–604.

40. Kaku T, Tsukamoto N, Tsuruchi N, et al. Endometrial metaplasia associated with endometrial carcinoma. Obstet Gynecol 1992;80:812–16.

41. Jacques SM, Qureshi F, Lawrence WD. Surface epithelial changes in endometrial adenocarcinoma: diagnostic pitfalls in curettage specimens. Int J Gynecol Pathol 1995;14:191–97.

42. Ronnett BM, Kurman RJ. Precursor lesions of endometrial carcinoma. In: Kurman RJ, editor. Blaustein's pathology of the female genital tract. 5th edn. New York: Springer-Verlag; 2001. p. 484–93.

43. Lehman MB, Hart WR. Simple and complex hyperplastic papillary proliferations of the endometrium; a clinicopathologic study of nine cases of apparently localized papillary lesions with fibrovascular stromal cores and epithelial metaplasia. Am J Surg Pathol 2001;25:1347–54.

44. Gribaudi G, Alasio L. Cytological changes caused by intrauterine devices. Pathologica 1981;73:207–16.

45. Norimatsu Y, Shimizu K, Kobayashi TK, et al. Endometrial glandular and stromal breakdown, part 2: cytomorphology of papillary metaplastic changes. Diagn Cytopathol 2006;34:665–69.

46. Zaman SS, Mazur MT. Endometrial papillary syncytial change: a nonspecific alteration associated with active breakdown. Am J Clin Pathol 1993;99:741–45.

47. Tavassoli FA, Devilee P. Tumours of the breast and female genital organs. Pathology and genetics. World Health Organization Classification of Tumours. Lyon: IARC Press; 2003.

48. Sorosky JI. Endometrial cancer. Obstet Gynecol 2008;111:436–47.

49. Brown L. Pathology of uterine malignancies. Clin Oncol 2008;20:433–47.

50. Fadeare O, Zheng W. Endometrial glandular dysplasia (EmGD): morphologically and biologically distinctive putative precursor lesions of Type II endometrial cancers. Diagn Pathol 2008;3:6.

51. Jia L, Liu Y, Yi X, et al. endometrial glandular dysplasia with frequent p53 gene mutation: a genetic evidence supporting its precancer nature for endometrial serous carcinoma. Clin Cancer Res 2008;15:2263–69.

52. Trahan S, Tetu B, Raymond PE. Serous papillary carcinoma of the endometrium arising from endometrial polyps: a clinical, histological, and immunohistochemical study of 13 cases. Human Pathol 2005;36:1316–21.

53. Kobayashi H, Otsuki Y, Simizu S, et al. Cytological criteria of endometrial lesions with emphasis on stromal and epithelial cell clusters: result of 8 years of experience with intrauterine sampling. Cytopathology 2008;19:19–27.

54. Taddei GL, Buccoliero AM. Atlante di citologia endometriale. L'endometrio normale, iperplastico e neoplastico nella citologia in fase liquida. Florence: SEE Editrice; 2005.

55. Maksem JA, Meiers I, Robboy SJ. A primer of endometrial cytology with histological correlation. Diagn Cytopathol 2007;35:817–44.

56. Wright C, Leiman G, Burgess SM. The cytomorphology of papillary serous carcinoma of the endometrium in cervical smears. Cancer Cytopathol 1999;87:12–18.

57. Todo Y, Minobe S, Okamoto K, et al. Cytological features of cervical smears in serous adenocarcinoma of the endometrium. JPN J Clin Oncol 2003;33:636–41.

58. Lax SF. Molecular genetic pathways in various types of endometrial carcinoma: from a phenotypical to a molecular-based classification. Virchows Arch 2004;444:213–23.

59. Norimatsu Y, Kouda H, Kobayashi TK, et al. Utility of liquid-based cytology in endometrial pathology: diagnosis of endometrial carcinoma. Cytopathology 2009;20:395–402.

60. Meisels A, Jolicoeur C. Criteria for the cytologic assessment of hyperplasia in endometrial samples obtained by the Endopap endometrial sampler. Acta Cytol 1985;29:297–302.

61. PrepStain™ Slide Processor Operators Manual 780-B000-00 Rev. B Burlington, NC: Becton-Dickinson and Company; 2005.

62. Garbini F, Buccoliero AM, Castiglione F, et al. Gestational choriocarcinoma: morphological features in a liquid-based endometrial cytological sample. Diagn Cytopathol 2008;36:113–14.

63. Wappenschmidt B, Wardelmann E, Gehrig A, et al. PTEN mutations do not cause nuclear beta-catenin accumulation in endometrial carcinomas. Hum Pathol 2004;35:1260–65.

64. Norimatsu Y, Moriya T, Kobayashi TK, et al. Immunohistochemical expression of PTEN and beta-catenin for endometrial intraepithelial neoplasia in Japanese women. Ann Diagn Pathol 2007;11:103–8.

65. Norimatsu Y, Miyamoto T, Kobayashi TK, et al. Utility of thin-layer preparations in endometrial cytology: immunocytochemical expression of PTEN, beta-catenin and p53 for benign endometrial lesions. Diagn Cytopathol 2008;36:216–23.

66. Hech JL, Mutter GL. Molecular and pathologic aspects of endometrial carcinogenesis. J Clin Oncol 2005;24:4783–91.

67. Norimatsu Y, Miyamoto M, Kobayashi TK, et al. Diagnostic utility of phosphatase and tensin homolog, beta-catenin, and p53 for endometrial carcinoma by thin-layer endometrial preparations. Cancer 2008;114:155–64.

68. Yanoh K, Norimatsu Y, Hirai Y, et al. New diagnostic reporting format for endometrial cytology based on cytoarchitectural criteria. Cytopathology 2008; 24 July [Epub ahead of print].

69. Jimenez-Ayala M, Jimenez-Ayala Portillo B, Iglesias E, Vallejo MR. Endometrial adenocarcinoma: prevention and early diagnosis. Monogr Clin Cytol 2008;17:1–91.

# Ovaries, fallopian tubes and associated lesions

Sanjiv Manek and Vesna Mahovlić

## Chapter contents

## Introduction

The application of cytological techniques such as fine needle aspiration (FNA) in the routine diagnosis of ovarian lesions used to be limited, particularly for malignant neoplasms, but is now less so with the advent of accurate imaging and the introduction of key monoclonal antibodies for immunocytochemistry. When judiciously employed, FNA of cystic lesions in the pelvis can be valuable as a diagnostic, screening or therapeutic procedure and this is reflected by the increasing number of articles in the recent literature.[1–5] The majority of pelvic cysts that can be aspirated are ovarian in origin. However, other 'cysts' in the vicinity may be misinterpreted as ovarian, and aspirated accordingly. These include peritoneal inclusion cysts, paratubal cysts, colon reduplication cysts and hydrosalpinges. As has already been described, malignant cells of ovarian origin are also occasionally identified in vaginal, cervical and endometrial samples (see Chs 23, 24, 25).

## Obtaining cytological material

### FNA technique

Cystic lesions in the pelvis can be approached through the vagina or rectum, transabdominally, during laparoscopy and at the time of laparotomy.[6] The transvaginal route is generally favoured as the vagina can be cleansed before puncture and is the preferred route for aspirations performed in the infertility unit, in conjunction with transvaginal ultrasonography. Transrectal aspirates are usually performed in conjunction with examination of the patient under general anaesthesia. Ovarian cysts and solid lesions, especially those that extend

into the abdomen or are associated with omental lesions, can be readily aspirated via the transabdominal route. Laparoscopic visualisation and aspiration can also be safely and effectively employed in the diagnosis and management of ovarian cysts. Occasionally, pelvic cysts are found incidentally during laparotomy undertaken for other reasons. Aspiration of these cysts can provide useful diagnoses to ascertain further management. Transvaginal aspiration of ovarian cysts has been advocated as a viable alternative to surgery in patients who are high-risk surgical candidates.[7] Lee et al. performed aspiration curettage of the inner surface of the cyst present during aspiration to facilitate cytological diagnosis.[8]

The laboratory procedure is also crucial in determining the diagnostic potential of a given sample. The fluid can be smeared directly or cytocentrifuged depending on its viscosity. It can also be processed via the liquid-based cytology (LBC) technique.[9] It is useful to have at least two air-dried May-Grünwald Giemsa (MGG) and two wet-fixed Papanicolaou (PAP) preparations to improve the diagnostic yield as quite often only one slide contains the relevant cells. It is also advisable to prepare spare slides for immunocytochemistry.

## Peritoneal washings

Peritoneal washing cytology (PWC) is a useful indicator of ovarian surface involvement and peritoneal dissemination by ovarian tumours. It may identify subclinical peritoneal spread and thus provide valuable staging and prognostic information, particularly for non-serous ovarian tumours.[10,11] The role of PWC as a prognostic indicator for endometrial carcinoma is less clear, due in part to the questionable significance of identifying endometrial tumour cells in the peritoneum. Detection of metastatic carcinoma in PWC is based on the recognition of non-mesothelial cell characteristics. However, a number of conditions such as reactive mesothelial cells, endometriosis and endosalpingiosis may mimic this appearance. Cells from these conditions may have a similar presentation in PWC to that of serous borderline tumours and low-grade serous carcinoma.[12] The presence of cilia, lack of single atypical cells, prominent cytoplasmic vacuolation, marked nuclear atypia or two distinct cell populations are features favouring a benign process. Attention to these features along with close correlation with clinical history and the results of surgical pathology should help avoid errors. Additional assistance may be provided by the use of cell blocks and special stains.

Any free fluid or PWC are obtained intraoperatively, immediately after entering the abdominal cavity by using a small

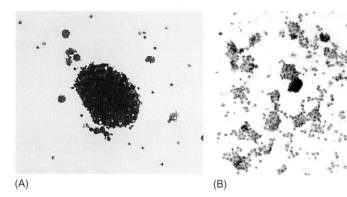

(A)          (B)

**Fig. 27.1** Tightly packed clusters of follicular cells with round to oval nuclei and scanty cytoplasm. FNA of ovary (A, MGG; B, PAP).

amount of normal saline (100–150 mL). The material is prepared in a standard manner as soon as possible after collection, in order to avoid degenerative changes, allowing sufficient material for standard and special stains including immunocytochemistry (see Ch. 3).[13] In addition, cytological examination of peritoneal washing is applied during 'second look' procedures (laparotomy, laparoscopy) as a method of assessing the response to treatment.

## Ovaries

### Non-neoplastic cystic lesions

Prior to the cytological interpretation of ovarian FNA smears, cytopathologists should be thoroughly familiar with the aspiration route and with clinical and radiological findings, in particular, if the investigation is part of the infertility treatment.[2,3] Knowledge of the route is essential as normal cells from various sites may be inadvertently aspirated during the passage of the needle towards the ovary.[1] These contaminants include squamous epithelial cells from vaginal mucosa, columnar cells from rectal mucosa and mesothelial cells from the peritoneum.

The clinical and radiological features are extremely important in order to formulate a differential diagnosis and determine if the findings are representative of the aspirated lesion.[1,6] The decision to aspirate an ovarian lesion is usually determined by the radiological findings, especially ultrasonography.[6,14] FNA of cystic and solid lesions present different problems and opinions concerning its use in diagnosis and treatment are not unanimous.[2,3,15–17]

Ultrasound can generally distinguish unilocular cysts from those that are multiloculated, which have thick septa or contain solid areas.[2,3] Unilocular cysts, especially when present in young or pregnant women, are usually benign, while multiloculated cysts could be associated with a more serious lesion. Unilocular ovarian cysts measuring <5 cm in diameter and containing <20 mL fluid are usually functional and resolve spontaneously. Those 5–10 cm in size are more likely to be symptomatic and associated with a more significant condition, including a neoplastic process, and these are more often investigated by FNA.[18]

In the appropriate clinical setting, if the FNA from one of these cysts is straw coloured or clear, most patients are managed conservatively. A high fluid level of unconjugated oestradiol-17β ($E_2$) favours a functional follicular cyst rather than a neoplastic process.[16] However, certain ovarian neoplasms such as granulosa cell tumour also produce oestrogen and the

measurement may therefore be of limited significance. A high CA125 level in the fluid may indicate a neoplastic process.[19] If, however, the cyst recurs after aspiration or the aspirated fluid is haemorrhagic, removal may be necessary. When necrotic material or pus is aspirated, distinction between abscess and necrotic tumour may be cytologically difficult.[3]

The use of immunocytochemical techniques enables the distinction between functional and neoplastic cysts in most cases, as the latter are usually lined by epithelial cells.[20] Positivity of cells with the antibody to the α-subunit of inhibin, and to a lesser extent to the β-subunit, indicates follicular cells of a functional cyst.[21] Positivity with BerEP4 or CA125 indicates epithelial cells and hence a neoplasm, but can include endometriotic cysts.[20]

Non-neoplastic cystic lesions of the ovary include follicular, corpus luteal and germinal inclusion cysts. In most aspirates from benign unilocular cysts with clear fluid the specimens are usually sparsely cellular, containing lymphocytes and macrophages. It is often not possible to make a definitive diagnosis or differentiate the various types of cysts on the basis of the cytological findings alone.[2,16]

### Cytological findings: non-neoplastic cysts

#### Follicular cysts

- Watery straw-coloured fluid which may be blood stained
- Moderate cellularity
- May include numerous granulosa cells arranged singly and in tight clusters (Fig. 27.1)[2,22]
- The cells generally have round and sometimes oval nuclei, some of which have longitudinal nuclear grooves, producing a coffee bean appearance
- The nuclei have coarsely granular chromatin rendering a pepper-pot appearance and there is a small rim of distinct cytoplasm (Fig. 27.2)
- Mitotic figures may be present.

The existence of ciliated bodies (detached ciliary tufts in fluids of ovarian cysts) indicates the presence of ciliated columnar epithelial cells in the wall of the cyst, which would exclude a follicular origin.[23]

#### Luteinised follicular cysts

- Large polyhedral luteinised granulosa cells
- Abundant granular or vacuolated cytoplasm and slight anisocytosis (Fig. 27.3)[22]
- The nuclei are often eccentric and have finely granular chromatin with one or two small prominent nucleoli.[22]

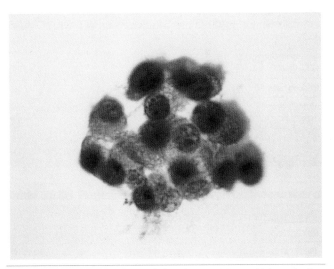

**Fig. 27.2** Follicular cells with rounded nuclei containing multiple nucleoli and coarse chromatin rendering a pepper-pot appearance. FNA of ovary (PAP).

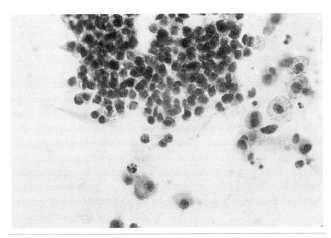

**Fig. 27.3** Luteinised follicular cyst of ovary. A cluster of granulosa cells with round to oval nuclei and small rim of cytoplasm surrounded by larger luteinised granulosa cells with ample foamy cytoplasm. FNA of ovary (PAP).

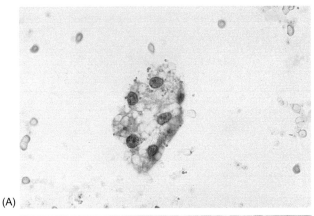

(A)

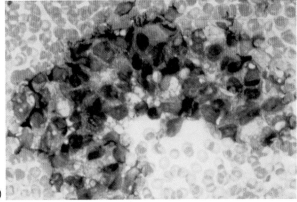

(B)

**Fig. 27.4** Corpus luteum cyst of ovary. A loose cluster of luteinised granulosa cells containing round to oval nuclei with small prominent nucleoli. The cytoplasm is abundant with vacuolisation. FNA of ovary (A, PAP; B, MGG).

Such cells are commonly seen during IVF treatment when the ovary is being stimulated with hormones. There may also be anisonucleosis in these circumstances.[24]

### Corpus luteum and luteal cysts

- Numerous luteinised granulosa cells in a background of fresh blood, fibrin and haemosiderin-laden macrophages (Fig. 27.4)[22]
- The granulosa cells are often in small clusters, unlike the macrophages which are dispersed
- Macrophages with haematoidin pigment and numerous fibroblasts suggest a regressing corpus luteum.

### Luteinised follicular cysts of pregnancy

- Aspirates from luteinised follicular cysts of pregnancy and the puerperium may yield cells with atypical cytological features[24]

- These atypical luteinised granulosa cells exhibit an increased nuclear/cytoplasmic ratio
- Enlarged nuclei with granular chromatin, chromocentres and prominent nucleoli
- In some cells chromatin clearing and irregular nucleoli are present.

Similar findings of cytological atypia, however, have been reported in cellular follicular cysts not associated with current or recent pregnancy.[25] Accurate clinical correlation is essential in order to minimise rendering a false positive diagnosis of malignancy.

### Endometriotic cysts

- Aspirates usually macroscopically haemorrhagic, brown fluid and contain numerous haemosiderin-laden macrophages (Fig. 27.5)
- In the background of degenerate blood, there is quite often cellular debris including wisps of cytoplasm admixed with degenerate nuclear material, both generally of small size, but of variable shapes
- Occasionally collagenous bodies are noted[26,27]
- Intact endometrial cells are seldom seen.[22] These cells are isolated or arranged in tight clusters. The cytoplasm is scanty and the nuclei are round or oval with finely granular chromatin (Fig. 27.6).

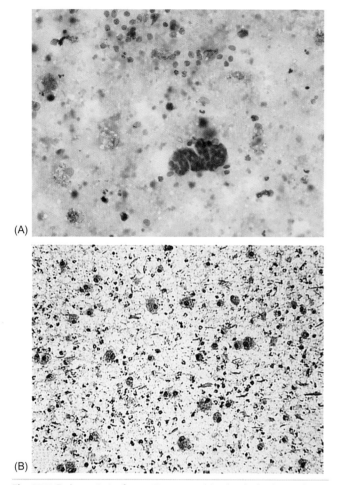

(A)

(B)

**Fig. 27.5** Endometriosis of ovary. Degenerate blood in the background with haemosiderin-laden macrophages, indicative of old haemorrhage into cyst, with cytonuclear debris. Other types of cysts may also show old and recent haemorrhage. FNA of ovary (A, MGG; B, PAP).

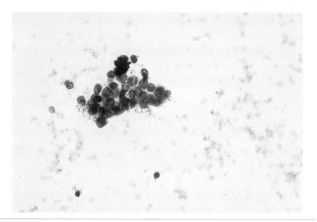

**Fig. 27.6** Endometriosis of ovary. A tight cluster of small uniform endometrial cells. The background usually shows numerous haemosiderin-laden macrophages as illustrated in Figure 27.5. FNA of ovary (PAP).

### Diagnostic pitfalls: non-neoplastic ovarian cysts

- Haemorrhage, recent or old, may be seen in many types of cysts, e.g. mucinous cysts and does not always indicate endometriosis

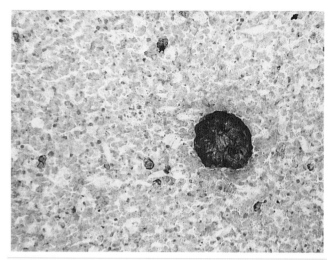

**Fig. 27.7** BerEP4 positivity in cytoplasmic debris and scanty endometrioid cells in ovarian endometriosis. FNA of ovary.

- In the absence of characteristic luteinised granulosa cells or intact endometrial cells, aspirates from haemorrhagic luteal cysts are difficult to distinguish from endometriosis[1,2,5,28,29]
- Aspirates of cellular follicular cysts may mimic granulosa cell tumours.[25]

### Immunocytochemistry of non-neoplastic ovarian cysts

As mentioned earlier, immunocytochemistry helps in distinguishing between haemorrhagic functional (corpus luteal or follicular) cysts and endometriotic cysts. Inhibin positivity indicates the former and BerEP4/CA-125 positivity, particularly in the cytoplasmic debris (Fig. 27.7) indicates the latter, although with BerEP4 positivity, it is not possible to exclude a neoplastic epithelial cell-lined cyst.[20]

Occasional cases of clinically unsuspected endometriosis may be diagnosed by examining ovarian cyst fluid cytology as part of an *in vitro* fertilisation (IVF) protocol.[30]

### Management of non-neoplastic ovarian cysts

Most non-neoplastic cysts are treated conservatively. Many do not reaccumulate after initial aspiration and others regress spontaneously. Endometriotic cysts are generally removed to exclude neoplastic changes and to relieve symptoms. Many are now removed laparoscopically.[31,32]

## Benign ovarian tumours

Ovarian tumours are classified according to the WHO histological classification.[33] In this chapter, we present the cytological findings of the most common ovarian tumours,

Most benign epithelial tumours of ovary are cystic, filled with fluid and appear distended, tense and multilocular. They are therefore seldom aspirated. In general, the finding of epithelium with or without atypia in FNA smears warrants surgical intervention.

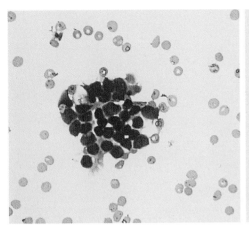
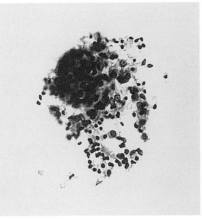

**Fig. 27.8** Serous cystadenoma of ovary. A cluster of uniform cuboidal cells with round to oval nuclei and amphophilic cytoplasm, some of which are ciliated. FNA of ovary (A, MGG; B, PAP).

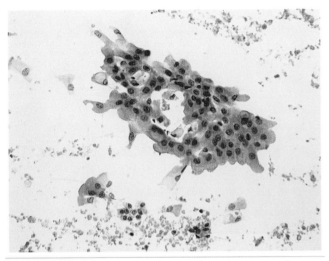

**Fig. 27.9** Mucinous cystadenoma of ovary. A sheet of mucin secreting epithelial cells displaying both a honeycomb pattern and a picket-fence arrangement at the edges. FNA of ovary (MGG).

## Cytological findings: benign ovarian tumours (general)

- Watery or mucoid clear or straw-coloured fluid
- Usually hypocellular
- Background may be blood stained
- Macrophages and other inflammatory cells may predominate.

## Cytological findings: serous cystadenoma[34]

- Occasional single epithelial cells or papillary aggregates
- Epithelial cells uniform cuboidal or columnar lacking atypia
- Cells are usually ciliated (Fig. 27.8).[1,3,29,32]

## Cytological findings: mucinous cystadenoma

- Usually macroscopically gelatinous mucoid fluid
- Microscopically mucinous background
- Columnar mucin-secreting cells, arranged in honeycomb or picket-fence configurations (Fig. 27.9)[1,32]
- The cytoplasm contains either many small vacuoles or a single large vacuole displacing the nucleus to the periphery

- The nuclei are homogeneous and have finely granular evenly distributed chromatin.

## Cytological findings: Brenner tumour (Fig. 27.10)

- May contain both epithelial and mesenchymal cells[35]
- Epithelial cells are polygonal or cuboidal and occur singly or in sheets
- The nuclei are ovoid and often have a linear groove giving them a coffee bean appearance
- Eosinophilic amorphous globules can be seen at the centre of the cell groups or lying free in the background. These correspond to the inspissated colloid material that is often present at the centre of epithelial islets in histological sections.[32]

## Cytological findings: fibrothecomatous tumours

- Sparse spindle cells, either isolated or in bundles, with scant cytoplasm (Fig. 27.11A)
- Elongated nuclei in which coarsely granular, but evenly distributed chromatin is seen (Fig. 27.11B)
- In some cases, luteinised cells with more abundant, finely vacuolated cytoplasm may be present (Fig. 27.12).

## Cytological findings: benign mature cystic teratoma (dermoid cyst)

- Macroscopically usually viscous, oily aspirates, sometimes containing hair
- Amorphous debris, numerous anucleate squames, superficial squamous cells and hair (Figs 27.13, 27.14). If hair is identified in smears and contamination can be ruled out, this is pathognomonic for teratoma[36]
- Other epithelial components such as respiratory and intestinal epithelium may occasionally be present
- Occasionally colloid and thyroid follicular cells can be identified if there is a large component of struma ovarii.

## Cytological findings: sex cord tumour with annular tubules

- Relatively uniform cells that are predominantly isolated but also occur in solid, follicular and trabecular arrangements[37]

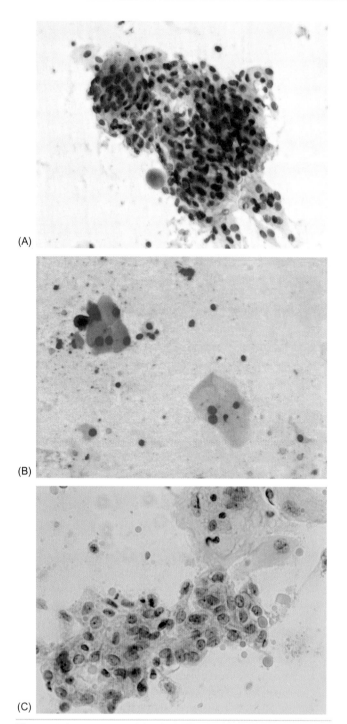

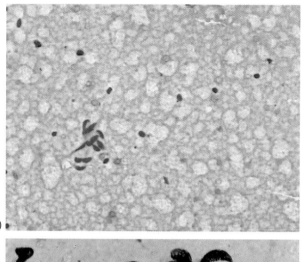

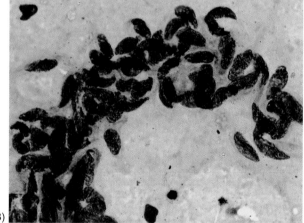

**Fig. 27.11** Fibroma. (A) Few spindle cells like fibrocytes and few bare oval nuclei. Scanty material. (B) Bundle of elongated cells with elongated coarsely granular, but evenly distributed chromatin and scanty cytoplasm (MGG × 600). Imprint of the ovary.

**Diagnostic pitfalls: benign ovarian tumours**

- Colonic cells contaminating transrectal aspirates can simulate the appearance of cells derived from mucinous cystadenomas
- Aspirates from fibrothecomas can be misinterpreted as leiomyomas
- Transvaginal aspirates contaminated with vaginal squamous cells can sometimes simulate a dermoid cyst
- Sampling from benign locules with a multilocular mucinous carcinoma may render a false negative diagnosis
- Haemorrhagic aspirates from benign neoplasms with degenerate epithelium may be interpreted as endometriotic.

## Borderline tumours[33]

**Cytological findings: borderline tumours**

- Greater cellularity and cytological features of malignancy (Fig. 27.15)
- The cells are seen singly or more frequently in groups with sheet-like or papillary configurations
- Slightly to markedly atypical nuclei which may contain nucleoli

**Fig. 27.10** Brenner tumour. (A) A sheet of transition type epithelial cells and cell-free body (MGG); (B) umbrella-like cells with binucleation (MGG); (C) transition type epithelial cells and umbrella like cells (PAP). Imprint of the ovary.

- The tumour cells have a small to medium amount of pale cytoplasm
- The nuclei are round to oval with evenly distributed chromatin, a small nucleolus and occasional nuclear grooving
- Round or oval shaped hyaline bodies with palisading producing rosette or ring-like arrangements of the nuclei at their periphery are typically present.

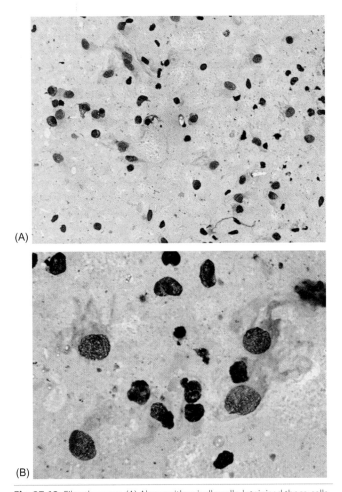

(A)

(B)

**Fig. 27.12** Fibrothecoma. (A) Along with spindle cells, luteinised theca cells are seen (B). Imprint of the ovary (A, MGG; B, MGG).

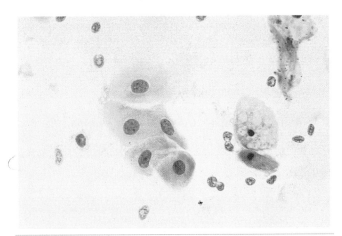

**Fig. 27.13** Benign mature cystic teratoma of ovary. Mature superficial squamous cells are present. FNA of ovary (PAP).

- Serous and endometrioid tumours include columnar cells with eosinophilic cytoplasm; some of the cells are ciliated
- Mucinous tumours show columnar cells with vacuoles of different sizes.

Tumours with marked cellular atypia are almost invariably classified as carcinomas whereas tumours with mild atypia may be difficult to distinguish from benign cystadenomas.

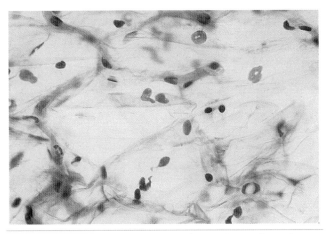

**Fig. 27.14** Benign mature cystic teratoma of ovary. Mature adipose tissue. Abundant cellular and keratin debris were also present. FNA of ovary (PAP).

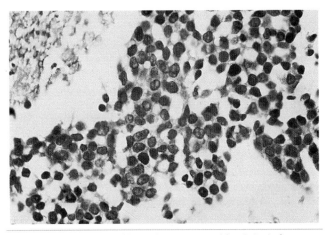

**Fig. 27.15** Serous tumour of low malignant potential (borderline) of ovary. A loose cluster of cuboidal to columnar cells with irregular arrangement, nuclear hyperchromasia and an irregular chromatin pattern. FNA of ovary (PAP).

The presence or absence of invasion cannot be determined from the cytology alone; thus borderline tumours are not cytologically distinguishable from invasive malignant tumours.[2]

Patients with a borderline mucinous tumour may have associated pseudomyxoma peritonei. Pseudomyxoma peritonei (PMP) is a rare disease that is characterised by a large amount of mucinous ascites with peritoneal and omental implants. The etiology of the disease remains unclear. Histologically, two main categories have been described: disseminated peritoneal adenomucinosis (DPAM) and peritoneal mucinous carcinomatosis (PMCA). It is commonly diagnosed incidentally at laparotomy. The optimal management of the disease remains controversial. The role of intraoperative and intraperitoneal chemotherapy has been evaluated by a number of authors. The clinical outcomes vary widely between the benign and the malignant forms and between the different treatment modalities.[38,39]

Needle aspirate smears of pseudomyxoma peritonei are characterised by the presence of macroscopically gelatinous fluid that contains a dual population of mesothelial and fibroblastic cells in a background of fibrillary mucin. A few epithelial cells may be admixed.[40] The tumour may be appendiceal in origin.[41]

## Box 27.1 WHO Histological Classification of Tumours of the Ovary[33]

**I    Surface epithelial–stromal tumours**

- Serous tumours
  - Serous cystadenoma, (cyst)adenofibroma
  - Borderline serous tumour, (cyst)adenofibroma
  - Serous (cyst)adenocarcinoma
- Mucinous tumours
  - Mucinous cystadenoma, (cyst)adenofibroma
  - Borderline mucinous tumour
  - Mucinous (cyst)adenocarcinoma
- Endometrioid tumours
  - Endometrioid cystadenoma, (cyst)adenofibroma
  - Borderline cystic tumour, (cyst)adenofibroma
  - Endometrioid (cyst)adenocarcinoma
- Clear cell tumours
  - Clear cell cystadenoma, (cyst)adenofibroma
  - Borderline clear cell tumour, (cyst)adenofibroma
  - Clear cell adenocarcinoma
- Transitional cell tumours
  - Brenner tumour
  - Borderline Brenner tumour
  - Malignant Brenner tumour
- Undifferentiated carcinoma

**II    Sex cord–stromal tumours**

- Granulosa – stromal cell tumours
  - Granulosa cell tumour (adult, juvenile)
  - Thecoma (fibrothecoma)
  - Fibroma
- Sertoli–Leydig cell tumour group

**III    Germ cell tumours**

- Dysgerminoma
- Yolk sac tumour
- Embryonal carcinoma
- Choriocarcinoma
- Teratoma
  - Mature (dermoid cyst, solid teratoma)
  - Immature teratoma (malignant)
  - Monodermal teratoma (struma ovarii, carcinoid)
- Others
  - Germ cell sex cord-stromal tumours (gonadoblastoma, mixed)

**IV    Unclassified tumours**

**V    Secondary (metastatic) tumours**

**VI    Tumour-like conditions**

Modified from Tavassoli and Devilee 2003.[33]

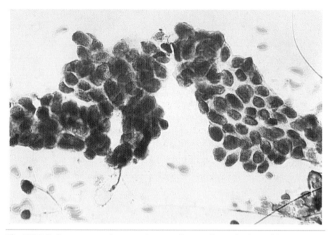

**Fig. 27.16** Serous cystadenocarcinoma of ovary. Irregular branching group of malignant columnar cells with syncytial and papillary configurations. FNA of ovary (PAP).

sites and in most instances do not present a diagnostic problem.[1,2,42]

It is important to realise that a negative cytology result in the presence of a lesion suspicious of malignancy does not exclude the possibility. In these situations another aspirate or a surgical biopsy should be undertaken as the initial aspirate may have sampled a benign component of the tumour.[1,42] Subclassification of ovarian carcinomas on the basis of the cytological findings is possible in low and intermediate grade neoplasms; however, subtyping may be extremely difficult in high-grade tumours (Box 27.1).[2,33,42]

### Cytological findings: malignant ovarian tumours (general)

- The aspirates are cellular and usually blood stained or frankly haemorrhagic
- Variable amounts of debris and often evidence of necrosis is seen in carcinomas
- Presence of inflammatory cells.

### Cytological findings: serous adenocarcinoma

- Cuboidal to low columnar cells arranged in syncytial and branching papillary groups (Fig. 27.16)[2,42]
- Moderate amounts of homogeneous basophilic cytoplasm
- The nuclei tend to be eccentric and are hyperchromatic with irregularly distributed chromatin
- Nuclear pleomorphism and nucleoli are usually conspicuous
- Psammoma bodies (Fig. 27.17) are infrequent.

### Cytological findings: mucinous adenocarcinoma

- Numerous clusters of abnormal columnar cells surrounded by mucus (Fig. 27.18). The cells can occur singly, in papillary groups, and in a picket-fence or honeycomb arrangement in low-grade tumours[42,29]
- The tumour cells from low-grade lesions have abundant cytoplasm with single or multiple vacuoles

## Malignant ovarian tumours

Ovarian carcinomas are usually predominantly multicystic with a solid component and in roughly three-quarters of patients peritoneal tumour seeding is present at the time of diagnosis.[1] Aspirates may be obtained from primary, recurrent or metastatic

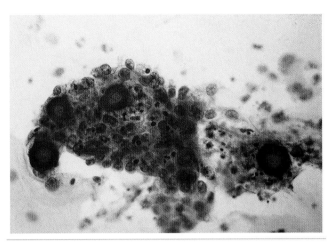

**Fig. 27.17** Serous cystadenocarcinoma of ovary. Clusters of atypical cells centred around psammoma bodies. FNA of ovary (PAP).

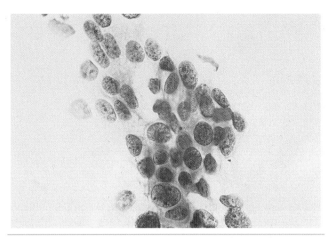

**Fig. 27.19** Metastatic colonic adenocarcinoma to ovary. The cytological features are those of a mucinous adenocarcinoma and are indistinguishable from those of primary ovarian mucinous adenocarcinoma. The clinical findings were those of metastatic disease to the ovary. FNA ovary (PAP).

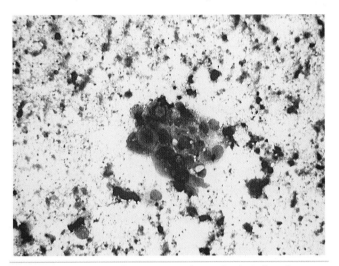

**Fig. 27.18** Mucinous cystadenocarcinoma of ovary. Cytologically malignant mucin-secreting cells in a vague picket-fence arrangement. FNA of ovary (MGG).

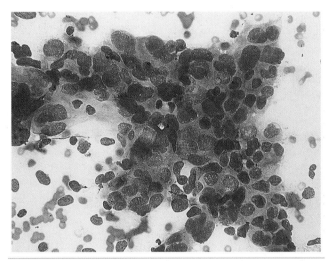

**Fig. 27.20** Endometrioid adenocarcinoma of the ovary. Syncytial sheets of malignant cells with moderate amounts of granular cytoplasm and atypical nuclei (MGG).

- High-grade tumour cells have a high nuclear/cytoplasmic ratio and the enlarged nuclei are eccentrically placed and are often indented by the vacuoles. They have irregularly distributed chromatin material and nucleoli are seen.

Metastatic mucin secreting carcinomas involving the ovary can have the same cytological appearances as primary mucinous ovarian carcinomas (Fig. 27.19).[1] In such cases, using a panel of antibodies, it may be possible to suggest a primary site of the tumour if the ovary itself is not considered to be the source of the malignant cells.[13,20,21]

### Cytological findings: endometrioid adenocarcinoma

- Abundant cells in syncytial groups and cell clusters with frequent acinar arrangements (Fig. 27.20)
- Papillary groups are occasionally seen
- Individual cells are cuboidal to polygonal and have small amounts of homogeneous to finely granular cytoplasm
- Multiple small vacuoles and large single vacuoles may be present
- The nuclei are round to oval, eccentric in position and have finely granular irregularly distributed chromatin with prominent nucleoli

- They can be difficult to distinguish from serous carcinomas.[1,31]

### Cytological findings: clear cell carcinoma

- Cells with abundant pale staining, finely granular, vacuolated cytoplasm (Fig. 27.21)[43–45]
- Often an acinar arrangement
- May have eosinophilic debris in the background.

### Cytological findings: mixed müllerian tumour

- Aspirates mostly comprise the malignant epithelial component that appears as an adenocarcinoma (Figs 27.22, 27.23)[46]
- The sarcomatous component can present with isolated or small groups of spindle cells with features of malignancy, or as predominantly isolated large cells with bizarre configurations, dense cytoplasm and markedly abnormal nuclei.

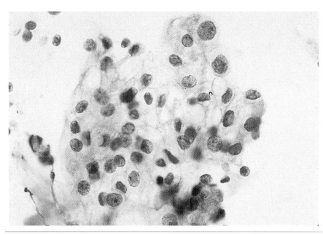

**Fig. 27.21** Clear cell carcinoma of ovary. Malignant cells with abundant, granular or vacuolated clear cytoplasm and round nuclei with prominent nucleoli. FNA of ovary (PAP).

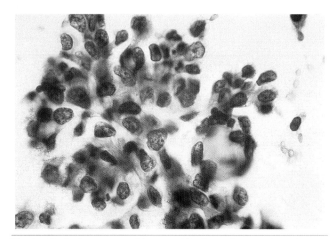

**Fig. 27.22** Carcinosarcoma of the ovary. This figure illustrates the malignant epithelial component, which is poorly differentiated with features of adenocarcinoma. FNA of ovary (PAP).

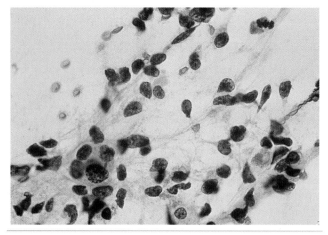

**Fig. 27.23** Carcinosarcoma of the ovary. This illustrates a malignant spindle cell mesenchymal component from the same case as Fig. 27.17. FNA of ovary (PAP).

If both epithelial and stromal elements are present an accurate diagnosis can be achieved; otherwise, the tumours are classified as adenocarcinomas or less frequently as sarcomas.

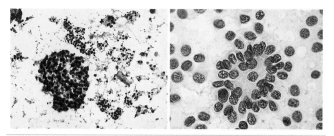

**Fig. 27.24** Granulosa cell tumour of ovary. (A) Tumour cells in a cluster with a vague acinus-like arrangement (PAP). (B) Scattered nuclei show nuclear grooves. FNA of ovary (PAP).

## Granulosa cell tumours

| Cytological findings: granulosa cell tumour |
| --- |

- Many tumour cells, which are arranged in solid, trabecular or follicular patterns (Fig. 27.24)[2,42,47,48]
- Sometimes small acinar-like structures with centrally placed amorphous, reddish violet bodies. They correspond to the Call-Exner bodies which are characteristic of this type of tumour
- The individual cells of granulosa cell tumour are homogeneous in appearance and have scanty cytoplasm
- The nuclei are round to oval with granular evenly distributed chromatin and small nucleoli. Nuclear grooves can be seen in a number of nuclei.

The cell pattern and the presence of Call-Exner bodies on aspirated cyst fluid aid in distinguishing cystic granulosa cell tumour from a follicular cyst.[22,25] The presence of cells with nuclear grooving, giving a coffee bean appearance and also, extracellular hyaline bodies may make the distinction between granulosa cell and Brenner tumour difficult, although immunocytochemistry is useful in resolving this.[20] Immunohistochemical stains for markers which have known variable specificity for sex cord-stromal lineage [inhibin, calretinin, MART-1/melan-A, CD99, steroidogenic factor 1 (SF-1, adrenal 4-binding protein), and WT1] can be used as an aid in diagnosis of sex cord stromal tumours.[49]

The juvenile granulosa cell tumour differs cytologically from its adult counterpart by the lack of prominent grooved nuclei, absence of Call-Exner bodies and the presence of mucin and prominent lipid vacuoles in granulosa cells.[33] Granulosa cell tumours can rarely be found outside the ovary.[50]

| Cytological findings: germ cell tumours |
| --- |

Germ cell tumours are the group of malignant neoplasms which primarily occur in the gonads (male and female). They are curable at all stages of disease.[51]

Germ cell tumours may be also occur in a variety of extragonadal locations (retroperitoneum, mediastinum, pineal gland, sacrococcygeal region) and therefore may be encountered in a routine cytology practice.[52,53]

The classification of germ cell tumours is based on their presumed resemblance to primitive germ cells or various embryonic and extraembryonic tissues in a fertilised ovum. FNA is an extremely useful procedure for the diagnosis of germ cell tumours. Most of the subtypes can be recognised and differentiated from other subtypes.[54]

## Cytological findings: dysgerminoma (Fig. 27.25)

- Numerous large poorly cohesive cells, with relatively abundant delicate pale staining cytoplasm
- The nuclei are large with clumped, irregularly distributed chromatin and macronucleoli
- Mitotic figures can be numerous
- Mature lymphocytes and occasional multinucleated giant cells of trophoblastic origin are usually present in the background
- These cells are usually positive on staining immunocytochemically with placental alkaline phosphatase (PLAP).

## Yolk sac tumour

Yolk sac tumour is common among the germ cell tumours of paediatric age group which presents a spectrum of cytomorphologic features having important differences with other germ cell neoplasm, e.g. embryonal carcinoma. Clinicoradiological features and tumour markers, such as alpha-fetoprotein (AFP) and β-human chorionic gonadotropin (βHCG) are additionally helpful for an accurate cytological diagnosis.

## Cytological findings: yolk sac tumour

- Cellular smears with a combination of morphological patterns
- Characteristically, tumour cells are arranged in papillary groups
- Tight cell clusters
- Acinar structures
- Enlarged, moderately pleomorphic, hyperchromatic nuclei
- Moderate amount of cytoplasm, some of which display cytoplasmic vacuolation or granularity, displacing the nuclei eccentrically
- Cells positive on staining immunocytochemically with alpha-fetoprotein (AFP).

## Immature teratoma

Immature teratoma displays an extremely diverse array of characteristics. It is composed of differentiated as well as immature cellular elements, predominantly of neuroglial tissue.[55] Proper cytological classification is possible due to the combination of benign and malignant neuroglial elements in the same smear. Primitive neuroectodermal element of the tumour is composed of highly anaplastic cells with high N:C ratio and marked hyperchromasia.

## Immunocytochemistry of ovarian tumours

The advent of immunocytochemistry has altered the potential for cytological diagnoses in ovarian cysts. There has been a surge of research into inhibin, not least in cytology.[21,16] The availability of monoclonal antibodies to the subunits of inhibin has enabled confident detection of follicular (granulosa) cells in aspirates (Figs 27.26, 27.27),[10] and when used in conjunction with epithelial markers such as BerEP4, CA125 and cytokeratin (CK) 7 (the latter two are relatively specific for ovary), it allows the distinction between functional, non-neoplastic cysts and neoplastic epithelial cell-lined cysts which require removal.[20]

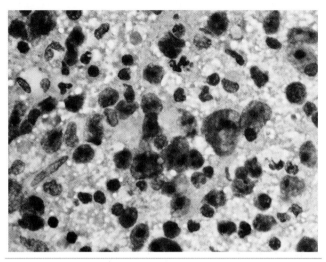

**Fig. 27.25** Dysgerminoma. Large poorly cohesive cells in 'tigroid' background with mature lymphocytes. Nuclei with irregularly, distributed chromatin and prominent macronucleoli. Imprint of ovary (MGG).

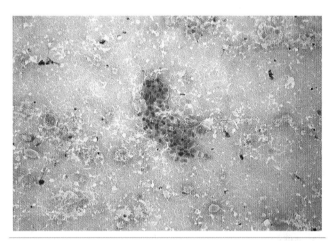

**Fig. 27.26** Follicular cells from a functional cyst staining positively with α-inhibin immunocytochemistry. FNA of ovary (immunoalkaline phosphatase).

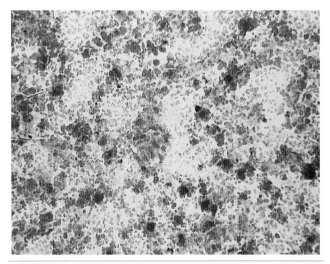

**Fig. 27.27** Corpus luteal cells from an haemorrhagic cyst staining positively with α-inhibin immunocytochemistry. FNA of ovary (immunoalkaline phosphatase).

Granulosa cell tumours are usually inhibin and steroidogenic factor 1 (SF-1, adrenal 4-binding protein) positive.[20,49] SF-1 is the most sensitive sex cord–stromal marker among the most common types of sex cord–stromal tumours. The most informative sex cord–stromal markers to be used for the distinction from non-sex cord–stromal tumours are inhibin, calretinin, SF-1, and Wilms tumour gene 1 (WT1).[49]

Although it has long been appreciated that ovarian carcinoma subtypes (serous, clear cell, endometrioid, and mucinous) are associated with different natural histories, most ovarian carcinoma biomarker studies and current treatment protocols for women with this disease are not subtype specific.[56]

In cases of metastatic carcinoma, it may be possible to determine the site of origin of the malignant cells. For example, gastrointestinal tumours are generally positive on staining with antibodies to carcinoembryonic antigen (CEA), CDX2 and CK20 (Fig. 27.28). These tumours are CK7 negative.[20]

In germ cell tumours, it may be possible to diagnose dysgerminomas (PLAP positive), yolk-sac tumours (AFP positive) and choriocarcinomas (βHCG positive).

WT1 and GCDFP-15 could be useful markers for the differential diagnosis of ovarian and peritoneal serous papillary adenocarcinoma versus breast invasive micropapillary adenocarcinoma.[57]

## Fallopian tubes

The application of cytological techniques for detection of fallopian tube lesions is limited. Malignant cells from the fallopian tubes are occasionally accidentally detected in endometrial, cervical or vaginal samples and peritoneal washings. The distal fallopian tube is emerging as an established source of many early serous carcinomas in women with BRCA mutations (BRCA+). Protocols examining the fimbrial end have revealed a non-invasive but potentially lethal form of tubal carcinoma, designated tubal intraepithelial carcinoma. Tubal intraepithelial carcinoma is present in many women with presumed ovarian or peritoneal serous cancer.[58]

Peritoneal washings cytology has an important place in diagnosis and staging of tubal carcinoma (see p. 733).

### Benign fallopian tube lesions

Occasionally aspiration of a hydrosalpinx is undertaken either in the IVF unit or at laparoscopy/laparotomy.[59] The fluid obtained from such aspirates is generally hypocellular and comprises of macrophages, lymphoid cells and scanty epithelial cells, which are variably degenerate. A diagnosis of hydrosalpinx can only be proffered or confirmed if these epithelial cells are ciliated. In such circumstances, it may not be possible to exclude a benign serous cystadenoma of the ovary, although the ovarian lesion is often more cellular.

Endosalpingiosis is defined as the presence of multiple glandular cystic inclusions on the surface of the ovary, fallopian tubes, uterine serosa and elsewhere in the pelvic peritoneum, omentum and even in pelvic lymph nodes. Cystic inclusions are lined by cuboidal or columnar epithelial cells some of which are ciliated.[60]

Tubal sterilisation is a common method of contraception in some countries. Imprint cytology can be suitable method to exclude erroneous ligation of structures that mimic tube shape

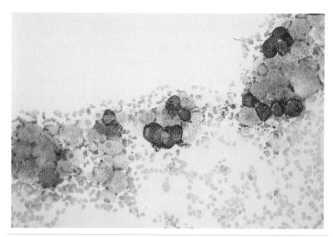

**Fig. 27.28** Metastatic colonic carcinoma in the ovary. These cells stain positively with CK20 immunocytochemistry. FNA of ovary (immunoalkaline phosphatase).

during small incision made for tubectomy, distinguishing tubal from non-tubal structures. To avoid false negative reports, it is recommended the preparation of smears from the ampulla promptly after excision of the tissue.[61]

## Malignant fallopian tube lesions

Although a common site of metastases, primary fallopian tube carcinoma comprises only 0.3% of all gynaecological malignancies.[62] Presenting symptoms are variable and non-specific, with preoperative diagnosis rarely entertained. The FIGO system assigns nearly two-thirds of patients to stage I or II and is based on surgical staging criteria similar to those for ovarian cancer. Likewise, management is based on that for ovarian cancer-radical debulking followed by platinum-based combination chemotherapy. Five-year survival for patients with disease confined to the tube at diagnosis (stage I) is only about 60% and only 10% of patients with advanced disease will be cured.[62]

### Cytological findings: malignant fallopian tube lesions

- The cytopathological features of adenocarcinoma of the fallopian tube are not distinctive or unique to the site
- Usually a clean background
- Paucity of cellular material, features noted in cervicovaginal smears that contain malignant tumour cells from any other extrauterine origin
- The malignant cells are most commonly glandular in origin and occur singly or in clusters
- The cells are medium sized, with round to oval nuclei, coarse chromatin, nucleoli and variably vacuolated cytoplasm.

The neoplastic cells from fallopian tube adenocarcinoma are histopathologically and cytopathologically similar to those from ovarian, endometrial and endocervical carcinomas. In the absence of diagnostic features, the cytopathologist is more likely to suggest an origin from these more common sites than from the fallopian tube. In general, fallopian tube carcinoma should be suspected when malignant cells are noted in patients with unremarkable pelvic examination and negative endometrial curettings.[86]

Malignant tumour cells from fallopian tube adenocarcinoma may also be encountered in ascitic fluid or peritoneal washings (see Ch. 3).

## Pelvic serous carcinoma of the peritoneum

Pelvic serous carcinoma of the peritoneum (PSCP) has traditionally been viewed as a rapidly evolving malignancy, due principally to its late stage at diagnosis and tendency for poor outcome, both in the endometrium and the upper genital tract. The incidence of PSCP has increased dramatically during the past decade in the USA with the greatest rise (>13% per year) among non-Hispanic and white women. This trend was more pronounced among older women and women with early stage disease.[63] Recently, studies of women with BRCA1 or BRCA2 mutations (BRCA+) undergoing risk reducing salpingo-oophorectomy have highlighted the distal fallopian tube as a common (80%) site of tumour origin and additional studies of unselected women with pelvic serous carcinoma have demonstrated that serous tubal intraepithelial carcinoma may precede a significant percentage of these tumours.[64,65]

Cytological material is obtained from the initial diagnostic paracenteses or exploratory laparotomies. These show mostly three-dimensional tumour cell clusters, as well as single malignant cells, with occasional papillae. The cytoplasm is abundant and often vacuolated. The cytomorphological features of PSCP enabled differentiation from other conditions involving the peritoneal surface, including mesothelial hyperplasia, malignant mesothelioma, endometriosis and endosalpingiosis. However, there are no characteristic features that differentiated PSCP from metastatic serous carcinoma of the ovary.[66]

## Other pelvic cysts

Occasionally cysts in the vicinity of the fallopian tubes and ovaries may be mistaken for ovarian cysts and aspirated for diagnostic and therapeutic purposes. These include peritoneal inclusion cysts which may occur spontaneously but are more common after abdominal surgical procedures. Aspirates from such cysts are usually paucicellular and contain mesothelial cells which are reasonably easy to recognise. Very occasionally, paratubal cysts may develop in a Walthard's rest. Aspirates from these are also paucicellular and contain bland cuboidal cells. Very rarely colon reduplication cysts can mimic ovarian cysts if they are in the appropriate location.[67]

## The role of peritoneal washings

Cytological examination of peritoneal washings taken during surgery enables the initial as well as the 'second-look' clinical staging of the ovarian carcinoma and influences the prognosis of the disease, further management and response to therapy.[11,68,69] The sensitivity and specificity of cytological analysis depends on the quality of the sample, histological type of the tumour and the stage of disease.[12,70] Cytological findings need to be evaluated in the light of clinical, serological and intraoperative findings.[71,72] Using peritoneal histology as a standard, peritoneal cytology is highly specific (98.1%) but less sensitive (82.9%) in detecting intraperitoneal involvement.[12] Sensitivity decreases with further surgical procedures due to adhesions which prevent a reliable peritoneal sampling during the 'second-look' procedure. A false positive finding[69] represents an exceptionally serious problem because it implies a higher clinical stage at first surgery or unnecessary continuation of treatment after the 'second-look' operation. In order to improve diagnostic accuracy, peritoneal washing cytology is supplemented by immunocytochemistry and flow cytometry as well as the use of the cell block and ThinPrep cell preparations.[73-76]

## The role of cytology in management of ovarian lesions

Given the advances in imaging techniques in the last decade, FNA of the ovary is nowadays performed relatively rarely. The indication for a cytological investigation is usually a clinically benign cystic lesion found during the course of gynaecological investigation, often associated with fertility treatment. Cytological evaluation of non-neoplastic ovarian cysts is important for women who want to retain their fertility as well as in the clinical management of women with neoplastic lesions.

Wojcik et al. evaluated the cytomorphological features of cystic ovarian lesions[32] from 103 cases and found 82% to be benign, predominantly non-neoplastic entities which included follicular, corpus luteum and endometriotic cysts. Neoplastic cystic lesions included serous, mucinous, and Brenner tumours, germ cell neoplasms, a sex cord–stromal tumour, and an undifferentiated carcinoma. Borderline tumours could not be distinguished from well-differentiated cystadenocarcinomas.

All neoplastic cysts are removed surgically for symptom relief, treatment and subtyping. Malignant cysts are removed with the uterus, opposite tube and ovary, omentum, peritoneal fluid sampling ± peritoneal biopsies for full staging, which is discussed at multidisciplinary-team meetings. All malignancies greater than stage IC are usually treated with adjuvant chemotherapy. In more advanced cases, there may be initial treatment with chemotherapy which is followed by interval debulking and further chemotherapy. FNA cytology may be useful in assessing new lesions which may be recurrences without the need for major intervention. The multidisciplinary-team setting requires a cytohistopathologist to offer the most appropriate diagnosis, prognosis and advise on further tests that can be performed.

Diagnostic accuracy of FNA ovary depends on acquiring a satisfactory sample. However, the rate of unsatisfactory samples ranges from 18%,[32] 43%,[4] to 74%[28] and mainly relates to benign lesions, although they also occur in malignant lesions.[42] Associated with these findings are the false negative diagnoses ranging from 4% to 74%.[18,77,78] Additional material may be obtained by aspiration curettage of the inner surface of the cyst during aspiration.[8]

An adequate, technically well prepared FNA sample, as well as the experience of the cytopathologist, account for the high sensitivity and diagnostic accuracy (>90%) of the ovarian lesions diagnosed in this way.[2,79] The false positive cytology findings are rare, usually associated with a particularly cellular follicular cysts[80] or serous cystadenoma and endometriosis with atypia.[81]

The application of ancillary techniques to FNA material such as immunocytochemistry,[13,20,21,49] measurement of tumour markers in cyst fluids, flow cytometry[74,82] and static cytometry, morphometry[83] and nucleolar organiser regions, can yield diagnostic and prognostic information in ovarian tumours.[84]

Two new technologies of proteomics, mass spectrometry and protein array analysis, have advanced the proteomic characterisation of ovarian cancer. Mass spectrometry may in the future allow identification of the elusive 'needle in the haystack', heralding ovarian cancer. Proteomic profiling of tumour tissue samples can survey molecular targets during treatment (see Ch. 34).[85] The evolution of proteomic technologies has the capacity to rapidly advance our understanding of ovarian cancer at a molecular level and thus elucidate new directions for the treatment of this disease.

Ovarian cytology can be used in conjunction with ultrasound imaging and CA125 biochemistry as part of screening for ovarian tumours in at risk women (usually BRCA-1 and BRCA-2 carriers).

In summary, under appropriate conditions FNA cytology of the ovary is useful in the diagnosis of ovarian lesions. It is especially helpful in the diagnosis and management of benign cysts and in the diagnosis of recurrent ovarian cancer. It is also ideal in rare cases where laparoscopy cannot be performed because of poor physical condition of the patient. These days most primary ovarian carcinomas can be distinguished from metastatic carcinoma to the ovary on the basis of the cytological findings and ancillary methods. Full knowledge of the clinical and radiological findings and the implications of the cytological diagnosis on management cannot be overemphasised. Regular attendance by cytopathologists at the multidisciplinary-team meetings for discussion of individual patient management is essential.

# REFERENCES

1. Zajicek J. Cytology of infradiaphragmatic organs. 3. Ovary. Monogr Clin Cytol 1979;7:54–56.

2. Ganjei P, Dickinson B, Harrison T, et al. Aspiration cytology of neoplastic and non-neoplastic ovarian cysts: is it accurate? Int J Gynecol Pathol 1996;15:94–101.

3. Papathanasiou K, Giannoulis C, Dovas D, et al. Fine needle aspiration cytology of the ovary: is it reliable? Clin Exp Obstet Gynecol 2004;31:191–93.

4. Martinez-Onsurbe P, Ruiz Villaespesa A, Sanz Anquela JM, et al. Aspiration cytology of 147 adnexal cysts with histologic correlation. Acta Cytol 2001;45:941–47.

5. Allias F, Chanoz J, Blache G, et al. Value of ultrasound-guided fine-needle aspiration in the management of ovarian and paraovarian cysts. Diagn Cytopathol 2000;22:70–80.

6. Hemalatha AL, Divya P, Mamatha R. Image-directed percutaneous FNAC of ovarian neoplasms. Indian J Pathol Microbiol 2005;48:305–9.

7. Duke D, Colville J, Keeling A, et al. Transvaginal aspiration of ovarian cysts: long-term follow-up. Cardiovasc Intervent Radiol 2006;29:401–5.

8. Lee CL, Lai YM, Chang SY, et al. The management of ovarian cysts by sono-guided transvaginal cyst aspiration. J Clin Ultrasound 1993;21:511–14.

9. Lu D, Davila RM, Pinto KR, et al. ThinPrep evaluation of fluid samples aspirated from cystic ovarian masses. Diagn Cytopathol 2004;30:320–24.

10. Shield P. Peritoneal washing cytology. Cytopathology 2004;15:131–41.

11. Benedet JL, Bender H, Jones H, et al. FIGO staging classifications and clinical practice guidelines in the management of gynecologic cancers. FIGO Committee on Gynecologic Oncology. Int J Gynaecol Obstet 2000;70:209–62.

12. Zuna RE, Behrens A. Peritoneal washing cytology in gynecologic cancers: long-term follow-up of 355 patients. J Natl Cancer Inst 1996;88:980–87.

13. McCluggage WG, Young RH. Immunohistochemistry as a diagnostic aid in the evaluation of ovarian tumors. Semin Diagn Pathol 2005;22:3–32.

14. Guariglia L, Conte M, Are P, et al. Ultrasound-guided fine needle aspiration of ovarian cysts during pregnancy. Eur J Obstet Gynecol Reprod Biol 1999;82:5–9.

15. Mathevet P. DD, Nov; 30. Role of ultrasound guided puncture in the management of ovarian cysts. J Gynecol Obstet Biol Reprod (Paris) 2001;30:S53–58.

16. Mulvany NJ. Aspiration cytology of ovarian cysts and cystic neoplasms. A study of 235 aspirates. Acta Cytol 1996;40:911–20.

17. Trimbos JB, Hacker NF. The case against aspirating ovarian cysts. Cancer 1993;72:828–31.

18. Higgins RV, Matkins JF, Marroum MC. Comparison of fine-needle aspiration cytologic findings of ovarian cysts with ovarian histologic findings. Am J Obstet Gynecol 1999;180:550–53.

19. Candido Dos Reis FJ, Moreira de Andrade J, Bighetti S. CA 125 and vascular endothelial growth factor in the differential diagnosis of epithelial ovarian tumors. Gynecol Obstet Invest 2002;54:132–36.

20. Manek S. The role of immunohistochemistry in gynaecological diseases. CPD Bull Cell Pathol 1999;1:162–66.

21. McCluggage WG, Patterson A, White J, et al. Immunocytochemical staining of ovarian cyst aspirates with monoclonal antibody against inhibin. Cytopathology 1998;9:336–42.

22. Selvaggi SM. Cytology of nonneoplastic cysts of the ovary. Diagn Cytopathol 1990;6:77–85.

23. Rivasi F, Gasser B, Morandi P, et al. Ciliated bodies in ovarian cyst aspirates. Acta Cytol 1993;37:489–93.

24. Selvaggi SM. Fine-needle aspiration cytology of ovarian follicle cysts with cellular atypia from reproductive-age patients. Diagn Cytopathol 1991;7:189–92.

25. Dejmek A. Fine needle aspiration cytology of an ovarian luteinized follicular cyst mimicking a granulosa cell tumor. A case report. Acta Cytol 2003;47:1059–62.

26. Fulciniti F, Caleo A, Lepore M, et al. Fine needle cytology of endometriosis: experience with 10 cases. Acta Cytol 2005;49:495–99.

27. Hemachandran M, Nijhawan R, Srinivasan R, et al. Collagenous bodies in endometriotic cysts. Diagn Cytopathol 2004;31:330–32.

28. de Crespigny LC, Robinson HP, Davoren RA, et al. The 'simple' ovarian cyst: aspirate or operate?. Br J Obstet Gynaecol 1989;96:1035–39.

29. Petrovic N, Arko D, Lovrec VG, et al. Ultrasound guided aspiration in pathological adnexal processes. Eur J Obstet Gynecol Reprod Biol 2002;104:52–57.

30. Greenebaum E, Mayer JR, Stangel JJ, et al. Aspiration cytology of ovarian cysts in in vitro fertilization patients. Acta Cytol 1992;36:11–18.

31. Ghezzi F, Cromi A, Bergamini V, et al. Should adnexal mass size influence surgical approach? A series of 186 laparoscopically managed large adnexal masses. Br J Obstet Gynaecol 2008;115:1020–27.

32. Wojcik EM, Selvaggi SM. Fine-needle aspiration cytology of cystic ovarian lesions. Diagn Cytopathol 1994;11:9–14.

33. Tavassoli FA, Devilee P. Pathology and genetics of tumours of the breast and female genital organs (WHO Classification of Tumours). Lyon: IARC Press; 2003 114–115.

34. Diamantopoulou S, Sikiotis K, Panayiotides J, et al. Serous cystadenoma with massive ovarian edema. A case report and review of the literature. Clin Exp Obstet Gynecol 2009;36:58–61.

35. Ahr A, Arnold G, Gohring UJ, et al. Cytology of ascitic fluid in a patient with metastasizing malignant Brenner tumor of the ovary. A case report. Acta Cytol 1997;41:S1299–304.

36. Miller SJ, Waddell CA, Rollason TP, et al. Perplexing findings in a cystic teratoma. Cytopathology 2001;12:49–53.

37. Premalata CS, Amirtham U, Devi G, et al. Ovarian sex cord tumour with annular tubules diagnosed by fine needle aspiration cytology – a case report. Indian J Pathol Microbiol 2005;48:358–60.

38. Smeenk RM, Bruin SC, van Velthuysen ML, et al. Pseudomyxoma peritonei. Curr Probl Surg 2008;45:527–75.

39. Jackson SL, Fleming RA, Loggie BW, et al. Gelatinous ascites: a cytohistologic study of pseudomyxoma peritonei in 67 patients. Mod Pathol 2001;14:664–71.

40. Leiman G, Goldberg R. Pseudomyxoma peritonei associated with ovarian mucinous tumors. Cytologic appearance in five cases. Acta Cytol 1992;36:299–304.

41. Bradley RF, Stewart JH, Russell GB, et al. Pseudomyxoma peritonei of appendiceal origin: a clinicopathologic analysis of 101 patients uniformly treated at a single institution, with literature review. Am J Surg Pathol 2006;30:551–59.

42. Granados R. Aspiration cytology of ovarian tumors. Curr Opin Obstet Gynecol 1995.

43. Atahan S, Ekinci C, Icli F, et al. Cytology of clear cell carcinoma of the female genital tract in fine needle aspirates and ascites. Acta Cytol 2000;44:1005–9.

44. Rust MM, Susa J, Naylor R, et al. Clear cell carcinoma in a background of endometriosis. Case report of a finding in a midline abdominal scar 5 years after a total abdominal hysterectomy. Acta Cytol 2008;52:475–80.

45. Vrdoljak-Mozetic D, Stankovic T, Krasevic M, et al. Intraoperative cytology of clear cell carcinoma of the ovary. Cytopathology 2006;17:390–95.

46. Donat EE, McCutcheon JM, Alper H. Malignant mixed müllerian tumor of the ovary. Report of a case with cytodiagnosis by fine needle aspiration. Acta Cytol 1994;38:231–34.

47. Ozkara SK TG. Cystic fluid and fine needle aspiration cytopathology of cystic adult granulosa cell tumor of the ovary: a case report. Acta Cytol 2008;52:247–50.

48. Lal A, Bourtsos EP, Nayar R, et al. Cytologic features of granulosa cell tumors in fluids and fine needle aspiration specimens. Acta Cytol 2004;48:315–20.

49. Zhao C, Vinh TN, McManus K, et al. Identification of the most sensitive and robust immunohistochemical markers in different categories of ovarian sex cord-stromal tumors. Am J Surg Pathol 2009;33:354–66.

50. Hameed A, Coleman RL. Fine-needle aspiration cytology of primary granulosa cell tumor of the adrenal gland: a case report. Diagn Cytopathol 2000;22:107–9.

51. Pectasides D, Pectasides E, Kassanos D. Germ cell tumors of the ovary. Cancer Treat Rev 2008;34:427–41.

52. Gupta R, Mathur SR, Arora VK, et al. Cytologic features of extragonadal germ cell tumors: a study of 88 cases with aspiration cytology. Cancer 2008;114:504–11.

53. Yang GC, Hwang SJ, Yee HT. Fine-needle aspiration cytology of unusual germ cell tumors of the mediastinum: atypical seminoma and parietal yolk sac tumor. Diagn Cytopathol 2002;27:69–74.

54. Akhtar M, al Dayel F. Is it feasible to diagnose germ-cell tumors by fine-needle aspiration biopsy? Diagn Cytopathol 1997;16:72–77.

55. Ramalingam P, Teague D, Reid-Nicholson M. Imprint cytology of high-grade immature ovarian teratoma: a case report, literature review, and distinction from other ovarian small round cell tumors. Diagn Cytopathol 2008;36:595–99.

56. Kobel M, Kalloger SE, Boyd N, et al. Ovarian carcinoma subtypes are different diseases: implications for biomarker studies. PLoS Med 2008;5:e232.

57. Moritani S, Ichihara S, Hasegawa M, et al. Serous papillary adenocarcinoma of the female genital organs and invasive micropapillary carcinoma of the breast. Are WT1, CA125, and GCDFP-15 useful in differential diagnosis? Hum Pathol 2008;39:666–71.

58. Crum CP, Drapkin R, Miron A, et al. The distal fallopian tube: a new model for pelvic serous carcinogenesis. Curr Opin Obstet Gynecol 2007;19:3–9.

59. Matsushima T, Kaseki H, Ishihara K, et al. Assessment of fallopian tube cytology for the diagnosis of endometriosis and hydrosalpinx. J Nippon Med Sch 2002;69:445–50.

60. Kobayashi TK, Moritani S, Urabe M, et al. Cytologic diagnosis of endosalpingiosis with pregnant women presenting in peritoneal fluid: a case report. Diagn Cytopathol 2004;30:422–25.

61. Aali BS, Malekpour R, Nakheii N, et al. Utility and diagnostic accuracy of fallopian tube touch imprint cytology. Cytopathology 2005;16:252–55.

62. Ng P, Lawton F. Fallopian tube carcinoma – a review. Ann Acad Med Singapore 1998;27:693–97.

63. Goodman MT, Shvetsov YB. Rapidly increasing incidence of papillary serous carcinoma of the peritoneum in the United States: fact or artifact? Int J Cancer 2009;124:2231–35.

64. Folkins AK, Jarboe EA, Roh MH, et al. Precursors to pelvic serous carcinoma and their clinical implications. Gynecol Oncol 2009;113:391–96.

65. Roh MH, Kindelberger D, Crum CP. Serous tubal intraepithelial carcinoma and the dominant ovarian mass: clues to serous tumor origin? Am J Surg Pathol 2009;33:376–83.

66. Tauchi PS, Caraway N, Truong LD, et al. Serous surface carcinoma of the peritoneum: useful role of cytology in differential diagnosis and follow-up. Acta Cytol 1996;40:429–36.

67. Meyberg-Solomayer GC, Buchenau W, Solomayer EF, et al. Cystic colon duplication as differential diagnosis to ovarian cyst. Fetal Diagn Ther 2006;21:224–27.

68. Anastasiadis PG, Romanidis KN, Polichronidis A, et al. The contribution of rapid intraoperative cytology to the improvement of ovarian cancer staging. Gynecol Oncol 2002;86:244–49.

69. Kudo R, Takashina T, Ito E, et al. Peritoneal washing cytology at second-look laparotomy in cisplatin-treated ovarian cancer patients. Acta Cytol 1990;34:545–48.

70. Spriggs A. Cytology of peritoneal aspirates and washings. Br J Obstet Gynaecol 1987;94:1–3.

71. Bibbo M, Wood MD, Fitzpatrick BT. Peritoneal washings and ovary. In: Bibbo M, Wilbur DC, editors. Comprehensive cytopathology. Philadelphia: Saunders, Elsevier Inc; 2008. p. 291–301.

72. Audy-Jurkovi S. Cytology in the diagnosis of ovarian cancer today and tomorrow. Gynecol Perinatol 1992;1:170–72.

73. Weir MM, Bell DA. Cytologic identification of serous neoplasms in peritoneal fluids. Cancer 2001;93:309–18.

74. Risberg B, Davidson B, Dong HP, et al. Flow cytometric immunophenotyping of serous effusions and peritoneal washings: comparison with immunocytochemistry and morphological findings. J Clin Pathol 2000;53:513–17.

75. Selvaggi SM. Diagnostic pitfalls of peritoneal washing cytology and the role of cell blocks in their diagnosis. Diagn Cytopathol 2003;28:335–41.

76. Sadeghi S, Ylagan LR. Pelvic washing cytology in serous borderline tumors of the ovary using ThinPrep: are there cytologic clues to detecting tumor cells? Diagn Cytopathol 2004;30:313–19.

77. Moran O, Menczer J, Ben-Baruch G, et al. Cytologic examination of ovarian cyst fluid for the distinction between benign and malignant tumors. Obstet Gynecol 1993;82:444–46.

78. Sheombar ES, Logmans A, Verhoeff A, et al. Ovarian cysts, cytology and histology: a conflicting story. Eur J Obstet Gynecol Reprod Biol 1993;52:41–44.

79. Larsen T, Torp-Pedersen ST, Ottesen M, et al. Abdominal ultrasound combined with histological and cytological fine needle biopsy of suspected ovarian tumors. Eur J Obstet Gynecol Reprod Biol 1993;50:203–9.

80. Nunez C, Diaz JI. Ovarian follicular cysts: a potential source of false positive diagnoses in ovarian cytology. Diagn Cytopathol 1992;8:532–36. discussion 536–537.

81. Davila RM. Cytology of benign cystic uterine adnexal masses. Acta Cytol 1993;37:385–90.

82. Krishan A, Ganji-Azar P, Jorda M, et al. Detection of tumor cells in body cavity fluids by flow cytometric and immunochemical analysis. Diagn Cytopathol 2006;34:528–41.

83. Stemberger-Papic S, Stankovic T, Vrdoljak-Mozetic D, et al. Morphometry and digital AgNOR analysis in cytological imprints of benign, borderline and malignant serous ovarian tumours. Cytopathology 2006;17:382–89.

84. Versa-Ostojc D, Stankovic T, Stemberger-Papic S, et al. Nuclear morphometry and AgNOR quantification: computerized image analysis on ovarian mucinous tumor imprints. Anal Quant Cytol Histol 2008;30:160–68.

85. Annunziata CM, Azad N, Dhamoon AS, et al. Ovarian cancer in the proteomics era. Int J Gynecol Cancer 2008;18:S1–S6.

86. Pusiol T, Piscioli F, Morelli L, et al. Cervicovaginal smears in the diagnosis of asymptomatic primary fallopian tube carcinoma. Cytopathology 2009;20:409–11.

# Section 13

## Skin, Soft Tissues and Musculoskeletal System

# Skin

Anna M. Bofin and Eidi Christensen

## Chapter contents

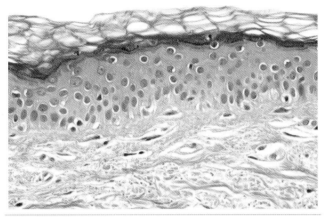

**Fig. 28.1** Normal skin showing the epidermis and the upper dermis. Biopsy (H&S).

## Introduction

Skin cytology is a rapid, relatively non-invasive diagnostic technique. In many cases, it is sufficient for definitive diagnosis,[1] and preferable to biopsy from areas such as the face to avoid or minimise scarring, particularly in conjunction with topical treatment modalities in some types of skin cancer. Furthermore, cytological material is well suited for certain ancillary tests. It is a simple, inexpensive diagnostic method and is especially helpful when resources are limited.

Skin cytology offers cytopathologists a wide range of lesions, some of which are well documented with robust diagnostic criteria, whereas others are encountered only occasionally by the individual cytopathologist, with merely case reports offering descriptions of their cytological characteristics.

## Normal skin

Histologically, the skin can be divided into three main areas:

1. The epidermis is derived from the primitive ectoderm and is composed of multilayered squamous cells (keratinocytes) and dendritic cells. Squamous cells, which form the bulk of cells in epidermis, possess intercellular bridges. The main dendritic cells found are Langerhans cells and melanocytes (Fig. 28.1).
2. The dermis is divided into papillary and reticular areas. The papillary dermis is superficial, interdigitating with the rete pegs of the epidermis.

3. Skin appendages including the pilosebaceous unit comprising hair follicles, sebaceous glands and arrector pili muscles; apocrine and eccrine sweat glands are situated in the deeper layer of the dermis.

### Cytological findings: normal skin

- Under normal conditions, only squamous cells of the horny layer exfoliate
- Cells from the horny layer are large, polyhedral and anucleate with a certain degree of folding
- Granular layer: cells are smaller than those in the horny layer; they contain deeply basophilic keratohyaline granules
- Squamous cell layer: cells vary in size according to their degree of maturity; in clusters of cells intercellular bridges may be seen. Nuclei have well-defined, lacy chromatin
- Basal cell layer: this is composed of immature, germinative cells, seen histologically as a single row of small regular cells lying perpendicular to the underlying basement membrane, which anchors them (palisading). The nuclear/cytoplasmic ratio is high
- Melanocytes, conspicuous with their clear cytoplasm and small, dark nuclei, are scattered along the basal layer but are rarely seen in smears
- Langerhans cells, part of the immune system, are scarce and difficult to identify. A few inflammatory cells including lymphocytes, histiocytes and mast cells may also be seen in skin smears.[2]

*We acknowledge the following for kindly providing pictures: Dr M. Baba, Dr M. Durdu, Dr R. Hannula and Professor T. Sauer.*

## Technical procedures

Various methods for obtaining and staining cytological material from skin lesions include skin scrape, brush cytology, touch imprint and fine needle aspiration (FNA) cytology.

### Direct skin scrape

The skin scrape was first employed in the late 1940s by Tzanck in the differential diagnosis of bullous diseases, and is still mainly used for sampling superficial lesions.[3]

A blunt or sharp curette, a double-ended elevator or a scalpel blade can be used. The skin should be cleansed before the procedure. The keratotic surface and any crusts must be removed completely to obtain a satisfactory representative smear.[4] Samples from superficial, crusted lesions should be taken from the periphery of the lesion, as the centre may be inflamed and necrotic. It is important to avoid scraping unnecessarily deep as this will lead to bleeding and possibly also scarring. In non-crusted nodular lesions, it is possible to cut into the lesion, either removing the top and scraping the exposed surface, or scraping the incision area to obtain an adequate sample (skin slit smear).[5]

The material is deposited on a glass slide and spread directly with a second slide. If material is abundant, several slides should be prepared. It is important that the cells are evenly spread on the slide so that a thin layer of material is achieved (Fig. 28.2). Small fragments of tumour tissue can be placed on one slide and a second slide then placed directly on top. Firm vertical pressure is applied and the slides are separated horizontally, spreading the cells evenly.[2]

### Brush sampling

Brush cytology is also used for sampling superficial lesions.[6] A gynaecological cytobrush may be used. The material is deposited on the slide avoiding vigorous brushing backwards and forwards which may damage the cells.

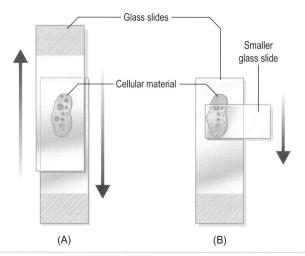

**Fig. 28.2** (A) The cellular material is placed between two glass slides. The slides are then drawn apart horizontally making two smears. (B) The cellular material is placed on a glass slide and smeared with a smaller glass slide.

### Touch imprint cytology

This technique may be used successfully in ulcerating lesions and the cut surface of biopsies. A clean, dry microscope slide should be firmly pressed against the lesion after removal of any crusts. Slight abrasion of the surface exposes viable tissue, freeing up tissue fragments and individual cells.

Imprints can also be made from shave or punch biopsies. Excess blood should be carefully removed and the biopsy gently pressed or rolled on the slide.[2]

### Fine needle sampling

Fine needle sampling with aspiration (FNA) or without aspiration (FNS) may be employed to sample skin nodules and deeper lesions. The procedure does not require sterile conditions. Local anaesthetic is not necessary and may, in some instances, make it difficult to obtain adequate cellular material. A narrow gauge needle, <0.7 mm (22–23G) in diameter, is used. The needle is moved back and forth, sometimes almost tangentially to the skin surface, aiming at the raised edges of an ulcer or centre of a nodule. The needle contents are ejected and smeared in a thin layer on a glass slide (Fig. 28.2).[7] Material may also be deposited in a variety of media for special procedures such as liquid-based cytology (LBC) flow cytometry, polymerase chain reaction (PCR), or microbiology.

Sampling without aspiration, allowing the material to enter the needle by capillary attraction, is particularly suitable for cellular nodules such as lymph nodes or melanoma metastases.

### Staining techniques

The Papanicolaou stain (PAP) requires immediate fixation in alcohol. Nuclear chromatin patterns are easily discerned and the degree of maturation/keratinisation of squamous cells is readily appreciated. Mucin may not be seen so easily.

May-Grünwald Giemsa (MGG) staining is used on air-dried smears. Nuclear detail is less readily discerned though mucin and other extracellular substances may be easily seen. Modified MGG stains are available for rapid staining.

Wet films may be also stained immediately with a drop of 0.5% methylene blue followed by coverslipping to spread the stain (Tzanck's stain).[3] Ideally, smears should be prepared for PAP and MGG staining and air-dried smears or cell suspensions should be kept for special tests.

### Special techniques

Immunocytochemistry can be performed on cytological smears or cytospin preparations, preferably on coated glass slides. Cells from stained or unstained smears may be used for PCR and may be particularly useful in lymphoma diagnostics (see Chs 13, 14, 34). Cell suspensions may be utilised for PCR or flow cytometry. Air-dried smears are eminently suited for *in situ* hybridisation techniques with either fluorescent or chromogenic markers.[8]

# Infections

## Bacterial lesions

It is unusual for a pustular lesion clinically considered to be a primary or secondary bacterial infection to be sampled for cytological diagnosis. However, when a scraping or aspirate of pus is taken, samples should be sent for bacterial culture, PCR and extra smears made for special stains such as Gram or Ziehl Neelsen.

## Mycobacterial infections

### Leprosy

Leprosy is a slowly progressive, highly infectious disease caused by *Mycobacterium leprae* predominantly affecting the skin and peripheral nerves. It is mostly found in warm tropical countries. According to the immune status of the patients, leprosy is classified in five clinically and histologically recognisable groups with tuberculoid and lepromatous variants at either pole of the scale and the unstable form (borderline) between.

Skin lesions usually appear early, varying from sharply demarcated, hypopigmented, hypoaesthetic maculae with elevated borders in tuberculoid leprosy to papules, plaques or nodules and diffuse thickening of the skin in lepromatous leprosy.

Serological tests for anti-PGL antibodies and PCR are available in some centres but in the field the diagnosis and classification of leprosy have been based on clinical examination and cytology. The specificity of the cytological diagnosis is close to 100% but sensitivity is only 50%.[9,10] In cases with few acid-fast bacilli in the smear multiple lesions should be sampled and biopsy for histology should be performed.[11] Skin scraping is suitable in flat lesions whereas needle aspiration is better in raised or nodular lesions.[10]

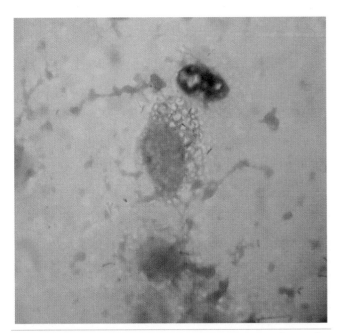

**Fig. 28.3** Leprosy. Acid-fast bacilli in bundles in a foamy macrophage and scattered in the background. Smear (Ziehl Neelsen).

**Cytological findings: leprosy**

- Foamy macrophages containing bundles of acid-fast bacilli in Ziehl Neelsen stained preparations (Fig. 28.3)
- Loosely cohesive epithelioid cell granulomas, macrophages and varying amounts of lymphocytes.

**Diagnostic pitfalls: leprosy**

- The smear may sometimes resemble sarcoidosis
- The bacterial index may vary widely in mid-borderline leprosy and in many cases no bacteria are found.

### Tuberculosis

Cutaneous tuberculosis is relatively uncommon and has a range of clinical presentations. It is caused by *Mycobacterium tuberculosis*. Direct infection of the skin may, after an incubation period of about 1 month, present as a firm, inflamed papule, which rapidly ulcerates. FNA is preferable to skin scrape cytology in tubercular ulcers and sinuses of the skin because FNA enables sampling of more viable parts of the lesion whereas skin scrape cytology is likely to result in a smear containing only necrotic debris.[12] PCR has improved the detection of the mycobacterium bacillus which is difficult to demonstrate by microscopy and culture.[13]

**Cytological findings: tuberculosis**

- Granulomas or epithelioid cells, multinucleated giant cells, lymphocytes and necrotic material.

## Protozoan lesions

### Leishmaniasis

Leishmaniasis is endemic in many countries, mainly in the developing world. However, it may occasionally be seen in other geographic areas, mostly among immigrants or troops stationed away from their home countries.[14] It is caused by a number of protozoa of the genus *Leishmania*. The disease is a chronic, inflammatory response to intracytoplasmic parasites in activated macrophages. In later stages granulomas develop. Cutaneous leishmaniasis presents in several clinical forms, affecting exposed areas on the body as a single papule or plaque which increases in size. The nodular form can develop crusted, soft ulceration and multiple lesions may occur.

The diagnosis of leishmaniasis is made by measuring serum antibody levels, bacterial culture or detection of parasite DNA by PCR. However, these techniques are not always available in the parts of world afflicted by the disease, leaving cytology as the most common diagnostic method. Scraping or FNA from both the centre and the margin of the lesion is widely employed for detecting the parasite (Fig. 28.4).[14–16]

**Cytological findings: leishmaniasis**

- Macrophages containing intracytoplasmic amastigotes (Leishman bodies)
- Extracellular amastigotes in the background
- The amastigotes are spherical or ovoid, 2–3 μm in size. It may be possible to detect the nucleus and the rod-shaped kinetoplast in some of the amastigotes.

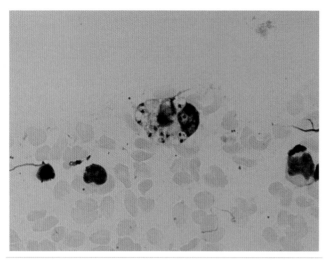

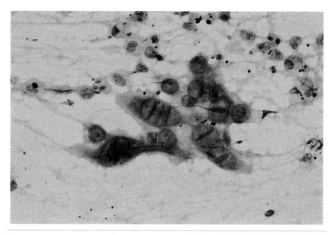

**Fig. 28.6** Herpes virus infection. Multinucleated giant cells with ground glass nuclei and nuclear moulding. Skin scrape (PAP).

**Fig. 28.4** Leishmaniasis. Macrophage with amastigotes in its cytoplasm. From an ulcerated lesion. Smear (MGG).

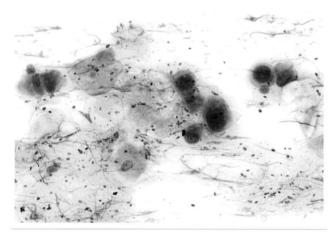

**Fig. 28.5** Budding yeast forms in actinic keratosis. Skin scrape (PAP).

### Diagnostic pitfalls: leishmaniasis

- Secondary bacterial infection may obscure the diagnostic amastigotes.

## Superficial fungal lesions

Fungal elements are usually a coincidental finding in skin smears (Fig. 28.5). However, cases of fungal cutaneous lesions diagnosed by FNA have been reported in the literature.[17,18]

### Cytological findings: superficial fungal lesions

- Fungal spores, hyphae or pseudohyphae.

## Viral lesions

At least five groups of viruses can affect the skin; two groups produce lesions with characteristic cytological features that can be reliably diagnosed by skin cytology: the herpes virus group

and the poxvirus group. Human papillomavirus causes skin warts. However, these are seldom sampled for cytology except when they occur in the vulvar region. The cytological changes are similar to those of human papillomavirus infection of the lower genital tract (see Chs 21, 23).

## Herpes virus infection

The herpes virus group comprises *Herpes simplex* types 1 and 2 and *Varicella zoster*. Despite clinical differences, early stages show grouped or isolated vesicles on an inflamed base, that later become covered by crusts. It is impossible to distinguish these entities cytologically; however, a number of diagnostic tests, including PCR, may be used. Samples should be taken from the vesicle at an early stage to avoid degenerative changes and superimposed infection (Fig. 28.6).[2,9]

### Cytological findings: herpes virus

- Multinucleated cells measuring between 20 and 30 μm in diameter with up to 30 nuclei
- Nuclear moulding and margination of chromatin
- Pale, eosinophilic, ground glass-like intranuclear inclusion bodies
- Inflammatory cells.

### Diagnostic pitfalls: herpes virus

- The large eosinophilic inclusions may be confused with nucleoli
- Multinucleated giant cells in pemphigus vulgaris lack nuclear inclusions and moulding and are accompanied by acantholytic cells.

## Molluscum contagiosum

Molluscum contagiosum is caused by a pox-type virus causing isolated, hard, dome-shaped papules with umbilicated centres, occurring mostly in children. Specimens can be obtained either by compression of the lesion to extrude the central keratinous material or, preferably, by removing cells from the top of the papule with a small curette. Vaccinia and Orf share cytological features with molluscum contagiosum (Fig. 28.7).[20]

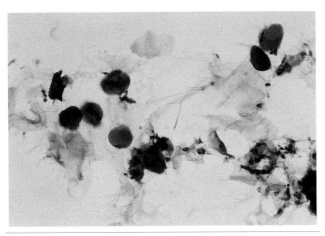

**Fig. 28.7** Molluscum contagiosum. Squamous cells with eosinophilic 'molluscum bodies'. Skin scrape (PAP).

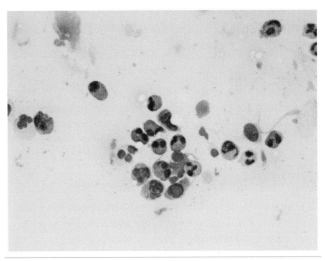

**Fig. 28.8** Bullous pemphigoid. Eosinophils and neutrophils. Skin scrape (MGG).

## Cytological findings: molluscum contagiosum

- Numerous single, round squamous cells with large eosinophilic (PAP), intracytoplasmic aggregates of viral particles ('molluscum bodies') giving a mosaic appearance to the cytoplasm
- The nucleus is pushed to the periphery of the cell and is crescent-shaped.

## Parasitic infections

### Demodex folliculitis

Demodex folliculitis may present with extensive, erythematous pustular skin lesions. Examination of scraped smears obtained from the pustules reveals numerous parasitic organisms typical of *Demodex folliculorum*.[21]

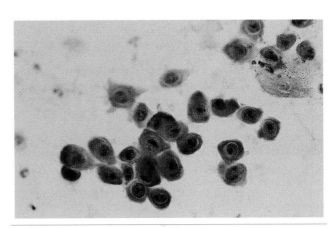

**Fig. 28.9** Pemphigus. Rounded single cells with perinuclear halos. Skin scrape (PAP).

## Bullous lesions

The Tzank test was first used in the differential diagnosis of bullous lesions to demonstrate dissolution of intercellular bridges in acantholytic cells. These findings are also typical of the intraepidermal bullae in pemphigus diseases. However, in subepidermal bullae as in bullous pemphigoid, the blisters rather contain inflammatory cells with variable numbers of neutrophils and eosinophils (Fig. 28.8). Smears should preferably be made from an early, intact vesicle or bulla; scraping the floor of a bulla will result in a more cellular smear. The test is non-specific and it may be difficult to differentiate between the various bullous diseases and other lesions presenting with acantholytic blisters. It is probably more appropriate to biopsy an early bulla and demonstrate antibody binding by immunological techniques.

## Pemphigus vulgaris

Pemphigus vulgaris can appear in all areas of the skin and mucosa. Bullae form as the cells lose their prickles and intercellular clefts form into which fluid from the underlying corium passes. The disease presents as thin, loose blisters with serous content which easily break leaving an eroded surface with crust formation. Direct immunofluorescence on a Tzank smear has been shown to be comparable to biopsy in diagnosing early pemphigus vulgaris and is particularly useful in lesions in the oral cavity (Fig. 28.9).[22]

## Cytological findings: pemphigus vulgaris

- Numerous single, rounded acantholytic cells with cyanophilic cytoplasm
- Large hyperchromatic nuclei with pronounced nucleoli and perinuclear halos
- Neutrophils, eosinophils and lymphocytes in the background.

## Diagnostic pitfalls: pemphigus vulgaris

- Acantholytic cells may be misinterpreted as suspicious of malignancy.

## Benign and malignant tumours of the surface epithelium

### Seborrhoeic keratosis

Seborrhoeic keratosis is a common benign pigmented hyperplastic and keratotic skin lesion occurring as multiple oval brown-to-black plaques, mainly on the trunk in adults. Clinically they may be mistaken for malignant melanoma (Fig. 28.10).

### Cytological findings: seborrhoeic keratosis

- Anucleate squames with sheets of squamous and basal cells
- A wet film preparation reveals intercellular bridges which is useful in excluding a pigmented basal cell carcinoma.

### Keratoacanthoma

Keratoacanthoma develops from hair follicles and presents as a rapidly growing hard dome-shaped papule evolving to a tumour with a central horny plug, covered by a crust concealing a keratin-filled crater. It occurs on sun-exposed areas and in solitary, multiple and eruptive forms. It involutes spontaneously leaving a depressed scar. It can be difficult to differentiate between keratoacanthoma and squamous cell carcinoma on histopathological examination and even more difficult cytologically.[23]

### Cytological findings: keratoacanthoma

- Anucleate and keratinised mature squamous cells.

Reactive change and foreign body reaction to keratin may result in a worrisome cytological picture in smears from deeper parts of the lesion.

### Actinic keratosis

Actinic keratosis is very common and widely regarded as a premalignant lesion comprising abnormal keratinocyte proliferation and differentiation. It carries a low risk of progression to squamous cell carcinoma. Actinic keratosis occurs most often on sun-exposed skin of head, face and hands, predominantly in fair-skinned individuals and prevalence increases with age. It varies clinically from scaly, erythematous, sometimes confluent, patches with poorly defined borders to rough, thickened keratotic lesions, usually less than 1 cm in diameter and often multiple. The PAP stain is useful for differentiating between keratinising and non-keratinising cells (Figs 28.11–28.13).[24]

### Cytological findings: actinic keratosis

- Cellular smears
- Single cells and groups of dyskaryotic keratinocytes with uneven or 'feathery' edges
- Intercellular bridges often seen
- Polyhedral or spindle-shaped cells
- Raised nuclear/cytoplasmic ratio
- Nuclei are enlarged and may have vesicular chromatin
- Nucleoli may be seen.

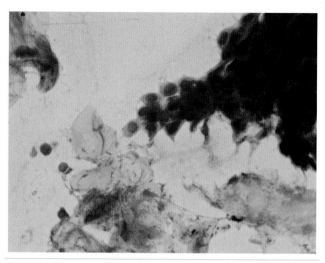

**Fig. 28.10** Seborrhoeic keratosis. Sheets of basal and squamous cells and anucleate squames. Skin scrape (PAP).

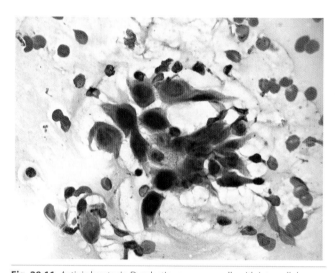

**Fig. 28.11** Actinic keratosis. Dysplastic squamous cells with intercellular bridges, enlarged nuclei. Clean background. Skin scrape (PAP).

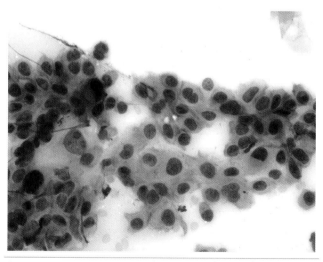

**Fig. 28.12** Actinic keratosis. Dysplastic squamous cells with enlarged nuclei with nucleoli. Same case as Figure 28.11 (MGG).

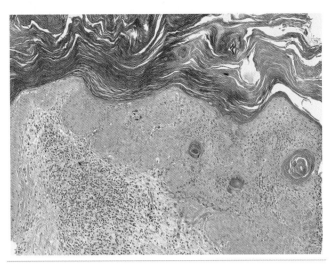

**Fig. 28.13** Actinic keratosis. Hyperkeratosis, atypical squamous cells with enlarged, hyperchromatic nuclei and a chronic inflammatory infiltrate in the upper dermis. Punch biopsy (H&S).

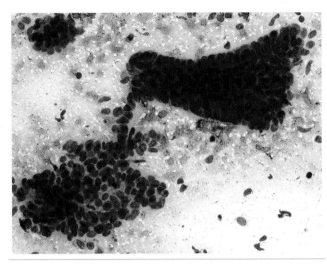

**Fig. 28.14** Basal cell carcinoma. Smooth-edged fragments and atypical basal cells with peripheral palisading. Skin scrape (MGG).

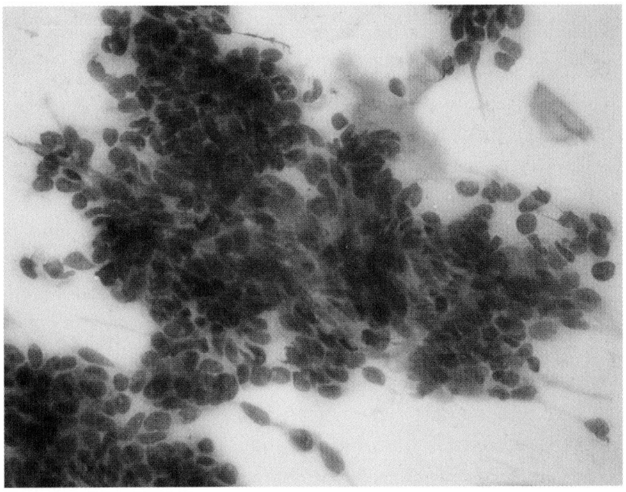

## Bowen's disease

The typical lesions of Bowen's disease (carcinoma *in situ*) are similar to actinic keratosis, although lesions are usually solitary and may occur in skin not exposed to sunlight. It often presents as an enlarging well-demarcated erythematous plaque with an irregular border covered by a scale or crust. The risk of invasive cancer is low.[25]

### Cytological findings: Bowen's disease

- Cellular smear
- Single cells or sheets of cells
- Atypical squamous cells with basophilic cytoplasm
- Atypical keratinised cells are unusual.

## Basal cell carcinoma

Basal cell carcinoma (BCC) is the most frequent of all cancers in fair-skinned populations, and occurs most often on sun-exposed areas. It is a malignant, locally aggressive epithelial tumour that very rarely metastasises. The tumour has a variable clinical appearance presenting as superficial, nodular or morphoeic types. Cytological diagnosis of either air-dried or alcohol-fixed scrapes or FNA smears is reliable if sufficient material is obtained (Figs 28.14–28.17).[24,26,27]

### Cytological findings: basal cell carcinoma

- Cellular smear
- Tightly cohesive sheets of small uniform hyperchromatic cells with scanty cytoplasm and indistinct cell borders
- Well-defined, club-like groups of atypical cells
- Focal peripheral palisading in sheets and club-like structures
- Hyperchromatic round or oval nuclei with fine granular chromatin
- Little variation in nuclear size and shape
- Scattered tumour cells seldom seen.

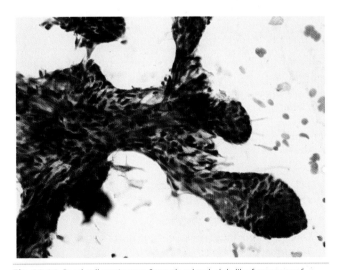

**Fig. 28.15** Basement cell carcinoma. Groups of atypical basal cells with fragments of pink-staining basal membrane matrix. Skin scrape (MGG).

**Fig. 28.16** Basal cell carcinoma. Smooth-edged, club-like fragments of atypical basal cell with peripheral palisading. Skin scrape (PAP).

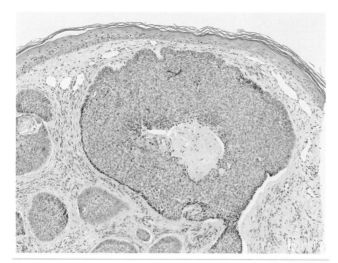

**Fig. 28.17**  Basal cell carcinoma. Sheets of atypical basal cells with peripheral palisading of the nuclei. Punch biopsy (H&S).

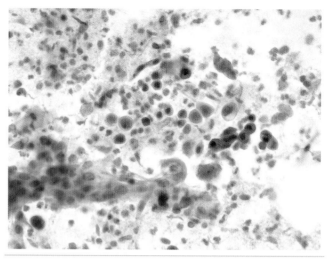

**Fig. 28.18**  Squamous cell carcinoma. Atypical keratinised cells, fragments of atypical cells with large, vesicular nuclei and bizarre ('tadpole') cells. Skin scrape (PAP).

Occasionally, fragments of pink-staining (MGG) basal membrane matrix may be seen close to the palisading edges. In some cases melanin or keratinised whorls may be observed. These findings reflect some of the subtypes of basal cell carcinoma.

### Diagnostic pitfalls: basal cell carcinoma

- Metastatic small cell carcinoma may resemble BCC. However, the atypical cells will be more dispersed and can be distinguished by the nuclear pleomorphism and chromatin pattern. Nuclear moulding is seen and probably also necrotic debris
- The basaloid cell component of pilomatrixoma may resemble BCC. However, it differs in clinical presentation and contains 'ghost' cells and multinucleate giant cells
- The basosquamous type may be difficult to differentiate from keratoacanthoma and squamous cell carcinoma
- Basaloid cells in smears from sebaceous gland tumours may be difficult to distinguish from BCC
- Merkel cell carcinoma may pose problems but has greater cellular dissociation and lacks club-like structures.

## Squamous cell carcinoma

Squamous cell carcinoma (SCC) arises from the epithelial cells of the epidermis. UV-radiation, chronic inflammatory skin changes, chemical carcinogens, immunosuppression and viral infections are associated with the development of SCC. The tumour begins as a small, slightly raised, grey or brownish lesion with irregular margins. It progresses rapidly and may present as a shallow ulcer or an exophytic tumour (Fig. 28.18).[1,28]

### Cytological findings: squamous cell carcinoma

- Single cells due to loss of cohesion
- Often highly orangeophilic cells due to abnormal keratinisation (PAP)
- Solid fragments of less differentiated tumour cells
- Bizarre cell shapes, e.g. tadpole cells

- Large irregular nuclei with nucleoli
- Polymorphs and occasional eosinophils.

The cytological findings depend on the degree of cell differentiation. Since over 80% of squamous cell carcinomas are well differentiated, keratinised cells are usually found.

### Diagnostic pitfalls: squamous cell carcinoma

- Actinic (solar) keratosis and Bowen's disease show some of the features of SCC but lack the extremes of cytoplasmic and nuclear pleomorphism typical of SCC
- Regenerative squamous epithelium at the edge of an ulcer shows hyperchromatic nuclei with nucleoli, mitoses and polymorphs. However, the squamous cells are cohesive and the nuclear/cytoplasmic ratio is low
- Scrapings from a keratoacanthoma may be difficult to differentiate from a highly differentiated SCC.

## Melanocytic naevi and malignant melanoma

### Naevi

Benign melanocytic naevi may be present at birth or may develop during the course of life. They are benign proliferations of melanocytes found in the epidermis, dermis or both. Scrape cytology is rarely performed and is not recommended because the smears are seldom diagnostic.

### Malignant melanoma

Malignant melanoma is the major cause of death from skin cancer. It arises from melanocytes and is associated with genetic susceptibility and exposure to UV-radiation.[29] About 75% are superficial spreading melanomas, while 15% are nodular. Superficial spreading melanomas are usually diffusely pigmented, indurated, irregular lesions, sometimes with nodular areas, whereas nodular melanomas are associated with more rapid growth and may ulcerate. Clinically suspicious lesions should be surgically removed with free resection margins. FNA cytology is almost exclusively used in the diagnosis of metastatic melanoma in the skin rather than in the primary diagnosis of the disease.[28,30]

### Cytological findings: malignant melanoma

- Cellular smears
- Dissociated single cells with occasional loosely cohesive groups of cells
- Cells may vary considerably in size and shape
- Variable nuclear/cytoplasmic ratio
- Hyperchromatic eccentric nuclei
- Large nucleoli (often macronucleoli), often multiple
- Atypical mitoses
- Binucleate or multinucleated cells
- Cytoplasmic pigment may be seen
- Fine cytoplasmic vacuolation
- Peripheral condensation of the cytoplasm, often well defined.

As in histology, the cytological appearance of malignant melanoma is quite variable. Some smears show large, undifferentiated cells. The nuclei may vary greatly in size and shape and may contain macronucleoli. Some have intranuclear vacuoles. Others contain spindle-shaped cells, singly and in sheets, or round cells. The amount of pigment is variable and may be in the cytoplasm or the background of the smear. Blood and/or necrotic debris may be present (Figs 28.19, 28.20).

Immunocytochemical staining with a melanoma associated antigen, such as HMB-45, confirms the diagnosis (Fig. 28.21).

## Tumours of the skin adnexae

A variety of adnexal tumours may be encountered in cytological specimens. They include those originating from hair follicles, sebaceous glands and sweat glands. Although adnexal tumours show considerable clinical and morphological overlap, a correct diagnosis can be made.[31]

## Pilomatrixoma

Pilomatrixoma (calcifying epithelioma of Malherbe) is regarded as a benign tumour arising from cells resembling those of the hair matrix, usually located to head, neck and upper extremities. It usually presents as a single, slow growing, firm tumour a few millimetres to a few centimetres in diameter in the deep dermal or subcutaneous layer of the skin. Malignancy has been described but is very rare.

Pilomatrixoma may occur at any age but appears usually in children and young adolescents, especially females.[32]

The classical cytological findings of pilomatrixoma, when present are diagnostic. However, diagnosis can be difficult and clinical data, particularly age and location, may be helpful in the interpretation of the smear (Fig. 28.22).[33]

### Cytological findings: pilomatrixoma

- Clusters of basaloid cells with small- to medium-sized, round, vesicular nuclei with distinct nucleoli and peripheral condensation of the cytoplasm, often well defined

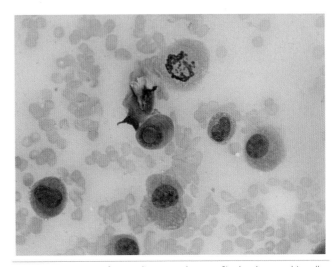

**Fig. 28.19** Metastasis from malignant melanoma. Single, pleomorphic cells with macronuclei and one cell in mitosis. FNA (MGG).

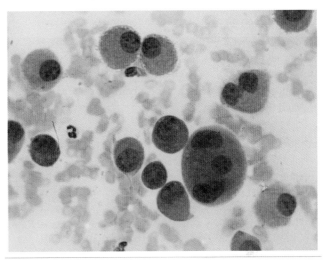

**Fig. 28.20** Metastasis from malignant melanoma. Single cells with multiple nuclei, abundant cytoplasm. FNA (MGG).

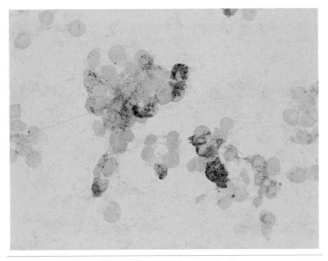

**Fig. 28.21** Metastasis from malignant melanoma. Positive immunocytochemical staining for HMB-45. FNA.

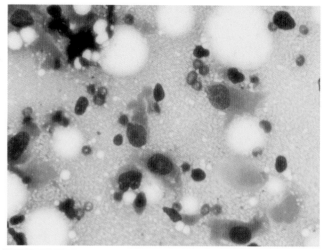

**Fig. 28.22** Pilomatrixoma. Clusters of basaloid cells and squamous cells with ghost-like nuclei from nodule in the scalp. FNA (PAP).

**Fig. 28.23** Sebaceous carcinoma. Poorly differentiated, atypical cells. Varying nuclear size. Small lipid droplets in the background. Skin metastasis from sebaceous carcinoma. FNA (MGG).

- Nuclear moulding may be present among basaloid cells
- Sheets of squamous 'ghost' cells
- Calcium deposits
- Scattered naked nuclei from basal cells
- Fibrillary pink material enveloping basaloid cells
- Multinucleated giant cells.

### Diagnostic pitfalls: pilomatrixoma

- Pilomatrixoma may be mistaken for various types of carcinoma particularly when only one or two of the classical findings are present in the smear
- Groups of basal cells in BCC show peripheral palisading. The nuclei in BCC are smaller with less prominent nucleoli. Occasionally, sparse pink fibrillary background material may be seen in BCC
- Anucleate keratinised cells are seen in well-differentiated squamous carcinoma but clearly malignant cells will also be found
- Anucleate keratinised squamous cells and multinucleated giant cells are seen in smears from epidermal cysts but groups of basaloid cells are not seen
- The nuclei in Merkel cell carcinoma have more prominent nuclear moulding and rather granular chromatin pattern.

## Sebaceous gland lesions

Sebaceous lesions include hyperplasia, adenoma and carcinoma and occur most frequently in the skin of the head and neck. The extent of the basal cell component in benign sebaceous neoplasia varies, giving rise to a number of subtypes.

### Sebaceous carcinoma

Sebaceous carcinoma is rare and its clinical presentation may be indistinguishable from several forms of non-melanoma skin cancer. It usually occurs in the ocular region and presents as an erythematous nodule or plaque.

Sebaceous carcinoma is highly aggressive with significant metastatic potential (Fig. 28.23).[1,34]

### Cytological findings: sebaceous carcinoma

- Often abundantly cellular samples with single and clustered atypical cells with foamy or vacuolated cytoplasm
- Nuclei are central, large and pleomorphic with coarse chromatin
- Variably sized but often prominent nucleoli
- Occasional atypical keratinised cells
- Mitotic figures are easily identified.

### Diagnostic pitfalls: sebaceous carcinoma

- May be confused with SCC but vacuolated or foamy cytoplasm is not a feature of keratinising SCC
- Cells from chalazion may have foamy cytoplasm, but have smaller, benign nuclei
- Some BCCs show areas of sebaceous differentiation.

## Eccrine tumours

Eccrine gland tumours comprise a large, fairly common group of appendage lesions arising from eccrine ducts and pores. There are few reports describing the cytomorphological findings of this group of tumours. FNA smears may contribute to differentiating sweat gland tumours from other adnexal neoplasms and malignant from benign tumours.[35]

## Primary mucinous carcinoma of the skin

Primary mucinous carcinoma of the skin is a rare neoplasm of sweat gland origin usually occurring on the scalp and eyelids. Smears contain loosely cohesive groups of atypical epithelial cells and abundant extracellular mucinous material. Tumours cells are small and monotonous in appearance with round or oval nuclei. It may not be possible to exclude metastatic mucinous carcinoma.[36]

## Cutaneous lymphomas

The usefulness of cytology in the diagnosis and classification of lymphomas is controversial. However, recent classification systems place more emphasis on cell morphology, thus more readily accommodating cytology.[37,38] Primary cutaneous lymphomas are a heterogeneous group of diseases comprising clonal accumulations of lymphocytes originating in the skin. Cutaneous lymphoma should always be considered in the presence of atypical lymphoid cells in smears from skin lesions. Diagnosis is based on the clinical and histological findings in addition to immunophenotyping and genotyping of the neoplastic lymphocytes.

Apart from primary cutaneous lymphomas, systemic non-Hodgkin lymphomas may also involve the skin.

## Mycosis fungoides

Mycosis fungoides (MF) is the most common variant of cutaneous T-cell lymphoma.[39] Skin lesions of MF may have a chronic, variable and often slowly progressive course with erythematous patches, plaques and/or accompanied by pruritus. The disease can, in advanced stages, involve the peripheral nodes and further extracutaneous sites. FNA in conjunction with immunophenotyping and PCR has been found to be useful in evaluation of lymphadenopathy in patients with MF (Fig. 28.24).[40]

### Cytological findings: mycosis fungoides

- Atypical lymphocytes with enlarged hyperchromatic nuclei and irregular cerebriform nuclear contours
- The degree of nuclear folding relates to the stage of the disease
- Eosinophils may been seen
- Fragile atypical nuclei are often subject to smearing artefacts resulting in thread-like tails of nuclear material.

## CD30 positive lymphoproliferative conditions of the skin

Atypical, CD30 positive lymphoid cells can be seen in a number of conditions ranging from lymphomatoid papulosis, which is usually benign, to anaplastic large cell lymphoma (ALCL). Definitive diagnosis is usually not possible but a CD30 lymphoproliferative condition may be suggested if the clinical history and additional tests are in agreement (Fig. 28.25).[41]

## Soft tissue lesions affecting the skin and subcutis

## Dermatofibroma

Dermatofibroma is a benign, relatively common lesion often occurring after microtrauma to skin and most often appearing on the extremities. It usually presents as an asymptomatic, solitary, firm, grey-red-brown, small nodule in the mid-dermis extending into the upper subcutaneous fatty tissue. Cytology is rarely performed and smears are generally quite paucicellular.

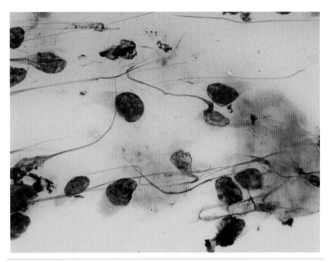

**Fig. 28.24** Mycosis fungoides. Atypical lymphoid cells with enlarged, cerebriform nuclei between anucleate squamous cells. Note fragile nuclei with smearing artefacts. Skin scrape (MGG).

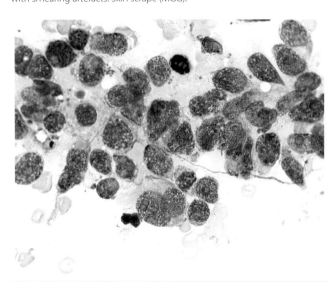

**Fig. 28.25** Anaplastic large cell lymphoma, cutaneous type. Large anaplastic cells with pleomorphic nucleus. Some multinucleated cells may also present, resembling Reed-Sternberg cells. Reactive neutrophils and macrophages infiltrate the lymphomatous lesion. Unlike systemic CD30+ ALCL, the expression of the ALK protein is not found in primary cutaneous tumours. Skin FNA.

## Dermatofibrosarcoma protuberans

Dermatofibrosarcoma protuberans (DFSP) is a nodular cutaneous mesenchymal tumour that is locally aggressive but rarely metastasises. It most often appears on the trunk and presents initially as a plaque in which multiple broad based, blue-red, painless nodules develop. Diagnosis may be difficult on cytological smears, as it shares some features with other spindle cell lesions occurring in the skin and soft tissue. Tumour cells in DFSP have been shown to be positive for CD34.[42]

## Kaposi sarcoma

Kaposi sarcoma has an aetiological linkage with human herpes virus 8 and is more often evident in immunosuppressed patients. It is a multifocal neoplastic proliferation of capillaries and

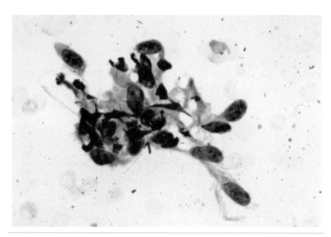

**Fig. 28.26** Kaposi sarcoma. Loosely cohesive clusters of bland spindle cells with cytoplasmic vacuoles and fusiform nuclei. Skin FNA (MGG).

perivascular connective tissue cells of the skin, mucous membranes and internal organs. The diagnosis can be made by FNA of skin lesions or lymph nodes (Fig. 28.26 and see Ch. 16).[43]

### Cytological findings: Kaposi sarcoma

- Loosely cohesive clusters of bland spindle cells arranged radially
- Fusiform nuclei sometimes with nuclear crush artefacts
- Red blood cells.

## Other conditions

### Merkel cell carcinoma

Merkel cell carcinoma (MCC) is an aggressive neuroendocrine carcinoma of the skin. It usually appears as an asymptomatic, flesh-coloured or bluish-red nodule, often on sun-exposed areas in fair-skinned individuals; most often face, head or neck. Patients are usually over 50. MCC tends to grow rapidly, metastasise early and is associated with immunosuppression.[44] Recently, a new virus called Merkel cell polyomavirus (MCV or MCPyV) has been demonstrated in MCC tumours.[45]

Cytologically, the overall impression is that of a poorly differentiated small blue cell neoplasm resembling metastasis from a small cell carcinoma, lymphoma or BCC. Air-dried smears should be prepared for immunocytochemistry. Positive staining for cytokeratins and neuroendocrine markers is seen in MCC.[46] Although not diagnostic of MCC, it has been shown that, in the absence of specific molecular markers, detection of trisomy 6 and/or trisomy 8 could help in identifying this tumour (Figs 28.27, 28.28).[47]

### Cytological findings: Merkel cell carcinoma

- Cellular smears usually composed of small atypical non-cohesive cells
- Small clusters forming rosette-like structures may also be seen
- Fragile cells often resulting in crush artefact
- Numerous apoptotic bodies and occasional mitotic figures
- Nuclei relatively uniform in size, round or oval with minimal nuclear irregularities
- Nuclear chromatin finely dispersed, with an occasional visible nucleolus

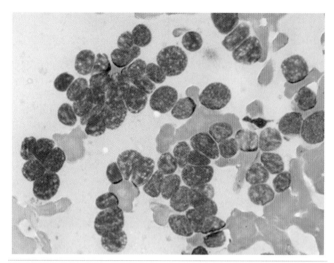

**Fig. 28.27** The overall impression is that of a poorly differentiated small blue cell neoplasm resembling metastasis from a small cell carcinoma, lymphoma or BCC (MGG).

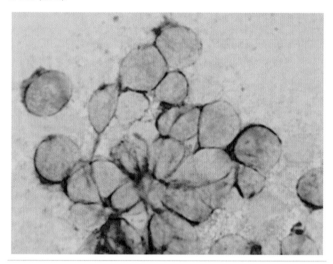

**Fig. 28.28** Merkel cell carcinoma stains positively with neuroendocrine markers and cytokeratins, as shown here, distinguishing it from lymphoma (CD56).

- Lack of discernible cytoplasm (rare cells may show eccentric dense cytoplasm with a hyaline appearance indenting the nucleus, particularly evident in MGG staining)
- Cell-to-cell moulding and nuclear moulding
- Necrotic dirty background with occasional tingible body macrophages.

### Diagnostic pitfalls: Merkel cell carcinoma

- BCC may be difficult to differentiate from MCC. BCC shows less cell dissociation and has club-like epithelial structures
- MCC may resemble small cell carcinoma. However, rosette-like structures are not usually a feature of small cell carcinoma.

### Paget's disease of the nipple

Paget's disease of the breast nipple is an eczematous skin change of the nipple-areola complex often associated with an underlying *in situ* or invasive ductal carcinoma of the breast. The crust should be scraped off and imprint cytology made of the surface

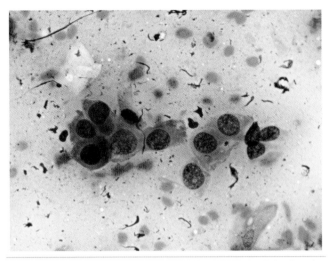

**Fig. 28.29** Paget's disease of the nipple. Large, atypical epithelial cells and proteinaceous background material. Imprint cytology (MGG).

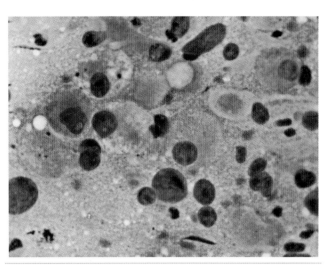

**Fig. 28.31** Plasmacytoma. Atypical plasma cells in a necrotic background from a tumour in skin and underlying tissue. FNA (MGG).

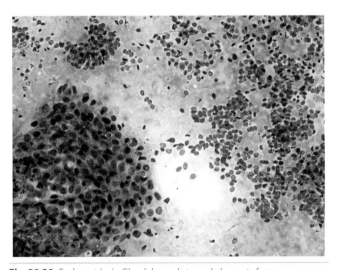

**Fig. 28.30** Endometriosis. Glandular and stromal elements from endometriosis in the skin of the abdomen. FNA (MGG).

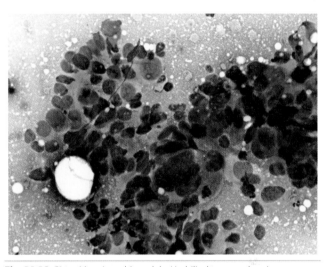

**Fig. 28.32** Sister Mary Joseph's nodule. Umbilical tumour showing metastasis from gastric adenocarcinoma. FNA (MGG).

beneath. Alcohol-fixed and air-dried smears may be prepared for staining with Papanicolaou or MGG (Fig. 28.29).[48]

### Cytological findings: Paget's disease of the nipple

- Large malignant cells with irregular nuclei and prominent nucleoli are seen in a proteinaceous background.

### Diagnostic pitfalls: Paget's disease of the nipple

- Bowen's disease and melanoma of the nipple are rare and the cytological appearances of these two lesions are described elsewhere
- Imprints from true eczema of the nipple reveal reactive epithelial cells and inflammatory cells.

## Endometriosis

Endometriosis may occur in skin, sometimes near an incisional scar on the abdominal wall. Typically, smears show groups of glandular and stromal cells accompanied by some inflammatory cells and haemosiderin-laden macrophages (Fig. 28.30).[49]

## Metastatic tumours

Cutaneous metastases from tumours of internal organs do occur; although they are relatively infrequent. Cancer arising in the breast, stomach, uterus, lung, kidney and prostate are among the most common. Occasionally plasmacytoma may occur as a solitary tumour (Fig. 28.31). Clinical history and immunocytochemistry contribute to making a more precise diagnosis in a number of cases.

Occasionally, skin metastases are the first sign of malignancy. The famous Sister Mary Joseph's nodule is a metastasis to the umbilical area from an intraabdominal tumour usually arising in the endometrium, ovary, gastrointestinal tract or prostate (Fig. 28.32).[50]

## The role of skin cytology in clinical management

Cytology may be used as a diagnostic tool in a wide range of dermatological conditions. It enables rapid diagnosis at low cost and swift referral of the patient for appropriate treatment. The procedures are well tolerated by the patient and complications are rare. In addition to its role in the diagnosis of disease, cytology is useful in monitoring disease progress and detecting relapse.

In many cases, a specific diagnosis can be given and treatment can be initiated. Special tests including immunocytochemistry and PCR further contribute to the diagnostic potential of skin cytology. In developing countries clinical information supported by cytodiagnosis is valuable in the investigation of various infectious diseases. Furthermore, cytology can provide highly reliable information concerning a variety of skin tumours in situations where biopsy is to be avoided.

Cytological sampling techniques result in minimal tissue injury compared with biopsy. With the increasing use of new, non-invasive topical treatment modalities for non-melanoma skin cancer cytology may become the diagnostic method of choice.

A comprehensive knowledge of the cytological features of primary skin neoplasms is particularly important in establishing the precise origin of a skin tumour and to distinguish it from metastasis from another site. Close cooperation between dermatologist and cytopathologist is essential to ensure a correct diagnosis and to exploit fully the potential of dermatological cytology.

## REFERENCES

1. Layfield LJ, Glasgow BJ. Aspiration biopsy cytology of primary cutaneous tumours. Acta Cytol 1993;37:679–88.

2. Barr RJ. Cutaneous cytology. Dermatology 1984;10:163–79.

3. Tzanck A. Le cytodiagnostic immédiat en dermatologie. Ann de Dermat et Syph 1948;8:205–18.

4. Gordon LA, Orell SR. Evaluation of cytodiagnosis of cutaneous basal cell carcinoma. J Am Acad Dermatol 1984;11:1082–86.

5. Bindu B, Kurien A, Shenoi SD, et al. Role of slit skin smear examination in cutaneous T-cell lymphomas and other chronic dermatoses. Dermatol Online J 2006;12:22.

6. Tamiolakis D, Proimos E, Skoulakis CE, et al. Brushing cytology in cutaneous lesions of the head and neck. J Laryngol Otol 2007;121:676–79.

7. Koss LG. Aspiration biopsy: a tool in surgical pathology. Am J Surg Pathol 1988;12:43–53.

8. Bofin AM, Ytterhus B, Martin C, et al. Detection and quantitation of her2 gene amplification and protein expression in breast carcinoma. Am J Clin Pathol 2004;122:110–19.

9. Moschelle SL. An update on the diagnosis and treatment of leprosy. J Am Acad Dermatol 2004;51:417–26.

10. Jaswal TS, Jain VK, Jain V, et al. Evaluation of leprosy lesions by skin smear cytology in comparison to histopathology. Indian J Pathol Microbiol 2001;44:277–81.

11. Singh N, Manucha V, Bhattacharya SN, et al. Pitfalls in the Cytological Classification of Borderline Leprosy in the Ridley-Jopling Scale. Diagn Cytopathol 2004;30:386–88.

12. Bhambhani S, Das DK, Luthra UK. Fine needle aspiration cytology in the diagnosis of sinuses and ulcers of the body surface (skin and tongue). Acta Cytol 1991;35:320–24.

13. Quirós E, Bettinardi A, Quirós A, et al. Detection of mycobacterial DNA in papuolonecrotic tuberculid lesions by polymerase chain reaction. J Clin Lab Anal 2000;14:133–35.

14. Faulde M, Schrader J, Hayl G, et al. Zoonotic cutaneous leishmaniasis outbreak in Mazar-e Sharif, Northern Afghanistan: An epidemiological evaluation. Int J Med Microbiol 2008;298:543–50.

15. Mashhood AA, Khan IM, Nasir S, et al. Fine needle aspiration cytology versus histopathology in the diagnosis of cutaneous leishmaniasis in Pakistan. J Coll Physicians Surg Pak 2005;15:71–73.

16. Tareen I, Qazi A, Kasi PM. Fine-needle aspiration cytology in the diagnosis of cutaneous leishmaniasis. Ann Saud Med 2004;24:93–97.

17. Barboza-Quintata O, Garza-Guajardo R, Assad-Morel C, et al. Pseudomycetoma for microsporum canis: report of a case diagnosed by fine needle aspiration biopsy. Acta Cytol 2007;51:424–28.

18. Deshpande AH, Agarwal S, Kelkar AA. Primary cutaneous rhinosporidiosis diagnosed on FNAC: a case report with review of literature. Diagn Cytopathol 2009;37:125–27.

19. Ozcan A, Senol M, Saglam H, et al. Comparison of the Tzanck test and polymerase chain reaction in the diagnosis of cutaneous herpes simplex and varicella zoster virus infections. Int J Derm 2007;47:1177–79.

20. Jain S, Das DK, Malhotra V, et al. Molluscum contagiosum. A case report with fine needle aspiration cytologic diagnosis and ultrastructural features. Acta Cytol 2000;44:63–66.

21. Dong H, Duncan LD. Cytologic findings in Demodex folliculitis: a case report and review of the literature. Diagn Cytopathol 2006;34:232–34.

22. Aithal V, Kini U, Jayaseelan E. Role of direct immunofluorescence on Tzanck smears in Pemphigus Vulgaris. Diagn Cytopathol 2007;35:403–7.

23. Cribier B, Asch PH, Grosshans E. Differentiating squamous cell carcinoma from keratoacanthoma using histopathological criteria is it possible? A study of 296 cases. Dermatology 1999;199:208–12.

24. Christensen E, Bofin A, Gudmundsdóttir I, et al. Cytological diagnosis of basal cell carcinoma and actinic keratosis, using Papanicolaou and May-Grünwald-Giemsa stained cutaneous tissue smear. Cytopathology 2008;19:316–32.

25. Cox NH, Eedy DJ, Morton CA. Therapy guidelines and audit subcommittee, British Association of Dermatologists guidelines for management of Bowen's disease: 2006 update. Br J Dermatol 2007;156:11–21.

26. García-Solano J, Garíía-Rojo B, Sánchez-Sánchez C, et al. Basal-cell carcinoma: cytologic and immunocytochemical findings in fine-needle aspirates. Diagn Cytopathol 1998;18:403–8.

27. Bakis S, Irwig L, Wood G, et al. Exfoliative cytology as a diagnostic test for basal cell carcinoma: a meta-analysis. Br J Dermatol 2004;150:829–36.

28. Vega-Memije E, De Larios NM, Waxtein LM, et al. Cytodiagnosis of cutaneous basal and squamous cell carcinoma. Int J Dermatol 2000;39:116–20.

29. Hussein MR. Ultraviolet radiation and skin cancer: molecular mechanisms. J Cutan Pathol 2005;32:191–205.

30. Perry MD, Gore M, Seigler HF, et al. Fine needle aspiration biopsy of metastatic melanoma. A morphologic analysis of 174 cases. Acta Cytol 1986;30:385–96.

31. Rege J, Shet T. Aspiration cytology in the diagnosis of primary tumors of skin adnexa. Acta Cytol 2001;45:715–22.

32. Lemos LB, Brauchle RW. Pilomatrixoma: a diagnostic pitfall in fine needle aspiration biopsies. A review from a small country hospital. Ann Diagn Pathol 2004;8:130–36.

33. Singh S, Gupta R, Mandal AK. Pilomatrixoma: a potential diagnostic pitfall in aspiration cytology. Cytopathology 2007;18:260–62.

34. Stern RC, Liu K, Dodd LG. Cytomorphologic features of sebaceous carcinoma of fine-needle aspiration. Acta Cytol 2000;44:760–64.

35. Gangane N, Joshi D, Sharma SM. Cytomorphological diagnosis of malignant eccrine tumours: report of two cases. Diagn Cytopathol 2008;36(Nov):801–4.

36. Reid-Nicholson M, Iyengar P, Friedlander MA, et al. Fine needle aspiration biopsy of primary mucinous carcinoma of the skin. Acta Cytol 2006;50:317–22.

37. Hehn ST, Grogan TM, Miller TP. Utility of fine-needle aspiration as a diagnostic technique in lymphoma. J Clin Oncol 2004;22:3046–52.

38. Wakely PE. Fine-needle aspiration cytopathology in diagnosis and classification of malignant lymphoma: accurate and reliable? Diagn Cytopathol 1999;22:120–25.

39. Olsen E, Vonderheid E, Pimpinelli N, et al. Revisions to the staging and classification of mycosis fungoides and Sézary syndrome: a proposal of the International Society for Cutaneous Lymphomas (ISCL) and the cutaneous lymphoma task force of

the European Organization of Research and Treatment of Cancer (EORTC). Blood 2007;110:1713–22.

40. Pai RK, Mullins FM, Kim YH, et al. Cytologic evaluation of lymphadenopathy associated with mycosis fungoides and Sézary syndrome: role of immunophenotypic and molecular ancillary studies. Cancer 2008;114:323–32.

41. Kempf W, Kutzner H, Cozzio A, et al. MUM1 expression in cutaneous CD30+ lymphoproliferative disorders: a valuable tool for the distinction between lymphomatoid papulosis and primary cutaneous anaplastic large-cell lymphoma. Br J Dermatol 2008;158:1280–87.

42. Domanski HA. FNA diagnosis of dermatofibrosarcoma protuberans. Diagn Cytopathol 2005;32:299–302.

43. Gamborino E, Carrilho C, Ferro J, et al. Fine-needle aspiration diagnosis of Kaposi's sarcoma in a developing country. Diagn Cytopathol 2000;23:322–25.

44. Becker JC, Schrama D, Houben R. Merkel cell carcinoma. Cell Mol Life Sci 2009;66:1–8.

45. Feng H, Shuda M, Chang Y, et al. Clonal integration of polyomavirus in human Merkel cell carcinoma. Science 2008;319:1096–100.

46. Soloman RK, Lundeen SJ, Hamlar DD, et al. Fine-needle aspiration of unusual neoplasms of the scalp in HIV-infected patients: a report of two cases and review of the literature. Diagn Cytopathol 2001;24:186–92.

47. Suciu V, Botan E, Valant A, et al. The potential contribution of fluorescent in situ hybridization analysis to the cytopathological diagnosis of Merkel cell carcinoma. Cytopathol 2008;19:48–51.

48. Gupta RK, Simpson J, Dowle C. The role of cytology in the diagnosis of Paget's disease of the nipple. Pathology 1996;28:248–50.

49. Pathan SK, Kapila K, Haji BE, et al. Cytomorphological spectrum in scar endometriosis: a study of eight cases. Cytopathology 2005;16:94–99.

50. Handa U, Garg S, Mohan H. Fine-needle aspiration cytology of Sister Mary Joseph's (paraumbilical) nodules. Diagn Cytopathol 2008;36:348–50.

# Soft tissue and musculoskeletal system

Henryk A. Domanski, Måns Åkerman and Jan Silverman

## Chapter contents

## Introduction

There are two main indications for fine needle aspiration (FNA) of soft tissue and bone lesions: the diagnosis before the definitive treatment and the investigation of lesions clinically suspicious of tumour recurrence or metastasis. The use of FNA to verify a recurrent tumour or a metastasis has never been controversial. However, the use of FNA and cytodiagnosis as the diagnostic method, obviating open biopsy, before definitive treatment of soft tissue and bone tumours, has been intensively debated and called in question. However, at present, the use of FNA as the diagnostic pre-treatment method for musculoskeletal tumours is accepted in many orthopaedic tumour centres, provided that certain requirements are fulfilled and that the final cytological diagnosis is based on the combined evaluation of clinical data, radiographic findings and cytomorphology.

One important reason why FNA might replace open surgical biopsy in the pre-treatment diagnosis, apart from the usual

advantages with FNA as a diagnostic method, is the nature of the main treatment of soft tissue tumours. Primary radical surgery is the treatment of choice for the majority of such tumours in many orthopaedic tumour centres. When this is the case, the type of surgical procedure depends more on the site of the tumour (cutaneous, subcutaneous, intra- or intermuscular), the tumour size and the relationship of the tumour to fasciae, blood vessels, nerve bundles and periosteum, than on its histological subtype. Thus the most important preoperative information for the orthopaedic surgeon is whether the lesion is a true soft tissue tumour, either benign or malignant. The histotype of a sarcoma is of secondary importance. However, paradoxically in cases of benign soft tissue tumours, the cytopathologist must be able to differentiate correctly between benign lipomatous tumours, nerve sheath tumours, the so-called pseudosarcomas and fibrous tumours such as desmoid fibromatosis. Not all benign soft tissue tumours are primarily surgically removed. For example, expectancy and clinical follow-up is often suggested to patients with nodular fasciitis or pseudomalignant myositis ossificans as these tumours often spontaneously regress or totally disappear after some weeks. Extra-abdominal desmoid fibromatosis, although a non-metastasising tumour, may be locally invasive and destructive or may spontaneously cease to enlarge or may be favourably treated with interferon. In many cases these tumours are not primarily surgically removed but followed-up clinically. In these cases a correct diagnosis is mandatory.

On the other hand, when the optimal treatment is considered to be neoadjuvant therapy (radiotherapy or chemotherapy) followed by surgery, the FNA diagnosis must equal that of a histopathological examination with regard to histotype and the malignancy grade. At present, this is the case with small round-cell sarcomas such as rhabdomyosarcoma, neuroblastoma and Ewing family of tumours, but variably so in synovial sarcoma and in large high-grade malignant intramuscular sarcoma.

With bone lesions, FNA may also replace open biopsy in the primary diagnosis. It is the task of the cytopathologist to distinguish benign and malignant primary bone tumours from metastatic deposits and from the range of benign reactive and inflammatory conditions of bone. Furthermore, the cytopathologist must give a confident type-diagnosis of the various benign bone tumours and sarcomas if open biopsy is to be avoided.[1–10]

## Technical procedures

### Soft tissue

FNA of soft tissue tumours is performed in the same way as for epithelial tumours. It is usually not necessary to use a local anaesthetic. A syringe holder, 10 mL syringe and needles of varying lengths are recommended. Needles wider than 22 gauge are seldom needed. For deep-seated intramuscular or intermuscular tumours, a needle with a stylet is preferable to avoid sampling subcutaneous fat and other tissue surrounding the tumour.

All passes with the needle should go through the same site in the skin but the direction of the needle should be changed with each pass to cover different parts of the tumour. In most cases, it is not necessary to make more than five passes.

As a general rule, the orthopaedic surgeon ought to decide the site of the insertion point, but if this is not possible, the vertex of the tumour is the best choice. Tattooing of the skin area at the insertion point is valuable if the surgeon wishes to include the needle tract in the surgical specimen. Core needle biopsy for immunohistochemistry can also be taken.

## Bone

Skeletal aspirations do not differ from other FNAs, but it is important to remember that it is not possible to penetrate intact cortical bone with thin needles. However, partly destroyed or eroded bone can usually be penetrated quite easily with a 22-gauge needle. If the cortical bone is almost intact, an 18-gauge needle can be used, through which a 23-gauge needle may be inserted into the lesion and multiple aspirations performed. In this case, local anaesthetic must be used before aspiration.

Many malignant bone tumours have palpable soft tissue involvement and are aspirated with the aid of the palpatory findings. As a general rule, it is strongly recommended that the cytopathologist is familiar with the radiological findings, eventually discusses the best approach to the tumour with the radiologist and that aspirations of impalpable lesions are guided by the use of imaging techniques. Fluoroscopy and computerised tomographic (CT) scanning may be used. With CT scanning, it is possible to select specific small areas within the lesion for sampling.

## Staining methods

Alcohol-fixed and air-dried smears should be prepared from soft tissue and bone lesions, staining by Papanicolaou or haematoxylin and eosin (H&E) and by May–Grünwald Giemsa (MGG), respectively. For rapid evaluation of air-dried smears, Diff-Quik staining is recommended.

MGG staining is superior for evaluation of cytoplasmic details and background matrix while the wet-fixed staining methods are the best choice in the evaluation of nuclear structures.

## Ancillary methods in the diagnosis of soft tissue and bone tumours

Fine needle aspirates, when cellular and technically satisfactory, provide suitable material for use of specialised techniques to assist in the diagnosis. Essentially the same techniques used for histopathological diagnosis are applicable on fine needle aspirates. Many centres use cell blocks or core needle biopsies for ancillary techniques (see Ch. 34).

## Electron microscopy

Electron microscopic (EM) examination of fine needle aspirates was the first ancillary diagnostic method applied. At present EM has been largely replaced by immunocytochemistry and molecular genetic analyses but it is still an important adjunct for selected diagnoses such as the demonstration of Birbeck granules in Langerhans' cell histiocytosis.

## DNA-ploidy analysis

Flow cytometry and static cytometry have been applied to fine needle aspirates with regard to analysis of ploidy status and proliferation. Despite numerous investigations, however, analysis of tumour cell DNA has not proved to be of major help in diagnosis or prognosis of soft tissue tumours. In the FNA diagnosis of bone tumours, however, DNA ploidy analysis is, in our experience, helpful in the diagnosis of high-grade chondrosarcoma and osteosarcoma.

## Immunocytochemistry

Immunocytochemistry is at present the most common ancillary method used. When aspirates are used for immunocytochemistry, different preparation methods have been tried and used (Table 29.1).

## Cytogenetics

Cytogenetics, especially molecular genetic techniques such as RT-PCR and FISH have during recent years been important diagnostic aids. FNA preparations are suitable for both these techniques. The diagnostic use of the ancillary techniques listed above is given when the various tumours are suspected.

**Table 29.1** Different preparation methods of fine needle aspirates for immunocytochemistry. Advantages and disadvantages

| Preparation method | Advantages | Disadvantages |
|---|---|---|
| Direct smear | No preparation | Stripped nuclei and cytoplasmic background make evaluation of cytoplasmic antibodies difficult. No problem with nuclear antibodies |
| Cytospin preparation | For many years the most common method for immunocytochemistry | False negative results may happen when the expression of antibodies is focal |
| Cell block preparation | A cell block preparation is to compare with a histological 'mini-biopsy'. Easy to compare results with IC on histological samples and to perform controls | At times difficult to aspirate sufficient material for preparation |
| Liquid based cytology (ThinPrep) | Monolayer of cells. 'Clean' background. Material can be saved | All antibodies not yet tested and evaluated |

## Complications of FNA of soft tissue and bone tumours

In our experience of FNA over more than 30 years in the primary diagnosis of soft tissue and bone tumours we have never recorded any severe complications. Patients have complained of tenderness, and in case of subcutaneous tumours, of small haemorrhages. We have not experienced cases of infection or severe haemorrhage. At the Musculoskeletal Tumour Centre, Lund University Hospital, the orthopaedic surgeons always ask for the tattooing of the needle insertion point in the case of a clinically suspected sarcoma. The needle insertion area is always part of the surgical specimen and investigated histologically; we have never experienced microscopic evidence of sarcoma cell seeding.

## Cytological findings in normal and reactive soft tissues

### Cytological findings: normal soft tissues

#### Fibrous tissue
Normal fibroblasts are spindle-shaped cells with slender contours. Cytoplasmic borders may be indistinct but unipolar or bipolar processes can usually be seen. The nuclei are ovoid, rounded or elongated with regular chromatin distribution and small or absent nucleoli. Stripped nuclei are a common finding. Fibroblasts are seen either dispersed or in groups or runs of loosely cohesive cells (Fig. 29.1).

#### Adipose tissue
Normal adipose tissue cells are found in fragments or clusters in smears showing large fat cells with abundant univacuolated cytoplasm and small dark regular nuclei. In the larger fragments a discrete network of slender capillaries may be observed. Dissociated fat cells are quite uncommon. The larger fragments resemble adipose tissue in histological sections and look like microbiopsies (Fig. 29.2).

#### Striated muscle
Fragments of muscle fibres are pink or amphophilic on Papanicolaou staining, eosinophilic with H&E and deep blue in MGG-stained preparations. The peripherally placed nuclei are small, rounded and dark (Fig. 29.3). Cross-striations may be observed.

### Cytological findings: reactive soft tissues

#### Fibroblasts
Reactive fibroblasts/myofibroblasts show wide variation in size and shape irrespective of the aetiology. The cells became fusiform, rounded or triangular, with abundant cytoplasm, which may display one or several processes or angulated cytoplasmic extensions. The nuclei vary in size and take on rounded, ovoid, spindly or irregular contours. The chromatin is often irregularly distributed and nucleoli may be prominent. Binucleated cells are common (Fig. 29.4). Typical examples of reactive fibroblasts/myofibroblasts are present in smears from posttraumatic states and in the benign pseudosarcomatous soft tissue lesions.

#### Fat
Reactive adipose tissue fragments may show a myxoid background and the capillary network is often more prominent. The fragments are more cellular than normal

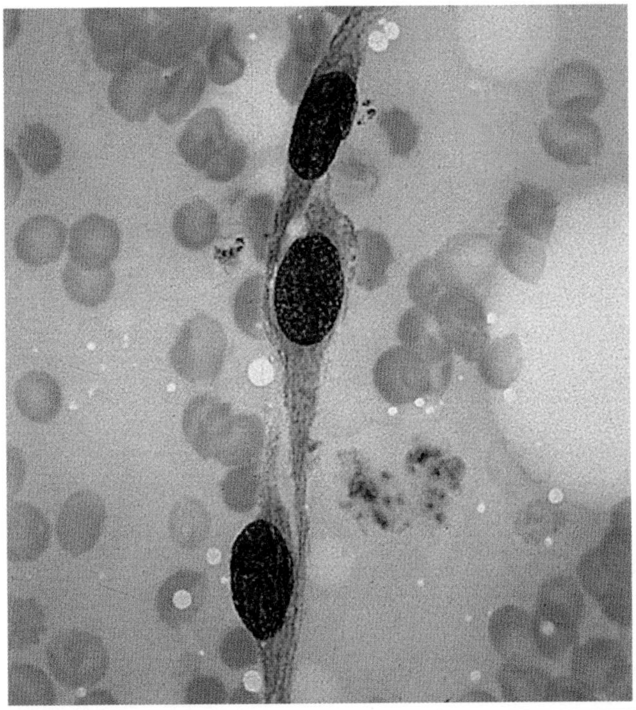

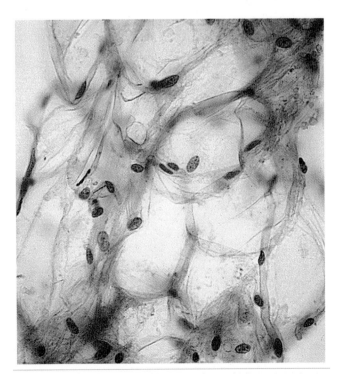

**Fig. 29.1** Fibroblasts. Spindle-shaped cells with ovoid uniform nuclei and cytoplasmic processes (MGG).

**Fig. 29.2** Adipose tissue. Part of a fragment of normal adipose tissue. Large univacuolated fat cells with small regular nuclei (H&E).

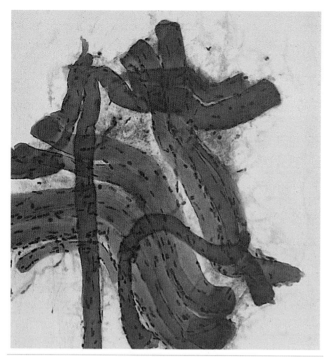

**Fig. 29.3** Striated muscle. A group of striated muscle fibres. The fibres have eosinophilic faintly striated cytoplasm and small rounded dark uniform nuclei. Cross-striation is not evident in this group (H&E).

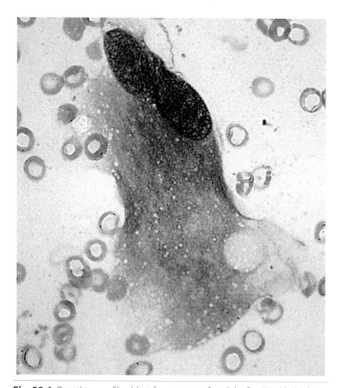

**Fig. 29.4** Reactive myofibroblast from a case of nodular fasciitis. Marked reactive changes showing binucleation, prominent nucleoli and abundant cytoplasm (MGG).

due to reactive increase in fibroblasts, endothelial cells and sometimes also due to the presence of histiocytes. Adipocytes may show a multivacuolated cytoplasm. Between the fragments histiocytes with vacuolated or foamy cytoplasm are observed (Fig. 29.5). Reactive adipose tissue is found in

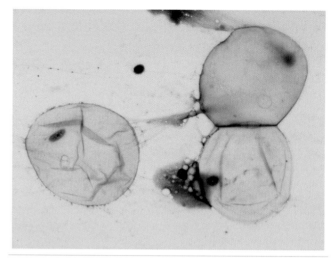

**Fig. 29.5** Reactive adipose tissue. Histiocyte with vacuolated cytoplasm close to normal fat cells (H&E).

posttraumatic states and in adipose tissue surrounding non-adipose tumours.

### Striated muscle

The principal reactive changes observed in striated muscle are regenerative in origin. Regenerating striated muscle fibres usually appear as large multinucleated cells with varying shapes including spindly, rounded and straplike forms. They are known as 'muscle giant cells.' The dense cytoplasm is deeply eosinophilic on H&E or Papanicolaou (PAP) staining and dark blue on MGG. The multiple nuclei are rounded or ovoid in shape, and often arranged in rows or eccentrically placed. Nucleoli may be large and prominent. Occasionally regenerating muscle fibres appear as tadpole-like cells with large eccentrically placed nuclei with prominent nucleoli (Fig. 29.6). Regenerating muscle fibres are seen in aspirates from tumours and lesions infiltrating striated muscle. Typical examples are fibromatosis colli and desmoid fibromatosis.

## Cytological findings in normal and reactive bone

## Cytology of the normal bone

### Osteoblasts

Osteoblasts are most often seen as single cells but small clusters or rows are also encountered. They are uniform cells of rounded or triangular shape, with abundant cytoplasm, which contains a characteristic clear area or 'Hof' adjacent to the nucleus or midway in the cytoplasm. The nuclei are round with a central nucleolus and are situated very close to the cytoplasmic membrane, almost protruding through it (Fig. 29.7).

### Osteoclasts

Osteoclasts appear as scattered single large cells with abundant cytoplasm and multiple uniform rounded nuclei arranged closely together. In MGG-stained smears, a characteristic cytoplasmic red granulation is seen (Fig. 29.8).

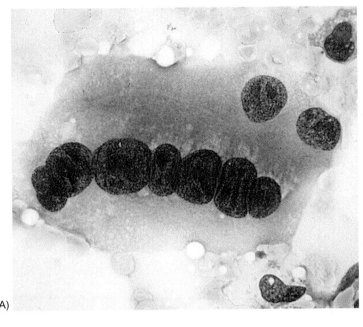

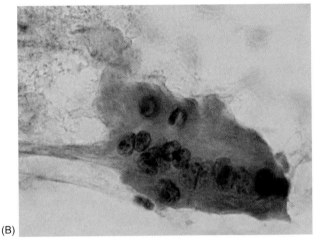

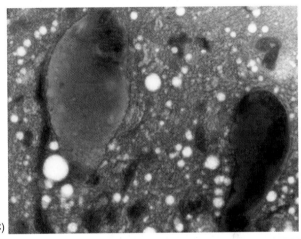

**Fig. 29.6** Regenerating muscle fibres. (A) A 'muscle giant cell' with dense blue cytoplasm and multiple rounded nuclei in a row. Note prominent nucleoli (MGG). (B) In wet-fixed smears, the cytoplasm is deeply eosinophilic (H&E). (C) Uninucleated regenerating muscle fibres may appear as tadpole-like cells with eccentric nuclei (H&E).

## Chondrocytes

Normal chondrocytes are almost never seen as dissociated cells, but may be observed in lacunae in cartilaginous fragments. These are composed of a hyaline matrix, which is reddish-blue to violet with MGG, or pink with H&E staining. In Papanicolaou-stained preparations the matrix has a pale greyish red amphophilic fibrillary appearance (Fig. 29.9).

## Bone marrow cells

Bone marrow is not an uncommon finding in aspirates from ribs, vertebrae and sacrum and it is important not to mistake the immature cells and megakaryocytes for malignant cells. A mixture of erythropoietic and myelopoietic cells and megakaryocytes

is characteristic. The bone marrow cells are best visualised with MGG stain.

## Mesothelial cells

Occasionally aspirates from vertebral lesions include small flat sheets of pavemented mesothelial cells. It is important not to diagnose reactive mesothelial cells for carcinoma cells in cases where FNA is performed for suspected vertebral metastases.

## Cytological findings in reactive changes

Reactive changes in bone aspirates are seen only in osteoblasts and are found in smears from lesions such as fracture callus,

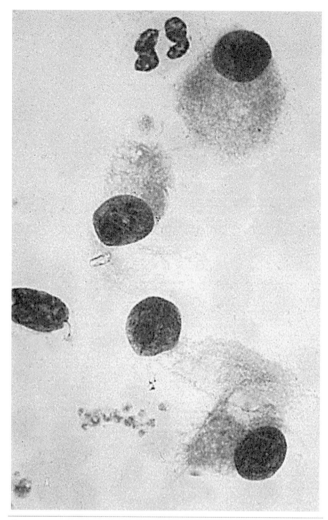

**Fig. 29.7** Osteoblasts. The typical osteoblast is rounded or triangular with a round eccentrically placed nucleus and a perinuclear clear 'Hof' (MGG).

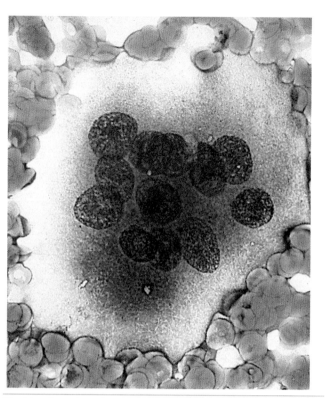

**Fig. 29.8** Osteoclast. A large cell with abundant cytoplasm showing red granules and multiple uniform nuclei (MGG).

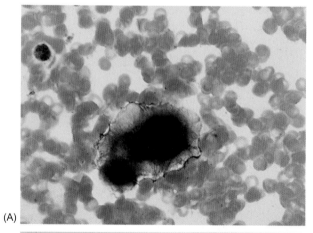

(A)

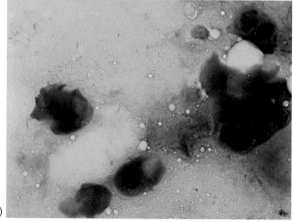

(B)

**Fig. 29.9** Chondrocytes. Small fragments of strongly stained hyaline matrix with chondrocytes. (A: H&E; B: MGG).

proliferative periostitis and pseudomalignant myositis ossificans. The reactive osteoblasts resemble normal osteoblasts with eccentric nuclei and a clear cytoplasmic 'Hof', but they are often larger and more variable in size and shape. Their nuclei may also be large with prominent nucleoli (Fig. 29.10). These reactive osteoblasts may be embedded in small fragments of a faintly fibrillary background matrix staining reddish violet with MGG stains. This material probably represents osteoid (Fig. 29.11).

A lesion which demonstrates the typical reactive changes found in soft tissue as well as bone is pseudomalignant myositis ossificans (PMO).

This is a rapidly proliferating soft tissue lesion, which has been mistaken clinically as well as radiologically and histologically for a malignant tumour. In most false positive diagnoses PMO has been diagnosed as osteosarcoma. It generally arises in the subcutaneous tissues or musculature of the extremities of young adults, forming a tender swelling which undergoes ossification in a zonal pattern after 2–3 weeks.

### Cytological findings: reactive changes

- Proliferating fibroblasts/myofibroblasts
- Proliferating osteoblasts, often with reactive changes

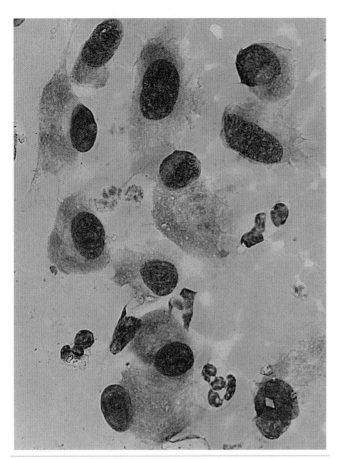

**Fig. 29.10** Reactive osteoblasts. Reactive osteoblasts have the same cytological features as normal osteoblasts, including eccentric nuclei and a perinuclear 'Hof', but they vary in size and shape and anisocytosis may be marked (MGG).

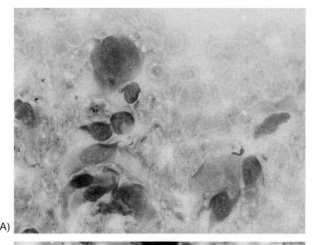

(A)

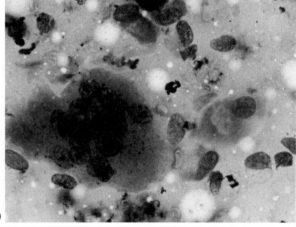

(B)

**Fig. 29.12** Pseudomalignant myositis ossificans. (A) A mixture of proliferating fibroblasts/myofibroblasts and reactive osteoblasts (MGG). (B) An osteoclast-like giant cell and proliferating osteoblasts. Note the clear cytoplasmic 'Hof' (MGG).

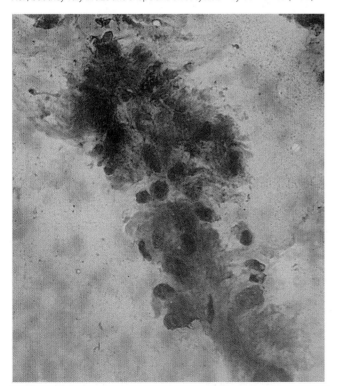

**Fig. 29.11** Reactive osteoblasts. Reactive osteoblasts embedded in a reddish violet background substance which is osteoid. From a case of proliferative periostitis (MGG).

- Osteoclastic giant cells
- Occasionally small calcifications.

The characteristic findings are the mixture of proliferating fibroblasts/myofibroblasts, osteoblasts and osteoclastic giant cells (Fig. 29.12).[11] When striated muscle is involved, regenerating muscle fibres ('muscle giant cells') are also observed. Experience indicates that a correct diagnosis of PMO may be rendered from the combined evaluation of clinical history, radiological features and FNA findings. Computed tomography is especially valuable for visualising the typical changes. In our experience, PMO may resolve spontaneously a number of weeks after needling.

## Soft tissue tumours

Modern histological classification of soft tissue tumours is based on the presumptive cell of origin of the tumour. Continuous modification is needed to incorporate newly recognised tumour variants and respond to new information on cell derivation. The most recent classifications are found in the World Health Organization fascicle Tumours of Soft Tissue and Bone 2002[12] and in Weiss and Goldblum's *Soft Tissue Tumours* 2007.[13]

Benign soft tissue tumours are far more common than sarcomas. It is important to note that while most tumour types have benign and malignant counterparts, almost all sarcomas arise *de novo* rather than from malignant transformation of a benign tumour. One exception is the nerve cell tumours in von Recklinghausen's disease. At times, a neurofibroma is diagnosed in one part of the tumour, while a malignant peripheral nerve sheath tumour is present in another area.

There is usually no clear indication of any risk factors, although putative agents such as industrial carcinogens, chronic trauma and viruses are thought to be involved in the pathogenesis of certain sarcomas. Factors which have been considered important are previous radiation treatment of a malignant tumour (lymphangiosarcoma after irradiation of breast carcinoma), liver angiosarcoma after exposure to vinyl chloride or thorium dioxide and with regard to epidemiological forms of Kaposi sarcoma, human herpesvirus (KS-associated herpesvirus, HHV8).

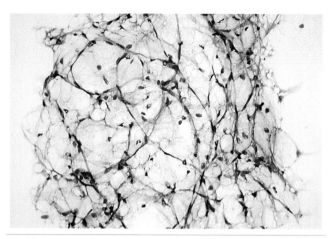

**Fig. 29.13** Lipoma. Part of a fragment of adipose tissue. Large fat cells with small, dark nuclei. Thin capillary strands intersect the fragment (MGG).

## Benign soft tissue tumours

The incidence of different benign soft tissue tumours is broadly reflected in the rate of referral of various tumour types for aspiration. At the Orthopaedic Oncology Group at Lund University Hospital in Sweden with an uptake area comprising slightly more than 1.7 million inhabitants, benign lipomatous tumours are the most common and have been recorded most frequently since the Group started more then 30 years ago.

Neurilemmoma is a fairly common lesions as well as ganglion and haemangioma while desmoid fibromatosis, intramuscular myxoma and nodular fasciitis are encountered somewhat less often. Benign fibrous histiocytoma, although a rather common soft tissue tumour, is infrequently aspirated. A number of rare tumours such as elastofibroma dorsi, ossifying fibromyxoid tumour, granular cell tumour, soft tissue leiomyoma and rhabdomyoma are only occasionally referred for aspiration.

## Benign adipocytic tumours

### Lipoma

Usually slow growing asymptomatic tumours of adults, lipomas may be subcutaneous (superficial lipoma) or deeply placed (intramuscular or intermuscular lipoma), solitary or multiple and vary enormously at presentation. Their histological structure is also variable. They are composed of mature adipose tissue, but may include other connective tissue elements and may show evidence of trauma or degeneration.

### Cytological findings: lipoma

- Fatty tissue fragments
- Few dissociated adipocytes
- Fragments of striated muscle or regenerating muscle fibres ('muscle giant cells') in inter/intramuscular lipoma.

Aspirates from lipomas have virtually the same appearance as aspirates from normal adipose tissue. It is therefore important to know that the needle was actually placed within the mass. If a needle with a stylet is used for deep-seated tumours, contamination with normal subcutaneous fat is avoided.

Typically, smears from lipoma consist of fragments of adipose tissue composed of large cells containing a single vacuole of fat and a small dark peripheral nucleus. Within the fragments a few capillary strands are usually observed (Fig. 29.13). Dispersed lipocytes are uncommon. Inter/intramuscular lipomas often include fragments of ordinary striated muscle. Intramuscular lipoma often infiltrates surrounding striated muscle and in those cases multinucleated regenerating muscle fibres may be observed.

Lipomas with chondroid metaplasia include fragments of acellular myxoid matrix stained bluish red with MGG, along with the adipose tissue fragments. Occasionally rounded chondrocytes are observed in lacunae in this matrix. Aspirates from lipomas with myxoid degeneration often yield a few drops of colourless stringy fluid. Smears show a blue or bluish red myxoid background matrix containing isolated lipocytes or small clusters of fat cells, in addition to the usual fragments of adipose tissue.

### Lipoblastoma/lipoblastomatosis

This tumour of infancy, most commonly involving the extremities, is well circumscribed as a subcutaneous tumour (lipoblastoma) but as a deep-seated lesion diffusely infiltrates striated muscle (lipoblastomatosis). Composed of immature fat histologically, with mesenchymal, myxoid and fibrotic areas, the tumour is thought to be capable of maturing to a common lipoma. The cytological findings in FNA have been described.[14] Typical features are the presence of small uniform adipocytes with vacuolated cytoplasm and rounded regular nucleoli, set in a myxoid background matrix, which also contains branching strands of capillaries (Fig. 29.14). In our experience smears at times may be dominated by large ordinary univacuolated adipocytes.

### Angiolipoma

Angiolipomas are subcutaneous and often multiple and tender at palpation. The majority of angiolipomas are smaller than 2 cm. An angiolipoma should be suspected when the tumour is small, tender at palpation and numerous branching capillary vessel fragments are seen in the fat tissue fragments. Occasionally fibrin thrombi are present in scattered vessels.

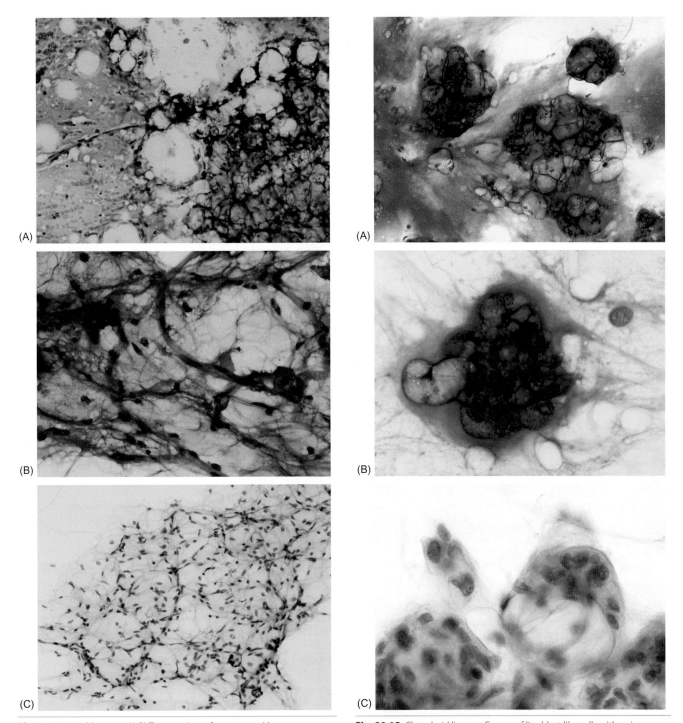

**Fig. 29.14** Lipoblastoma. (A,B) Tumour tissue fragments with a more or less abundant myxoid background, vacuolated adipocytes and intersecting capillaries (A: MGG; B: MGG). (C) The numerous intersecting capillaries are evident in wet-fixed material (H&E).

**Fig. 29.15** Chondroid lipoma. Groups of lipoblast-like cells with uni-or multivacuolated cytoplasm within a myxoid matrix (A: MGG; B: MGG). The tumour cell nuclei are irregular and lobulated (C: H&E).

## Chondroid lipoma

Chondroid lipoma, an infrequent benign lipomatous tumour, was fully categorised about 15 years ago.[15] Chondroid lipoma is a well-defined, predominantly subcutaneous tumour in the extremities, trunk and head and neck region.

Histologically it is composed of an admixture of normal adipocytes, chondroblast-like cells and vacuolated, lipoblast-like cells in a myxochondroid matrix.

### Cytological findings: chondroid lipoma (Fig. 29.15)

- More or less abundant myxochondroid background matrix
- Groups and clusters of ordinary fat cells
- Groups and clusters of uni-or multivacuolated, lipoblast-like cells with irregular nuclear shape, scalloped nuclei and multivacuolated cytoplasm
- Nuclei are often irregular, lobulated or coffee bean shaped.

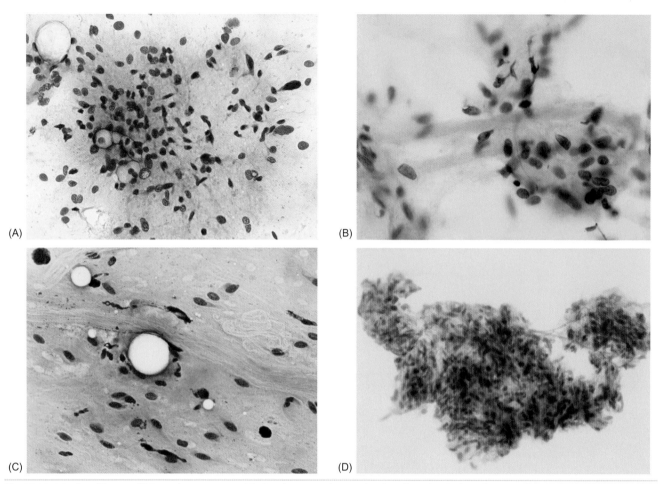

**Fig. 29.16** Spindle cell lipoma. (A) Smear from a tumour with abundant myxoid matrix, few fat cells and multiple uniform spindle cells (MGG). (B) Spindle cells and fragments of collagen-hyaline fibres (H&E). (C) Mast cells are often present (MGG). (D) ThinPrep preparation stained with CD34 (immunoperoxidase).

Although rarely a target for FNA, the cytologic features of chondroid lipoma have been recorded in case reports.[16,17]

In spite of the variation in size and shape, the nuclei are benign-looking. One important feature in the differential diagnosis from myxoid liposarcoma is the lack of a plexiform capillary network in the cell clusters.

### Spindle cell and pleomorphic lipoma

These two examples of benign lipomatous tumours share clinical, morphological and cytogenetic features. For both tumours the typical clinical setting is a subcutaneous tumour in the neck region, upper back and shoulders in middle-aged men.

The microscopic appearance of spindle cell lipoma in sections varies; lipomatous tissue is more or less replaced by bundles or fascicles of uniform spindle cells in a myxoid background matrix. Eosinophilic hyaline collagen fibres are a typical finding. Mast cells are often present.

Aspirates contain a mixture of adipose tissue fragments and sheets or clusters of spindle cells with elongated, uniform nuclei and poorly demarcated cytoplasm in a myxoid background matrix. A diagnostically important but variable sign is fragments of eosinophilic (H&E) collagen-hyaline fibres. Mast cells are often present in the myxoid matrix (Fig. 29.16A–C).

Due to the variable tissue pattern, aspirates from spindle cell lipoma may show a predominance of adipose tissue fragments or a predominance of spindle cell fascicles and abundant myxoid back ground matrix. The spindle cells are strongly positive for CD34 (Fig. 29.16D). The various cytological features of spindle cell lipoma have been described in a series of 12 tumours.[18]

The characteristic findings of pleomorphic lipoma on histology are the so-called floret cells. They are multinucleated giant cells with a moderate amount of cytoplasm and multiple marginally placed hyperchromatic nuclei with indistinct chromatin. These cells are easily observed in aspiration smears within and between adipose tissue fragments (Fig. 29.17). Pleomorphic lipomas may feature collagen fibres and areas of myxoid stroma similar to spindle cell lipoma and transitional forms between spindle and pleomorphic lipoma are not uncommon.

### Hibernoma

Hibernoma derived from brown (foetal) fat is a rare tumour not only situated in the interscapular region, back or chestwall (sites of normal deposits of brown fat), but also on the extremities. Hibernomas are usually subcutaneous but they may be deep-seated (intramuscular). Hibernomas are easily identified

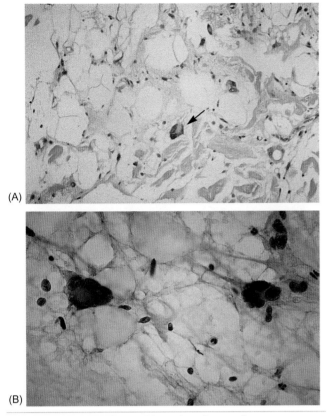

(A)

(B)

**Fig. 29.17** Pleomorphic lipoma. (A) Histological section from a pleomorphic lipoma. One typical multinucleated floret cell (arrow) (H&E). (B) Floret cells in FNA of pleomorphic lipoma. Large multinucleated cells with abundant cytoplasm and with overlapping nuclei along the cytoplasmic border (H&E).

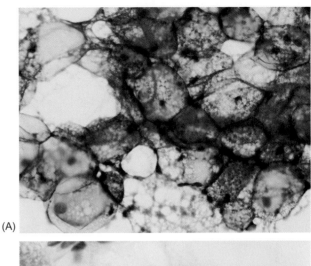

(A)

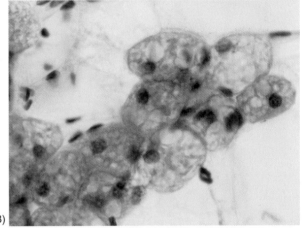

(B)

**Fig. 29.18** Hibernoma. Small tumour fragments composed of vacuolated fat cells with small nuclei (A: MGG; B: H&E).

histologically as lobulated tumours with a tan brown cut surface. The tumour cells are mainly small and rounded with multiple cytoplasmic vacuoles or granular cytoplasm surrounding a central nucleus. They are vascular and contain numerous capillaries. The aspiration cytology of hibernoma has been reported.[19] In smears, clusters or fragments of ordinary large lipocytes are intermingled with small rounded cells with vacuolated or granulated cytoplasm and centrally placed small uniform nuclei. The tissue fragments often contain numerous capillary vessels (Fig. 29.18). In the hibernoma lobules, ordinary, large adipocytes may predominate and the typical cells may be in minority. FNA from hibernomas may thus be made up of lipoma-like fat cells and 'hibernoma' cells.

### Extra-adrenal myelolipoma

Myelolipoma is a tumour-like lesion composed of bone marrow cells and mature fat in the adrenals (see Ch. 18). Myelolipoma may also arise in retroperitoneum and in the pelvic region. For the cytopathologist, extra-adrenal myelolipoma is one of differential diagnoses when tumours or tumour-like masses are needled in those sites. Whether myelolipoma is a true neoplasm or not is not clarified, although one theory is that it originates from rests of haemopoietic stem cells. In FNA smears, myelolipoma consists of cluster of normal adipocytes mixed with bone marrow cells. It is often possible to identify cells from all three cell-lines (Fig. 29.19).

> ### Diagnostic pitfalls: benign adipose tumours
>
> The main clinical problem is to differentiate the various benign variants from liposarcoma. The main clue to a benign diagnosis is the absence of atypical lipoblasts, but clinical details such as age, site and size are also of importance.
> In Table 29.2 the various variants of benign lipomatous tumours and the main differential diagnoses for each type is summarised.

## Benign fibroblastic/myofibroblastic and fibrohistiocytic tumours

### Nodular fasciitis

Nodular fasciitis is the commonest of the so-called benign pseudosarcomatous lesions. It affects all age groups but is most common in young adults. It is usually subcutaneous and the predilection sites are the upper extremities, trunk and the head and neck region. It grows with great rapidity over a few weeks, but usually not reaching more than about 3 cm in diameter. Nodular fasciitis is composed of fibroblasts and myofibroblasts showing variable grades of anisocytosis and anisokaryosis. The stroma is often myxoid, at least in the early phase.

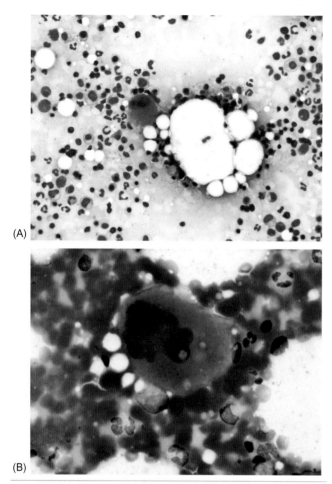

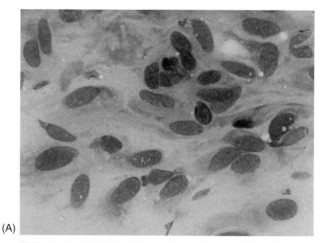

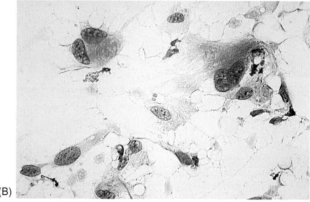

(A)

(B)

**Fig. 29.19** Myelolipoma. (A) An adipose tissue fragment surrounded by bone marrow cells (MGG). (B) Megakaryocyte and myelopoietic cells (MGG).

(A)

(B)

**Fig. 29.20** Nodular fasciitis. (A) A myxoid background matrix with dispersed fibroblasts/myofibroblasts displaying moderate variation in shape and size (MGG). (B) Two binucleate cells, closely resembling ganglion cells, and one normal fibroblast (H&E).

**Table 29.2** Various variants of benign lipomatous tumours and the main diagnostic pitfalls

| Tumour type | Main pitfalls |
| --- | --- |
| Common lipoma | Normal adipose tissue. Important to certify that the needle is within the target |
| | Well-differentiated liposarcoma |
| Lipoblastoma/lipoblastomatosis | Common lipoma |
| | Myxoid liposarcoma (extremely rare in children) |
| Spindle cell lipoma | Neurilemmoma |
| | Myxoid liposarcoma |
| | Low-grade myxofibrosarcoma |
| Pleomorphic lipoma | Well-differentiated liposarcoma |
| Hibernoma | Common lipoma |
| | Granular cell tumour |
| | Adult rhabdomyoma |
| | Liposarcoma |
| Chondroid lipoma | Myxoid liposarcoma |
| | Extraskeletal myxoid chondrosarcoma |

## Cytological findings: nodular fasciitis

- Cellular aspirates
- Myxoid background matrix
- Dispersed cells are mixed with clusters or closely packed sheets of cells
- More or less marked anisocytosis and anisokaryosis
- Cells resembling ganglion cells
- Admixture of leucocytes and histiocytes.

The cytological appearance of nodular fasciitis has been previously described.[20] The more than 70 examples of nodular fasciitis from the author's files reveal remarkable similarity from case to case (Åkerman and Domanski, unpublished work, 2007). The most important feature is the wide variation in size and shape of the proliferating fibroblasts and myofibroblasts. Spindle-shaped cells with cytoplasmic processes and fusiform nuclei are the commonest type seen, but plump cells with ovoid, rounded, kidney-shaped or irregular nuclei are also always found.

A further typical finding is the presence of polyhedral or triangular cells with abundant cytoplasm. They have one or two rounded nuclei at the periphery near the cytoplasmic membrane, and closely resemble ganglion cells. In spite of the pleomorphism throughout the smear, the chromatin in all of the cells is finely granular and, although their nucleoli may be very large, it is always possible to identify normal looking fibroblasts and fibroblasts with minor reactive changes (Fig. 29.20).

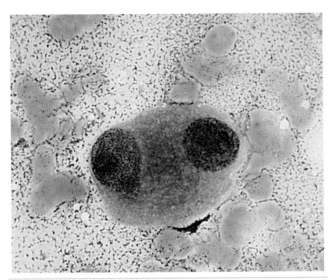

**Fig. 29.21** Proliferative myositis. A characteristic cell; large, rounded and binucleate with abundant cytoplasm and nuclei opposite each other (MGG).

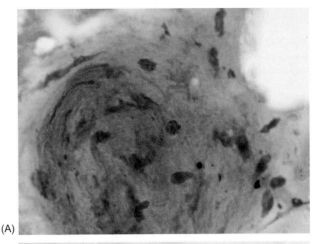

(A)

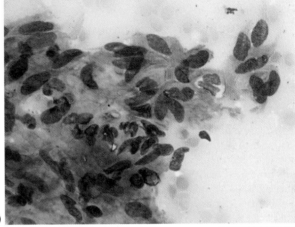

(B)

**Fig. 29.22** Desmoid fibromatosis. (A) Part of a fragment of collagenased stroma with faintly outlined fibrillar background and scattered nuclei (MGG). (B) A cluster of loosely attached fibroblast-like cells with ovoid nuclei and greyish-blue cytoplasm (MGG).

This rapidly growing lesion is often painful and tender and most cases are needled in the early phase of growth. Experience indicates that nodular fasciitis often decreases in size or even vanishes in 3 or 4 weeks. When the clinical findings are of a rapidly growing, tender, firm subcutaneous tumour, and the cytological appearances are typical, our policy at present is clinical observation, thereby avoiding surgical intervention.

Two other less common and occasionally needled benign pseudosarcomatous lesions are proliferative myositis/fasciitis. They predominantly develop in adults, proliferative myositis occurring mainly on the trunk, while fasciitis is more common on the extremities. These two lesions share cytological findings with nodular fasciitis, although the myxoid background matrix is less prominent and the large mono- or binucleated cells resembling ganglion cells are numerous and often feature large prominent nucleoli (Fig. 29.21).

## Desmoid fibromatosis

Almost all cases collected from our files are abdominal and extraabdominal. The rare intra-abdominal fibromatoses are, in our experience, almost never needled. Extra-abdominal desmoid fibromatosis, which arises from connective tissue associated with muscle or fascia, typically affects young adults. Most common sites are around the shoulder and pelvic girdle and proximal parts of the extremities. Histologically, desmoid fibromatosis is a poorly defined lesion with an infiltrative growth. It is composed of bundles or fascicles of elongated fibroblasts with bland fusiform nuclei. Abundant intercellular collagen is present and a myxoid matrix may be found focally. Due to the tendency to infiltrate, desmoid fibromatosis may behave aggressively and local recurrence is not uncommon.

---

### Cytological findings: desmoid fibromatosis

- Variable cell yield
- Cell clusters and dispersed cells
- Fragments of collagenised stroma

---

- The fibroblasts are spindle shaped with fusiform nuclei with moderate anisokaryosis.
- Preserved cells show cytoplasmic processes
- Stripped nuclei common
- When smears originate from an infiltrative area of striated muscle, 'muscle giant cells' are found.

The cytological appearance of desmoid fibromatosis has been described in a series of 69 cases.[21] The cases from our files have all shown similar features as described. Due to the often abundant collagenous stroma, desmoid fibromatoses are very firm to palpate and a rubbery resistance is felt when needling. Often vigorous aspirations are needed to collect sufficient material for examination. A finding common to all our cases has been the presence of quite numerous fragments of collagenised stroma staining bluish-grey with MGG and showing a faintly fibrillary background (Fig. 29.22A). Stripped nuclei are also commonly seen. The nuclei are elongated or ovoid with finely granular chromatin and small nucleoli (Fig. 29.22B). Preserved cells have well-demarcated pale cytoplasm, often with unipolar or bipolar cytoplasmic processes. The cells appear in small cohesive clusters or are dissociated. Sometimes faintly outlined nuclei are seen in the stromal fragments. When infiltration of striated muscle occurs, 'muscle giant cells' are found.

## Diagnostic pitfalls: desmoid fibromatosis

Important diagnostic pitfalls arise when the cellular yield is poor and stromal fragments are lacking. Monophasic synovial sarcoma and low-grade malignant peripheral nerve sheath tumour (MPNST) as well as low-grade fibromyxoid sarcoma may be cytologically misdiagnosed as desmoid tumour and vice versa. Other differential diagnoses include nodular fasciitis, neurilemmoma and soft tissue leiomyoma. The uniform spindle cell population, fragments of collagenised stroma, absence of a myxoid background and ganglion-like cells exclude nodular fasciitis; while tumour tissue fragments with elongated or comma-shaped nuclei in a fibrillar background are the hallmarks of neurilemmoma rather than desmoid tumour.

## Extrapleural solitary fibrous tumour and haemangiopericytoma

According to the recent WHO classification of soft tissue tumours, these two fibroblastic neoplasms are closely related, possibly representing two variants of the same entity.[12]

### Haemangiopericytoma

Haemangiopericytoma is most common in deep soft tissue, with a predilection for the pelvic retroperitoneum. The typical histological pattern includes numerous, thin walled, branching vessels similar to stag horns. The tumour cells have ovoid or rounded, bland nuclei. The diagnosis of haemangiopericytoma is at present considered as a diagnosis of exclusion as some other tumours, notably monophasic synovial sarcoma, deep fibrous histiocytoma and mesenchymal chondrosarcoma may exhibit the same type of vascularity. Haemangiopericytomas most often show positivity for CD34 and CD99.

## Cytological findings: haemangiopericytoma (Fig. 29.23)

- The aspirates are often haemorrhagic
- Dispersed cells are mixed with small tissue fragments
- In the tissue fragments, a branching network of vessels is often present

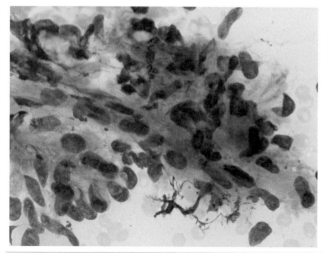

**Fig. 29.23** Haemangiopericytoma. A vessel fragment surrounded by tumour cells with ovoid or rounded bland nuclei (MGG).

- Stripped nuclei not uncommon
- The tumour cells feature small cytoplasmic processes and ovoid or rounded bland nuclei with inconspicuous nucleoli.

### Extrapleural solitary fibrous tumour

Morphologically extrapleural solitary fibrous tumour resembles its pleural counterpart (see Ch. 2). The essential histological features are alternating hypercellular and hypocellular sclerotic areas of bland looking short spindly or ovoid cells with poorly defined, scanty cytoplasm. Thick or thin collagen fibrils are intimately mixed with the spindle cells. Branching vessels of the same type as seen in haemangiopericytoma ('staghorn pattern') are often present. The most diagnostically important feature, similar to haemangiopericytoma, is CD34 positivity of the spindle cells. In some cases, the cells are also CD99 and bcl-2 positive.[22,23]

The cytological features of solitary fibrous tumour have been described in small series.[24] The cytological appearance is the same as its pleural counterpart.

## Cytological findings: extrapleural solitary fibrous tumour (Fig. 29.24)

- Variable cellularity
- Stripped nuclei
- Cells in tight, at times fascicle-like clusters, or dispersed
- Bland chromatin structure
- Inconspicuous nucleoli.

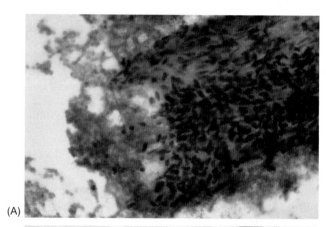

(A)

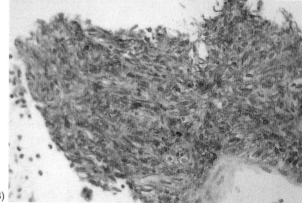

(B)

**Fig. 29.24** Solitary fibrous tumour of soft tissue. (A) A fascicle of tightly packed cells with bland looking fusiform nuclei (H&E). (B) Cell block preparation stained with CD34 (immunoperoxidase).

### Diagnostic pitfalls: desmoid fibromatosis

With regard to haemangiopericytoma as well as extrapleural solitary fibrous tumour, the most important pitfall is monophasic synovial sarcoma, other differential diagnoses are low-grade fibromyxoid sarcoma and low-grade malignant peripheral nerve sheath tumour. A clue to a correct diagnosis is the immunophenotype CD34+, CD99+, bcl-2+ (Fig. 29.24B). As is evident from the cytological findings tabulated above and the common immunophenotype, the distinction between haemangiopericytoma and solitary fibrous tumour in FNA is very difficult, sometimes impossible.

## Elastofibroma

Elastofibroma is a slow growing fibroelastic tumour-like lesion arising in elderly individuals. The typical site for elastofibroma is a deep-seated lesion beneath the scapula. Elastofibroma is made up of hypocellular collagenous tissue and elastic fibres associated with fat cells. The characteristic of this lesion is faulty elastin fibrillogenesis. The elastic fibres are large, eosinophilic and fragmented appearing as globuli or serrated fragments.

### Cytological findings: elastofibroma

- Variably cellular smears, often poor yield
- Variable amount of clustered fat cells
- Fibroblast-like, uniform spindly cells, dispersed or in small clusters
- Fragments of degenerate elastic fibres appearing as small globules or as fragments with serrated edges.

The cytology of elastofibroma has been described in a small series of five patients.[25] The most important clue to the diagnosis is the presence of the degenerate elastic fibres (Fig. 29.25).

## Fibrous histiocytoma

This common tumour occurs in young adults, especially on the extremities. The lesions may be solitary or multiple, and either subcutaneous or deep. They are composed of cells resembling histiocytes and fibroblasts with a storiform pattern of growth, likened to a cartwheel. There are usually some inflammatory cells and deposits of iron within the tumour.

### Cytological findings: fibrous histiocytoma

- Solid cell clusters and dispersed cells
- Fibroblast-like and histiocyte-like cells
- Multinucleated giant cells of Touton type
- Phagocytosis with haemosiderin deposits in histiocytes.

The variable histological features of fibrous histiocytomas are reflected in the cytological findings in aspirated smears. A common picture is the dual presence of fibroblastic cells with ovoid or elongated nuclei and histiocytic cells, which have rounded or irregular nuclei and rather abundant cytoplasm. Giant cells of Touton type, with their characteristic peripheral circle of nuclei, are almost always found, as are deposits of haemosiderin in the histiocytic cells (Fig. 29.26). Capillary strands may be observed. One large series of the cytology of the various types of benign fibrous histiocytoma has been published.[26]

## Localised tumour of tendon sheath (giant cell tumour of tendon sheath)

A relatively common lesion. Most tumours arise in the fingers, less common sites are hands, wrists and feet. The tumours usually are less than 3–4 cm in size and slow-growing.

Histologically, they are composed of mononuclear rounded cells, histiocytic cells as xanthoma cells and siderophages and multinucleated giant cells resembling osteoclasts.

In some tumours the stroma can be hyalinised.

### Cytological findings: localised tumour of tendon sheath (Fig. 29.27)

- Variable yield
- Dispersed and clustered mononuclear rounded cells at times plasma-cell-like
- Rounded, uniform nuclei
- Moderate cellular pleomorphism
- Multinucleated osteoclast-like giant cells
- Histiocytes, often with haemosiderin deposits.

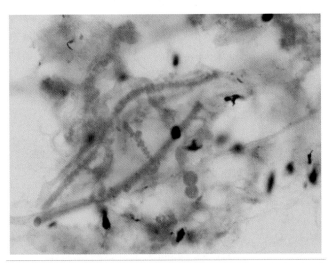

**Fig. 29.25** Elastofibroma. Degenerated elastic fibres with serrated edges (H&E).

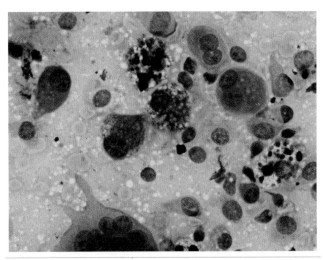

**Fig. 29.26** Fibrous histiocytoma. A group of loosely attached fibroblast-like cells mixed with histiocytes with cytoplasmic haemosiderin deposits (MGG).

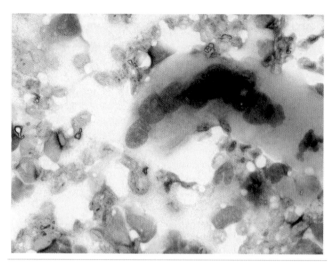

**Fig. 29.28** Fibromatosis colli. A regenerating muscle fibre with multiple nuclei surrounded by fibroblast-like cells (MGG).

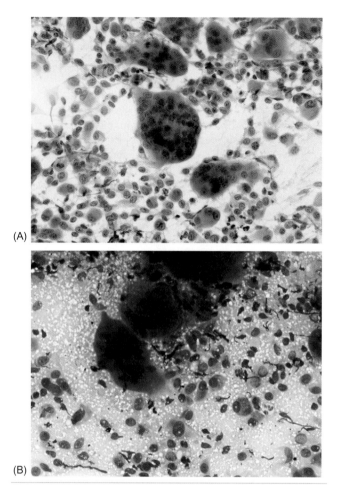

**Fig. 29.27** Localised tumour of tendon sheath. Dispersed rounded cells with rounded nuclei exhibiting moderate cellular pleomorphism and two osteoclast-like giant cells (A: H&E; B: MGG).

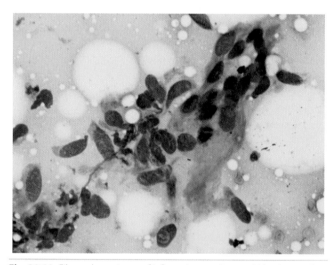

**Fig. 29.29** Fibrous hamartoma of infancy. In a partly myxoid background normal adipose tissue mixed with clusters of spindly cells (MGG).

Various benign fibroblastic/myofibroblastic tumours in infancy and childhood are described in the current literature. The two of these entities most often sampled by FNA are fibromatosis colli and fibrous hamartoma of infancy.

## Fibromatosis colli (torticollis)

Fibromatosis colli is a firm lesion arising in the sternocleidomastoid muscle in infants. Histologically there is a diffuse proliferation of fibroblasts within the muscle tissue. The entrapped muscle fibres are atrophic with numerous regenerating multinucleated fibres.

### Cytological findings: fibromatosis colli

- Small amounts of myxoid back ground matrix
- Dispersed and clustered uniform, bland-looking fibroblasts
- Often stripped nuclei
- Often numerous regenerating muscle fibres appearing as 'muscle giant cells' or tadpole-like cells.

The mixture of fibroblasts and regenerating muscle fibres is typical (Fig. 29.28). Most cases of fibromatosis colli regress spontaneously; conservatory treatment as physiotherapy and stretching is recommended and surgical intervention

is not necessary in most cases. The cytological features of fibromatosis colli have been investigated in two series, comprising 16 tumours.[27,28]

## Fibrous hamartoma of infancy

Fibrous hamartoma of infancy is a rare subcutaneous mass composed of a mixture of mature fat, trabeculae of fibrous tissue and areas of primitive mesenchymal cells. The predilection sites are the upper arms, axillary region and shoulder. The majority of cases are seen up to 2 years of age.

### Cytological findings: fibrous hamartoma of infancy

- Fragments of normal adipose tissue mixed with clusters, groups or runs of spindle cells
- Small tufts of myxoid matrix
- The spindle cells have bland nuclei with inconspicuous nucleoli.

The cytological features of fibrous hamartoma of infancy have been reported in case reports[29] and we have one case recorded in our files (Fig. 29.29).

## Tumours of peripheral nerves

This group of tumours, derived from the Schwann cells, which myelinate and protect all peripheral nerves, includes neurilemmoma, also known as Schwannoma, and neurofibroma, the tumour type seen classically in von Recklinghausen's disease. Granular cell tumours are also believed be of neural origin.

## Neurilemmoma

These are the commonest of the group, occurring in adults on limbs, head and neck. Encapsulated histologically, they are composed of alternating structured areas of palisaded spindle-shaped cells (Antoni A) and loose myxoid areas (Antoni B). Degenerative changes are common, earning the title of ancient neurilemmoma when large lesions of long duration exhibit the marked nuclear pleomorphism characteristic of this variant.

### Cytological findings: neurilemmoma

- Variable cellularity
- Tumour tissue fragments vary in size and cellularity
- Cohesive cells, rarely single tumour cells
- Occasional palisades of cells
- Indistinct cytoplasm, elongated nuclei, pointed ends
- Small rounded cells with rounded nuclei occasionally seen in the fragments
- Moderate nuclear pleomorphism
- Myxoid background matrix occasionally
- Fragmented fibrillary background fragments.

There are numerous reports of the typical cytological features of neurilemmoma and there is also one correlative cytohistological study of 116 tumours.[30] A characteristic clinical sign is the sharp, sometimes radiating pain experienced by the patient on needling. Smears vary in cellularity, usually consisting of numerous tissue fragments of different size. The fragments also vary in cellularity and have irregular borders, so that at low magnification they have been compared with pieces of a jigsaw puzzle (Fig. 29.30A). The cytological findings generally correspond to Antoni A tissue: the fragments consist of cohesive cells with very indistinct cell borders and spindle-shaped nuclei with pointed ends. Small cells with rounded 'lymphocyte-like' or ovoid nuclei are also seen (Fig. 29.30B). A number of the elongated nuclei are comma-shaped or have one end bent like a fishhook. Variation in nuclear size is always seen and may be marked. Palisading of nuclei and Verocay body structures are sometimes observed. Dispersed cells are uncommon and mitoses are almost never seen. Another typical feature is a fibrillary background substance in which the cells are embedded. This background is best visualised by H&E staining (Fig. 29.30C). Some neurilemmomas yield a small amount of cystic fluid when aspirated. In other cases dispersed cells are embedded in a myxoid background and the tumour fragments are small with less cohesive tumour cells mingling with histiocytes. These findings correspond to Antoni B areas on histology.

Aspirates from neurofibromas may have an abundant myxoid background and dispersed cells are often more common than tumour tissue fragments. Other than this, the findings are similar to those of neurilemmomas.

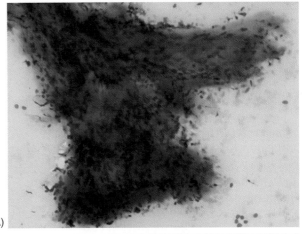

(A)

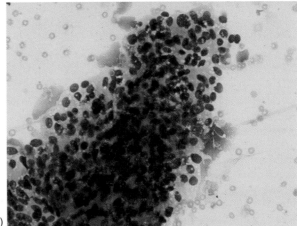

(B)

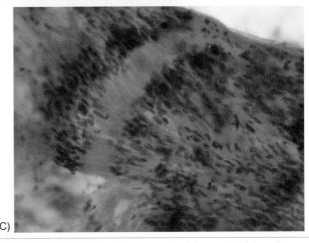

(C)

**Fig. 29.30** Neurilemmoma. (A) A tumour tissue fragment with irregular borders with varying cellularity. (MGG ). (B) Small cells with rounded 'lymphocyte-like' nuclei are occasionally seen in the tumour fragments (MGG). (C) A Verocay body like structure. Note the fibrillar back ground (H&E).

## Granular cell tumour

The granular cell tumour, described by Abrikosoff in 1926 and originally considered to be of myogenic origin, is now regarded as a tumour of peripheral nerve derivation. Much more common in adults than in children, it is mainly situated subcutaneously but occasionally found in muscle and skin, and more rarely in internal organs. Breast and tongue are quite common sites. Histologically, there is a tendency to packaging of the tumour cells. They are rounded with central nuclei and coarsely granular cytoplasm, with some smaller period acid Schiff (PAS)-positive cells between.

### Cytological findings: granular cell tumour

- Dispersed cells and clusters
- Naked nuclei common
- Round nuclei, bland chromatin, prominent nucleoli
- Abundant granular cytoplasm, when preserved.

The cellular yield is usually good, consisting of tumour cells with abundant but fragile cytoplasm and stripped nuclei are therefore common. In preserved cells, the cytoplasm is typically granular, staining eosinophilic with H&E and blue with MGG (Fig. 29.31). The chromatin structure in the rounded nuclei is uniformly regular and nucleoli are quite small but prominent. A study of the cytological features of 17 granular cell tumours has been published.[31]

### Diagnostic pitfalls: benign nerve sheath tumours

The most difficult problem lies in correctly diagnosing the so-called ancient neurilemmoma, which is easily mistaken for sarcoma. The large cells with pleomorphic, hyperchromatic sometimes bizarre nuclei typical of an ancient neurilemmoma are deceptively like sarcoma cells. However, careful inspection of the enlarged nuclei reveals degenerative changes, including the so-called 'kern-loche', which are large intranuclear vacuoles usually present if looked for carefully (Fig. 29.32A). Mitoses are not observed cytologically. According to our experience, leiomyosarcoma and malignant peripheral nerve sheath tumour (MPNST) are the most common false positive diagnoses of sarcoma with regard to neurilemomas with Antoni A features and ancient neurilemmoma.[30] Neurilemmoma and neurofibromas with a myxoid background matrix in smears may be misdiagnosed as a number of other soft tissue tumours exhibiting a similar background. These are listed in Table 29.3.

A correct diagnosis of neurilemmoma and granular cell tumour can be confirmed by immunocytochemical staining with S-100-protein and anti-desmin. Ancient neurilemmoma and granular cell tumour display strong S-100 positivity and are desmin negative (Fig. 29.32B, C). MPNSTs usually show only focal S-100 positivity or are negative in contrast to diffuse staining of neurilemmoma and neurofibroma.

The rich cellular yield of granular cell tumour and large numbers of naked nuclei with prominent nucleoli seen in these lesions have been misinterpreted as malignant in smears. In fact, malignant granular cell tumours are very rare, and the key to the correct diagnosis lies in awareness of the characteristic cellular features of the benign lesion.[31]

The most important differential diagnosis is adult rhabdomyoma. Immunocytochemically granular cell tumour is characterised by positivity for S 100-protein, NSE and inhibin.

## Tumours of smooth muscle

Benign smooth muscle tumours, leiomyomas, can be divided into visceral and extravisceral types. The main extravisceral lesions needled are angioleiomyoma and the rare deep-seated soft tissue leiomyoma.

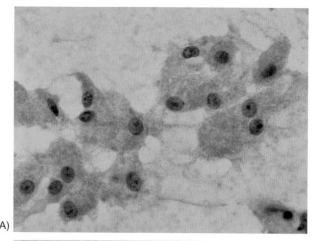

(A)

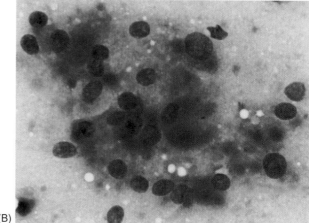

(B)

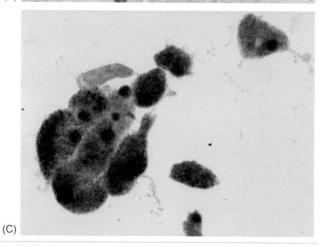

(C)

**Fig. 29.31** (A,B) Granular cell tumour. The tumour cells have abundant granular cytoplasm and rounded bland nuclei with prominent nucleoli (A: H&E; B: MGG). (C) ThinPrep-preparation stained with S 100 protein (immunoperoxidase).

## Angioleiomyoma

Angioleiomyoma is a deep dermal or subcutaneous, most often small (at most 2 cm) and distinctly painful tumour on palpation. Most angioleiomyomas occur in the extremities. They are composed of bundles of uniform smooth muscle cells and thick-walled vessels.

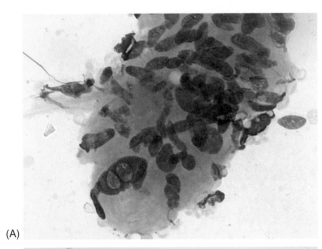

(A)

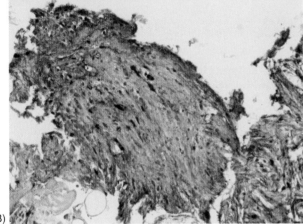

(B)

**Fig. 29.32** Ancient neurilemmoma. (A) Tumour cells with anisokaryosis and a typical bizarre cell with degenerative nuclear changes ('kern-loche') in lower left corner (MGG). (B) Cell block preparation from the same case stained with S 100 protein. (Immunoperoxidase).

**Table 29.3** Soft tissue tumours with a myxoid background matrix. Important cytological features in the differential diagnosis

| Tumour | Cytological findings |
| --- | --- |
| Nodular fasciitis | Marked anicytosis and anisokaryosis in proliferating fibroblasts/myofibroblasts. Single and binucleated cells resembling ganglion cells |
| Neurilemmoma | Mainly tissue fragments, dispersed cells uncommon. Fibrillary background in fragments. Nuclei with pointed ends, comma or fish-hook shaped. Nuclear palisading. Infrequently Verocay body structures |
| Neurofibroma | Mixture of dispersed cells and cell clusters. Cell morphology as neurilemmoma |
| Intramuscular myxoma | Abundant myxoid background. Rather poor cellularity. Slender tumour cells with long cytoplasmic processes and elongated nuclei. Occasional vessel fragments and 'muscle giant cells' in background |
| Ganglion | Abundant myxoid background. Poor cellularity. Scattered round cells with rounded nuclei |
| Myxofibrosarcoma | Abundant myxoid background. Tumour tissue fragments mixed with dispersed cells. Curvilinear vessel fragments in the myxoid matrix. Variable cellular and nuclear atypia |
| Low-grade fibromyxoid sarcoma | Variable pattern, often myxoid background. Dispersed cells mixed with cell clusters. Spindle cells with slight to moderate atypia. Occasionally curvilinear vessel fragments in the myxoid matrix |
| Myxoid liposarcoma | Abundant myxoid background. Tumour tissue fragments with myxoid matrix and a distinct branching capillary network. Slight to moderately atypical lipoblasts |
| Extraskeletal myxoid chondrosarcoma | Varying amount of myxoid matrix. Cell clusters, cell balls and branching cells mixed with dispersed cells. Rounded, elongated cells. Rounded, ovoid or spindly nuclei. Slight to moderate atypia |

### Cytological findings: angioleiomyoma (Fig. 29.33)

- The yield is more often poor than moderate or rich
- Predominantly dissociated cells, small groups or runs of cells may be seen
- Uniform spindle cells with bland chromatin and small nucleoli. Nuclei occasionally blunt-ended or cigar-shaped
- Collagenous matrix fragments with embedded tumour cells are occasionally present.

According to our experience, angioleiomyoma is difficult to diagnose correctly in FNA smears. Only one study comprising 10 cases has been published and none of these cases were correctly diagnosed as angioleiomyoma, the majority having been diagnosed as a benign soft tissue lesion or tumour of other histotype.[32]

## Leiomyoma of deep soft tissue

Leiomyoma of deep soft tissue is a relatively rare tumour predominantly arising in the extremities or in the abdominal cavity and pelvic peritoneum. The abdominal tumours almost always occur in women.

Histologically, these leiomyomas are composed of interlacing bundles of spindly eosinophilic cells closely resembling normal smooth muscle cells with little nuclear pleomorphism. Degenerative changes such as fibrosis, hyalinisation and myxoid change are common in large tumours. The mitotic activity is very low, with the number of mitoses not exceeding 1/50 high power fields.

### Cytological findings: leiomyoma of deep soft tissue

- Dispersed cells, clusters, occasionally small tissue fragments
- Naked nuclei common
- Low to moderate anisokaryosis
- Blunt-ended elongated or truncated nuclei
- Small nucleoli
- Abundant grey or blue cytoplasm (MGG) in dispersed cells
- Fragments have a bluish red background matrix (MGG).

FNA features of deep-seated leiomyoma are limited. In our experience, the most important clue to the diagnosis is the

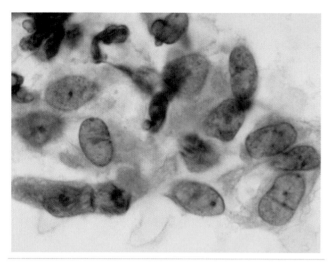

**Fig. 29.33** Angioleiomyoma. A small group of spindle cells with blunt-ended bland nuclei with small nucleoli (H&E).

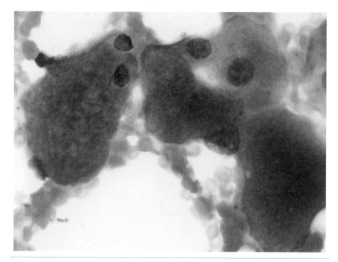

**Fig. 29.35** Adult rhabdomyoma. Large cells with abundant granulated cytoplasm and rounded nuclei with prominent nucleoli (MGG).

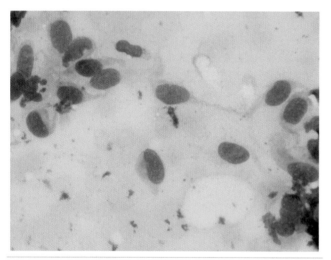

**Fig. 29.34** Soft tissue leiomyoma. The tumour cells have faintly stained grey-blue cytoplasm and blunt-ended uniform nuclei (MGG).

characteristics typical of smooth muscle cells including blunt-ended, 'cigar-shaped', elongated or ovoid nuclei of varying size, nuclei are often truncated and sometimes contain vacuoles. The chromatin is finely granular and nucleoli small. The cytoplasm in preserved dispersed cells is light grey to blue on MGG staining (Fig. 29.34). Mitoses should not be present.

There are two important differential diagnoses: low-grade malignant leiomyosarcoma and extra-abdominal desmoid fibromatosis. At low power magnification, the overall pattern in smears is similar in leiomyosarcoma and desmoid fibromatosis; a mixture of dispersed cells and cell clusters, many stripped nuclei and stromal fragments. The presence of single mitotic figures and/or focally more than marked anisokaryosis should warn the cytopathologist against making a definitive diagnosis of deep leiomyoma.

## Tumours of striated muscle

An exception to the generalisation that the benign soft tissue tumours outnumber their malignant counterparts, rhabdomyoma

is a rare neoplasm compared with rhabdomyosarcoma. Two main variants, adult and foetal, are distinguished, and a third similarly rare tumour, the genital type, develops in the vagina. Descriptions of the cytological features have been published.[33] Similar findings have been described; the smears including large elongated cells resembling muscle fibres, with large nuclei and prominent nucleoli. The cytoplasm is abundant and granulated, cross-striation is a rare feature (Fig. 29.35). Naked nuclei are a common find. The most important differential diagnosis is granular cell tumour. Rhabdomyomas typically express desmin and myoglobin.

## Tumours of blood vessels

Localised haemangiomas are extremely common, particularly in childhood. Structurally, they are difficult to distinguish from hamartomas, malformations and reactive vascular proliferations, such as pyogenic granuloma, since all of these lesions are composed of well-formed blood vessels. Capillary and cavernous patterns are recognised microscopically, and there are other less common variants.

Aspirations of any type of haemangioma invariably yield copious blood. The smears are usually poor in cells, but often include cells with spindle-shaped or ovoid nuclei with a varying amount of indistinct cytoplasm (Fig. 29.36). Macrophages containing haemosiderin pigment may be found. In our experience, aspirates are not characteristic and are usually non-diagnostic. However, clinical findings in case of intramuscular haemangiomas may be highly suggestive since these are deep-seated tumours, which increase in size and become painful during exercise, yielding abundant blood on aspiration, with few cells.

## Tumours of uncertain histogenesis

### Intramuscular myxoma

The intramuscular myxoma is a benign soft tissue tumour of uncertain histogenesis which generally occurs in the middle-aged or elderly. Most common sites are the thigh, shoulder

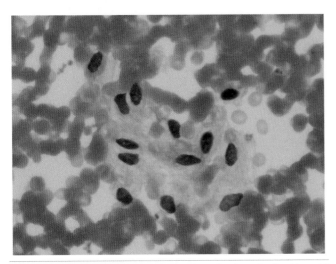

**Fig. 29.36** Haemangioma. A small cluster of spindle-shaped cells with ovoid nuclei in a haemorrhagic back ground (MGG).

region and buttock. Because of the deep location and a rather firm consistency intramuscular myxoma may be suspicious of a sarcoma clinically.

Histologically, the intramuscular myxoma is a paucicellular lesion with an abundant myxoid and poorly vascularised stroma. The tumour cells have bland nuclei and long, slender cytoplasmic processes. The cells are elongated or triangular. Macrophages with vacuolated cytoplasm are often present. The myxoma infiltrates the striated muscle and myxoma cells together with regenerating muscle fibres are seen peripherally.

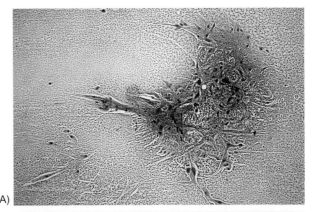

(A)

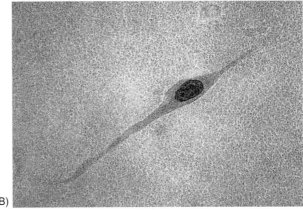

(B)

**Fig. 29.37** Intramuscular myxoma. (A) Overview: an abundant myxoid background matrix and myxoid tumour fragment containing spindle cells with bipolar cytoplasm (MGG). (B) The typical myxoma cell has very long, thin cytoplasmic processes (H&E).

### Cytological findings: intramuscular myxoma

- Colourless, stringy, glue-like fluid on aspiration
- Abundant myxoid background
- Predominantly dispersed cells intermingled with scanty tissue fragments
- Occasionally vessel fragments in the background matrix
- Slender tumour cells, long thin uni-or bipolar cytoplasmic processes
- Elongated nuclei, uniform chromatin
- Scattered large macrophage-like cells with abundant vacuolated cytoplasm.

The cytological findings on FNA have been published[34] and in our files we have FNA smears from more than 30 tumours. Characteristically, the aspirate consists of a few drops of stringy myxoid colourless fluid, not easily spread. This fluid is blue or violet on MGG and faintly eosinophilic on H&E stains. The cellularity is generally poor. Dispersed cells mingle with a few tissue fragments of loosely attached cells in the myxoid background matrix (Fig. 29.37A). The cells are usually elongated, with cytoplasmic processes which may be extremely long (Fig. 29.37B). They have ovoid, elongated or sometimes rounded nuclei. Cells with rounded nuclei may have abundant triangular or polyhedral cytoplasm, blue or violet with MGG stains, and which may contain a single large vacuole or sometimes several. Binucleated cells may also be found. The chromatin texture is uniformly finely granular and nucleoli, if any, are small. A few vessel strands may be observed in the background matrix.

### Diagnostic pitfalls: intramuscular myxoma

A number of benign and malignant soft tissue tumours with abundant myxoid background in smears must be considered in the differential diagnosis. Benign nerve sheath tumours, deep-seated nodular fasciitis, ganglion, myxoid liposarcoma, low-grade myxofibrosarcoma, low-grade fibromyxoid sarcoma and extraskeletal myxoid chondrosarcoma are important diagnostic pitfalls (Table 29.3).

## Ossifying fibromyxoid tumour

This is a rare tumour, first described in 1989. It is a subcutaneous tumour, predominantly arising in adults. Common sites are the extremities but it has been observed in other sites such as the head and neck region and the trunk.

It is a well-circumscribed, lobulated lesion with a fibrous capsule. The lesional cells are rounded, ovoid or spindle shaped with a pale or eosinophilic cytoplasm and uniform rounded nuclei containing small nucleoli. In the majority of tumours, a shell of mature bone, more or less complete is seen within the fibrous capsule. Immunohistochemically, the tumour cells express S-100 protein in most cases and smooth muscle actin in about 50% of cases.

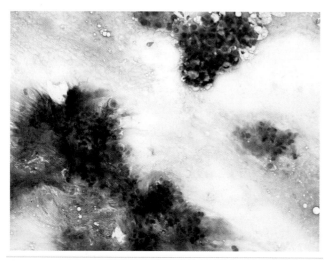

**Fig. 29.38** Mixed tumour of soft tissue. In a myxoid, partly fibrillar background matrix groups and clusters of rounded epithelial-like cells (MGG).

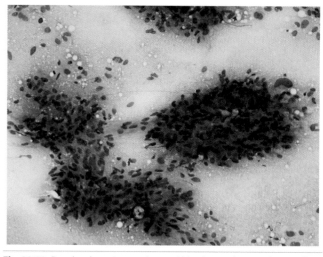

**Fig. 29.39** Parachordoma. In a partly myxoid background matrix clusters of more or less tightly packed rounded epithelial-like cells. Note the similarity between mixed tumour of soft tissue and parachordoma in FNA-material (MGG).

## Cytological findings: ossifying fibromyxoid tumour

- Variable cellularity
- Dispersed cells, cell clusters and acinar structures in variable amount of myxoid matrix
- Epithelioid-like cells with rounded or ovoid nuclei with slight anisokaryosis
- Often paracentral nuclei in rather abundant cytoplasm.

The cytological features of ossifying fibromyxoid tumour have not been sufficiently evaluated. The cytologic findings have so far been described in one case.[35] We have one case of ossifying fibromyxoid tumour in our files. The diagnostic pitfalls include tumours with rounded epithelioid-like cells set in a myxoid matrix such as mixed tumour of soft tissue and chondroid syringoma.

## Mixed tumour/myoepithelioma of soft tissue

These tumours, recently categorised, are well circumscribed lesions made up of epithelial-and/or myoepithelial-like cells set in within a chondromyxoid or hyalinised stroma. When myoepithelial cells predominate they resemble salivary pleomorphic adenomas or chondroid syringoma.

Most cases are subcutaneous tumours of the extremities in middle-aged adults. We have had the opportunity to study FNA samples from two tumours and their cytomorphology was similar to that of pleomorphic adenoma or chondroid syringoma (Fig. 29.38). The most important differential diagnosis of subcutaneous tumours is chondroid syringoma and in deep-seated tumours extraskeletal myxoid chondrosarcoma.

## Parachordoma

Parachordoma is a rare soft tissue tumour. It was first described in 1951. Parachordoma is included because it is an important differential diagnosis to extraskeletal myxoid chondrosarcoma. It is debated whether parachordoma is a peripheral chordoma or should be considered as a variant of mixed tumour of soft tissue. At present, parachordoma is presented and discussed

together with myoepithelioma and mixed tumour of soft tissue.[12]

Histologically, parachordomas display a myxoid and/or hyaline background matrix in which cords or acinar-like structures of cells are embedded. The tumour cells are epithelioid, rounded or spindle shaped; vacuolated cells resembling the physaliferous in chordoma are occasionally present. Parachordomas express S-100 protein and high-molecular weight cytokeratins. We have had the opportunity to study two cases of this rare tumour. Common to both was an abundant myxoid background matrix. The tumour cells were rounded or elongated with rounded or ovoid bland nuclei. Some tumour cells had a vacuolated cytoplasm and paracentral nuclei. The cellular pleomorphism was moderate and the cells were both dispersed and arranged in groups or cords (Fig. 29.39).

## Malignant soft tissue tumours

Sarcomas represent up to 1% of all malignant tumours, at present more than 50 different histotypes have been recognised.[12] Of these, liposarcoma, leiomyosarcoma together with pleomorphic sarcoma (malignant fibrous histiocytoma) are considered to be the most common entities. Other relatively frequent sarcomas are myxofibrosarcoma, synovial sarcoma and malignant peripheral nerve sheath tumour (MPNST) and dermatofibrosarcoma protuberans. Rhabdomyosarcoma, the Ewing family of tumours (ES/PNET), neuroblastoma and angiosarcoma are less frequent while extraskeletal myxoid chondrosarcoma, clear cell sarcoma, epithelioid sarcoma, low-grade fibromyxoid sarcoma, extrarenal rhabdoid tumour and alveolar soft part sarcoma are rare histotypes. These data are in accord with data from the Central Soft Tissue Sarcoma Registry of the Scandinavian Sarcoma Group (a multidisciplinary association of the Nordic Countries) and related to registered sarcomas from 1995 to March 2008; about 5000 sarcomas were registered during this 13-year period. At present, the most common sarcomas referred to the Musculoskeletal Tumour Centre, Lund University Hospital and primarily needled are leiomyosarcoma, liposarcoma, myxofibrosarcoma, pleomorphic sarcoma (malignant fibrous histiocytoma) and synovial sarcoma. Rhabdomyosarcoma, the Ewing family of tumours, MPNST and low-grade fibromyxoid sarcoma are occasionally needled and rare sarcomas such as clear cell sarcoma, epithelioid sarcoma, angiosarcoma, extrarenal rhabdoid tumour and alveolar soft part sarcoma are very rarely referred for FNA.

## Malignant tumours of adipose tissue

In the WHO classification (Box 29.1) of soft tissue tumours,[12] liposarcomas are divided in the following subtypes.

### Atypical lipomatous tumour/well-differentiated liposarcoma

The term atypical lipomatous (ATL) tumour is used when the tumours are localised to the subcutis or musculature of the extremities because they follow a benign clinical course and do not recur or metastasise provided that they are removed with a clear margin. When these tumours arise in retroperitoneum, mediastinum or the spermatic cord they often recur and after multiple recurrences may dedifferentiate and metastasise. Thus it is the anatomical site and not the cytological appearance on FNA which determines the prognosis. The risk of dedifferentiation has been estimated to be 20% for retroperitoneal tumours and less than 2% for extremity tumours. The important cytological findings in smears from these tumours is the mixture of ordinary lipoma-like fragments (often with different-sized-adipocytes) and a varying number of atypical cells with large, irregular hyperchromatic nuclei. Atypical lipoblasts with cytoplasmic vacuoles and scalloped nuclei may be present but are not necessary for the diagnosis (Fig. 29.40).

Dedifferentiated liposarcoma is diagnosed when a well-differentiated liposarcoma also displays cellular material from a high-grade malignant sarcoma, spindle type or pleomorphic. The clue to the diagnosis, cytological as well as histological, is that it is possible to diagnose a well-differentiated liposarcoma and a high-grade sarcoma in the same tissue specimen or smear.

### Myxoid liposarcoma

Myxoid liposarcoma is the commonest subtype, consisting of a mixture of round or ovoid uniform mesenchymal cells and small lipoblasts in a prominent myxoid stroma with anastomosing capillaries. A subset of myxoid liposarcoma are hypercellular with numerous atypical rounded cells with sparse cytoplasm

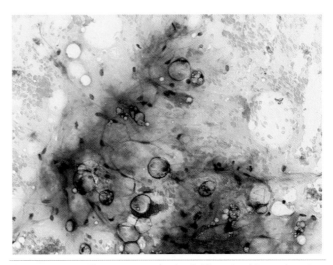

**Fig. 29.40** Atypical lipomatous tumour/well-differentiated liposarcoma. In this case, slight to moderately atypical, uni-and multivacuolated lipoblasts predominate (MGG).

mixed with atypical lipoblasts. The stroma is less myxoid and the capillary network less prominent. This hypercellular variant was formerly diagnosed as round cell liposarcoma. One reason to re-name the former round cell liposarcoma is that myxoid liposarcoma as well as round cell sarcoma were found to harbour the same chromosomal aberration, the reciprocal translocation t(12;16(q13;p11)) (see Table 34.1, p. 892).

**Cytological findings: myxoid liposarcoma (Fig. 29.41)**

- Abundant myxoid back ground substance
- Vacuolated tumour tissue fragments with myxoid matrix and branching capillary network
- Almost no dispersed cells
- Uni-or multivacuolated slightly atypical lipoblasts, often alongside the capillary fragments
- Spindly or rounded uniform mesenchymal cells other than lipoblasts
- No mitoses.

**Cytological findings: hypercellular myxoid liposarcoma (round cell liposarcoma) (Fig. 29.42)**

- Less conspicuous myxoid matrix and capillaries compared to myxoid liposarcoma
- Often rich yield of rounded or ovoid tumour cells with variable atypia
- Atypical lipoblasts
- Mitotic figures may be present.

### Pleomorphic liposarcoma

Pleomorphic liposarcoma is a high-grade malignant sarcoma with markedly atypical cells. Giant multinucleated tumour cells are often numerous and hyaline cytoplasmic droplets are occasionally present in the tumour cells. The most important clue to the diagnosis is the presence of highly atypical uni-or multinucleated lipoblasts. Mitoses are numerous and foci of necrosis common.

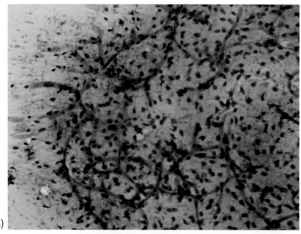

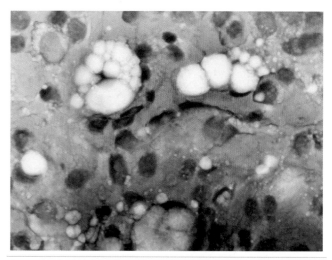

**Fig. 29.42** Hypercellular myxoid liposarcoma (round cell liposarcoma). In a myxoid background numerous uni-and multivacuolated lipoblasts exhibiting moderate cellular atypia (MGG).

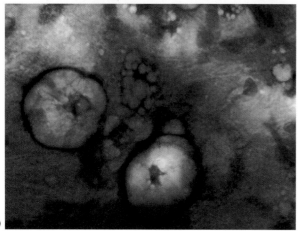

**Fig. 29.41** Myxoid liposarcoma. (A) A moderately cellular tissue fragment with a myxoid background matrix and a network of branching capillaries. A few univacuolated lipoblasts are seen (MGG). (B) Detail from the tumour fragment in (A). Multivacuolated lipoblasts with scalloped nuclei (MGG).

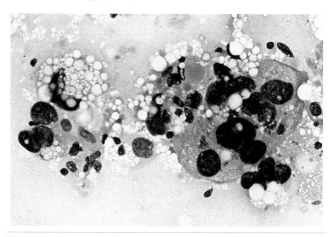

**Fig. 29.43** Pleomorphic liposarcoma. Highly atypical lipoblasts some of which are multinucleated (MGG).

### Cytological findings: liposarcoma (Fig. 29.43)

- A mixture of cell clusters and dispersed cells
- Pleomorphic tumour cells, often multinucleated
- More or less numerous highly atypical lipoblasts
- Tumour cells with multiple hyaline cytoplasmic droplets occasionally present
- Foci of necrotic tumour not uncommon.

The cytological appearance of the various subtypes of liposarcoma has been described in retrospective studies.[34,36–39] Important cytological features in liposarcoma are summarised in Table 29.4.

### Diagnostic pitfalls: pleomorphic liposarcoma

The most important benign tumours, which may be misdiagnosed as liposarcoma, are lipoma with regressive changes, hibernoma, chondroid lipoma and intramuscular myxoma. The two former tumours are bland, while myxomas do not include lipoblasts.

Among sarcomas, high-grade pleomorphic sarcoma (malignant fibrous histiocytoma), myxofibrosarcoma and extraskeletal

myxoid chondrosarcoma are the most frequent pitfalls. Soft tissue metastases from renal clear cell carcinoma has been misdiagnosed as hypercellular myxoid liposarcoma (personal observation). The best clue to a correct diagnosis of myxoid and pleomorphic liposarcoma is the identification of true lipoblasts.

## Malignant fibroblastic/myofibroblastic and fibrohistiocytic tumours

The most important sarcomas for the cytopathologist are pleomorphic malignant fibrous histiocytoma (undifferentiated high-grade pleomorphic sarcoma), myxofibrosarcoma, dermatofibrosarcoma protuberans and low-grade fibromyxoid sarcoma. Classical adult fibrosarcoma is very seldom the target for FNA as low-grade myofibroblastic sarcoma and atypical fibroxanthoma. Of the paediatric sarcomas, infantile fibrosarcoma is very infrequently aspirated.

### Pleomorphic malignant fibrous histiocytoma (undifferentiated high-grade pleomorphic sarcoma)

Malignant fibrous histiocytoma (MFH) was recognised as a distinctive sarcoma of soft tissue and bone of probable histiocytic

**Table 29.4** Important cytological findings in liposarcoma

| Type | Background | Cytology |
|------|-----------|----------|
| Atypical lipomatous tumour/well-differentiated | | |
| liposarcoma | No background | Lipoma-like fragments with different-sized fat cells. In and between fragments large atypical cells with hyperchromatic nuclei. Occasionally lipoblast-like cells |
| Myxoid, paucicellular | Granular myxoid, bluish red (MGG) | Tissue fragments with myxoid matrix with distinct capillary network. Rounded cells with slight atypia. Uni- or multivacuolated slightly atypical lipoblasts |
| Myxoid, cellular (round cell) | Myxoid or none | Numerous dissociated cells mixed with highly cellular tissue fragments. Numerous atypical lipoblasts. Capillary network not prominent |
| Pleomorphic | Necrosis and cell debris may be seen | Dispersed cells and cell clusters. Marked cellular and nuclear atypia. Multinucleated tumour cells. Highly atypical lipoblasts |
| Spindle cell | Not evaluated | Not evaluated |

origin in 1963. Over the years several subtypes were described. However, around 1970, MFH as a specific tumour entity was questioned for several reasons; consensus was never reached on the histogenesis and furthermore the various subtypes (pleomorphic, myxoid, giant cell, angiomatoid and inflammatory) proved to show obvious clinical and morphological heterogeneity.

According to the WHO fascicle 'Tumours of soft tissue and bone', published in 2002, pleomorphic MFH is at present defined as 'a small group of undifferentiated pleomorphic sarcomas. Current technology does not show a definable line of differentiation'.[12]

Angiomatoid and myxoid MFH (myxofibrosarcoma) are regarded as specific tumour entities.

The most important criterion for diagnosis is the failure to demonstrate any line of differentiation in spite of thorough histological examination supplemented with ancillary techniques. In the re-evaluation of various materials, a surprisingly high number of pleomorphic MFH proved to exhibit lipogenic, myogenic and Schwann cell differentiation as well as non-mesenchymal histogenesis.[40,41] Due to this new knowledge, we do not use the diagnosis MFH. Instead, we suggest descriptive diagnoses such as pleomorphic sarcoma, high-grade spindle cell sarcoma or high-grade spindle and pleomorphic sarcoma.

### Cytological findings: pleomorphic sarcoma of MFH type

- Often highly cellular yield
- Tissue fragments, cell clusters, dispersed tumour cells
- Spindle-shaped fibroblast-like cells
- Pleomorphic, histiocyte-like tumour cells
- Tumour cells of indeterminate origin

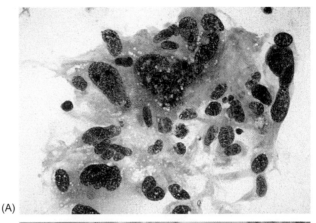

(A)

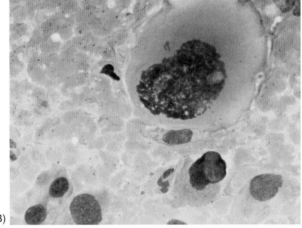

(B)

**Fig. 29.44** Pleomorphic sarcoma of MFH type (A,B). (A) A cluster of loosely attached pleomorphic cells with marked anisokaryosis (MGG). (B) Atypical mitosis (MGG).

- Large multinucleated tumour cells
- Often marked nuclear pleomorphism and atypia. Large irregular nucleoli
- Mitotic figures, often atypical.

Smears are generally cellular, but necrosis, cystic degeneration or haemorrhage occasionally dominate the picture. In such cases, very few preserved tumour cells may be found, despite thorough screening.

Marked anisocytosis and anisokaryosis are the rule in high-grade malignant tumours. However, it is always possible to recognise fibroblast-like cells with fusiform or ovoid atypical nuclei and elongated cytoplasm, as well as cells resembling histiocytes with abundant cytoplasm and large eccentric rounded or irregular nuclei. The cytoplasm in the histiocyte-like cells is occasionally vacuolated. Multinucleated giant cells are always found and bizarre nuclei often seen. Normal and atypical mitoses are common (Fig. 29.44).

The cytomorphology of pleomorphic sarcoma of MFH type has been described in detail.[42]

### Diagnostic pitfalls: pleomorphic sarcoma of MFH type

Pleomorphic sarcoma of the MFH type may be difficult to distinguish from other pleomorphic sarcomas, such as pleomorphic liposarcoma, high-grade pleomorphic leiomyosarcoma and pleomorphic MPNST. The presence of

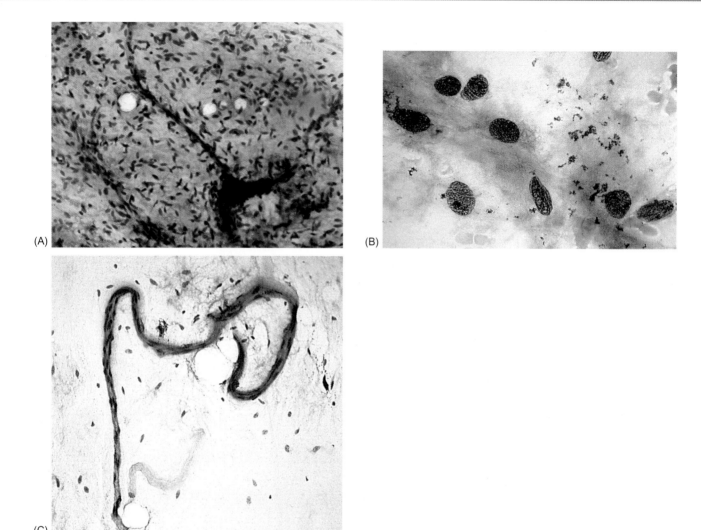

**Fig. 29.45** Myxofibrosarcoma. (A) A moderately cellular tissue fragment with myxoid back ground matrix and curved vessel fragments (MGG). (B) Spindle shaped moderately atypical cells in a myxoid background matrix (MGG). (C) Vessel fragment in the myxoid background (MGG).

highly atypical lipoblasts favours liposarcoma as the presence of cigar-shaped, often segmented nuclei leiomyosarcoma.

Clinically, the most important pitfall is to distinguish pleomorphic sarcoma from the soft tissue presentation of malignant pleomorphic tumours of non-mesenchymal histogenesis. Primary soft tissue presentation of anaplastic large cell lymphoma as well as soft tissue metastases from anaplastic carcinoma and sarcoma-like malignant melanoma are the most important differential diagnoses. When sufficient material for routine staining as well as immunocytochemistry is aspirated, a battery of antibodies often resolves the diagnostic problem as staining with cytokeratin markers, S-100 protein, HMB45 and Melan A to diagnose metastatic carcinoma and malignant melanoma, respectively. Positive immunolabelling with CD30, EMA, and often ALK-1 is typical for anaplastic large cell lymphoma.

## Myxofibrosarcoma

Myxofibrosarcoma (MFS), earlier designated myxoid type of MFH, is typically a subcutaneous extremity tumour of elderly patients, although it may occur in skeletal muscle and retroperitoneum. Histologically, myxofibrosarcoma is a lobulated tumour with a more or less abundant myxoid back ground matrix. A typical feature is the presence of numerous thin-walled curvilinear vessels in the myxoid matrix. In low-grade tumours fibroblast/myofibroblast-like cells with slight to moderate atypia predominate, while high-grade tumours exhibit a marked atypia with the presence of multinucleated tumour cells. Tumour cells with vacuolated cytoplasm (pseudolipoblasts) may be found.

### Cytological findings: myxofibrosarcoma (Fig. 29.45)

- Abundant myxoid back ground. Macroscopically aspirates resemble aspirates from intramuscular myxoma
- Mixture of dispersed cells, cell clusters and small tumour tissue fragments
- Curved vessel fragments in the myxoid matrix
- Predominance of slightly to moderately atypical fibroblast-like cells in low-grade tumours
- Marked nuclear pleomorphism and atypia in high-grade tumours.

From the clinical point of view, the most important differential diagnoses are nodular fasciitis and intramuscular myxoma with regard to the low-grade malignant MFS. The tumour vasculature is a discriminating factor. In nodular fasciitis as well as in smears from intramuscular myxoma only a few vessel fragments are present in the myxoid matrix while aspirates from myxofibrosarcoma almost always exhibit rather numerous curved rather coarse vessel fragments. The vasculature is also important in the differential diagnosis versus myxoid liposarcoma; where in myxoid liposarcoma the branching capillary network is mainly seen in the tumour tissue fragments in contrast to MFS, where the vessels are embedded in the myxoid matrix. The cellular features of myxofibrosarcoma have been thoroughly evaluated in two publications.[34,43]

## Dermatofibrosarcoma protuberans

Dermatofibrosarcoma protuberans (DFSP) is a slowly growing low-grade malignant spindle cell sarcoma, most commonly seen in adults. DFSP is a dermal/subcutaneous tumour and predominantly arising in the extremities. Histologically, the common features are a storiform pattern composed of bland, slightly atypical spindle cells, infiltrating the subcutaneous fat. The tumour cells typically stain for CD34.

### Cytological findings: dermatofibrosarcoma protuberans (Fig. 29.46)

- Variable cellular yield
- Clusters or three-dimensional tumour fragments of cohesive spindle cells embedded in a collagenous matrix, occasionally with focal myxoid changes
- Dispersed cells not uncommon as naked nuclei
- Slight to moderate cellular and nuclear atypia.

Clinically, the most important differential diagnoses are cellular benign fibrous histiocytoma and neurilemmoma. Smears from DFSP are difficult to discriminate from other types of subcutaneous low-grade spindle cell sarcoma. The positivity for CD34 excludes fibrous histiocytoma and neurilemmoma. Apart from single case reports one series of 12 cases has been published.[44]

## Low-grade fibromyxoid sarcoma (LGFMS)

Low-grade fibromyxoid sarcoma, first described in 1987 is a rare variant of fibrosarcoma. Most cases occur in the extremities in patients of any age, most commonly in young adults. Histologically LGFMS is characterised by a mixture of collagenous and myxoid areas, often low cellularity, bland spindle cells and curvilinear vessels predominantly in myxoid areas. In up to 40% of LGFMS, rosette-like structures made up of hyalinised collagen surrounded by plump fibroblasts are present. Immunohistochemical stains only demonstrate vimentin-positivity. Apart from single case reports, the cytologic features of LGFMS have been extensively studied in a report of eight cases.[45]

### Cytological findings: low-grade fibromyxoid sarcoma (Fig. 29.47)

- Loosely cohesive cell clusters and three-dimensional tumour tissue fragments admixed with dispersed cells and stripped nuclei
- Alternating a collagenous or myxoid back ground matrix
- Variable presence of curvilinear vessel fragments
- Infrequently rosette-like structures
- Slight to moderate atypia in spindled fibroblast-like cells.

Due to the alternating tissue pattern of collagenous and myxoid matrix in varying proportions in FNA smears and the

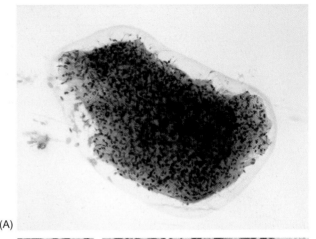

(A)

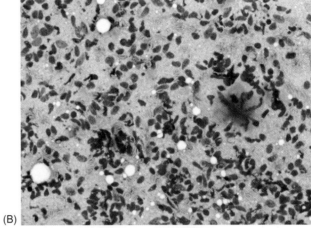

(B)

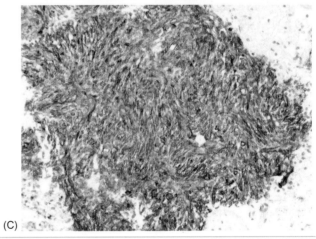

(C)

**Fig. 29.46** Dermatofibrosarcoma protuberans. (A) A cellular tumour fragment of tightly packed, cohesive spindle cells (H&E). (B) The occasionally myxoid collagenous matrix is best visualised in MGG. Numerous, irregularly distributed moderately atypical spindle cells (MGG). (C) Cell block preparation. The spindle cells are typically positive for CD34. (Immunoperoxidase).

rather bland spindle tumour cell population, LGFMS is easily mistaken for a number of benign as well as mesenchymal tumours in FNA material. In one series a correct diagnosis was not rendered, with neurilemmoma, desmoid fibromatosis and myxofibrosarcoma suggested as differential diagnoses.[45] In our opinion, it is not possible to diagnose LGFMS specifically on FNA and often difficult to prove that it is a low-grade spindle cell sarcoma (see Table 34.1, p. 892).

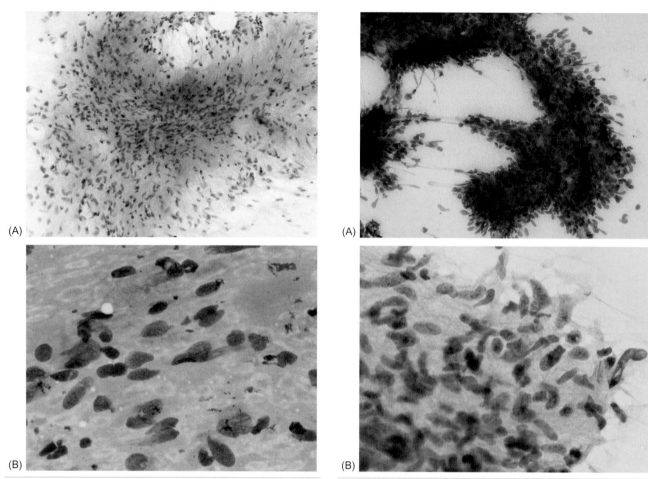

**Fig. 29.47** Low-grade fibromyxoid sarcoma. (A) A tumour fragment with unevenly distributed spindly cells in a collagenous back ground matrix (H&E). (B) In this case the moderately atypical spindle cells are embedded in a myxoid back ground matrix (MGG).

**Fig. 29.48** Infantile fibrosarcoma. (A) A cellular cohesive fascicle of spindle cells (MGG). (B) The tumour cells are fibroblast-like with fusiform or ovoid bland nuclei (H&E).

## Atypical fibroxanthoma

The superficial cutaneous atypical fibroxanthoma is histologically indistinguishable from pleomorphic malignant fibrous histiocytoma and is at present regarded as a cutaneous variant of this lesion. In FNA material, too, the cell pattern resembles that of pleomorphic malignant MFH.

## Low-grade myofibroblastic sarcoma

Low-grade myofibroblastic sarcoma is at present considered as a distinct entity composed of atypical myofibroblasts. It occurs predominantly in adults and most common sites are the extremities and head and neck region. Histologically, the lesional cells are elongated with ill-defined cytoplasm and fusiform nuclei. The cellular pleomorphism and atypia is slight to moderate and the spindled tumour cells show a storiform or fascicular pattern. Immunohistochemically the tumour cells display an immunophenotype typical for myofibroblasts; variably smooth muscle actin positive and desmin negative or vice versa.

The cytological features of this sarcoma are not specific, with single cases in our files diagnosed as low-grade malignant spindle cell sarcoma.

The rare infantile fibrosarcoma is predominantly seen before the age of two. Congenital tumours have been reported. Most arise in the extremities and present as large tumours. Histologically, the main feature is fascicles of fibroblasts with slight atypia. Mitoses may be numerous. A haemangiopericytoma-like vascular pattern as well as a myxoid background matrix may be seen. We have had the opportunity to study FNA material from one case, a large tumour in the lower leg. The predominant cytological findings were streaky and cohesive fascicles and clusters of fibroblast-like uniform cells with bland nuclei (Fig. 29.48). The most important differential diagnosis is fibrous hamartoma of infancy.

## Malignant tumours of peripheral nerves

This group of tumours (MPNST) includes those malignant nerve sheath tumours, which develop in patients with von Recklinghausen's disease, as well as those arising spontaneously in peripheral nerves. About 5–10% of soft tissue sarcomas originate from peripheral nerves. Most patients are adults, but MPNST can also occur in children. Common sites are upper extremities, buttock, thigh, brachial plexus and from paraspinal nerves. MPNST usually arise from large- and medium-sized nerves. Histologically, most MPNST appear as spindle cell sarcomas featuring fascicles, a storiform pattern or a whorled arrangement of the tumour cells. The tumour cells are spindly with fusiform nuclei which often are comma-shaped, wavy or buckled. Pleomorphic cells as well as multinucleated tumour cells are found in some cases. Islands of heterotopic elements, such as mature bone and cartilage, with glandular elements and striated muscle less often seen, are present in 10–15 % of tumours. S-100 protein is reported to be focally positive in up to 70% and CD57 stains a large number of MPNST. However, CD57 also stains other histotypes of spindle cell sarcomas and is less valuable in the diagnostic evaluation.

The cytological findings on FNA have been reported in single cases, but also in one relatively large series.[46] The majority of cases in our files produced cellular smears composed of a mixture of fascicles of tightly packed sarcoma cells, dispersed cells and stripped nuclei. The cells within the fascicles had indistinct cytoplasm and elongated nuclei, often with pointed ends or wavy configuration (Fig. 29.49A). The tumour cells were often embedded in a fibrillary background substance similar to the background in neurilemmoma aspirates (Fig. 29.49B). The extent of nuclear and nucleolar atypia varied considerably and a uniform appearance of the sarcoma cells with only slight atypia was not uncommon. Less commonly, the smears featured pleomorphic or multinucleated tumour cells.

### Diagnostic pitfalls: malignant tumours of peripheral nerves

With regard to benign tumours, ancient neurilemmoma and cellular Schwannoma are the most important pitfalls. However, both these tumours demonstrate strong, diffuse staining with S-100 protein while the staining in MPNST is typically focal or negative. Among sarcomas, leiomyosarcoma, synovial sarcoma and fibrosarcoma may be diagnostic problems. High-grade MPNST featuring pleomorphic and multinucleated tumour cells may be difficult to distinguish from other pleomorphic sarcomas (Fig. 29.49C) (see Table 34.1, p. 892).

## Malignant tumours of smooth muscle

### Leiomyosarcoma

Leiomyosarcomas occur in adults, most frequently arising in the extremities, abdomen and retroperitoneum. A rare subset of leiomyosarcoma arises from larger veins. The histology of these tumours is diverse regardless of the site of origin, but the cutaneous and subcutaneous varieties are usually moderately differentiated. The tumour cells have a fascicular growth pattern and the nuclei are typically elongated, blunt-ended, cigar-shaped or segmented. Sometimes intranuclear vacuoles occur. High-grade pleomorphic leiomyosarcoma show marked cellular atypia with multinucleated giant tumour cells and often scattered osteoclast-like multinucleated giant cells. Epithelioid changes occur within some leiomyosarcomas with rounded cells showing clear or vacuolated cytoplasm.

### Cytological findings: leiomyosarcoma

- Very variable cell yield
- Cohesive clusters, tissue fragments or large fascicular tumour fragments
- Rather few dissociated cells
- Blue or magenta background matrix in clusters and fascicles
- Abundant cell cytoplasm with indistinct borders
- Degenerate bare nuclei
- Blunt ended or cigar-shaped elliptic nuclei, sometimes segmented or with nuclear vacuoles

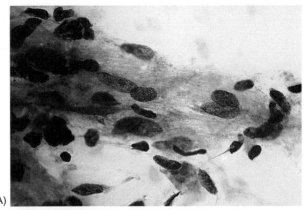

(A)

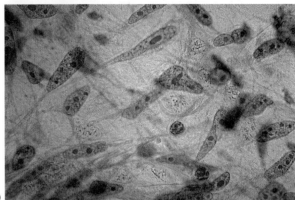

(B)

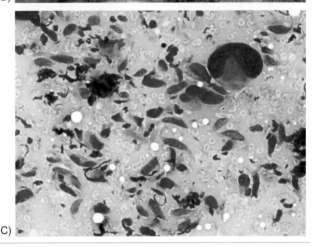

(C)

**Fig. 29.49** Malignant peripheral nerve sheath tumour. (A) Atypical spindle cells in a fibrillary background matrix. Note the nuclei with pointed ends (MGG). (B) Atypical spindle cells with fibrillar cytoplasm; nuclei have coarse chromatin and prominent nucleoli (H&E). (C) Occasionally in high-grade tumours marked cellular pleomorphism (MGG).

- Occasionally rounded epithelioid-like cells with rounded nuclei
- Marked pleomorphism in high-grade tumours with the presence of multinucleated osteoclast-like cells.

A typical smear includes tissue fragments, clusters or fascicles of cohesive cells mixed with a few dispersed cells, the latter often appearing as naked degenerate nuclei (Fig. 29.50A). The cells in fragments and clusters are embedded in a dense matrix, which is blue or magenta with MGG staining (Fig. 29.50B). Cell borders are indistinct and the cytoplasm dense, staining greyish-blue with MGG stains. The nuclei are cigar shaped or blunt ended

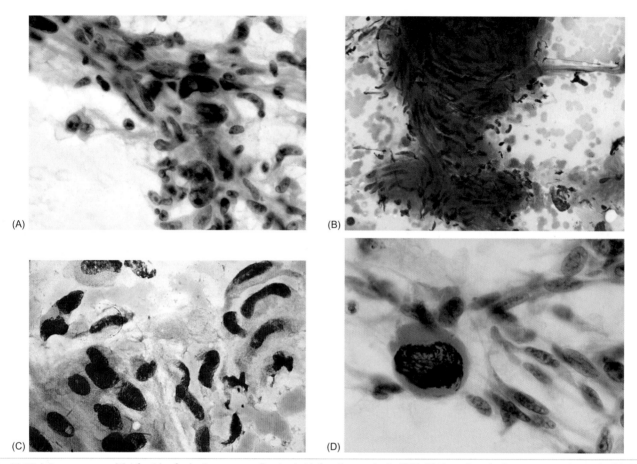

**Fig. 29.50**  Leiomyosarcoma. (A) A fascicle of cohesive tumour cells mixed with few dispersed cells (H&E). (B) The cells in the fragments are often embedded in a dense matrix (MGG). (C) Part of a fascicle of elongated cells with blunt-ended nuclei (MGG). (D) In high-grade tumours, mitotic figures may be found (H&E).

and often appear segmented or vacuolated (Fig. 29.50C). Pleomorphism is more marked in high-grade leiomyosarcomas and in these tumours multinucleated tumour giant cells can be seen. Occasionally in high-grade pleomorphic leiomyosarcomas scattered osteoclast-like cells are present in the smears. On careful screening, usually mitotic figures may be found (Fig. 29.50C). The FNA cytology of leiomyosarcoma has been described in one large series.[47]

### Diagnostic pitfalls: leiomyosarcoma

Leiomyosarcoma of low-grade malignancy with only moderate cellular atypia may be misdiagnosed as soft tissue leiomyoma or neurilemmoma. However, cigar-shaped segmented nuclei are not a feature of neurilemmoma and the presence of mitotic figures is not consistent with FNA aspirates from leiomyoma. Among sarcomas MPNST may be difficult to distinguish from leiomyosarcoma in FNA material, and high-grade leiomyosarcoma with marked cellular pleomorphism is easily mistaken for other pleomorphic sarcomas as pleomorphic malignant fibrous histiocytoma, pleomorphic PNST or pleomorphic liposarcoma. The presence of scattered highly atypical lipoblasts favour liposarcoma and immunocytochemistry can be helpful in problematic cases. Leiomyosarcoma stain positively with smooth muscle actin (SMA) and most often in FNA material at least focally with desmin and/or caldesmon (Fig. 29.51).The cytology of leiomyosarcoma with extensive epithelioid morphology is not well defined and it may be difficult to distinguish those tumours from poorly differentiated carcinoma.

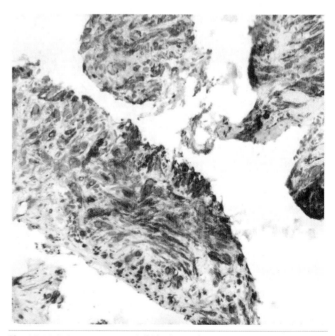

**Fig. 29.51**  Leiomyosarcoma. Cell block preparation stained with desmin (Immunoperoxidase).

Immunocytochemistry is of diagnostic help in those cases when positivity for SMA and desmin or caldesmon is present, however, it must be remembered that leiomyosarcoma may be focally cytokeratin positive.

## Malignant tumours of striated muscle

### Rhabdomyosarcoma

Rhabdomyosarcoma is an aggressive tumour predominantly of young adults and children, widely distributed anatomically, but found principally in the head and neck region, the genitourinary tract and retroperitoneum, and in the extremities. The classical main histological types in order of frequency are:

1. *Embryonal rhabdomyosarcoma*, composed of tumour tissue of variable cellularity which resembles developing muscle in the early embryo with some recognisable racquet-shaped rhabdomyoblasts. This is the commonest type and includes the botryoid sarcoma, a lobulated oedematous tumour that protrudes into various body cavities as the site of origin, particularly in the vagina as well as the spindle type predominantly occurring in the peritesticular area.
2. *Alveolar rhabdomyosarcoma*, showing an ill-defined alveolar pattern of packaging of tumour cells which cling to the surrounding fibrous tissue septa, mimicking an adenocarcinoma. In the solid type of alveolar rhabdomyosarcoma the alveolar pattern is replaced by sheets of tumour cells.
3. *Pleomorphic rhabdomyosarcoma*, a tumour of elderly adults, consisting of a mixture of rounded and pleomorphic tumour cells including bizarre rhabdomyoblasts. The classification of rhabdomyosarcoma in children and adolescents has been debated due to the need for an accepted and reproducible histopathological classification with prognostic significance. In 1995, the 'International Classification of Rhabdomyosarcoma' was introduced.[48] This classification scheme is based on prognostically verified histopathological subgroups. As is evident from the classification, alveolar rhabdomyosarcoma belongs to the poor prognosis group. Furthermore, it was proposed that any degree of alveolar pattern or cytomorphology in a rhabdomyosarcoma would imply a bad prognostic sign. This is of interest in the FNA diagnosis of rhabdomyosarcoma when the diagnosis also includes subtyping.

### Cytological findings: rhabdomyosarcoma

- Cell rich aspirates
- Stripped nuclei in cytoplasmic background
- Predominantly dissociated cells
- Variable pleomorphism
- Myoblast like cells
- Cytoplasmic vacuolation
- Binucleated and multinucleated cells.

The cytological appearance of the various subtypes of rhabdomyosarcoma has been addressed in several reports.[49–51] Although rhabdomyosarcoma is grouped with the so-called small round cell malignancies the overall pattern in embryonal rhabdomyosarcoma, apart from the spindle type, is predominantly pleomorphic (Fig. 29.52). Broad-spectrum tumour cells having fusiform, rounded, tadpole and strap-like shapes, occasionally embedded in a variably myxoid matrix, are often the rule. The alveolar rhabdomyosarcoma, however, is a true small cell malignant tumour.

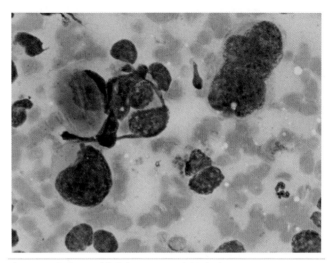

**Fig. 29.52** Embryonal rhabdomyosarcoma. Marked variation in size, preserved cells often myoblast-like with eccentric nuclei (MGG).

Dispersed cells are more common than cell clusters or fragments and the cytoplasm is fragile. Stripped nuclei in a blue-grey background of smeared cytoplasm are not uncommon, often demonstrating a 'tigroid' appearance. The typical cells resemble small rounded primitive myoblasts with eosinophilic cytoplasm on H&E (Fig. 29.53A) or greyish blue with MGG staining and with rounded paracentral nuclei and prominent nucleoli. The cytoplasm is often vacuolated due to dissolved glycogen. Multinucleated tumour cells are found (Fig. 29.53B). Our experience as well as that of other investigators has shown that definitive typing of alveolar and embryonal rhabdomyosarcoma is possible in most cases (see Ch. 33, p. 882 and Table 34.1, p. 892).[49]

We have also had the opportunity to study a case of the spindle cell variant of embryonal rhabdomyosarcoma. In a cellular aspirate the majority of cells were spindle shaped with fusiform or elongated nuclei. The nuclei had alternating pointed or blunt ends and showed moderate pleomorphism (Fig. 29.54). The pleomorphic rhabdomyosarcoma may be difficult to distinguish from other types of pleomorphic sarcomas. Highly atypical, often bizarre, myoblast-like cells with eosinophilic cytoplasm on H&E may be present in the smears (Fig. 29.55).

### Diagnostic pitfalls: rhabdomyosarcoma

The most important diagnostic difficulties lie in distinguishing between the different histological types of small round cell malignant tumours. These include rhabdomyosarcoma, neuroblastoma, the Ewing family of tumours, desmoplastic small round cell sarcoma and precursor lymphoma/leukaemia (Table 29.5). The immunocytochemical hallmarks of the various subtypes of rhabdomyosarcoma are the positive stainings with muscle specific actin, desmin and the specific markers for striated muscle, myogenin and Myo-D1 (Fig. 29.56). Myoglobin is occasionally present in more differentiated myoblasts. Almost all cases of alveolar rhabdomyosarcoma present with the chromosomal aberration t(2;13)(q35;q14), resulting in a fusion transcript between the PAX3 and FKHR genes. Cytogenetic investigation of FNA samples to diagnose the typical aberration have been published.[52]

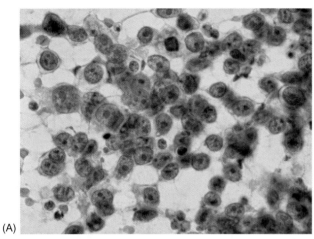

(A)

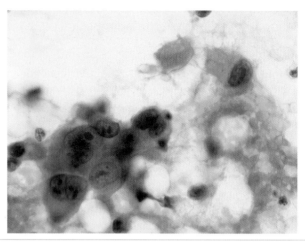

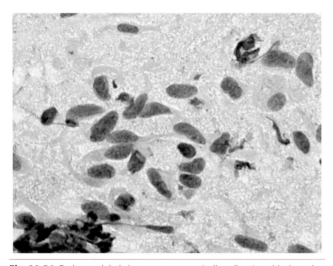

(B)

**Fig. 29.53** (A,B) Alveolar rhabdomyosarcoma. The typical cells are small, rhabdomyoblast-like with eosinophilic cytoplasm and rounded paracentral nuclei with prominent nucleoli (H&E). (B) The small cell population often mixed with multinucleated tumour cells (H&E).

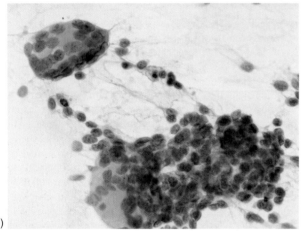

**Fig. 29.54** Embryonal rhabdomyosarcoma, spindle cell variant. Moderately pleomorphic spindly cells with fusiform nuclei with alternating pointed or blunt ends (H&E).

**Fig. 29.55** Pleomorphic rhabdomyosarcoma. One clue to the diagnosis is the presence of highly atypical myoblast-like cells with eosinophilic cytoplasm and eccentric atypical nuclei (H&E).

**Table 29.5** Important cytological findings in the differential diagnosis of small cell malignant tumours in childhood and adolescence

| Tumour | Cytology |
|---|---|
| Embryonal rhabdomyosarcoma | Occasionally myxoid background matrix. Often marked anisocytosis and anisokaryosis. Fusiform, strap-shaped, ribbon-like, triangular or rounded myoblast-like cells. Predominance of fusiform cells in the spindle cell type |
| Alveolar rhabdomyosarcoma | Predominantly small cell pattern. Rounded or pear-shaped primitive myoblast-like cells with eccentric nuclei. Cytoplasm eosinophilic in H&E and grey-blue in MGG. Cytoplasmic vacuolation. Occasionally multinucleated giant cells with small nuclei |
| Neuroblastoma | Small cell pattern. Occasionally large cells resembling ganglion cells. Mixture of dispersed cells and cell clusters of loosely attached cells. Moulded cell clusters. Neuropil background. Occasional rosettes. Dark rounded or irregular nuclei. In preserved cells often long thin cytoplasmic processes connecting one cell to another |
| Classical, conventional Ewing sarcoma | Mixture of dispersed cells and groups of cells. Often stripped nuclei and cytoplasmic background |
|  | Double cell population. Large light cells with rounded nuclei and abundant thin cytoplasm with vacuoles or clear spaces. Small dark cells with scanty cytoplasm and irregular hyperchromatic nuclei. Bland nuclear morphology. Inconspicuous nucleoli |
| Atypical Ewing sarcoma/PNET | Variable anisocytosis and anisokaryosis. Double cell population less evident. Often rosettes. Rounded or spindly cells with small cytoplasmic processes. In PNET often marked nuclear pleomorphism (rhabdomyoblast-like cells, cells with rhabdoid morphology) |
| Desmoplastic small round cell tumour | Mixture of dispersed cells and clusters of loosely attached cells. Rounded or ovoid cells with scant cytoplasm and rounded, ovoid nuclei with finely granular chromatin and small nucleoli |

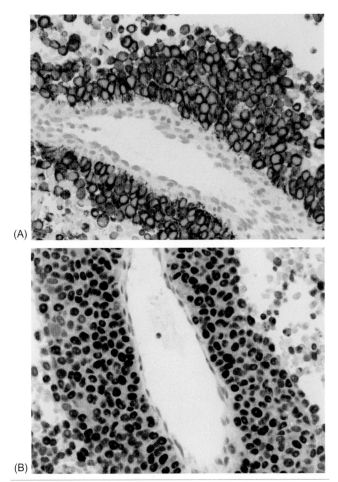

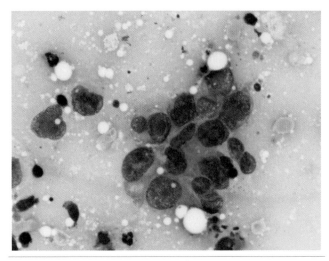

**Fig. 29.57** Angiosarcoma. The cytological features in FNA are very variable. In this case, the tumour cells are epithelioid-like featuring an acinar-like structure (MGG).

**Fig. 29.56** Cell block preparation of alveolar rhabdomyosarcoma. (A) Cytoplasmic positivity for desmin (Immunoperoxidase). (B) Nuclear positivity for Myo-D1 (immunoperoxidase).

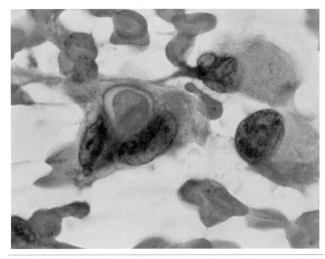

**Fig. 29.58** Angiosarcoma. An important, although rather infrequent sign, is the presence of atypical cells with vacuolated cytoplasm containing erythrocytes as a sign of primitive angiogenesis (H&E).

## Malignant tumours of blood vessels

Different types of sarcoma are known to arise from blood vessels as angiosarcoma and Kaposi sarcoma. Angiosarcoma is a relatively rare target for FNA.

The histological pattern of angiosarcoma is variable, with the more differentiated tumours composed of vascular channels lined by tumour cells showing variable pleomorphism and atypia. Papillary extensions and cell tufts are rather common. Obvious vessel-like structures are often difficult to find in poorly differentiated angiosarcoma and tumour cells with paracentral nuclei and cytoplasmic vacuoles with single or small groups of erythrocytes may be the only sign to indicate a vascular origin. In a subset of angiosarcoma, the epithelioid angiosarcoma have tumour cells with large and epithelial type of shape. Most angiosarcoma stain for CD31, with other useful markers being CD34 and Fli-1.

About 50% of epithelioid angiosarcomas stain for cytokeratins. The cytological features of angiosarcoma in FNA material is very variable corresponding to those in histological sections. Atypical spindle cells, rounded and polygonal cells featuring variable pleomorphism and atypia are common (Fig. 29.57). Less frequently vacuolated atypical cells with erythrocytes in the vacuoles are found (Fig. 29.58). Important pitfalls are spindle cell sarcoma and pleomorphic sarcoma of other lines of differentiation, metastatic carcinoma and melanoma. Most often

the cell population of angiosarcoma is diagnosed as malignant in smears. A specific diagnosis, however, is very difficult or impossible to render based on routinely stained smears and requires immunocytochemical stainings (Fig. 29.59). The cytological features of angiosarcoma have been described in three relatively large series.[53–55]

## Neuroectodermal tumours

Neuroblastoma and extraskeletal Ewing family of tumours are the most important for the cytopathologist.

### Neuroblastoma

This aggressive malignant tumour of infancy and childhood occurs mainly in the adrenal gland but is occasionally encountered as a soft tissue mass at sites of sympathetic nerve trunks or as a metastatic tumour. It is not uncommon that the first

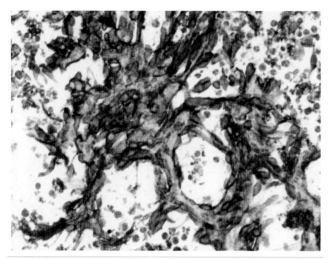

**Fig. 29.59** Angiosarcoma, cell block preparation. A specific diagnosis in FNA material most often requires adjunctive immunocytochemical staining, in this case with CD31 (immunoperoxidase).

target for the cytopathologist is a metastatic deposit. Common sites for metastatic neuroblastoma are lymph nodes, liver and bone.

Histologically, sheets of small round undifferentiated tumour cells are found, sometimes showing rosette formations around foci of delicate neurofibrillary matrix known as neuropil. If maturation of the tumour occurs, large ganglion cells are seen.

### Cytological findings: neuroblastoma

- Dissociated cells and clusters of loosely attached cells
- Neuropil in the background of cell clusters
- Tumour cells arranged in Indian file or in molded clusters
- Tumour cells with small, hyperchromatic irregular nuclei and unipolar or bipolar cytoplasmic processes connecting adjacent cells
- Rosette formations with central fibrillary material
- Occasional cells resembling ganglion cells.

Neuroblastoma smears are generally very cellular with a mixture of dispersed cells and clusters of loosely cohesive cells. In the clusters, the cells are arranged in rosettes with a fibrillary centre of neuropil sometimes observed (Fig. 29.60A). At times, the clusters are embedded in neuropil (Fig. 29.60B). Neuroblastoma cells are small to medium sized with dark irregular nuclei, a coarse chromatin structure and insignificant nucleoli. Their cytoplasm is scanty but drawn out in long thin processes connecting one cell to another (Fig. 29.60C). Arrangement of cells in Indian file or moulded clusters is a common finding. Ganglion cell differentiation is sometimes seen in the form of large cells with abundant cytoplasm and eccentric nuclei with prominent nucleoli. In aspirates from primitive neuroblastoma, rosettes are not found and the tumour cells are small with scanty cytoplasm devoid of processes. The diagnostic pitfalls are the other tumours belonging to the small round cell malignancies of childhood and adolescence, Ewing family of tumours, alveolar rhabdomyosarcoma, precursor lymphoma and desmoplastic small round cell tumour. Important cytological features in the differential diagnosis are listed in Table 29.5.

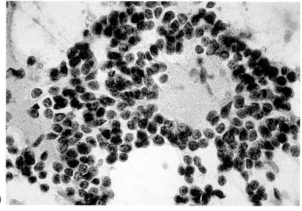

(A)

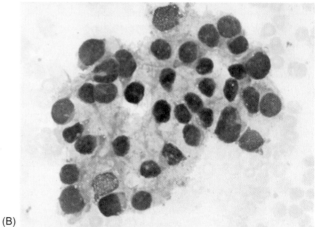

(B)

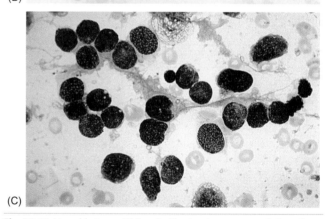

(C)

**Fig. 29.60** Neuroblastoma. (A) Rosette-like structure composed of small cells around a fibrillary centre (H&E). (B) The cell clusters often embedded in fibrillary neuropile (MGG). (C) Neuroblastoma cells have fragile fibrillar cytoplasm; the cells are often connected by thin cytoplasmic strands (MGG).

The cytomorphology of neuroblastoma has been evaluated elsewhere.[56–58] Immunocytochemistry and/or molecular studies can often be useful in making a specific diagnosis of a small round cell sarcoma (see Chs 33, 34).

### Extraskeletal Ewing family of tumours (ES/PNET)

ES/PNET comprises a number of tumours of presumed neuroectodermal origin, involving extraskeletal and skeletal sites. ES/PNET includes classic Ewing sarcoma, atypical Ewing sarcoma, the so-called Askin tumour and peripheral neuroepithelioma. The rationale for lumping these neoplasms together and diagnosing them as belonging to the Ewing family of tumours is because all share the same chromosomal abnormality t(11;22)(q24;q12). This translocation fuses the EWS gene in chromosome 22 with the FLI1 gene in chromosome 11 and detection of the fusion protein is an important diagnostic sign in this family of tumours. Classical ES is considered to be the least differentiated and atypical ES and PNET are the more differentiated varieties (see Table 34.1, p. 892).

Extraskeletal ES/PNET not only has been reported to arise in the extremities, retroperitoneum, mediastinum and pelvis but has also been diagnosed as a cutaneous and subcutaneous tumour and in parenchymatous organs such as kidney and breast. Some years ago, we had the opportunity to study an ES/PNET tumour primarily diagnosed in the heart. ES/PNET is most frequent diagnosed in older children and adolescents but has been reported in elderly patients. The oldest patient on our files is a male, aged 73. Histologically, classical EC cells are rather uniform with a pale cytoplasm, rounded or ovoid nuclei with bland chromatin and insignificant nucleoli and deposits of cytoplasmic glycogen. In the more differentiated tumours cellular pleomorphism and atypia are more marked, the nuclear chromatin coarser and nucleoli more prominent. Rosettes with a fibrillary centre are occasionally seen in classical ES but this is a characteristic diagnostic feature in atypical ES and PNET. Cytoplasmic glycogen is less often present in the tumour cells of atypical ES and PNET. Immunohistochemically, positive staining for CD99 and the FLI-1 antibody is common to all variants. Neuroectodermal antibodies such as NSE, synaptophysin and chromogranin are present in the more differentiated tumours. The cytology of classical ES as well as the other variants has been documented in several series.[58–61]

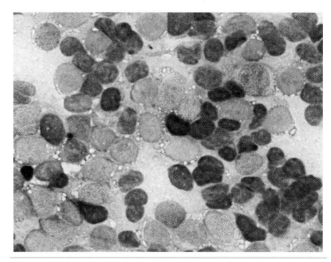

**Fig. 29.61** Classic Ewing sarcoma. Typical double cell population with large light cells featuring vacuolated cytoplasm and small dark cells with irregular dark nuclei (MGG).

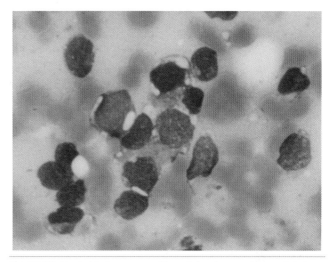

**Fig. 29.62** Atypical Ewing sarcoma. The cellular pleomorphism and nuclear atypia more marked than in classic Ewing sarcoma. In this case a few cells resemble 'large light' cells with vacuolated cytoplasm (MGG).

## Cytological findings: classical ES

- As a rule cellular smears
- A mixture of dissociated cells and cell clusters and groups
- Naked nuclei and a cytoplasmic background common
- A double cell population; large cells with abundant cytoplasm with vacuoles or clear spaces (dissolved glycogen) and rounded bland nuclei with finely granular chromatin
- Small nucleoli (large light cells) and smaller cells with scanty cytoplasm and irregular dark nuclei (small, dark cells).
- The dark cells often in moulded groups within the cell clusters.

## Cytological findings: atypical ES and PNET

- As a rule, cellular pleomorphism and atypia more marked than in classical ES
- The double cell population less evident, often not present in PNET
- Atypical cells forming rosette-like structures
- Presence of fusiform or spindly cells with thin cytoplasmic processes
- In PNET occasionally rhabdomyoblast-like cells or cells with rhabdoid morphology.

Smears from classical ES are surprisingly very similar in all cases (Fig. 29.61) in contrast to the cellular population in atypical ES and PNET (Fig. 29.62). From the clinical point of view, the distinction between the different variants is not of decisive importance as all variants are treated alike in most centres. In our reports, we diagnose these tumours as ES/PNET or as a Ewing family tumour.

## Diagnostic pitfalls: atypical ES and PNET

As in the case of neuroblastoma, the important pitfalls are other small round cell malignancies of childhood and adolescence as neuroblastoma, rhabdomyosarcoma, precursor lymphoma and desmoplastic small round cell tumour (Table 29.5). Immunocytochemistry is a valuable adjunctive diagnostic method. However, even if CD99 and FLI-1 are present in many tumours and therefore are not specific for this tumour entity requiring staining with a battery of other antibodies is required to make a diagnosis. The most important ancillary method is, however, cytogenetic/molecular genetic analysis. Experience has shown that karyotyping is less diagnostically valuable than RT-PCR or FISH.[62–64]

## Extragastrointestinal stromal tumour

Tumours with the same immunophenotype as gastrointestinal stromal tumours (GISTs) may occur in the retroperitoneum, omentum and mesentery (see Ch. 7). Extragastrointestinal GISTs are rather uncommon targets for FNA but are important in the differential diagnosis versus other mesenchymal tumours in the abdomen. Histologically, these tumours have a variable morphology, with two predominant patterns; spindle cell and epithelioid. In a small subset a marked cellular pleomorphism is evident. The diagnostic specific immunophenotype is a positive reaction for c-kit (CD117) and CD34. CD117 is positive in approximately 95% and CD34 in about 50% of cases. SMA is also expressed in some tumours.

Smears from extragastrointestinal GISTs are often cellular, made up of clusters or fascicles of cohesive cells. Dissociated stripped nuclei are common.

The spindle cells feature nuclei which are either spindly, ovoid or cigar-shaped with finely granular chromatin and scanty cytoplasm (Fig. 29.63A). In epithelioid GISTs, the cells are ovoid, rounded or polygonal with rounded or ovoid nuclei and relatively abundant cytoplasm (Fig. 29.63B). The most important differential diagnoses are leiomyosarcoma, peripheral nerve sheath tumours and carcinoma. Based on the cellular morphology, it may be impossible to distinguish GIST from the above-mentioned tumours; therefore, the diagnosis should be based on the combined evaluation of routinely stained smears and a positivity for preferably CD117 (Fig. 29.63C), and CD34. Several articles of FNA of GIST have been published, including mutational analysis of the c-kit gene in FNA smears.[65,66]

## Malignant tumours of uncertain, unknown or debated origin

Apart from synovial sarcoma, most tumours are rare and very infrequently needled including alveolar soft part sarcoma, clear cell sarcoma, epithelioid sarcoma and extraskeletal myxoid chondrosarcoma.

## Synovial sarcoma

Synovial sarcoma may present in the vicinity of joints but most often occur in the extremities without any connection to joints and are also found at other sites as trunk wall, the abdominal wall and pharyngeal region. Most synovial sarcomas are deep-seated. Young and middle-aged adults are most often affected but synovial sarcoma may also occur in children and the elderly. Histologically, synovial sarcomas are divided into biphasic tumours, monophasic fibrous, monophasic epithelial and poorly differentiated tumours. Poorly differentiated areas may also occur in any of the other types. Three different histological variants have been described in the poorly differentiated tumours: a small cell variant resembling the tumour cells in classical Ewing sarcoma, a spindle cell variant resembling high-grade malignant fibrosarcoma or MPNST and, finally, a type composed of epithelioid-like large cells with rounded nuclei with prominent nucleoli.

### Cytological findings: synovial sarcoma

- Cellular aspirates
- Dispersed cells and tissue fragments
- Stripped nuclei
- Branching capillaries with attached tumour cells
- Spindly or ovoid bland nuclei
- In biphasic tumours, occasionally small acinar-like structures
- Mitotic figures common in the tissue fragments
- The presence of mast cells in many aspirates.

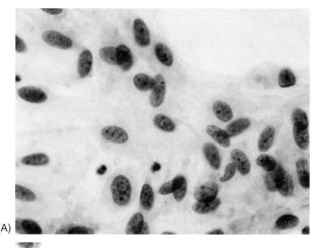

(A)

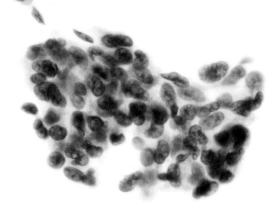

(B)

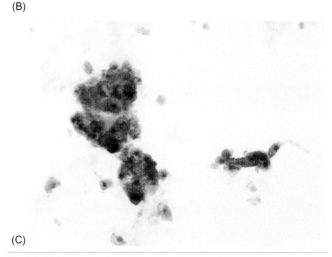

(C)

**Fig. 29.63** Extra-gastrointestinal stromal tumour. (A) In this case the tumour cell population is spindly with ovoid, almost blunt-ended nuclei (H&E). (B) The cell population can be epithelioid-like with the presence of rounded cells with rounded nuclei (H&E). (C) A specific diagnosis is often not possible without immunochemical staining. ThinPrep stained with CD117 (Immunoperoxidase).

The cytology of synovial sarcoma has been described in some large series of tumours.[67,68] As a rule, the smears are rich in cells, with a mixture of dispersed cells and different-sized fragments of tightly packed cells (Fig. 29.64A). Small glandular-type structures are infrequently seen in biphasic tumours (Fig. 29.64B). The most common cells are small to medium sized with scanty unipolar or bipolar cytoplasm. They have spindly

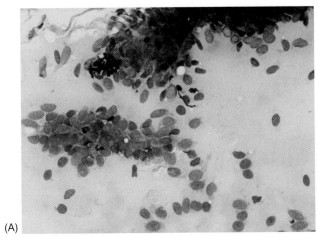

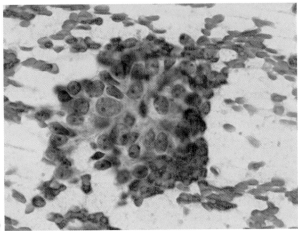

**Fig. 29.64** Synovial sarcoma. (A) The typical smear is composed of a mixture of fragment of tightly packed cells and dispersed cells of which stripped nuclei are common (MGG). (B) In biphasic tumours, glandular-like structures may be present (H&E).

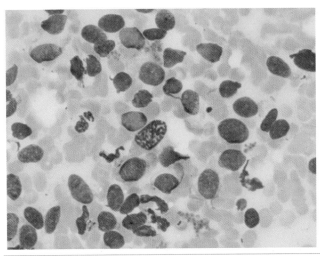

**Fig. 29.65** Synovial sarcoma. The lesional cells are most often medium-sized with uni-or bipolar cytoplasm and spindly or ovoid nuclei (H&E). A common find is mitotic figures (MGG).

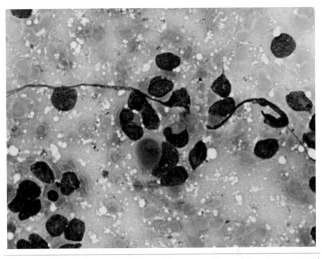

**Fig. 29.66** Poorly differentiated synovial sarcoma. One subtype is composed of atypical epithelioid-like cells, at times rhabdoid-like (MGG).

to ovoid to rounded nuclei with finely granular chromatin and insignificant nucleoli (Fig. 29.64C). Mitoses are not uncommon (Fig. 29.65). In the majority of our cases mast cells were a common finding.

The cells in the poorly differentiated variants or in aspirates from poorly differentiated areas may be Ewing sarcoma cell-like, appearing as highly atypical spindle cells or as atypical large rounded epithelioid-like cells with prominent nucleoli, at times rhabdoid-like (Fig. 29.66). The poorly differentiated variant has been described in single case reports.[69,70]

### Diagnostic pitfalls: synovial sarcoma

Synovial sarcoma may be very difficult to distinguish from other spindle cell tumours including solitary fibrous tumour and spindle cell sarcomas such as fibrosarcoma. Sparsely cellular aspirates from monophasic fibrous synovial sarcoma have been misdiagnosed as desmoid tumours. The poorly differentiated type may be difficult to distinguish from high-grade fibrosarcoma or MPNST, the Ewing family of tumours and extrarenal rhabdoid tumour. To correctly diagnose a synovial sarcoma in routinely stained smears is most often difficult. Ancillary techniques are almost always necessary to reach a confident diagnosis. Most synovial sarcomas stain positively for EMA and cytokeratins 7 and 19 although the

staining may be focal in poorly differentiated tumours (Fig. 29.67). A substantial number of tumours are positive for CD99 and Bcl-2.[71]

Cytogenetic examination of aspirated material to diagnose the t(X;18)(p11;q12) translocation or the two major gene fusion products, SYT/SSX1 and SYT/SSX2, is probably the most effective adjunctive method for achieving a correct diagnosis (see Table 34.1).[68]

## Alveolar soft part sarcoma

This rare sarcoma, occurring mainly in young adults and adolescents develops in the deep soft tissues of the lower extremities or in soft tissues internally. It is aspirated infrequently and the cytomorphology has only been described in case reports.[72,73] Common to all descriptions is the presence of large tumour cells with abundant often granular cytoplasm, and rounded nuclei with prominent nucleoli. Binucleate or multinucleated cells are uncommon. The cells appear singly or in cluster containing a

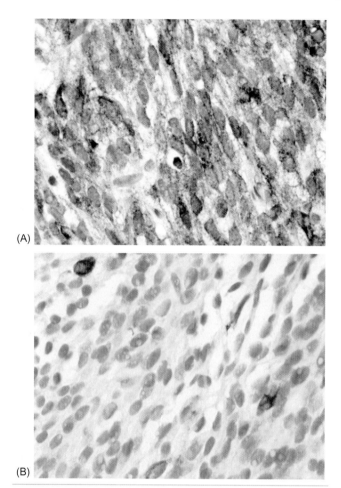

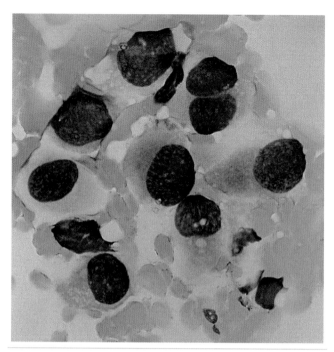

**Fig. 29.69** Clear cell sarcoma. A group of cells of epithelial appearance with sharp cytoplasmic borders and rounded nuclei (MGG).

**Fig. 29.67** Synovial sarcoma. (A) Cell block preparation. Most tumour cells stain for EMA (Immunoperoxidase). (B) Cell block preparation. The tumour cells are focally positive for CK7 (immunoperoxidase).

## Clear cell sarcoma

Clear cell sarcoma was first described in 1965 by Enzinger and, although controversial at first, it is now accepted as a clinico-pathological entity. Another term proposed for the tumour is malignant melanoma of soft parts. It is prone to occur in relation to tendons and aponeuroses in young adults. Based on the authors' experiences of two cases and those reported in two small series[74,75] of this relatively rare tumour, the sarcoma cells are mostly dissociated, but small clusters of loosely attached cells are also present. The cells are spindle shaped or polygonal with abundant pale cytoplasm and rounded or ovoid large nuclei. The nucleoli are prominent and the cytoplasmic borders sharp (Fig. 29.69). Immunocytochemically, most clear cell sarcomas stain positively for S-100 and HMB-45. (Metastatic) melanoma is the most important diagnostic pitfall with cytological and immunocytochemical findings the same as clear cell sarcoma. However, characteristic translocation (t12;22) is seen only in clear cell sarcoma (see Table 34.1, p. 892).

## Epithelioid sarcoma

Epithelioid sarcoma, first reported by Enzinger, is a peculiar tumour of unknown histogenesis developing mainly in adolescents and young adults. The sarcoma usually involves subcutaneous tissues or fascial planes and tendon sheaths of deeper soft tissues and appears as a multinodular growth, frequently showing central necrosis of nodules. An inflammatory cell infiltrate around the tumour nodules is common, as is hyalinisation. The cytological appearance of epithelioid sarcoma on FNA is reported in small series.[76,77] In our files, two cases are reported, but the most important feature was the difficulty in aspirating sufficient tumour material for microscopic examination. Because of necrosis, hyalinisation and the presence of inflammatory cells

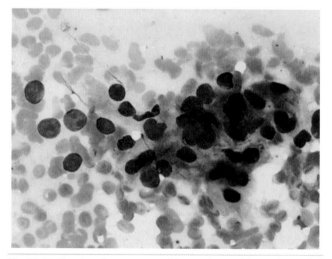

**Fig. 29.68** Alveolar soft part sarcoma. Often a mixture of clustered and dispersed cells. Stripped nuclei with prominent nucleoli is a common find (MGG).

capillary network. Another typical finding is stripped nuclei and a cytoplasmic background. Two cases are recorded in our files and the cellular features corresponded to previously described findings (Fig. 29.68). The most important differential diagnoses are granular cell tumour and metastasis from renal carcinoma (see Table 34.1, p. 892).

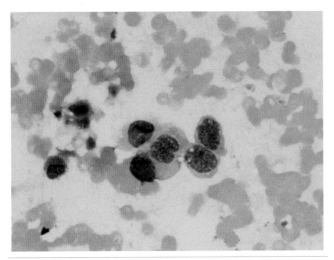

**Fig. 29.70** Epithelioid sarcoma. Large cells with abundant cytoplasm and irregular nuclei (MGG).

consisting of lymphocytes, plasma cells and histiocytes, the sarcoma cells were sparse. The tumour cells were spindly, polygonal or rounded, with fragile cytoplasm and rounded, ovoid or irregular nuclei (Fig. 29.70). Small tight clusters of cells can look like cell aggregates from large cell carcinoma, reflecting their epithelioid appearance on histology. The clinically most important pitfall is not to diagnose the smears as originating from a granulomatous lesion.

## Extraskeletal myxoid chondrosarcoma (EMC)

EMC as a clinicopathologic entity was first described in 1972. It has been diagnosed in children and adults, predominantly in the middle-aged and the elderly.

The extremities and trunk are the sites of predilection. EMCs display an abundant matrix and are variably cellular. The tumour cells are arranged in strands and rings, and appear as small tumour balls embedded in the myxoid background or show a reticular and/or cribriform growth pattern. The tumour cells are variably shaped, spindly, epithelioid-like or rounded, with ovoid or spindle-shaped nuclei with finely granular chromatin and small nucleoli. Well developed hyaline cartilage is not present. There is no typical immunohistochemical profile, although 30–40% of cases have been reported to be S-100 positive. EMA is positive in 20–25% of cases. Cytogenetics has been considered useful in the diagnosis; the t(9;22) translocation is typical for EMC. Recently, yet another translocation t(9;17(q22;q12) has been described, probably connected with neuroendocrine differentiation (see Table 34.1, p. 892).[78] The cytological findings in our cases of EMC are similar to those described.[34,79]

### Cytological findings: extraskeletal myxoid chondrosarcoma (Fig. 29.71)

- Abundant myxoid background
- Tumour cells arranged in cell-balls, branching strands or clusters or dispersed
- Rounded or spindly cells with rounded or ovoid nuclei
- Bland nuclear chromatin and small nucleoli.

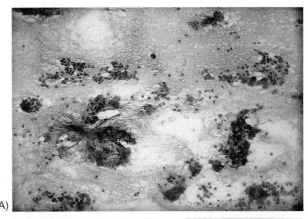

(A)

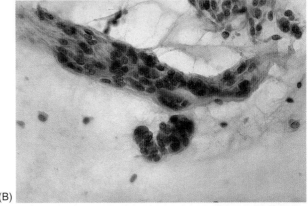

(B)

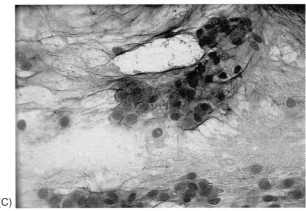

(C)

**Fig. 29.71** Extraskeletal myxoid chondrosarcoma. (A) Strands and clusters as well as dispersed cells embedded in an abundant, partly fibrillar myxoid background substance (MGG). (B) Cell-balls and cluster of rounded cells with ovoid rather bland nuclei (H&E). (C) The myxoid background is better visualised in MGG (MGG).

### Differential diagnosis

Of all tumours exhibiting an abundant myxoid background matrix, myxoid liposarcoma, low-grade myxofibrosarcoma, low-grade fibromyxoid sarcoma and mixed myoepithelial tumour are the most important.

## Extrarenal rhabdoid tumour

Extrarenal rhabdoid tumours have been described as having a wide anatomical distribution in the soft tissues. The age range is broad, although most cases occur in children. The histological features common to all these tumours irrespective of site are rather large cells with various amount of cytoplasm, eccentric large vesicular nuclei with prominent nucleoli and paranuclear hyaline globular inclusions. Very few reports have been published on the cytological findings in FNA smears.[80,81] The cytological features of the single case in our files correspond with published reports. Clusters of loosely attached cells were mixed with dispersed cells. The tumour cells were elongated, rounded or polygonal with vesicular nuclei exhibiting prominent nucleoli. A number of cells displayed rounded cytoplasmic inclusions. To confirm the diagnosis, the tumour cells stain for vimentin, cytokeratins and neuroectodermal antibodies such as NSE. Extrarenal rhabdoid tumour is easily diagnosed as a malignant tumour in FNA smears, but the diagnostic pitfalls are other malignant tumours exhibiting a rhabdoid morphology, such as rhabdomyosarcoma, poorly differentiated synovial sarcoma, epithelioid sarcoma and malignant melanoma.

## Intra-abdominal desmoplastic small round cell tumour

Intra-abdominal desmoplastic small round cell tumour (DSRCT) is of uncertain histogenesis but its predilection for serosal involvement may suggest that it is a primitive mesothelial tumour. It occurs predominantly in male adolescents and young adults. The typical histopathological pattern is that of well-defined nests and trabeculae of small- to medium-sized tumour cells with a desmoplastic stroma. The tumour cells are uniform with scanty cytoplasm and rounded or ovoid hyperchromatic nuclei. Nucleoli are small (Fig. 29.72A). The immunohistochemical profile indicates a multilinear phenotype with positive staining for keratin antibodies, neuroendocrine markers, desmin and vimentin (Fig. 29.72B, C). Cytogenetic analysis has revealed a unique translocation t(11;22)(p13;q12), involving the EWS gene on chromosome 22 and the WT1 gene on chromosome 11, thus a gene fusion product different from that found in the Ewing family of tumours (see Table 34.1, p. 892). A polyclonal anti-WT1 antibody, detecting the WT1 protein, is available and is reported to stain most cases. The cytological features have been described in a few cases.[58,82,83] Most important differential diagnoses are other small round cell malignancies such as Ewing family of tumours, small cell carcinoma and precursor lymphoma (Table 29.5).

## Skeletal tumours/lesions

Definition of the cytological criteria for interpreting aspiration samples from primary bone tumours is at present largely confined to malignant neoplasms, since FNA findings in very few benign tumours have been thoroughly documented (Table 29.6). Nevertheless, as was emphasised in the introduction to this chapter, a combination of cytological diagnosis and careful evaluation of clinical and radiographic data can be the basis of definitive treatment in a substantial number of primary benign and malignant bone tumours. FNA will also frequently diagnose inflammatory and lymphohistiocytic lesions and distinguish primary bone tumours from metastatic deposits.

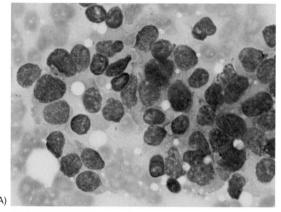

(A)

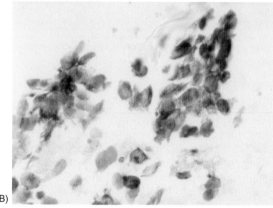

(B)

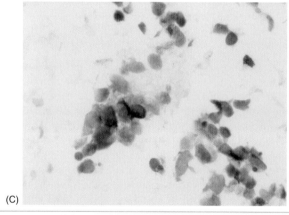

(C)

**Fig. 29.72** Intra-abdominal desmoplastic small round cell tumour. (A) Small tumour cells with scanty cytoplasm and rounded or ovoid nuclei (MGG). (B,C) Intra-abdominal desmoplastic small round cell tumour has a multi-lineage immunophenotype. Cell block preparation stained with cytokeratin (B) and desmin (C) (Immunoperoxidase).

**Table 29.6** Primary bone tumours/lesions with clearly defined cytological features enabling a specific diagnosis to be made

| Benign | Malignant |
|---|---|
| Giant cell tumour | Osteosarcoma |
| Osteoblastoma | Chondrosarcoma |
| Chondroblastoma | Ewing family of tumours |
| Langerhans cell histiocytosis | Chordoma |

References are given with the presentation of respective tumour/lesion

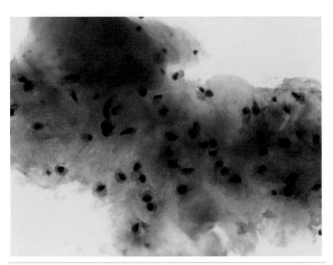

**Fig. 29.73** Chondroma. A cartilaginous fragment, strongly blue-violet with irregularly distributed small cells with bland nuclei (MGG).

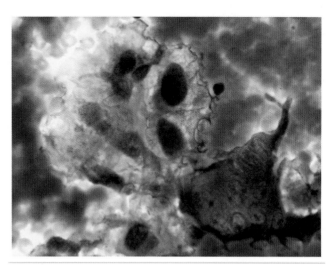

**Fig. 29.74** Chondroblastoma. A small group of chondroblast-like cells embedded in a red-blue chondroid matrix + one osteoclast-like cell (MGG).

## Chondroblastic tumours

The main chondroblastic tumours of interest for the cytopathologist are chondroma, chondroblastoma, chondromyxoid fibroma and chondrosarcoma.

### Chondroma

Chondromas are evenly distributed throughout life and also occur in children. They may be single or multiple and are composed of mature hyaline cartilage interspersed with areas of degeneration. Chondromas are the most common tumours in the small bones of the hand and feet.

### Cytological findings: chondroma

- Cartilaginous fragments with cells in lacunar spaces
- Cells with small regular nuclei
- Cellular pleomorphism not uncommon.

It is usually not difficult to aspirate tumour tissue from chondromas. Characteristically, the smears are made up of numerous fragments of cartilage with dispersed cells being uncommon. The fragments stain strongly violet or blue with MGG and faintly pink with H&E. Within fragments small rounded uniform cells with regular nuclei are seen in lacunar spaces (Fig. 29.73). Binucleated cells are not found but the fragments may be highly cellular and exhibit cellular pleomorphism, especially in chondromas of small peripheral bones. The cytological features of chondroma in FNA smears have been investigated in single reports.[84]

### Chondroblastoma

Chondroblastomas occur most often in young people, especially in the second decade, but are commoner in males, and are often painful. The most usual site is the epiphysis of the long bones, but they may also be found in small tubular and flat bones. Histologically, the tumour is composed of immature chondroblasts and osteoclast-like giant cells, with focal calcification. Areas resembling an aneurysmal bone cyst may be present.

### Cytological findings: chondroblastoma

- Mononuclear cells, well formed cytoplasm, round nuclei
- Multinucleated osteoclast-like cells
- Fragments of chondroid matrix.

Although a rare tumour, the cytological findings of chondroblastoma have been published.[85] The findings described are similar to those of the few cases in our files. Diagnostic features in FNA smears are the mixed pattern of chondroid matrix fragments, cells of chondroblastic type and multinucleated osteoclast-like cells. The most characteristic finding is the presence of chondroblasts. These are typically monomorphic and rounded with well-demarcated cytoplasm and round or occasionally lobulated or reniform nuclei. Nuclei are generally central and vary in size; binucleated forms are not uncommon and mitotic figures may be found. The chondroblastic cells are either dissociated or often seen in small ill-defined clusters embedded in chondroid matrix (Fig. 29.74). The chondroid matrix fragments are usually acellular and fibrillary, and stain red to reddish blue with MGG and faintly eosinophilic in H&E preparations.

### Chondromyxoid fibroma

A benign cartilaginous tumour of young adults, chondromyxoid fibroma is rare, being less common than chondroblastoma. Patients are most often in second and third decades and the tumours typically arise in the metaphyseal region of long tubular bones and especially the tibia. Histologically, lobular masses of myxochondroid tissue are seen, surrounded by cellular areas with a mixture of spindle cells of fibroblastic type and osteoclasts.

### Cytological findings: chondromyxoid fibroma

- Myxoid background matrix
- Cartilaginous fragments (with chondroblast-like cells in lacunae)
- Dispersed or clustered spindle-shaped fibroblastic cells
- Osteoclastic giant cells.

Only single cases of FNA from chondromyxoid fibroma have been published[86,87] and our experience is limited to three cases.

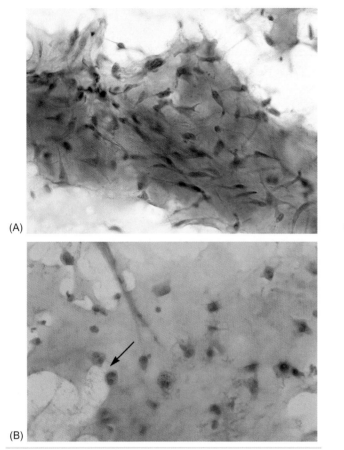

(A)

(B)

**Fig. 29.75** Chondromyxoid fibroma. (A) Spindle-shaped fibroblast-like cells within a myxoid back ground matrix (MGG). (B) In wet-fixed smears the cartilaginous fragments are faintly stained and the tumour cells better visualised than with MGG. Note slight anisokaryosis and binucleated cell (arrow) (H&E).

Smears show fragments of cartilaginous matrix, fusiform spindle cells and osteoclastic cells embedded in a myxoid background matrix. The spindle cells vary in size and have elongated nuclei. They appear either singly or in ill-defined groups. In the cartilaginous fragments rounded chondroblast-like cells in lacunar spaces may be found. Both chondroblastic and spindle-shaped cells may show a certain polymorphism with plump nuclei and small but prominent nucleoli. Binucleated chondroblast-like cells are not uncommon (Fig. 29.75). In our cases the most striking finding was the presence of cartilaginous fragments.

## Chondrosarcoma

This group of tumours occurs in adults, in the fourth to seventh decades. Predominant sites are the bones of the trunk and upper ends of femur and humerus, and a few are extraskeletal. Histologically, cartilage forming tumour cells permeate the local tissues, often engulfing normal or reactive bone. Thus chondrosarcomas may include bone, but bone is never formed by the tumour cells themselves, in contrast to osteosarcomas, which may produce bone and cartilage.

### Cytological findings: chondrosarcoma

- Fragments of hyaline cartilage
- Myxoid background matrix
- Mononuclear and binucleated tumour cells often in lacunae

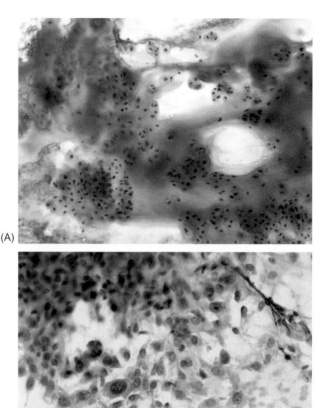

(A)

(B)

**Fig. 29.76** Chondrosarcoma. (A) Low-grade malignant chondrosarcoma. Cartilaginous fragments with irregularly dispersed uniform cells. Note the variable cellularity (MGG). (B) High-grade malignant chondrosarcoma. A highly cellular tumour fragment exhibiting marked nuclear atypia (H&E).

- Large rounded individual cells with well-defined cytoplasm
- Nuclei rounded or irregular and lobulated.

Most chondrosarcomas are easy targets for FNA. A surprisingly rich yield may be obtained and fragments or 'microbiopsies' of tumour tissue are found relatively commonly in smears.

The cytology of chondrosarcoma has been described in three rather large series.[4,88,89] The cytological findings depend on the grade of malignancy. In most textbooks, chondrosarcomas are graded in a three-tiered scale of 1–3.[12] Grade 1 tumours are considered low-grade, Grades 2 and 3 as high-grade malignant. Most primary chondrosarcoma are Grade 1 or 2. Results from several studies confirm that grading is important in predicting prognosis. It is important for the cytopathologist to be able to separate Grade 1 tumours from tumours of higher grades as it has been shown that Grade 1 chondrosarcomas have a prognosis similar to chondromas in extremities.[90] Chondrosarcoma of low-grade malignancy yields tumour cells in fragments of variable size, cell dissociation being infrequent. The fragments are of variable cellularity, with some cells lying in lacunar spaces. A myxoid background matrix is not prominent and individual tumour cells display a slight to moderate atypia. Some tumour cells are binucleate (Fig. 29.76A).

Smears from high-grade (Grades 2 and 3) chondrosarcoma are generally cellular with cellular tissue fragments and more

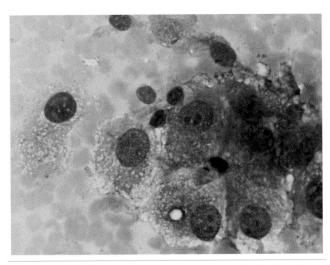

**Fig. 29.77** Clear cell chondrosarcoma. Large tumour cells with abundant finely vacuolated cytoplasm and rounded nuclei (MGG).

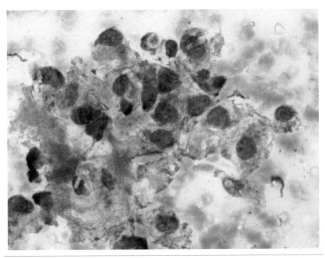

**Fig. 29.78** Mesenchymal chondrosarcoma. Monomorphic, small cells with rounded or ovoid nuclei within a partly fibrillar matrix (MGG).

prominent myxoid background matrix, especially in Grade 3 tumours. As a rule the number of fragments is lower than in low-grade tumours and dissociated cells more common. The cellular and nuclear atypia is marked and occasional mitoses may be found, mostly in Grade 3 tumours (Fig. 29.76B).

The histological subtypes clear cell chondrosarcoma, mesenchymal chondrosarcoma and dedifferentiated chondrosarcoma are rare and their FNA cytology has rarely been described.

## Clear cell chondrosarcoma

The only case reported[91] showed a cellular smear dominated by large tumour cells. The cells had an abundance of finely vacuolated cytoplasm with a central nucleus and prominent nucleoli. The only case in our files showed similar features (Fig. 29.77).

## Mesenchymal chondrosarcoma

The cytological features of mesenchymal chondrosarcoma in FNA smears have been reported in a few cases.[88] Small, monomorphic tumour cells in cohesive clusters have been described as a fibrillar matrix encircling cells (Fig. 29.78). A cartilaginous matrix may be observed as osteoclast-like giant cells. The extra

skeletal myxoid chondrosarcoma is not related to mesenchymal chondrosarcoma of the bone.[92]

## Dedifferentiated chondrosarcoma

Dedifferentiated chondrosarcoma is a rare subtype, comprising about 10% of all chondrosarcoma. Histologically, it has the characteristics of a low-grade chondrosarcoma, which contains areas of high-grade malignant non-chondroid sarcoma such as osteosarcoma or pleomorphic sarcoma of the MFH-type. A report of four cases has been published.[93]

### Diagnostic pitfalls: chondrosarcoma

Chondroma may be difficult to distinguish from low-grade malignant chondrosarcoma on histology and the same problem is present in FNA material.[4] This is due to the presence of only insignificant atypia in low-grade chondrosarcomas and cellular pleomorphism in some chondromas, especially in those arising in the small tubular bones on hands and feet. Chondromyxoid fibroma may also be difficult to distinguish from chondrosarcoma when the smears are predominated by a myxoid background matrix and cartilaginous cells are binucleated and slightly pleomorphic.

Chondrosarcoma cells may be epithelioid and hence mistaken for carcinoma cells if only alcohol-fixed smears are examined. This is because the characteristic background matrix and cartilaginous fragments are weakly stained unless MGG is used. There is a similarity between high-grade chondrosarcoma and chondroblastic osteosarcoma which may lead to a false interpretation of the chondrosarcoma smears. As has been emphasised by Rinas et al.[93] sampling error in the needling of dedifferentiated chondrosarcoma might give a false impression of a high-grade sarcoma of non-cartilaginous origin.

When situated in the vertebral column, chordoma is another differential diagnosis because of the similar myxoid background matrix, but the tumour cell morphology in chordoma is different from that of chondrosarcoma.

The small cell population in mesenchymal chondrosarcoma may be misdiagnosed as another type of small cell tumour if the cartilaginous component is not represented in the smear.

## Ancillary techniques

Adjunctive methods, such as immunocytochemistry using S-100 protein[4] may help to prove the chondromatous nature of a tumour but do not assist in distinguishing between chondroma and chondrosarcoma, although cytokeratin positivity is seen only in chordoma. DNA-ploidy analysis may be helpful when the cytological findings are inconclusive with regard to benignity or malignancy. A non-diploid histogram strongly suggests a chondrosarcoma (see Table 34.1, p. 892).[4,94]

## Osteogenic tumours

The osteogenic tumours which are predominantly needled are osteoblastoma and the different variants of osteosarcoma.

## Osteoblastoma

This benign bone-forming tumour has a definitive predilection for males in the first three decades of life and may be difficult

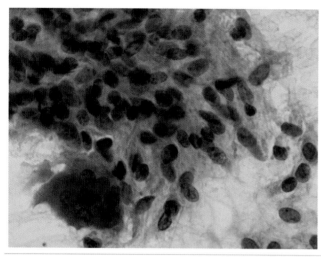

**Fig. 29.79** Osteoblastoma. A group of tightly packed spindly cells and osteoblast-like cells and one osteoclast-like cell (H&E).

to distinguish from osteosarcoma. The majority of cases occur in the vertebral column, long bones being next in frequency. Structurally, there are close similarities to related tumour osteoid osteoma, with a central nidus of osteoid and vascular osteoblastic tissue, surrounded by sclerotic bone. Some cases have bizarre tumour cells but mitoses are not a prominent feature.

### Cytological findings: osteoblastoma

- Cells of osteoblastic type, mononuclear and binucleated
- Clusters of spindle cells
- Osteoclastic cells.

Only single cases of the cytology of osteoblastoma have been reported[95] and our experience is limited to a few tumours. These few cases were characterised by a mixed cell pattern. The diagnostic cells resembled osteoblasts, with eccentric rounded nuclei and a more or less distinct clear space or 'Hof' in the cytoplasm of many of the cells. Cell and nuclear size were variable and binucleated cells were observed. These osteoblast-like cells were either dispersed in the smear or arranged in small groups or rows. A blue to red or pink matrix was seen between the cells in some groups on MGG. A few clusters of tightly packed spindle cells with elongated nuclei were found in all smears and there were also scattered osteoclastic multinucleated cells (Fig. 29.79).

## Osteosarcoma

Osteosarcoma is the commonest of all primary malignant bone tumours. Little is known of the pathogenesis, although there are associations with pre-existing bone lesions as Paget's disease, and with exposure to radiation or chemotherapeutic agents. The majority of patients are in the second and third decades of life, but osteosarcoma has been reported in children below 10 years and in middle-aged or elderly patients. There is a slight male preponderance. The metaphysis of long bones is the site of predilection, especially the distal femur and proximal tibia.

The osteosarcoma classification can be according to site, including conventional intramedullary with cortical destruction, parosteal, periosteal and exclusively intramedullary, or

by morphology, the histological findings being osteoblastic, chondroblastic, fibroblastic, telangiectatic or of small cell type. Mixed forms, especially osteoblastic/chondroblastic occur.

### Cytological findings: osteosarcoma

- Mixture of cell clusters and dispersed cells
- Pleomorphic pattern of obviously malignant cells
- Relatively frequent mitoses, including atypical forms
- Intercellular tumour matrix of osteoid within clusters
- Benign osteoclastic giant cells
- Epithelioid tumour cells, which may be of osteoblastic type or resemble chondroblasts in osteoblastic or chondroblastic variants, respectively
- Atypical spindle-shaped fibroblast-like cells in fibroblastic types.

The FNA cytology of osteosarcoma has been thoroughly described in two large series.[96,97] The results of these reports correspond well with the author's experience of 59 cases.[98]

### Intramedullary osteosarcoma

Conventional intramedullary osteosarcoma with cortical destruction is the commonest subtype histologically and on cytology, and may be osteoblastic, chondroblastic or mixed. Smears from these tumours are obviously malignant, with dispersed cells mixed with cell clusters or cohesive groups of variable size. The cell pattern is pleomorphic in the pure osteoblastic type, the majority of tumour cells having rounded or polygonal shape with sharp cytoplasmic borders and eccentric nuclei. The nuclei are rounded, oval or occasionally irregular, with coarse chromatin and prominent large nucleoli. Many cells resemble osteoblasts but the clear 'Hof' is not always visible (Fig. 29.80A).

In the cell clusters and groups thin strands of a tumour matrix stained red or purple by MGG is occasionally observed between the cells (Fig. 29.80B). Small clumps of similar matrix may also be found in the background. This matrix, which is difficult to detect in wet-fixed smears, is considered to represent osteoid[4] and is an important diagnostic sign, especially when observed between the tumour cells in clusters or groups.

In the pure chondroblastic type, the predominant cell is mainly rounded with sharp cytoplasmic borders and a central rounded nucleus with relatively small nucleoli. In general, the cellular pleomorphism is less pronounced in the chondroblastic than in the osteoblastic type. A myxoid background and fragments of cartilaginous matrix staining blue or purple on MGG are common in chondroblastic osteosarcoma, while the thin strands of osteoid are less frequent (Fig. 29.81). In the cartilage fragments, tumour cells are sometimes seen in lacunar spaces.

Both types contain multinucleated tumour cells and scattered benign osteoclastic cells are a common finding. Mitotic figures, including atypical mitoses, are seen, especially in the osteoblastic type (Fig. 29.82). Aspiration smears from osteosarcoma are usually blood stained. In the telangiectatic type, which is very haemorrhagic, the cell yield may be poor.

### Fibroblastic osteosarcoma

Experience of the fibroblastic type is limited to single cases. Atypical spindle-shaped cells with fusiform nuclei predominate with moderately cellular pleomorphism (Fig. 29.83).

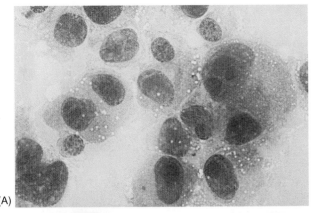

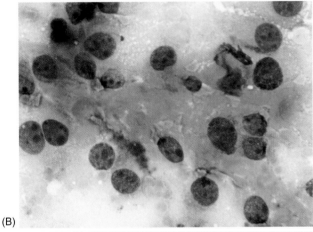

Fig. 29.80 Osteoblastic osteosarcoma. (A) Mostly rounded tumour cells with eccentric nuclei and abundant cytoplasm (MGG). (B) Thin strands of tumour osteoid encircling a group of tumour cells (MGG).

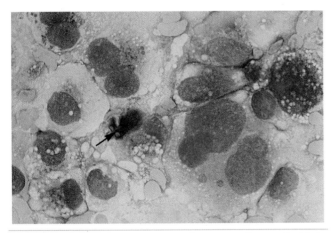

Fig. 29.81 Chondroblastic osteosarcoma. The tumour cells are embedded in a myxoid background matrix and a small fragment of purple-stained cartilage matrix is seen (arrow). MGG.

## Small cell osteosarcoma

The rare small cell osteosarcoma has been only briefly described.[97,99]

The main cytological features were a mixture of cohesive fragments and dispersed small- to medium-sized cells, having rounded or spindle-shaped nuclei, but the smears demonstrating less pleomorphism than other types (Fig. 29.84).

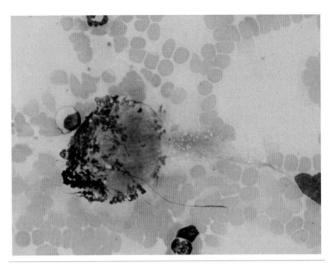

Fig. 29.82 Osteoblastic osteosarcoma. Atypical mitotic figures are often present (MGG).

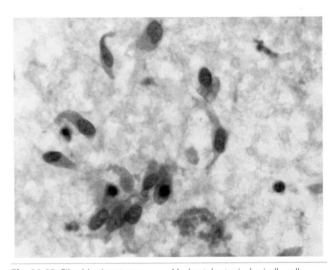

Fig. 29.83 Fibroblastic osteosarcoma. Moderately atypical spindle cells predominate the smears (H&E).

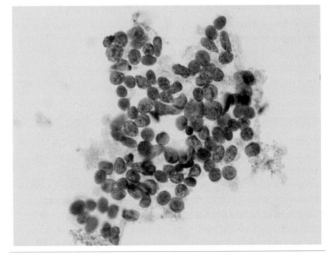

Fig. 29.84 Small cell osteosarcoma. A cluster of small to medium-sized, rather uniform cells, with rounded nuclei (MGG).

## Box 29.2  Differential diagnoses of osteosarcoma in FNA

- Benign tumours/lesions
- Reactive osteoblastic proliferations (pseudomalignant myositis ossificans)
- Fracture callus
- Aggressive osteoblastoma
- Giant cell tumour
- Malignant tumours
- Primary pleomorphic sarcoma of bone (MFH-like)
- High-grade malignant chondrosarcoma
- Dedifferentiated chondrosarcoma
- Metastatic anaplastic carcinoma
- Anaplastic large cell lymphoma
- Ewing family of tumours (small cell osteosarcoma)

### Parosteal osteosarcoma

FNA of the parosteal type is only documented in two cases.[98] The yield was very poor, consisting of scattered atypical spindle cells and small fragments of cartilage. In the authors' limited experience, parosteal osteosarcomas are less suitable for FNA than other types since it is difficult to aspirate sufficient material by thin needle.

### Diagnostic pitfalls: osteosarcoma

The principal differential diagnoses are listed in Box 29.2. Reactive osteoblasts exhibit a wide range of shapes and sizes, their nuclear size is variable and nucleoli may be large and prominent. The chromatin pattern is, however, uniformly regular and a clear 'Hof' is most often visible. In pseudomalignant myositis ossificans, multinucleated tumour cells with atypical nuclei are never encountered nor are there any atypical mitoses.

Typical osteoblastomas are composed of spindle cell fragments, cells resembling osteoblasts with slight atypia and osteoclastic cells, producing a cell pattern different from that of a typical osteosarcoma. Predictably, the rare aggressive osteoblastoma and osteoblastoma with bizarre cells, both of which have pleomorphic hyperchromatic nuclei, do pose diagnostic problems.

Giant cell tumour has been regarded as another pitfall in diagnosis, especially versus osteoclast-rich osteosarcoma. However, the mononuclear cells of giant cell tumours never show the pleomorphism and nuclear atypia found in osteosarcoma and atypical mitoses are never present.

Primary pleomorphic sarcoma of the malignant fibrous histiocytoma (MFH) type can occur primarily in bone, and the cell pattern may resemble that of an osteosarcoma.

However, osteoblastic tumour cells are not found in the former tumour, nor are there intercellular strands of osteoid matrix. Osteosarcomatous tumour cells of either osteoblastic or chondroblastic type may have an epithelioid appearance and, therefore, may be mistaken for carcinoma cells when seen in cohesive groups. Yet another, albeit rare, diagnostic pitfall is anaplastic large cell lymphoma primary arising in bone. The correct diagnosis of entities considered in the differential diagnosis can be resolved by the use immunocytochemical markers as described in the next section.

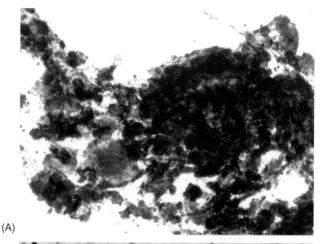

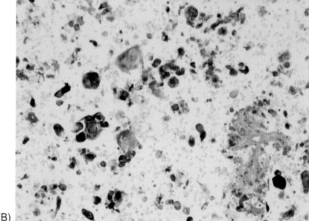

**Fig. 29.85** Osteoblastic osteosarcoma. (A) Strong cytoplasmic staining for alkaline phosphatase (Air-dried smear). (B) Cell block preparation stained with osteocalcin (Immunoperoxidase).

The most difficult of all the differential diagnoses is between chondroblastic osteosarcoma and high-grade malignant chondrosarcoma and between dedifferentiated chondrosarcoma with a high-grade osteosarcoma component and pure osteosarcoma when there are no fragments of low-grade chondrosarcoma in aspirated material.

The small cell variant of osteosarcoma has been considered to cause confusion with the Ewing family of tumours primary in bone. This diagnostic problem can be resolved by means of ancillary techniques.

Those osteosarcomas that are pure intramedullary often show bland-looking tumour cells that may also give diagnostic problems. However, pure intra-medullary osteosarcomas are not usually subjected to FNA because of overlying intact cortical bone.

### Ancillary techniques

Aspirated material may be used for a number of ancillary methods as an aid to diagnosis. Osteoblasts as osteosarcoma cells are strongly positive when stained for alkaline phosphatase (ALP). In our experience, ALP-staining is of great help in the differential diagnosis of high-grade malignant chondrosarcoma versus metastatic carcinoma and anaplastic large cell lymphoma.[98] All histological subtypes of osteosarcoma including chondroblastic, fibroblastic and small cell variants, stain for ALP (Fig. 29.85A).

During recent years, immunohistochemical staining with antibodies against osteonectin and osteocalcin has proved to be important in the diagnosis of osteosarcoma.[100] In our experience, immunocytochemical staining with these antibodies on aspirated material is of diagnostic help (Fig. 29.85B).

Apart from the parosteal type, the majority of osteosarcomas are aneuploid on DNA- ploidy analysis.[4] Unequivocal aneuploidy on DNA analyses excludes a benign osteoblastic proliferation.

## Benign bone tumours/lesions with osteoclast-like giant cells

Apart from chondroblastoma and osteoblastoma, several tumours/lesions exhibit more or less numerous osteoclast-like giant cells (Box 29.3). Of interest for the cytopathologist is above all giant cell tumour, aneurysmal bone cyst and osteitis fibrosa cystica (brown tumour of hyperparathyroidism).

### Giant cell tumour

An easy target for FNA, giant cell tumour is the primary benign bone tumour which has been most thoroughly investigated by cytology.[4,101,102] Giant cell tumour is most common in the second and third decades of life and the majority of cases occur in females. The epiphyses of long bones are common sites, especially on either side of the knee joint.

Histologically, the tumour is composed of stromal cells, probably neoplastic, and osteoclastic giant cells, which are probably reactive. The cortical bone is either very thin and weakened, or destroyed over the lesion and therefore not difficult to aspirate with a 22-gauge needle.

### Cytological findings: giant cell tumour

- Easy to needle, abundant yield
- Mixture of cell clusters and dispersed cells
- Double cell population
- Elongated mononuclear (sometimes bi- or trinucleated) cells variable in size
- Regular rounded or ovoid nuclei, inconspicuous nucleoli
- Large multinucleated cells of osteoclastic type
- Osteoclast-like cells attached to periphery of cell clusters.

Typically, the smears are richly cellular, consisting of a mixture of cell clusters and dissociated cells. A double cell population

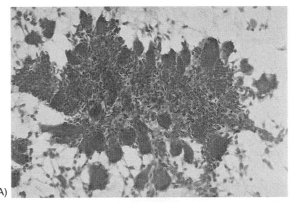

(A)

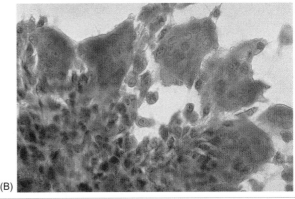

(B)

**Fig. 29.86** Giant cell tumour. (A) A typical cell cluster with the osteoclast-like giant cells attached to the periphery (H&E). (B) detail from (A). Tightly packed mononuclear cells with uniform nuclei and a peripheric row of giant cells (H&E).

is always obvious. The majority of tumour cells are elongated and mononuclear with moderate to abundant cytoplasm and sharp cytoplasmic borders. The nuclei are round or ovoid and of uniform appearance. Chromatin is regularly distributed and one or two small nucleoli are common. The other cell type resembles an osteoclast with abundant cytoplasm and numerous uniform rounded nuclei. Fine red granules are often observed in the cytoplasm on MGG. A typical cell cluster has irregular borders along which the osteoclast-like cells are attached, the central part being composed of tightly packed mononuclear cells (Fig. 29.86). Among the dispersed cells bi- or trinucleated forms may be found, suggesting a transition to the multinucleated forms. In cell-poor aspirates the clusters are few, small or absent. The smears consist of a mixture of dispersed mononuclear and multinucleated cells. Occasionally mitoses, although never atypical, are found in the mononuclear cells.

### Diagnostic pitfalls: giant cell tumour

The radiological features of aneurysmal bone cyst are similar those seen in giant cell tumour and combinations of the two have been described. The most characteristic finding in FNA material from aneurysmal bone cyst is the very large amount of blood obtained, such that the syringe fills with blood immediately on sampling. The cellular yield is usually sparse; consisting of scattered osteoclastic cells, spindle-shaped fibroblastic cells and haemosiderin laden macrophages are typical findings. Single reports of the cytological findings in aneurysmal bone cyst have been recorded.[103] Similar cytology has been described in FNA material of osteitis fibrosa cystica, also known as the 'brown tumour' of hyperparathyroidism, in which osteoclasts, spindly mononuclear cells and macrophages are also found.[104] One author has seen a case of brown tumour consisting of fragments of tightly packed spindle cells with numerous giant cells attached to the periphery, an appearance almost indistinguishable from that of a typical giant cell tumour. Non-ossifying fibroma or metaphyseal fibrous defect is a rare lesion on FNA and only one cytology case reported.[105] The most important finding was the presence of groups or clusters of fibroblast-like spindle cells. histiocytic cells with foamy or vacuolated cytoplasm and osteoclastic cells were also found.

## Notochordal tumours

## Chordoma

Chordoma is a slow growing malignant tumour which arises from cells of the notochord, which are foetal remnants found in vertebral bodies and intervertebral disks. The tumour is more common in males than females and very uncommon before 30 years of age. Chordomas are found in the midline of the body, usually in the sacrococcygeal and spheno-occipital regions but may also appear in vertebral bodies in the neck region. They form gelatinous masses composed of large and small, often epithelioid, tumour cells arranged in ribbons or lobules set in mucinous material. Some of the cells, referred to as physaliferous cells, are variably sized, with abundant clear, eosinophilic, or multivacuolated cytoplasm and large vesicular nuclei.

### Cytological findings: chordoma

- Abundant myxoid background
- Tumour cells singly or in groups or cords
- Network of myxoid material round single cells and groups
- Many tumour cells have vacuolated cytoplasm
- Physaliferous cells.

Because of their ability to destroy bone and invade soft tissues, chordomas are often easy to needle and the yield is usually good. The cytology of chordomas has been described in a number of studies.[106–108] The findings in the neoplasms from our file are similar to other reports.[4]

An abundant myxoid, often fibrillary, background matrix is the rule. Within this, dispersed tumour cells are mixed with cells in groups or cords. The myxoid matrix is difficult to identify in alcohol-fixed smears, but easily detected in air-dried MGG-stained preparations (Fig. 29.87A).

The predominant tumour cell is medium sized to large, with rounded well-demarcated cytoplasm and central nucleus. The cytoplasm is often vacuolated or bubbly (Fig. 29.87B). Cells may occasionally look like signet ring cells with a large cytoplasmic vacuole pushing the nucleus to the periphery, at times producing nuclear indentation. Generally, some cells are very large, with abundant foamy or vacuolated cytoplasm and central prominent nuclei, corresponding to the typical physaliferous cells seen in tissue section. Binucleated cells are found and there are also small uniformly rounded cells with scanty cytoplasm. In the dedifferentiated chordoma a population of large highly atypical, mono or multinucleated cells are present besides the typical cellular pattern.[109]

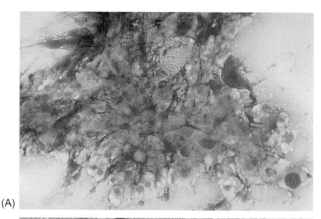

(A)

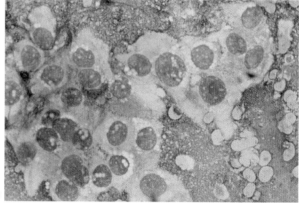

(B)

**Fig. 29.87** Chordoma. (A) The myxoid matrix encircles single cells as well as groups of tumour cells (MGG). (B) Cytoplasm-rich tumour cells with rounded nuclei and vacuolated cytoplasm (MGG).

### Diagnostic pitfalls: chordoma

The main pitfalls are chondrosarcoma and metastatic clear cell carcinoma or mucus producing carcinoma, especially in alcohol-fixed smears in which the typical fibrillary myxoid matrix is easily overlooked (Fig. 29.88). In other cases where the myxoid tissue component is dominant, it may be interpreted as a true soft tissue tumour if the cytopathologist is unaware of the radiological findings. A number of myxoid soft tissue sarcomas then become important in the differential diagnosis, such as myxofibrosarcoma and extraskeletal myxoid chondrosarcoma. Chordomas show typically a double positivity for S-100 protein and cytokeratin and immunocytochemical staining may help in the differential diagnosis between chordoma and chondrosarcoma and metastatic carcinoma.

## Neuroectodermal tumours

## Skeletal Ewing family of tumours

The Ewing family of tumours has been presented above.

## Lymphohistiocytic lesions

Primary Hodgkin lymphoma in bone is extremely rare. Primary non-Hodgkin lymphoma is also quite uncommon. The most

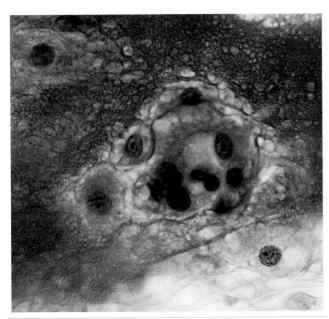

**Fig. 29.88** Chordoma. The myxoid matrix is almost non-visible in wet-fixed smears and cell clusters may be misinterpreted as coming from clear cell carcinoma metastasis (H&E).

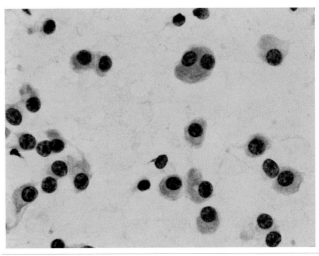

**Fig. 29.89** Solitary plasmocytoma. Numerous slightly atypical plasma cells, including binucleated forms (H&E).

frequent variants encountered are diffuse large B-cell lymphoma, precursor lymphoma, small lymphocytic lymphoma and anaplastic large cell lymphoma. The cytological features are identical to those described in FNA of lymph nodes (see Ch. 13).

## Solitary plasmacytoma

Solitary plasmacytoma is a lesion that is often difficult to diagnose radiologically and the findings are often misdiagnosed as metastatic carcinoma. Aspirates from plasmacytoma are often very haemorrhagic, containing a variable number of normal-looking and atypical plasma cells. Slightly atypical plasma cells may resemble osteoblasts. Poorly differentiated plasmacytomas are composed of markedly atypical plasma cells, resembling carcinoma cells (Fig. 29.89). For the most part clinical data are not helpful in diagnosis as the sedimentation rate often is within normal limits and light chain restriction is not found in the blood. In doubtful cases immunocytochemical staining is helpful. Positive staining with CD138 combined with negative cytokeratin staining strongly suggests plasmacytoma in cases of poorly differentiated plasmacytoma and light chain restriction helps to identify a plasmacytoma composed of normal-looking plasma cells (see Ch. 13, p. 425).

## Langerhans cell histiocytosis

Langerhans cell histiocytosis, also known as eosinophilic granuloma, is a benign lesion characterised by proliferation of histiocytic cells of Langerhans type, with a variable number of eosinophils, neutrophils, lymphocytes and plasma cells. Most cases occur before the age of 20 and the majority of lesions are monostotic. The most frequent sites are skull, vertebrae, ribs, clavicle and scapula. Radiologically, the main differential diagnosis are osteomyelitis in the younger age group and metastasis in adults. The cytological findings on FNA have been well

described,[110,111] and the author's experience of 15 cases is in agreement with these reports.[4]

### Cytological findings: Langerhans cell histiocytosis

A rich cellular yield is common. Smears are composed of a mixed population of eosinophils, neutrophils, lymphocytes, plasma cells, osteoblasts and osteoclasts in addition to the Langerhans histiocytes. The latter are large- to medium-sized cells with plentiful cytoplasm and rounded, bean- or kidney-shaped nuclei. Characteristically, the nuclei are irregular and lobulated or show folded nuclear membranes, having a 'coffee-bean' shape (Fig. 29.90). Some of the cells are binuclear or multinucleated.

In the authors' opinion, osteomyelitis is the most important differential diagnosis. Immunocytochemistry using markers as S-100 protein and CD1(a) are of value to establish a reliable diagnosis. Another important diagnostic adjunct is to identify the specific Birbeck granulas in electron microscopical preparations.

## Inflammatory lesions of bone

## Osteomyelitis

Although much less common today in the developed world, cases of osteomyelitis are, nevertheless, still seen in underdeveloped countries, especially in children. The metaphyses of long bones is the classical site for lesions to develop in childhood and staphylococci are the commonest infecting organism. Histologically, there is an acute inflammatory reaction with necrosis of bone and regenerative changes. In cases of tuberculous osteomyelitis a more chronic inflammatory picture is seen, including giant cell granuloma formation with lymphocytes and caseation necrosis. The radiological appearance of bacterial osteomyelitis may be difficult to differentiate from classical Ewing sarcoma in children. However, the cytological findings are distinctive and when combined with microbiological culture are often diagnostic.

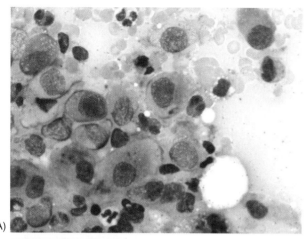

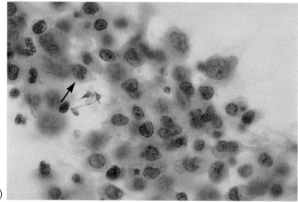

**Fig. 29.90** Langerhans cell histiocytosis. (A) A mixed population of Langerhans histiocytes, eosinophils and neutrophils (MGG). (B) The typical nuclear morphology, irregular nuclei with folded nuclear membrane is better visualised in wet-fixed smears. Note the 'coffee-bean' nucleus to the upper left (arrow) (H&E).

### Cytological findings: osteomyelitis

- Highly cellular yields
- Neutrophils
- Debris
- Histiocytes
- Epithelioid histiocytes in granulomatous inflammation.

Aspirates are cellular and dominated by neutrophils and cellular debris, with a variable proportion of macrophages. The smears look like purulent material aspirated from any abscess.

Tuberculous osteomyelitis must be suspected when clusters of epithelioid histiocytes are mixed with the neutrophils. These histiocytes are often arranged in granuloma-like clusters in FNA material. They have pale greyish-blue cytoplasm with indistinct cell borders and their elongated kidney-shaped nuclei are also pale staining. Small lymphocytes may also be noted but typical giant cells of Langerhans type as found histologically are seldom observed and caseation necrosis is not easily recognised.

## Metastatic tumours

In hospitals other than those specialising in the diagnosis and treatment of musculoskeletal tumours, metastatic lesions

**Table 29.7** Important antibodies to apply to suggest the primary site when a bone metastasis is the first sign of the tumour

| Primary site | Antibody | Comment |
|---|---|---|
| Kidney | CK8/18; CK7/20; CD10,RCC | CK8/18 + ; CD10 + ; CK7/20− |
| Lung | Squamous cell carcinoma: CK5/6; CK7 | CK5/6 + ; CK7 +/− |
| | Adenocarcinoma: CK7/20; TTF-1 | CK7 + ; TTF-1 + ; CK20− |
| | Small cell carcinoma: CK7/20; TTF-1, synaptophysin, CD 56 | TTF-1 + ; CK7/20− |
| Breast | CK7/20; ER; PGR, G6PD-15, mammoglobin | CK7 + ; CK20− |
| Thyroid | Thyroglobulin; TTF-1, calcitonin | |
| Prostate | CK8/18; CK7/20; PSA | CK8/18 + ; CK7/20− |
| Liver | Hepar-1; pCEA; CK7/20 | CK7/20− |
| Malignant melanoma | S-100 protein; HMB45; Melan A | |

are the malignant tumours most commonly encountered in bone. Carcinomatous metastases in the skeleton are mainly derived from the breast, kidney, lung, prostate thyroid and liver. Cutaneous and extracutaneous malignant melanoma are another important source of metastases.

The cytological features in skeletal metastases are the same as those of the primary tumours. When bone deposits are the first manifestation of the tumour, immunocytochemistry may help to disclose the primary site. In Table 29.7 the most important antibodies to apply to pinpoint the primary are listed.

## The role of FNA cytology in management of soft tissue lesions

### Diagnostic accuracy and grading

The clinical usefulness of FNA depends on the ability to aspirate sufficient material for diagnostic evaluation, to diagnose true sarcomas and to separate benign tumours and other lesions (including other types of malignant tumours and inflammatory lesions) from sarcomas. In general these requirements can be achieved in the diagnostic evaluation of soft tissue as well as bone tumours by FNA.

Due to the rarity of soft tissue sarcomas and the relative inexperience of many practising pathologists in dealing with the morphological diversity of sarcomas, many centres have traditionally obtained diagnostic material from either open biopsies or core needle biopsies (CNB). Further apprehension by pathologists in making a soft tissue sarcoma diagnosis with FNA cytology is that the incidence is higher in children than in adults and a misdiagnosis can potentially lead to debilitating treatments such as amputation.[112,113] Accordingly, FNA cytology has been underutilised in most centres, which is compounded by the requirement of accurate histological subtyping for enrolment of paediatric patients in specific therapeutic protocols.[113] However, there have been a number of studies comparing the accuracy of FNA cytology with CNBs that demonstrate that with adequate cellularity and the use of ancillary studies, there is a similar accuracy rate, approaching 95% for establishing a benign versus a malignant diagnosis.[1,2,3,114–124] In a retrospective 20-year study of 517 soft tissue tumours (295 benign tumours and 202 sarcomas) from the Musculoskeletal Tumour Centre, Lund University Hospital, there were 5% false diagnoses (14 false positive and 14 false negative), an inconclusive diagnosis was given in 3% and the aspirated material was insufficient for diagnosis in 6% of cases.[1] The accuracy figures for bone tumours are essentially the same.[4–6]

A number of studies have evaluated the accuracy rate of subtyping soft tissue sarcomas by FNA cytology with an accuracy range of 50–70%,[117,118,124–126,127] Kilpatrick et al. found the accuracy rate of 92% for subtyping pediatric sarcomas when ancillary studies are employed, which was a higher rate than that achieved in adults (52%).[125] However, in 83% of the patients with soft tissue sarcomas, Kilpatrick et al. report that the diagnosis was sufficient to begin definitive therapy.[124,125] In contrast, the small round cell tumours in the paediatric age group require specific histological subtyping for enrolment in specific treatment protocols. Kilpatrick et al. reported a series of 18 paediatric patients eligible for specific treatment protocols and demonstrated an accurate diagnosis by FNA cytology in 17 of 18 patients (94%).[125]

In order to achieve these results, we recommended that an on-site, experienced cytopathologist, should be present for both the immediate interpretation and determination of the need for obtaining additional specimens for ancillary studies.

There are four main limitations of FNA in the diagnosis of soft tissue and bone tumours: (1) the tumour is not sampled with the needle; (2) insufficient material is obtained from the tumour (poor yield or technically inferior smears due to inadequate smearing, necrosis or haemorrhage) for evaluation; (3) misinterpretation of the cellular material; and (4) inaccurate tumour grading.

Grading for soft tissue sarcomas can also be challenging in FNA cytology since accurate grading is based on a number of factors, including tissue necrosis and mitotic activity, which often cannot be adequately assessed in the FNA specimen. Therefore, a number of studies have recommended a classification in FNA cytology based on dividing soft tissue sarcomas into five major subgroups, reflecting the predominant cytomorphological phenotype identified (Table 29.8).[19,20,113] Following establishing a cytomorphological phenotype, a corresponding histological grade can often be determined.[19,124] A two-tier grading system has been shown to work best (low grade and high grade), since certain cytomorphological phenotypes such as round cell, pleomorphic and epithelioid/polygonal subgroups are by definition high-grade sarcomas (Table 29.9).[19,124] In a study from Lund, the cytological malignancy grade, low grade versus high grade, was assessed in 127 sarcomas and was correct in 103 (81%) and inconclusive in 24 (19%).[1] Cellular pleomorphism, abnormalities of chromatin, nucleolar structure, presence of necrosis and mitoses (mitotic rate and atypical mitoses) are the most important criteria used for malignancy grading.

## The cytological report

On the basis of clinical data and radiological findings alone, it may be difficult even for experienced orthopaedic surgeons and

**Table 29.8** Soft tissue tumours/lesions with definitive cytological features making diagnosis of tumour type possible

| Benign | Malignant |
|---|---|
| Nodular fasciitis | Leiomyosarcoma |
| Proliferative fasciitis/myositis | Liposarcoma |
| Myositis ossificans | Synovial sarcoma |
| Lipoma | Rhabdomyosarcoma |
| Neurilemmoma | Ewing family of tumours |
| Desmoid fibromatosis | Neuroblastoma |
| Elastofibroma | Low-grade fibromyxoid sarcoma |
| Solitary fibrous tumour | Myxofibrosarcoma |
| Intramuscular myxoma | Angiosarcoma |
| | Malignant peripheral nerve sheath tumour (MPNST) |
| | Extraskeletal myxoid chondrosarcoma |
| | Epithelioid sarcoma |

References are given with the presentation of respective tumours.

**Table 29.9** Soft tissue sarcoma classification and grading based on predominant cytomorphological phenotypes

| Small round cell sarcomas | Spindle cell sarcomas |
|---|---|
| Ewing sarcoma/primitive neuroectodermal tumour (PNET) | Fibrosarcoma |
| Rhabdomyosarcoma (childhood types) | Leiomyosarcoma |
| Neuroblastoma | Synovial sarcoma |
| Mesenchymal chondrosarcoma | Malignant peripheral nerve sheath tumour |
| Desmoplastic small round cell tumour | Gastrointestinal stromal tumour (GIST) |
| Pleomorphic sarcomas | Epithelioid/polygonal cell sarcomas |
| Pleomorphic malignant fibrous histiocytoma (MFH) | Epithelioid sarcoma |
| | Clear cell sarcoma (melanoma of soft parts) |
| Pleomorphic liposarcoma | Alveolar soft part sarcoma |
| Extraskeletal osteosarcoma | Malignant schwannoma |
| Pleomorphic rhabdomyosarcoma | Malignant granular cell tumour |
| Pleomorphic leiomyosarcoma | |
| Angiosarcoma | |
| Myxoid sarcoma | |
| Myxoid liposarcoma | |
| Myxofibrosarcoma (myxoid MFH) | |
| Low-grade fibromyxoid sarcoma | |
| Extraskeletal myxoid chondrosarcoma | |

(Modified from Singh HK, Kilpatrick SE, Silverman JF. Fine needle aspiration biopsy of soft tissue sarcomas: utility and diagnostic challenges. Adv Anat Pathol 2004; 11:24–37.)

radiologists to decide whether a soft tissue tumour is benign or malignant or even if the lesion is a true soft tissue tumour. This is especially the case with deep-seated tumours. In these circumstances, the cytological diagnosis becomes the most important parameter in determining further management. To avoid misleading diagnoses and misinterpretation of reports, we have for many years, in agreement with the orthopaedic surgeons, summarised our FNA diagnoses as follows:

- Sarcoma, including highly suspicious of sarcoma
- Malignant tumour other than sarcoma
- Benign
- Non-diagnostic, including insufficient material for diagnosis and inconclusive findings with regard to benignity or malignancy.

With regard to soft tissue, as well as bone lesions it is very important to realise that the final diagnosis is based on a combined evaluation of clinical data, including patient's age, the site of the tumour and duration of the lesion, together with the radiological and cytological findings. Above all, in all cases of bone lesions it is unwise to render a definitive diagnosis without knowledge of the radiological data.

## Future trends in the diagnosis of soft tissue and bone tumours

Demand for minimally invasive diagnostic techniques has resulted in an increasing use of core needle biopsy (CNB) with needles having an outer diameter of 1.2–1.4 mm instead of open surgical biopsy. One acknowledged disadvantage of FNA is the occasional difficulty in obtaining sufficient material when various ancillary diagnostic methods are necessary. An approach to overcome this difficulty and still benefit by the advantages of FNA in the primary diagnosis is when the cytopathologist at the same first encounter performs the FNA, rapidly assesses an immediately stained smear and, based on this immediate diagnostic evaluation, decides whether a CNB should be performed to certify that sufficient material is at hand for ancillary techniques. At our musculoskeletal tumour centre, this double approach has proved to be successful.[10]

## REFERENCES

1. Åkerman M, Willén H. Critical review on the role of fine needle aspiration in soft tissue tumours. Pathol Case Rev 1998;3:111–17.

2. Maitra A, Ashfaq R, Saboorian MH, et al. The role of fine-needle aspiration biopsy in the primary diagnosis of mesenchymal lesions. Cancer (Cancer Cytopathol) 2000;90:178–85.

3. Kumar S, Chowdhury N. Accuracy, limitations and pitfalls in the diagnosis of soft tissue tumors by fine needle aspiration cytology. Indian J Pathol Microbiol 2007;50:42–45.

4. Åkerman M, Domanski HA. Fine needle aspiration (FNA) of bone tumours: with special emphasis on definitive treatment of primary malignant bone tumours based on FNA. Curr Diagn Pathol 1998;5:82–92.

5. Jorda M, Rey L, Hanly A, et al. Fine-needle aspiration cytology of bone. Cancer (Cancer Cytopathol) 2000;90:47–54.

6. Söderlund V, Skoog L, Kreicbergs A. Combined radiology and cytology in the diagnosis of bone lesions: a retrospective study of 370 cases. Acta Orthop Scand 2004;75:492–99.

7. Åkerman M. Fine-needle aspiration cytology of soft tissue sarcoma: benefits and limitations. Sarcoma 1998;2:155–61.

8. Kilpatrick SE, Geisinger KR. Soft tissue sarcoma. The usefulness and limitations of fine-needle aspiration biopsy. Am J Clin Pathol 1998;110:50–68.

9. Domanski HA. Fine-needle aspiration cytology of soft tissue lesions: diagnostic challenges. Diagn Cytopathol 2007;12:768–73.

10. Domanski HA, Åkerman M, Carlén B, et al. Core-needle biopsy performed by the cytopathologist. A technique to complement fine-needle aspiration of soft tissue and bone lesions. Cancer (Cancer Cytopathol) 2005;105:229–239-.

11. Dodd LG, Martinez S. Fine-needle aspiration cytology of pseudosarcomatous lesions of soft tissue. Diagn Cytopathol 2001;24:28–35.

12. Fletcher DM, Unni KK, Mertens F. World Health Organization Classification of Tumours. Pathology and Genetics. Tumours of soft tissue and Bone. Lyon: IARC Press; 2001.

13. Weiss SW, Goldblum JR. Soft tissue tumors. 5th edn St Louis: Mosby; 2008.

14. Klobowes-Prevodnik VV, Us-Krasovec M, Gale N, et al. Cytologic features of lipoblastoma: A report of three cases. Diagn Cytopathol 2005;33. 195–120.

15. Meis JM, Enzinger FM. Chondroid lipoma. A unique tumor simulating liposarcoma and myxoid chondrosarcoma. Am J Surg Pathol 1993;17:1103–12.

16. Gisselson D, Domanski HA, Höglund M, et al. Unique cytological features and chromosome aberrations in chondroid lipoma: a case report based on fine-needle aspiration cytology, histopathology, electron microscopy, chromosome banding, and molecular cytogenetics. Am J Surg Pathol 1999;23:1300–4.

17. Yang YJ, Damron TA, Ambrose JL. Diagnosis of chondroid lipoma by fine-needle aspiration biopsy. Arch Pathol Lab Med 2001;125:1224–26.

18. Domanski HA, Carlén B, Jonsson K, et al. Distinct cytologic features of spindle cell lipoma. A cytologic-histologic study with clinical, radiologic, electron microscopic, and cytogenetic correlations. Cancer (Cancer Cytopathol) 2001;93:381–89.

19. Lamos MM, Kindblom L-G, Meis-Kindblom JM, et al. Fine-needle aspiration characteristics of hibernoma. Cancer (Cancer Cytopathol) 2001;93:206–10.

20. Kong CS, Cha I. Nodular fasciitis: diagnosis by fine needle aspiration biopsy. Acta Cytol 2004;48:473–77.

21. Dalén BP, Meis-Kindblom JM, Sumathi VP, et al. Fine-needle aspiration cytology and core needle biopsy in the preoperative diagnosis of desmoid tumors. Acta Orthop 2006;77:926–31.

22. Mentzel T, Bainbridge TC, Katenkamp D. Solitary fibrous tumour: clinicopathological, immunohistochemical, and ultrastructural analysis of 12 cases arising in soft tissues, nasal cavity and nasopharynx, urinary bladder and prostate. Virchows Arch 1997;430:445–53.

23. Chilosi M, Facchettti F, Dei Tos AP, et al. bcl-2 expression in pleural and extrapleural solitary fibrous tumours. J Pathol 1997;181:362–67.

24. Clayton AC, Diva RS, Gary LK, et al. Solitary fibrous tumor. A study of cytologic features of six cases diagnosed by fine-needle aspiration. Diagn Cytopathol 2001;25:172–76.

25. Domanski HA, Carlén B, Sloth M, et al. Elastofibroma has distinct cytomorphologic features making diagnostic surgical biopsy unnecessary: cytomorphologic study with clinical, radiologic, and electron microscopic correlations. Diagn Cytopathol 2003;29:327–33.

26. Klijanienko J, Caillaud J-M, Lagacé R. Fine-needle aspiration of primary and recurrent benign fibrous histiocytoma: classic, aneurysmal, and myxoid variants. Diagn Cytopathol 2004;31:387–91.

27. Pereira S, Tani E, Skoog L. Diagnosis of fibromatosis colli by fine needle aspiration (FNA) cytology. Cytopathology 1999;10:25–29.

28. Sharma S, Mishra K, Khanna G. Fibromatosis colli in infants. A cytological study of eight cases. Acta Cytol 2003;47:359–62.

29. Jadushing IH. Fine needle aspiration cytology of fibrous hamartoma of infancy. Acta Cytol 1997;41(Suppl 4):1391–93.

30. Domanski HA, Åkerman M, Engellau J, et al. Fine-needle aspiration of neurilemmoma. A clinicocytopathologic study of 116 patients. Diagn Cytopathol 2006;34:403–12.

31. Wieczorek TJ, Krane JK, Domanski HA, et al. Cytologic findings in granular cell tumors, with emphasis on the diagnosis of malignant granular cell tumor by fine-needle

aspiration biopsy. Cancer (Cancer Cytopathol) 2001;93:398–408.

32. Domanski HA. Cytologic features of angioleiomyoma: cytologic-histologic study of 10 cases. Diagn Cytopathol 2002;27:161–66.

33. Domanski HA, Dawiskiba S. Adult rhabdomyoma in fine needle aspiration. A report of two cases. Acta Cytol 2000;44:223–26.

34. Wakely PE. Myxomatous soft tissue tumors: correlation of cytopathology and histopathology. Ann Diagn Pathol 1999;3:227–42.

35. Lax S, Langsteger W. Ossifying fibromyxoid tumor misdiagnosed as follicular neoplasia. A case report. Acta Cytol 1997;41:1261–64.

36. Nemanqani D, Mourad WA. Cytomorphologic features of fine-needle aspiration of liposarcoma. Diagn Cytopathol 1999;20:67–69.

37. Dey P. Fine needle aspiration cytology of well-differentiated liposarcoma. A report of two cases. Acta Cytol 2000;44:459–62.

38. Vicandi B, Jimenez-Heffernan J, Lopez-Ferrer P, et al. Cytologic features of round cell liposarcoma. Cancer (Cancer Cytopathol) 2003;99:28–32.

39. Klijanienko J, Caillaud J-M, Lagacé R. Fine-needle aspiration in liposarcoma: cytohistologic correlative study including well-differentiated, myxoid, and pleomorphic variants. Diagn Cytopathol 2004;30:307–12.

40. Meis-Kindblom J, Bjerkehagen B, Böhling T, et al. Morphologic review of 1000 soft tissue sarcomas from the Scandinavian Sarcoma Group (SSG) register. The peer-review committee experience. Acta Orthop Scand 1999;70(Suppl 285):18–26.

41. Fletcher CDM, Gustafson P, Rydholm A, et al. Clinicopathologic re-evaluation of 100 malignant fibrous histiocytomas: prognostic relevance of subclassification. J Clin Onc 2001;19:3045–50.

42. Klijanienko J, Caillaud JM, Lagacé R, et al. Comparative fine-needle aspiration and pathologic study of malignant fibrous histiocytoma: cytodiagnostic features of 95 tumors in 71 patients. Diagn Cytopathol 2003;29:320–26.

43. Kilpatrick SE, Ward WG. Myxofibrosarcoma of soft tissues: cytomorphologic analysis of a series. Diagn Cytopathol 1999;20:6–9.

44. Domanski HA, Gustafson P. Cytologic features of primary, recurrent, and metastatic dermatofibrosarcoma protuberans. Cancer (Cancer Cytopathol) 2002;96:351–61.

45. Domanski HA, Mertens F, Panagopoulos I et al. Low-grade fibromyxoid sarcoma is difficult to diagnose by fine needle aspiration cytology: a cytomorphological study of eight cases. Cyropathology 2008; 14 July. [Epub ahead of print].

46. Klijanienko J, Caillaud J-M, Lagacé R, et al. Cytohistologic correlation of 24 malignant peripheral nerve sheath tumors (MPNST) in 17 patients: the Institut Curie experience. Diagn Cytopathol 2002;27:103–8.

47. Domanski HA, Åkerman M, Rissler P, et al. Fine needle aspiration of soft tissue leiomyosarcoma. An analysis of the most common cytologic findings and the value of ancillary techniques. Diagn Cytopathol 2006;34:597–604.

48. Coffin CM. The new international rhabdomyosarcoma classification, its progenitors, and considerations beyond morphology. Adv Anat Pathol 1997;4:1–16.

49. Atahan S, Aksu O, Ekinici C. Cytologic diagnosis and subtyping of rhabdomyosarcoma. Cytopathology 1998;9:389–97.

50. Daneshbod Y, Monabati A, Kumar PV, et al. Paratesticular spindle cell rhabdomyosarcoma diagnosed by fine needle aspiration cytology: A case report. Acta Cytol 2005;49:331–34.

51. Klijanienko J, Caillaud JM, Orbach D, et al. Cyto-histological correlations in primary, recurrent and metastatic rhabdomyosarcoma: the Institut Curie experience. Diagn Cytopathol 2007;35:482–87.

52. Udayakumar AM, Sundareshan TS, Appaji L, et al. Rhabdomyosarcoma: cytogenetics of five cases using fine-needle aspiration samples and review of the literature. Ann Genet 2002;45:33–37.

53. Boucher LD, Swanson PE, Stanley MW, et al. Cytology of angiosarcoma. Findings in fourteen fine needle aspiration biopsy specimens and one pleural fluid specimen. Am J Clin Pathol 2000;114:210–19.

54. Minimo C, Zakowski M, Lin O. Cytologic findings of malignant vascular neoplasms: A study of twenty-four cases. Diagn Cytopathol 2002;26:349–55.

55. Klijanienko J, Caillaud J-M, Lagacé R, et al. Cytohistologic correlations in angiosarcoma including classic and epithelioid variants: the Institute Curie experience. Diagn Cytopathol 2003;29:140–45.

56. Åkerman M, Carlén B. Diagnosis of neuroblastoma in fine needle aspirates. Acta Orthop Scand 1997;68(Suppl 274):72.

57. Fröstad B, Tani E, Kogner P, et al. The clinical use of fine needle aspiration cytology for diagnosis and management of children with neuroblastic tumours. Eur J Cancer 1998;34:529–36.

58. Das DK. Fine-needle aspiration (FNA) cytology diagnosis of small round cell tumors: value and limitations. Indian J Pathol Microbiol 2004;47:309–18.

59. Guiter GE, Gamboni MM, Zakowski MF. The cytology of extraskeletal Ewing sarcoma. Cancer 1999;87:141–48.

60. Sahu K, Pai RR, Khadilkar UN. Fine needle aspiration cytology of the Ewing's sarcoma family of tumors. Acta Cytol 2000;44:332–336-.

61. Fröstad B, Tani E, Brosjö O, et al. Fine needle aspiration cytology in the diagnosis and management of children and adolescents with Ewing sarcoma and peripheral primitive neuroectodermal tumor. Med Pediatr Oncol 2002;38:33–40.

62. Åkerman M, Dreinhöfer K, Rydholm A, et al. Cytogenetic studies on fine-needle aspiration samples from osteosarcoma and Ewing's sarcoma. Diagn Cytopathol 1995;15:17–22.

63. Fröstad B. Fine needle aspiration cytology in diagnosis and management of childhood small round cell tumours. Thesis, Stockholm; 2000.

64. Udayakumar AM, Sundareshan TS, Goud TM, et al. Cytogenetic characterisation of Ewing tumors using fine needle aspiration samples, a 10-year experience and review of the literature. Cancer Genet Cytogenet 2001;127:42–48.

65. Li SQ, O'Leary TJ, Buchner SB, et al. Fine needle aspiration of gastrointestinal stromal tumors. Acta Cytol 2001;45:9–17.

66. Rader AE, Avery A, Wait CL, et al. Fine-needle aspiration biopsy diagnosis of gastrointestinal stromal tumors using morphology, immunocytochemistry and mutational analysis of c-kit. Cancer (Cancer Cytopathol) 2001;93:269–75.

67. Klijanienko J, Caillaud J-M, Lagacé R, et al. Cytohistological correlations in 56 synovial sarcomas in 36 patients: the Institut Curie's experience. Diagn Cytopathol 2002;27:96–102.

68. Åkerman M, Ryd W, Skytting B. Fine-needle aspiration of synovial sarcoma: criteria for diagnosis: retrospective examination of 37 cases, including ancillary diagnostics. AA Scandinavian Sarcoma Group study. Diagn Cytopathol 2003;28:232–38.

69. Kwon MS. Aspiration cytology of pulmonary small cell variant of poorly-differentiated synovial sarcoma metastatic to the tongue: a case report. Acta Cytol 2005;49:92–96.

70. Åkerman M, Domanski HA. The complex cytological features of synovial sarcoma in fine needle aspirates, an analysis of four illustrative cases. Cytopathology 2007;18:234–40.

71. Nilsson G, Ming MD, Weide J, et al. Reverse transcriptase polymerase chain reaction on fine needle aspirates for rapid detection of translocations in synovial sarcoma. Acta Cytol 1998;42:1317–24.

72. Logrono R, Wojtowycs MM, Wunderlich DW, et al. Fine needle aspiration cytology and core biopsy in the diagnosis of alveolar soft part sarcoma presenting with lung metastases. A case report. Acta Cytol 1999;43:464–70.

73. Lopez-Ferrer P, Jimenez-Heffernan JA, Vicandi B, et al. Cytologic features of alveolar soft part sarcoma: report of three cases. Diagn Cytopathol 2002;27:115–19.

74. Creager AJ, Pitman MB, Geisinger KR. Cytologic features of clear cell sarcoma (malignant melanoma) of soft parts: a study of fine needle aspirates and exfoliative specimens. Am J Clin Pathol 2002;117:217–24.

75. Tong TR, Chow TC, Chan OW, et al. Clear cell sarcoma diagnosis by fine-needle aspiration: cytologic, histologic, and ultrastructural features; potential pitfalls; and literature review. Diagn Cytopathol 2002;26:174–80.

76. Cardillo M, Zakowski MF, Lin O. Fine-needle aspiration of epithelioid sarcoma. Cytology findings in nine cases. Cancer (Cancer Cytopathol) 2001;93:246–51.

77. Yildiz I, Onder S, Kutlay L, et al. Cytology of epithelioid sarcoma. Cytopathology 2006;17:305–7.

78. Domanski HA, Carlén B, Mertens F, et al. Extraskeletal myxoid chondrosarcoma with neuroendocrine differentiation: a case report with fine-needle aspiration biopsy, histopathology, electron microscopy, and cytogenetics. Ultrastructural Pathology 2003;27:363–68.

79. Jakowski JD, Wakely PE. Cytopathology of extraskeletal myxoid chondrosarcoma. Report of 8 cases. Cancer (Cancer Cytopathol) 2007;111:298–305.

80. Pogacnik A, Zidar N. Malignant rhabdoid tumor of the liver diagnosed by fine needle aspiration cytology. A case report. Acta Cytol 1997;41:539–43.

81. Drut R, Drut RM. Renal and extrarenal congenital rhabdoid tumor: diagnosis by fine-needle aspiration biopsy and FISH. Diagn Cytopathol 2002;27:32–34.

82. Ali SZ, Nicol TL, Port J, et al. Intraabdominal desmoplastic small round cell tumor: Cytopathologic finding in two cases. Diagn Cytopathol 1998;18:449–52.

83. Ferlicot C, Coue O, Gilbert E, et al. Intraabdominal desmoplastic small round cell tumor: report of a case with fine needle aspiration, cytologic diagnosis and molecular confirmation. Acta Cytol 2001;45:617–21.

84. Dhawan SB, Aggarwal R, Mohan K, et al. Cytodiagnosis of enchondroma. Cytopathology 2003;14:157–59.

85. Kilpatrick SE, Pike EJ, Geisinger KR, et al. Chondroblastoma of bone: use of fine-needle aspiration biopsy and potential diagnostic pitfalls. Diagn Cytopathol 1997;16:65–71.

86. Layfield LJ, Ferreiro JA. Fine-needle aspiration cytology of chondromyxoid fibroma: a case report. Diagn Cytopathol 1988;4:148–51.

87. Gupta S, Dev G, Marya S. Chondromyxoid fibroma: a fine-needle aspiration diagnosis. Diagn Cytopathol 1993;9:63–65.

88. Lerma E, Tani E, Brosjö O, et al. Diagnosis and grading of chondrosarcoma on FNA biopsy material. Diagn Cytopathol 2003;28:13–17.

89. Dodd LG. Fine needle aspiration of chondrosarcoma. Diagn Cytopathol 2006;34:413–18.

90. Bauer HC, Brosjö O, Kreicbergs A, Lindholm J. Low risk of recurrence of enchondroma and low grade chondrosarcoma in extremities. Acta Orthop Scand 1995;66:283–88.

91. Walaas L, Kindblom L-G, Gunterberg B, et al. Light and electron-microscopic examination of fine-needle aspiration in the preoperative diagnosis of cartilaginous tumours. Diagn Cytopathol 1990;6:396–408.

92. Antonescu C, Argani P, Erlandson R, et al. Skeletal and extraskeletal myxoid chondrosarcoma. A comparative clinicopathologic, ultrastructural, and molecular study. Cancer 1998;83:1504–21.

93. Rinas AC, Ward WG, Kilpatrick SE. Potential sampling error in fine-needle aspiration biopsy of dedifferentiated chondrosarcoma: a report of 4 cases. Acta Cytol 2005;49:554–59.

94. Kreicbergs A, Söderberg G, Zetterberg A. Prognostic significance of nuclear DNA content in chondrosarcoma. Anal Quant Cytol 1980;4:271–78.

95. Rhode MG, Lucas DR, Krueger CH, et al. Fine-needle aspiration of spinal osteoblastoma in a patient with lymphangiomatosis. Diagn Cytopathol 2006;34:295–97.

96. Dodd LG, Scully SP, Cothran RL, et al. Utility of fine-needle aspiration in the diagnosis of primary osteosarcoma. Diagn Cytopathol 2002;27:350–53.

97. Klianienko J, Caillaud J-M, Orbach D, et al. Cytohistological correlations in primary, recurrent and metastatic bone and soft tissue osteosarcoma: the Institut Curie's experience. Diagn Cytopathol 2007;35:270–75.

98. Domanski HA, Åkerman M. Fine-needle aspiration of primary osteosarcoma: a cytological-histological study. Diagn Cytopathol 2005;32:269–75.

99. Park SH, Kim I. Small cell osteosarcoma of the ribs: immunohistochemical, and ultrastructural study with literature review. Ultrastruct Pathol 1999;23:133–40.

100. Fanburg JC, Rosenberg AE, Weaver DL, et al. Osteocalcin and osteonectin immunoreactivity in the diagnosis of osteosarcoma. Am J Clin Path 1997;108:464–73.

101. Sneige N, Ayala GA, Carrasco CH, et al. Giant cell tumor of bone. A cytologic study of 24 cases. Diagn Cytopathol 1985;1:111–17.

102. Vetrani A, Fulciniti F, Boschi R, et al. Fine needle aspiration biopsy diagnosis of giant-cell tumor of bone. Acta Cytol 1990;34:863–67.

103. Yamamato T, Nagira K, Akisu T, et al. Fine-needle aspiration biopsy of solid aneurysmal bone cyst in the humerus. Diagn Cytopathol 2003;28:159–62.

104. Gupta RK, Voss DM, McHutchinson AG, et al. Osteitis fibrosa cystica (brown tumor) in a patient with renal transplantation. Acta Cytol 1992;36:555–58.

105. Troncone G, Vetrani A, Boschi R. Il difetto fibroso metafisario (DFM) in biopsia per ago sottile. Istocitopatologia 1988;10:113–18.

106. Finley JL, Silverman JF, Dabbs DJ, et al. Chordoma: diagnosis by fine-needle aspiration with histologic, immunocytochemical, and ultrastructural confirmation. Diagn Cytopathol 1998;2:330–37.

107. Crapanzano JP, Ali SZ, Ginsberg MS, et al. Chordoma: a cytologic study with histologic and radiologic correlation. Cancer (Cancer Cytopathol) 2001;93:40–51.

108. Kay PA, Nasciemento AG, Unni KK, et al. Chordoma. Cytomorphologic findings in 14 cases diagnosed by fine needle aspiration. Acta Cytol 2003;47:202–8.

109. Bergh P, Kindblom L-G, Gunterberg B, et al. Prognostic factors in chordoma of the sacrum and mobile spine. Cancer 2000;88:2122–34.

110. Pohar-Marinsek Z, Us-Krasovec M. Cytomorphology of Langerhans cell histiocytosis. Acta Cytol 1996;40:1257–64.

111. Kilpatrick SE. Fine needle aspiration biopsy of Langerhans cell histiocytosis: are ancillary studies necessary for a 'definitive diagnosis'. Acta Cytol 2002;42:820–23.

112. Geisinger KR, Silverman JF, Wakely P. Pediatric Cytopathology. Chicago: American Society of Clinical Pathologists; 1994.

113. Singh HK, Kilpatrick SE, Silverman JF. Fine needle aspiration biopsy of soft tissue sarcomas: utility and diagnostic challenges. Adv Anat Pathol 2004;11:24–37.

114. Kilpatrick SE, Ward WG, Chauvenet AR, et al. The role of fine needle aspiration biopsy in the initial diagnosis of pediatric bone and soft tissue tumors: an institutional experience. Mod Pathol 1998;11:923–28.

115. Abdul-Karim FW, Rader AE. Fine needle aspiration of soft-tissue lesions. Clin Lab Med 1998;18:507–40.

116. Costa MJ, Campman SC, David R, et al. Fine-needle aspiration cytology of sarcoma: retrospective review of diagnostic utility and specificity. Diagn Cytopathol 1996;15:23–32.

117. Wakely PE Jr, Kneisl JS. Soft tissue aspiration cytopathology. Cancer 2000;90:292–98.

118. Bommer KK, Ramzy I, Mody D. Fine-needle aspiration biopsy in the diagnosis and management of bone lesions: a study of 450 cases. Cancer 1997;81:148–56.

119. Kilpatrick SE, Cappellari JO, Bos GD, et al. Is fine-needle aspiration biopsy a practical alternative to open biopsy for the primary diagnosis of sarcoma? Experience with 140 patients. Am J Clin Pathol 2001;115:59–68.

120. Jones C, Liu K, Hirschowitz S, et al. Concordance of histopathologic and cytologic grading in musculoskeletal sarcomas: can grades obtained from analysis of the fine-needle aspirates serve as the basis for therapeutic decisions? Cancer 2002;96:83–91.

121. Bennert KW, Abdul-Karim FW. Fine needle aspiration cytology vs. needle core biopsy of soft tissue tumors: a comparison. Acta Cytol 1994;38:381–84.

122. Kilpatrick SE, Ward WG, Cappellari JO, et al. Fine-needle aspiration biopsy of soft tissue sarcomas: a cytomorphologic analysis with emphasis on histologic subtyping, grading, and therapeutic significance. Am J Clin Pathol 1999;112:179–88.

123. Kilpatrick SE, Geisinger KR. Soft tissue sarcomas: The usefulness and limitations of fine-needle aspiration biopsy. Am J Clin Pathol 1998;110:50–68.

124. Singh HK, Volmar KE, Elsheikh TM, et al. The diagnostic utility of fine-needle aspiration biopsy of soft-tissue sarcomas in the core needle biopsy era. Pathol Case Rev 2007;12:36–43.

125. Kilpatrick SE. Histologic prognostication in soft tissue sarcomas: grading versus subtyping or both? A comprehensive review of the literature with proposed practical guidelines. Ann Diagn Pathol 1999;3:48–61.

126. Pollock RE. The National Cancer Data Base report on soft tissue sarcoma. Cancer 1996;78:2247–57.

127. Ladanyi M. The emerging molecular genetics of sarcoma translocation. Diagn Mol Pathol 1995;4:162–73.

128. Fletcher JA. Cytogenetics and molecular biopsy of soft tissue tumors. In: Weiss SW, Brooks JSJ, editors. Soft Tissue Tumors. Philadelphia: Williams & Wilkins; 1996. p. 37–64.

# Synovial fluid

Anthony J. Freemont and John Denton

## Chapter contents

## Introduction

### Normal synovial fluid

Synovial or diarthrodial joints are the most sophisticated in the body. Unlike fibrous or cartilaginous joints in which the bone ends are effectively tethered together with bands of motion-limiting fibrous tissue or cartilage, in synovial joints each bone end is covered by an independent layer of hyaline cartilage. The two cartilage-covered bone ends are separated by a narrow space containing the lubricant, synovial fluid. This arrangement allows two adjacent bones the freedom to move in multiple directions.

The downside of increased movement is decreased stability and as a consequence, all diarthrodial joints are inherently unstable. Stability comes from the joint capsule, ligaments and muscle tone. The capsule consists of dense fibrous tissue which, rather than joining the bone ends, forms a strong flexible sleeve that surrounds the joint and envelops the peripheral segments of the two bones. This creates a cavity inside the joint which, except for the cartilage, is completely lined by a specialised form of connective tissue called synovium. The synovium is covered by an incomplete layer of cells – the synoviocytes. There are two main types of synoviocyte: type A, derived from macrophages that phagocytose any debris that falls into the fluid from the joint lining, and type B, derived from synovial fibroblasts with a synthesising function.

Synovial fluid is a transudate of plasma supplemented with high-molecular-weight saccharide-rich molecules, notably hyaluronans, and a molecule called lubricin, produced by the type B synoviocytes.

Synovial fluid differs from all other body fluids in that the surfaces of synovium and cartilage (the tissues in immediate contact with the synovial fluid) are covered by an incomplete layer of cells. This means that there is no intact basement membrane, which in other tissues is a significant physical and chemical barrier to the movement of molecules and cells. It also means that the matrix of cartilage and synovium are in contact with the synovial fluid, allowing a relatively homogeneous chemical environment to develop within the joint. Because of this unusual arrangement it is perhaps better to regard the synovial fluid as a semi-liquid, avascular, hypocellular connective tissue rather than a true body fluid, such as may form in the pericardial, abdominal or pleural cavity.

### Synovial fluid in diseased joints

Variations in the volume and composition of synovial fluid reflect pathological processing occurring within the joint. Because of the relationship between the tissues within the joint, chemically mediated events such as inflammation or enzyme-mediated degradation occurring within the synovium and cartilage are reflected in changes within the synovial fluid. These changes include the production of factors responsible for the accumulation of different cell types within the fluid, and it is this that explains why the complement of cells within the joint varies between diseases.

## Synovial fluid cytology

Cytology of synovial fluid differs in three important regards from that of other body fluids. First, synovial joints are very rarely affected by neoplastic processes. Second, 'cytology' of synovial fluid is better described as 'microscopy', as accurate recognition of non-cellular particulate material, such as crystals and matrix fragments, is essential to an understanding of the disease process within the joint. Third, the greatest diagnostic information comes not only from the recognition of cell types but also from their quantification.[1–3]

## The basic approach to synovial fluid microscopy

It is normal for samples to pass through a 4 step sequential analysis after receipt in the laboratory:

1. Gross analysis
2. The nucleated cell count
3. The 'wet prep'
4. The cytocentrifuge preparation.

## Gross analysis

Because synovial fluids from inflamed joints have a tendency to clot, they should be received in the laboratory in anticoagulant. Choosing the most appropriate anticoagulant is problematic. Because one of the key elements of synovial fluid analysis is examination for crystals, crystalline anticoagulants have to be avoided, as do chelating anticoagulants, which destroy crystals by removing core structural metal ions such as $Ca^{2+}$. We find lithium heparin to be the best anticoagulant.

It is not possible to fix synovial fluid and the specimen therefore represents fresh tissue, and should be treated as such in every case. Even with refrigeration the optimum cytological information can only be extracted if the sample is examined within 48 hours of aspiration, and preferably as soon as possible within the first 24 hours.

Upon arrival in the laboratory the synovial fluid should be examined macroscopically. Macroscopic analysis involves a subjective assessment of colour, clarity and viscosity.

### Colour

Synovial fluid is normally pale yellow. In haemarthroses it will be red or orange and in inflammatory arthropathies may appear cream or white. Occasionally in septic arthritis it may be coloured by bacterial chromogens.

### Clarity

Normal synovial fluid is clear. As the number of particles and/or cells it contains increases so it passes through a phase of opalescence to one of being frankly opaque. Examination of the clarity therefore gives a clue to the cellularity and/or crystal content of the fluid specimen.

### Viscosity

Normal synovial fluid has a thick mucoid consistency because of complex interactions between proteins and proteoglycans. These interactions are fundamental to the lubricating properties of synovial fluid. In inflammatory joint disease, the viscosity of the fluid falls due to enzymatic digestion and altered synthesis of these molecules.

## The nucleated cell count

A sample of synovial fluid, agitated to achieve the most uniform distribution of cells, is diluted to a known concentration with normal saline containing methyl violet as a supravital stain. A count of the number of nucleated cells is then performed, either 'manually,' using a haemocytometer chamber or by machine using an automated cell counting instrument such as a Coulter Counter.[4] The number of cells is expressed per unit volume (usually /mm$^3$). To convert this to cell counts per mL necessitates multiplying the cell count by 1000. Normal synovial fluid contains approximately 200 cells/mm$^3$. In inflammatory joint disease the cell count exceeds 1000 cells/mm$^3$ and in non-inflammatory arthropathies is usually less than 1000 cells/mm$^3$. Cell counts in excess of 30 000 cells/mm$^3$ are found predominantly in three clinical settings: rheumatoid arthritis, septic arthritis and reactive arthritis (a form of arthropathy associated with infection at an extra-articular site and caused by the presence of, and reaction to, epitopes of the organism, but not the whole organism, within the joint).

## The 'wet prep'

Synovial fluid often contains small particles that can be recognised with the naked eye. In making the 'wet prep' the specimen is agitated and a small aliquot containing as many of these particles as possible is aspirated into a glass pipette, then placed as a large drop onto a microscope slide. The drop is gently squeezed flat beneath a coverslip and viewed unstained with a conventional microscope. For optimal results the microscope condenser diaphragm should be nearly closed to produce diffused light in which the unstained cells and particles are more clearly seen. In addition to particulate matter including crystals and fragments of tissues from joint associated structures such as cartilage, meniscus and ligament, the preparation is examined for one type of cell, the ragocyte.

## Crystals

Several classes of crystalline material are found in joints.[5,6] They consist of the following:

### Monosodium urate

These are typically needle-shaped, highly birefringent crystals usually 5–30 μm long (Fig. 30.1). They can be distinguished from other crystals in that they are negatively birefringent when

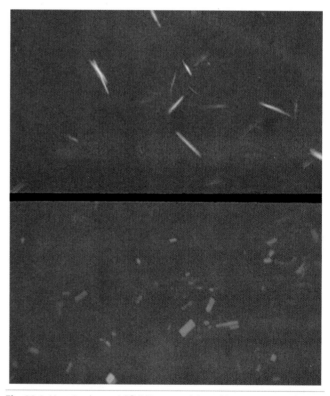

**Fig. 30.1** Unstained synovial fluid 'wet prep' viewed between crossed polarisers with an interference plate in the light path giving the magenta background. The upper picture is of highly birefringent needle-shaped urate crystals and the lower of less birefringent rhomboidal CPPD. Note that crystals with their long axis running top left to bottom right are yellow in the top image and blue in the lower. This allows crystals to be distinguished easily from one another.

viewed in polarised light with an interposed quarter wave plate. These crystals are diagnostic of gout. If found within the background of a high cell count fluid their presence usually signifies acute gout,[6] but even if the cell count is low the diagnosis is beyond doubt.

### Calcium pyrophosphate dihydrate (CPPD)

These crystals accumulate naturally within certain connective tissues with advancing age, where they are most commonly seen as white deposits. In joints, they are found predominantly in fibrocartilage. Histologically, they appear as grey-brown aggregates in which crystals can be identified by polarising microscopy.

There are three main clinical settings in which CPPD deposition occurs in tissues and in many cases this is reflected in the synovial fluid:

- Most commonly the patients are asymptomatic and are identified radiologically as having chondrocalcinosis. These patients rarely, if ever, have joint aspiration consequent upon their chondrocalcinosis
- Some patients have an acute crystal monoarthritis caused by the presence of CPPD within the joint. The clinical picture mimics gout, and in the synovial fluid the cell count is high. Intra and extra cellular CPPD crystals are readily seen. This is acute pseudogout (Fig. 30.1)
- CPPD may be found in association with otherwise characteristic features of osteoarthritis (OA). This is typical of the more common form of degenerative joint disease – hypertrophic OA.

### Hydroxyapatite

Crystals of hydroxyapatite within synovial fluid indicate damage either to the calcified zone of cartilage or underlying subarticular bone. Loss of cartilage sufficient to expose these structures to the synovial fluid is seen in the non-inflammatory disorder osteoarthritis and in the erosive inflammatory arthropathies of which easily the most common is rheumatoid arthritis. Sometimes the crystals are too small and amorphous to be seen with the conventional light microscope but staining with Alizarin red stain produces a birefringent bright red product (calcium alizarate) which is easily visualised (Fig. 30.2).[7] Some patients have an aggressive destructive arthropathy caused by the presence of hydroxyapatite crystal spheroids within the joint. This was first described in the shoulder[8] (Milwaukee shoulder) in association with calcification in the tendons of the rotator cuff, but has since been described in most large joints.

### Lipids

Lipids enter the synovial fluid from the blood in inflammatory joint disease, intra-articular haemorrhage and following trauma.[9] Different lipids have different crystalline shapes varying from the notched plates of cholesterol to the spherical liquid crystals of cholesterol esters (Fig. 30.3).[10]

### Steroids

Intra-articular injection of depot steroids is conventional management of certain arthropathies. Unfortunately, the crystalline steroid preparation may remain within the joint for up to 10 weeks and may mislead the unwary if the characteristic appearance is not recognised.[11]

### Others

Numerous other crystals may be found within the synovial fluid specimen but they are too numerous and rare to describe here. A more exhaustive analysis is given by Freemont and Denton.[3]

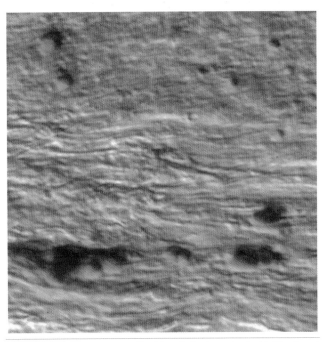

**Fig. 30.2** Hydroxyapatite crystalloids in a fibrin clot stained with Alizarin red.

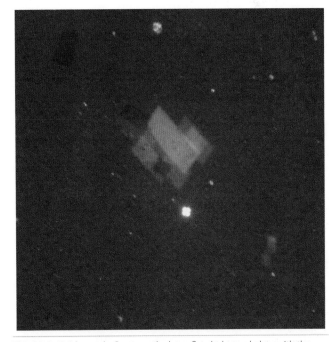

**Fig. 30.3** Lipid crystals. Compare the large flat cholesterol plate with the smaller brighter Maltese cross of a lipid liquid crystal.

## Non-crystalline, non-cellular particulate material

The inside of conventional synovial joints is lined by cartilage and synovium, and may be crossed by ligaments and bands of fibrocartilage. Damage caused by trauma or inflammation may lead to small fragments of these tissues appearing free within the synovial fluid. Most common are fragments of cartilage, or following trauma, particularly to the knee, fragments of cruciate ligament and meniscal fibrocartilage.

Cartilage can be recognised by the silken sheen of its matrix. In osteoarthritis, the most common disorder in which fragments of cartilage are found in the joint, cartilage fragments have many of the characteristics of osteoarthritic cartilage seen in tissue sections. In particular, they may show surface crimping of early fibrillation and contain clustered chondrocytes (Fig. 30.4). Large quantities of cartilage and bone are typical of avascular bone necrosis. Sometimes nodules of cartilage from patients with synovial chondromatosis may be small enough to be aspirated. These are hypercellular and may have stellate cells on their surface.

Fragments of meniscal fibrocartilage can be recognised by the curved arrays of collagen fibres and flattened chondrocytes they contain. They are typically found within traumatised knee and shoulder joints.

In the knee in both twisting trauma and in rheumatoid disease small fragments of ligament may be found within synovial fluid. These fragments usually consist of long thin fibrils made up of highly organised arrays of collagen fibres which are quite distinctive when viewed in polarised light.

With the advent of prosthetic surgery, and particularly as the number of ageing prostheses increases, wear of implants leads to the presence of prosthesis-derived debris within the joint. Many of the modern plastics such as high-density polyethylene used for articular surfaces, methyl methacrylate used as a cement, and fibres such as Dacron and carbon fibre used as replacement ligaments can mimic crystals as they fragment. Metal debris from metal-based prostheses can be shed or abraded and appear as tiny black particles. These may be harbingers of imminent prosthetic failure.[12,13]

Occasionally, peculiar extraneous material is found within the synovial fluid, usually introduced by a clinician. We have found structures as diverse as paper, pollen and mites.

## Ragocytes

Ragocytes is the term for cells of various lineages, most often polymorphs but also macrophages and lymphocytes, which are recognised by the presence within their cytoplasm of refractile granules that vary from apple-green to black (depending on the focus) when viewed with a microscope with a partially closed condenser diaphragm. The granules are larger than 'conventional' neutrophil granules and can be distinguished on the basis of their size and refractivity (Fig. 30.5). The cells are called 'ragocytes' as they were first described in patients with rheumatoid arthritis (RA).[14] It is now recognised that ragocytes are frequently found in many inflammatory arthropathies. Extensive study of these cells shows them to contain immune complexes, including rheumatoid factors.

Ragocytes are counted and their number expressed as a proportion of all nucleated cells seen in the 'wet preparation'. Ragocytes are found in many inflammatory arthropathies but the percentage of nucleated cells containing ragocyte granules is usually low (5–30%). However, in rheumatoid arthritis the proportion of ragocytes is typically greater than 70% of all nucleated cells, and, in diagnostic terms, a ragocyte count of 70–95% is typical of, and specific to, rheumatoid arthritis. A ragocyte count above 95% usually indicates septic arthritis and can be used to suggest this diagnosis even in the absence of detectable organisms.

## The cytocentrifuge preparation

Synovial fluid cytoanalysis is best conducted on cytocentrifuge preparations stained with a modified Jenner–Giemsa stain.

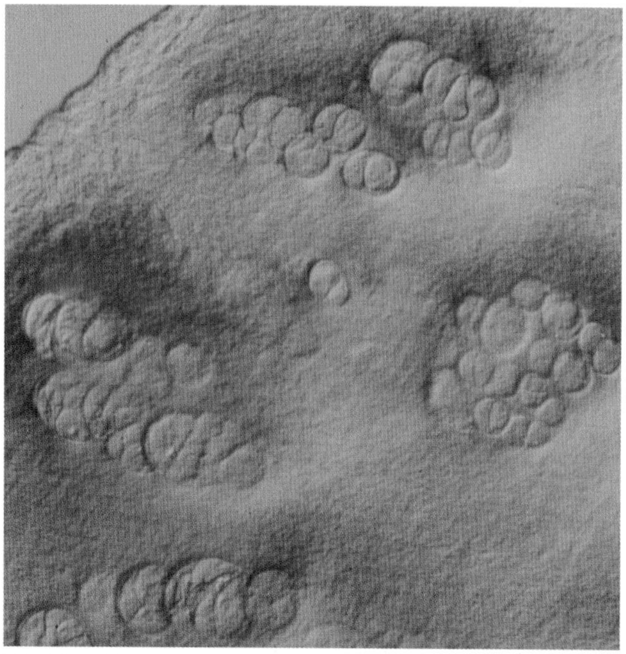

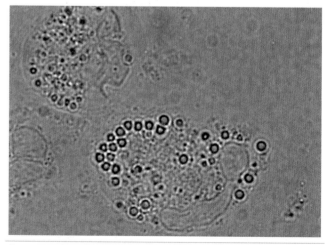

**Fig. 30.4** A fragment of osteoarthritic cartilage showing the characteristic chondrocyte clusters.

**Fig. 30.5** Ragocytes showing characteristic granules with apple green colouration in diffused transmitted light. Unstained 'wet preparation'.

Optimal cytocentrifuge preparations are made by diluting the fluid down to 400 cells/mm$^3$ with isotonic saline. The one exception is when septic arthritis is suspected, when the greatest likelihood of identifying organisms is afforded by diluting the fluid to a concentration of 1200 cells/mm$^3$.

## Organisms

As most infective arthritis is caused by Gram-positive bacteria (Fig. 30.6); careful microscopic examination of Gram-stained synovial fluid cytocentrifuge preparations allows microorganisms to be identified in approximately 80% of instances of clinical infective arthritis.[15] This means, however, that even careful evaluation misses one in eight cases of septic arthritis.

The greatest problems in diagnosing infective arthritis are first, the recognition of Gram-negative organisms and organisms rendered Gram-negative by incomplete antibiotic therapy, and second, distinguishing contaminating organisms from those that are truly pathogenic. The latter is made more difficult because synovial fluid is a live tissue and accidental contamination of the fluid by organisms may lead to those organisms becoming intracellular, one of the features often said to be pathognomonic of infection.

Most bacterial infections result in a neutrophil response, however, in contrast to this, infection resulting from *Mycobacteria* spp are characteristically lymphocyte-rich fluids.

With an increase in the number of patients who are immunosuppressed, either as a consequence of disease, or through therapy, there is an increasing incidence of non-suppurative infective arthritis, particularly caused by *Mycobacteria* and fungi. Although it is often possible to see organisms in these cases, close cooperation between clinician and cytopathologist is necessary to achieve the optimal detection rate.

Care must also be taken in patients who have a pre-existing arthropathy, particularly rheumatoid arthritis. These patients are both at a greater risk of developing a superimposed infective arthritis and of receiving treatment that may mask the presence of infection.

Possibly the greatest recent advance in the diagnosis of infective arthritis has come in the most difficult bacterial infections to diagnose: infections in joints containing a prosthesis. In 2004, a paper appeared from the Mayo Clinic which has heralded a step change in diagnosis.[16] The authors investigated the cell count and differential polymorph count (see below) in patients with infected knee prostheses. They showed that: 'A leukocyte count of >1.7 × 10$^3$/μL [1700 cells/mm$^3$], had a sensitivity of 94% and a specificity of 88% for diagnosing prosthetic joint infection; a differential of >65% neutrophils had a sensitivity of 97% and a specificity of 98%'.

## Cells

For reasons that are not clearly understood primary neoplastic disease is exceptionally rare in joints. Occasionally, leukaemic cells may be found in synovial fluid, but there are only a handful of cases of other neoplastic processes involving joints. Malignant cells are therefore so rare as to be disregarded in everyday practice.

The cells that are found most frequently in synovial fluid are a reflection of the two major groups of joint diseases, namely the inflammatory arthropathies such as septic arthritis, gout, seronegative spondyloarthropathies and rheumatoid disease, and the non-inflammatory arthropathies resulting from trauma or due to osteoarthritis.

The cells most commonly encountered in synovial fluid are polymorphs, lymphocytes, macrophages and synoviocytes (Fig. 30.7). In very general terms, in inflammatory arthropathies polymorphs dominate the cytological picture and in non-inflammatory arthropathies macrophages, lymphocytes and synoviocytes are the most commonly encountered cells. Although making up the overwhelming majority of the cells within diseased joints, these four groups represent only a small proportion of the cell types that can be identified regularly within diseased joints. Most of these cell types are identifiable on morphological grounds in conventional Jenner–Giemsa stained cytocentrifuge

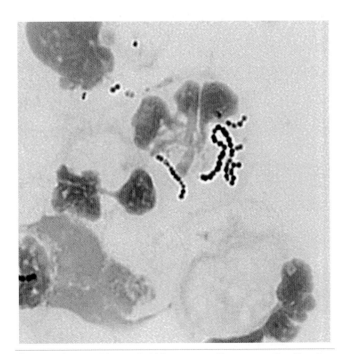

**Fig. 30.6** Gram-positive cocci within a cytocentrifuge preparation (Gram).

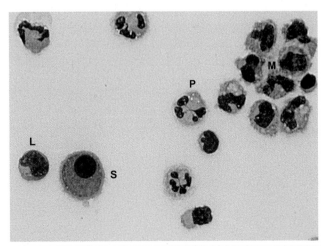

**Fig. 30.7** The four main cell types in a cytocentrifuge preparation. P, polymorphs; L, lymphocytes; M, macrophages; S, synoviocyte (Jenner–Giemsa).

preparations. The following are the most useful cells from a diagnostic perspective in synovial fluid.

## Neutrophil polymorphs

These cells are recognised by their characteristic nuclear morphology. They are the predominant cells in inflammatory arthropathies and in intra-articular haemorrhage (in both accounting for 60–80% of nucleated cells). In septic arthritis, they frequently amount to more than 95% of the total nucleated cells. Even in the absence of detectable organisms, finding a ragocyte count of >95% together with >95% polymorphs is a good basis for suggesting that the patient has a septic arthritis.

## Small lymphocytes

These are up to 12 μm in diameter with a nuclear/cytoplasmic ratio greater than 9:1. They predominate (i.e. account for more than 50% of the nucleated cells) in approximately 10% of all cases of inflammatory arthritis. In patients with rheumatoid arthritis finding >50% lymphocytes in the synovial fluid indicates a better long-term prognosis for that joint.[17] When seen in the company of LE cells, a high proportion of lymphocytes strongly suggests the diagnosis of systemic lupus erythematosus (SLE).

## Rieder cells

These cells are up to 15 μm in diameter with a nuclear/cytoplasmic ratio of 6:1. The nuclei are lobed, the lobes showing symmetry about a pale, attenuated, central region (Fig. 30.8). This peculiar morphology is almost certainly a consequence of cytoskeletal abnormalities brought about by a toxic extracellular environment. They are seen almost exclusively in rheumatoid disease.

## Macrophages

These form one of the three morphologically distinct categories of large mononuclear cells encountered in synovial fluid. They are common in all types of arthritis and are frequently the most common cell found in non-inflammatory arthropathies, particularly in some cases of osteoarthritis and in joints in which previously implanted prostheses are breaking down. True viral arthritis (i.e. one in which the virus is present in the joint) is the main type of inflammatory arthropathy in which macrophages predominate.

## Cytophagocytic mononuclear cells (CPM)

CPM are mononuclear cells that have phagocytosed apoptotic polymorphs (Fig. 30.9). The cells are normally seen wherever apoptosis is occurring and, as this is the usual way in which polymorphs are removed from joints, they are common in tissues. They are, however, most abundant in synovial fluid in the seronegative spondylarthropathies.[18] These are a group of diseases which includes: the peripheral arthritis associated with psoriasis, inflammatory bowel disease and ankylosing spondylitis; reactive arthritis, which is an oligoarthropathy occurring in association with extra-articular infection, notably of the gastrointestinal and genitor-urinary tracts; the arthritis which follows vaccination and viral infection; and the major group of arthritides in childhood, juvenile idiopathic arthritis.[19]

In rheumatoid arthritis, apoptosis occurs in the absence of CPM formation, a feature of such universal occurrence that it can be used diagnostically.

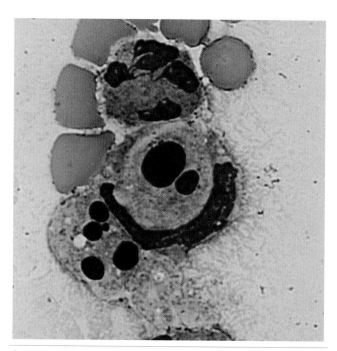

**Fig. 30.9** CPM. Note the apoptotic polymorphs, one inside and the other outside the macrophage. They have the same cytoplasm as the viable polymorph (12 o'clock) (Jenner–Giemsa).

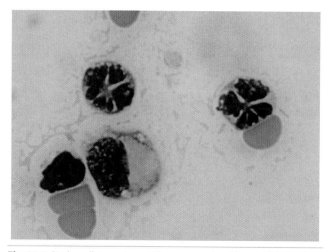

**Fig. 30.8** Rieder cells in a cytocentrifuge preparation. Note the lobulated nuclei with the pale attenuated centre (Jenner–Giemsa).

## Synoviocytes

These are a morphologically distinct subgroup of the large mononuclear cells, with a low nuclear/cytoplasmic ratio, round eccentrically placed nuclei and a 'pericellular frill'. They are shed from the surface of the synovium and are found most commonly in non-inflammatory arthropathies where multinucleate forms may occur.[20]

## Eosinophils

Eosinophils are seen following intra-articular haemorrhage and arthrography, as well as in the rare parasitic infestations of joints and in type I hypersensitivity-type reactions to injected material.

## Mast cells

Although mast cells (Fig. 30.10) can be found in most arthropathies they are seen most commonly in inflammatory arthritis in patients with a seronegative spondyloarthropathy and in non-inflammatory arthropathies associated with trauma.

## LE cells

Phagocytes containing a cytoplasmic inclusion of nuclear material are not uncommon and do not have the same significance in synovial fluid as they do in blood. In the presence of a fluid rich in lymphocytes, however, they are strongly suggestive of SLE.

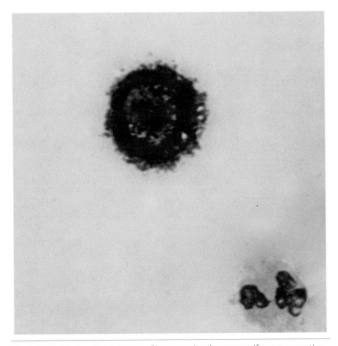

**Fig. 30.10** Mast cell in a Jenner–Giemsa stained cytocentrifuge preparation.

## Clinical applications of synovial fluid microscopy and the value of diagnostic algorithms

The features described above represent a short analysis of the important microscopic findings in synovial fluid. By retrospective analysis of proven cases, it is possible to recognise patterns of microscopic features specific for certain of the arthropathies. These form the basis of a series of diagnostic algorithms that can be used diagnostically.[3] A practical version of value in everyday cytological diagnosis is given below.

The starting point for each of these algorithms is the nucleated cell count. The first (Fig. 30.11) has a low cell count. By following the algorithm it is possible to distinguish between the various non-inflammatory arthropathies. There are two important elements to this algorithm of particular note:

- Because of the short duration of disease, by the time some patients with gout reach the clinic, the signs of inflammation have subsided. In this setting the diagnosis of gout can still be made by identifying urate crystals
- Joints with failing prostheses often contain prosthetic debris, which should not be confused with pathogenic crystals. Fluids from these joints are frequently sent for analysis to distinguish aseptic loosening (low cell count fluid) from infection (cell count >1700 cell/mm$^3$; see Organisms, above).

The second and third (Figs 30.12, 30.13) have high cell counts. As can be seen from the crystal and infected arthritides, there is considerable diagnostic overlap between the two but it is helpful to have a way of handling very high cell count fluids (>30 000 cells/mm$^3$).

Figure 30.12 gives a useful approach to the inflammatory fluid. Like the other algorithms, it incorporates data from the wet prep and the cytocentrifuge preparation, and its diagnostic yield is reliant upon the ability of the observer to recognise and record features in both these preparations. That said, a failure to recognise any one feature does not result in a false positive diagnosis but rather drops the accuracy of the analysis from a specific diagnosis to the more general diagnosis of 'an inflammatory arthropathy'.

Figure 30.13 outlines a coping strategy for the alarming situation of the high cell count fluid. These appear 'purulent' to the clinician who immediately suspects infection. This may well be the case, and while there is little harm in giving most patients antibiotics on suspicion of infection, giving any drug unnecessarily is not considered good medical practice and the alternative approach of joint washout under general anaesthetic has attendant risks. If the pathologist can help the patient to avoid such unnecessary interventions, she/he should. There are four main causes of very high cell counts, acute crystal arthritis, septic arthritis, reactive arthritis and an acute rheumatoid flare. The last is, however, extremely rare nowadays because of the changing nature of rheumatoid disease and the availability of over-the-counter medications; except in one modern setting which occurs when a patient's disease 'breaks away' from control with anti-TNF drugs, when an acute rheumatoid flare may be seen.

These algorithms have been tested in several trials. In randomised anonymous trials conducted in ignorance of clinical data it proved possible to produce an accurate diagnosis

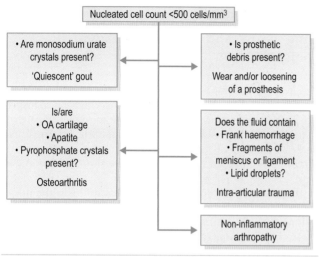

**Fig. 30.11** Diagnostic algorithm for a 'low cell count' fluid.

(e.g. crystal arthropathies, rheumatoid disease, septic arthritis, osteoarthritis and meniscal/ligamentous injury) in approximately 45% of cases. In a further 25% a short differential diagnosis (e.g. seronegative spondyloarthropathy, trauma) can be produced and in all but 4% of the remainder it proves possible to say whether the patient has an inflammatory or non-inflammatory basis to their joint disease.

The overall diagnostic rate in synovial fluid cytoanalysis is therefore 96%, although it is true that in half of these the diagnosis is not precise. Providing the diagnostic criteria are not over-interpreted and the cytopathologist recognises that in a significant proportion of cases the most accurate diagnosis possible is 'inflammatory' or 'non-inflammatory' arthropathy, the false positive rate is almost zero and, as such, synovial fluid cytoanalysis represents the most selective and specific of all rheumatological and orthopaedic investigations.

Even a relatively imprecise diagnosis may be of considerable clinical value to non-specialist physicians and general practitioners for whom referral policy to a specialist can be influenced by whether the disease in the joint is inflammatory or non-inflammatory, which is a surprisingly difficult distinction for

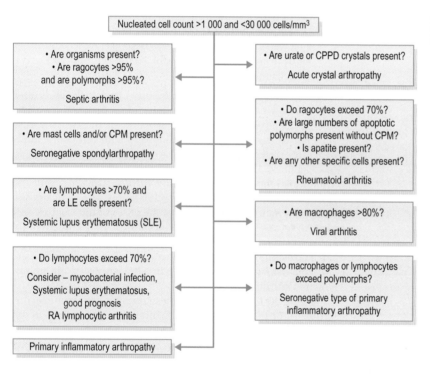

**Fig. 30.12** Diagnostic algorithm for a 'conventional inflammatory arthropathy'.

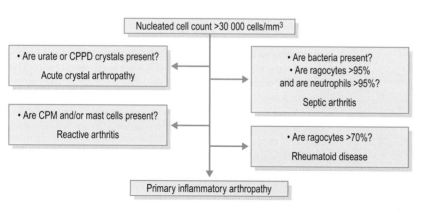

**Fig. 30.13** Diagnostic algorithm for a 'high cell count' fluid. There are four main causes of very high cell counts: acute crystal arthritis, septic arthritis, reactive arthritis and an acute rheumatoid flare. However, the last is extremely rare nowadays because of the changing nature of rheumatoid disease and the availability of over-the-counter medications.

even experienced rheumatologists to make clinically in some patients.

A short list of differential diagnoses may be equally important, particularly where further clinical information, unknown to the pathologist, is available to the clinician. For instance, the presence of mast cells and CPM is typical of the seronegative spondyloarthropathies. This appears imprecise but just making this diagnosis excludes the patient having rheumatoid arthritis, which is reassuring for the patient and also leads the clinician into a new line of investigation that could reveal hidden psoriatic plaques, evidence of inflammatory bowel disease or undiagnosed venereal infection.

## The place of synovial fluid microscopy in clinical management

Histopathologists have very limited access to tissue from diseased joints. The articular surfaces are rarely biopsied except in end-stage disease when they are removed, usually as part of joint replacement surgery. These specimens offer little of diagnostic value.

Synovium is not infrequently biopsied. Synovial biopsy is the investigation of choice in joint diseases with specific appearances, such as granulomatous inflammation and pigmented villonodular synovitis. However, most biopsies are performed for the diagnosis of one of the inflammatory or non-inflammatory arthropathies. Even very experienced histopathologists can have difficulty in distinguishing inflammatory from non-inflammatory arthropathies since the latter frequently have a moderate lymphocytic infiltrate in the synovium. Even if a distinction can be made it is usually impossible to be more specific because there are few microscopic differences between disorders in the same broad group.

By contrast, synovial fluid microscopy is of greatest value in those disorders which are most difficult for the clinician to diagnose. It is of great value in distinguishing inflammatory from non-inflammatory arthropathies; and in the differential diagnosis of acute monoarthritis and oligoarthropathies.

It is also important in recognising specific inflammatory arthropathies early in the course of the disease, and often before the full-blown syndrome develops. In these cases, accurate early diagnosis often allows the initiation of specific therapy before irreversible joint damage has occurred.

Finally, it permits the very rapid diagnosis of joint disease, particularly disorders such as septic and crystal arthritis, where the prognosis is inversely related to delay in diagnosis.

## Summary

The simple observations described above are based on conventionally stained and illuminated preparations. These can represent a simple addition to the diagnostic armamentarium of the cytopathologist, but one of considerable importance to rheumatologists, orthopaedic surgeons, accident and emergency physicians and general practitioners.

By necessity, this chapter has been unable to cover all aspects of synovial fluid microscopy, giving only a flavour of the important areas in the subject. For more detailed discussions, other texts are available.[3]

## REFERENCES

1. Swan A, Amer H, Dieppe P. The value of synovial fluid assays in the diagnosis of joint disease: a literature survey. Ann Rheum Dis 2002;61:493–98.

2. Brannan SR, Jerrard DA. Synovial fluid analysis. J Emerg Med 2006;30:331–39.

3. Freemont AJ, Denton J. Atlas of synovial fluid cytopathology, Vol 18. Current histopathology. Dordrecht: Kluwer Academic; 1991.

4. de Jonge R, Brouwer R, Smit M, et al. Automated counting of white blood cells in synovial fluid. Rheumatol 2004;43:170–73.

5. Lumbreras B, Pascual E, Frasquet J, et al. Analysis of the crystals in synovial fluid: training of the analysts results in high consistency. Ann Rheum Dis 2005;64:612–15.

6. Chen LX, Clayburne G, Schumacher HR. Update on identification of pathogenic crystals in joint fluid. Curr Rheumatol Rep 2004;6:217–20.

7. Paul H, Reginato AJ, Schumacher HR. Alizarin red-S staining as a screening test to detect calcium compounds in synovial fluid. Arth Rheum 1983;26:191–200.

8. McCarty DJ, Halverson PB, Carrera Gf, et al. Milwaukee shoulder: association of microspheroids containing hydroxyapatite crystals, active collagenase, and neutral protease with rotator cuff defects II. Synovial fluid studies. Arth Rheum 1981;24:474–83.

9. Freemont AJ, Denton J. Synovial fluid findings early in traumatic arthritis. J Rheumatol 1988;15:881–82.

10. Riordan JW, Dieppe PA. Cholesterol crystals in shoulder synovial fluid. Br J Rheumatol 1987;26:430–32.

11. Kahn CB, Hollander JL, Schumacher HR. Corticosteroid crystals in synovial fluid. JAMA 1970;211:807–9.

12. Peterson C, Benjamin JB, Szivek JA, et al. Polyethylene particle morphology in synovial fluid of failed knee arthroplasty. Clin Orthop Relat Res 1999;359:167–75.

13. Niki Y, Matsumoto H, Otani T, et al. Phenotypic characteristics of joint fluid cells from patients with continuous joint effusion after total knee arthroplasty. Biomaterials 2006;27:1558–65.

14. Rawson AJ, Abelson NM, Hollander JL. Studies of the pathogenesis of rheumatoid joint inflammation. II. Intracytoplasmic particulate complexes in rheumatoid synovial fluids. Ann Int Med 1965;62:281–84.

15. Ryan MJ, Kavanagh R, Wall PG, et al. Bacterial joint infections in England and Wales: analysis of bacterial isolates over a four year period. Br J Rheumatol 1997;36:370–73.

16. Trampuz A, Hanssen AD, Osmon DR, et al. Synovial fluid leukocyte count and differential for the diagnosis of prosthetic knee infection. Am J Med 2004;117:556–62.

17. Davies MJ, Denton J, Freemont AJ, et al. Comparison of serial synovial fluid cytology in rheumatoid arthritis; delineation of subgroups with prognostic implications. Ann Rheum Dis 1988;47:559–62.

18. Freemont AJ, Denton J. The disease distribution of synovial fluid mast cells and cytophagocytic mononuclear cells in inflammatory arthritis. Ann Rheum Dis 1985;44:312–15.

19. Nash P, Mease PJ, Braun J, et al. Seronegative spondyloarthropathies: to lump or split? Ann Rheum Dis 2005;64(Suppl 2):ii9–ii13.

20. Iwanaga T, Shikichi M, Kitamura H, et al. Morphology and functional roles of synoviocytes in the joint. Arch Histol Cytol 2000;63:17–31.

# Section **14**

## Central Nervous System

# Brain and cerebrospinal fluid

Malcolm Galloway and Maria Thom

## Chapter contents

## INTRAOPERATIVE CYTOLOGY OF THE CENTRAL NERVOUS SYSTEM

*Malcolm Galloway*

## Introduction

Tumours of the central nervous system (CNS) account for 1.6% of cancers in England and Wales; however, due to the high mortality of many of the common brain tumours, they account for a substantial burden in years of life lost. The annual incidence of primary CNS tumours in adults in England and Wales is approximately 6500, of which 58% are reported to be 'malignant' (WHO grade III or IV).[1,2]

The current national guidelines for CNS tumours recommend that all patients with brain tumours are cared for by a multidisciplinary team (MDT) with core members including a neuropathologist.[1] Patients should be discussed where possible by the MDT prior to surgery to allow selection of cases for intraoperative neuropathological assessment. Intraoperative assessment can be particularly useful when stereotactic biopsies are being taken, to ensure adequate material has been obtained for subsequent definitive histology. Intraoperative pathology can also assist the surgeon in the management of the patient during the operation. In rare cases, the intraoperative assessment may be used to guide postoperative management, while awaiting definitive paraffin section histological diagnosis.

## Intraoperative neuropathological techniques

A variety of techniques may be used, including frozen section histology and smears or imprint cytology. Frozen section is superior to smear cytology for the assessment of architectural features; however, smear cytology allows better demonstration of nuclear morphology, which can be particularly useful in distinguishing astrocytic and oligodendroglial neoplasms.[3] A danger of using frozen sections is that, although the block used to prepare a frozen section can be retained for subsequent formalin-fixed, paraffin wax embedded sections, tissue that has been previously frozen can show substantial freezing artefact. Cytological techniques are more rapid than frozen sections, and use relatively little tissue. Where there is sufficient material to perform both techniques, they should be considered to be complementary.

Occasionally, brain smears may be used for postmortem diagnosis allowing a more accurate assessment of underlying neuropathology than gross examination alone.

## Intraoperative neuropathological cytology techniques

This chapter focuses on smear preparations, which are the most widely used cytological technique in intraoperative neuropathology. An alternative technique is the touch (imprint) cell preparation, which can be useful particularly when the cells within the lesion are discohesive.[4]

The cytological assessment of fluid from cystic brain lesions may also be performed intraoperatively. However, this has been shown to have a high false negative rate, and, therefore, is not used routinely.[5]

*Malcolm Galloway wishes to thank Dr J McLaughlan, who originally performed many of the smears in the departmental archive, some of which are included here and Dr WR Timperley, the author of this chapter in the previous edition, from which several figures have been retained. Maria Thom wishes to acknowledge Steve Durr, Andy Beckett, Derek Marsden and Indran Davagnanam for their help in preparing her part of the chapter.*

The smear technique involves placing samples of tissue at one end of a glass slide, pressing on to the tissue with another slide, and sliding it over to produce a thin trail of cellular material. The challenge with the technique is to provide enough pressure on the tissue to produce material as close to a monolayer of cells as is possible, without crushing the cells and producing too much artefact. With experience, the skill of applying the appropriate level of pressure for different types of tumour is acquired. For example a pituitary adenoma usually spreads into a monolayer of cells with minimal pressure, whereas a schwannoma requires considerable pressure and often cutting the sample into small pieces prior to smearing in order to produce an interpretable preparation.

The quantity of tissue used on each smear, and the number of smears made depends on the quantity of tissue available for assessment. If the smear is too thick, the cellularity of the lesion is difficult to assess and nuclear detail is obscured. The more tissue examined, the more likely the examination is to be representative of the whole lesion. However, this may mean that less tissue is available for final histological diagnosis.

Various stains may be suitable for intraoperative smear cytology, the two most commonly used stains are haematoxylin and eosin (H&E) and toluidine blue. H&E staining demonstrates cytoplasmic features, such as astrocytic cell processes well. Toluidine blue is particularly useful for fine nuclear detail, but demonstrates cytoplasmic features less well. Individual preference, experience and local practice will determine whether either or both stains are used.

The tissue used for smear cytology is initially unfixed. This raises health and safety concerns. The procedure should only be carried out in an environment that is suitable for handling potentially infectious material, and appropriate safety clothing should be worn. The smear itself should be made with caution, as occasionally slides may break during the procedure. Rubbery lesions, such as schwannomas and some meningiomas may 'ping' out from the slide when compression is applied, potentially posing an ocular hazard.

## Cytology of the normal brain

When looking at a brain smear, it is essential to know the approximate location of the lesion. Different parts of the normal brain have very different appearances on smear cytology, and it is important not to misinterpret these as pathological findings. For example, the granular cell layer of the cerebellum smears out as a monolayer of small cells with round nuclei and scanty cytoplasm. This appearance could mimic a lymphocytic infiltrate (Fig. 31.1A). Normal white matter will usually produce a relatively even smear, with low cellularity and evenly spaced out cells (Fig. 31.1B). Smears from the cortex or from deep grey nuclei will show similar features, with interspersed neurones, the size and shape of which will vary depending on the location (Fig. 31.1C). The neuropil in grey matter tends to have a 'fluffy' appearance.

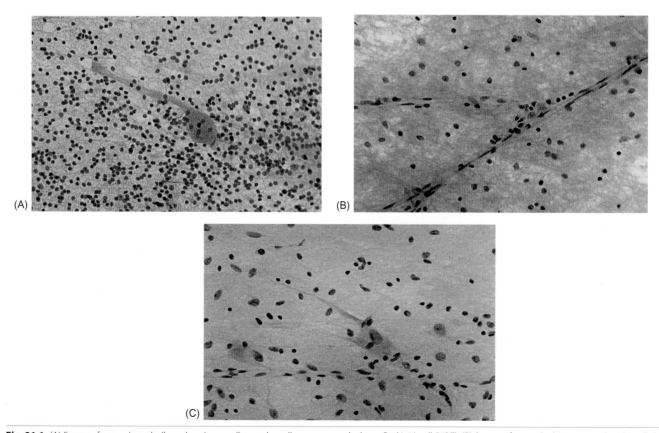

(A)  (B)  (C)

**Fig. 31.1**  (A) Smear of normal cerebellum showing small granular cell neurones and a large Purkinjé cell (H&E). (B) Smear of normal white matter showing glial cells and capillaries (H&E). (C) Smear showing normal grey matter with neurones and glial cells (H&E).

## Neurones

Neurones usually have a prominent nucleolus. In distinguishing normal neurones from neoplastic cells, the smooth outline of the nucleus and the fine chromatin can be helpful. The cytoplasm is easily lost during the smearing process, but if present Nissl substance, lipofuscin and sometimes a pyramidal shape may be noted.

## Astrocytes and oligodendrocytes

Astrocytes and oligodendrocytes are the other main cellular constituent of brain tissue. It is not always possible on a smear to determine with certainty the identity of individual cells. Oligodendrocytes tend to have small round nuclei with dense chromatin.[6] Astrocytic nuclei tend to be larger, round to ovoid, and have less dense chromatin.[5] Sometimes the cytoplasm of an astrocyte and its associated cellular processes will be visible (Fig. 31.2A).

In practice, it is very rare to smear entirely normal brain, as brain biopsy is only performed in patients with suspected underlying pathology. A stereotactic biopsy may miss the lesion and sample non-neoplastic brain tissue; however, this usually shows some reactive changes in response to the adjacent lesion.

## Reactive processes

Reactive astrogliosis is a non-specific phenomenon, occurring in reaction to almost any neuropathological process, including neoplasms, infections, infarction, demyelination and trauma. Reactive astrogliosis produces a mildly hypercellular smear in which astrocytes are prominent, evenly spaced and have complex cytoplasmic processes. The nuclei may be larger than normal, but should still have a delicate chromatin pattern and smooth nuclear membrane (Fig. 31.2A, B). The glial stroma is dense.

The presence of numerous macrophages or other inflammatory cells should always raise the suspicion of a non-neoplastic diagnosis. Reactive brain tissue may be difficult to distinguish from low-grade diffusely infiltrating astrocytoma (see below).

## Non-neoplastic conditions

## Infections

Infections are an important differential diagnosis for intracranial lesions, particularly in immunocompromised patients. Such patients present a particular challenge as abscesses, tumours and progressive multifocal leukoencephalopathy may all produce a similar radiological pattern of a ring-enhancing lesion.

The range of infections that may affect the central nervous system includes parasites, fungi, bacteria, viruses and prions.

### Bacterial abscess

Bacterial abscesses are an important clinical and radiological mimic of neoplastic lesions. A mature bacterial abscess typically has a central necrotic region, a rim of reactive tissue with fibrosis and a peripheral zone of gliotic brain tissue with oedema. Smear cytology findings will depend on which region of an

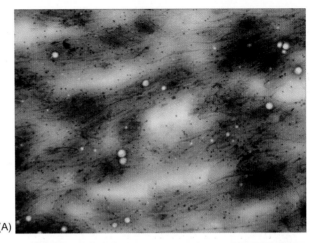

(A)

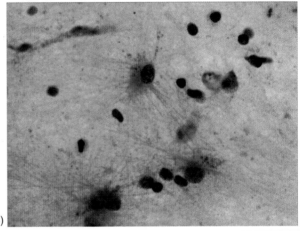

(B)

**Fig. 31.2** (A) Smear of reactive brain tissue (toluidine blue). (B) Smear of reactive brain tissue, high power, showing astrocytes with complex finely branching processes (toluidine blue).

abscess is sampled; however, neutrophils tend to be prominent in all areas (Fig. 31.3A). The central zone will contain pus. The reactive rim will contain newly formed capillaries and macrophages in addition to acute inflammatory cells. A sampling of the surrounding reactive tissue may not be diagnostic.

### Cytological findings: bacterial abscess

- Neutrophils and necrotic debris in the core
- Reactive gliosis in reactive margin.

### Diagnostic pitfalls: bacterial abscess

- The presence of necrosis and astrocytes with reactive atypia may lead to an erroneous diagnosis of glioblastoma.

### Tuberculosis

Tuberculosis is an important cause of infection of the central nervous system. Suspected cases should not usually undergo frozen section, due to the risk to laboratory staff; however, smear cytology with appropriate health and safety precautions may be undertaken. Necrotic tissue, epithelioid macrophages, and multinucleated giant cells may be seen (Fig. 31.3B,C). Epithelioid macrophages may resemble the epithelial cells of a metastatic carcinoma.[7]

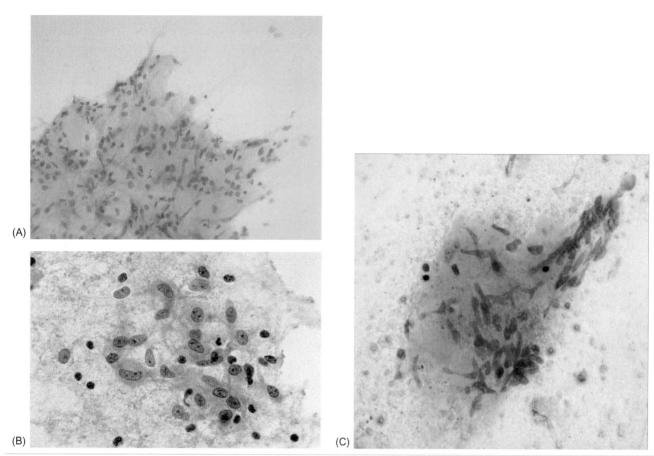

**Fig. 31.3** (A) Smear of the wall of a bacterial abscess, showing infiltration of neutrophils (toluidine blue). (B) Smear of cerebral tuberculosis showing epithelioid macrophages (H&E). (C) Smear of cerebral tuberculosis showing multinucleated giant cell (toluidine blue).

### Cytological findings: tuberculosis

- Epithelioid macrophages
- Multinucleated giant cells
- Necrosis.

### Diagnostic pitfalls: tuberculosis

- Epithelioid macrophages may be misinterpreted as metastatic carcinoma or meningioma.

## Other infections

Parasitic cysts may contain fragments of the parasite which may be of diagnostic utility intraoperatively. The cyst fluid in such cysts will usually contain macrophages and eosinophils.

Toxoplasmosis, due to infection by the parasite *Toxoplasma gondii*, results in a necrotising infection, usually in immuno-compromised patients. On imaging, it produces ring-enhancing lesions that may be mistaken for a neoplasm. On smear, the edge of the lesion may show reactive gliosis and contain chronic inflammatory cells. More central smears also include necrotic debris and neutrophils. If found, the bradyzoites, swollen cells containing numerous Toxoplasma organisms, are diagnostic.

Fungal infection may produce a granulomatous pattern of inflammation. The presence of a mixed inflammatory infiltrate including multinucleated giant cells in a smear should raise the possibility of fungal infection. Although typically the organism will be identified on paraffin sections rather than cytological specimens, fungal elements may be seen on smear. Fungi that infect the central nervous system may produce hyphae (*Aspergillus*, *Mucor*), pseudohyphae (*Candida*), or yeasts (*Cryptococcus*).[7] In histoplasmosis the organisms are characteristically found within macrophages.

The most frequently seen viral infection on intraoperative smear is progressive multifocal demyelinating leukoencephalopathy (see below).

Patients with suspected prion infection should not routinely undergo intraoperative neuropathological assessment, and the tissue should be handled with appropriate decontamination protocols.

### Diagnostic pitfalls: other infections

- Reactive astrocytes and macrophages in an infectious disease may mimic neoplastic astrocytes
- Epithelioid macrophages may mimic metastatic epithelial cells.

## Demyelination

Progressive multifocal leukoencephalopathy (PML) is a particular challenge intraoperatively, and correlation with clinical and radiological findings is critical. PML is a demyelinating condition caused by the *JC papovavirus* in immunocompromised patients. A wide spectrum of pathology may be seen, including reactive astrocytosis and foamy macrophage infiltration, atypical virally transformed astrocytes and infected oligodendrocytes with enlarged glassy nuclei. A population of lymphocytes may also be seen. A rare eosinophil rich variant also exists. Given the associated astrocytic atypia, it is easy to misdiagnose PML as a malignant astrocytic tumour if the diagnosis is not considered.

Non-infectious demyelinating diseases may also occasionally mimic a tumour, radiologically and clinically, and lead to a biopsy. For example, there is a rare hyperacute form of multiple sclerosis which may mimic a tumour, and the presence of necrosis and reactive astrocytes may cause confusion with an astrocytic tumour intraoperatively. The presence of abundant foamy macrophages should always be taken as a signal that a non-neoplastic diagnosis should be carefully sought.

### Cytological findings: demyelination

- Macrophages are abundant
- Reactive astrocytes
- Lymphocytes without nuclear atypia.

### Diagnostic pitfalls: demyelination

- Macrophages and reactive astrocytes may resemble neoplastic astrocytes.

## Infarction

A typical infarct would not be subject to biopsy; however, infarcts occasionally clinically and radiologically mimic a neoplasm, and may be encountered as intraoperative smears. Approximately 12 hours after an infarct, ischaemic changes can be seen in neurones. These cells become shrunken and eosinophilic. The nuclei of glial cells also degenerate. Within the first 5 days, there is an infiltrate of neutrophils. Later, there will be an infiltrate of foamy macrophages (Fig. 31.4), and adjacent astrocytes will undergo reactive changes. The infarct induces ingrowth of newly formed capillaries.

The smear findings will depend on the age of the lesion, and the region of the lesion sampled. The central necrotic zone will smear as poorly cohesive necrotic material. The edge of a well-established lesion will show prominent reactive astrocytes set within a fibrillary stroma.

There is a danger of misidentifying macrophages as neoplastic astrocytes. The presence of foamy, vacuolated cytoplasm suggests that the cells are macrophages.

### Cytological findings: infarction

- Shrunken neurones and neutrophil infiltrate (early)
- Foamy macrophages, proliferating capillaries, reactive gliosis (later).

### Diagnostic pitfalls: infarction

- Proliferating capillaries may be misinterpreted as hyperplastic endothelial proliferation in glioblastoma or pilocytic astrocytoma
- Macrophages and reactive astrocytes may resemble neoplastic astrocytes.

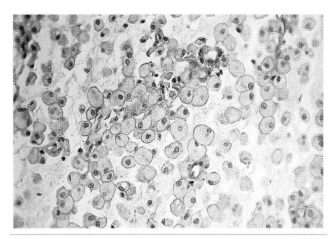

**Fig. 31.4** Smear of an infarct showing prominent foamy macrophages (H&E).

## Tumours

The WHO Classification[2] divides tumours of the central nervous system into four grades, with grade I having the most benign natural history, and grade IV the most aggressive. Unfortunately, the traditional concepts of benign and malignant can be difficult to apply meaningfully to tumours of the central nervous system. The adult brain is housed in the bony cranium, with relatively little capacity for deformation by underlying tumour, resulting in the potential for raised intracranial pressure and compression of vital structures, regardless of the degree of histological atypia of the underlying tumour. Thus the prognosis for an individual patient depends on the location of the lesion as well as the histological type and grade. Most glial tumours have an infiltrative nature, which precludes surgical cure.

### Diffusely infiltrating astrocytic tumours

Astrocytic tumours are the most common gliomas. They vary enormously in morphological features and clinical outcome, ranging from the relatively benign pilocytic astrocytoma (WHO grade I), a circumscribed childhood tumour, to the most frequent type of astrocytic tumour, glioblastoma (WHO grade IV).

Grade II, III and IV astrocytic tumours typically have an infiltrative biology, and by the time of presentation have usually crept along nerve fibre pathways far beyond what appears to be the edge of the tumour on imaging. The diffusely infiltrating astrocytic tumours are not usually amenable to curative therapy.

Glioblastoma may arise de novo (primary glioblastoma) without any previous history to suggest a lower grade precursor tumour, or may evolve from a diffusely infiltrating astrocytoma (WHO grade II) or anaplastic astrocytoma (WHO grade III) (Fig. 31.5). It is very rare for pilocytic astrocytoma to transform into a higher grade lesion, and if the clinical history suggests such a transformation, cautious review of the original biopsy would be warranted.

#### Glioblastoma

Glioblastoma, also known as glioblastoma multiforme is, as its name suggests, a tumour characterised by a wide variety of morphologies, both between different tumours, and within the same tumour. It is defined as a WHO grade IV, diffusely infiltrating

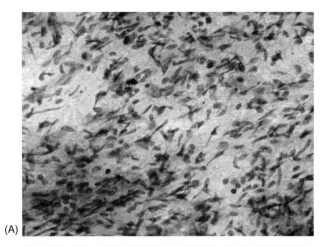

(A)

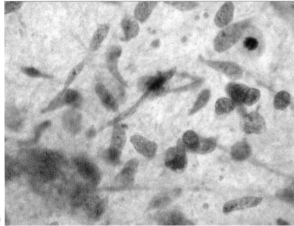

(B)

**Fig. 31.5** (A) Smear of anaplastic astrocytoma, showing high cellularity (toluidine blue). (B) Smear of anaplastic astrocytoma at higher power, showing mitotic activity (toluidine blue).

astrocytic tumour with nuclear pleomorphism, mitotic activity and necrosis and/or vascular endothelial hyperplasia.

Glioblastomas range from tumours composed of small cells with high nuclear/cytoplasmic ratio and relatively little specific evidence of differentiation (Fig. 31.6A), to giant cell forms with abundant GFAP-positive cytoplasm (Fig. 31.6B). Many are somewhere between these two extremes, consisting of moderate sized cells with elongated nuclei set within a fibrillary stroma (Fig. 31.6C). On intraoperative smear the full range of morphology seen on histology can be represented. Polarisation may help to reveal a fibrillary stroma, which should have a finer texture than the vessel associated collagen, which may be more prominent. Mitotic activity, necrosis and vascular endothelial hyperplasia are all supportive features (Fig. 31.6D); however, such features may not be seen, which may be due to sampling artifact, and their absence is not diagnostic of a low-grade tumour. In some cases it may only be possible to diagnose an astrocytic tumour, with grading awaiting paraffin sections.

### Cytological findings: glioblastoma

- Atypical astrocytic cells set within a fibrillary stroma
- Nuclei often elongated
- Great variability of size and shape of cells occurs between different glioblastomas, and within the same tumour.

### Diagnostic pitfalls: glioblastoma

- Small cell glioblastoma may have poorly differentiated cells with scanty glial stroma, leading to misdiagnosis as carcinoma or lymphoma
- Anaplastic oligodendroglioma and glioblastoma may look very similar
- Primitive neuroectodermal tumours (PNET) may mimic glioblastoma; however, glioblastoma is typically seen in older adults and PNET in children
- Reactive astrocytes associated with infections or inflammatory conditions may look atypical and be misinterpreted as malignant. Be very cautious of diagnosing glioblastoma in a macrophage-rich smear
- Radiation necrosis, in which there may be considerable astrocytic nuclear pleomorphism, may mimic a malignant glial tumour.

## Diffuse astrocytoma, WHO grade II

Grade II diffusely infiltrating astrocytomas are usually slowly growing tumours in young adults. They tend to transform to anaplastic astrocytoma or glioblastoma.

There are several morphological variants of diffuse astrocytoma: fibrillary astrocytoma, gemistocytic astrocytoma and protoplasmic astrocytoma. The most common form is fibrillary astrocytoma, in which astrocytic cells with mildly atypical nuclei and poorly discernible cytoplasm are set within a fibrillary stroma (Fig. 31.7A). The stroma is often microcystic. Mitotic activity is minimal, and necrosis and vascular endothelial hyperplasia absent. On smear, the fibrillary stroma is prominent. The cellularity may be only slightly greater than that of normal brain, and in some cases it may be necessary to wait for paraffin sections to confirm neoplasia.

Gemistocytic astrocytomas contain prominent astrocytes with abundant eccentric eosinophilic cytoplasm. This subtype of astrocytoma, while remaining grade II, has a more aggressive natural history than other types of grade II astrocytoma. The gemistocytic cells are prominent in smears (Fig. 31.7B).

Protoplasmic astrocytoma is a rare subtype composed of astrocytes with monomorphous rounded nuclei and scanty cytoplasm with few processes, set within a stroma rich in mucoid microcysts.[2]

### Cytological findings: diffuse astrocytoma, WHO grade II

- Neoplastic astrocytes with fibrillary processes[5]
- Mild hypercellularity
- Mild nuclear pleomorphism and atypia
- Mitotic activity absent or minimal.

### Diagnostic pitfalls: diffuse astrocytoma, WHO grade II

- The distinction between a grade II diffuse astrocytic tumour and reactive gliosis is often difficult, even on paraffin embedded material. The nuclei in an astrocytic tumour are usually more irregular in shape and hyperchromatic.

## Anaplastic astrocytoma, WHO grade III

Anaplastic astrocytoma, WHO grade III, shows features of a diffusely infiltrating astrocytic tumour, set within a fibrillary stroma; however, mitotic activity is more prominent than in

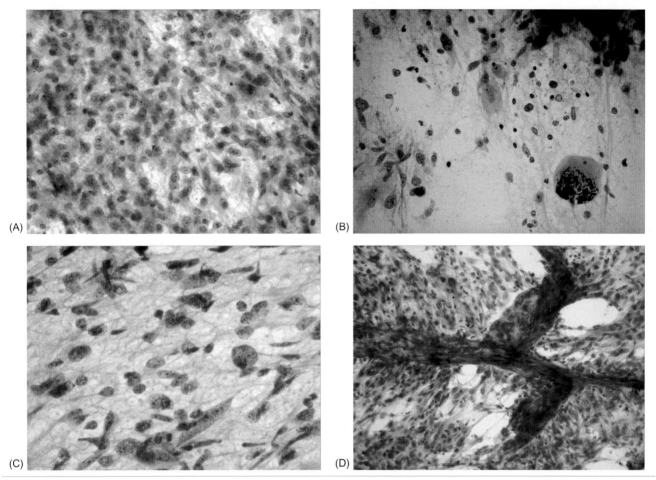

**Fig. 31.6** Different examples highlighting the range of morphology that may be seen in smears of glioblastoma. (A) A tumour composed of relatively small cells. (B) A tumour containing large neoplastic cells. (C) A typical glioblastoma showing atypical elongated nuclei set within a fibrillary stroma. (D) A glioblastoma with vascular endothelial hyperplasia (toluidine blue).

a grade II astrocytoma (Fig. 31.7). The WHO Classification is vague about the mitotic rate cut-off between grade II and III astrocytic tumours (which may be reasonable as the distinction is an arbitrary definition within a spectrum of malignancy). Finding any identifiable mitotic figures in a smear should raise concern regarding atypia, and if more than one or two mitoses are seen, I would regard this as favouring anaplasia. Necrosis and vascular endothelial hyperplasia (in the absence of previous intervention) are not present by definition.

### Cytological findings: anaplastic astrocytoma, WHO grade III

- Similar to grade II astrocytoma, although may be more cellular and show greater nuclear atypia
- Mitotically active (although mitoses may be hard to find on smear compared with paraffin sections)
- Vascular endothelial hyperplasia and necrosis are absent.

### Diagnostic pitfalls: anaplastic astrocytoma, WHO grade III

- Necrosis may be difficult to recognise on a smear, leading to an undergrading of a glioblastoma.

## Circumscribed astrocytic tumours

Unfortunately, the most common glial tumours are diffusely infiltrative and not amenable to curative treatment. A less frequent group of gliomas (including pilocytic astrocytoma and pleomorphic xanthoastrocytoma) have a circumscribed growth pattern, and a much more favourable prognosis. Recognition of these entities is vital in order to reliably predict prognosis and offer appropriate therapy.

The circumscribed gliomas are often difficult to distinguish from diffusely infiltrative gliomas intraoperatively on cytological grounds alone, however, the age of the patient and the radiological findings should encourage consideration of a lower grade diagnosis.

### Pilocytic astrocytoma

Pilocytic astrocytoma is a slowly growing, frequently cystic WHO grade I tumour most frequently found in children and adolescents. The posterior fossa is a common site of origin. The tumour tends to have a biphasic architecture, with areas of differing cellularity. This may be reflected in the smear. The neoplastic cells of pilocytic astrocytoma have fine bipolar processes. The nuclei are usually relatively monomorphous and

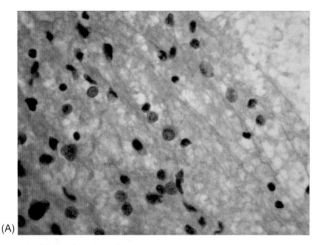

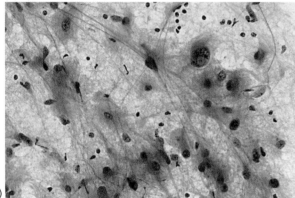

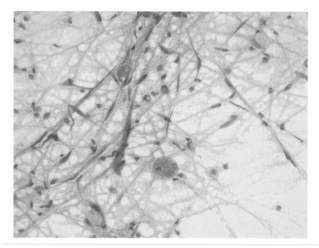

**Fig. 31.8** Smear of pilocytic astrocytoma showing bipolar astrocytic cells with minimal nuclear atypia, and a granular eosinophilic body (Toluidine blue).

**Fig. 31.7** (A) Smear of a diffuse fibrillary astrocytoma (H&E). (B) Smear of gemistocytic astrocytoma showing neoplastic astrocytes with abundant eosinophilic cytoplasm (H&E).

Eosinophilic granular bodies may be seen. A useful feature to help avoid overdiagnosing such tumours is the discrepancy between the pleomorphic cytology and the paucity of mitotic activity.

**Cytological findings: pleomorphic xanthoastrocytoma**

- Prominent nuclear pleomorphism and hyperchromasia[10]
- Multinucleated neoplastic giant cells
- Fibrillary stroma
- Eosinophilic granular bodies.

### Subependymal giant cell astrocytoma (SEGA)

Subependymal giant cell astrocytoma (SEGA) is a rare WHO grade I periventricular tumour found in patients with tuberous sclerosis. The neoplastic cells are large and intermediate in morphology between astrocytes and neurones.[11] These cells will be conspicuous on intraoperative smear.

**Diagnostic pitfalls: circumscribed astrocytic tumours**

Vascular endothelial hyperplasia and/or nuclear pleomorphism may lead to misdiagnosis as a malignant glial tumour.[6]

Rosenthal fibres may be seen in reactive brain adjacent to a variety of lesions particularly in association with cerebellar haemangioblastomas and suprasellar craniopharyngiomas. The presence of Rosenthal fibres is not diagnostic of a circumscribed glioma.

The degree of nuclear pleomorphism in pleomorphic xanthoastrocytoma may lead to misdiagnosis of a malignant astrocytic tumour. Monstrocellularity in the absence of other features suggestive of malignancy should at least raise the suspicion of a low-grade intrinsic tumour.

have a delicate chromatin pattern;[5] however, in longstanding lesions nuclear pleomorphism may be prominent, and is not of prognostic significance.

Rosenthal fibres are eosinophilic on H&E stained smears, and stain blue with toluidine blue. They are frequent in pilocytic astrocytomas. Granular eosinophilic bodies are also supportive of the diagnosis of a circumscribed astrocytoma (Fig. 31.8).

The vascular pattern of a pilocytic astrocytoma may cause confusion. Although in diffusely infiltrating astrocytomas vascular endothelial hyperplasia is an indicator of a grade IV diagnosis, in pilocytic astrocytoma it is of no prognostic significance.

**Cytological findings: pilocytic astrocytoma**

- Cells with fine bipolar processes
- Bland, oval, rounded or elongated nuclei[8,9]
- Occasional multinucleated giant cells
- Rosenthal fibres and granular eosinophilic bodies.

### Pleomorphic xanthoastrocytoma

Pleomorphic xanthoastrocytoma (PXA) is a rare circumscribed WHO grade II tumour found predominantly in children and adolescents. The lesion is usually superficial and supratentorial. Always consider PXA in the differential of a young patient with a superficial glioma. It is easy to mistake for a malignant astrocytic tumour, as the astrocytes are large and pleomorphic. The cells may have foamy cytoplasm, but this may be inconspicuous.

## Oligodendroglioma

Oligodendrogliomas are less common than astrocytic tumours. They are typically cerebral tumours in adults. Most oligodendrogliomas are WHO grade II tumours; however, they may evolve into, or present de novo, as anaplastic oligodendroglioma, WHO grade III. Oligodendrogliomas are frequently calcified, which can produce a gritty feel when performing the smear;[9] however, calcification is not seen in all oligodendrogliomas, and not all calcified gliomas are oligodendroglial.

The characteristic hallmark of oligodendroglioma in paraffin sections is the prominent zone of perinuclear clearing. This is a fixation artefact, and is not usually seen in smears or frozen sections, making diagnosis more difficult. The smear should, however, show a fine network of thin-walled capillaries with a wide branching angle, tumour cells with rounded nuclei and mildly clumped chromatin, and (in contrast to astrocytic tumours) little fibrillary stroma (Fig. 31.9A). The tumour cells usually have scanty cytoplasm; however, a population of 'mini-gemistocytes', cells with rounded nuclei and a bulge of glial fibrillary acidic protein containing cytoplasm without extensive processes may be seen. Oligodendrogliomas are frequently calcified; however, calcification is not seen in all oligodendrogliomas, and not all calcified gliomas are oligodendroglial.

Typical grade II oligodendrogliomas do not show necrosis or vascular endothelial hyperplasia, and mitotic activity is minimal. Anaplastic oligodendrogliomas, WHO grade III have more irregular, hyperchromatic nuclei with coarser chromatin, show substantial mitotic activity, and may show necrosis and/or vascular endothelial hyperplasia. The cytoplasm may be more prominent in anaplastic oligodendrogliomas, and the nuclei less round, and there is a spectrum of smear morphology between anaplastic oligodendroglioma and malignant astrocytic tumours (Fig. 31.9B). Definite diagnosis in such cases may require paraffin sections, and may depend on cytogenetic testing for loss of regions of chromosomes 1p and 19q (a pattern typical of oligodendroglial tumours).

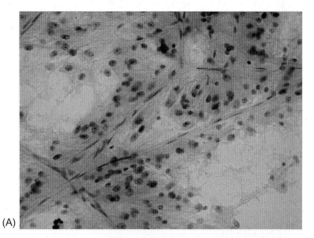

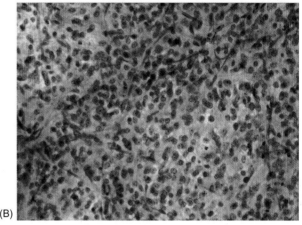

**Fig. 31.9** (A) Smear of oligodendroglioma. Note the absence of the fixation artifact induced perinuclear clearing typical of paraffin sections of oligodendroglioma (toluidine blue). (B) Smear of anaplastic oligodendroglioma showing increased cellularity (toluidine blue).

### Cytological findings: oligodendroglioma

- High cellularity
- Discohesive cells with scanty cytoplasm
- Monomorphous rounded nuclei with condensed chromatin
- Nucleoli may be prominent
- Calcification
- Fine capillary network.

A subset of gliomas, including oligoastrocytoma WHO grade II, anaplastic oligoastrocytoma WHO grade III, and glioblastoma with oligodendroglioma component WHO grade IV, either contain a mixed population of neoplastic astrocytic and oligodendroglial cells, or cells intermediate in morphology between astrocytic and oligodendroglial neoplastic cells. The interobserver variability in the diagnosis of these lesions is very high and, although such a diagnosis might be suggested intraoperatively, paraffin sections will be essential to categorise these lesions as reliably as is currently possible.

### Diagnostic pitfalls: oligodendroglioma

- Mini-gemistocytes in oligodendroglial tumours resemble astrocytic gemistocytes[6]
- Pleomorphic cells in anaplastic oligodendroglioma resemble neoplastic astrocytes.

## Ependymoma

Ependymomas are typically slowly growing tumours in children and young adults, arising around the ventricles or in the spinal cord. They are usually WHO grade II; however, an anaplastic grade III variant occurs, as do the grade I variants myxopapillary ependymoma (in the cauda equina region) and subependymoma.[2]

The ependymal rosette is a specific structure in which columnar cells are arranged around a central lumen; however, this structure is not seen on paraffin sections in the majority of ependymomas, and is even less frequently identified intraoperatively. Perivascular pseudorosettes, in which processes from tumour cells converge on blood vessels, are much more frequently seen, but are less specific.

Ependymomas are usually moderately cellular, and have monomorphous oval nuclei with granular chromatin. Nuclear grooves have been reported to be more frequent in ependymoma than in other common brain tumours.[12]

There are subtypes of ependymoma which may cause difficulties on smear diagnosis. Papillary ependymomas could be mistaken for carcinomas or choroid plexus tumours. Clear cell ependymomas may be mistaken for oligodendrogliomas or central neurocytomas. Tanycytic ependymomas may closely resemble astrocytomas.

### Cytological findings: ependymoma

- High cellularity
- Uneven spread of cells[9]

- Uniform cells with oval to rounded nuclei and dense chromatin[5,12]
- Small nucleoli may be present
- Pseudorosettes around vessels
- Ependymal rosettes (tumour cells with processes running towards a lumen).

### Diagnostic pitfalls: ependymoma

- May be misdiagnosed as an astrocytic tumour, particularly when ependymal rosettes are not present
- Ependymomas usually have more uniform nuclei than astrocytic tumours.

## Tumours showing neuronal differentiation

Tumours consisting entirely or partially of cells showing neuronal differentiation range from highly malignant tumours containing cells with a primitive appearance, such as medulloblastoma, to relatively indolent tumours with large, well-differentiated ganglion cells such as gangliocytoma and ganglioglioma.

### Primitive neuroectodermal tumours

Primitive neuroectodermal tumours (PNETs) are WHO grade IV tumours predominantly found in children. The most frequent subtype is the cerebellar medulloblastoma; however, supratentorial PNETs are also found, and PNETs are occasionally seen in adults.

PNETs are highly cellular, malignant tumours, with immunocytochemical and sometimes morphological evidence of primitive neuronal differentiation. They may also concurrently show evidence of glial differentiation.

PNETs usually smear as densely cellular monolayers with oval or carrot-shaped nuclei and scanty cytoplasm (Fig. 31.10).[13] The chromatin pattern is finely granular, and the nuclei are moderately pleomorphic. Mitotic activity may be prominent, and necrosis may be seen. Neuroblastic rosettes may be identified.

Given the cerebellar location of many PNETs great care should be taken not to confuse cerebellar granular cell neurones

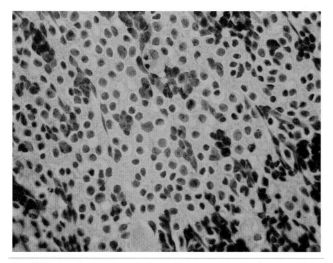

**Fig. 31.10** Smear of medulloblastoma. (Courtesy of Dr T S Jacques, Institute of Child Health, London.)

with neoplastic medulloblastoma cells. The cells of a medulloblastoma are usually larger than cerebellar granule cell neurones, more pleomorphic, and mitotically active.

In older adult patients metastatic small cell carcinoma and small cell glioblastoma may produce a similar appearance, and are statistically much more frequent than PNET in this age group.

### Cytological findings: primitive neuroectodermal tumours

- Highly cellular smears
- Even spread of cells[9]
- Round, oval or irregular carrot-shaped nuclei, which may have multiple nucleoli
- Nuclear moulding and 'cannibalism' (cells wrapping around tumour cell nuclei[14]
- Homer–Wright rosettes
- Mitotic figures and apoptotic bodies.

### Diagnostic pitfalls: primitive neuroectodermal tumours

Atypical teratoid/rhabdoid tumours are malignant paediatric tumours. They are most common in the posterior fossa, and radiologically resemble medulloblastoma. A population of rhabdoid cells should raise the suspicion of this entity.[15]

Granular cell neurons of the cerebellum may be misinterpreted as neoplastic PNET cells; however, cerebellar granule cells are smaller, round, and do not show nuclear atypia.

Vascular endothelial hyperplasia may be seen in PNETs. Such vascular changes are not exclusive to astrocytic tumours.

### Ganglioglioma/gangliocytoma, WHO grade I

Tumours partially or exclusively composed of neurons with a mature appearance are typically found in the cerebral cortex of young patients with seizures. The neurons are usually large, atypical, and may be binucleate. In gangliocytomas the neoplastic ganglion cells are the only neoplastic component of the tumour. Gangliogliomas contain an additional neoplastic glial component. Calcification and a perivascular chronic inflammatory reaction are often seen. There is frequent subarachnoid involvement of the tumour, which can induce a fibrous response, making smearing difficult.

It may be difficult on a smear to differentiate between an astrocytic tumour infiltrating grey matter and a ganglioglioma. Often the cytoplasm of the neoplastic neurons will be damaged by the smearing process, leaving large bare nuclei with prominent nucleoli. If preserved, the cytoplasm of the ganglion cells may be abundant, and abnormal processes may be seen.

There is a rare malignant variant of ganglioglioma in which there is frank anaplasia of the neoplastic glial component (anaplastic ganglioglioma, WHO grade III).

### Cytological findings: ganglioglioma/gangliocytoma

- Neoplastic ganglion cells, which are often multinucleated
- Perivascular lymphocytic infiltrate
- Eosinophilic granular bodies
- Neoplastic glial component in ganglioglioma.

It may be difficult to differentiate between entrapped non-neoplastic neurones and neoplastic ganglion cells. Consider the morphology of the neurones that would be expected to be present at the site of the biopsy.

## Central neurocytoma

Central neurocytoma is a tumour composed of sheets of monomorphous small neuronal cells resembling granular cell neurons with rounded nuclei, delicate chromatin, and scanty cytoplasm set within a variably abundant neuropil stroma.[16] It is usually found in the lateral ventricles, is associated with a good prognosis, and is a WHO grade II lesion.

Central neurocytomas tend to spread evenly on smearing, and the monomorphic nature of the cells is prominent. Cytoplasm is inconspicuous.

Although there may be rosette-like fibrillary areas, the neuronal nature of the lesion may be easier to appreciate with immunocytochemical staining than on morphological grounds. The morphology may closely resemble oligodendroglioma.

**Cytological findings: central neurocytoma**

- Monomorphous small cells
- Rounded nuclei with delicate speckled chromatin[17]
- Homer–Wright rosettes may be seen.

**Diagnostic pitfalls: central neurocytoma**

- Can mimic oligodendroglioma or pituitary adenoma. Intraventricular location favours central neurocytoma.

## Dysembryoplastic neuroepithelial tumour

Dysembryoplastic neuroepithelial tumour (DNET) is a benign tumour characteristically found in the temporal cortex of children and younger adults with partial seizures. The characteristic feature of the tumour is the 'specific glioneuronal element', in which parallel bundles of axons are surrounded by cells with small rounded nuclei, resembling oligodendrocytes. 'Floating neurons' are present in the matrix between these columns. Many cases are associated with cortical dysplasia in adjacent cortex.

DNET has been divided into simple and complex forms depending on the architecture. The simple form shows the glioneuronal element, without additional cellular elements. The complex form includes both the glioneuronal element and glial nodules. The tumour may include areas with astrocytic, oligodendroglial and/or neuronal differentiation.

Given the vast range of architecture and morphology that can be associated with the diagnosis of DNET, the diagnosis may be difficult to make on small biopsies. The differential diagnosis may include oligodendroglioma, astrocytic tumours and ganglioglioma.

The situation is even more difficult on intraoperative smear. In an appropriate clinical and radiological context finding a population of small, round oligodendroglial-like cells associated with spaces containing 'floating neurons' on a smear would be supportive of a diagnosis of DNET.[17] Great caution should be exercised in making such a diagnosis in the absence of supportive clinical/radiological features. It is very difficult to reliably establish intraoperatively whether a neurone is a 'floating neurone' in a DNET, or whether the neurone is an entrapped non-neoplastic neurone at the edge of a diffusely infiltrating glioma.

**Cytological findings: dysembryoplastic neuroepithelial tumour**

- The variability of elements that may be found in a DNET makes diagnosis intraoperatively extremely difficult, unless the characteristic radiological and clinical findings are recognised.

## Choroid plexus

Choroid plexus tumours in adults are typically benign papillomas. In contrast, in infants a much higher proportion are high-grade malignant tumours.

A well-differentiated choroid plexus papilloma will look similar to normal choroid plexus, so care should be taken not to misinterpret a fragment of non-neoplastic choroid plexus as part of a choroid plexus tumour. On smear choroid plexus papillomas usually show bland epithelial cells surrounding fibrovascular cores (Fig. 31.11).[18]

Choroid plexus carcinoma will have smear features of a papillary carcinoma.

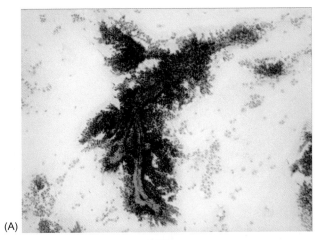

(A)

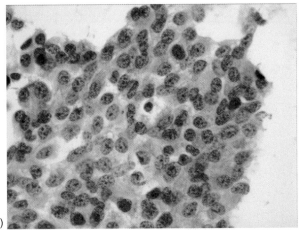

(B)

**Fig. 31.11** (A) Smear of choroid plexus papilloma (H&E). (B) Higher power view of choroid plexus papilloma smear (H&E).

## Cytological findings: choroid plexus papilloma

- Papillary structure
- Cuboidal epithelial cells overlying fibrovascular core
- Rounded nuclei, fine chromatin, inconspicuous nucleoli.

## Diagnostic pitfalls: choroid plexus papilloma

- Normal choroid plexus may be misinterpreted as choroid plexus papilloma. Correlation with radiology is essential
- Other papillary tumours may be misinterpreted as choroid plexus papilloma, including papillary ependymoma, papillary meningioma and metastatic papillary carcinoma.

## Meningioma

A durally attached tumour compressing the brain or spinal cord, without directly infiltrating the brain will usually be a meningioma. Most meningiomas are low-grade (WHO grade I) tumours, which if surgically accessible can be cured by excision. In some cases, either due to recurrence, higher grade, brain invasion and/or incomplete excision, radiotherapy may be necessary. A minority of meningiomas are considered histologically atypical, and are associated with a more aggressive natural history, and regarded as WHO grade II. A very small minority show histological features of frank anaplasia, mimicking carcinoma, sarcoma, melanoma or lymphoma, and are regarded as WHO grade III lesions.

There are currently 15 histological subtypes of meningioma recognised by the WHO Classification.[2] Nine of the subtypes are by definition WHO grade I (meningothelial, fibrous, transitional, psammomatous, angiomatous, microcystic, secretory, lymphoplasmacyte-rich, metaplastic). Three subtypes are defined as grade II (chordoid, clear cell, atypical), and three as WHO grade III (papillary, rhabdoid, anaplastic).

Particularly useful features on smear are lobules (Fig. 31.12A) and whorls of meningothelial cells (Fig. 31.12B) and psammoma bodies (Fig. 31.12C).

The features used to define atypia (WHO grade II) are increased mitotic activity (four or more mitoses/10×40 high-power fields) or three or more of the following: foci of small cells with a high nuclear/cytoplasmic ratio, prominence of nucleoli, sheet-like architecture, and focal necrosis.

It should be noted that nuclear pleomorphism, a feature that may be striking in some meningioma smears, is not part of the diagnostic criteria for atypia. Figure 31.12D shows a smear of a durally-based tumour which had prominent nuclear pleomorphism, raising the possibility of a sarcoma, metastatic tumour, or of a higher grade meningioma. Although there was a hint of lobularity in this case, nucleoli were only small, and mitotic activity was inconspicuous. In such a case it is not possible to give a definite report of meningioma intra-operatively, and paraffin sections are required to judge the architecture and immunophenotype. In this case paraffin sections confirmed a microcystic meningioma, WHO grade I.

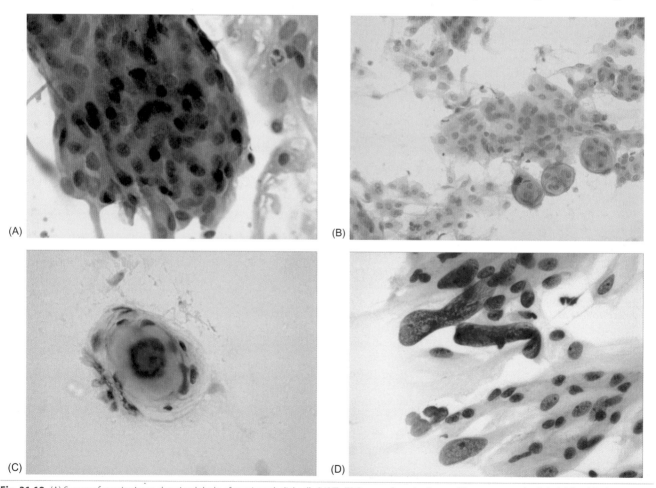

(A)  (B)  (C)  (D)

**Fig. 31.12** (A) Smear of meningioma showing lobule of meningothelial cells (H&E). (B) Smear of meningioma with numerous whorls (toluidine blue). (C) Psammoma body, toluidine blue. (D) Smear of microcystic meningioma showing prominent nuclear pleomorphism (toluidine blue).

It is common for microcystic and angiomatous meningiomas to show a greater degree of nuclear pleomorphism than would be expected for their grade or degree of mitotic activity.

Intranuclear pseudoinclusions are often described as typical of meningiomas, and are frequently encountered in meningiomas, both in intraoperative smears, and in histological sections; however, they may not be either as specific or as sensitive as appears to be generally believed. Not all meningiomas have intranuclear pseudoinclusions, and some other tumours (including gliomas and extraskeletal myxoid chondrosarcoma) may contain them.

The reactive lymphocytic and plasma cell infiltrate in a lymphoplasmacytic meningioma may almost entirely obscure the neoplastic component, and may mimic a lymphoma or an infectious/inflammatory process.

A chordoid background and architecture would be expected in chordoid meningioma, although there should also be areas of tumour with a more typically meningioma-like morphology. Such a tumour may mimic chordoma and, depending on location, chordoid glioma.

Papillary meningiomas are a rare subtype characterised by pseudopapillary architecture, and aggressive behaviour, leading to systemic metastasis in approximately 20% of patients.[2] Papillary meningiomas may mimic other papillary/pseudopapillary tumours (such as metastatic papillary carcinoma and choroid plexus tumours). Intraoperatively it would usually only be possible to report such a lesion as a papillary tumour, which, given the location, would be compatible with a papillary meningioma, and await paraffin sections and immunocytochemistry for further assessment.

### Cytological findings: meningioma

- Oval nuclei usually without significant pleomorphism[15]
- Nuclear pseudo-inclusions
- Spindle-shaped cells in some meningioma subtypes
- Polygonal to spindle-shaped cells with oval monomorphous nuclei in syncytial fragments (in meningothelial meningioma)[19]
- Psammoma bodies (psammomatous meningioma)
- Microcystic spaces within clusters or sheets of cells (microcystic meningioma)[19]
- Eosinophilic intracytoplasmic inclusions ('pseudopsammoma bodies') in secretory meningioma.

### Diagnostic pitfalls: meningioma

- Spindle-shaped cells may mimic nerve sheath tumour
- Meningothelial hyperplasia adjacent to another pathological process may mimic meningioma
- Secretory meningioma may mimic adenocarcinoma, as the inclusions may mimic lumina in breast, gastric or hepatocellular carcinoma[21]
- The cytoplasmic processes of meningiomas may mimic the fibrillary processes of an astrocytic tumour.

## Schwannoma

Schwannomas are benign nerve sheath tumours occurring most frequently on the vestibular nerve. Schwannomas are typically difficult to smear and the bulk of the material sticks together as impenetrable lumps on the slide. Usually a small amount of material escapes from the tumour with firm smearing to demonstrate fascicles of spindle-shaped cells (Fig. 31.13). Haemosiderin is often present.

Malignant peripheral nerve sheath tumours occasional occur in neuropathological practice but are much less frequent than schwannomas. Schwannomas usually have a low mitotic rate, so the finding of a spindle cell tumour with a high mitotic rate should raise concern.

### Cytological findings: schwannoma

- Difficult to smear
- Cohesive fragments of tissue
- Spindle-shaped cells
- Little or no mitotic activity.

### Diagnostic pitfalls: schwannoma

- The spindle-shaped cells in fibroblastic meningioma and neurofibroma resemble those seen in schwannoma.

## Lymphoma

Most lymphomas biopsied in the central nervous system are diffuse large B-cell lymphomas. These characteristically have tumour cells concentrated around blood vessels, producing an onion-skin-like perivascular reticulin pattern (Fig. 31.14A). In contrast to a reactive infiltrate of inflammatory cells, there is more nuclear pleomorphism in most lymphomas. In a smear the perivascular regions are densely cellular, and the neoplastic cells are trapped within the reticulin framework. Away from the vessels, discohesive neoplastic lymphoid cells spread out, often in a necrotic background (Fig. 31.14B).

### Cytological findings: lymphoma

- Perivascular infiltrate of neoplastic lymphocytes
- Discohesive neoplastic cells spread away from vessels
- Atypical hyperchromatic lymphocytes with scanty cytoplasm
- Mitotic activity
- Necrosis.

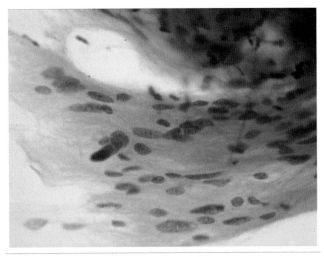

**Fig. 31.13** Smear of schwannoma (toluidine blue).

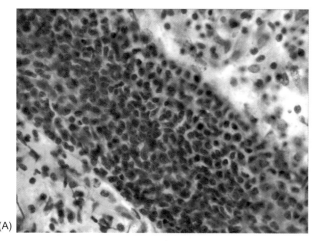

(A)

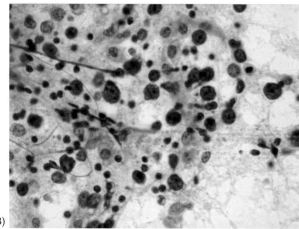

(B)

**Fig. 31.14** (A) Smear of diffuse large B-cell lymphoma (toluidine blue). (B) Smear of diffuse large B-cell lymphoma, higher power (toluidine blue).

### Diagnostic pitfalls: lymphoma

The perivascular distribution may raise the possibility of an inflammatory process, particularly in a low-grade lymphoma; however, the monomorphous nature of the infiltrate should suggest a neoplastic diagnosis

Some diffuse large B cell lymphomas have a substantial amount of cytoplasm, and the differential diagnosis includes small cell glioblastoma and poorly differentiated carcinomas or melanoma. It may not be possible to make a definite intraoperative diagnosis in this group of tumours (see Chs 13, 14).

## Germ cell tumours

Central nervous system germ cell tumours are typically midline lesions, usually in the pineal gland or suprasellar areas. There is a marked geographical variation in the incidence of CNS germ cell tumours, being more than ten times more frequent in Japan than in Western countries.[2] They are most common in male children and adolescents.

Germ cell tumours of the CNS are divided into germinoma, embryonal carcinoma, yolk sac tumour, choriocarcinoma, teratoma and mixed germ cell tumours.

Germinomas are histologically equivalent to seminomas of the testis. They are composed of two distinct cell populations, which may be clearly defined on smear. The neoplastic cells are large polygonal or rounded cells with large central vesicular nuclei with finely granular chromatin and a prominent central nucleus.[20] The nucleoli may be irregular in shape and angulated. The tumour cells are admixed with a reactive population of small lymphocytes. A granulomatous reaction may be seen.

Teratomas contain a variety of different tissue types, sometimes including teeth, hair and bone, which can make smearing difficult. The tissues may be well differentiated in a mature teratoma, or primitive in immature forms.[22] Multinucleated giant cells may be prominent in a smear of choriocarcinoma.

### Cytological findings: germinoma

- Large polygonal or rounded cells
- Vesicular nuclei and a prominent central nucleus
- Admixed reactive lymphocytes.

### Diagnostic pitfalls: germinoma

- If the large neoplastic cells are overlooked or not represented in the sample, the lymphocytic population may be misinterpreted as reflecting an inflammatory process or a low-grade lymphoid neoplasm
- A granulomatous reaction to a germinoma may be misinterpreted as an infectious process.

## Haemangioblastoma

Haemangioblastomas are tumours usually of the cerebellum, brainstem, or spinal cord, which may be found in patients with von Hippel–Lindau syndrome, or may be sporadic. They are composed of vacuolated neoplastic stromal cells in a richly vascular background. Haemangioblastomas do not smear well, producing clumps of cells. The tumour cells have medium-sized to large oval nuclei and vacuolated cytoplasm.

Patients with von Hippel–Lindau syndrome are at risk of both haemangioblastoma and metastatic renal cell carcinoma, both of which may look very similar on smear. It is reasonable to await immunocytochemical exclusion of a metastatic carcinoma, rather than making a definite diagnosis of haemangioblastoma intraoperatively.

### Cytological findings: haemangioblastoma

- Vacuolated neoplastic stromal cells
- Richly vascular lesion.

### Diagnostic pitfalls: haemangioblastoma

- The brain tissue adjacent to a haemangioblastoma may contain prominent Rosenthal fibres as a reactive phenomenon.

## Pituitary

The most common lesion encountered in the region of the pituitary gland is the pituitary adenoma. These are usually relatively simple to diagnose on smear, although the immunophenotype can only rarely be predicted on smear cytology alone.

## Pituitary adenoma

Pituitary adenomas typically spread on a slide as a monolayer of cells with rounded nuclei, finely granular chromatin, and inconspicuous cytoplasm. There is often perinuclear clearing.

An important distinction between non-neoplastic and neoplastic anterior pituitary glandular tissue may need to be made. One of the most distinctive features of pituitary adenomas is the effacement of the normal architecture of the anterior pituitary gland, which is composed of nests of cells surrounded by a reticulin framework. Non-neoplastic anterior pituitary tissue tends to retain some degree of nesting of its architecture on smear. The monomorphism of a tumour is also a useful diagnostic feature.

Differential diagnoses of pituitary adenomas include other lesions which may show perinuclear clearing, such as oligodendroglioma, clear cell meningioma, clear cell ependymoma and other lesions which are composed of small cells with a high nuclear/cytoplasmic ratio, such as lymphoma and small cell carcinoma. The location needs to be considered, and usually makes an intrinsic glial tumour unlikely. The fine granularity of the chromatin favours pituitary adenoma rather than a malignant tumour.

The histological and cytological degree of anaplasia in pituitary adenomas shows little correlation with clinical outcome, and malignancy is determined primarily by clinical/radiological evidence of metastasis, thus cannot usually be reliably determined by a biopsy of the pituitary region alone.

### Cytological findings: pituitary adenoma

- Discohesive cells with mildly pleomorphic rounded nuclei and scanty cytoplasm
- A single population of cells
- Paranuclear fibrous bodies (a paranuclear collection of intermediate filaments in sparsely granulated somatotroph adenomas).[23]

### Diagnostic pitfalls: pituitary adenoma

- A variety of cell types can be seen in smears of non-neoplastic anterior pituitary gland tissue, in contrast to the single population of tumour cells in pituitary adenomas
- Lymphomas, plasma cell tumours and oligodendrogliomas can produce smears with appearances similar to those seen in pituitary adenoma; however, these would be very uncommon in the seller region.

## Other lesions of the pituitary region

Craniopharyngiomas are histologically benign, WHO grade I cystic epithelial tumours of the sellar region. They are thought to arise from Rathke pouch remnants. These lesions are frequently calcified. The intraoperative findings depend on whether the epithelium, the cyst contents, or both are sampled. If the epithelium is present in the smear, clusters of squamous cells may be identified.[24] The cyst fluid is dark and proteinaceous. 'Wet keratin' (keratinised squamous cells showing the ghost outline of dead nuclei) is often present. A giant cell foreign body type reaction with cholesterol clefts in the surrounding tissue may also be prominent.[25] Occasional cases have focal ciliation of the epithelium.

Rathke cleft cysts are benign cystic structures lined by simple columnar or cuboidal ciliated epithelium.[26] The epithelium may be attenuated, or may show squamous metaplasia.

Metastatic carcinomas may present as pituitary region masses. Very occasionally a pituitary adenoma may contain a metastatic adenocarcinoma.

### Diagnostic pitfalls: other lesions of the pituitary region

- Craniopharyngiomas may induce a prominent piloid gliosis in the surrounding brain tissue, with prominent Rosenthal fibre formation.

## Chordoma

Chordoma is a slowly growing midline tumour predominantly affecting the skull base and lower spine. Although the tumour is relatively paucicellular, and the neoplastic cells are only mildly pleomorphic and show little mitotic activity, due to the difficult location of the tumours, they have a slow but relentless tendency to locally recur. The tumour cells are set in cords and strands, within a rich myxoid stroma (Fig. 31.15A). The stroma is prominent on smear, and deeply metachromatic with toluidine blue staining. The neoplastic cells are often described on paraffin sections as 'physalipherous' (containing bubbles). The vacuolated nature of these cells may or may not be readily identifiable on smear (Fig. 31.15B).

### Cytological findings: chordoma

- Myxoid stroma
- Polyhedral vacuolated physaliphorous cells with rounded nuclei in cords and strands.[5]

### Diagnostic pitfalls: chordoma

- May be difficult to distinguish from chondrosarcoma intraoperatively.

## Metastatic tumours

Metastatic carcinomas will often show aggregation of atypical cells in sheets and nests (Fig. 31.16A). The architecture can be a useful diagnostic feature; however, it should be noted that meningiomas and occasional gliomas may show similar architecture. The nucleoli are often prominent, and the background may be necrotic.[6] Glandular structures in adenocarcinomas (Fig. 31.16B) and papillary structures in papillary carcinomas may also be seen in smears.

Metastatic small cell carcinomas (typically arising from the lung) produce poorly cohesive smears in which the neoplastic cells have little discernible cytoplasm (Fig. 31.16C).

Squamous differentiation is not usually identified on intraoperative smear. Diagnosis of a well-differentiated metastatic squamous tumour should be made with caution, and entities such as craniopharyngioma, dermoid and epidermoid cysts, and teratomas should be considered.

The differential diagnosis for a papillary tumour includes metastatic carcinoma, papillary meningiomas, papillary ependymomas, choroid plexus tumours and the very rare papillary

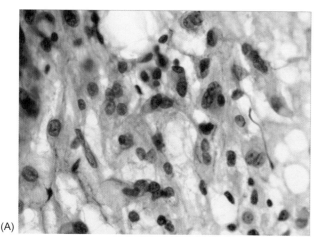

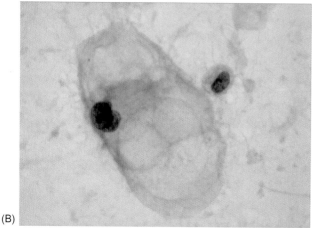

**Fig. 31.15** (A) Smear of chordoma (toluidine blue). (B) Higher power image of physaliphorous cell in chordoma (H&E).

glioneuronal tumours. Necrotic tumours may give a pseudo-papillary appearance on smear due to the greater viability of perivascular tumour cells.

Although metastatic tumours typically form sheets and nests of cells within brain tissue, some metastatic tumours may have a more diffusely infiltrating architecture. This makes differentiation from an astrocytic tumour difficult. In such cases areas of sheet-like architecture should be carefully sought.

Metastatic tumours may appear deceptively benign on intraoperative smear (Fig. 31.16D,E). This is frequently the case with metastatic renal cell carcinomas, in which mitotic activity and nuclear pleomorphism may be minimal.

Metastatic melanoma is an important differential to consider, particularly if the tumour cells are discohesive and have a prominent nucleolus (Fig. 31.16F).[6] Melanin pigment may or may not be present.

**Cytological findings: metastatic tumours**

- The cytological features depend on the primary site
- Carcinomas form cohesive sheets and nests of atypical cells
- Nucleolar prominence
- Necrotic background
- Adenocarcinomas may have intracytoplasmic mucin droplets and form glandular structures

- Squamous carcinomas have single cells and sheets of cells with focal keratinisation and hyperchromatic, and atypical nuclei.[27]

**Diagnostic pitfalls: metastatic tumours**

- Small cell carcinomas may mimic small cell glioblastoma or lymphoma
- Metastases from some primary sites, particularly renal, may look deceptively benign
- Squamous cells may derive from non-metastatic lesions, such as craniopharyngioma, dermoid and epidermoid cysts
- Intracytoplasmic 'pseudopsammoma bodies' in secretory meningiomas can mimic adenocarcinoma
- Metastatic melanoma may be amelanotic and the primary lesion may be unrecognised at the time of surgery.

## New techniques

Immunocytochemical staining is not currently in routine use for brain smears. Polymerase chain reaction and *in situ* hybridisation studies are plausible on microdissected smears, and due to the presence of whole cells rather than parts of cells in histological sections, there may be theoretical advantages over histological sections.[28] For details of new techniques, see Chapter 34.

## The role of CNS intraoperative cytology in patient management

### Accuracy of intraoperative smear

There is evidence that intraoperative neuropathological assessment to confirm the adequacy of a biopsy can be of benefit to the patient. One study has shown an increase in the adequacy rate of CT-guided biopsy from 87% to 94%, by the addition of intraoperative cytological assessment.[29] There is a danger that an inadequate biopsy may lead to repeat surgery, which is not without risk to the patient. A recent study of 5000 radiologically guided stereotactic biopsies reported a mortality rate of 0.7%, and a persistent deficit rate of 1.3%.[30]

There is wide variation in the published rates of discordance between intraoperative findings and final histological results for neurosurgical stereotactic biopsies, ranging between 5% and 92%[3,9] the results depending much on the definition of 'accuracy' and inclusion of inadequate samples in the final figures. If defined as differentiation between neoplastic and non-neoplastic lesions, accuracy is not necessarily of great value intraoperatively for a neurosurgeon, as the intraoperative management of a meningioma and a glioblastoma will be vastly different, despite both being neoplastic processes. Studies using more stringent definitions of 'accuracy' show a complete correlation in 81.3–89.8% of cases.[31,32] The intraoperative cytological diagnosis is reported to be correct in a high proportion of meningiomas, metastases and glioblastomas, but is less accurate in cases of oligodendroglioma and ependymoma. A report from India, including a relatively high proportion of infective cases, showed a diagnostic accuracy rate 84.2%.[32]

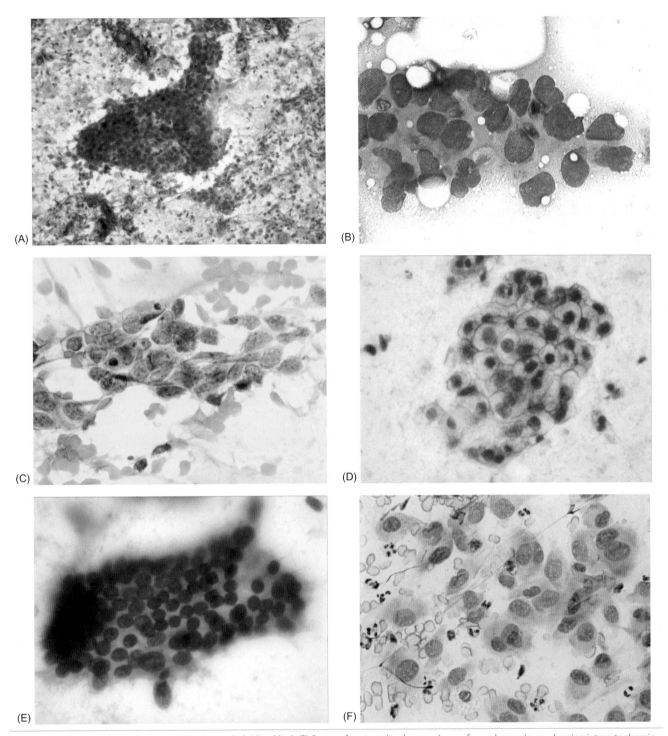

**Fig. 31.16** (A) Smear of metastatic breast carcinoma (toluidine blue). (B) Smear of metastatic adenocarcinoma from a lung primary showing intracytoplasmic vacuolation (MGG). (C) Smear of small cell carcinoma metastasis. The cells have scanty cytoplasm, and tend to form small clusters (MGG). (D) Smear of metastatic renal cell carcinoma, showing clusters of deceptively bland cells with clear cytoplasm (toluidine blue). (E) Smear of peri-spinal metastatic prostatic carcinoma. The lobules of cells with relatively bland nuclei could mimic meningioma (toluidine blue). (F) Smear of metastatic melanoma. Melanin production may be scanty or absent (MGG).

An international survey of neuropathologists published in 1999[33] showed that for the intraoperative assessment of stereotactic brain biopsies 64% used a combination of frozen section and cytological techniques, 23% used frozen section alone, and 13% only used cytological techniques. The majority used H&E and/or toluidine blue stains.

There is evidence that a combination of both intraoperative cytology and frozen section may improve the intraoperative diagnostic yield and increase diagnostic accuracy from 87% to 91% when comparing imprint cytology combined with frozen section against frozen section alone.[6] However, there is considerable local variation in use of intraoperative neuropathology, based partly on availability of suitably accredited neuropathologists and laboratory facilities, and partly on the preferences of individual neurosurgeons.

Published rates of discrepancy of diagnosis of imaging techniques compared with final histological diagnosis range between 10% and 33%.[34,35] It is of note that in one study a single confident presumptive diagnosis could be made by the neurosurgeon prior to biopsy in 90% of cases, and in 95% of this group the diagnosis was confirmed by biopsy, or subsequent clinical outcome.[35]

If auditing diagnostic accuracy of intraoperative smear cytology the diagnostic practice of an institution needs to be taken into account. At an institution in which only the most clinically challenging biopsies are subject to intraoperative assessment, the anticipated accuracy rate would be expected to be much lower than in an institution in which intraoperative assessment is routine in all cases.

## The role of intraoperative smear in patient management

Before undertaking an intraoperative neuropathological smear, the key question that should be asked is why is it being performed? It is critical to be aware of the question that the neurosurgeon needs answering from the procedure, since smearing the small amount material available may preclude further histological assessment. If there is no good reason to perform the intraoperative smear, it is advisable to fix all available tissue for histology.

Usually the most important question the smear can answer is whether the tissue from a stereotactic biopsy is likely to be adequate for providing a histological diagnosis and avoiding re-operation. Nonetheless, it has been demonstrated that even in a major neurosurgical unit with routine intraoperative smear cytology support, 10.7% of stereotactic biopsies failed to provide a histological diagnosis.[36] In cases where either the smear shows exclusively necrotic or reactive tissue, the neurosurgeon may wish to have a second, and if necessary multiple further smears until suitable material has been biopsied to ensure reliable neuropathological diagnosis.

The presence of exclusively or predominantly necrotic tissue may be suggestive in the appropriate clinical/radiological context of origin from the necrotic component of a malignant glial tumour; however, it should not be regarded as diagnostic, as necrosis is also seen in other neoplastic and non-neoplastic conditions (including infarction, acute demyelination, infections, radiation necrosis). If the smear is necrotic, the biopsy can be taken from a more peripheral area, more likely to contain viable cells.

Conversely, an intraoperative smear may show relatively paucicellular glial tissue with a reactive pattern. The possibilities in this situation would include biopsy from tissue adjacent to a tumour, or at the edge of an infiltrative glioma, or a reaction to another disease process.[37] The differential diagnosis may also include low-grade gliomas, which can be difficult to distinguish from reactive gliosis. A finding of reactive appearing glial tissue needs to be discussed by the pathologist and surgeon in the light of clinical/radiological findings. If, for example there is radiological evidence of a malignant tumour, it is likely that the biopsy has missed the lesional tissue and the surgeon may wish to rebiopsy at another site.

In some cases more specific information regarding the diagnosis may be required to guide intra-operative management, e.g. to guide the extent of excision.[38] Occasionally a precise intraoperative diagnosis is required prior to the insertion of intra-tumoural chemotherapeutic agents. In such a case, I would recommend combined frozen section and smear cytology, and that the degree of uncertainty involved in the diagnosis should be clearly communicated to the surgeon.

Sometimes an intraoperative finding may be used to guide postoperative management prior to availability of definitive histology.[6] This should be done with caution. Given the approximately 5–10% error rate, unless there is a clinical emergency, it is usually safer to wait for the final histological diagnosis.

Smear cytology has an important role in the intraoperative management of selected neurosurgical patients under the care of an experienced team of specialist pathologists, radiologists, neurosurgeons and oncologists. It is essential that those performing brain smears, and those interpreting the results, are aware of the potential pitfalls in intraoperative neuropathological diagnosis, in order to provide a safe and effective service.

# THE CYTOLOGY OF CEREBROSPINAL FLUID

*Maria Thom*

## Introduction

Cytological examination of the cerebrospinal fluid (CSF) in the investigation of neurological disease remains a basic tool in clinical practice, despite the rapid advancement in the last decades of non-invasive methods, particularly neuroimaging. As such, familiarity with the normal cell constituents, contaminants and abnormal cell types remains an essential requirement for the trainee and practising pathologist. CSF examination may be carried out by either neuropathology specialists, cytopathologists or in some cases haematologists. Disease processes involving the ventricular system and leptomeninges are particularly amenable for cytological analysis and more likely to yield positive results. The role of CSF cytology examination is in the identification of an infection or an underlying cerebral neoplasm which may aid the clinician in planning future investigations and management (Fig. 31.17).

## Cerebrospinal fluid production and flow

Cerebrospinal fluid is actively produced at the rate of 500 mL/day (or 350 μL/min). CSF is secreted from the choroid plexus, is circulated through the ventricles, subarachnoid space and is absorbed into the venous system (Fig. 31.18). In the intracranial compartment the total volume of CSF is around 100 mL. The ventricular system is lined by ependymal cells, which form a leaky barrier between CSF and the cerebral interstitium and bear cilia which may contribute to CSF movement. In the subarachnoid space the outer arachnoid barrier is formed by closely packed meningothelial cells with cell junctions and basal lamina.

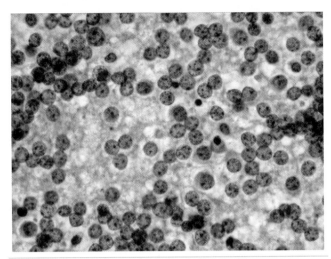

**Fig. 31.17** CSF. Smear of thyroid stimulating hormone producing pituitary adenoma (toluidine blue).

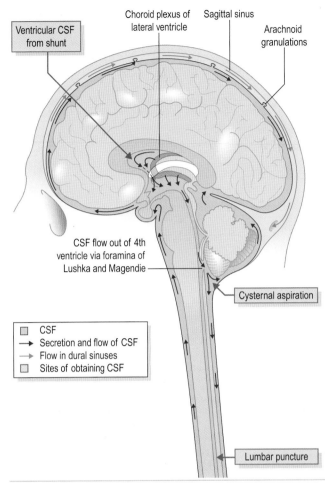

**Fig. 31.18** CSF secretion, circulation and common sites of collection.

## Source of CSF samples

In general, 10–15 mL of CSF is collected for laboratory testing, usually through a spinal tap, which, although a seemingly large volume, will be renewed in the patient within 30 minutes.[39] An average of 2–3 mL of CSF is typically reserved for cytological analysis but larger volumes of 10 mL are recommended where there is a clinical suspicion of malignancy. CSF may also be obtained from a ventricular shunt (inserted as a surgical procedure for the treatment of hydrocephalus) or more rarely aspirated from the cisterna magna.[39] Occasionally fluid from a suspected CSF leak or cystic fluid from a tumour may also be received as 'CNS fluid', although the latter is not strictly speaking CSF.

## Laboratory testing on CSF and when cytology is appropriate

CSF samples are of limited volume and aliquots are shared between neurochemistry, microbiology and neuropathology laboratories as appropriate. Common tests carried out in addition to cytology include glucose, protein, lactate, electrophoresis, culture, ELISA (enzyme-linked immunoabsorbent assay) and polymerase chain reaction (PCR) for viral studies.[39] It has been argued that the principal value of CSF cytology is in the identification of malignant cells and it is of limited value in the investigation of inflammatory and non-neoplastic disease of the CSF where the findings are generally non-specific,[40] apart from the identification of some fungal organisms.[41,42] In general, although there are exceptions, if the CSF cell count or protein is not abnormally raised or the clinical suspicion of tumour is low, then CSF cytology is unlikely to provide useful information. Automated cell analysis of CSF for differential cell counts may become more widely used in the future.[43]

### Key points: when CSF cytology examination is likely to be diagnostic

- Clinical or radiological suspicion of involvement of the sub-arachnoid space or ventricular system by cellular infiltrative process
- Raised CSF cell count or protein
- Previous history of CNS or other tumour.

## Slide preparation and laboratory methods

CSF samples should be transported to the laboratory without delay, within at least 2 hours (ideally 30 minutes) following the lumbar puncture, as cell deterioration and precipitation, which begin immediately, could interfere with the cell count.[39] Samples should be stored at 4°C. Cytocentrifugation of CSF is a widely employed and suitable method due to the low cellularity and volume of these samples, the rapidity of the preparation and the broad range of staining methods that can be applied, including preparations for immunohistochemistry and special stains for organisms.[42] Alternative preparatory methods employ membrane filtration methods, such as Millipore filter systems, Nucelopore[42] or Schleicher and Schuell filters with pore size of 3 μm, which efficiently collect a high percentage of cells of all size in the CSF. Most laboratories include a Papanicolaou in addition to a Giemsa-based stain (Wright–Giemsa, Romanowsky or Diff-Quik methods) for analysis (Fig. 31.19).

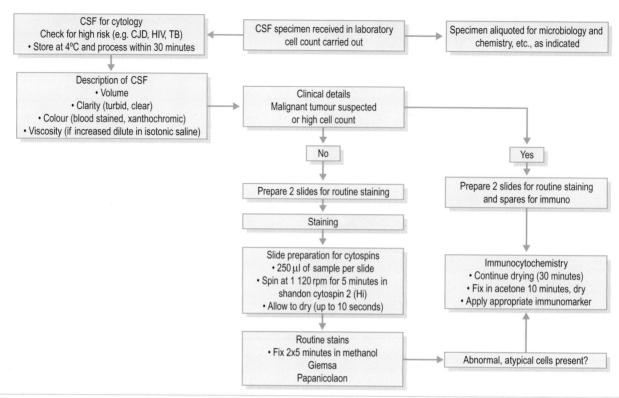

**Fig. 31.19** Flow diagram of standard procedures for handling and processing of CSF specimens in neurocytology laboratory.

## Cytological examination of the CSF

The interpretation of CSF cytology should be carried out in the knowledge of the CSF cell count, differential cell count, protein analysis and the source of the sample, for example whether it was obtained by lumbar puncture or from another other site. In addition relevant clinical information is required, in particular the age of the patient, clinical signs of meningeal disease (e.g. cranial nerve dysfunction), a history of CNS or systemic neoplasm, any MRI findings of cranio-spinal abnormalities. It is also important to ascertain if there has been any recent neurosurgical procedure when interpreting findings.

## Normal cell types, contaminants and artefacts

Normal CSF contains only a few lymphocytes and monocytes with total cell counts of $0-4/mm^3$ or $\mu L$ (excluding red blood cells) (Fig. 31.20A,B). A raised CSF cell count is often taken as $>5/mm^3$ after correction for any blood contamination.[39,40] The normal ratio of lymphocytes to monocytes is about 2–3:1. This ratio is reversed in newborns and there is less consensus on normal CSF values in children less than 1 year.

Additional cells, such as chondrocytes and fibroblasts, may be seen as cellular contaminants introduced during the lumbar puncture procedure (Fig. 31.20C,D).[42]

A 'traumatic tap' occurs when a small blood vessel is punctured introducing red blood cells and leucocytes into the CSF sample. In these situations the white blood cell count can be

corrected by subtracting one white cell for every 700–1000 red blood cells/$mm^3$ (Fig. 31.20E).[39,44] If the red blood cells are lysed during processing this may give a false impression of raised white cell count in the CSF.

Clusters of cuboidal or columnar cells of choroid plexus or ependymal origin may occasionally be shed into the CSF (Fig. 31.20F). These are more commonly seen with ventricular samples and in CSF taken from small children and in patients with hydrocephalus.[45] Often it is not possible on morphological grounds to distinguish normal choroid plexus from ependymal cells in the CSF but it is considered likely that the majority are of choroid plexus origin.

Meningothelial cells of leptomeningeal origin (Fig. 31.20H) are occasionally seen in addition to squamous cell contaminants.

Fragments of brain (neuroglial) tissue may also be encountered, the latter more particularly following a ventricular tap (Fig. 31.20I).[42] Islands of neuropil containing elongated astrocytes should not be misinterpreted as a glial tumour. Similarly isolated neurones dislodged from the parenchyma in shunt or ventriculostomy CSF samples can be misinterpreted as large atypical cells with prominent nucleoli suggestive of underlying tumour (Fig. 31.20J).

Corpora amylacea may be occasionally shed into the CSF and identified, which may relate to their frequent accumulation in the subpial region with aging.

Epithelioid histiocytes and giant cells may occasionally be observed in shunt samples, more likely to suggest a foreign body response to the shunt rather than a primary granulomatous disease.[42]

Artefacts in CSF specimens including poor cell preservation and viability may arise, including as a result of delayed processing and sample deterioration. Specimens which are unsuitable

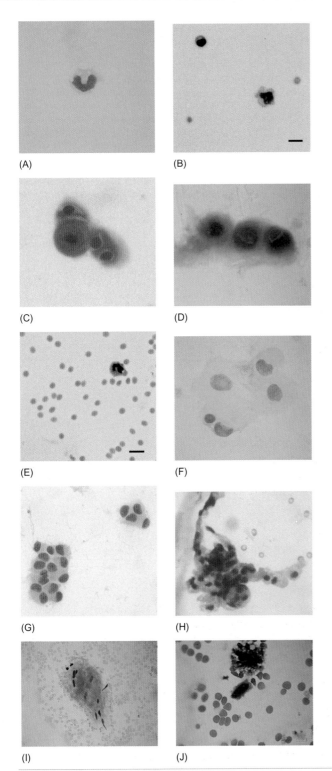

(A)

(B)

(C)

(D)

(E)

(F)

(G)

(H)

(I)

(J)

**Fig. 31.20** Normal cells and contaminants in the CSF. (A) Normal macrophage and lymphocyte (B) in a CSF specimen on Giemsa stain. (C,D) Introduction of chondrocytes either singly or in clusters into the CSF may occur during a lumbar puncture procedure. (E) Traumatic LP tap with the introduction of a few red blood cells into the CSF in this case. (F, G) Normal cells shed from the choroid plexus or ventricular surface showing a benign cuboidal morphology may be seen in the CSF occasionally. Their preservation may vary. (H) Clusters of normal meningothelial cells are rarely seen in the CSF, in this case demonstrating a typical cell whorl formation. (I) Fragments of normal brain parenchyma may be introduced into the CSF during a ventriculostomy or shunt insertion for the treatment of hydrocephalus. (J) Large neuronal cells with prominent nucleoli, sometimes with a pyramidal, may be mistaken for atypical cells including germ cell tumours.

for cytology should be retaken if the clinical suspicion for tumour is high.

## CSF cytology in non-neoplastic conditions

### Infectious diseases

It is debatable how useful CSF cytology is overall in the investigation of inflammatory and infectious diseases of the CNS[40,46] as the findings are non-specific. The main justifications for CSF cytology in this clinical situation are, therefore:

- Confirmation of an inflammatory CNS disorder
- To help exclude an underlying tumour
- Differential white cell counts to distinguish acute from chronic inflammatory responses and identification of eosinophils
- Identification of fungi in some infections.

#### Bacterial infections

##### Pyogenic infection

Leptomeningitis from a pyogenic infection (bacterial meningitis) typically has an acute presentation, characterised by turbid or cloudy CSF with a high polymorph count typically >1000/mm$^3$ (Fig. 31.21A). There are acute, recurrent and chronic forms of bacterial meningitis, each showing a typical pattern and time course of differential white cell counts in the CSF. High polymorph counts in the CSF are seen in acute bacterial meningitis and organisms may be seen on gram stain (Fig. 31.21B), but specific diagnosis is confirmed by CSF microbiological investigations. Low glucose and high lactate levels (>3.5 mmol/L),[39] particularly where Gram stain is negative, are helpful in the diagnosis of acute bacterial meningitis. In partially treated bacterial meningitis, macrophages become the dominant cell type over polymorphs. Acute infection and ventriculitis can also occur in patients with cerebrospinal fluid shunts which can lead to shunt failure.[47]

##### Tuberculous meningitis

Tuberculosis (TB) involving the CNS, including TB meningitis, is an important and serious type of extra-pulmonary TB. The bacilli reach the CNS though haematogenous routes and the non-specificity as well as variation in the severity of the symptoms can lead to a wide differential diagnosis including viral infections or other inflammatory disease processes.[48] CSF findings on admission typically show elevated opening pressure (>200 mm H$_2$O), lymphocytosis (>10/mm$^3$), high protein levels (>40 mg/dL) and low CSF/serum glucose ratios (<0.6). In up to 20–25% of the patients, neutrophilic predominance can be present at first presentation; this usually changes into a lymphocytic predominance over the following 24–48 hours (Fig. 31.21C).[48] Following the initiation of therapy, a lymphocytic pleocytosis may briefly change in the direction of neutrophilic predominance. This therapeutic paradox may be associated with clinical deterioration and has been regarded by some as being most likely due to an uncommon hypersensitivity reaction to the sudden release of large amounts of tuberculin proteins into the subarachnoid space.

More rarely epithelioid cells are also seen or clusters of macrophages in the CSF (Fig. 31.21D). Organisms may be detected on ZN stain[48] but more often identified by culture or PCR.

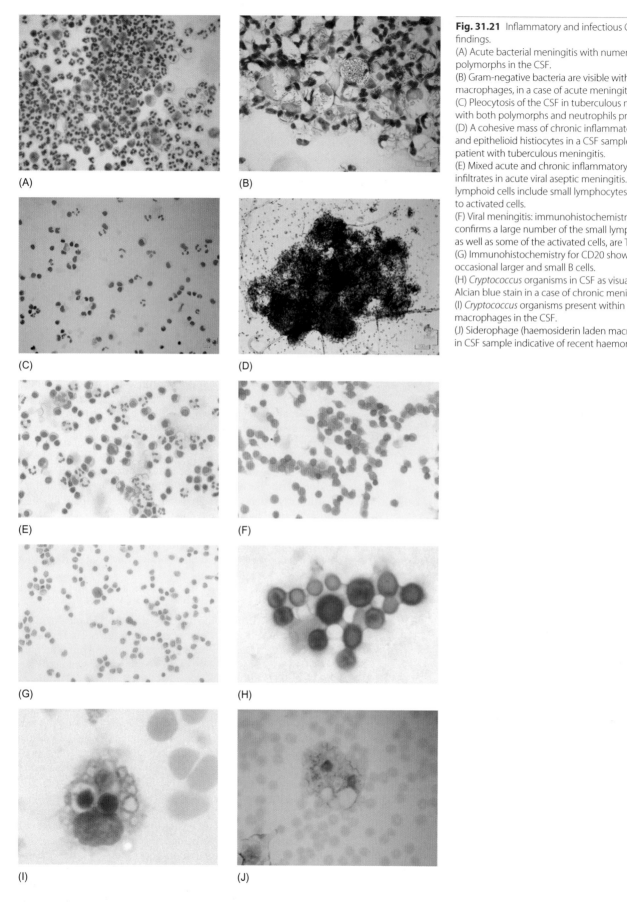

**Fig. 31.21** Inflammatory and infectious CSF findings.
(A) Acute bacterial meningitis with numerous polymorphs in the CSF.
(B) Gram-negative bacteria are visible within macrophages, in a case of acute meningitis.
(C) Pleocytosis of the CSF in tuberculous meningitis with both polymorphs and neutrophils present.
(D) A cohesive mass of chronic inflammatory cells and epithelioid histiocytes in a CSF sample from a patient with tuberculous meningitis.
(E) Mixed acute and chronic inflammatory cell infiltrates in acute viral aseptic meningitis. The lymphoid cells include small lymphocytes in addition to activated cells.
(F) Viral meningitis: immunohistochemistry for CD3 confirms a large number of the small lymphocytes, as well as some of the activated cells, are T cells.
(G) Immunohistochemistry for CD20 shows occasional larger and small B cells.
(H) *Cryptococcus* organisms in CSF as visualised with Alcian blue stain in a case of chronic meningitis.
(I) *Cryptococcus* organisms present within macrophages in the CSF.
(J) Siderophage (haemosiderin laden macrophage) in CSF sample indicative of recent haemorrhage.

Tumours infiltrating the meninges may be misdiagnosed as TB meningitis clinically. Therefore, care should be exercised to exclude an unsuspected underlying neoplastic meninigitis, especially in cases with limited clinical response to anti-tuberculous treatment.

## Cytological findings: tuberculous meningitis

- Increased lymphocytes (small and reactive cells)
- Increased neutrophils may be present in the early stages not to be confused with pyogenic bacterial meningitis
- More rarely clumps of epithelioid cells and giant cells may be seen
- ZN stains should be performed on spare cytospin slide.

## Viral infections

### Viral lymphocytic meningitis

The term 'aseptic meningitis' denotes a clinical syndrome of meningitis associated with a predominance of lymphocytes in the cerebrospinal fluid (CSF) with no common bacterial agents identified in the CSF. Viral meningitis is considered the main cause of lymphocytic meningitis and the terms 'aseptic' and viral meningitis are often used synonymously. Other infectious causes of lymphocytic meningitis are detailed in Table 31.1.[39,49,50] In acute viral meningitis, raised white cell counts of 500–1000/mm$^3$ are seen with counts of usually <500/mm$^3$ in more chronic cases (defined as persisting disease for 1 month or longer).[51]

A predominance of polymorphs (>50%) in the CSF may occur in the initial stages (the first 6 hours[39]) of an acute aseptic meningitis,[52] although a lymphocytic reaction is a more typical finding occurring within 8–48 hours.[49]

Typically, a range in lymphocyte differentiation and reactivity is seen with a spectrum from small lymphocytes, to larger activated lymphocytes together with a few plasma cells. Overall there is a predominance of small lymphocytes.

In viral meningitis, as well as encephalitis associated with high CSF cell counts (including *Herpes simplex* and in *Japanese encephalitis*), atypical lymphocytes have been noted in the CSF and the differential diagnosis from lymphoma arises.[42,53] Such atypical lymphocytes include large cells with basophilic cytoplasm and coarse chromatin and prominent nucleoli, similar to cells observed in peripheral blood in infectious mononucleosis[53] and CD4-positive cells with multilobulated or clover-leaf nuclei have been reported. Mitotic figures may be present in a reactive lymphocytosis and should not be interpreted as supporting a neoplastic process.

Immunophenotyping can support reactive changes through the demonstration of mixed, non-clonal lymphocytic populations, often with T cell predominance (Fig. 31.21E–G). In addition, cytological interpretation should always be correlated with virology results using PCR, serology and ELISA,[39,49] particularly in suspicious cases.[54] The more common viruses associated with meningitis are listed in Table 31.1.

## Cytological findings: aseptic meningitis

- Predominance of polymorphs can occur in first 6 hours
- Lymphocytosis with reactive lymphocytes and occasional plasma cells
- Spectrum of size and activation of lymphocytes supports a reactive process

**Table 31.1** Causes of chronic lymphocytic meningitis

| |
|---|
| Infection (non-viral)[39] |
| TB |
| Syphilis |
| *Cryptococcus* |
| *Listeria* |
| *Brucella* |
| *Mycoplasma* |
| *Neurocysticercosis* |
| *Toxoplasmosis* |
| Viral meningitis |
| Common: Enteroviruses (Coxsackie virus A and B, Echovirus[49]), Arbovirus, West Nile virus,[50] HIV, HSV-2 and 1 |
| Rare: Mumps, measles, EBV, CMV, VZV |
| Inflammatory conditions |
| Collagen vascular disorders, e.g. SLE |
| Sarcoidosis |
| Vasculitis, e.g. Behçet's |
| Chemical meningitis |
| Response to intrathecal medical treatments, e.g. antibiotics, chemotherapy, contrast chemicals. |
| Rupture of cystic contents, e.g. craniopharyngioma |
| Following subarachnoid haemorrhage |
| Neoplasms |
| Carcinomatous meningitis |
| Lymphoma |

- Immunocytochemistry may be helpful in the differential diagnosis with lymphoma in specimens with atypical cells
- Interpret cytology in context of any virology results
- Suggest a repeat CSF examination after an interval if both cytological and clinical suspicion of lymphoma
- Mollaret's macrophages may be identified in recurrent aseptic meningitis.

### Herpes simplex virus

Herpes encephalitis (HSE) may be associated with a meningitis and abnormal CSF in 97% of cases.[39] There is an increase in white blood cells from 5 to 500 cells/mm$^3$ with a lymphocytic predominance and is often associated with xanthochromia. PCR for HSV is more likely to be positive in the first 2 weeks of the illness and demonstration of intrathecal antibody production may be a useful retrospective test.[55] More rarely, a specific diagnosis of HSV and CMV encephalitis are made by the identification of intracellular inclusions in cells shed into the CSF.

### Mollaret's meningitis

Mollaret's meningitis is also known as idiopathic recurrent meningitis. It is a rare and benign disease associated with acute episodes of headache and meningism lasting around 5–7 days.[56] The CSF findings include marked pleocytosis with neutrophils, and mononuclear cell infiltrates including large macrophages with vacuolated cytoplasm ('Mollaret cells') which often characterise this disease process.[57] Ghost cells have also been described. The large monocytic cells have a characteristic bean-shaped or bi-lobed nuclei with deep nuclear cleft, in some cases resembling footprints.[56] Plasma cells may also be seen and, similar to HSV meningitis, haemosiderin laden macrophages may be present. In a proportion of cases with Mollaret's meningitis, HSV 2 has been identified as the causative agent.[56,58] It has been proposed, however, that the term Mollaret's meningitis be reserved for idiopathic cases of recurrent aseptic meningitis.[55]

### West Nile virus

West Nile virus infection, which is seasonally epidemic in the USA can present with a meningitic illness. The CSF typically shows elevated white cells including neutrophils and lymphocytes. The lymphocytes are reactive varying from small to transformed lymphocytes and, in one study, plasma cells were seen in 11% of cases.[50] The lymphoid atypia can suggest a diagnosis of an underlying lymphoproliferative disorder; however, studies have confirmed a non-clonal pleocytosis.[50] Protein is typically elevated but glucose is normal.

### Human immunodeficiency virus (HIV)

Around 5–10% of HIV-positive patients have meningitis at any phase of their infection, but it is more common at the point of seroconversion.[39] Frequencies of epitope-specific CD8(+) T cells are higher in CSF than in blood, while HIV RNA concentrations are lower.[120] In patients with AIDS, the CSF can show non-specific chronic inflammatory infiltrates in HIV encephalitis. Chronic meningeal inflammation in AIDS, however, should only be attributed to HIV after the exclusion of other pathogens[51] and opportunistic infections such as Cryptococcus and CMV should be considered. Rarely, viral inclusions of JC virus in cases of PML have been reported in cells in the CSF.[59] The presence of atypical lymphocytes in inflammatory conditions in immunosuppressed patients may be misinterpreted as lymphoma and immunophenotyping should be carried out in such cases.[42]

## Fungal CNS infections

Cryptococcus neoformans is the most common cause of chronic infectious meningitis in immunosuppressed patients, particularly HIV, but can occur in immunocompetent patients. The CSF abnormalities can resemble TB meningitis.[51] The CSF white cell count is typically raised in immunocompetent patients, with a predominance of lymphocytes. In HIV-associated cryptococcal meningitis, the CSF white cell count is lower and may even be normal. CSF protein is usually elevated but CSF glucose may be normal.

The organism has a characteristic thick mucopolysaccharide capsule which is a major virulence factor and the substrate detected by the cryptococcal antigen tests (Fig. 31.21H). The yeasts are spherical to oval cells, 5–10μm in diameter. Cryptococcus neoformans is an intracellular as well as an extracellular pathogen, and can survive and replicate within acidic macrophage phagolysosomes; occasionally these organisms are seen outside or within macrophages in CSF specimens (Fig. 31.21I) usually as refractile round structures with pale haloes on routine MGG staining. Alcian blue or mucicarmine stains are useful to confirm their presence.[60] The India Ink stain is also traditionally used to demonstrate these organisms and is positive in 70–90% of AIDS patients but in only ~50% of non-HIV

patients. The most rapid test is the cryptococcal antigen in CSF and serum,[51] which has a high sensitivity and specificity.[60]

In HIV patients Cryptococcus infection is histologically characterised by a lack of granulomata, a higher incidence of involvement of brain parenchyma and greater numbers of yeast cells which tend to be extra- rather than intracellular.[60] In non-HIV-associated disease, especially in apparently immunocompetent patients, cultures and antigen tests may sometimes be negative; large-volume CSF samples with repeat lumbar punctures may be required to reach the diagnosis.

### Cytological findings: fungal meningitis

- Lymphocytosis in CSF
- Cryptococcal organisms demonstrated with MGG or PAP stains and confirmed with Alcian blue or India Ink stains
- There may be a paucity of lymphocytes in immunosuppressed patients
- The organisms may be intracellular within macrophages.

## Other infectious causes of chronic meningitis

Lyme disease caused by the spirochete Borrelia burgdorferi is associated with a mild increase in lymphocytes in the CSF in patients who develop a meningitic illness. In one study it was associated with a significantly lower neutrophilic cell count in the CSF compared to viral meningitis, one of the main clinical differential diagnosis.[61] Acanthamoeba and toxoplasmosis infections are associated with mononuclear pleocytosis[51] but these organisms are best demonstrated through tissue needle biopsy.[42,46] Echinococcal components have rarely been reported in the CSF examination of patients with intracranial hydatidosis.[62]

# Inflammatory conditions of unknown cause

## Neurosarcoidosis

Sarcoidosis is a multisystem granulomatous disorder, characterised histologically by non-caseating epithelioid granulomas. It is said to affect the CNS in less than 10% of cases, although this is likely to be an under-representation based on autopsy studies.[63] Primarily, it results in parenchymal granulomatous masses or a granulomatous meningitis. CSF is characterised by a mild to moderate increase in lymphocytes (range 10–200/mm³) and increase of protein.[51] An increased ratio of helper-suppressor T cells (CD4:CD8 > 5) has been proposed as an aid to the differentiation of neurosarcoid from multiple sclerosis.[63] CSF oligoclonal bands (in 30–40% of cases) are associated with the presence of raised protein. Serum ACE (angiotensin converting enzyme) levels may be abnormal but this is considered a non-specific finding.

## Multiple sclerosis (MS)

MS is an autoimmune demyelinating disorder. There is no diagnostic test and a lumbar puncture is often carried out to obtain evidence of CNS inflammation to correlate with clinical symptoms and the MRI demonstration of multifocal white matter lesions on T2-weighted sequences. It is typically associated with a moderate increase in lymphocytes and monocytes in the CSF (10–20/mm³), although they may be normal. High white cell counts (>50/mm³) and polymorph infiltrates have been reported however, in some forms of MS, such as Devic's neuromyelitis optica.[64] Plasma cells are a characteristic finding.[65] In healthy individuals, B cells are rarely present in the CSF, while in MS patients, a clonally expanded B-cell population is detected. This consists of memory B cells, centroblasts and antibody-secreting plasma blasts and plasma cells that are responsible for intrathecal immunoglobulin G production and oligoclonal band formation in more than 90% of MS patients.[66] An excess of apoptotic lymphocytes was not shown in MS compared with other inflammatory diseases.[67] In the future, biomarkers in the CSF, such as antimyelin IgG antibodies are promising, specific markers and correlate to MR measures of disease activity.[68,69] The differential diagnosis of MS includes ADEM (acute disseminated encephalomyelitis), which typically follows an upper respiratory or febrile illness. In ADEM, the CSF cell count can be as high as 270 cell/mm³.[70]

### Systemic autoimmune and vasculitic disorders

It is estimated that SLE may involve the CNS in around 50% of patients, one neuropsychiatric manifestation of which is lymphocytic meningitis. CNS involvement, including parenchymal vasculitis may rarely be the presenting symptom.[71]

Meningoencephalitis may be a manifestation of neuro-Behçet's with a lymphocytic pleocytosis, although in some cases a high percentage of polymorphs have been noted.[51,72] A CSF lymphocytosis may also be present in primary angiitis and hypertrophic pachymeningitis.[73]

### Chemical meningitis

Chemical meningitis is a form of lymphocytic or chronic meningitis following the introduction of an irritant into the subarachnoid space. This can include therapeutic agents as well as contrast material (Table 31.1). Craniopharyngioma, or other cyst rupture,[74] can induce a chemical meningitis and CSF analysis commonly reveals a neutrophil pleocytosis, raised protein, fat and cholesterol and sometimes crystals in the CSF. This is usually associated with symptoms of meningism but occasionally may be clinically silent.[75]

## Cerebral haemorrhage

Subarachnoid haemorrhage (SAH), usually caused by rupture of a saccular aneurysm, is diagnosed by CT imaging in 98% of patients. Measurement of bilirubin in the CSF, a breakdown product of haemoglobin, which imparts a yellow tinge to the CSF (xanthochromia), can be measured using spectrophotometry after 12 hours of symptom onset.[76] Cytological analysis of CSF during the period following a subarachnoid haemorrhage may reveal siderophages (haemosiderin-laden macrophages, Fig. 31.21J), which can be confirmed with Perls stain; however, their identification is not a specific or sensitive test for spontaneous SAH. Siderophages, for example, may also be observed following a previous traumatic lumbar puncture and in other conditions.[42]

Superficial siderosis is caused by repeated small bleeds into the subarachnoid space with resulting haemosiderin deposition in the parenchyma. In many cases the cause of the bleeding is not identified. It may be related to previous trauma with friable vessels in a dural defect. In the majority of the patients xanthochromia or red blood cells in the CSF are identified.[77]

## Cytological examination of shunt fluid in the management of hydrocephalus

Patients with hydrocephalus may have an intraventricular shunt inserted for the management of raised intracranial pressure. Fluid aspirated from shunt may be sent for cytological analysis for the investigation of suspected infection or in the investigation of shunt failure. Neuropil fragments are commonly encountered following insertion. Epithelioid histiocytes and giant cells may occasionally be observed in patients with long-standing shunts, more likely to suggest a foreign body response rather than a primary granulomatous disease.[42] In the case of ventriculitis due to pyogenic organisms, many polymorphs are seen in shunt fluid with a shift to increased numbers of lymphocytes and macrophages in partially treated cases. In some cases, cytology may requested for the exclusion of recurrent tumour.

## CSF cytology in the investigation of neurodegenerative diseases

CSF cytology is of limited value in the investigation of suspected neurodegenerative disease. Insoluble proteins which accumulate in neurodegenerative diseases, such as PrP$^{sc}$ and Aβ in Creutzfeldt-Jakob disease (CJD) and Alzheimer's disease, respectively, accumulate in the interstitial space in addition to limited elimination through CSF drainage.[78] CSF biomarkers, for example, tau/Aβ42 ratios have been shown of value in the discrimination of dementia type[79] and α-synuclein levels in the investigation of dementia with Lewy bodies.[80]

## CSF cytology for tumour diagnosis

Despite the fact that primary CNS tumours account for around two-thirds of all brain neoplasms, overall, the main tumour types diagnosed in the CSF are metastases from solid tumours or lymphomas and leukaemias (Table 31.2).[40,46,81–83] Neoplastic or malignant meningitis defines the process of multifocal seeding of the leptomeninges by malignant cells. Neurological signs and symptoms are varied but common symptoms include headache, cranial nerve palsies, myelopathy or radiculopathy. Often, neurological signs are more prominent than reported symptoms. The clinical differential diagnosis includes infectious causes of chronic meningitis. MRI features can be virtually diagnostic, with diffuse meningeal and cranial nerve enhancement. However, identification of atypical cells in CSF still remains the 'gold standard' as the most definitive laboratory test.

The overall incidence of neoplastic meningitis is around 3–8% of cancer patients but it is becoming more common due to a combination of increased detection using MRI and more effective therapies for systemic cancer resulting in longer survival times and increased incidence of late-CNS spread.[84] It often presents in patients with known disseminated tumours, but can present after a disease-free interval, or even more rarely as the presenting symptom of the tumour. Tumour cells reach the meninges through vascular channels (venous plexus or arteries), via direct extension from a tumour mass (around 30–40% of patients will have cerebral parenchymal disease) or

**Table 31.2** Common tumour types identified in some of the larger CSF series (%)

| CSF series | Carcinoma | | | Melanoma | Primary CNS tumour | | | Leukaemias and lymphoma (primary and secondary) |
|---|---|---|---|---|---|---|---|---|
| Tumour type | Breast: adeno-carcinoma | Lung: adeno-carcinoma | Other primary site | | PNET | Glial | Other | ALL, B cell NHL, others |
| Mackenzie (1996)[40] | 20 | 14 | 11 | 6 | 12 | 2 | 6 | 20 |
| Prayson and Fischler (1998)[46] Adults | 41.3 (all adenocarcinoma) | | | 2.9 | | 2.5 | | 40.3 |
| Children | | | | | 77 | | 9.6 | 13 |
| Gupta et al. (2004)[81] | 22 | 8 | | 16 | 7 | 9.5 | 2 | 11 |
| Chamberlain (2006)[82] ('Solid' metastatic tumours only) | 27–50 | 50–56 | 9 | 12 | | | | |
| van Oostenbrugge (1997)[83] | 24 | 24 | 13 | | 2 | | 2 | 33 (22 NHL; 11 ALL) |

PNET, primitive neuroectodermal tumour; ALL, acute lymphoblastic lymphoma; NHL, non-Hodgkin lymphoma.

along perineural routes. Once within the subarachnoid space there may be dissemination throughout the neuroaxis via the CSF resulting in multiple seedings.

## CSF cytology in diagnosis of primary CNS tumours

Primary CNS tumours form only 10–20% of positive CSF specimens.[40,45] Many CNS primary tumours, particularly diffuse astrocytomas and glioblastoma multiforme (GBM), have a propensity to infiltrate the brain parenchyma, particularly the white matter (see p. 825). When these tumours are identified on MRI the most certain approach for tissue confirmation is stereotactic biopsy or tumour resection rather than lumbar puncture, which in fact may be contraindicated if there is raised ICP and a risk of precipitating herniation. Therefore, the proportion of patients with primary glial tumours that undergo lumbar puncture is small. As a result, there are no precise data on the percentage that have positive CSF cytology, but it is estimated to be around 15–20%.[81] Gliomas seen to involve the leptomeninges or extend into the ventricle, particularly ependymomas, are more likely to be detectable by CSF. Some tumour types, such as embryonal tumours (PNET), pineal tumours and germ cell tumours, have a predilection to seed through the CSF.

### Glial tumours

Oligodendrogliomas and astrocytomas of varying grade, but particularly grade IV astrocytomas (GBM), may occasionally disseminate in the subarachnoid space.[85] However, as a result of cohesive properties, cells exfoliate poorly in the CSF. As mentioned earlier, cytological examination of CSF in patients with gliomas is not routinely carried out and they are usually seen in particular clinical settings, for example during the examination of aspirated cyst fluid and in the investigation of postoperative infection, CSF leaks, inoperable tumours, spinal tumours and meningeal seeding.

### Gliomas: key cytopathology features

*Malignant astrocytomas and glioblastoma multiforme (GBM):* Cells in the CSF form loose clusters or occasionally single cells are seen. Unlike intraoperative smear preparations (see p. 825, Figs 31.5–31.8) or histological sections, cellular processes are not clearly defined, although overall astrocytic morphology may be retained (Fig. 31.22). In GBM, the appearances of cells may be 'multiform' and variable as in histological sections with pleomorphic, irregular nuclear membranes, coarse chromatin and prominent nucleoli (Fig. 31.23). Apoptosis and mitosis may be evident. The cytoplasm may be variable in amount but can be prominent on both Giemsa and Papanicolaou (PAP) stains or vacuolated.[45] Multinucleation in GBM[81] as well as cells with gemistocytic morphology may be a feature. The differential diagnosis includes epithelial tumours, melanoma and sarcomas. Small cell glioblastomas in the CSF may have appearances similar to PNET and small cell carcinomas. Knowledge of any prior history of malignancy as well as age will be helpful in formulating the differential diagnosis.

*Oligodendrogliomas* may shed cells into the CSF. The cells show nuclear atypia and are larger than lymphocytes but specific features to distinguish them from other glial tumours are lacking (Figs 31.9, 31.24).[42]

*Ependymomas* (WHO grade II) tend to form tightly cohesive groups and in some cases may appear cuboidal or columnar[45,81] with mild nuclear atypia; the differential diagnosis is with normal shed ependymal cells (see p. 829). Malignant (WHO grade III) ependymomas, particularly those arising in the fourth ventricle, may shed clusters of anaplastic cells with a high nuclear/cytoplasmic ratio which may be difficult to differentiate from PNET and other high-grade small cell tumours (Fig. 31.25).

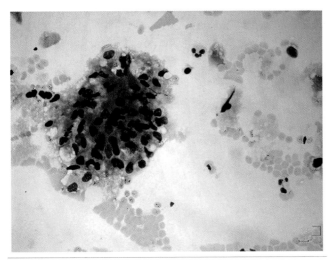

**Fig. 31.22** Shunt specimen containing fragments of hypercellular glial tissue with pleomorphic ovoid to elongated and fibrillary cells. The patient had a grade III anaplastic astrocytoma.

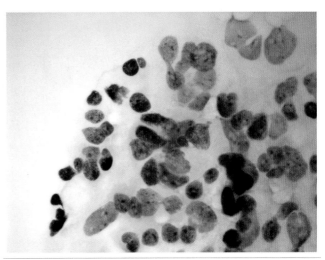

**Fig. 31.24** Oligodendroglioma grade III with clusters and single tumour cells in the CSF. The nuclei show pleomorphism, fine chromatin and overall roundness of nuclei is appreciated reminiscent of oligodendroglia in tissue sections.

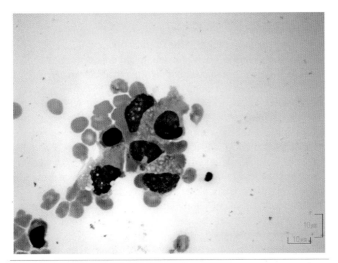

**Fig. 31.23** A cluster of pleomorphic cells in the CSF on Giemsa stain with irregular nuclei and moderate amounts of cytoplasm, forming a cohesive cluster in a patient with biopsy-proven glioblastoma multiforme (GBM).

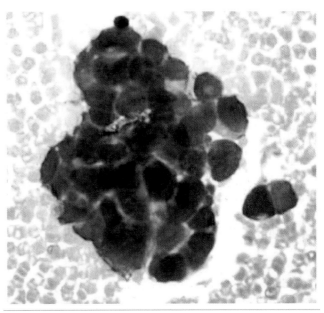

**Fig. 31.25** Clusters of cohesive cells shed from an anaplastic ependymoma.

### Immunocytochemistry

Most tumours usually retain expression of GFAP and this can be helpful in the determination of glial-cell lineage. GFAP may in some cases be phagocytosed by macrophages in necrotic glial tumours. The application of other common markers, such as S100, MAP2, vimentin and nestin in CSFs have not been fully assessed.

## Leptomeningeal gliomatosis (LG)

'Gliomatous meningitis' or 'leptomeningeal gliomatosis' (LG) describes the process where there is diffuse and extensive involvement of the leptomeningeal compartment. This may be associated with an extension from a variety of parenchymal glial tumour types, including oligodendrogliomas (grades II and III), astrocytomas (grades II and III), GBM as well as gliomatosis cerebri,[86,87] but in some cases may be a primary leptomeningeal process (Fig. 31.26).

*Primary LG* is very rare and rapidly fatal disease.[88] It has been described more frequently around the spinal cord.[86,88] MRI on T1-weighted images may show enhancing intradural, extramedullar nodules along nerve roots and at base of the brain but an absence of an intra-axial lesion. One possibility is that primary LG may arise from heterotopic meningeal glial rests and an association with spinal cord dysraphism has been shown.

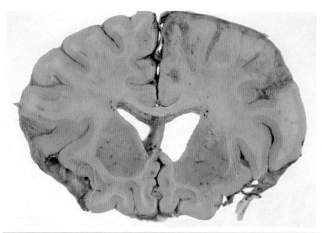

**Fig. 31.26** Primary leptomeningeal tumour. Macroscopic coronal section from a patient with a cerebral tumour which was primarily leptomeningeal based with no evidence of parenchymal infiltration, although focal cortical infarction was present due to compression of tumour around leptomeningeal blood vessels. The histological sections confirmed that the tumour, with a marked desmoplastic response, was confined to the leptomeninges. Although there was a paucity of GFAP expression and focal vimentin positivity (CD34 negative, EMA weakly positive) primary leptomeningeal gliomatosis remained one possible diagnosis.

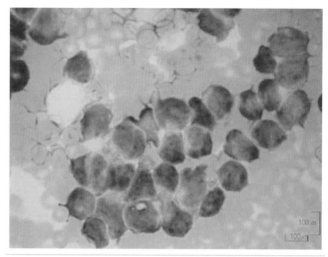

**Fig. 31.27** PNET/medulloblastoma with pleomorphic cells with little cytoplasm and nuclear moulding.

### Cytological findings: leptomeningeal gliomatosis

- The pathological confirmation is often difficult despite the presence of extensive disease. CSF cytology samples may be negative for tumour cells, even with repeat testing, but show lymphocytosis or pleocytosis and elevated protein.[86,88,89] As a result these cases are often misdiagnosed as infectious or inflammatory meningitis, for example TB
- Tissue biopsy is often necessary. Tumour types in LG include: astrocytoma (grades II and IV), oligoastrocytomas, oligodendroglioma (grades II and III) and rarely pilocytic astrocytoma.[89]

## Medulloblastoma and PNET

PNET, including medulloblastomas, the commonest type of which arises in the cerebellum, spread readily through the CSF and tumour cells may be detected in 25% of cases.[90] This is the commonest primary CNS tumour seen in the CSF, particularly in the paediatric age group,[40,45,46] where they can represent over 70% of tumour-positive CSF cases (Table 31.2).[46] CSF cytological examination, as well as MRI, has a role in the routine post-surgical follow-up of patients with medulloblastoma for the detection of cranio-spinal seeding.

### Cytological findings: primitive neuroectodermal tumours

- Tumour cells are small- to medium-sized cells with high nuclear: cytoplasmic ratios, occurring singly but often in clumps (Figs 31.10, 31.27)
- Nuclear moulding is frequently observed and occasional rosette-like arrangements within cell clusters may be appreciated (Fig. 31.27)[81]
- Nuclear pleomorphism and anaplasia may be pronounced and cell necrosis and mitosis often apparent

- Overall, cell preservation may be poor rendering confirmation of neoplasia problematic. Furthermore, in some cases, the tumour infiltrate may be accompanied by a florid inflammatory reaction, obscuring the tumour cells.

The main differential diagnosis is with other malignant small cell tumours: pineoblastoma, retinoblastoma, ependymoblastoma, Ewing tumour in children and small cell carcinoma or small cell glioblastoma in adults. In atypical teratoid/rhabdoid tumour (AT/RT), positive CSF cytology has also been reported and may show similarities to PNET.[91] The most consistent cytological features in AT/RT are the large size of the tumour cells, eccentricity of the nuclei and prominent nucleoli. Distinction of PNET from lymphomas in the CSF is often less problematic. Lymphomas are less likely to form cell clusters than PNET. When clusters of small primitive cells are seen in an infant, particularly a neonate, this may represent a remnant of normal germinal matrix.

### Immunocytochemistry

Immunoreactivity for synaptophysin or other neuronal markers (e.g. MAP2, neurofilaments) are typically positive in PNET (Fig. 31.28), which can support the diagnosis together with an absence of cytokeratin and lymphocyte marker expression. GFAP expression may be present in PNET as evidence of divergent differentiation.

## Germ cell tumours

Germinomas typically show a biphasic cell population in CSF with large atypical round to polygonal cells with prominent nucleoli and delicate cytoplasm,[81] together with smaller populations of lymphocytes (Fig. 31.29). Along with the neuroimaging findings of a mid-axial space occupying lesion, immunohistochemistry for placental alkaline phosphatase can support this diagnosis and its distinction from other tumours, such as melanoma and carcinoma.

## Choroid plexus tumours

With regard to the CSF cytological diagnosis in choroid plexus tumours, difficulty may be encountered in the distinction of papillomas (see Fig. 31.11) from normal choroid plexus epithelium, as

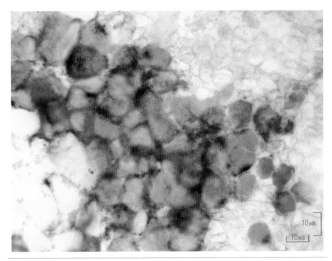

**Fig. 31.28** PNET with focal synaptophysin positivity.

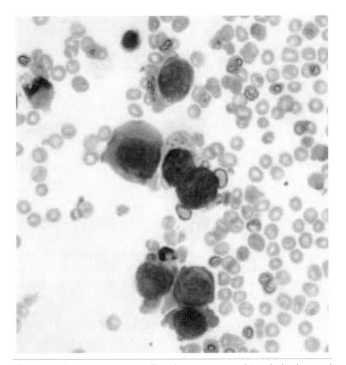

**Fig. 31.29** Germinoma: Large cells with prominent nuclei and a background of red blood cells and small lymphocytes.

the degree of nuclear pleomorphism may be minimal. However, abundant cells with papillary formations are seen with tumours in positive CSF samples. It is important to confirm in such cases if an intraventricular mass is present. With choroid plexus carcinomas an increasing degree of cytological anaplasia is present in diagnostic CSF samples. Although the majority of these tumours occur in a younger age group, their distinction from other malignant epithelial tumours should be considered. Cerebrospinal metastasis from a choroid plexus papilloma is a rare occurrence but likely to be the result of tumour seeding through the CSF; in reported cases, cytology of CSF was, however, negative.[92]

## Pineal tumours

Tumours of the pineal region represent a diverse collection and due to difficulties in surgical accessibility the initial evaluation

often commences with MRI and examination of the CSF for atypical exfoliated cells.[93] Pineoblastomas have a tendency to spread in the CSF which is morphologically indistinguishable from other PNET, including medulloblastoma.

## Other primary CNS tumours

Meningiomas have a superficial location with a dural attachment; however, shedding or exfoliation of tumour cells into the CSF is infrequent in practice[45] and the diagnosis if meningioma is rarely made through CSF examination as for other meningeal-based mesenchymal tumours, including haemangiopericytoma.

There are reports of detection of central neurocytoma in the CSF with clusters and individual, medium-sized cells, an absence of mitotic activity and synaptophysin positivity.[94] As these tumours are often adjacent to the ventricular system, detection in the CSF may not necessarily herald the widespread metastatic dissemination that is rarely reported with neurocytoma.

## CSF cytology in the investigation of secondary CNS tumours

### Carcinomatous meningitis

Neoplastic meningitis as a result of spread from a solid tumour is commonly termed 'carcinomatous meningitis' and in most cases identified at CSF the diagnosis is suspected clinically.[40] MRI findings typically show a fine signal-intense layer that follows the gyri and the superficial sulci and also the ventricles (Fig. 31.30).[95] CSF circulation is also frequently abnormal with

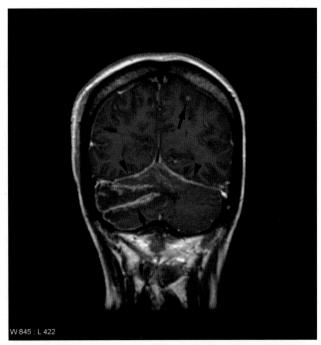

**Fig. 31.30** Carcinomatous meningitis – MRI features. Post gadolinium-enhanced sequences demonstrating diffuse nodular enhancement of the leptomeninges of the right cerebellar fissures (arrow) and tentorium cerebelli (arrowheads). Nodular leptomeningeal enhancement is apparent in the left parietal sulcal space (arrow with asterisk). A lumbar puncture confirmed malignant cells. (Courtesy of Dr Indran Davagnanam, Senior Neuroradiology Fellow, National Hospital for Neurology and Neurosurgery, London).

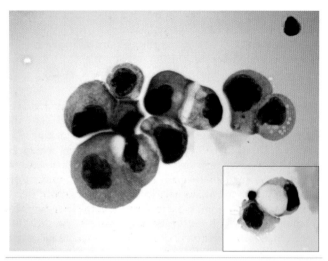

**Fig. 31.31** Clusters of cohesive, atypical cells with epithelial morphology and marked nuclear pleomorphism. The patient has a history of lung adenocarcinoma (inset) cytoplasmic vacuolation of atypical cells.

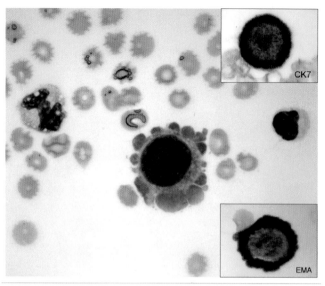

**Fig. 31.32** Giemsa-stained preparations illustrating atypical cells with ruffled outer borders and cytoplasmic vacuolation in the CSF from a patient with known breast carcinoma and hydrocephalus with shunt dysfunction. Insets: immunocytochemistry was positive for CK7 and EMA.

flow obstruction. Postmortem studies have shown that 5–20% of cancer patients with neurological symptoms have evidence of meningeal involvement.[42,96,97] More rarely, it is the initial presentation of a cancer with no prior history of neoplasia.

Carcinoma cells probably enter the subarachnoid space through blood vessels, or less often form direct extension of a neoplasm. They may remain floating free in the CSF with little evidence of involvement of CNS tissues. Lung and breast adenocarcinoma and melanoma are the commonest tumours (Table 31.2), but leptomeningeal disease from other tumours, such as GI tract, bladder, kidney, female genital tract and prostate, can occur.

The overall outlook in carcinomatous meningitis is generally poor with average survival times of 3–4 months,[98] although long-term survival is occasionally observed in patients with metastatic breast cancer with a 6% 2-year survival reported.[84] Poor prognostic factors include age over 60 years, encephalopathy or cranial nerve deficits, high initial CSF protein levels and bulky meningeal deposits.[84]

### Cytological findings: carcinomatous meningitis

- Single or clusters of large, pleomorphic cells are seen in contrast to smaller lymphocytes also often present as a reactive cellular component. In breast carcinoma, the cells are often single rather than clustered in a 'morula'
- In adenocarcinoma, cytoplasmic vacuolation may be prominent and mucin secretion demonstrated with appropriate stains as diastase PAS. The cells may have a frilly or ruffled cytoplasmic border (Fig. 31.31)
- In squamous cell carcinomas involving the CSF, Cytospin preparations are typically hypercellular with numerous malignant cells occurring singly, in loose sheets, and in tight clusters. Tumour cells exhibit large, irregular nuclei with clumped chromatin, irregular nuclear membranes, hyperchromasia, anisonucleosis, anisocytosis and keratinisation of the cytoplasm is identified
- Infrequent atypical cells present in the CSF cytology with a high index of suspicion for an underlying neoplasm: in situations where there is no previous tumour diagnosis and immunohistochemistry is not available, further classification

is not possible.[81] In some instances, although suspicious, the diagnosis falls short of confirmed malignancy and a further CSF sample may be necessary.

#### Immunohistochemistry

Immunomarkers such as cytokeratins and EMA can provide confirmation and aid in delineation of tumour type (Fig. 31.32).

## Other investigations

In clinically suspicious cases with repeatedly negative CSF samples, if there is histologically proven primary neoplasm and radiological and clinical evidence of leptomeningeal disease, treatment for meningeal carcinomatosis is usually commenced.[99,100] CSF tumour biomarkers have been evaluated as an adjunct to cytology but in general show poor specificity and sensitivity. Cytogenetic techniques such as FISH may become more widely used in the detection of metastatic malignant cells in the CSF.[83]

### Melanoma

The incidence of CNS involvement in patients with disseminated melanoma at the time of death is said to approach 90%.[42] Melanoma, or melanocytoma, may more rarely arise as a primary leptomeningeal tumour which accounts for 1% of all CNS cases.[101]

The cytological diagnosis of melanoma in the CSF is based on the presence of large dissociated cells with mainly eccentric nuclei and macronucleoli (Fig. 31.33).[81] The cytoplasm may be scant or abundant. Infrequently melanin granules may be visible in the cell cytoplasm.[81] Melanophages may also be present. When melanin is not present, distinction of these cells from carcinoma may not be possible. Immunohistochemistry for S100, HMB45 and MelanA can be helpful. As with other leptomeningeal tumours, CSF cytology analysis may be negative, even with widespread leptomeningeal disease.[101]

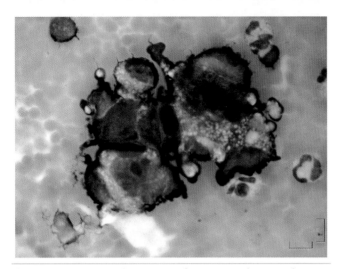

**Fig. 31.33** Giemsa-stained preparation of metastatic malignant melanoma. Pleomorphic cells with large nuclei compared to adjacent small lymphocyte (top left) and prominent nucleoli.

## Lymphomas and leukaemias

Haematological malignancies such as leukaemias and lymphomas can frequently involve the CNS,[42] forming between 11% and 40% of all malignant CSFs (Table 31.2). Lumbar puncture is often a practical way to diagnose as well as monitor disease progression in terms of CNS recurrence or response to treatment. Meningeal leukaemia or lymphoma more often arises in a patient either with known haematological malignancy or a primary CNS lymphoma (PCNSL). PCNSL accounts for 5% of brain tumours and 1% of all NHL[102] and leptomeningeal involvement is estimated to occur in around 5–10% of all NHL.[103] Lymphomatous meningitis in association with PCNSL was found in 65% of cases in one study. Rarely, primary leptomeningeal lymphomas have been reported representing 7% of all PCNSL.[104] In practice, in a patient with no previous diagnosis, the presence of atypical lymphoid cells in the CNS should prompt further investigations, including bone marrow trephine and lymph node sampling, neuroimaging and HIV status (see Chs 13,14). Leptomeningeal lymphoma can mimic other neurological conditions, including TB meningitis, vasculitis and sarcoidosis.[105]

### Leukaemias

In the acute childhood leukaemias, such as acute lymphoblastic leukaemia (ALL), frequent involvement of the CNS occurs. Identification of patients with cytological evidence of CSF involvement, regardless of symptoms, has implications in guiding appropriate treatment.[106] Prior to CNS prophylaxis, 70% of ALL patients had evidence of leptomeningeal involvement at postmortem examination.

The definition of meningeal leukaemia in ALL has been given as the presence of more than 5 white blood cells/mm³ in the CSF together with the identification of morphological blasts.[106] Blast cells of ALL have a high nuclear cytoplasmic ratio, smooth chromatin and prominent nucleoli. In some smaller blast cell types, nucleoli are not prominent. Mitotic figures may be present. In addition, an irregular nuclear membrane is a striking feature and overall increase in size of the cell,[107] being up to twice the size of normal small lymphocytes. In T-cell type ALL, the nuclei may be more convoluted.[42] The cytopathological features of blasts are better visualised with Giemsa-based stains.

In ALL, periodic examination of the CSF for typical blast cells may be undertaken, even in patients with normal cell counts and no CNS symptoms,[42] to monitor for relapse. Normal CSF cell counts do not exclude the diagnosis of leukaemia,[108] although some studies suggest that the presence of blasts in the absence of a raised cell count is not associated with an adverse prognosis.[106] Symptomatic CNS relapse is usually paralleled by an increased blast cell count in the CNS when the cytological diagnosis becomes more obvious. The distinction of reactive lymphocytes from blast cell can be aided using Tdt (terminal deoxytransferase) staining.[107] Blast cells in the CSF may also be introduced from blood contamination following a traumatic lumbar puncture.[106]

Acute myelogenous leukaemia (AML) less rarely results in leptomeningeal dissemination compared to ALL. AML involvement of the CSF is characterised by more heterogenous cell types than in ALL. Immature myeloid cells with large nuclei and scant cytoplasm are often accompanied by more mature cells, including granulocytes and eosinophils. The cell types are best visualised with Giemsa stains.

CNS spread in chronic lymphocytic leukaemia (CLL) is an uncommon complication.[109] When patients with CLL develop meningeal signs, an underlying infection due to their immunocompromised status should be excluded first. The cells of CLL are morphologically indistinguishable from small mature lymphocytes. Lymphocyte marker studies or flow cytometry studies are essential to confirm the diagnosis of CSF involvement as the majority of CLL are clonal B-cell neoplasms. Involvement of the CNS in CML can occasionally occur, but more often during blast crisis. CNS including CSF involvement can occur in the course of adult T-cell leukaemia-lymphoma (ATLL), which may occasionally present as CNS disease.[110]

### Lymphomas

Lymphomatous involvement of the leptomeninges is a result of systemic disease (lymphomatous meningitis), spread of an parenchymal PCNSL or primary leptomeningeal involvement. Of the lymphoma subtypes, high-grade tumours are more often encountered in the CSF[42,46] as diffuse large B-cell lymphoma (systemic or PCNSL), Burkitt's lymphoma, lymphoblastic lymphoma or mantle cell lymphoma.[108] T-cell lymphomas form between 3.6% and 8.5% of PCNSL,[102] with some studies suggesting a predilection for involvement of the leptomeninges.[105] Low-grade systemic lymphomas and Hodgkin's diseases rarely involve the CNS. CNS disease in a patient with systemic lymphoma is usually predictive of a poor clinical outcome; risk factors include high lymphoma stage or grade, extranodal disease, young age and HIV-positive status.

---

**Cytological findings: lymphoma**

- In virtually all patients with meningeal involvement by a lymphoma, the CSF is abnormal, even where the cytology is negative

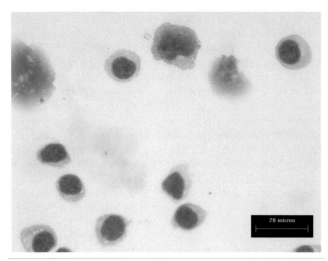

**Fig. 31.34** Cellular CSF with a mixed population of small lymphocytes and interspersed single large atypical lymphoid cells.

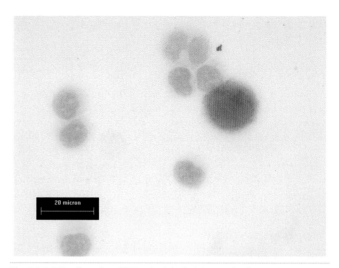

**Fig. 31.36** B-cell marker CD79a also labelled the atypical large lymphoid cells.

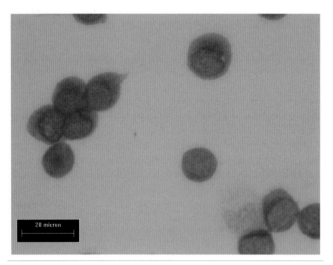

**Fig. 31.35** Immunotyping in the above case showed frequent CD3 positive small T-lymphocytes.

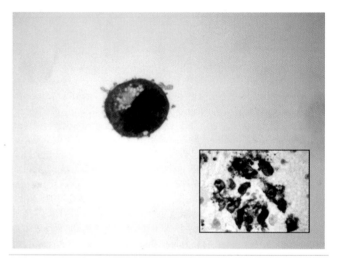

**Fig. 31.37** Anaplastic large cell lymphoma in the CSF (Giemsa). Inset: histology was carried out of a region of cortex with abnormal imaging on MRI to confirm the CSF impression of lymphoma with atypical lymphoid cells which were CD30 positive in tissue section following cortical biopsy. Immunohistochemistry for ALK1 was also positive confirming the diagnosis of anaplastic large cell lymphoma (primary CNS lymphoma).

- In diagnostic cases, a population of atypical large lymphoid blast cells is seen, with prominent nucleoli, abnormal chromatin and irregular nuclear contours (Figs 31.34–31.37). These cells often stand out as a distinct population from the background of accompanying smaller lymphocytes. Mitotic activity may be present. For diagnosis of lymphoma, see Chapter 13. CSF biomarkers may help in the discrimination of lymphoma from non-malignant inflammatory conditions. Elevated IL10 to IL6 ratio of more than 1.0 in the CSF is associated with lymphoma.[39]

### Other investigations of CSF in lymphomas

CSF flow cytometry, for example using a FACScan flow cytometer, is a useful adjunct to cytological examination in the detection of malignant haematopoietic cells,[108,111] particularly in CSFs with low cell counts. The detection rates of tumours using flow cytometry in conjunction with cytology are around 40–50% higher than that of cytology alone.[108,112]

## Diagnostic pitfalls in CSF tumour cytology

### False negative diagnosis

The diagnosis of leptomeningeal neoplasia is based on a combination of clinical symptoms, features on gadolinium-enhanced MRI, a history of neoplasia and detection of atypical cells in the CSF. Although regarded as the 'gold standard' test, the precise sensitivity and specificity of CSF cytology is difficult to determine.

It is quoted that in 10–20% of patients with leptomeningeal malignancy the CSF cytology is persistently negative. In another study of autopsy proven leptomeningeal tumour, CSF examination in life was positive in 59% of cases.[96] However, lumbar CSF cytology has been reported as diagnostic in 30–75%

of patients with neoplastic meningitis and normal MRI.[113] Therefore, cytology should be used in conjunction with MRI.[114]

*Specimen handling.* False-negative rates can be reduced by quick processing of the CSF and the examination of larger volumes of CSF (up to 10 mL).

*Source of CSF.* Obtaining specimens from a site nearest to the known leptomeningeal disease may increase detection of tumours. In paediatric tumours, CSF obtained from lumbar puncture was more sensitive than that obtained from shunt fluid.[113] Other studies suggest cisternal CSF should be obtained if lumbar puncture is negative.[115] In the study of lymphomas in the CSF, variability in the level of protein and presence of malignant cells was noted, depending on which level of the neuroaxis the sample was taken, even in the absence of obstruction to CSF flow.

*Repeated samples.* It has been shown that for autopsy confirmed leptomeningeal tumour in a series of 90 patients,[116] the initial CSF was positive in only 54% of cases but this had increased to 90% by the third lumbar puncture over the clinical course of the disease. Although this may be a reflection of disease progression, it also confirms that repeat LPs where the clinical suspicion is high may be appropriate.[83] For example some recommend repeating the procedure twice or three times if the first result is negative.[44]

Treatment with steroids, which are lymphocytotoxic, could affect the positive cytology rates in the detection of CSF lymphomas.[117]

In one study, concurrent use of immunocytochemistry with cytology was demonstrated to increase detection rates of tumours in the CSF.[118]

## False positive CSF diagnosis

False positive diagnoses in CSF are considered less frequent than false negatives.[40] False positive calls are more common for lymphoid or haematological malignancies than primary brain neoplasms and carcinomas.[42,119] Atypical lymphoid cells as a result of a viral infection, such as EBV, can be misinterpreted as lymphoma. Correlation with viral serology, judicious use of immunocytochemistry and flow cytometry to exclude clonal B- or T-cell populations can eliminate such false positives.[54] Neuroglial contaminants and clusters of normal ependymal cells in CSF specimens may be misinterpreted as primary tumours.

## REFERENCES

1. National Institute for Health and Clinical Excellence. Service guidance for improving outcomes for people with brain and other central nervous system tumours. CSG Brain. London: National Institute for Health and Clinical Excellence 2006.

2. Louis DN, Ohgaki H, Wiestler OD, et al. WHO Classification of tumours of the central nervous system. World Health Organization 2007.

3. Plesec TP, Prayson RA. Frozen section discrepancy in the evaluation of central nervous system tumours. Arch Pathol Lab Med 2007;131:1532–40.

4. Brommeland T, Lindal S, Straume B, et al. Does imprint cytology of brain tumours improve intraoperative diagnoses? Acta Neuro Scand 2003;108:146–153.

5. Hernandez O, Zagzag D. Kelly P, et al. Cytologic diagnosis of cystic brain tumours: a restrospective study of 88 cases. Diagn Cytopathol 2004;31:221–28.

6. Powell SZ. Intraoperative consultation, cytologic preparations, and frozen section in the central nervous system. Arch Pathol Med 2005;129:1635–52.

7. Heper AO, Erden E, Savas A, et al. An analysis of stereotactic biopsy of brain tumors and nonneoplastic lesions: A prospective clinicopathologic study. Surg Neurol 2005;64:S282–88.

8. Ghosal N, Sridhar M, Satish R, et al. Visual pathway glioma presenting as suprasellar mass with extension into the retrosellar region – a diagnosis by smear preparation. Cytopathology 2004;15:237–40.

9. Iqbal M, Shah A, Wani MA, et al. Cytopathology of the central nervous system. Part 1. Utility of crush smear cytology in intraoperative diagnosis of central nervous system lesions. Acta Cytol 2006;50:608–16.

10. Kobayashi S, Hirakawa E, Haba R. Squash cytology of pleomorphic xanthoastrocytoma mimicking glioblastoma, a case report. Acta Cytol 1993;43:652–58.

11. Kim SH, Lee K-G, Kim TS. Cytologic characteristics of subependymal giant cell astrocytoma in squash smears. Morphometric comparisons with gemistocytic astrocytoma and giant cell glioblastoma. Acta Cytol 2007;51:375–79.

12. Kumar PV. Nuclear grooves in ependymoma. Cytologic study of 21 cases. Acta Cytol 1997;41:1726–31.

13. Kumar PV, Hosseinzadeh M, Bedayat GR. Cytologic findings of medulloblastoma in crush smears. Acta Cytol 2001;45:542–46.

14. Takei H, Dauser RC, Adesina AM. Cytomorphologic characteristics, differential diagnosis and utility during intraoperative consultation for medulloblastoma. Acta Cytol 2007;51:183–92.

15. Yachnis AT. Intraoperative consultation for nervous system lesions. Sem Diagn Pathol 2002;19:192–206.

16. Sugita Y, Tokunaga O, Morimatsu M, et al. Cytodiagnosis of central neurocytoma in intraoperative preparations. Acta Cytol 2005;48:194–98.

17. Bleggi-Torres LF, de Noronha L, Schneider Gugelmin E, et al. Accuracy of the smear technique in the cytological diagnosis of 650 lesions of the central nervous system. Diagn Cytopathol 2001;24:293–95.

18. Radha RP, Kini H, Rao VS, et al. Choroid plexus papilloma diagnosed by crush cytology. Diagn Cytopathol 2001;25:165–67.

19. Siddiqui MT, Mahon BM, Cochran E, et al. Cytologic features of meningiomas on crush preparations: a review. Diagn Cytopathol 2008;36:202–6.

20. Ng H-K. Cytologic diagnosis of intracranial germinomas in smear preparations. Acta Cytol 1995;39:693–97.

21. Hinton DR, Kovacs K, Chandrasoma PT. Cytologic features of secretory meningioma. Acta Cytol 1999;43:121–25.

22. Adesina AM. Intraoperative consultation in the diagnosis of pediatric brain tumors. Arch Pathol Lab Med 2005;129:1653–60.

23. Ng H-K. Smears in the diagnosis of pituitary adenomas. Acta Cytol 1998;42:614–18.

24. Daneshbod Y, Monabati A, Kumar P, et al. Intraoperative cytologic crush preparation findings in craniopharyngioma. A study of 12 cases. Acta Cytol 2005;49:7–10.

25. Paul Z, Yee WJ. Cytology of common primary midline brain tumours. Acta Cytol 1980;24:384–90.

26. Smith Alan R, Elsheikh Tarik M, Silverman Jan F. Intraoperative cytologic diagnosis of suprasellar and sellar cystic lesions. Diagn Cytopathol 1999;20:137–47.

27. Parwani AV, Taylor DC, Burger PC, et al. Keratinized squamous cells in fine needle aspiration of the brain. Cytopathologic correlates and differential diagnosis. Acta Cytol 2003;47:325–31.

28. Walker C, Joyce K, Du Plessis D, et al. Molecular genetic analysis of archival gliomas using diagnostic smears. Neuropathol Appl Neurobiol 2000;26:441–47.

29. O'Neill KS, Dyer PV, Bell BA, et al. Is preoperative smear cytology necessary for stereotactic surgery? Br J Neurosurg 1992;6:421–27.

30. Tilgner J, Herr M, Ostertag C, et al. Validation of intraoperative diagnoses using smear preparations from stereotactic brain biopsies: Intraoperative versus final diagnosis – influence of clinical factors. Neurosurgery 56:257–65.

31. Roessler K, Dietrich W, Kitz K. High diagnostic accuracy of cytologic smears of central nervous system tumours. A 15-year experience based on 4,172 patients. Acta Cytol 2002;46:667–74.

32. Goel D, Sundaram C, Paul TR, et al. Intraoperative cytology (squash smear) in neurosurgical practice – pitfalls in diagnosis experience based on 3057 samples from a single institution. Cytopathology 2007;18:300–8.

33. Firlik KS, Martinez AJ, Lundsord LD. Use of cytological preparations for the intraoperative diagnosis of stereotactically obtained brain biopsies: a 19-year experience and survey of neuropathologists. J Neurosurg 1999;91:454–58.

34. Aker FV, Hakan T, Karadereler S, et al. Accuracy and diagnostic yield of stereotactic biopsy in the diagnosis of brain masses: comparison of results of biopsy and resected surgical specimens. Neuropathology 2005;25:207–13.

35. Vaquero J, Martinez R, Manrique M. Stereotactic biopsy for brain tumors: Is it always necessary?. Surg Neurol 2000;53:432–38.

36. Shastri-Hurst N, Tsegaye M, Robson DK, et al. Stereotactic brain biopsy: an audit of sampling reliability in a clinical case series. Br J Neurosurg 2006;20:222–26.

37. Joseph JT. Diagnostic Neuropathology Smears. Philadelphia: Lippincott Williams and Wilkins; 2007.

38. Moss TH, Nicoll JAR, Ironside JW. Intraoperative Diagnosis of CNS Tumours. London: Edward Arnold; 1997.

39. de Almeida SM, Nogueira MB, Raboni SM, et al. Laboratorial diagnosis of lymphocytic meningitis. Braz J Infect Dis 2007;11:489–95.

40. MacKenzie JM. Malignant meningitis: A rational approach to cerebrospinal fluid cytology. J Clin Pathol 1996;49:497–99.

41. Weatherall MW, Chatterjee KM, Tan AT, et al. Audit can reduce inappropriate requests for cytological examination of cerebrospinal fluid. Cytopathology 2004;15:119–20.

42. Bigner SH. Cerebrospinal fluid (CSF) cytology: current status and diagnostic applications. J Neuropathol Exp Neurol 1992;51:235–45.

43. Strik H, Luthe H, Nagel I, et al. Automated cerebrospinal fluid cytology: limitations and reasonable applications. Anal Quant Cytol Histol 2005;27:167–73.

44. Glantz MJ, Cole BF, Glantz LK, et al. Cerebrospinal fluid cytology in patients with cancer: minimizing false-negative results. Cancer 1998;82:733–39.

45. Chhieng DC, Elgert P, Cohen JM, et al. Cytology of primary central nervous system neoplasms in cerebrospinal fluid specimens. Diagn Cytopathol 2002;26:209–12.

46. Prayson RA, Fischler DF. Cerebrospinal fluid cytology: an 11-year experience with 5951 specimens. Arch Pathol Lab Med 1998;122:47–51.

47. Browd SR, Ragel BT, Gottfried ON, et al. Failure of cerebrospinal fluid shunts: part I: Obstruction and mechanical failure. Pediatr Neurol 2006;34:83–92.

48. Sutlas PN, Unal A, Forta H, et al. Tuberculous meningitis in adults: review of 61 cases. Infection 2003;31:387–91.

49. Kumar R. Aseptic meningitis: diagnosis and management. Indian J Pediatr 2005;72:57–63.

50. Rawal A, Gavin PJ, Sturgis CD. Cerebrospinal fluid cytology in seasonal epidemic West Nile virus meningo-encephalitis. Diagn Cytopathol 2006;34:127–29.

51. Hildebrand J, Aoun M. Chronic meningitis: still a diagnostic challenge. J Neurol 2003;250:653–60.

52. Negrini B, Kelleher KJ, Wald ER. Cerebrospinal fluid findings in aseptic versus bacterial meningitis. Pediatrics 2000;105:316–19.

53. Sato Y, Hachiya N, Kuno H, et al. Cerebrospinal fluid atypical lymphocytes in Japanese encephalitis. J Neurol Sci 1998;160:92–95.

54. Manucha V, Zhao F, Rodgers W. Atypical lymphoid cells in cerebrospinal fluid in acute Epstein Barr virus infection: a case report demonstrating a pitfall in cerebrospinal fluid cytology. Acta Cytol 2008;52:334–36.

55. Tyler KL. Herpes simplex virus infections of the central nervous system: encephalitis and meningitis, including Mollaret's. Herpes 2004;11(Suppl 2):57A–64A.

56. Chan TY, Parwani AV, Levi AW, et al. Mollaret's meningitis: cytopathologic analysis of fourteen cases. Diagn Cytopathol 2003;28:227–31.

57. Stoppe G, Stark E, Patzold U. Mollaret's meningitis: CSF-immunocytological examinations. J Neurol 1987;234:103–6.

58. Picard FJ, Dekaban GA, Silva J, et al. Mollaret's meningitis associated with herpes simplex type 2 infection. Neurology 1993;43:1722–27.

59. Katz RL, Alappattu C, Glass JP, et al. Cerebrospinal fluid manifestations of the neurologic complications of human immunodeficiency virus infection. Acta Cytol 1989;33:233–44.

60. Bicanic T, Harrison TS. Cryptococcal meningitis. Br Med Bull 2004;72:99–118.

61. Tuerlinckx D, Bodart E, Garrino MG, et al. Clinical data and cerebrospinal fluid findings in Lyme meningitis versus aseptic meningitis. Eur J Pediatr 2003;162:150–53.

62. Sherwani RK, Abrari A, Jayrajpuri ZS, et al. Intracranial hydatidosis. Report of a case diagnosed on cerebrospinal fluid cytology. Acta Cytol 2003;47:506–8.

63. Joseph FG, Scolding NJ. Sarcoidosis of the nervous system. Pract Neurol 2007;7:234–44.

64. Wingerchuk DM, Hogancamp WF, O'Brien PC, et al. The clinical course of neuromyelitis optica (Devic's syndrome). Neurology 1999;53:1107–14.

65. von Budingen HC, Harrer MD, Kuenzle S, et al. Clonally expanded plasma cells in the cerebrospinal fluid of MS patients produce myelin-specific antibodies. Eur J Immunol 2008;38:2014–23.

66. Fraussen J, Vrolix K, Martinez-Martinez P, et al. B cell characterization and reactivity analysis in multiple sclerosis. Autoimmun Rev 2009.

67. Goertsches R, Knappe S, Mix E, et al. Detection of apoptotic cells in cerebrospinal fluid of patients suffering from neurological disease. J Neuroimmunol 2007;188:175–80.

68. Vogt M, Teunissen CE, Iacobaeus E, et al. CSF anti-myelin antibodies are related to MR measures of disease activity in multiple sclerosis. J Neurol Neurosurg Psychiatry 2008.

69. Teunissen CE, Dijkstra C, Polman C. Biological markers in CSF and blood for axonal degeneration in multiple sclerosis. Lancet Neurology 2005;4:32–41.

70. Waldman A, O'Connor E, Tennekoon G. Childhood multiple sclerosis: a review. Ment Retard Dev Disabil Res Rev 2006;12:147–56.

71. Joseph FG, Lammie GA, Scolding NJ. CNS lupus: a study of 41 patients. Neurology 2007;69:644–54.

72. Joseph FG, Scolding NJ. Neuro-Behçet's disease in Caucasians: a study of 22 patients. Eur J Neurol 2007;14:174–80.

73. Kupersmith MJ, Martin V, Heller G, et al. Idiopathic hypertrophic pachymeningitis. Neurology 2004;62:686–94.

74. Kaido T, Okazaki A, Kurokawa S, et al. Pathogenesis of intraparenchymal epidermoid cyst in the brain: a case report and review of the literature. Surg Neurol 2003;59:211–16.

75. Yasumoto Y, Ito M. Asymptomatic spontaneous rupture of craniopharyngioma cyst. J Clin Neurosci 2008;15:603–6.

76. Cruickshank A, Auld P, Beetham R, et al. Revised national guidelines for analysis of cerebrospinal fluid for bilirubin in suspected subarachnoid haemorrhage. Ann Clin Biochem 2008;45:238–44.

77. Kumar N, Cohen-Gadol AA, Wright RA, et al. Superficial siderosis. Neurology 2006;66:1144–52.

78. Weller RO. How well does the CSF inform upon pathology in the brain in Creutzfeldt-Jakob and Alzheimer's diseases? J Pathol 2001;194:1–3.

79. Bian H, Van Swieten JC, Leight S, et al. CSF biomarkers in frontotemporal lobar degeneration with known pathology. Neurology 2008;70(19 Part 2):1827–35.

80. Aarsland D, Kurz M, Beyer M, et al. Early discriminatory diagnosis of dementia with Lewy bodies. The emerging role of CSF and imaging biomarkers. Dement Geriatr Cogn Disord 2008;25:195–205.

81. Gupta RK, Naran S, Lallu S, et al. Cytodiagnosis of neoplasms of the central nervous system in cerebrospinal fluid samples with an application of selective immunostains in differentiation. Cytopathology 2004;15:38–43.

82. Chamberlain MC. Neoplastic meningitis. Neurologist 2006;12:179–87.

83. van Oostenbrugge RJ, Hopman AH, Lenders MH, et al. Detection of malignant cells in cerebrospinal fluid using fluorescence in situ hybridization. J Neuropathol Exp Neurol 1997;56:743–48.

84. Jaeckle KA. Neoplastic meningitis from systemic malignancies: diagnosis, prognosis and treatment. Semin Oncol 2006;33:312–23.

85. Strik HM, Effenberger O, Schafer O, et al. A case of spinal glioblastoma multiforme: immunohistochemical study and review of the literature. J Neurooncol 2000;50:239–43.

86. Debono B, Derrey S, Rabehenoina C, et al. Primary diffuse multinodular leptomeningeal gliomatosis: case report and review of the literature. Surg Neurol 2006;65:273–82. discussion 282.

87. Poisson M, Stragliotto G, Davila G, et al. [Gliomatous meningitis of hemispheric tumors. Study of 22 cases in adults]. Rev Neurol (Paris) 1995;151:177–89.

88. Baborie A, Dunn EM, Bridges LR, et al. Primary diffuse leptomeningeal gliomatosis predominantly affecting the spinal cord: case report and review of the literature. J Neurol Neurosurg Psychiatry 2001;70:256–58.

89. Bohner G, Masuhr F, Distl R, et al. Pilocytic astrocytoma presenting as primary diffuse leptomeningeal gliomatosis: report of a unique case and review of the literature. Acta Neuropathol 2005;110:306–11.

90. Jereb B, Reid A, Ahuja RK. Patterns of failure in patients with medulloblastoma. Cancer 1982;50:2941–47.

91. Lu L, Wilkinson EJ, Yachnis AT. CSF cytology of atypical teratoid/rhabdoid tumor of the brain in a two-year-old girl: a case report. Diagn Cytopathol 2000;23:329–32.

92. Jinhu Y, Jianping D, Jun M, et al. Metastasis of a histologically benign choroid plexus papilloma: case report and review of the literature. J Neurooncol 2007;83:47–52.

93. Blakeley JO, Grossman SA. Management of pineal region tumors. Curr Treat Options Oncol 2006;7:505–16.

94. Jacques TS, Galloway MJ, Scaravilli F. Cerebrospinal fluid findings in central neurocytoma. Cytopathology 2006;17:301–3.

95. Maroldi R, Ambrosi C, Farina D. Metastatic disease of the brain: extra-axial metastases (skull, dura, leptomeningeal) and tumour spread. Eur Radiol 2005;15:617–26.

96. Glass JP, Melamed M, Chernik NL, et al. Malignant cells in cerebrospinal fluid (CSF): the meaning of a positive CSF cytology. Neurology 1979;29:1369–75.

97. Grossman SA, Krabak MJ. Leptomeningeal carcinomatosis. Cancer Treat Rev 1999;25:103–19.

98. Blaney SM, Poplack DG. Neoplastic meningitis: diagnosis and treatment considerations. Med Oncol 2000;17:151–62.

99. Chamberlain MC. Leptomeningeal metastases: a review of evaluation and treatment. J Neurooncol 1998;37:271–84.

100. DeAngelis LM, Boutros D. Leptomeningeal metastasis. Cancer Invest 2005;23:145–54.

101. Levidou G, Korkolopoulou P, Papetta A, et al. Leptomeningeal melanoma of unknown primary site: two cases with an atypical presentation of acute meningitis. Clin Neuropathol 2007;26:299–305.

102. Shenkier TN, Blay JY, O'Neill BP, et al. Primary CNS lymphoma of T-cell origin: a descriptive analysis from the international primary CNS lymphoma collaborative group. J Clin Oncol 2005;23:2233–39.

103. Nolan CP, Abrey LE. Leptomeningeal metastases from leukemias and lymphomas. Cancer Treat Res 2005;125:53–69.

104. Lachance DH, O'Neill BP, Macdonald DR, et al. Primary leptomeningeal lymphoma: report of

9 cases, diagnosis with immunocytochemical analysis, and review of the literature. Neurology 1991;41:95–100.

105. Levin N, Soffer D, Grissaru S, et al. Primary T-cell CNS lymphoma presenting with leptomeningeal spread and neurolymphomatosis. J Neurooncol 2008;90:77–83.

106. te Loo DM, Kamps WA, van der Does-van den Berg A, et al. Dutch Childhood Oncology Group. Prognostic significance of blasts in the cerebrospinal fluid without pleocytosis or a traumatic lumbar puncture in children with acute lymphoblastic leukemia: experience of the Dutch Childhood Oncology Group. J Clin Oncol, 2006;24:2332–36.

107. Desai K, Fallon MA, Willard-Smith D, et al. Improving the diagnostic accuracy of cytologic cerebrospinal fluid examinations in acute lymphoblastic leukemia using high-power microscopy and terminal deoxynucleotidyl transferase determinations. Diagn Cytopathol 1997;16:413–19.

108. Roma AA, Garcia A, Avagnina A, et al. Lymphoid and myeloid neoplasms involving cerebrospinal fluid: comparison of morphologic examination and immunophenotyping by flow cytometry. Diagn Cytopathol 2002;27:271–75.

109. Morrison C, Shah S, Flinn IW. Leptomeningeal involvement in chronic lymphocytic leukemia. Cancer Pract 1998;6:223–28.

110. Marshall AG, Pawson R, Thom M, et al. HTLV-I associated primary CNS T-cell lymphoma. J Neurol Sci 1998;158:226–31.

111. Schinstine M, Filie AC, Wilson W, et al. Detection of malignant hematopoietic cells in cerebral spinal fluid previously diagnosed as atypical or suspicious. Cancer 2006;108:157–62.

112. Bromberg JE, Breems DA, Kraan J, et al. CSF flow cytometry greatly improves diagnostic accuracy in CNS hematologic malignancies. Neurology 2007;68:1674–79.

113. Gajjar A, Fouladi M, Walter AW, et al. Comparison of lumbar and shunt cerebrospinal fluid specimens for cytologic detection of leptomeningeal disease in pediatric patients with brain tumors. J Clin Oncol 1999;17:1825–28.

114. Fouladi M, Gajjar A, Boyett JM, et al. Comparison of CSF cytology and spinal magnetic resonance imaging in the detection of leptomeningeal disease in pediatric medulloblastoma or primitive neuroectodermal tumor. J Clin Oncol 1999;17:3234–37.

115. Rogers LR, Duchesneau PM, Nunez C, et al. Comparison of cisternal and lumbar CSF examination in leptomeningeal metastasis. Neurology 1992;42:1239–41.

116. Wasserstrom WR, Glass JP, Posner JB. Diagnosis and treatment of leptomeningeal metastases from solid tumors: experience with 90 patients. Cancer 1982;49:759–72.

117. Fischer L, Jahnke K, Martus P, et al. The diagnostic value of cerebrospinal fluid pleocytosis and protein in the detection of lymphomatous meningitis in primary central nervous system lymphomas. Haematologica 2006;91:429–30.

118. Oschmann P, Kaps M, Volker J, et al. Meningeal carcinomatosis: CSF cytology, immunocytochemistry and biochemical tumor markers. Acta Neurol Scand 1994;89:395–99.

119. Olson ME, Chernik NL, Posner JB. Infiltration of the leptomeninges by systemic cancer. A clinical and pathologic study. Arch Neurol 1974;30:122–37.

120. Sadagopal S, Lorey SL, Barnett L, et al. Enhancement of human immunodeficiency virus (HIV)-specific CD8+ T cells in cerebrospinal fluid compared to those in blood among antiretroviral therapy-naive HIV-positive subjects. J Virol 2008;82(21):10418–28.

# Eyelids, orbit and eye

Pio Zeppa and Lucio Palombini

## Chapter contents

## Introduction

The eyelids, orbit and eye probably represent one of the most complex and difficult anatomical regions to investigate, and one where cytopathologists are rarely requested to make a diagnosis. In fact, non-invasive diagnostic procedures such as optical coherence tomography (OCT) or A/B scan ultrasonography have significantly reduced the need to examine tissues or cells.[1] This is mainly the case for the ocular globe and some of the orbital masses. Complexity and difficulties arise also from other factors: indeed, despite the anatomical unity (Fig. 32.1), every component of this region presents its own peculiarities in terms of anatomy, variety of pathologies, diagnostic requests and technical approaches to obtain cytological samples. Moreover,

anatomical and clinical peculiarities require close cooperation between ophthalmologists and cytopathologists. The sampling is usually, but not exclusively, the task of ophthalmologists. The role of the cytopathologist is to manage the diagnostic material, evaluate the adequacy, including the choice of ancillary techniques, and make the final diagnosis. Cytopathologists may deal with scanty cellular samples from different and sometimes complex or rare pathologies. The samples may range from exfoliative cytology for conjunctival smears, to cytology of fluids for aqueous paracentesis and fine needle aspiration (FNA) for choroid or orbital masses. Finally, ancillary techniques, such as immunocytochemistry (ICC),[2] flow cytometry (FC)[3] fluorescence *in situ* hybridisation (FISH)[4] and molecular techniques[5,6] may be applied. The only advantage for ophthalmic cytopathologists is the existence of excellent books in this field[7–9] including the previous edition of this book.

This chapter will summarise the anatomy of the eye, eyelid and orbit and try to focus on its relationship with sampling methods. The cytopathological features of the different pathological entities in each anatomical region will then be described.

## Eyelids

### Skin

The eyelids are lined by the skin externally and the conjunctiva on the inner surface. Eyelid skin, its cytological sampling and microscopic examination are similar to those of other sites. Scraping is the most commonly used technique for cytological diagnosis and may be performed by skilful cytopathologists, whereas lesions of the canthus or the rim should be performed by ophthalmologists. Scrapings may be performed without anaesthesia using a small platinum spatula (Swedish Dissector) or the blunt side of a scalpel blade. When suspected lesions are not ulcerated, it may be necessary to lift or remove the external epidermal layer covering the lesion. This can be achieved by using the sharp edge of a scalpel blade to gently cut the superficial layer of the epidermis and allow the scraping of the deeper one. FNA has also been used to diagnose eyelid masses.[10] Smears are prepared as previously described and may be fixed in alcohol and stained by the Papanicolaou method or air-dried and stained with May-Grünwald Giemsa (MGG) or Diff-Quik. As in other regions, MGG or Diff-Quik staining are generally preferable for the demonstration of bacteria and to diagnose lymphoid and mesenchymal tumours, while the Papanicolaou (PAP) method is preferable for epithelial or melanocytic tumours.

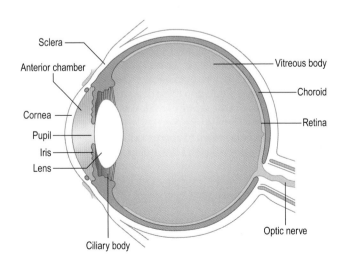

Sclera

Anterior chamber

Cornea

Pupil

Iris

Lens

Ciliary body

Vitreous body

Choroid

Retina

Optic nerve

**Fig. 32.1** Diagram representing the main parts of the eye.

*The authors would like to thank Dr R Aricò, Dr I Cozzolino, Professor G. Troncone, Professor A. Vetrani, Dr L. Zeppa and Dr M. Zeppa for their support and suggestions, and to dedicate the chapter to Dr Rosario Zeppa, ophthalmologist, master of life and culture.*

## Squamous papillomas

Squamous papillomas are the most frequent benign tumours of the eyelid. They may be sessile or pedunculated and are composed of finger-like projections of acanthotic and parakeratotic epithelium arising from a fibro-vascular stalk. Cells may show atypical nuclei with koilocytotic modifications, as observed in HPV infections.

## Benign adnexal tumours

The cytological features of adnexal tumours are described in Chapter 28. Eyelid hidroadenomas[11] and eccrine poromas[12] diagnosed by FNA have been reported. Strangely enough, the cytological features of sebaceous adenoma, which represents the most frequent adnexal tumour of this area, have not been described.

## Basal cell carcinoma

Basal cell carcinoma (BCC) is the most frequent malignant tumour of the eyelid. It arises as a single lesion after prolonged exposure to sunlight or as multiple lesions in patients with xeroderma pigmentosum. The clinical presentation of BCC may be nodular and/or ulcerative or sclerosing (morphea type). BCCs rarely metastasise, but grow slowly, eroding surrounding tissues, proximal structures and even the globe. Timely diagnosis and treatment are therefore mandatory because a large BCC may present surgical problems as far as excision and plastic reconstruction are concerned; conversely, small lesions may be conveniently treated by cryotherapy, photodynamic therapy or pharmacologically (imiquimod, fluorouracil). Adequate scraping has to reach the dermis; prompt or disproportionate bleeding may suggest the presence of a tumour. Smears (Fig. 32.2) generally show the following:

### Cytological findings: basal cell carcinoma

- Dense compact overlapping cell groups
- Cytological details observable only at the edges of fragments

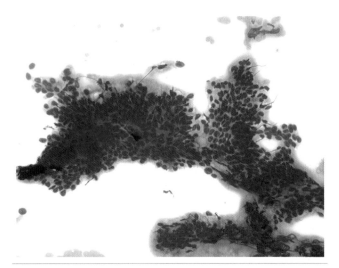

**Fig. 32.2** Basal cell carcinoma of the eyelid. Scraping cytology sample shows dense groups of small basal cells; note the nuclear cohesion, the hyperchromasia and the partial peripheral palisading arrangement of the nuclei (Diff-Quik).

- Nuclei at times organised in regular lines perpendicular to the group, producing a 'palisading' pattern
- Presence of isolated cells
- Poorly differentiated cells with scanty cytoplasm and oval nuclei
- Nuclei with dense, compact, chromatin without nucleoli
- Scanty mitoses if any at all.

In some cases, macrophages containing haemosiderin or melanin are distributed across the background, representing the cytological aspect of 'pigmented' BCC. In others, some nuclei are larger, with coarse chromatin and evident nucleoli, the cytoplasm is larger, denser than usual and stains orange with the Papanicolaou stain. In these cases, the differential diagnosis includes Bowen disease and squamous-cell carcinoma. It would be wise to remember that the eyelids, as other areas exposed to sunlight, have a high incidence of precancerous lesions, squamous cell carcinomas and melanomas. As the cytological diagnosis of BCC is often requested when non-surgical treatment is being considered, cytopathologists should be aware that these lesions might be destroyed *in situ*. It would therefore be wise to reach a definite cytological diagnosis only when all cytological criteria are fulfilled and to request repetition or suggest surgical biopsy in any scanty cellular, unclear or doubtful case.

## Squamous cell carcinoma

Squamous cell carcinoma is less frequent than BCC. Scraping samples are better observed with Papanicolaou-stained smears.

### Cytological findings: squamous cell carcinoma

- Cell dissociation
- Nuclear polymorphism and squamous cytoplasmic differentiation
- Cytological pattern varying according to cellular differentiation, ranging from extremely well differentiated to anaplastic.

When almost all cells show indirect signs of parakeratosis, such as wide and extremely keratinising cytoplasm with retention of small pyknotic nuclei, mainly in clinically suspected carcinomas, the cytological diagnosis should be delayed if the smear lacks cells representative of a possible underlying lesion. A variable number of neutrophils may also be present in the smears, depending on the presence of necrosis. Inflammatory infiltrate may also characterise non-tumoural ulcerated lesions in which scraping may be requested. In these cases it is advisable to scrape the edges instead of the centre of the lesion. It may also be useful to remember that benign ulcerated lesions are generally more painful than tumours when scraped, produce less cellular smears and obviously yield cells with a lesser degree of atypia.

## Malignant melanoma

Malignant melanomas are less frequent than squamous cell carcinomas and their cytological diagnosis is requested less frequently. Cytological features and diagnostic criteria of melanoma are reported in Chapter 28. Pigmentation of the eyelid margins, occurring in association with conjunctival melanoma, is an ominous clinical sign.

## Sebaceous carcinoma

Sebaceous carcinomas are found almost exclusively in eyelid skin and arise from the meibomian or other local sebaceous glands, more frequently on the upper eyelid. They appear clinically as firm subcutaneous nodules resembling a chalazion or other lesions, thus delaying the diagnosis and resulting in relatively high morbidity and mortality. Sometimes the tumour growth results in a pagetoid or carcinoma *in situ*-like involvement of the conjunctiva causing persisting unilateral conjunctivitis before the correct diagnosis is made. The tumour has a lobular pattern and is formed by cells with variable sebaceous differentiation depending on their grade of differentiation. Sebaceous carcinomas may involve adjacent structures or metastasise to cervical or preauricular lymph nodes. FNA shows hyperchromatic nuclei, prominent nucleoli and abundant cytoplasm which contains small fat vacuoles.[13] FNA of lymph node metastases from sebaceous carcinomas has also been described.[14]

## Conjunctiva

### Histology

Conjunctival epithelium is a stratified non-keratinising epithelium formed by cuboid-columnar cells and containing mucus-producing goblet cells (Fig. 32.3). These cells, together with lachrymal and meibomian glands, maintain hydration and lubrication of the cornea and conjunctiva by producing the tear film. Conjunctival epithelium starts from the eyelid rim, lines the inner eyelid layer, turns at the bottom and continues covering the sclera up to the limbus where the cornea merges with the sclera. The limbus is an important clinical area as it is the point of insertion of the needle for anterior chamber paracentesis. Cytological samples may be obtained by scraping, brushing or imprint cytology.

Conjunctival scraping requires local anaesthesia and should be performed by trained ophthalmologists. Conjunctival brush may also be used under local anaesthesia using a small cytobrush (Cytobrush- S, Medscand, Malmo, Sweden).[15] Imprint cytology of the conjunctiva can be performed by placing cellulose acetate strips on the surface of the conjunctiva or the cornea and pressing gently.[16] The strip is then removed, fixed in absolute ethanol or glacial acetic acid and stained using PAS/Papanicolaou stain.[16] More recently, Biopore membranes have been used[17–19] and specific training in interpreting the corresponding samples has been suggested.[20]

## Conjunctival inflammatory lesions

Allergic and vernal conjunctivitis are quite common and characterised by a prevalence of eosinophils in the inflammatory infiltrate. Bacterial and viral infections are generally diagnosed on the basis of the clinical presentation or sometimes by microbiology. Nonetheless, cytological features may be helpful for a presumptive diagnosis, mainly in clinically unexpected cases. Infections by *Verruca vulgaris*, measles and herpes may be suggested by specific cytological features as described in Chapter 21. Exhaustive descriptions of the cytological features of the most frequent viral infections are available in the literature.[7–9,21] Trachoma is a 'historical' bacterial conjunctival infection caused by *Chlamydia trachomatis*; it has almost disappeared but may still be a cause of blindness in underdeveloped countries. The cytological features are almost the same as those described in the female genital tract and are characterised by cytoplasmic basophilic inclusions with halos (Fig. 32.4). Cytological features of *Candida*, *Aspergillus*, mucormycosis and phycomycetes conjunctivitis have also been described;[7–9] diagnosis and treatment must be timely and effective because of the risk of corneal damage.

## Conjunctival epithelial tumours

Benign epithelial tumours are principally represented by papillomas, which are composed of a fibrovascular stalk covered by acanthotic squamous epithelium. Cytological diagnosis is rarely requested; papillomas often recur after surgical excision.

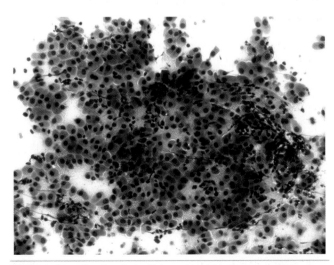

**Fig. 32.3** Normal conjunctival cells in conjunctivitis. Scrape cytology sample showing loosely attached conjunctival cells with wide and well defined cytoplasm. Crashed granulocytes are interspersed among the cells (Diff-Quik).

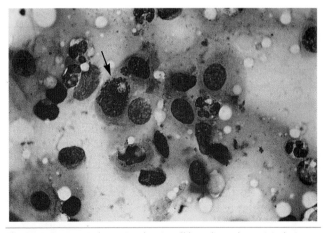

**Fig. 32.4** Conjunctival scraping showing *Chlamydia trachomatis* inclusion bodies forming a dark granular cluster in the cytoplasm, partly surrounding the nucleus (arrow) (MGG).

Malignant conjunctival tumours are principally represented by squamous cell carcinoma and its precursors; the term ocular surface squamous neoplasia (OSSN) is generally used to describe a spectrum of lesions, ranging from mild dysplasia to carcinoma *in situ*, which may arise on the conjunctiva and cornea. Carcinogenetic factors are mainly represented by human papillomavirus types 16 and 18, which have been detected in many of these lesions by PCR. Exposure to ultraviolet light or mustard gas, as observed in exposed soldiers,[22] may induce squamous cell carcinoma or precancerous lesions; conjunctival and corneal carcinomas are also more frequent among patients with acquired immune deficiency syndrome (AIDS).[7,8] Squamous cell carcinomas are often observed on the bulbar conjunctiva, mostly at the limbus, and the clinical presentation is not always clear. Pre-invasive lesions show increased vascularity and thickening of the epithelium, which may be initially misdiagnosed as inflammatory or degenerative processes. Sometimes they may be present without any clinical evidence[20] or appear as gelatinous and ill-defined lesions. Smears show immature cells with increased nucleus/cytoplasm ratio; the nuclei are enlarged and hyperchromatic with irregular contours, coarse chromatin and prominent nucleoli. Many high-grade lesions and some invasive carcinomas may show superficial keratinisation, which makes the cytological diagnosis more difficult (Fig. 32.5), mainly on Biopore membrane samples.[17,19] Therefore, the presence of hyperkeratotic cells and a few dysplastic cells may suggest intramucosal high-grade lesion or squamous cell carcinoma. The differential diagnosis must include conjunctival squamous metaplasia (abundant cytoplasm, reduced nuclear/cytoplasmic ratio, pyknotic nuclei) and parakeratosis (dyskeratotic cells and keratohyaline granules). A relatively high correlation between cytology and the corresponding histological diagnoses has been found, while the greatest probability of false negatives is in keratinising squamous cell carcinoma.[16,20]

## Conjunctival lymphoma

Lymphomas may arise from conjunctiva-associated lymphoid tissue (CALT); cytopathological features are similar to those of other mucosa-associated lymphomas (MALT) (see Chs 5, 14).

*Chlamydia psittaci* has recently been associated with ocular adnexal lymphomas.

## Conjunctival melanocytic tumours

Melanocytic naevi of the conjunctiva are classified in almost the same way as those of the skin, i.e. as junctional, sub-epithelial and compound. Microscopically they are formed by pigmented polygonal cells and are more cellular than their epidermal counterparts. Conjunctival naevi may increase in size, as may occur in puberty, or change shape, as in the case of 'irritated' naevi or in malignant transformation. Primary acquired melanosis (PAM) may be considered as the conjunctival counterpart of cutaneous Hutchinson lentigo. The histological features of PAM are quite variable even within the same lesion, and range from small monomorphous melanocytes, which line the basal layer, to atypical nucleolated epithelioid cells. Pagetoid infiltration of the epithelium is indicative of malignant transformation in most cases. Malignant melanomas may arise de novo or by transformation of pre-existing naevi (Fig. 32.6) or acquired melanosis.

### Cytological findings: conjunctival melanoma[23]

- Dispersed tumour cells with eccentric nuclei
- Coarsely granular chromatin and prominent nucleoli
- Occasional or prominent cytoplasmic melanic granules
- Occasional spindle-shaped cells.

Imprint cytology and Biopore membrane have given excellent diagnostic results, predicting the histological diagnosis by detection of superficial atypical melanocytes and their proportion relative to the conjunctival cells (Fig. 32.7).[24]

## Cornea

The cornea represents the transparent anterior part of the globe. It is lined with stratified, non-keratinised squamous epithelium and continues into the sclera at the limbus, where epithelial stem cells proliferate centripetally in a vortex-like fashion, pushing mature and more transparent cells toward the centre.

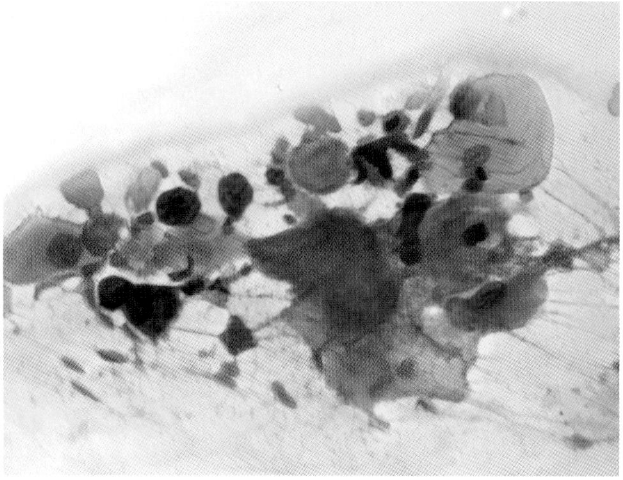

**Fig. 32.5** Ocular surface squamous neoplasia. Conjunctival scraping cytology showing isolated malignant nuclei interspersed among superficial keratinising cells (PAP).

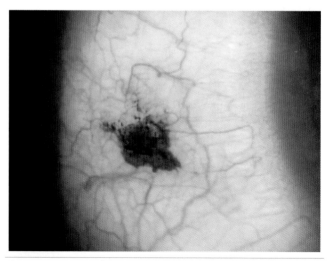

**Fig. 32.6** Superficial melanoma of the scleral conjunctiva showing dyschromia and irregular borders. (Courtesy of Dr L Zeppa, Benevento, IT.)

Normal corneal cells strongly resemble the intermediate squamous cell of the female genital tract. Corneal inflammation is generally diagnosed and treated on the basis of the clinical presentation. Cytology has been used to diagnose unusual clinical presentations or rare infections such as actinomycosis, blastomycosis or acanthamoebic keratitis,[8,9] especially when the organisms are superficial. Corneal neoplasia is represented by OSSN as reported in the conjunctiva.

## Ocular globe

### Anatomy of the globe

The globe is divided into two segments: the anterior segment, which comprises the anterior and posterior chambers, and the posterior segment, containing the vitreous (humor vitreous), called the vitreal chamber.

The wall of the globe consists of three concentric layers: the external layer is the sclera, composed of scantily vascular collagen tissue, which in the anterior part of the globe, at the limbus, is in continuity with the cornea. An important anatomical point of the sclera is the pars plana, which is located at 3–4 mm from the limbus and is the point of insertion of needles for vitrectomy or FNA of the vitreal chamber. The intermediate layer is the uvea, formed by the choroid, which surrounds the whole posterior chamber and is in continuity anteriorly with the ciliary body and iris. The choroid is composed of a pigmented fibrous stroma containing dendritic melanocytes and fenestrated vessels which supply the retinal pigmented epithelium. The retina has an inner layer, the neuroretina, which consists of complex multilayered neuronal tissue, and an outer layer, the retinal pigment epithelium (RPE), which maintains the neuroretina and extends anteriorly into the pigmented epithelium of the iris. The crystalline lens, which separates the two segments of the eye, consists of a single layer of epithelium, a basal membrane and a collagenous nucleus. Interposed between the crystalline lens and the sclera are the ciliary muscles and suspensory ligaments, which regulate the accommodative movements of the crystalline lens.

### Ocular FNA

The cytological diagnosis of intraocular pathology is rather complex both because of sampling and interpretation problems. FNA of the ocular globe was first introduced in the fifties and was successfully used to diagnose different tumours.[8] Because of reported complications such as bleeding and seeding of malignant cells, ocular and anterior segment FNA were almost abandoned. However, in the last few years the accurate identification of ever smaller lesions, mainly choroidal melanomas, and the development of localised therapeutic procedures has allowed a conservative approach to tumour treatment. FNA again represents an attractive tool for obtaining material useful for diagnosis and prognosis. Further improvements in FNA technique and the use of thinner needles (27–30G) have reduced the risk of complications and raised the credibility of ocular FNA. FNA is used also in this case, mainly for collecting cells from choroidal melanomas for cytogenetic evaluations using FISH (Fig. 32.8) and high-density genome array or microsatellite assay (see Ch. 34).[4–6,25]

Ocular FNA is a complex procedure which must be performed by a qualified ophthalmologist. Retrobulbar or peribulbar anaesthesia is required and the procedure is performed at the slit lamp or under operating microscope guidance. Needles of 30 or 27 G are inserted via the limbus to sample the anterior segment and via the pars plana, at 3–4 mm posterior to the limbus, to sample the vitreal chamber. The needles may be connected to an automatic aspiration system to allow the ophthalmologist to place and move them with both hands. In order to make the wound self-healing, the needle is inserted with a slight cut in the sclera and pressure is applied after its withdrawal. If these precautions are taken, FNA is safe and the above-mentioned complications are extremely rare or absent.[5]

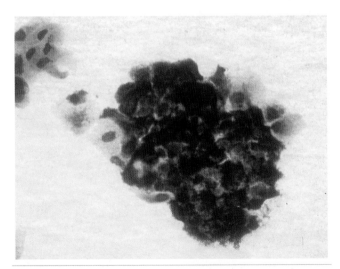

**Fig. 32.7** Conjunctival melanoma. Biopore membrane sample showing numerous hyperpigmented melanoma cells and few conjunctival cells in the upper left corner. Atypical nuclei are recognisable only in the lower right part of the group because of the abundance of melanin (MGG). (Courtesy of Dr S Keijser, Leiden, NL.)

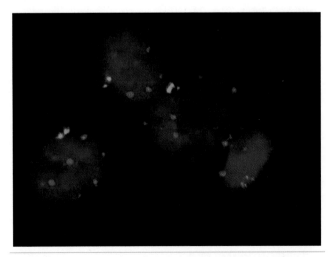

**Fig. 32.8** FISH on nuclei of uveal melanoma obtained by FNA. Nuclei are hybridised with probes for centromere 3 (green) and centromere 8 (red). Note the presence of one copy of chromosome 3 (split spot) and chromosome 8 again in three cells. (Courtesy of Dr A de Klein, Rotterdam, NL.)

## Anterior segment

### Inflammations

FNA of the anterior chamber has been mainly used for paracentesis and microbiological diagnosis of ocular infections (endophthalmitis). Bacterial endophthalmitis may be a post-surgical complication and is characterised by an inflammatory infiltrate including mono and multinucleated histiocytes and lymphocytes. In HIV patients, infections from rare and/or opportunistic agents such as aspergillosis and coccidiomycosis have become more common.[7,8] An aseptic inflammatory response may rarely be the result of the phacotoxic response to the release of lens proteins; more frequently the cause is surgical or prosthetic material such as silicon oil or artificial crystalline constituents. A granulomatous inflammation with macrophages and foreign body giant cells may be caused by phacoanaphylaxis, in which an inflammatory infiltrate and fragments of the lens may be observed in FNA samples. It is clinically important to differentiate phacoanaphylaxis from bacterial endophthalmitis because the latter requires prompt antibiotic therapy.

### Tumours

Tumours of the anterior segment are rather rare and are represented by melanocytic tumours of the iris, tumours of the posterior segment extending into the anterior segment, and metastases.

Melanocytic lesions of the iris include a spectrum of lesions ranging from naevi to aggressive naevi and melanomas. Both clinical and pathological diagnosis may be quite complex. Amelanotic naevi may be misdiagnosed as melanomas and aggressive naevi may grow and occlude the angle causing glaucoma. A case of melanocytoma of the ciliary body diagnosed by FNA has been reported;[26] the cytopathological features of the melanocytoma are summarised in the paragraph dealing with the choroid.

### Melanoma

Melanomas are by far the most common primary tumours of the iris. As with all uveal melanomas, they are classified as epithelioid, spindle or mixed cell type.

#### Cytological findings: melanoma

- Dispersed epithelioid cells with large, polygonal, dense, well-defined cytoplasm and one or more eccentrically located nuclei, with coarse chromatin and large nucleoli. A variable number of intranuclear cytoplasmic inclusions may be present. Melanic pigment may be present in the cytoplasm of tumoural cells as well as that of macrophages
- Spindle cell type with oval or even spindle nuclei and bipolar cytoplasmic processes. Spindle cell melanomas generally show a less dispersed pattern and are more monomorphous than the epithelioid variant.

One report claims that it is possible to distinguish cytologically aggressive iris naevi from melanomas or metastatic carcinoma,[27] but this differential diagnosis can be extremely difficult even in histological sections.

### Metastases

Metastatic tumours occur less frequently in the anterior chamber than in the posterior chamber; breast, lung and prostate are the most frequent primary tumours. Identification of primary tumours on FNA samples may be difficult or impossible and immunocytochemistry (ICC) can be applied to determine the possible source of the tumour. Tumours of the posterior chamber, such as retinoblastoma and melanoma, may extend into the anterior chamber and FNA of the anterior chamber has been used for their diagnosis.[7,8] Cytological features of a solitary extramedullary plasmacytoma arising in the ciliary body have been described.[28] FNA has also been used to diagnose ectopic lachrymal gland tissue of the iris[29] and corresponding tumours such as pigmented pleomorphic adenoma of the ciliary body.

## Posterior segment

### FNA of the posterior segment

Posterior segment pathologies may be investigated cytologically either by using FNA or cytological examination of vitrectomy samples.[30] Posterior segment FNA was first considered as a diagnostic tool in the seventies when pars plana vitrectomy was described.[7] This technique was first assessed for therapeutic purposes, i.e. the removal of non-resorbed vitreous haemorrhages, fibrous strands or membranes which mainly represent complications of diabetes mellitus. Vitrectomy has since also been used diagnostically; in fact vitrectomy samples may be used for microbiological or cytological examination. Microbiological diagnosis of calcofluor white staining and subsequent immunofluorescent microscopy (Fig. 32.9) may be used in the differential diagnosis of an inflammatory vitreitis. The technical details of ocular FNA have been described earlier; although some studies have reported excellent results in terms of diagnostic accuracy and safety,[5,31] FNA has not been extensively used for the diagnosis of retinal and choroidal tumours. Again, this is due to the fear of complications, but also because of the development of highly sensitive and very accurate non-invasive diagnostic tools. At the same time, the identification

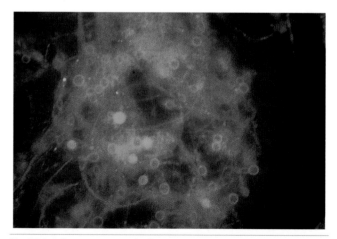

**Fig. 32.9** Infective vitreitis. Calcofluor white immunofluorescent demonstration of spores and filaments of *Candida albicans* obtained by vitrectomy with cytocentrifugation.

of increasingly smaller tumours and the possibility to manage them with conservative therapeutic measures such as plaque radiotherapy or transpupillary thermotherapy has reduced the need for enucleation and hence the possibility of histological confirmation and of studying prognostic factors. FNA has therefore been utilised once more for cytological diagnosis[5,6,32] and to perform genetic assessment using FISH or DNA amplification and microsatellite assay (see Ch. 34).[4,25]

## Retinoblastoma

Retinoblastoma is the most common ocular tumour of childhood. A highly malignant tumour, it arises in the retina and may be unilateral or bilateral; white pupil (leukoria) is the most common clinical sign. Retinoblastoma is genetically determined by the loss of both alleles of the tumour suppressor (Rb) gene on the long arm of chromosome 13. Thanks to timely diagnoses and appropriate therapeutic procedures, retinoblastoma, previously a fatal disease, has become curable in many cases. Bilaterality, optic nerve involvement and invasion of surrounding tissues are the only features significantly associated with an unfavourable prognosis. Microscopically, retinoblastoma is an undifferentiated neuroectodermal tumour; Flexner–Wintersteiner rosettes lined by tall cells with basal nuclei and cytoplasmic fibrillary processes orientated towards the lumen are a classical feature. The cytological characteristics (Fig. 32.10) are those of an undifferentiated small round cell tumour of infancy (see Ch. 33).[1,33]

### Cytological findings: retinoblastoma

- Small undifferentiated cells
- Basophilic nuclei and scanty or absent cytoplasm.

FNA of tumours that have invaded the anterior chamber is generally not used because of the risk of spreading, whereas retinoblastoma cells may be obtained from the anterior chamber tap. ICC positivity for neurogenic markers such as neuron-specific enolase (NSE) may confirm the neurogenic histogenesis, whereas the neoplasia is cytologically indistinguishable from neuroblastoma. Cytology of cerebrospinal fluid may also have a role in preoperative staging and postoperative treatment, because it may be involved in cases of retinoblastoma (see Ch. 31).

## Melanoma

Choroidal melanoma is the most common primary intraocular malignant tumour (Fig. 32.11). It arises most frequently in the choroid, and a visual deficit is its usual clinical manifestation. The incidence of choroidal melanoma is higher in blue-eyed blond individuals with prevalence in adult males and the Caucasian race. Several cytogenetic changes have been described, with chromosome 8 polysomy and chromosome 3 monosomy being the most frequent and having prognostic significance in terms of survival.[5]

Melanomas are classified as epithelioid (Fig. 32.12), spindle-cell and mixed type; the cytological features have been reported earlier. Prognostic factors are classically represented by tumour size, vascular pattern, levels of infiltration and histological pattern. It has been proven that monosomy of chromosome 3 and the presence of additional copies of chromosome 8 correlate with reduced survival; these chromosomal anomalies may be

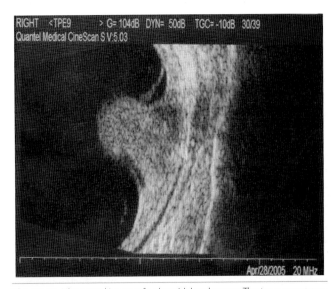

**Fig. 32.11** Ultrasound image of a choroidal melanoma. The tumour appears as a nodular lesion protruding in the vitreal chamber. The hypo-echoic area beneath the tumour indicates scleral infiltration. (Courtesy of Dr L Zeppa, Benevento, IT.)

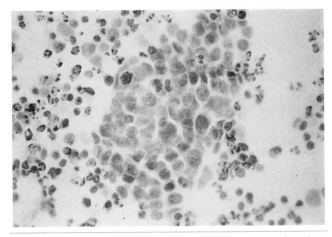

**Fig. 32.10** Retinoblastoma. Undifferentiated primitive neuroectodermal cells from anterior chamber tap. Inflammatory cells may also be seen (PAP).

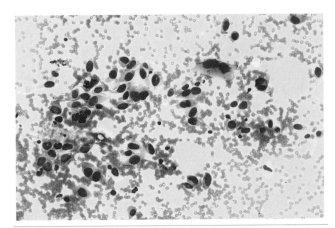

**Fig. 32.12** Choroidal melanoma. FNA trans pars plana showing atypical dispersed cells with elongated cytoplasm. Note a binucleate cell (Diff-Quik).

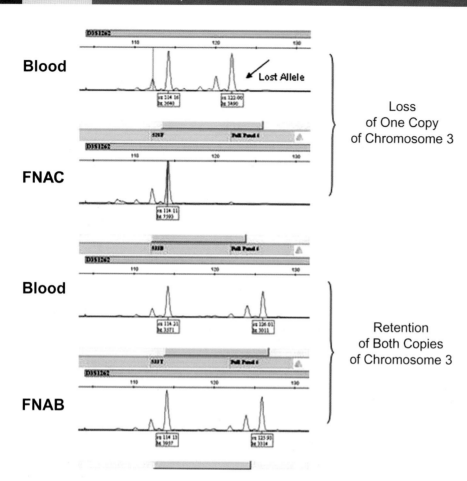

**Blood**

Lost Allele

**FNAC**

Loss
of One Copy
of Chromosome 3

**Blood**

Retention
of Both Copies
of Chromosome 3

**FNAB**

**Fig. 32.13** Microsatellite assay displaying two different samples. The top sample shows blood results (normal lymphocytes DNA) with both the copies of chromosome 3 and FNA of choroidal melanoma showing loss of 1 copy (monosomy 3). The bottom sample shows both the copies of chromosome 3 in the lymphocytes and in a choroidal melanoma (disomy 3). (Courtesy of Dr CL Shields, Philadelphia, USA.)

demonstrated using the microsatellite assay technique on fine-needle cytology samples (Fig. 32.13) (see Ch. 34).

## Melanocytoma

Melanocytoma is a rare pigmented tumour which may arise along the spinal neuraxis in association with nerve roots. The tumour is well-circumscribed, brown or black and composed microscopically of spindle cells organised in fascicles or whorls; nuclei are round-oval with prominent eosinophilic nucleoli. A melanocytoma arising near the optic nerve and with cytological features similar to those previously reported[29] has been described in vitrectomy cytology.[34]

## Astrocytoma

Retinal gliomas are extremely rare and almost exclusively represented by juvenile pilocytic astrocytoma. This tumour generally arises in the proximal part of the optic nerve, may be congenital and develops slowly through childhood. There is a slight female predominance. Neurofibromatosis type 1 patients represent half of the cases, although neurofibromatosis is often diagnosed after pilocytic astrocytoma. Loss of vision is the main clinical sign which differentiates pilocytic astrocytoma from meningioma involving the optic nerve; differential diagnosis includes retinoblastoma when the tumour grows in the anterior chamber. The cytological features of vitreus seeding from retinal

pilocytic astrocytoma have been described as showing astrocytic cells with a typical 'stringy' configuration (see Ch. 31).[35]

## Lymphoma

Intraocular lymphoma may be considered as two different diseases: primary intraocular lymphoma (PIOL) and intraocular manifestation of systemic lymphoma.

PIOL is a large B-cell lymphoma, often bilateral, which primarily involves the retina and vitreous and has a poor prognosis.[3] It is generally characterised by necrosis and highly aggressive behaviour, with frequent intracerebral and CNS involvement. Correct diagnosis is often delayed because of atypical presentations mimicking vasculitis or viral retinitis and may require multiple sampling as vitrectomy, vitreal aspiration and cytological examination of the CNS before the diagnosis can be confirmed and treatment (orbital radiotherapy and corticosteroids) begun. Cytological diagnosis may be hampered by scant cellularity, polymorphous presentation and difficulties in applying ancillary techniques.

Cytological features of intraocular lymphoma are similar to those of high-grade lymphomas described elsewhere (see Chs 13, 14). Immunocytochemistry, such as CD20 and CD45RO can be useful to demonstrate the lymphoid nature of malignant cells (Fig. 32.14).[36] More recently, flow cytometry (FC) evaluation of cell suspension and polymerase chain reaction (PCR) applied to FNA samples have also obtained excellent results. This is an important achievement because timely diagnosis and

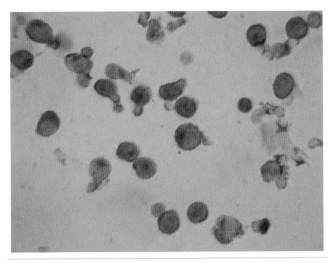

**Fig. 32.14** Primary intraocular lymphoma. Cytospin of a vitrectomy specimen showing isolated large lymphoid cells immunostained for CD20 (L26).

treatment can prevent or reduce the risk of CNS involvement. Systemic lymphomas may involve the eye, the uvea being the most frequent site of involvement; they are generally unilateral and show less aggressive biological behaviour than PIOL. Diagnosis may be made from cytological samples;[3,30,36] further cytological details are reported in Chapters 13 and 14.

## Metastases

Ocular metastases are more common in the posterior chamber than in the orbit and anterior chamber. The most frequent primary tumours are breast carcinoma in women and lung and prostate carcinomas in men. When the primary tumour is unknown, ICC may be used on smears or cell blocks. Metastases from adenoid cystic carcinoma of the lung,[37] mucinous adenocarcinoma of the ovary,[38] follicular thyroid carcinoma[39] and carcinoid tumours[40] have been reported.

## Orbit

### Anatomy and FNA

The orbit is a bony cavity with medial and lateral walls, roof and floor, which contains the globe, the lachrymal glands in the upper lateral parts and fibrous and fatty tissue in the posterior cone. The orbit also contains the orbital muscles, branches of the cranial nerves, a small number of lymphocytes and vessels. Although the globe is strongly protected by the bony consistency of the orbit, intracranial expansive processes or masses of the sinuses may invade the orbital cavity by passing through the foramen caecum or interrupting the thin bony laminae which divide the sphenoidal sinuses from the orbit medially. In addition, inflammatory processes of the maxillary sinus, even caused from dental implants, can permeate the orbital floor. Orbital masses may cause eyelid ptosis, purulent secretions, dysfunction of ocular mobility, diplopia and proptosis such as in Graves' disease. They may be sampled by FNA using 21–23 G needles under US or CT-guidance or without guidance by a skilled orbital ophthalmologist. The approach may be

transcutaneous at the base of the eyelid. The ophthalmologist places a finger on the globe, exerts light pressure downwards or upwards with the fingertip and inserts the needle parallel to the nail through the eyelid skin. In this way the roof, floor and upper lateral area may be reached and sufficiently large masses may be easily aspirated. The inadequacy rate and possible complications such as haemorrhage represent the main disadvantage of the procedure. Considering the limited possibility of movement of the needle in this area and the fibrous matrix which is a feature of many orbital expansive processes, a larger needle could increase the cell yield but also the risk of complications. In our experience, aspiration is definitively more effective than capillary cytology. A 23G needle is thin enough to reduce possible complications and large enough to collect cells.

## Benign, non-neoplastic lesions and inflammatory processes

Infections caused by bacteria, fungi and other organisms may cause inflammatory lesions which rarely need cytological diagnosis. Aspiration may produce quite non-specific granulocyte-rich smears and necrotic tissue fragments. Orbital aspergillosis, cryptococcosis and cysticercosis have been described cytologically.[41] Granulomatous lesions (tuberculosis or sarcoidosis) may also occur; their cytological patterns are indistinguishable and do not differ from that seen at other sites.[42–44] Granulomatous (Wegener) vasculitis lesions may occur and reactive granulomatous infiltrates may be caused by the rupture of dermoid cysts or other foreign bodies.[45] Orbital involvement by Langerhans cell histiocytosis[46] or sinus histiocytosis with massive lymphadenopathy (SHML)[47] have also been reported. The presence of histiocytes exhibiting emperipolesis is the key element suggesting a diagnosis of SHMH.

## Benign tumours and tumour-like lesions

Cysts are represented by mucocele, dermoid cysts and the very rare 'enterogenous type' of cyst because of its high content of carcinoembryonic epithelial antigen (CEA). A mucocele is a mucoid or debris-filled cyst lined by mucous producing cells, which may arise from the lachrymal glands and the lachrymal sac or even as a result of chronic inflammation of the ethmoid sinus which may erode the wall expanding into the orbit. As with its salivary counterpart, the aspiration of mucoid material and bland mucus-producing cells may represent either a mucocele or a well-differentiated, low-grade mucoepidermoid carcinoma. In these cases, a diagnosis in which both possibilities are proposed should be considered.

Orbital encapsulated cystic lesions such as dermoid cysts generally require surgical treatment therefore FNA is rarely requested. FNA may show squamous cells or just debris. Papanicolaou stain may be helpful recognising the presence of keratin. Because of the risk of leakage with consequent foreign body reaction, the use of thin needles is recommended.

## Benign tumours of the lachrymal gland

These tumours are almost exclusively represented by pleomorphic adenoma, in which the cytological presentation and diagnostic problems are the same as those of their salivary gland counterparts (see Ch. 5).[41,43,48]

## Meningioma

Meningiomas of the orbit may arise from the meningoendothelial cells which envelop the intraorbital tract of the optic nerve or present as an orbital extension of intracranial meningiomas.[7,43,49]

### Cytological findings: meningioma

- Cells in clusters or whorls
- Polygonal or spindle-shaped cells with large cytoplasm
- Nuclear pseudoinclusions
- Psammoma bodies.

## Other benign orbital tumours

Schwannomas and haemangiomas are relatively common benign orbital tumours. Imaging diagnosis of both is relatively accurate and hence cytological diagnosis is seldom requested. The cytological features of schwannoma are almost identical to those described at other sites (see Ch. 29). FNA is not usually requested for vascular lesions because it is usually poorly cellular and carries the risk of haemorrhage; FNA of orbital leiomyoma has been described.[7] Pilocytic astrocytoma of the optic nerve may grow as an orbital mass; cytological smears show typical bipolar elongated or spindle cells in a fibrillary background (Fig. 32.15).

## Pseudotumours

Inflammatory pseudotumours represent a spectrum of orbital space-occupying inflammatory disorders. Acute inflammatory pseudotumours show specific clinical presentation whereas chronic idiopathic pseudotumours are more subtle. They may be formed by fibrosis, capillaries, inflammatory cells and granulomata making them cytologically indistinguishable from other specific or non-specific granulomatous processes (Fig. 32.16). More complex pseudotumours may show ambiguous imaging and cytological patterns composed of lymphoid cells in various stages of maturation, similar to the hyperplastic lymph nodes causing diagnostic problems such as those encountered in the differential diagnosis of lymphomas (see Chs 13, 14).[42–44] Provided that the yield of cells is sufficient, ICC and FC may be successfully used to distinguish lymphoid pseudotumour from non-Hodgkin lymphoma.

## Malignant orbital tumours

Malignant orbital tumours may arise from any of the anatomical components of the orbital region; they include tumours of the lachrymal glands, malignant lymphomas, sarcomas including paediatric tumours, tumours invading the orbit from adjacent sites and metastases. In general, the less-differentiated these tumours are, the less an accurate cytological diagnosis can be made, especially without the aid of ancillary techniques. Considering the wide range of possible lesions and the commonly scanty material available, the clinical information including clinical history are important before performing an orbital FNA in order to choose the appropriate ancillary technique where applicable. Imaging techniques have become highly informative and may help cytopathologists restrict the differential diagnosis.

## Malignant tumours of lachrymal glands

With the exception of Warthin's tumour, all of the salivary gland tumours have been observed in the lachrymal glands, having almost the same cytological features. Adenoid cystic carcinoma,[7,48] mucoepidermoid carcinoma and carcinoma ex-pleomorphic adenoma[41,48] diagnosed by FNA have been reported (see Ch. 5).

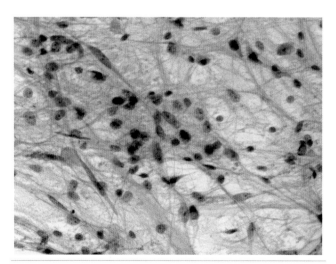

**Fig. 32.15** Pilocytic astrocytoma of the optic nerve growing as an orbital mass. FNA shows a dispersed cell population of bipolar oval or spindle cells in fibrillar back ground (PAP). (Courtesy of Professor ML De Caro, Napoli, IT.)

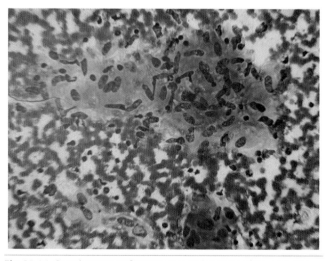

**Fig. 32.16** Granulomatous inflammatory pseudotumour of the orbit. FNA shows epithelioid cells in a granulomatous arrangement (this lesion was clinically suspected for lymphoma being positive on positron emission tomography) (Diff-Quik).

## Orbital lymphomas

Lymphomas represent the most frequent orbital malignancy whereas systemic lymphomas rarely involve the orbit. Primary lymphomas may occur in the lachrymal glands and they may arise *de novo* or as a result of the transformation of an inflammatory pseudotumour. Lymphomas arising from lachrymal glands are mainly represented by small-cell, monocytoid B-lymphocytic lymphomas, such as the mucosa associated lymphoid tissue (MALT) lymphomas seen at other extra-nodal sites (see Chs 13, 14), but other types of non-Hodgkin lymphoma, such as small lymphocytic lymphomas are also seen (Fig. 32.17). Cytological diagnosis improves when it is combined with ancillary techniques, mainly ICC or FC (Fig. 32.18).[42–44,50] Large cell lymphomas may arise de novo or as the result of the evolution of a pre-existing low-grade lymphoma. In the presence of large atypical lymphoid cells, the immunocytochemical demonstration of their lymphoid origin may be sufficient for a definitive diagnosis of lymphoma (see Chs 13, 14, 34).

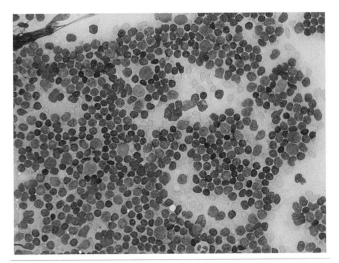

**Fig. 32.17** Small cell lymphoma of the orbit. FNA shows monomorphous dispersed small lymphocytes with dense chromatin and occasional plasma cells (Diff-Quik).

## Orbital soft tissue tumours

Orbital soft tissue tumours are represented by a wide spectrum of lesions almost identical to those found in other anatomical regions. Cytology is rarely used for diagnosis; nonetheless sporadic reports have documented the cytological features of different soft tissue tumours (see Ch. 29). As far as bone tumours are concerned, the cytological features of the orbital extension of a chondrosarcoma of the nasal cavity and sarcomatous transformation of orbital bone in Paget's disease diagnosed by FNA have been reported.[7] FNA of vascular tumours such as haemangioma and papillary endothelial hyperplasia[9] have also been reported. Embryonal rhabdomyosarcoma is the most frequent orbital soft tissue malignancy of infancy. The FNA features are those of a small round cell tumour of infancy and the cytological diagnostic criteria are reported in Chapter 33.

## Orbital metastases

Orbital metastases may appear in advanced phase of neoplastic diseases or may represent the first clinical evidence of a malignant tumour. Diagnosis may be made by FNA combined with ICC to identify the primary tumour (Fig. 32.19). Metastases from breast and lung carcinomas are those most frequently observed, although many other histotypes have been described, such as hepatocellular carcinoma, oesophageal adenocarcinoma,

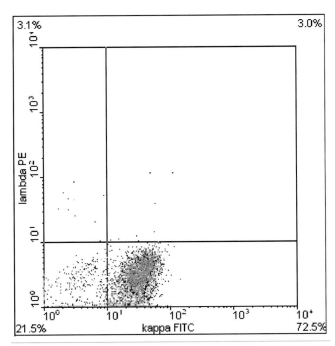

**Fig. 32.18** Flow cytometry evaluation of an orbital small cell lymphoma. FC shows: CD19 positive B-cells in the upper left quadrant and few CD5 positive, reactive T-lymphocytes, in lower right quadrant; CD19 positive B-cells in the upper left quadrant are CD10 negative (right quadrants empty); kappa light chain positivity in lower right quadrant (light chain restriction); CD19/kappa light chain co-expression in upper right quadrant.

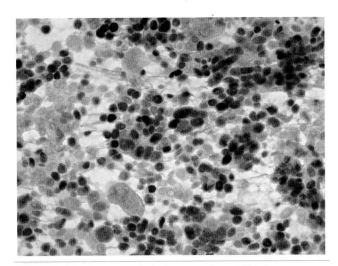

**Fig. 32.19** Orbital metastasis from a breast carcinoma. FNA shows a group of atypical epithelial cells immunostained with oestrogen receptors. (The patient had suffered from breast carcinoma 9 years before.) (Oestrogen receptors.)

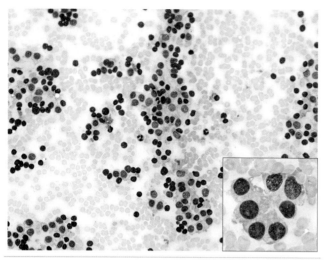

**Fig. 32.20** Olfactory neuroblastoma of the ethmoid sinus involving the orbit. FNA shows poorly differentiated neuroectodermal cells with irregularities of the nuclear membrane, dense chromatin and small nucleoli. Note a rudimental fleurette in upper right corner (Diff-Quik).

prostatic carcinoma, chordoma,[46] thymic carcinoma, ovarian adenocarcinoma[38] and various haematological processes[42–44] including Langerhans cell histiocytosis.[7] Metastatic neuroblastoma may occur in the eye, and olfactory neuroblastoma of the ethmoid sinus may infiltrate the orbit generating problems in differential diagnosis with retinoblastoma (Fig. 32.20). Microscopically, Flexner–Wintersteiner rosettes are more frequently associated with retinoblastoma than with neuroblastoma, although they are infrequently detected in cytological samples. Moreover, as these tumours share the same neuroectodermic origin, and hence the same antigenic and ICC pattern, the clinical context and imaging may be decisive in the differential diagnosis.

# REFERENCES

1. Karcioglu ZA. Fine needle aspiration biopsy (FNAB) for retinoblastoma. Retina 2002;22:707–10.

2. Faulkner-Jones BE, Foster WJ, Harbour JW, et al. Fine needle aspiration biopsy with adjunct immunohistochemistry in intraocular tumor management. Acta Cytol 2005;49:297–308.

3. Zaldivar RA, Martin DF, Holden JT, et al. Primary intraocular lymphoma: clinical, cytologic, and flow cytometric analysis. Ophthalmology 2004;111:1762–67.

4. Naus NC, Verhoeven AC, van Drunen E, et al. Detection of genetic prognostic markers in uveal melanoma biopsies using fluorescence in situ hybridisation. Clin Cancer Res 2002;8:534–39.

5. Shields CL, Ganguly A, Materin MA, et al. Chromosome 3 analysis of uveal melanoma using fine-needle aspiration biopsy at the time of plaque radiotherapy in 140 consecutive cases. Trans Am Ophthalmol Soc 2007;105:43–52.

6. Young TA, Burgess BL, Rao NP, et al. High-density genome array is superior to fluorescence in-situ hybridisation analysis of monosomy 3 in choroidal melanoma fine needle aspiration biopsy. Mol Vis 2007;13:2328–33.

7. Koss LG, ed. The eyelids, orbit and eye. In: Koss' Diagnostic Cytology, 5th edn. Philadelphia: Lippincott Williams & Wilkins; 2006: 1508–1522.

8. Rosenthal DL, Mandell DB, Glasgow BJ. Eye. In: Bibbo M, editor. Comprehensive Cytopathology. Philadelphia: WB Saunders; 1991. p. 484–501.

9. Glasgow BJ, Foos RY. Ocular Cytopathology. Boston: Butterworth-Heinemann; 1993.

10. Deshpande AH, Munshi MM. Fine needle capillary sampling of eyelid masses. A study of 70 cases. Acta Cytol 2003;47:349–58.

11. Agarwal S, Agarwal K, Kathuria P, et al. Cytomorphological features of nodular hidradenoma highlighting eccrine differentiation: a case report. Indian J Pathol Microbiol 2006;49:411–13.

12. Vu PP, Whitehead KJ, Sullivan TJ. Eccrine poroma of the eyelid. Clin Experiment Ophthalmol 2001;29:253–55.

13. Maheshwari R, Maheshwari S, Shekde S. Role of fine needle aspiration cytology in diagnosis of eyelid sebaceous carcinoma. Indian J Ophthalmol 2007;55:217–19.

14. Sadeghi S, Pitman MB, Weir MM. Cytologic features of metastatic sebaceous carcinoma: report of two cases with comparison to three cases of basal cell carcinoma. Diagn Cytopathol 1999;21:340–45.

15. Ersöz C, Ya mur M, Ersöz TR, et al. Preoperative brush and impression cytology in ocular surface squamous neoplasms. Acta Cytol 2003;47:13–15.

16. Mathew A, Stumpf T, McGhee C. Impression cytology: implications for ocular surface squamous neoplasia. Br J Ophthalmol 2008;92:157–58.

17. Tole DM, McKelvie PA, Daniell M. Reliability of impression cytology for the diagnosis of ocular surface squamous neoplasia employing the Biopore membrane. Br J Ophthalmol 2001;85:154–58.

18. Keijser S, Missotten GS, De Wolff-Rouendaal D, et al. Impression cytology of melanocytic conjunctival tumours using the Biopore membrane. Eur J Ophthalmol 2007;17:501–16.

19. Tananuvat N, Lertprasertsuk N, Mahanupap P, et al. Role of impression cytology in diagnosis of ocular surface neoplasia. Cornea 2008;27:269–74.

20. Nolan GR, Hirst LW, Bancroft BJ. The cytomorphology of ocular surface squamous neoplasia by using impression cytology. Cancer 2001;93:60–67.

21. Thiel MA, Bossart W, Bernauer W. Improved impression cytology techniques for the immunopathological diagnosis of superficial viral infections. Br J Ophthalmol 1997;81:984–88.

22. Safaei A, Saluti R, Kumar PV. Conjunctival dysplasia in soldiers exposed to mustard gas during the Iraq-Iran war: scrape cytology. Acta Cytol 2001;45:909–13.

23. Keijser S, Missotten GS, De Wolff-Rouendaal D, et al. Impression cytology of melanocytic conjunctival tumours using the Biopore membrane. Eur J Ophthalmol 2007; 17:501–6.

24. Gonidi M, Athanassiadou P, Drazinos S, et al. Primary malignant melanoma of the conjunctiva of the upper eyelid. A case report. Acta Cytol 1997;41:1790–92.

25. Midena E, Bonaldi L, Parrozzani R, et al. In vivo detection of monosomy 3 in eyes with medium-sized uveal melanoma using transscleral fine needle aspiration biopsy. Eur J Ophthalmol 2006;16:422–25.

26. El-Harazi SM, Kellaway J, Font RL. Melanocytoma of the ciliary body diagnosed by fine-needle aspiration biopsy. Diagn Cytopathol 2000;22:394–97.

27. Grossniklaus HE. Fine-needle aspiration biopsy of the iris. Arch Ophthalmol 1992;110:969–76.

28. Shields CL, Chong WH, Ehya H, et al. Sequential bilateral solitary extramedullary plasmacytoma of the ciliary body. Cornea 2007;26:759–61.

29. Kobrin EG, Shields CL, Danzig CJ, et al. Intraocular lacrimal gland choristoma diagnosed by fine-needle aspiration biopsy. Cornea 2007;26:753–55.

30. Liu K, Klintworth GK, Dodd LG. Cytologic findings in vitreous fluids. Analysis of 74 specimens. Acta Cytol 1999;43:201–6.

31. Dávila RM, Miranda MC, Smith ME. Role of cytopathology in the diagnosis of ocular malignancies. Acta Cytol 1998;42:362–66.

32. Augsburger JJ, Corrêa ZM, Schneider S, et al. Diagnostic transvitreal fine-needle aspiration biopsy of small melanocytic choroidal tumors in nevus versus melanoma category. Trans Am Ophthalmol Soc 2002;100:225–32.

33. Sen S, Singha U, Kumar H, et al. Diagnostic intraocular fine-needle aspiration biopsy. An experience in three cases of retinoblastoma. Diagn Cytopathol 1999;21:331–34.

34. Saro F, Clua A, Esteva E, et al. Cytologic diagnosis of ocular melanocytoma: a case report. Acta Cytol 2008;52:87–90.

35. Cohen VM, Shields CL, Furuta M, et al. Vitreous seeding from retinal astrocytoma in three cases. Retina 2008;28:884–88.

36. Farkas T, Harbour JW, Dávila RM. Cytologic diagnosis of intraocular lymphoma in vitreous aspirates. Acta Cytol 2004;48:487–91.

37. Finger PT, Marin JP, Berson AM, et al. Choroidal metastasis from adenoid cystic carcinoma of the lung. Am J Ophthalmol 2003;135:239–41.

38. Heerema A, Sudilovsky D. Mucinous adenocarcinoma of the ovary metastatic to the eye: report of a case with diagnosis by fine needle aspiration biopsy. Acta Cytol 2001;45:789–93.

39. Ritland JS, Eide N, Walaas L, et al. Fine-needle aspiration biopsy diagnosis of a uveal metastasis from a follicular thyroid carcinoma. Acta Ophthalmol Scand 1999;77:594–96.

40. Berman EL, Eade TN, Shields CL, et al. Choroidal metastasis from carcinoid tumour: diagnosis by fine-needle biopsy and response to radiotherapy. Australas Radiol 2007;51:398–402.

41. Rastogi A, Jain S. Fine needle aspiration biopsy in orbital lesions. Orbit 2001;20:11–23.

42. Zeppa P, Tranfa F, Errico ME, et al. Fine needle aspiration (FNA) biopsy of orbital masses: a critical review of 51 cases. Cytopathology 1997;8:366–72.

43. Tani E, Seregard S, Rupp G, et al. Fine-needle aspiration cytology and immunocytochemistry of orbital masses. Diagn Cytopathol 2006;34:1–5.

44. Nassar DL, Raab SS, Silverman JF, et al. Fine-needle aspiration for the diagnosis of orbital hematolymphoid lesions. Diagn Cytopathol 2000;23:314–17.

45. Iyer VK, Kapila K, Verma K. Fine-needle aspiration diagnosis of foreign body granulomatous reaction presenting as an orbital mass: case report and review of the literature. Diagn Cytopathol 1998;19:290–2922.

46. Bouvier D, Raghuveer CV. Aspiration cytology of metastatic chordoma to the orbit. Am J Ophthalmol 2001;131:279–80.

47. Malur PR, Bannur HB, Kodkany SB. Orbital Rosai-Dorfman disease: report of a case with fine needle aspiration cytology and histopathology. Acta Cytol 2007;51:581–82.

48. Sturgis CD, Silverman JF, Kennerdell JS, et al. Fine-needle aspiration for the diagnosis of primary epithelial tumors of the lacrimal gland and ocular adnexa. Diagn Cytopathol 2001;24:86–89.

49. Mehrotra R, Kumar S, Singh K, et al. Fine-needle aspiration biopsy of orbital meningioma. Diagn Cytopathol 1999;21:402–4.

50. Das DK. Fine needle aspiration cytology diagnosis of lymphoid lesions of the orbit. Acta Cytol 2007;51:367–69.

# Section 15

## Childhood Tumours

# Childhood tumours

Voichita Suciu, Monique Fabre, Jerzy Klijanienko, Ziva Pohar-Marinsek and Philippe Vielh

## Chapter contents

## Introduction

Despite a strong body of literature, the cytological approach for the diagnosis of paediatric tumours is not universally accepted among clinicians and pathologists. However, several studies have shown that in the hands of a well-trained team with good collaboration between paediatrician, radiologist and cytopathologist, fine needle aspiration (FNA) followed by cytological examination is a highly accurate approach for quickly rendering a preliminary or final diagnosis.[1,2] The definitive diagnosis may sometimes necessitate the use of ancillary studies such as immunocytochemistry and molecular genetic testing. In some cases, tissue examination by means of a needle core or an open surgical biopsy may be required.[3,4]

Childhood tumours are quite different from those observed in adults: (1) they are rare, corresponding to less than 1% of all malignancies and only one case of cancer is encountered annually among 10 000 children up to 15 years of age; (2) less than 5% are derived from respiratory, gastrointestinal and reproductive organs, whereas 80% of adult cancers are derived from these tissues; (3) most childhood tumours are embryonal and immature neoplasms.

## Role of the cytopathologist

Major contributions of diagnostic and prognostic value are to be gained by a detailed evaluation of the findings on cytology.[5-7] Cytological evaluation may be undertaken to determine the nature of a lesion (benign versus malignant) and attempt to define its histological subtype further. This is the case when the clinician deals with a child with lymphadenopathy or with a lesion which has to be treated by primary chemotherapy as

soon as possible. When a diagnosis has been previously established, cytological evaluation may be requested to define the anatomical extent of disease and identify tumour-related prognostic factors. This type of evaluation may provide important information for staging purposes, to help define prognosis and for monitoring response to therapy. Finally, in the follow-up of children with tumours, cytology can confirm the presence of recurrence, metastasis or secondary neoplasms.

Our policy in taking cytological samples from children is the following: (1) in palpable lesions, children are given local anaesthesia in the form of a cream which is applied over the area to be sampled a half to 1 hour prior to the procedure. Only babies are held down in order to ensure that they will not move during the procedure. With older children who recognise the doctor and injections, we ask them for cooperation and they usually do so perfectly. If they are unable to cooperate, the sample is taken under sedation or light general anaesthesia. In both cases the cytopathologist performs the procedure; (2) in non-palpable lesions, the sample is guided by image (usually ultrasound echography) and done either by the cytopathologist or the radiologist. The needles we use are 0.6–0.7 mm in diameter. It is important to emphasise that the presence of the cytopathologist is crucial for checking sample adequacy and ensuring proper handling of the specimen for smearing, fixation and triage for ancillary techniques.

## Main tumours

Some of the most frequently suspected diagnoses based on symptoms and locations are summarised in Table 33.1. Common tumour types in foetuses and newborns are listed in Box 33.1 and the distribution by percentage of malignant tumour types in children and adolescents is shown in Table 33.2.

In the foetal and neonatal periods (0–3 months of age), tumours are similar to those occurring in older infants. However, they differ in terms of frequency, sites of involvement, distribution, degree of differentiation and prognosis.

Tumours in children (3 months to 14 years of age) and adolescents (15–19 years of age) have distinct characteristics in terms of distribution. As shown above: (1) more than half of malignancies in children are acute leukaemias and central nervous system tumours; (2) Hodgkin disease and germ cell tumours are more frequent in adolescents than in children; (3) neuroblastoma, nephroblastoma and retinoblastoma are exceptional in adolescents. Other variations in incidence are also noted depending on gender and ethnicity.

*The authors wish to thank S. Vincent (CT) and A. Valent (PhD) for their help with the illustrations and M. P. Dupré (FRCPC) for text revision and editing.*

**Table 33.1** Presenting symptoms and commonly associated suspected diagnoses

| Usual presenting symptoms | Most frequent potential diagnoses |
|---|---|
| Lymphadenopathy | |
|   Localised | Infection (mononucleosis) |
| | Malignancy |
|   Generalised | Systemic infection (mononucleosis) |
| | Autoimmune, storage or metabolic disease |
| | Drug-induced hyperplasia |
| Thoracic mass | |
|   Anterior mediastinum | Acute lymphoblastic leukaemia (T cell) |
| | Lymphoblastic lymphoma |
|   Middle mediastinum | Lymphoma (Hodgkin) |
| | Metastases (from subdiaphragmatic tumours) |
| | Infections (tuberculosis, histoplasmosis) |
|   Posterior mediastinum | Neuroblastoma |
| | Ganglioneuroma |
| | Neurofibroma |
|   Chest wall | Ewing/pPNET |
| | Alveolar soft part sarcoma |
| | Langerhans' cell histiocytosis |
| Bone pain and/or mass | |
|   Localised | Osteomyelitis |
| | Ewing/pPNET |
| | Osteosarcoma |
| | Langerhans' cell histiocytosis |
| | Non-Hodgkin lymphoma |
|   Diffuse | Acute leukaemia |
| | Metastases (Ewing/pPNET, neuroblastoma) |
| Abdominal or pelvic mass | Congenital malformation (neonatal period) |
| | Nephroblastoma, neuroblastoma |
| | Lymphoma (Burkitt) |
| | Hepatic, germ cell and ovarian tumours |
| | Inflammatory process (abscess) |
| Lump or swelling | |
|   Extremities | Rhabdomyosarcoma |
|   Orbit | Rhabdomyosarcoma, retinoblastoma |
| | Lymphoma, neuroblastoma |
| | Langerhans' cell histiocytosis |
|   Sacrum | Sacrococcygeal teratoma |

pPNET, peripheral primitive neuroectodermal tumour (included in the Ewing's family of tumours).

**Table 33.2** Distribution (by percentage) of malignant tumour types in children (0–14 years) and adolescents (15–19 years)

| Type of malignancy | Children | Adolescents |
|---|---|---|
| Acute leukaemia | | |
|   Lymphoblastic | 23.7 | 5.8 |
|   Myeloid | 4.9 | 4.4 |
| Central nervous system tumours | 22.1 | 9.8 |
| Lymphomas | | |
|   Non-Hodgkin | 5.9 | 8.2 |
|   Hodgkin | 3.6 | 16.4 |
| Other solid tumours | | |
|   Neuroblastoma | 7.7 | 0.2 |
|   Nephroblastoma | 5.9 | 0.2 |
|   Non RMS-soft tissue tumours | 3.6 | 5.9 |
|   Rhabdomyosarcoma (RMS) | 3.4 | 1.9 |
|   Germ cell/gonadal tumours | 3.4 | 12.8 |
|   Retinoblastoma | 3.1 | 0.0 |
|   Osteosarcoma | 2.5 | 4.0 |
|   Ewing's/pPNET | 1.5 | 2.3 |
|   Hepatoblastoma | 1.4 | 0.0 |
|   Thyroid carcinoma | 1.2 | 8.2 |
|   Malignant melanoma | 1.2 | 7.6 |

RMS, rhabdomyosarcoma; pPNET, peripheral primitive neuroectodermal tumour (included in the Ewing family of tumours). (Adapted from Gurney JG, Bondy ML. Epidemiology of childhood cancer. In: Pizzo PA, Poplack DG (eds), Principles and Practice of Pediatric Oncology, 5th edn. Philadelphia: Lippincott Williams & Wilkins; 2006.)

---

**Box 33.1   Common tumours in the foetus and newborn**

- Teratoma (usually benign)
- Vascular malformations
- Sarcomas
- Brain tumours
- Neuroblastoma
- Retinoblastoma
- Leukaemias

---

## Non-Hodgkin and Hodgkin lymphomas

About 10% of all childhood neoplasms are lymphomas and most of these are of the non-Hodgkin type (Table 33.2).

Diagnosis and classification is based on morphology[8] and results of ancillary testing such as immunophenotyping by flow cytometry, cytogenetic studies (karyotype, FISH) and molecular genetic testing (PCR). Non-Hodgkin lymphoma (NHL) is rare in children less than 2 years of age and a peak incidence is observed between 5 and 15 years of age. More than 90% of NHL are high-grade lymphomas and include precursor and mature B-cell, T-cell or natural killer-cell neoplasms. High-grade

**Table 33.3** Most frequent non-Hodgkin lymphomas in children and adolescents

| Lymphoma type | Frequency | Main sites involved | Immunopheno-type |
|---|---|---|---|
| Burkitt (and Burkitt-like) | 40% | Cervical lymph nodes, tonsil, jaw, abdomen, kidneys, ovaries, bone marrow, CNS | B cell |
| Lymphoblastic | | | |
| Precursor T | 25% | Mediastinum, peripheral lymph nodes, liver, spleen, kidneys, retroperitoneum, testes, bone marrow, CNS | Pre-T cell |
| Precursor B | 5% | Cervical lymph nodes, skin, bone | Pre-B cell |
| Diffuse large B cell (includes mediastinal) | 20% | Peripheral lymph nodes, tonsil, bone, mediastinum, retroperitoneum, liver, bone marrow (rare), primary CNS | B cell |
| Anaplastic, large cell | 10% | Skin, soft tissue, bone, peripheral lymph nodes, mediastinum, liver, bone marrow, CNS (rare) | T cell or null cell |

CNS, central nervous system. (Adapted from Link MP, Weinstein HJ. Malignant non-Hodgkin lymphoma in children. In: Pizzo PA and Poplack DG (eds) Principles and Practice of Pediatric Oncology, 5th edn. Philadelphia: Lippincott Williams & Wilkins; 2006.)

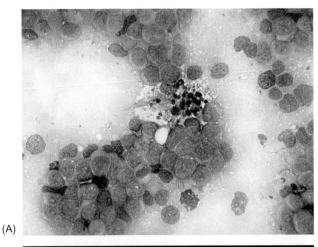

(A)

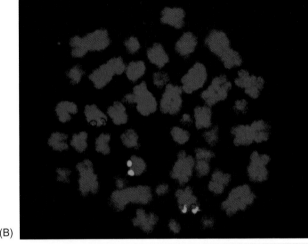

(B)

**Fig. 33.1** (A) Burkitt lymphoma. Medium-sized lymphoid cells with scanty blue cytoplasm showing lipid vacuoles. Note the dense chromatin and the presence of several mitoses and of a macrophage with tingible bodies (MGG). (B) Burkitt lymphoma. FISH on a metaphase with a c-myc «break apart» probe showing a translocation of part of cmyc gene to chromosome 14 (green spots). Part of the gene is still visible on chromosome 8 (red). The second-normal c-myc gene is composed of two overlapping parts on normal chromosome 8.

mature B-cell neoplasms are represented by Burkitt and diffuse large B-cell lymphomas, whereas high-grade mature T-cell tumours are most frequently anaplastic large cell lymphomas. The most frequently encountered lymphoma types in childhood are summarised in Table 33.3.

## Burkitt and Burkitt-like lymphomas[9,10]

### Background

Classical Burkitt (BL) and Burkitt-like lymphomas (BLL or atypical BL) (Fig. 33.1A) may present at extranodal sites or as an acute leukaemia. BL is mainly observed in equatorial Africa in its endemic form, with a peak incidence in children aged 4–7 years. The abdomen and jaw are the main sites of involvement in approximately 70% of children less than 5 years of age and in 25% of children over the age of 14 years. The sporadic form of BL is seen throughout the world, mainly arising in the abdomen and the Waldeyer's ring of children and young adults. A third form of BL is related to immunosuppression and may be the initial manifestation of the acquired immunodeficiency syndrome (AIDS) due to the human immunodeficiency virus (HIV) infection.

**Cytological findings: Burkitt and Burkitt-like lymphomas**

- Relatively uniform population of isolated medium-sized tumour cells
- Rounded nuclei with a high mitotic rate
- Granular or speckled chromatin with multiple small but prominent nucleoli
- Thin rim of dense blue cytoplasm with small lipid vacuoles
- Tingible body macrophages (producing a 'starry sky' pattern on histological sections) often prominent, apoptotic bodies in the background

- Variants: BL with plasmacytoid differentiation may show tumour cells with abundant blue cytoplasm and a single eccentric nucleus with central nucleolus. BLL usually exhibits a higher degree of pleomorphism in nuclear size and shape. Both of these variants are rare entities.

### Diagnostic pitfalls: BL and BLL

- B-cell lymphoblastic lymphoma
- Diffuse large B-cell lymphoma in BLL (atypical)
- Extramedullary myeloid malignancies (granulocytic or myeloid sarcoma)
- Other small round cell tumours (Box 33.2): CD45 may be absent in BL.

## Usefulness of ancillary techniques

Immunophenotyping of tumour cells demonstrates: (1) the absence of precursor markers (TdT negativity); (2) the presence of B-cell-associated antigens (CD19, CD20, and CD10); (3) expression of surface IgM with light chain (kappa or lambda) restriction; (4) over 95% of tumour cells express the Ki67 proliferative marker. Molecular genetic testing reveals a translocation of the MYC gene (Fig. 33.1B) at band q24 from chromosome 8 with the Ig heavy chain region on chromosome 14 at band q32 corresponding to t(8;14). Less commonly, translocations involve the MYC gene (8q24) and light chain loci on 2q11 (kappa chain) or on 22q11 (lambda chain) corresponding to t(2;8) and t(8;22), respectively. However, these translocations involving MYC may also be observed in other lymphomas, such as diffuse large B-cell lymphoma.

## Precursor T and B lymphoblastic lymphoma (LL) (Fig. 33.2)[11–13]

### Background

LL may present at nodal sites or as an acute lymphoblastic leukaemia (ALL) with bone marrow (>25%) and blood involvement. Precursor T-LL is the most frequent disease, usually affecting children >6 years and adolescents in a nodal form, and a mediastinal (thymic) mass is frequently present (85%), sometimes also with meningeal involvement. Precursor B-LL affects children <6 years and is more commonly seen in the leukaemic form.

### Cytological findings: precursor T and B lymphoblastic lymphoma

- Relatively uniform population of isolated medium-sized tumour cells
- Anisonucleosis and convoluted nuclei classically more prominent in T-cell than in B-cell variants
- Finely granular chromatin with inconspicuous nucleoli in the T-cell variant and granular or speckled chromatin with multiple small but prominent nucleoli in the B-cell variant
- Cytoplasm usually fragile and small cytoplasmic vacuoles may be seen.

### Diagnostic pitfalls: precursor T and B LL

- BL
- Distinction between T and B forms of lymphoblastic lymphoma
- Extramedullary myeloid malignancies (granulocytic or myeloid sarcoma)
- Other small round cell tumours (Box 33.2): CD45 may be negative in lymphoblastic lymphoma.

## Usefulness of ancillary techniques

Immunophenotyping of tumour cells demonstrates: (1) precursor markers (TdT positivity); (2) T-cell markers are identified in 85% of cases (CD3 and CD7 often present; CD4 and CD8 positivity variable and depends on degree of maturation), but aberrant T-cell populations with the loss of one or more pan-T-cell markers (CD2, CD3, CD5, CD7) can also be identified. B-cell markers are detected in 15% of cases (CD19 and CD79a

---

### Box 33.2  Main malignant round cell tumours

1. Lymphomas
   - Burkitt, lymphoblastic and centroblastic variant of diffuse large B cell (small cells)
   - Diffuse large B cell
2. Neuroblastoma (small and/or large cells)
3. Nephroblastoma (small and/or large cells)
4. Rhabdomyosarcoma of the alveolar type (small and/or large cells)
5. Germ cell tumours (large cells)
6. Other soft tissue sarcomas (small and/or large cells)
   - Malignant peripheral nerve sheath tumour
   - Liposarcoma
   - Malignant rhabdoid tumour
   - Desmoplastic small round cell tumour
7. Ewing family of tumours or pPNET (small cells)
8. Liver tumours (small or large cells)

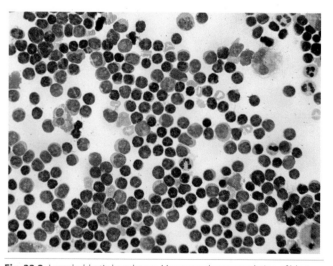

**Fig. 33.2** Lymphoblastic lymphoma. Monomorphous population of blasts with irregular or convoluted nuclei and dense finely granular chromatin (bone marrow) (MGG).

are almost always present; CD34, CD10 and cytoplasmic Ig positivity depends on the degree of maturation); (3) absence of surface Ig. A variety of molecular abnormalities of no currently defined clinical significance can be identified in precursor T-cell lymphoblastic lymphoma. However, some molecular abnormalities are of prognostic importance and are used to modify treatment in precursor B-LL. For example, hyperdiploidy with more than 50 chromosomes, corresponding to a DNA index of 1.16 to 1.60, or the presence of a t(12;21) translocation is associated with an improved prognosis, whereas hypodiploidy or detection of t(1;19), t(9;22) or t(4;11) is associated with a poor outcome.

## Diffuse large B-cell lymphoma (DLBCL)[14]

### Background

DLBCL constitutes a heterogeneous group of diseases representing a proliferation of large mature B cells equal or larger in size than macrophage nuclei or more than twice the size of a normal lymphocyte. A rapidly enlarging mass at a single nodal or extranodal site is typically the first symptom.

### Cytological findings: diffuse large B-cell lymphoma

- Centroblastic variant: isolated medium to large-sized lymphoid cells with round or irregular nuclei, fine chromatin, 2–4 membrane-bound nucleoli and scant cytoplasm
- Immunoblastic variant: pleomorphic population of large blasts, sometimes multinucleated, with a prominent centrally located nucleoli and an abundant blue cytoplasm (MGG staining)
- T-cell rich/histiocyte variant: small mature lymphocytes (over 90%), epithelioid histiocytes and scattered large tumour cells
- Anaplastic variant with very large cells and round, oval or pleomorphic nuclei.

### Diagnostic pitfalls: diffuse large B-cell lymphoma

- BL and BLL in the case of centroblastic variant
- Reactive lymphadenopathy, Hodgkin lymphoma, and metastatic carcinoma in the case of immunoblastic, T-cell rich/histiocyte and anaplastic variants
- Blastoid variant of mantle cell lymphoma (expressing cyclin D1)
- Extramedullary myeloid malignancies (granulocytic or myeloid sarcoma).

### Usefulness of ancillary techniques

Immunophenotyping of tumour cells demonstrates: (1) the presence of one or more B-cell associated antigens (CD19, CD20, CD79a), (2) monoclonal surface Ig in half of the cases; (3) the absence of precursor markers (TdT or CD34). Molecular studies show that most cases have Ig heavy and light chain gene rearrangements and a subset may show translocations of the BCL2 or of the BCL6 genes.

## Anaplastic large cell lymphoma (ALCL)[15–17]

### Background

ALCL (Fig. 33.3) is a mature T-cell or null cell lymphoma. It usually consists of large lymphoid cells frequently expressing CD30 (Ki-1) and the anaplastic large cell lymphoma kinase (ALK) protein. Most children present with lymphadenopathy and skin involvement may occur.

### Cytological findings: anaplastic large cell lymphoma

- Common variant (70%): large lymphoid cells with abundant cytoplasm and pleomorphic, often horseshoe-shaped nuclei (so-called hallmark cells)
- Lymphohistiocytic variant (10%): admixed histiocytes may obscure tumour cells
- Small cell variant (10%): small- to medium-sized plasmacytoid, spindle or tadpole cells, pale basophilic cytoplasm. Usually, diagnostic hallmark cells are admixed.

### Diagnostic pitfalls: ALCL

- Classic Hodgkin lymphoma (CD30 positive and ALK negative) in the case of T-cell common variant and the null cell form (CD15 and EBV negative)
- Malignant histiocytosis in the case of lymphohistiocytic variant
- Reactive lymphadenopathy in the case of small cell variant
- Metastatic carcinomas or melanomas are exceptional in children.

### Usefulness of ancillary techniques

Immunophenotyping of tumour cells shows: (1) frequent CD45 positivity, however a subset lacks CD45 expression; (2) positive T-cell markers (CD2, CD3 or CD5) in the mature T-cell form and negative T-cell markers with CD43 positivity in the null cell form; (3) frequent expression of CD30 (Ki-1) and ALK protein resulting from various gene fusions, the most frequent being t(2;5)(p23;q35) involving the NPM gene.

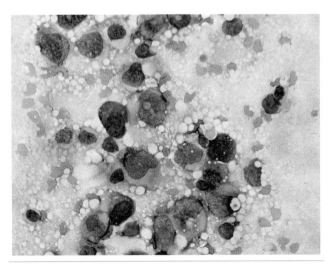

**Fig. 33.3** Anaplastic large cell lymphoma. Large isolated lymphoid cells (intense basophilic cytoplasm) showing pleomorphic and 'kidney-shaped' nuclei (MGG).

## Hodgkin lymphoma[18–22]

### Background

Hodgkin lymphoma (Fig. 33.4) is rare before the age of 5 years. Its frequency increases until the age of 11 years and remains high during adolescence and up to the age of 30. Two forms are described: classical Hodgkin lymphoma and nodular lymphocyte predominant Hodgkin lymphoma. The most frequent is classical Hodgkin lymphoma which usually presents with enlarged mediastinal lymph nodes and occurs more frequently in older children and adolescents. Further subclassification of classical Hodgkin lymphoma into nodular sclerosing, mixed cellularity, lymphocyte rich and lymphocyte depleted forms is of less clinical significance with current therapeutic approaches. Nodular lymphocyte predominant Hodgkin lymphoma is rare (5%), usually occurring in small children. It commonly involves cervical, axillary or inguinal lymph nodes and is of better prognosis than classical Hodgkin lymphoma.

### Cytological findings: Hodgkin lymphoma

- Classical Hodgkin lymphoma: characteristic Reed-Sternberg cells with abundant pale cytoplasm and lobulated nucleus with coarse irregularly distributed chromatin. Classic Reed-Sternberg cells are binucleate (mirror image nuclei) with prominent large eosinophilic nucleoli. A variable number of eosinophils, histiocytes, plasma cells and lymphocytes are associated. Atypical mononuclear variants, also termed Hodgkin cells and bizarre multinucleated cells may be seen
- Nodular lymphocyte predominant Hodgkin lymphoma: few tumour cells with abundant pale cytoplasm in a background of small lymphocytes. Nuclei and nucleoli are smaller than those of Reed-Sternberg cells and lobulated nuclei, corresponding to the popcorn cells seen in histological sections, are present. Some multinucleated forms may be seen

### Diagnostic pitfalls: Hodgkin lymphoma

- Reactive lymphadenopathy: infectious mononucleosis, toxoplasmosis
- Granulomatous lymphadenitis
- Mediastinal diffuse large B-cell lymphoma
- Anaplastic large cell lymphoma
- Undifferentiated metastatic carcinoma (nasopharyngeal).

### Usefulness of ancillary techniques

In classical Hodgkin lymphoma, immunophenotyping of Reed-Sternberg cells typically shows: (1) the presence of CD15 and CD30; (2) the absence of CD45 and T cell-associated antigens. Clonal episomal Epstein-Barr virus (EBV) genomes or EBV antigens may be detected in tumour cells, in a subset of neoplasms. Accompanying small lymphocytes are usually T lymphocytes. By contrast, in nodular lymphocyte predominant Hodgkin lymphoma, CD15 and CD30 are absent, CD45 is present, and small B lymphocytes express CD20.

## Neuroblastoma and nephroblastoma

### Neuroblastoma and related tumours[23–28]

### Background

Neuroblastoma is the third most common childhood malignancy and follows leukaemia/lymphomas and tumours of the central nervous system (Table 33.2). The male to female ratio is 1.1:1.0 and mean age at diagnosis is 2.5 years for both sexes. Around 75% of neuroblastomas are diagnosed after the neonatal period, and the vast majority of them (90%) are diagnosed by the age of 5 years. Derived from primordial neural crest cells populating the sympathetic nervous system, neuroblastomas may arise in the adrenal medulla or from any sympathetic ganglia within the retroperitoneum, posterior mediastinum, neck and sacral regions.

### Cytological findings: neuroblastoma and related tumours

- In well-differentiated neuroblastoma: small round cells (Fig. 33.5), variable number of Homer–Wright rosettes

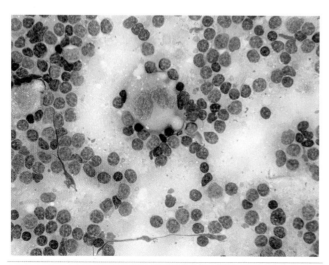

**Fig. 33.4** Hodgkin lymphoma (MGG).

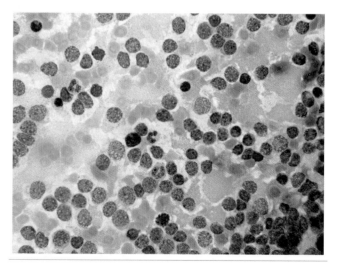

**Fig. 33.5** Neuroblastoma. Immature neuroblasts (MGG).

(Fig. 33.6) and neurofibrillary background (neuropil) (Fig. 33.7). Ganglion cells, which are large cells with one or more nuclei and prominent nucleoli are observed in ganglioneuroblastoma (Fig. 33.8). Ganglioneuroma shows only few mature ganglion cells admixed with spindled cells (Schwann cells) (Fig. 33.9). Neuroblasts and neurofibrillary background are lacking in these mature forms

- In poorly differentiated neuroblastoma: small round cells, nuclear moulding (Fig. 33.10A). Rosettes and neuropil are rare or absent.

### Diagnostic pitfalls: neuroblastoma and related tumours

- In contrast to the rosette-like structures sometimes observed in Ewing/peripheral primitive neuroectodermal tumour (pPNET), nephroblastoma, rhabdomyosarcoma, desmoplastic small round cell tumour, hepatoblastoma and melanotic progonoma, the Homer–Wright rosettes seen in well-differentiated neuroblastoma usually contain neuropil

- Ewing/pPNET, monophasic blastemal nephroblastoma may be confused with poorly differentiated neuroblastoma (Box 33.2)
- As these tumours are heterogeneous, the definite diagnosis of maturation into ganglioneuroma is not reliable on cytological specimens (a small neuroblastic component may not be sampled). This distinction requires extensive histopathological examination of the surgical specimen.

## Usefulness of ancillary techniques

Immunocytochemistry using an antibody against NB84 is positive in all well-differentiated neuroblastomas and in the majority of poorly differentiated tumours, but this antibody may also stain 25% of Ewing/pPNET tumours and 50% of desmoplastic small round cell tumours. Nephroblastomas are negative for NB84. Prognosis is predicted by the combination of: patient age, clinical stage, DNA ploidy and presence of *MYCN* (2p24) oncogene amplification as detected by fluorescence *in situ* hybridisation (FISH). Tumours which are near diploid

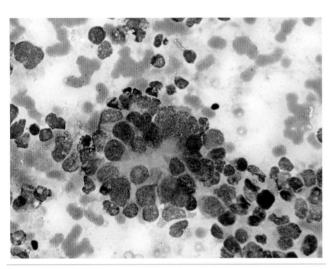

**Fig. 33.6** Neuroblastoma. Homer–Wright rosette (MGG).

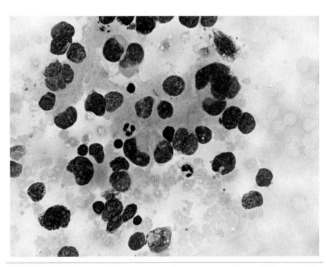

**Fig. 33.8** Ganglioneuroblastoma. Note the presence of large differentiated neuroblasts and of neuropil (MGG).

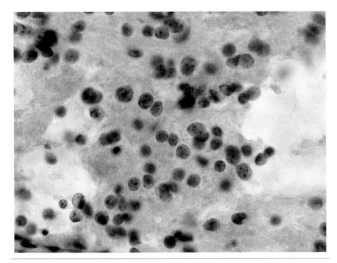

**Fig. 33.7** Neuropil (neurofibrillary background) in a poorly differentiated neuroblastoma (PAP).

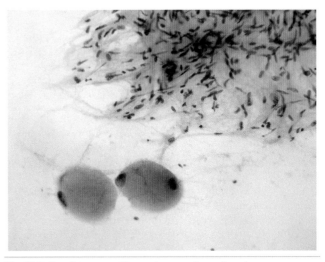

**Fig. 33.9** Ganglioneuroma. Two mature ganglion cells and numerous spindle-shaped (Schwann) cells (PAP).

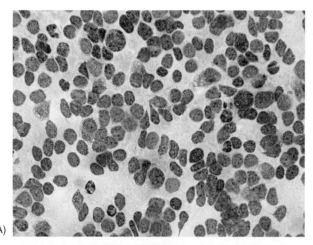

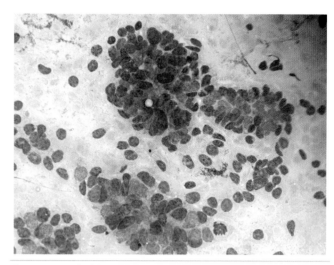

**Fig. 33.11**  Nephroblastoma. Epithelial component: small round or slightly irregular tumour cells arranged in tubular structures (MGG).

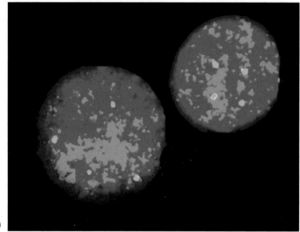

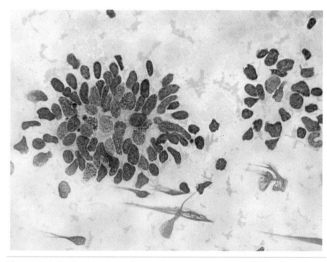

**Fig. 33.10**  (A) Neuroblastoma. Immature neuroblasts showing nuclear moulding (MGG). (B) FISH on interphase nuclei in neuroblastoma: amplification of the *MYCN* gene (red) in malignant immature neuroblasts showing a multiple copies pattern. The control probe is chromosome 2 centromere (green).

**Fig. 33.12**  Nephroblastoma. Stromal component: some spindle-shaped tumour cells arranged in loose sheets (MGG).

or near tetraploid and which harbour a *MYCN* amplification (Fig. 33.10B) correlate with a poor outcome.

## Nephroblastoma (Wilms' tumour)[29–32] and other renal tumours[33–39]

### Background

Nephroblastoma is the fourth most common childhood malignancy. The male to female ratio is 1.1:1.0 and mean age at diagnosis is 3 years for boys and 3.5 for girls. The rare tumours occurring during the neonatal period are usually associated with congenital and chromosomal abnormalities. Tumours are more often unilateral than bilateral. More than half of tumours occur before the age of 3 years and 90% are diagnosed before the age of 10 years. The other primitive renal tumours of childhood include: clear cell sarcoma of kidney (so-called 'bone-metastasising renal cell tumour of childhood'), rhabdoid tumour of the kidney, congenital mesoblastic nephroma (Bolande tumour) and renal cell carcinoma.

### Cytological findings: nephroblastoma (Wilms' tumour) and other renal tumours

- In the classic triphasic nephroblastoma: (1) epithelial elements: small round tumour cells with distinct cytoplasm, sometimes arranged in tubular structures (Fig. 33.11); (2) mesenchymal or stromal elements: spindle-shaped tumour cells arranged in loose sheets intermixed with a myxoid or collagenous matrix (Fig. 33.12); (3) undifferentiated blastemal elements: small and round tumour cells with little cytoplasm (Fig. 33.13). Anaplastic foci may be detected (Fig. 33.14)

- Recognition may be difficult in biphasic or even monophasic variants of nephroblastoma

- Other tumours: clear cell sarcoma, usually biphasic with round and spindle-shaped tumour cells; rhabdoid tumour of kidney composed of large cells with abundant eosinophilic cytoplasm, irregular nuclei and prominent nucleoli; congenital mesoblastic nephroma may be of classic type and contain spindle cells without mitoses or necrosis, reminiscent of infantile fibromatosis or, more frequently, of

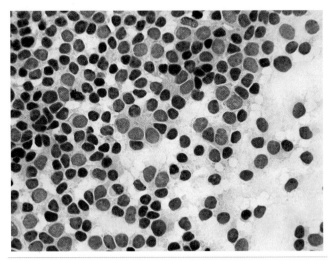

**Fig. 33.13** Nephroblastoma. Blastomatous component. Small round tumour cells without distinct cytoplasm (MGG).

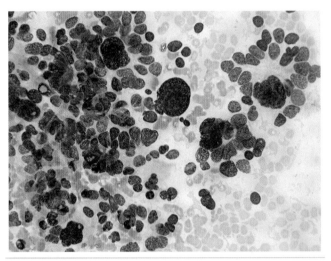

**Fig. 33.14** Anaplastic nephroblastoma. Note the at least three-fold enlarged hyperchromatic nuclei (MGG).

the cellular type and contain round cells with mitoses and necrosis, reminiscent of infantile fibrosarcoma.

### Diagnostic pitfalls: nephroblastoma (Wilms' tumour) and other renal tumours

- When epithelial cells predominate: multicystic nephroma, angiomyolipoma, renal cell carcinoma, clear cell sarcoma of the kidney, small round cell tumours (Boxes 33.2, 33.3)
- When mesenchymal (stromal) elements predominate: congenital mesoblastic nephroma, soft tissue tumours (ancient schwannoma), clear cell sarcoma of the kidney, rhabdoid tumour and rhabdomyosarcoma (Boxes 33.3, 33.4)
- When blastemal cells predominate: nephrogenic rests, nephroblastomatosis, and small round cell tumours (Box 33.2).

### Usefulness of ancillary techniques

Immunocytochemistry using an antibody against WT1 is positive in only 70% of nephroblastomas. Staining of

---

**Box 33.3  Main malignant round and spindle cell tumours**

1. Nephroblastoma (small and/or large cells)
2. Rhabdomyosarcoma (small and/or large cells)
3. Non-rhabdomyosarcoma soft tissue tumours (small and/or large cells)
   - Synovial sarcoma
   - Malignant peripheral nerve sheath tumour

---

**Box 33.4  Main malignant spindle cell tumours**

1. Nephroblastoma (small and/or large cells)
2. Rhabdomyosarcoma of embryonal type (small and/or large cells)
3. Non-rhabdomyosarcoma soft tissue tumours (small and/or large cells)
   - Synovial sarcoma
   - Malignant peripheral nerve sheath tumour
   - Fibrosarcoma
   - Leiomyosarcoma

---

nuclei may also be seen in desmoplastic small cell tumours, lymphoblastic lymphoma and neuroblastoma, and cytoplasmic staining can be present in rhabdomyosarcoma. The large cytoplasmic bellies of the malignant cells in rhabdoid tumour of the kidney are positive for various cytokeratins, epithelial-membrane antigen, desmin, and neurofilaments. Until now, no specific chromosomal translocation has been described in Wilms' tumour. Rhabdoid tumour of the kidney (as well as malignant extra-renal rhabdoid tumours) harbours a 22q11.12 chromosomal deletion (*hSNF5/INI1* gene). Cellular congenital mesoblastic nephroma consistently shows a t(12;15)(p13;q25) translocation (also observed in infantile fibrosarcoma). Subtypes of renal cell carcinomas exhibit a Xp11.2 translocation.

## Rhabdomyosarcoma and other soft tissue tumours

### Rhabdomyosarcoma[40–42]

#### Background

Rhabdomyosarcoma is the fifth most common childhood tumour and represents half of all malignant soft tissue tumours in infants and children. The male to female ratio is: 1.1:1.0. Median age at diagnosis is 5 years and almost 70% of children are diagnosed before the age of 10. At presentation, the most frequent sites of involvement are: head and neck region (35%), genitourinary tract (22%), and extremities (18%). According to the international classification, rhabdomyosarcomas are categorised with distinct prognostic significance into the following morphological types: (1) the embryonal type (65%) is stroma-rich, has a spindle cell appearance, and no evidence of an alveolar pattern. The embryonal type has an intermediate prognosis. Specific entities within this group are associated with a better prognosis. These specific types include: the botryoid variant (bladder, vagina or nasopharynx) and spindle cell or leiomyomatous variant (paratesticular region, orbit, extremities); (2) the alveolar type (20%) consisting of densely packed small round tumour cells lining septations. A solid variant is also recognised. Tumours of the alveolar category generally have a bad prognosis. Anaplastic foci may be present in embryonal and alveolar rhabdomyosarcoma and tumours with large anaplastic areas have a poor prognosis.

### Cytological findings: rhabdomyosarcoma

- Embryonal and alveolar rhabdomyosarcomas may only be suggested cytologically in 80% of the cases
- Embryonal rhabdomyosarcoma typically shows large and highly cellular tissue fragments with moderate or abundant stroma and a variable numbers of individual cells. Tumour cells are predominantly immature with uniform, slightly oval or round nuclei and small amounts of cytoplasm. Rare cells mimicking rhabdomyoblasts with single or multiple nuclei and variable amounts of cytoplasm may be observed (Fig. 33.15)
- Alveolar rhabdomyosarcoma usually yield high cellularity specimens. Individual tumour cells are small and round and the number of mature rhabdomyoblasts may vary from single to numerous (Fig. 33.16).

### Diagnostic pitfalls: rhabdomyosarcoma

- Large and highly cellular fragments in embryonal type should be differentiated from benign lesions such as: infantile myofibromatosis, haemangioendothelioma or neurofibroma (Boxes 33.3, 33.4)
- Small round tumour cells, mainly observed in the alveolar type: other small round cell tumours (Boxes 33.2, 33.3)
- Rhabdomyoblasts may mimic tumour cells observed in malignant rhabdoid tumours or in embryonal sarcoma (not otherwise specified).

## Usefulness of ancillary techniques

Immunocytochemistry using antibodies against muscle-specific (alpha smooth muscle antigen, desmin) and skeletal muscle (MyoD1, myogenin) proteins may be useful. However, the first two are not specific (desmin may be observed in some Ewing/pPNET) while nuclear detection of MyoD1 and myogenin may be difficult to detect on smears. In this context, the use of an antibody directed against WT1 showing strong cytoplasmic staining in rhabdomyosarcoma, nuclear staining in desmoplastic round cell tumour and only focal reactivity in Ewing/pPNET is helpful. Molecular genetic techniques are important for the diagnosis since alveolar rhabdomyosarcomas exhibit specific translocations between the *FKHR* gene located at 13q14 with members of the *PAX* family of genes coding for transcription factors (*PAX3* located at 2q35 or *PAX7* located at 1p36). The t(2;13)(q35;q14) translocation (*PAX3-FKHR* gene fusion), and the t(1;13)(p36;q14) translocation (*PAX7-FKHR* gene fusion) are detectable in 60% and 20% of alveolar rhabdomyosarcomas, respectively (Fig. 33.17). These two translocations may be observed by interphase FISH or detected by RT-PCR searching for the hybrid transcripts derived from the corresponding

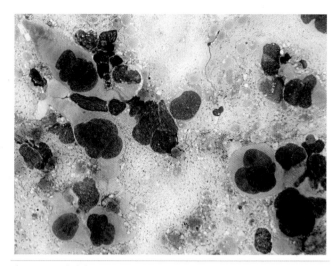

**Fig. 33.15** Rhabdomyosarcoma. Nuclear pleomorphism and multinucleated tumour cells with elongated cytoplasm (MGG).

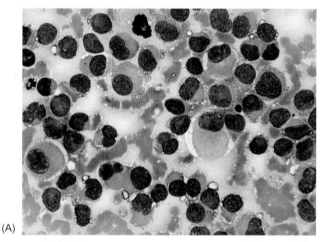

(A)

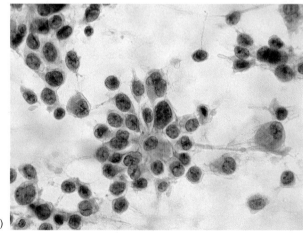

(B)

**Fig. 33.16** (A) Alveolar rhabdomyosarcoma. Dissociated small round tumour cells and a few elements with eccentric nuclei (MGG). (B) Alveolar rhabdomyosarcoma (PAP).

gene fusion. A loss of heterozygosity (LOH) at the 11p15 locus is consistently observed in embryonal rhabdomyosarcoma and, although still controversial, DNA diploidy seems to correlate with a poor outcome.

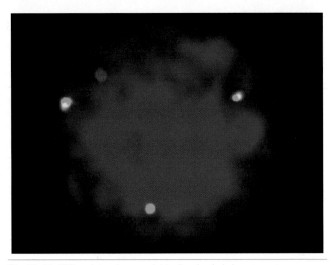

**Fig. 33.17** FISH on interphase nuclei in alveolar rhabdomyosarcoma: double fusion probe *FKHR* (red) and *PAX 3* (green) showing a translocation of these two genes. One 2-colour overlapping spot represents a derivative chromosome 2, the second represents the derivative chromosome 13.

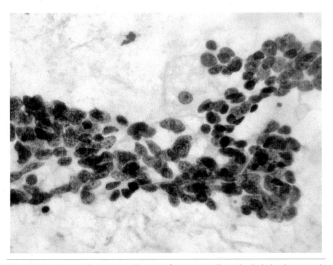

**Fig. 33.18** Synovial sarcoma. Cluster of tumour cells with slightly elongated nuclei (PAP).

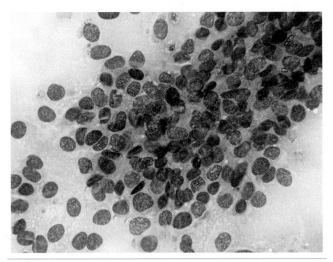

**Fig. 33.19** Synovial sarcoma. Dense cellular cluster of small round tumour cells (MGG).

## Other soft tissue tumours[43–48]

### Background

Benign soft tissue tumours are more common than soft tissue sarcomas at all ages. The incidence of specific histological types in sarcomas is age dependent: (1) rhabdomyosarcomas account for 60% of sarcomas in children <5 years and other sarcoma types represent more than three-quarters of all sarcomas in those aged 15–19 years; (2) fibrosarcoma is more common in infants, whereas synovial sarcoma and malignant peripheral nerve sheath tumour (MPNST) are more frequent in older children and adults.

### Cytological findings: other soft tissue tumours

- Biphasic (spindled and rounded tumour cells): usually synovial sarcoma
- Monophasic (spindled tumour cells): monophasic synovial sarcoma (Fig. 33.18), MPNST, congenital infantile fibrosarcoma, leiomyosarcoma
- Monophasic (rounded tumour cells): synovial sarcoma (Fig. 33.19), MPNST, liposarcoma, desmoplastic small round cell tumour (usually intra-abdominal), clear cell sarcoma (so-called melanoma of soft parts), malignant rhabdoid tumour and small cell osteosarcoma
- Pleomorphic: the very rare undifferentiated high-grade sarcoma (so-called malignant fibrous histiocytoma).

### Diagnostic pitfalls: other soft tissue tumours

- Spindle cells: benign lesions such as fibroblastic and myofibroblastic proliferations (Fig. 33.20), fibrous hamartoma of infancy, schwannoma (neurilemoma) (Box 33.4)
- Round cells: other small round cell tumours (Box 33.2).

### Usefulness of ancillary techniques

Immunocytochemistry is of limited value. By contrast, molecular techniques are potentially of great interest in a number of entities which are known to harbour specific genetic

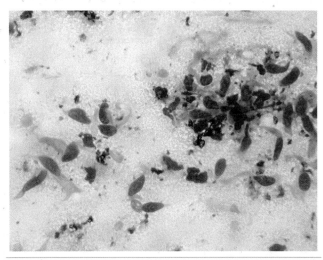

**Fig. 33.20** Myofibromatosis. Myofibroblasts showing elongated unipolar cytoplasm and regular oval shaped or elongated nuclei (MGG).

abnormalities detectable in both DNA (interphase FISH) and RNA (reverse transcriptase-PCR). This is the case for: (1) synovial sarcoma showing various translocations, namely t(X;18)(p11.23;q11); t(X;18)(p11.21;q11), leading to different fusion products (*SS18-SSX1* or *SS18-SSX4*; *SS18-SSX2*); (2) congenital infantile fibrosarcoma exhibiting the t(12;15)(p13;q25) leading to the *ETV-NTRK3* fusion product; (3) myxoid and round cell liposarcoma showing: t(12;16)(q13;p11) or t(12;22)(q13;q12), leading, respectively, to *FUS(TLS)-DDIT3(CHOP)* or *EWS-DDIT3* chimeric transcripts; (4) desmoplastic small round cell tumour with the t(11;22)(p13;q12), leading to the *EWS-WT1* hybrid; (5) clear cell sarcoma (so-called melanoma of soft parts) showing a t(12;22)(q13;q22) leading to *EWS-ATF1* gene fusion (see Table 34.1, p. 892).

## Ewing (sarcoma) family of tumours (pPNET)

### Background

The Ewing (sarcoma) family of tumours[49-52] are peripheral primitive neuroectodermal tumours (pPNET or peripheral neuroepitheliomas) comprising a spectrum of entities previously described as Ewing tumour (classical, atypical and peripheral neuroepithelioma), Askin's tumour (malignant small cell tumour of the thoracopulmonary region), malignant ectomesenchymoma, biphenotypic sarcoma, and olfactory neuroblastoma (esthesioneuroblastoma). These tumours commonly occur in bones but may also be seen in soft tissues. They represent the second most common malignant primary bone tumour in childhood, following osteosarcoma. The male to female ratio is 1.5:1.0 and 80% of tumours occur in patients younger than 20 years of age. Mean age at diagnosis is 15 years and incidence is higher in the white than in the black populations.

### Cytological findings: Ewing (sarcoma) family of tumours (pPNET)

- Cytological specimens are usually very cellular
- Clusters of loosely cohesive cells and single small round tumour cells. Tumour cells are fragile (naked or stripped nuclei are often observed) and two subtypes are frequently observed: one with hyperchromatic ('dark' cells) nuclei and scant cytoplasm corresponds probably to cells undergoing apoptosis, and the other is composed of cells with a larger amounts of cytoplasm containing glycogen vacuoles and round or ovoid nuclei with a finely granular chromatin and one to three small nucleoli ('light' cells) (Figs 33.21, 33.22)
- Rosettes may be seen (25%), but without detectable neuropil inside or outside the rosettes (Fig. 33.23). According to some authors, rosettes are never seen in the 'classic' Ewing tumour.

### Diagnostic pitfalls: Ewing (sarcoma) family of tumours (pPNET)

- Osteomyelitis
- Primary bone sarcomas (small cell osteosarcoma, mesenchymal chondrosarcoma)
- Langerhans' cell histiocytosis/eosinophilic granuloma of bone (formerly histiocytosis X) (Figs 33.24, 33.25)
- Other small round cell tumours (from soft tissues and metastatic neuroblastoma) (Box 33.2).

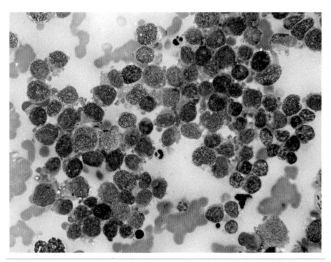

**Fig. 33.21** Ewing sarcoma. Loosely cohesive small round tumour cells with distinct cytoplasm. Some nuclei are smaller and hyperchromatic and correspond to apoptotic cells (MGG).

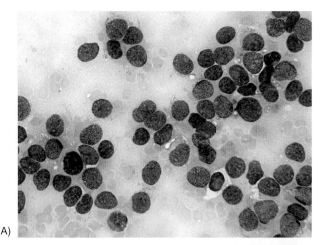

(A)

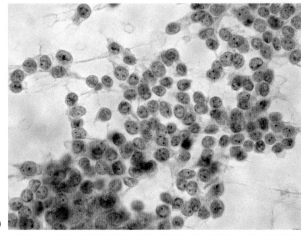

(B)

**Fig. 33.22** (A) Ewing sarcoma. Tumour cells showing vacuolated cytoplasm and monomorphous nuclei with slightly nuclear molding (MGG). (B) Ewing sarcoma (PAP).

### Usefulness of ancillary techniques

Immunocytochemistry using an antibody directed against CD99 stains the vast majority (90–100%) of tumour cells, but also stains a significant number of cells from other tumours within the differential diagnosis such as lymphoblastic

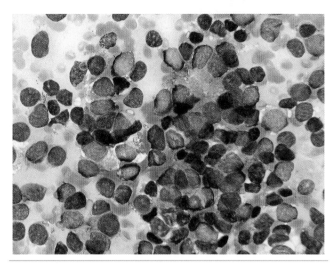

**Fig. 33.23** Rosette in a Ewing/pPNET (MGG).

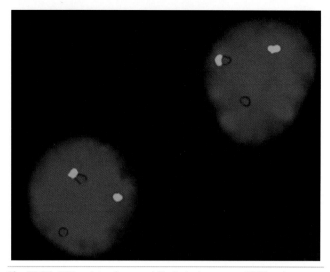

**Fig. 33.26** FISH on interphase nuclei in Ewing's sarcoma: *EWS* break apart probe which detect the split of *EWS* gene. Normal gene shows the double colour overlapping spots. The part of translocated gene (red) is on the other partner chromosome. This probe allows to detect the classical translocation t(11;22) but also all other translocation variants.

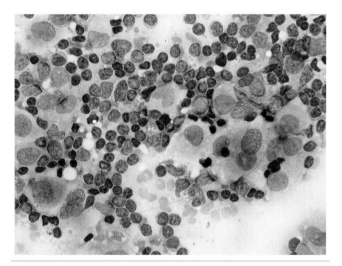

**Fig. 33.24** Eosinophilic granuloma. Admixture of histiocytes, eosinophils and lymphocytes (MGG).

lymphoma, neuroblastoma, rhabdomyosarcoma, desmoplastic small round cell tumours and synovial sarcomas. This is also the case for cytokeratins which are detectable in 10% of the Ewing sarcoma family of tumours as well as in poorly differentiated synovial sarcoma and in most cases of desmoplastic round cell tumours and malignant rhabdoid tumours. Molecular genetic techniques are very useful in this setting since the Ewing sarcoma family of tumours is characterised by reciprocal chromosomal translocations leading to various gene fusions between the *EWS* gene located on chromosome 22 (22q12) and a family of *ETS* genes (*FLI1*, *ERG*, and *ETV1* respectively located at 11q24, 21q22, and 7p22) which all code for different transcription factors. The t(11;22)(q24;q12) translocation (*EWS-FLI1* gene fusion) is observed in 85% of the cases, the t(21;22)(q22;q12) translocation (*EWS-ERG* gene fusion) in 10–15% of the cases, and the others types of gene fusions are very rare (Fig. 33.26).

## Other tumours

### Gonadal and extragonadal germ cell and sex-cord stromal tumours[53–56]

#### Background

Gonadal and extragonadal tumours are relatively infrequent in childhood. Most of them are derived from germ cells (germ cell tumours). Sex-cord stromal tumours derived from granulosa, Sertoli and Leydig cells are rare as are epithelial neoplasms derived from the coelomic epithelium covering the ovary. Germ cell tumours (Figs 33.27, 33.28) may develop in the ovary or the testis (gonadal tumours) or occur in extragonadal sites, usually midline sites (sacrum, retroperitoneum, mediastinum, pineal region) in young children. There are few cytological reports describing some of the most frequent entities: ovarian and extragonadal teratomas, yolk sac tumour (endodermal sinus tumour) of the testis, germinomas (dysgerminomas or

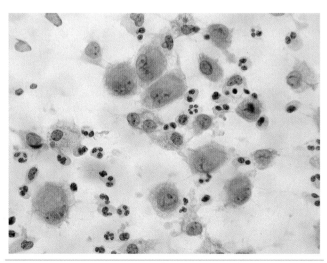

**Fig. 33.25** Eosinophilic granuloma. Reniform nuclei and linear nuclear groove in some histiocytes (PAP).

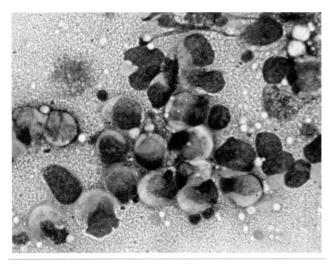

**Fig. 33.27** Seminoma. Large neoplastic cells and a few lymphocytes in a 'tigroid' background (MGG).

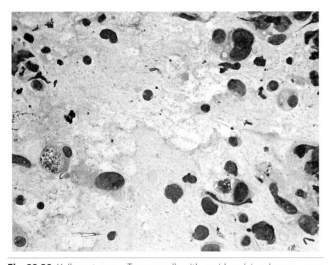

**Fig. 33.28** Yolk-sac tumour. Tumour cells with ovoid nuclei and one or more nucleoli. Note the cell with an intra-cytoplasmic inclusion (MGG).

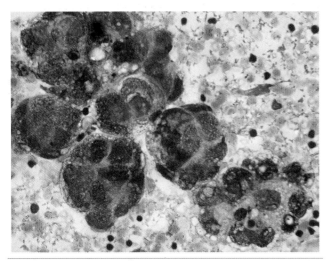

**Fig. 33.29** Embryonal carcinoma. Cohesive pseudo-papillary cluster of large pleomorphic cells with irregular nuclei (MGG).

seminomas) or mixed malignant germ cell tumour of the ovary including components of embryonal carcinoma (Fig. 33.29) or choriocarcinoma.

### Cytological findings: gonadal and extragonadal germ cell and sex-cord stromal tumours

- Dysgerminomas/seminomas contain dissociated medium- to large-size tumour cells with huge nuclei, prominent nucleoli and scant cytoplasm in a tigroid background. As lymphocytes and epithelioid cells are usually admixed with malignant cells, these tumours may be mistaken for lymphoma. Yolk sac tumours and embryonal carcinomas are cytologically similar to adenocarcinomas with well-formed, three-dimensional groups sometimes in the form of papillae
- Yolk sac tumours usually contain homogeneous matrix material in the background. Yolk sac tumours and embryonal carcinomas are cytokeratin and AFP positive and EMA negative
- Teratomas may be difficult to recognise in cytology. Mature tissues from benign teratomas may be regarded as non-representative especially if only one tissue type is sampled. The most frequently encountered cell type in mature teratomas is anucleated squamous cell. In immature teratomas the neural component is most common and smears may be similar to neuroblastoma or ganglioneuroblastoma. Smears are not always representative and do not contain immature cells and elements from two or even three germ layers. Wilms' tumour or rhabdomyosarcoma may finally also be a component of malignant teratoma and are the cause of false specific diagnoses if they are the only component sampled.

## Tumours of the liver[57–59]

Only one-third of all childhood liver masses are benign (hae-mangioendothelioma, mesenchymal hamartoma). Malignant tumours are mainly hepatoblastoma which occurs before the age of 3 years and hepatocellular carcinoma occurring after the age of 3 years. Hepatoblastomas (Figs 33.30, 33.31) are rarely composed of a single cell type: small undifferentiated tumours (co-expressing cytokeratin and vimentin) are rare as are 'pure' epithelial tumours such as the embryonal or the well-differentiated foetal types. Most often tumours are 'mixed' and contain epithelial and mesenchymal components some of which may be mature (heterologous elements). Hepatocellular carcinomas in children do not differ morphologically from those of adults. The fibrolamellar variant of HCC occurs more commonly in adolescents and young adults.

## Endocrine tumours[60–62]

Thyroid nodules in children are most frequently follicular adenomas. Two-thirds of thyroid carcinomas within the pae-diatric age group occur in girls with a peak incidence between ages 7 and 12 years. They are usually papillary thyroid carci-nomas (70%) and less frequently follicular carcinomas (20%). Medullary carcinomas represent 10% of cases and may occur

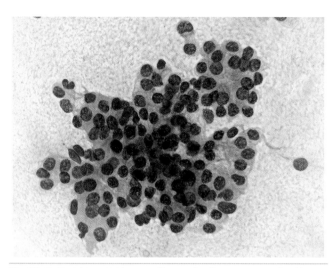

**Fig. 33.30** Foetal hepatoblastoma. Sheets of uniform tumour cells with pseudo-acinar formations. Note the round central placed nuclei and the moderate amount of cytoplasm (MGG).

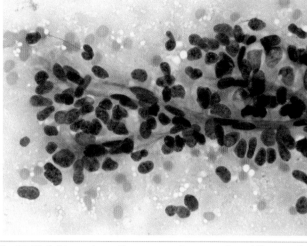

**Fig. 33.32** Solid pseudo-papillary tumour of pancreas. Central fibrovascular core surrounded by a layer of monomorphic tumour cells (MGG).

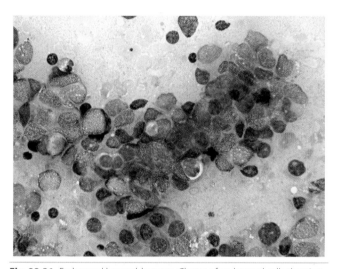

**Fig. 33.31** Embryonal hepatoblastoma. Cluster of embryonal cells showing a scant cytoplasm and a high nuclear:cytoplasmic ratio. The nuclei are irregularly shaped (MGG).

sporadically (70%) or in a familial context, as isolated tumours or associated with phaeochromocytoma in multiple endocrine neoplasia (MEN) syndromes IIA and IIB. Anaplastic carcinomas are extremely rare. Few reports discuss the cytology of parathyroid tumours (usually adenomas or hyperplasia), adrenal cortical tumours (adenomas and carcinomas) and tumours of the adrenal medulla (phaeochromocytomas).

## Miscellaneous

In contrast to adults, epithelial tumours are rare in childhood. On the other hand, pleuropulmonary blastoma, pancreatoblastoma, and solid pseudopapillary tumour of the pancreas (Fig. 33.32) are more frequent in children than in adults.[63,64]

## Conclusion

The cytopathologist has a crucial role in guiding the paediatrician for the adequate therapy of childhood tumours (see p. 873). Optimally, aspiration of the lesion should be performed by, or at least in the presence of, a cytopathologist who will verify the quality and the quantity of the material obtained by rapid staining and process the specimen according to the first 'on-site' diagnosis. This step, which we could name 'interventional cytopathology', is critical since in several childhood tumours, morphology currently needs to be confirmed by molecular assays easily performed from frozen cytological specimens and/or to be enriched at the molecular level (so-called 'molecular portraits') to help the clinician deliver personalised therapy or for predicting the outcome of a tumour in a given child. To achieve these aims it is essential that the cytopathologist is fully involved in the regular multidisciplinary team meetings for correlating the clinical, radiological, cytological and other laboratory findings, thus ensuring optimal patient management and also the necessary feedback between all of the specialists involved in the child's care.

## REFERENCES

1. Jereb B, Us-Krasovec M, Jereb M. Thin needle biopsy of solid tumors in children. Med Pediatr Oncol 1978;4:213–20.

2. Wakely PE Jr., Kardos TF, Frable WJ. Application of fine needle aspiration biopsy to pediatrics. Hum Pathol 1988;19:1383–86.

3. Pohar-Marinsek Z. Difficulties in diagnosing small round cell tumours of childhood from

fine needle aspiration cytology samples. Cytopathology 2008;19:67–79.

4. Barroca H. Fine needle biopsy and genetics, two allied weapons in the diagnosis, prognosis, and target therapeutics of solid pediatric tumors. Diagn Cytopathol 2008;36:678–84.

5. Rajwanshi A, Rao KL, Marwaha RK, et al. Role of fine-needle aspiration cytology in

childhood malignancies. Diagn Cytopathol 1989;5:378–82.

6. Silverman JF, Joshi VV. FNA biopsy of small round cell tumors of childhood: cytomorphologic features and the role of ancillary studies. Diagn Cytopathol 1994;10:245–55.

7. Drut R, Drut RM, Pollono D, et al. Fine-needle aspiration biopsy in pediatric oncology

patients: a review of experience with 829 patients (899 biopsies). J Pediatr Hematol Oncol 2005;27:370–76.

8. Skoog L, Tani E. Diagnosis of lymphoma by fine-needle aspiration cytology using the revised European-American classification of lymphoid neoplasms. Cancer 2000;90:320–23.

9. Das DK, Gupta SK, Pathak IC, et al. Burkitt-type lymphoma. Diagnosis by fine needle aspiration cytology. Acta Cytol 1987;31:1–7.

10. Stastny JF, Almeida MM, Wakely PE Jr, et al. Fine-needle aspiration biopsy and imprint cytology of small non-cleaved cell (Burkitt's) lymphoma. Diagn Cytopathol 1995;12:201–7.

11. Kardos TF, Sprague RI, Wakely PE Jr, et al. Fine-needle aspiration biopsy of lymphoblastic lymphoma and leukemia. A clinical, cytologic, and immunologic study. Cancer 1987;60:2448–53.

12. Jacobs JC, Katz RL, Shabb N, et al. Fine needle aspiration of lymphoblastic lymphoma. A multiparameter diagnostic approach. Acta Cytol 1992;36:887–94.

13. Wakely PE Jr, Kornstein MJ. Aspiration cytopathology of lymphoblastic lymphoma and leukemia: the MCV experience. Pediatr Pathol Lab Med 1996;16:243–52.

14. Hoda RS, Picklesimer L, Green KM, et al. Fine-needle aspiration of a primary mediastinal large B-cell lymphoma: a case report with cytologic, histologic, and flow cytometric considerations. Diagn Cytopathol 2005;32:370–73.

15. Shin HJ, Thorson P, Gu J, et al. Detection of a subset of CD30+ anaplastic large cell lymphoma by interphase fluorescence in situ hybridization. Diagn Cytopathol 2003;29:61–66.

16. Mourad WA, al NM, Tulbah A. Cytomorphologic differentiation of Hodgkin lymphoma and Ki-1+ anaplastic large cell lymphoma in fine needle aspirates. Acta Cytol 2003;47:744–48.

17. Ng WK, Ip P, Choy C, et al. Cytologic and immunocytochemical findings of anaplastic large cell lymphoma: analysis of ten fine-needle aspiration specimens over a 9-year period. Cancer 2003;99:33–43.

18. Das DK, Gupta SK, Datta BN, et al. Fine needle aspiration cytodiagnosis of Hodgkin disease and its subtypes. I. Scope and limitations. Acta Cytol 1990;34:329–36.

19. Das DK, Gupta SK. Fine needle aspiration cytodiagnosis of Hodgkin disease and its subtypes. II. Subtyping by differential cell counts. Acta Cytol 1990;34:337–41.

20. Fulciniti F, Vetrani A, Zeppa P, et al. Hodgkin disease: diagnostic accuracy of fine needle aspiration; a report based on 62 consecutive cases. Cytopathology 1994;5:226–33.

21. Chhieng DC, Cangiarella JF, Symmans WF, et al. Fine-needle aspiration cytology of Hodgkin disease: a study of 89 cases with emphasis on false-negative cases. Cancer 2001;93:52–59.

22. Jogai S, Al-Jassar A, Dey P, et al. Fine needle aspiration cytology of Hodgkin lymphoma: A cytohistologic correlation study from a cancer center in Kuwait. Acta Cytol 2006;50:656–62.

23. Akhtar M, Ali MA, Sabbah RS, et al. Aspiration cytology of neuroblastoma. Light and electron microscopic correlations. Cancer 1986;57:797–803.

24. Kumar PV. Fine needle aspiration cytologic diagnosis of ganglioneuroblastoma. Acta Cytol 1987;31:583–86.

25. Thiesse P, Hany MA, Combaret V, et al. Assessment of percutaneous fine needle aspiration cytology as a technique to provide diagnostic and prognostic information in neuroblastoma. Eur J Cancer 2000;36:1544–51.

26. Domanski HA. Fine-needle aspiration of ganglioneuroma. Diagn Cytopathol 2005;32:363–66.

27. Frostad B, Martinsson T, Tani E, et al. The use of fine-needle aspiration cytology in the molecular characterization of neuroblastoma in children. Cancer 1999;87:60–68.

28. Barroca H, Carvalho JL, da Costa MJ, et al. Detection of N-myc amplification in neuroblastomas using Southern blotting on fine needle aspirates. Acta Cytol 2001;45:169–72.

29. Akhtar M, Ali MA, Sackey K, et al. Aspiration cytology of Wilms' tumor: correlation of cytologic and histologic features. Diagn Cytopathol 1989;5:269–74.

30. Quijano G, Drut R. Cytologic characteristics of Wilms'' tumors in fine needle aspirates. A study of ten cases. Acta Cytol 1989;33:263–66.

31. Dey P, Radhika S, Rajwanshi A, et al. Aspiration cytology of Wilms' tumor. Acta Cytol 1993;37:477–82.

32. Sharifah NA. Fine needle aspiration cytology characteristics of renal tumors in children. Pathology 1994;26:359–64.

33. Drut R, Pomar M. Cytologic characteristics of clear-cell sarcoma of the kidney (CCSK) in fine-needle aspiration biopsy (FNAB): a report of 4 cases. Diagn Cytopathol 1991;7:611–14.

34. Iyer VK, Agarwala S, Verma K. Fine-needle aspiration cytology of clear-cell sarcoma of the kidney: study of eight cases. Diagn Cytopathol 2005;33:83–89.

35. Wakely PE Jr, Giacomantonio M. Fine needle aspiration cytology of metastatic malignant rhabdoid tumor. Acta Cytol 1986;30:533–37.

36. Drut R. Malignant rhabdoid tumor of the kidney diagnosed by fine-needle aspiration cytology. Diagn Cytopathol 1990;6:124–26.

37. Barroca HM, Costa MJ, Carvalho JL. Cytologic profile of rhabdoid tumor of the kidney. A report of 3 cases. Acta Cytol 2003;47:1055–58.

38. Drut R. Cytologic characteristics of congenital mesoblastic nephroma in fine-needle aspiration cytology: a case report. Diagn Cytopathol 1992;8:374–76.

39. Mansouri D, Dimet S, Couanet D, et al. Renal cell carcinoma with an Xp11.2 translocation in a 16-year-old girl: a case report with cytological features. Diagn Cytopathol 2006;34:757–60.

40. Akhtar M, Ali MA, Bakry M, et al. Fine-needle aspiration biopsy diagnosis of rhabdomyosarcoma: cytologic, histologic, and ultrastructural correlations. Diagn Cytopathol 1992;8:465–74.

41. Pohar-Marinsek Z, Anzic J, Jereb B. Topical topic: value of fine needle aspiration biopsy in childhood rhabdomyosarcoma: twenty-six years of experience in Slovenia. Med Pediatr Oncol 2002;38:416–20.

42. Klijanienko J, Caillaud JM, Orbach D, et al. Cyto-histological correlations in primary, recurrent and metastatic rhabdomyosarcoma: the Institut Curie experience. Diagn Cytopathol 2007;35:482–87.

43. Costa MJ, Campman SC, Davis RL, et al. Fine-needle aspiration cytology of sarcoma: retrospective review of diagnostic utility and specificity. Diagn Cytopathol 1996;15:23–32.

44. Domanski HA. Fine-needle aspiration cytology of soft tissue lesions: diagnostic challenges. Diagn Cytopathol 2007;35:768–73.

45. Klijanienko J, Caillaud JM, Lagace R, et al. Cytohistologic correlations of 24 malignant peripheral nerve sheath tumor (MPNST) in 17 patients: the Institut Curie experience. Diagn Cytopathol 2002;27:103–8.

46. Klijanienko J, Caillaud JM, Lagace R, et al. Cytohistologic correlations in 56 synovial sarcomas in 36 patients: the Institut Curie experience. Diagn Cytopathol 2002;27:96–102.

47. Insabato L, Di VD, Lambertini M, et al. Fine needle aspiration cytology of desmoplastic small round cell tumor. A case report. Acta Cytol 1999;43:641–46.

48. Ferlicot S, Coue O, Gilbert E, et al. Intraabdominal desmoplastic small round cell tumor: report of a case with fine needle aspiration, cytologic diagnosis and molecular confirmation. Acta Cytol 2001;45:617–21.

49. Akhtar M, Ali MA, Sabbah R. Aspiration cytology of Ewing's sarcoma. Light and electron microscopic correlations. Cancer 1985;56:2051–60.

50. Frostad B, Tani E, Brosjo O, et al. Fine needle aspiration cytology in the diagnosis and management of children and adolescents with Ewing sarcoma and peripheral primitive neuroectodermal tumor. Med Pediatr Oncol 2002;38:33–40.

51. Elsheikh T, Silverman JF, Wakely PE Jr, et al. Fine-needle aspiration cytology of Langerhans' cell histiocytosis (eosinophilic granuloma) of bone in children. Diagn Cytopathol 1991;7:261–66.

52. Shabb N, Fanning CV, Carrasco CH, et al. Diagnosis of eosinophilic granuloma of bone by fine-needle aspiration with concurrent institution of therapy: a cytologic, histologic, clinical, and radiologic study of 27 cases. Diagn Cytopathol 1993;9:3–12.

53. Assi A, Patetta R, Fava C, et al. Fine-needle aspiration of testicular lesions: report of 17 cases. Diagn Cytopathol 2000;23:388–92.

54. Garcia-Solano J, Sanchez-Sanchez C, Montalban-Romero S, et al. Fine needle aspiration (FNA) of testicular germ cell tumours; a 10-year experience in a community hospital. Cytopathology 1998;9:248–62.

55. Collins KA, Geisinger KR, Wakely PE Jr, et al. Extragonadal germ cell tumors: a fine-needle aspiration biopsy study. Diagn Cytopathol 1995;12:223–29.

56. Chao TY, Nieh S, Huang SH, et al. Cytology of fine needle aspirates of primary extragonadal germ cell tumors. Acta Cytol 1997;41:497–503.

57. Wakely PE Jr, Silverman JF, Geisinger KR, Frable WJ. Fine needle aspiration biopsy cytology of hepatoblastoma. Mod Pathol 1990;3:688–93.

58. Iyer VK, Kapila K, Agarwala S, et al. Fine needle aspiration cytology of hepatoblastoma. Recognition of subtypes on cytomorphology. Acta Cytol 2005;49:355–64.

59. Bakshi P, Srinivasan R, Rao KL, et al. Fine needle aspiration biopsy in pediatric space-occupying lesions of liver: a retrospective study evaluating its role and diagnostic efficacy. J Pediatr Surg 2006;41:1903–8.

60. Khurana KK, Labrador E, Izquierdo R, et al. The role of fine-needle aspiration biopsy in the management of thyroid nodules in children, adolescents, and young adults: a multi-institutional study. Thyroid 1999;9:383–86.

61. Amrikachi M, Ponder TB, Wheeler TM, et al. Thyroid fine-needle aspiration biopsy in children and adolescents: experience with 218 aspirates. Diagn Cytopathol 2005;32:189–92.

62. Hosler GA, Clark I, Zakowski MF, et al. Cytopathologic analysis of thyroid lesions in the pediatric population. Diagn Cytopathol 2006;34:101–5.

63. Pitman MB, Faquin WC. The fine-needle aspiration biopsy cytology of pancreatoblastoma. Diagn Cytopathol 2004;31:402–6.

64. Nadler EP, Novikov A, Landzberg BR, et al. The use of endoscopic ultrasound in the diagnosis of solid pseudopapillary tumors of the pancreas in children. J Pediatr Surg 2002;37:1370–73.

# Section **16**

## New Techniques

# New techniques

Victor Lee, Siok-Bian Ng and Manuel Salto-Tellez[1]

## Chapter contents

## Introduction

This chapter deals with two main aspects of modern cytopathology, namely (1) molecular diagnostic cytopathology and (2) other non-molecular technologies commonly used in cytopathology. It deals very succinctly with the technical background of these diagnostic approaches, and specifically focuses on applications in routine diagnostic practice.

## Diagnostic molecular cytopathology

Molecular diagnosis is the application of molecular biology techniques and knowledge of the molecular mechanisms of disease to the diagnosis, prognostication and treatment of patients, based on the use of cytological samples.[1] This chapter will consider techniques and technologies that are fully established in standard, routine molecular diagnostic laboratories and are therefore ones that are technically applicable to both tissues and cells. A plethora of information on molecular aspects of some diseases is generated in cytology samples, but with no proven direct diagnostic application. There are also upcoming techniques used in only a handful of laboratories. These will be briefly mentioned in a separate section at the end of the chapter, to distinguish them clearly from those tests that are widely accepted and translated into robust assays of general use.

The scope of molecular diagnostic cytopathology involves, primarily, those samples routinely analysed by cytomorphology and immunocytochemistry, and these are mainly from solid tumours (including lymphomas but excluding leukaemias), with a much smaller component of inherited and infectious disease testing.[2] Thus, this chapter will be mainly, although not exclusively, dealing with oncological molecular cytopathology.

Most of the tests considered here will be based on the two main technical approaches available in molecular diagnostic laboratories, namely the classical polymerase chain reaction (PCR) technique and variations thereof, such as reverse-transcriptase PCR, capillary electrophoresis and conventional sequencing, as well as fluorescent *in situ* hybridisation (FISH). Diagnostic PCR permits the amplification and subsequent detection and analysis of any short sequence of DNA (or RNA) with clinical significance. PCR and its variants have been technically optimised to work in all conventional cytology samples, including cytology smears, cytospins, cell suspensions, prepared cell blocks and even previously stained smears.[3] This is possible under two provisos. First, the validation of the tests in the individual laboratories must include appropriate documentation that the test can be confidently carried out in cytology samples. Second, it is recommended that there is an indication of the possible percentage of malignant versus non-malignant cells in the sample prior to the analysis, to make sure that the sample complies with the given sensitivity of the individual test. Most of these considerations do also apply to FISH-based testing. FISH is based on the binding of fluorescent probes to their complementary sequence on target DNA (cDNA) on standard preparations, which include fixed cells and tissues, enabling the detection of the two main FISH-related abnormalities of diagnostic significance, namely chromosomal translocations and gene amplification.

## Cervical cytology

It is now unquestionable that virtually all cases of cervical cancer are due to persistent infection by high-grade human papillomavirus (HPV) types, especially HPV types 16, 18, 31 and 45.[4] As a result, HPV testing is arguably the most important cytology-specific molecular diagnostic test. HPV is now recognised as a precursor of both squamous and glandular cervical pathology.[5,6]

The test is best suited for three main clinical scenarios: (1) for diagnostic triage of women with a conventional smear showing low-grade abnormalities, that is, low-grade dyskaryosis (low-dysk) or low-grade squamous intraepithelial lesion (LSIL);[7] (2) as a primary screening tool for women older than 30 years of age;[8] (3) as a follow-up test for patients after treatment of a high-grade abnormality.[9] Either by itself or as a complementary approach to conventional cervical smear cytology, HPV molecular testing can increase diagnostic accuracy and, importantly, do so in a more cost-effective manner. Large studies have shown that implementation of HPV DNA testing in cervical screening leads to earlier and higher detection rates of high-grade lesions[10] and greater sensitivity for detection of cervical intraepithelial neoplasia (CIN)[11,12] compared with conventional smear testing. Additionally, certain molecular HPV testing may be used as an effective triage for ASCUS or LSIL cervical smears, in detecting subsequent high-grade lesions during follow-up.[13] Further considerations on how to integrate HPV DNA testing in the routine diagnostic setting are discussed in Chapters 22 and 23.

[1]To Boon Peng, Eugene and Sharon.

There are various HPV detection modalities, based on different molecular techniques, such as signal amplification, target amplification, genotyping or *in situ* hybridisation, among others.[14] A literature meta-analysis[15] reveals two methods which are more commonly employed for routine diagnostic use, namely PCR-based studies using MY09/MY11 primers[16,17] and hybrid capture techniques.[18,19] However, these test modalities will only be useful if they achieve a practical balance between sensitivity and specificity to minimise unnecessary colposcopic intervention in high-risk HPV-positive patients without detectable lesions.[20]

Another approach is the identification of hypermethylated genes using quantitative methylation-specific PCR.[21] Aberrant promoter methylation of selective tumour suppressor genes has been detected in squamous intraepithelial lesions and invasive cervical cancer. Identification of methylation profiles of these genes in liquid-based cytology specimens can therefore be potentially useful to differentiate low-grade from high-grade lesions.[22] This is also discussed later in this chapter.

Finally, detection of p16(INK4A), a cyclin dependent kinase inhibitor, via immunocytochemical analysis has also been shown to increase the sensitivity of HPV testing. Compared with other biomarkers, p16(INK4A) was the most reliable marker for CIN.[23]

Although there is little doubt about the clinical utility of HPV molecular testing in routine diagnostic practice, its precise use may vary in the socioeconomic context of individual countries. This use may also be modified in the not-so-distant future once we see the impact of HPV vaccination in both developed and developing societies.

## Sarcoma and paediatric tumours

The main applications of molecular and cytogenetic testing in soft tissue tumours are:

- Diagnosis of problematic tumours with overlapping cytomorphology, for example, synovial sarcoma versus malignant peripheral nerve sheath tumour (Fig. 34.1) and overlapping immunocytochemical expression, for example, clear cell sarcoma versus melanoma
- Obtaining a definitive diagnosis with minimal tissue, as with fine needle aspiration (FNA) and other cytological preparations, especially in recurrent tumours, thereby avoiding invasive procedures[24]
- Prognostication of certain tumours by accurate subtyping, for example, alveolar rhabdomyosarcoma versus embryonal rhabdomyosarcoma (see Ch. 33, p. 882) or by detection of protein amplification, as with c-myc amplification in neuroblastoma (see Ch. 33, p. 878)
- Potential application for detection and monitoring of micrometastases or minimal residual disease, although the clinical significance for this is currently undetermined.[2]

In the diagnostic work-up of certain problematic tumours, the presence of recurrent or specific chromosomal translocations in many soft tissue tumours (Table 34.1) can be detected by various molecular testing modalities, including FISH, PCR, DNA sequencing and conventional cytogenetics. As well as conventional cytogenetic testing, which can be labour-intensive and slow, PCR and FISH are both suitable as first-line molecular investigations and nearly all forms of cytological preparations can be utilised for these tests, each with their inherent strengths and limitations.

In every case, interpretation of these molecular results should always be correlated with the clinical and pathological

**Table 34.1** The commonest molecular diagnostic targets associated to sarcomas

| | Translocation | Fusion protein | Prevalence |
|---|---|---|---|
| **Small round cell pattern** | | | |
| PNET/Ewing sarcoma | t(11;22)(q24;q12) | EWSR1-FLI1 | 90% |
| | t(21;22)(q22;q12) | EWSR1-ERG | 5% |
| | t(7;22)(p22;q12) | EWSR1-ETV1 | |
| | t(2;22)(q33;q12) | EWSR1-FEV | |
| | t(17;22)(q12;q12) | EWSR1-E1AF | |
| Desmoplastic small round cell tumour | t(11;22)(p13;q12) | EWSR1-WT1 | >95% |
| Alveolar rhabdomyosarcoma | t(2;13)(q35;q14) | PAX3-FOXO1a | 65% |
| | t(1;13)(p36;q14) | PAX7-FOXO1a | |
| Myxoid/round cell liposarcoma | t(12;16)(q13;p11) | FUS-CHOP | >95% |
| | t(12;22)(q13;q11) | EWSR1-CHOP | |
| Poorly differentiated synovial sarcoma | t(X;18)(p11.2;q11.2) | SYT-SSX1 | 65% |
| | | SYT-SSX2 | 35% |
| **Spindle cell pattern** | | | |
| Infantile fibrosarcoma | t(12;15)(p13;q26) | ETV6-NTRK3 | >95% |
| Synovial sarcoma | As above | As above | As above |
| Dermatofibrosarcoma protuberans/giant cell fibroblastoma | t(17;22)(q21;q13) | COL1A1-PDGFB | >90% |
| Low-grade fibromyxoid sarcoma | t(7;16)(q33;p11.2) | FUS-CREB3L2 | >95% |
| | t(11;16)(p13;p11.2) | FUS-CREB3L1 | |
| Angiomatoid fibrous histiocytoma | t(2;22)(q33;q12) | EWSR1-CREB1 | |
| | t(12;22)(q13;q12) | EWSR1-ATF | |
| Inflammatory myofibroblastic tumour | t with 2p23 | ALK fusions | >50% |
| **Other less common tumours** | | | |
| Alveolar soft part sarcoma | t(X;17)(p11;q25) | ASPL-TFE3 | >95% |
| Clear cell sarcoma | t(12;22)(q13;q12) | EWSR1-ATF1 | >90% |
| | t(2;22)(q33;q12) | EWSR1-CREB1 | |
| Extraskeletal myxoid chondrosarcoma | t(9;22)(q22-q3;q12) | EWSR1-NR4A3 | 75% |
| | t(9;17)(q22;q11) | TAF15-NR4A3 | 25% |

assessment as, very rarely, unrelated sarcomas (such as, for example, angiomatoid fibrous histiocytoma versus clear cell sarcoma), may possess similar translocations, that is, show chromosomal promiscuity[25] or aberrant chromosomal abnormalities including widely dispersed breakpoints and the variant translocations. Additionally, the use of molecular testing should be limited to a specific group of tumours, for instance recurrent translocations,

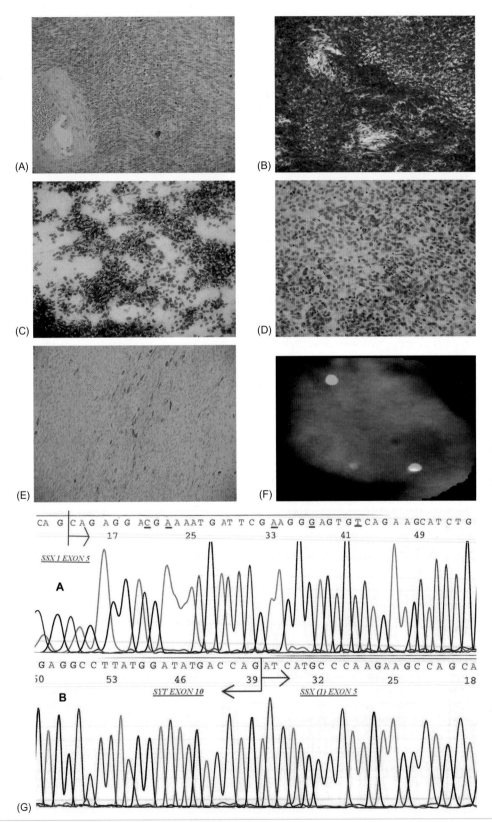

**Fig. 34.1** Molecular analysis of synovial sarcoma in a cytology sample (cell block). (A) H&E of a patient with monophasic synovial sarcoma showing tightly packed interlacing fascicles of spindle cells. (B) Diff-Quik stained smears of the fine needle aspirate demonstrate densely packed spindle cells with overlapping nuclei and interlacing fascicles. (C) Diff-Quik and (D) Papanicolaou stained smears showing relatively monomorphous spindle, oval and epithelioid-looking cells at higher power. (E) The spindle or epithelioid cells stain focally for cytokeratin 7. (F) A fluorescent *in situ* hybridisation study using a break apart probe demonstrates rearrangement of the *SYT* gene (indicated by the separation of the red and green signals). (G) Sequencing showing the site of translocation involving *SYT* exon 10 and *SSX* exon 5.

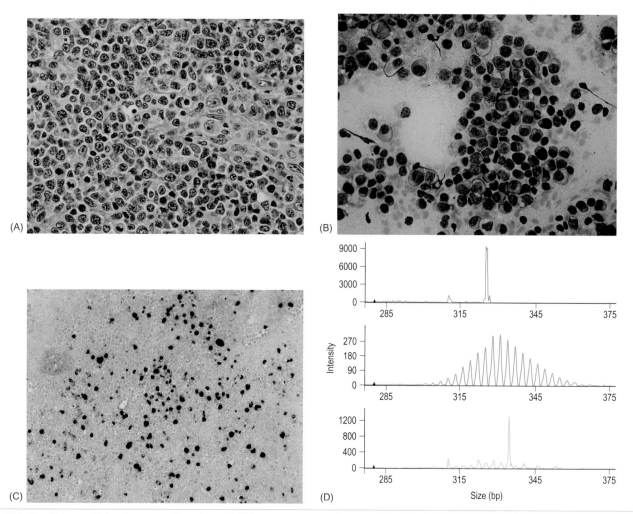

**Fig. 34.2** Tonsil biopsy with imprint smears of a patient with EBV-positive post transplant lymphoproliferative disorder, polymorphic subtype. The biopsy (A) and smear imprint (B) revealed a polymorphic lymphoid population including immunoblasts, small and intermediate-sized lymphocytes showing plasmacytic differentiation, and plasma cells. Many of the lymphoid cells in the biopsy were positive for EBER (C). Polymerase chain reaction for IgH gene rearrangement (D), performed using tissue scrapings from the imprint smears, identified a monoclonal B-cell population (top panel: monoclonal control; middle panel: polyclonal control; bottom panel: patient case).

and should be used only after appropriate initial work-up, so as to avoid unnecessary and costly testing or false results due to inherent problems with molecular tests such as false positive amplifications in PCR testing. Please also refer to Chapter 33 for further discussion on the cytogenetics and corresponding ancillary techniques of paediatric sarcomas and solid tumours.

## Lymphoma

The main applications of molecular and cytogenetic testing in the clinical context of lymphoma that are readily used in diagnostic cytopathology,[26] include: (1) establishing monoclonality to facilitate the initial diagnosis of a lymphoid malignancy; (2) identification of distinct entities within specific lymphoma subtypes to enable precise classification, prognostication and targeted personalised therapy; (3) detection and monitoring of minimal residual disease; (4) study of the clonal evolution during disease progression. Numerous analytical techniques are available for molecular testing and they can be applied on a variety of cytological specimens, including FNA, effusions, imprint smears and archival cytological material.[14,27]

Importantly, each of the techniques has its limitations and the data gleaned from them should be interpreted in the appropriate clinical context with consideration of the morphology and the immunophenotype.

Flow cytometry (FC) and immunocytochemistry (ICC) are complementary tests and the preference to utilise either one of them depends on the laboratory's expertise and experience and the resources available.[14] The uses of ICC in the diagnosis of lymphoma are well characterised[14,28,29] and the reader is referred to Chapter 13 for discussion of the immunophenotype of specific lymphoma subtypes. The primary advantage of FC over ICC is the multiparametric evaluation of single cells and the small sample requirement. In particular, the ability to evaluate antigen co-expression on the same cell, and simultaneous analysis of cytoplasmic and surface antigens confer distinct advantages to ICC. Other advantages include the determination of B-cell and T-cell clonality by analysis of immunoglobulin kappa and lambda light chains, and antibodies against the variable region of the TCR beta (V beta) chain, respectively.[14]

Polymerase chain reaction (PCR)-based assays are now the preferred tests in the assessment of clonality to differentiate between reactive and neoplastic lymphoid proliferations (Fig. 34.2).

**Table 34.2** Recurrent chromosomal abnormalities associated with specific non-Hodgkin lymphomas

| Lymphoma type | Chromosomal abnormalities | Frequency (%) | Mechanism of oncogene deregulation | Preferred detection method(s) |
|---|---|---|---|---|
| Follicular lymphoma (FL) | t(14;18)(q32;q21) | ~85 | BCL2/IgH fusion | PCR, FISH |
| Diffuse large B-cell lymphoma (DLBCL) | t(14;18)(q32;q21) | ~20 | BCL2/IgH fusion | PCR, FISH |
| | t(3;n)(q27;n)[b] | ~35 | Translocation of bcl-6 | FISH |
| Burkitt's lymphoma | t(8;14)(q24;q32) | ~80 | Fusion of C-MYC with IgH, IgK and IgL | FISH, PCR, CC, SB, |
| | t(8;22)(q24;q11) | ~5 | | |
| | t(2;8)(p12;q24) | ~15 | | |
| Mantle cell lymphoma (MCL) | t(11;14)(q13;q32) | 70–90 | CyclinD1/IgH fusion | IHC, FISH, RT-PCR, CC |
| Extranodal marginal zone lymphoma (MZL)(MALT) | t(11;18)(q21;q21) | ~35 | API2/MALT1 fusion | FISH, RT-PCR, IHC |
| | t(14;18)(q32;q21) | ~20 | IgH/MALT1 fusion | FISH, CC |
| | t(1;14)(p22;q32) | ~5 | IgH/BCL-10 fusion | CC, IHC |
| ALK+ Anaplastic Large cell lymphoma (ALCL) | t(2;5)(p23;q35) | ~75 | NPM-ALK fusion | IHC, FISH, CC, |
| Small lymphocytic lymphoma/chronic lymphocytic leukaemia (SLL/CLL) | del (13q14) | ~50 | [a] | FISH |
| | del (11q23) | ~20 | ATM deletion | FISH |
| | del (17p13) | ~7 | TP53 deletion | FISH |

PCR, polymerase chain reaction; FISH, fluorescent *in situ* hybridization; CC, conventional cytogenetics; SB, southern blot; IHC, immunohistochemistry.

[a]Several genes implicated, e.g. miRNA15, miRNA16.

[b]Many translocation partners with bcl-6 described.

Although clonality assays are powerful tools, it is important for clinicians and cytopathologists to be aware of the limitations, sensitivity and specificity of the assays. First, clonality does not necessarily equate with malignancy and the failure to detect clonality does not imply benignity. Second, false positive and false negative results can arise due to a combination of biological and technical factors and errors of interpretation. Third, IgH and TCR gene rearrangements are not necessarily restricted to B and T-cell lineages, respectively.[30]

The most common primary recurring genetic aberrations of non-Hodgkin lymphomas (NHL) are balanced chromosomal translocations leading to deregulation or activation of associated oncogenes (Table 34.2).[2,31] A variety of methods can be used to detect the translocations in cytological specimens and they include Southern Blot (SB), PCR and RT-PCR, conventional cytogenetics (CC), FISH and ICC. Of these, CC and SB techniques require fresh tissue for analysis. PCR-based assays are highly specific but are unable to detect the translocations with widely dispersed breakpoints and the variant translocations, unless multiple primer sets are used. Hence, in many pathology laboratories, interphase FISH and ICC are the preferred modalities because they can be readily applied on archival and imprint cytological preparations (Fig. 34.3).[14]

## Gastrointestinal tumours

With the abundant information related to the molecular basis of gastrointestinal pathology, cytology specimens are readily utilised for molecular testing in colorectal cancer (CRC) and gastrointestinal stromal tumours (GIST), as well as in pancreatic and pancreato-biliary oncology (see Chs 7 and 10).

CRC is arguably the neoplasm that is better understood from a molecular viewpoint. Of all the genetic information that is relevant to CRC, there are four tests that are of molecular diagnostic importance, namely *APC* mutations for the diagnosis of familial adenomatous polyposis, microsatellite instability and *BRAF* mutations as part of the molecular screening of hereditary non-polyposis colorectal cancer (HNPCC) and *KRAS* mutations for the use of *cetuximab* in the treatment of metastatic CRC. While the first test is primarily analysed in peripheral blood, the other three can be detected on various cytology samples and, on occasion, this may be the only sample available.

The microsatellite instability (MSI) test is used for both HNPCC diagnosis and for prognostication in the context of conventional therapy.[32] MSI analysis is possible on cytology samples[33] and, with the use of a mononucleotide repeat-only panel, no normal counterpart is needed for the analysis. Thus cytology samples with a good representation of neoplastic cells, that is at least 20–30% according to personal experience, are suitable for this analysis.[34] The MSI testing is complemented with the *BRAF* test for HNPCC diagnosis.[35] Mutation analysis of *BRAF*, easily done on cytology specimens in our experience, also offers additional information on sensitivity to newly developed MEK inhibitors.

One of the better established examples of personalised medicine is the detection of *KRAS* mutations in metastatic colorectal cancers.[36] Patients with wild-type *KRAS* are more likely to have disease control on Cetuximab therapy, while those with

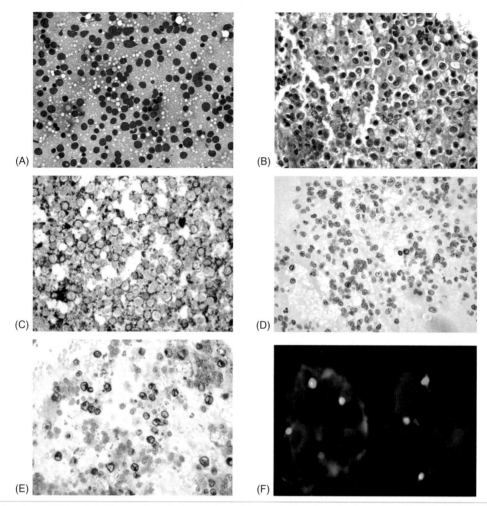

**Fig. 34.3** Follicular lymphoma FISH analysis. Fine needle aspiration cytology of the cervical lymph node of a 54-year-old man with follicular lymphoma and diffuse large B-cell lymphoma transformation. Diff-Quik smear (A) and cell block preparation (B) of the FNA cytology revealed a predominant population of large lymphoid cells resembling centroblasts and a minor population of centrocytes with grooved or folded nuclei. Immunohistochemistry was performed on the cell block. The tumour cells expressed CD20 (C) and bcl2 (E), and were negative for CD3 (D). Fluorescent *in situ* hybridisation performed on the cell block using IGH/BCL2 Dual Color, Dual Fusion Translocation Probe Set detected two orange/green (yellow) fusion signals in the cells, confirming the presence of t(14;18) (q32;q21) and hence the diagnosis of follicular lymphoma (F).

*KRAS* mutation may not benefit from this treatment. Our sensitivity studies show that a minimum of 20% of malignant cells in a cytology sample is sufficient to give a reliable analysis by direct sequencing.

GIST is molecularly characterised by mutations in the *c-kit* and *PDGFRA* genes. The detection of these mutations in cytology samples has diagnostic value when conventional immunocytochemistry does not allow a confident diagnosis as well as prognostic significance, since exon 11 mutations indicate a worse prognosis and also a better response to imatinib mesylate (Fig. 34.4, lower panels). This analysis can be demonstrated in material from cytology cell blocks, with prior careful confirmation of sufficient cells in the conventional H&E stain, see Ch. 7).[37]

FNA cytology is one of the preferred methods for the diagnosis of cystic lesions in the pancreas and the pancreaticobiliary system; this is, however, a difficult diagnostic area, particularly in assessing the benign or malignant nature of the cyst. Several PCR-based tests have been reported by many groups to be of help in this regard. Indeed, the detection of *KRAS* mutations and allelic losses of known tumour suppressor – linked microsatellite markers have shown adequate sensitivity and specificity.[38,39] Another marker found to be useful and sensitive in the detection of pancreaticobiliary malignancy in patients with indeterminate biliary strictures is the level of minichromosome maintenance protein 5 (Mcm5) in bile aspirates and biliary brushings (see Ch. 9).[40]

## Urothelial malignancies

Molecular testing can serve as a useful adjunctive tool for urine cytology and cystoscopy in early cancer detection, improving sensitivity and specificity. The main aim is to distinguish neoplastic urothelial cells, particularly low-grade or well-differentiated tumour cells, from other benign mimickers such as reactive changes or polyoma virus infected urothelial cells. This will also improve the surveillance of at risk patients, reducing the frequency of follow-up cystoscopies which are invasive and costly.

Currently, non-invasive biomarker assays utilising urine protein (e.g. NMP22, BTA TRAK), immunocytochemical (e.g. ImmunoCyt) and FISH assays are being used for surveillance and screening. FISH can detect genetic alterations of certain

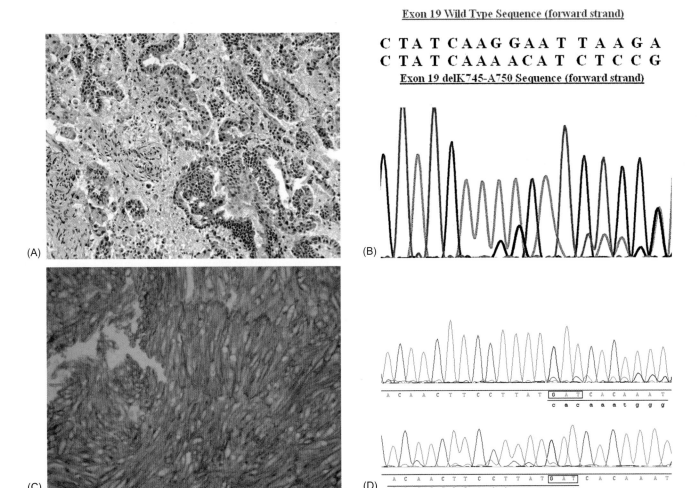

**Exon 19 Wild Type Sequence (forward strand)**

**C T A T C A A G G A A T T A A G A**
**C T A T C A A A A C A T C T C C G**

**Exon 19 delK745-A750 Sequence (forward strand)**

**Fig. 34.4** Detail of the cell block cytology of a FNAC lung sample showing an adenocarcinoma (A) and the corresponding mutation in *EGFR* exon 19 (B); detail of the cell block cytology of a FNA gastric sample showing CD117 expression in a gastrointestinal stromal tumour (C) and the corresponding mutation in c-kit exon 11 (D).

chromosomes (1, 3, 5, 7, 9, 11 and 17) associated with bladder cancer.[41] Some assays use multiple sets of probes which hybridise to the centromeres of chromosome 3, 7 and 17, and to the 9p21 locus of chromosome 9; indeed, the loss of 9p21 locus, which is the site of the p16 tumour suppressor gene, is the earliest and most frequent genetic aberration in bladder cancer.[42] FISH can be used independently or in combination with immunocytochemistry with fluorescent-labelled antibodies.[43] Recent published series on FISH assay have demonstrated results in the range of 68.6–100% and 65–96% for sensitivity and specificity.[44] A more detailed analysis of the sensitivities and specificities of the various markers is given in Chapter 11.

As in many molecular-based tests, major criticisms of these methods include the high-cost of probes, personnel and equipment and the lack of suitability for high-throughput screening.

## Lung cancer

The application of multi-target FISH approaches to bronchial specimens has shown the ability to detect gains in targeted areas of the genome such as chromosome 6 (CEP6), 5p15, 7p12 (EGFR) and 8q24 (C-MYC).[45] Furthermore, it is clear that distinct epigenetic events can be detected in exfoliative lung cytological samples.[46] Although this shows some diagnostic promise, the main molecular test applicable to lung cytology samples (and to lung samples in general) is the mutation detection of the epidermal growth factor receptor (*EGFR*) gene. *EGFR* tyrosine kinase mutations identify likely responders to the small molecule EGFR tyrosine kinase inhibitors (TKIs) gefitinib and erlotinib.[47,48] Studies have shown that small biopsies and cell blocks from FNA samples are an adequate source of DNA for the direct sequencing of the areas of the *EGFR* gene of therapeutic significance,[49,50] as well as previously stained FNA and brush cytology smears (personal experience, see Fig. 34.4 upper panel). A more detailed discussion is given in Chapter 2.

## Breast cancer

Assessment of HER-2/*neu* receptor status in breast cancer for therapeutic decision-making was one of the first and currently best established examples of personalised/predictive medicine. FISH is, arguably, the gold standard for the analysis of HER-2/*neu* amplification and therapeutic decision-making with trastuzumab. FISH allows reliable detection of Her-2/*neu* gene amplification on FNA samples.[51] HER-2/*neu* FISH or chromogenic *in-situ* hybridisation (CISH), which is a non-fluorescent and more affordable way of detecting gene amplification, is particularly useful in metastatic tumours, where the access to tissue-based sampling may be difficult,[52] thereby precluding the need for a core biopsy or excision. Furthermore, the HER-2/neu status may vary between the primary and metastatic lesion.

FISH can be also used in breast ductal lavage samples to detect molecular changes associated with malignant cells, the features of which may be not apparent morphologically.[53]

## Ovarian cancer

Although a significant amount of work has been done on cytology samples, primarily in peritoneal effusions, these approaches are still more in the realm of clinical research than routine molecular diagnostics. Studies have shown that cancer cells in effusions demonstrate increased intercellular adhesion and altered expression of many cancer-associated molecules, including adhesion molecules, proteases, angiogenic factors and tyrosine kinase receptors.[54,55] Examples of site-specific phenotypic alterations of ovarian cancer cells include the upregulation of adhesion molecules, such as the E-cadherin complex, in effusions and solid metastatic lesions when compared with primary carcinoma, and the downregulation of vascular endothelial growth factor, an angiogenic factor, in effusions when compared with solid tumours. The expression of NAC-1, a member of the bric-a-brac tram track broad complex/poxvirus and zinc domain family, is higher in ovarian carcinoma cells in effusions compared with their solid tumour counterparts.[14] Other interesting findings are mentioned later in this chapter and the application of molecular diagnostics to FNA samples from ovarian tumours is discussed further in Chapter 27.

## Thyroid

As with ovarian cancer, diagnostic molecular analysis of thyroid cytology samples is not widely utilised routinely, although recent reports are promising a future role as an adjunctive tool in the diagnosis of morphologically difficult lesions, especially indeterminate follicular, papillary and poorly differentiated neoplasms in preoperative FNA samples. For instance, mutations involving RET/PTC, TRK, BRAF and RAS oncogenes may occur in over 70% of papillary carcinomas, and these can be detected by RT-PCR and mutant allele-specific amplification techniques. The findings of these oncogenes therefore assist in determining definitive surgical management.[56,57] RET germline mutations are crucial for the development of heritable forms of medullary thyroid carcinoma (MTC), while somatic mutations of RET may be seen in sporadic MTCs.[58] CTNNB1 and p53 have been involved in the development and progression of poorly differentiated or anaplastic carcinomas.[58] Alternatively, an algorithm-based approach using a panel of various genes (TERT, TFF3, PPASR gamma, CITED1 and EGR2) has also been advocated to predict high-risk follicular thyroid disease, such as for discriminating adenomas from carcinomas.[59] The relevant thyroid cytology findings are discussed in Chapter 17.

## Oral lesions

The identification of high-risk oral pre-malignant lesions and intervention at pre-invasive stages is a significant step forward in reducing the mortality, morbidity and cost of treatment associated with oral squamous cell carcinoma.[60] A significant number of molecular diagnostic approaches have been postulated to complement traditional cytomorphological analysis, such as cytomorphometry,[61] nuclear DNA content and DNA-image cytometry,[62] and the detection of various genetic and epigenetic alterations such as loss of heterozygosity and microsatellite instability. Although some of these molecular approaches are enjoying a certain degree of acceptance in individual countries, there is no general consensus on the best molecular test to use in the routine setting. One of the tests used in some laboratories is DNA-image cytometry, which allows the detection of the cytometric equivalent of chromosomal aneuploidy (DNA-aneuploidy), and has shown improved diagnostic sensitivity and specificity in detecting early lesions in the oral cavity.[53] Further comments on the use of DNA-aneuploidy and the number of silver nitrate stained nucleolar organiser regions (AgNORs) as complementary diagnostic methods can be found in Chapter 6.

## Effusions: distinguishing benign from malignant and mesothelioma from carcinoma

The main clinical applications of molecular diagnostics in effusions include the detection of malignant cells in primary and metastatic tumours, as well as the distinction of mesothelioma from carcinoma.

Conventional cytogenetics (CC) refers to the culture of a suspension of cells in mitogenic media and the study of the characteristic banding patterns specific for each chromosome. It can be applied on fresh cells from effusions and is useful in distinguishing malignant from benign pleural effusions as numerical and structural chromosomal abnormalities are often seen in malignant epithelial cells and rarely encountered in reactive conditions.[63] It can also be applied in the differential diagnosis between mesothelioma and other carcinomas: recurrent chromosomal abnormalities on chromosome 6 (e.g. 6q-) are frequent in mesotheliomas, while adenocarcinomas often show aberrations on chromosome 8, such as gains or inversions of 8q. However, chromosomal abnormalities have also been described in reactive mesothelial cells and can be a pitfall in diagnosis. Loss of heterozygosity (LOH) is frequently associated with inactivation of tumour suppressor genes. Detection of LOH in specific cancer-associated loci using DNA-based PCR assay on cell blocks or ethanol-fixed smears from effusions can be used as an ancillary method for identifying metastatic disease in effusions, such as lung (LOH on 3p, 5q, 9p and 17p) and breast cancer (LOH of MycL1 and D7S486 loci).[63] FISH and CISH can be applied on effusions and archival cytological material to identify aneuploidy and aneusomy in malignant and suspicious effusions from patients with breast carcinomas. Furthermore, the detection of HER-2/neu amplification by FISH or CISH in metastatic effusions of HER-2/neu-negative primary tumours has important therapeutic implications and this can be used clinically to monitor patients with advanced breast carcinoma.[63] Details of such applications are discussed further in Chapter 3.

## Infectious diseases

Advances in molecular diagnostics with the development of assays aimed at rapid, specific and sensitive identification and

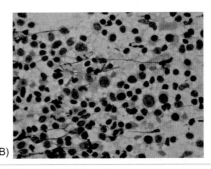
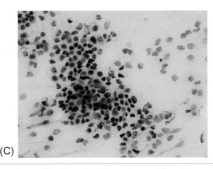

(A)　　　　　　　　　　(B)　　　　　　　　　　(C)

**Fig. 34.5** Imprint smears of a tonsil biopsy of a 16-year-old female with EBV-positive post-renal transplant lymphoproliferative disorder, polymorphic subtype. Diff-Quik (A) and Papanicolaou (B) stained smears revealed a polymorphic population of lymphoid cells with plasmacytic differentiation, and plasma cells. *In situ* hybridisation for EBER performed on PAP-stained imprint smears revealed positive nuclear staining in many of the lymphoid cells (C).

characterisation of DNA or RNA have expanded the diagnostic spectrum of infectious diseases in recent years. These include:

- Viruses, such as the hepatitis A, B, C, D and E viruses, HIV-1, HTLV, HHV-8, EBV
- Bacteria: such as *Mycobacterium tuberculosis, Chlamydia trachomatis, Helicobacter pylori, Mycoplasma pneumoniae*
- Fungi, such as *Candida* spp., *Cryptococcus* spp., *Pneumocystis carinii*
- Parasites, such as *Toxoplasma gondii* and *Entamoeba histolytica*.

Advances have also allowed the detection of genetic variants with potential implications for the treatment response and clinical course.[64] The molecular techniques include hybridisation analyses and PCR-based direct DNA sequencing, oligonucleotide ligation assays and branched DNA assays. A variety of cytological specimens are suitable for these tests, including FNA, effusions, imprint smears and archival cytological material.

The detection of the EBV-encoded small RNAs (EBER) via *in situ* hybridisation has become the standard method used to identify EBV infection in paraffin-embedded tissue sections; this can be similarly applied on imprint and stained archival cytological preparations (Fig. 34.5). The application of PCR-based methods has improved the sensitivity of detection of *Mycobacterium tuberculosis* in FNA smears. Mycobacterial-DNA was detected by PCR in 85% of cases, compared with detection of 15.3% and 24.4% of cases by Ziehl Neelsen stain and culture technique.[65] However, false positive PCR reaction is a potential pitfall. Despite limitations, FNA samples are easily amenable to PCR analysis for the detection of *Mycobacterium tuberculosis* and this is especially useful when conventional diagnostic modalities are equivocal, obviating the need for an excisional biopsy.

## New techniques

### Comparative genomic hybridisation (CGH)

CGH allows a genome wide analysis of a given tumour sample and provides an overview of the DNA sequences and copy number changes. CGH and high-resolution array-CGH can be applied on a variety of cytology samples including cell pellets, unstained slides, stained and imprint smears prepared from effusion specimens and FNA material. Currently performed by a few laboratories, because of its time-consuming and labour-intensive nature, CGH findings may be of importance in the near future.

CGH analysis of primary and metastatic ovarian carcinomas often shows chromosomal gains of 8q, 20q and 3q, and frequent losses of chromosomes 4q, 18q and 9q. Gain or high amplification of 8q24.1 is also reported to be associated with advanced-stage disease.[66] CGH has been applied to confirm the diagnosis of malignancy in the differentiation between benign mesothelial proliferation, malignant mesothelioma and metastatic adenocarcinoma in serous effusions; indeed, the presence of chromosomal imbalances argues against a reactive condition. Loss of 6q and 22q, as well as chromosomes 14 and 22 are some of the frequent and tumour-specific genetic imbalances in malignant mesothelioma. In contrast, loss of 22q is an uncommon finding in non-small cell lung carcinomas.[66] CGH can also be employed to document a relationship between a primary tumour and its metastatic deposits, especially if the metastatic tumour is poorly differentiated or undifferentiated.[14]

### Methylation

The detection of tumour-specific hypermethylation of *BRCA1* and *RAS* may enhance early detection of ovarian cancer.[67] Methylation studies may also be a promising tool to detect neoplastic urothelial cells; in fact, hypermethylation of at least one of three suppressor genes (*APC, RASSF1A* and *p14 arf*) can be found in the DNA of all tumour cells but not of normal or inflamed transitional cells.[68] Methylation studies on FNA and core biopsies of breast tissue can be potentially helpful to detect malignancy, as the methylation of certain genes (e.g. *RARbeta2, RASSF1A,* and *cyclin D2*) is present in almost in all cases of invasive carcinoma, while it has been uncommon in benign samples or *in situ* carcinoma.[69]

DNA methylation has a potential for use in liquid-based cytology samples of the uterine cervix in order to distinguish cervical intraepithelial neoplasia (CIN) from non-specific cytological changes and the normal cervix.[70] Apostolidou et al. demonstrated that methylation of *SOX1, HOXA11* and *CADM1* could discriminate between high-grade CIN cases and controls with high sensitivity and specificity. This is the first study that validates the results in an independent case/control set and presents *HOXA11*, a gene that is important for cervical development, as a potentially useful DNA marker in LBC samples.[71]

### Gene expression

Gene expression profiling (GEP) may identify genes that are essential determinants of tumour behaviour. Originally described in diffuse large B-cell lymphoma (DLBCL),[72] the feasibility of GEP using FNA from patients with non-Hodgkin lymphoma has been well documented.[73] GEP can be applied on fresh and formalin-fixed paraffin-embedded samples from effusions to distinguish lung adenocarcinoma from malignant mesothelioma in pleural effusions.[74] Overall, in the area of microarray analyses, both FNA and core biopsy of breast cancer specimens yield similar quality and quantity of total RNA and cDNA for analysis in approximately 70–75% of single pass samples, leading to similar transcriptional profiles.[75] Interestingly, individual gene expression may also be of help; for instance, MN/CA9, a cancer-related gene, is commonly activated in human cancers. In a recent study, MN/CA9 gene expression was detected in 89.8%, 72.2% and 8.3% of malignant effusions, cytologically negative effusions from cancer patients and effusions from control patients, respectively.[14]

## Technological advances (non-molecular)

Liquid-based cytology (LBC) has been introduced into cytopathology mainly in the field of cervical cytology with the aim of improving diagnostic accuracy. The advantages of thin-layer techniques compared with conventional smears include an optimal viewing of cellular features attributed to the reduction in air-drying artifact and obscuring background elements thus reducing the number of unsatisfactory smears.[76] Although several disadvantages have been reported with this technique, such as problems related to the reduction or alteration in background and extracellular material, disruption in architectural integrity and altered cellular morphology as well as increased cost of cell preparation, it is now widely accepted that the sensitivity of cervical LBC is similar to the conventional cervical smear, and is superior in high-risk populations.[77] Further information and considerations on LBC applied to cervical cytology, including semi-automated screening systems, is discussed in Chapters 1, 22 and 23.

The clinical utility of LBC has also been explored in non-gynaecological cytology with a relative degree of success. Brandao et al. evaluated the feasibility of grading follicular lymphoma using ThinPrep®(TP) slides and flow cytometry.[78] Counting centroblasts, either in 300 lymphoid cells or per 10 high-power fields in TP slides, represented a statistically significant method to separate different grades of follicular lymphoma in FNA samples. Flow cytometry analysis of cell size was less reliable, especially in differentiating grade 2 from grade 3 tumours.

Similarly, LBC has also been applied to thyroid cytopathology. The cytomorphological features of thyroid FNA on TP preparations have been studied and compared with those obtained and prepared by conventional methods. The sensitivity and specificity levels are higher for conventional smears than for TP (94% versus 81% and 67% versus 60%, respectively).[79] The lower specificity may be related to cytological alterations and reduction in the amount of colloid induced by methanol fixative. In addition, the diagnosis of Hashimoto's thyroiditis is more difficult on TP slides due to the limited number of lymphocytes.

Automated staining protocols for immunocytochemistry and FISH are now available[80] and, in the context of biomarkers with possible screening value, may become a laboratory tool of choice, provided that rigorous validation studies are carried out beforehand.[81] Similarly, automated scoring of immunohistochemistry and FISH are changing the presumed subjectivity of the qualitative or semi-quantitative analysis of biomarkers with diagnostic or therapeutic implications, and several such systems are available in the market.[82] These methods are beginning to be used for cytology samples as well and, together with strong molecular targets, may provide an automated molecular alternative to conventional screening, as shown recently in the context of sputum cytology.[83]

## The future of diagnostic molecular cytopathology

Molecular diagnostics has developed in the last two decades from a predominantly academic discipline into a medical specialty with significant and common applications. Cytopathology is not an exception. Indeed, the prospective role of diagnostic molecular cytopathology is enormous for the following reasons:[1]

- Molecular testing is sometimes indispensable to establish an unequivocal diagnosis on cell preparations
- Molecular testing provides extra information on the prognosis or therapy of diseases diagnosed by conventional cytology
- Molecular testing provides genetic information on the inherited nature of diseases that can be directly investigated in cytological samples, whether exfoliative, direct or fine needle aspiration cytology
- The cytopathology sample is sometimes the most convenient (or the only available) source of material for molecular testing
- Direct molecular interrogation of cells allows for a diagnostic correlation that would otherwise not be possible.

Parallel to these directly diagnostic applications, cytopathology is also assuming greater importance in the validation of biomarkers for specific diseases, and is therefore of significant impact in the overall translational research strategies.

The coming years will see the consolidation of diagnostic molecular cytopathology, a process that will lead to a change of many paradigms:[1]

- Diagnostic pathology departments will have to establish molecular testing as a cost-efficient operation
- Changes in sample preparation will have to be implemented for optimal preservation of nucleic acids
- The training of staff, the quality control and the quality assurance will have to include molecular diagnostics
- Pathologists opting for molecular diagnostics as a sub-specialty of choice will have to develop their professional expertise within the same framework of training currently in place for other sub-specialties.

Established pathologists with the expertise of combining clinical information and knowledge of morphological, immunocytochemical and molecular diagnostic interpretation will represent bona fide 'molecular cytopathologists', who will find themselves increasingly at the strategic centre of clinical decision-making.[84]

## REFERENCES

1. Salto-Tellez M, Koay ES. Molecular diagnostic cytopathology: definitions, scope and clinical utility. Cytopathology 2004;15:252–55.

2. Ng SB, Lee V, Salto-Tellez M. The relevance of molecular diagnostics in the practice of surgical pathology. Expert Opin Med Diagn 2008;2:1401–14.

3. Srinivasan M, Sedmak D, Jewell S. Effect of fixatives and tissue processing on the content and integrity of nucleic acids. Am J Pathol 2002;161:1961–71.

4. Lowy DR, Solomon D, Hildesheim A, et al. Human papillomavirus infection and the primary and secondary prevention of cervical cancer. Cancer 2008;113(7 Suppl):1980–93.

5. Castellsague X, Diaz M, de Sanjose S, et al. Worldwide human papillomavirus etiology of cervical adenocarcinoma and its cofactors: implications for screening and prevention. J Nat Cancer Inst 2006;98:303–15.

6. Brink AA, Zielinski GD, Steenbergen RD, et al. Clinical relevance of human papillomavirus testing in cytopathology. Cytopathology 2005;16:7–12.

7. Safaeian M, Solomon D, Wacholder S, et al. Risk of precancer and follow-up management strategies for women with human papillomavirus-negative atypical squamous cells of undetermined significance. Obstet Gynecol 2007;109:1325–31.

8. Grce M, Davies P. Human papillomavirus testing for primary cervical cancer screening. Expert Rev Mol Diagn 2008;8:599–605.

9. Kitchener HC, Walker PG, Nelson L, et al. HPV testing as an adjunct to cytology in the follow up of women treated for cervical intraepithelial neoplasia. Br J Obstet Gynecol 2008;115:1001–7.

10. Bulkmans NW, Berkhof J, Rozendaal L, et al. Human papillomavirus DNA testing for the detection of cervical intraepithelial neoplasia grade 3 and cancer: 5-year follow-up of a randomised controlled implementation trial. Lancet 2007;370:1764–72.

11. Mayrand MH, Duarte-Franco E, Rodrigues I, et al. Human papillomavirus DNA versus Papanicolaou screening tests for cervical cancer. New Engl J Med 2007;357:1579–88.

12. Naucler P, Ryd W, Tornberg S, et al. Human papillomavirus and Papanicolaou tests to screen for cervical cancer. New Engl J Med 2007;357:1589–97.

13. Molden T, Nygard JF, Kraus I, et al. Predicting CIN2+ when detecting HPV mRNA and DNA by PreTect HPV-proofer and consensus PCR: A 2-year follow-up of women with ASCUS or LSIL Pap smear. Int J Cancer 2005;114:973–76.

14. Schmitt FC, Longatto-Filho A, Valent A, et al. Molecular techniques in cytopathology practice. J Clin Pathol 2008;61:258–67.

15. Koliopoulos G, Arbyn M, Martin-Hirsch P, et al. Diagnostic accuracy of human papillomavirus testing in primary cervical screening: a systematic review and meta-analysis of non-randomized studies. Gynecol Oncol 2007;104:232–46.

16. Schneider A, Hoyer H, Lotz B, et al. Screening for high-grade cervical intra-epithelial neoplasia and cancer by testing for high-risk HPV, routine cytology or colposcopy. Int J Cancer 2000;89:529–34.

17. Oh YL, Shin KJ, Han J, et al. Significance of high-risk human papillomavirus detection by polymerase chain reaction in primary cervical cancer screening. Cytopathology 2001;12:75–83.

18. Costa S, Sideri M, Syrjanen K, et al. Combined Pap smear, cervicography and HPV DNA testing in the detection of cervical intraepithelial neoplasia and cancer. Acta Cytol 2000;44:310–18.

19. Kuhn L, Denny L, Pollack A, et al. Human papillomavirus DNA testing for cervical cancer screening in low-resource settings. J Nat Cancer Inst 2000;92:818–25.

20. Meijer CJ, Berkhof J, Castle PE, et al. Guidelines for human papillomavirus DNA test requirements for primary cervical cancer screening in women 30 years and older. Int J Cancer 2008;124:516–20.

21. Kang S, Kim JW, Kang GH, et al. Polymorphism in folate- and methionine-metabolising enzyme and aberrant CpG island hypermethylation in uterine cervical cancer. Gynecol Oncol 2005;96:173–80.

22. Kahn SL, Ronnett BM, Gravitt PE, et al. Quantitative methylation-specific PCR for the detection of aberrant DNA methylation in liquid-based Pap tests. Cancer 2008;114:57–64.

23. Murphy N, Ring M, Heffron CC, et al. p16INK4A, CDC6, and MCM5: predictive biomarkers in cervical preinvasive neoplasia and cervical cancer. J Clin Pathol 2005;58:525–34.

24. Chiu LL, Koay ES, Chan NH, et al. Sequence confirmation of the EWS-WT1 fusion gene transcript in the peritoneal effusion of a patient with desmoplastic small round cell tumor. Diagn Cytopathol 2003;29:341–43.

25. Rossi S, Szuhai K, Ijszenga M, et al. EWSR1-CREB1 and EWSR1-ATF1 fusion genes in angiomatoid fibrous histiocytoma. Clin Cancer Res 2007;13:7322–28.

26. Kocjan G. Best Practice No 185. Cytological and molecular diagnosis of lymphoma. J Clin Pathol 2005;58:561–67.

27. Mattu R, Sorbara L, Filie AC, et al. Utilization of polymerase chain reaction on archival cytologic material: a comparison with fresh material with special emphasis on cerebrospinal fluids. Mod Pathol 2004;17:1295–301.

28. Fowler LJ, Lachar WA. Application of immunohistochemistry to cytology. Arch Pathol Lab Med 2008;132:373–83.

29. Venkatraman L, Catherwood MA, Patterson A, et al. Role of polymerase chain reaction and immunocytochemistry in the cytological assessment of lymphoid proliferations. J Clin Pathol 2006;59:1160–65.

30. Spagnolo DV, Ellis DW, Juneja S, et al. The role of molecular studies in lymphoma diagnosis: a review. Pathology 2004;36:19–44.

31. Vega F, Medeiros LJ. Chromosomal translocations involved in non-Hodgkin lymphomas. Arch Pathol Lab Med 2003;127:1148–60.

32. Salto-Tellez M, Lee SC, Chiu LL, et al. Microsatellite instability in colorectal cancer: considerations for molecular diagnosis and high-throughput screening of archival tissues. Clin Chem 2004;50:1082–86.

33. Karatzanis AD, Samara KD, Zervou M, et al. Assessment for microsatellite DNA instability in nasal cytology samples of patients with allergic rhinitis. Am J Rhinol 2007;21:236–40.

34. Murphy KM, Zhang S, Geiger T, et al. Comparison of the microsatellite instability analysis system and the Bethesda panel for the determination of microsatellite instability in colorectal cancers. J Mol Diagn 2006;8:305–11.

35. Tan YH, Liu Y, Eu KW, et al. Detection of BRAF V600E mutation by pyrosequencing. Pathology 2008;40:295–98.

36. Lievre A, Bachet JB, Boige V, et al. KRAS mutations as an independent prognostic factor in patients with advanced colorectal cancer treated with cetuximab. J Clin Oncol 2008;26:374–79.

37. Pang NK, Chin SY, Nga ME, et al. Validation of c-kit exon 11 mutation analysis on cytology samples in gastrointestinal stromal tumours. Cytopathology 2009;20:297–303.

38. Khalid A, Nodit L, Zahid M, et al. Endoscopic ultrasound fine needle aspirate DNA analysis to differentiate malignant and benign pancreatic masses. Am J Gastroenterol 2006;101:2493–500.

39. Khalid A, Pal R, Sasatomi E, et al. Use of microsatellite marker loss of heterozygosity in accurate diagnosis of pancreaticobiliary malignancy from brush cytology samples. Gut 2004;53:1860–65.

40. Ayaru L, Stoeber K, Webster GJ, et al. Diagnosis of pancreaticobiliary malignancy by detection of minichromosome maintenance protein 5 in bile aspirates. Br J Cancer 2008;98:1548–54.

41. Hopman AH, Poddighe PJ, Smeets AW, et al. Detection of numerical chromosome aberrations in bladder cancer by in situ hybridization. Am J Pathol 1989;135:1105–17.

42. Daniely M, Rona R, Kaplan T, et al. Combined analysis of morphology and fluorescence in situ hybridization significantly increases accuracy of bladder cancer detection in voided urine samples. Urology 2005;66:1354–59.

43. Mian C, Lodde M, Comploj E, et al. Liquid-based cytology as a tool for the performance of uCyt+ and Urovysion Multicolour-FISH in the detection of urothelial carcinoma. Cytopathology 2003;14:338–42.

44. Budman LI, Kassouf W, Steinberg JR. Biomarkers for detection and surveillance of bladder cancer. Can Urol Assoc J 2008;2:212–21.

45. Halling KC, Rickman OB, Kipp BR, et al. A comparison of cytology and fluorescence in situ hybridization for the detection of lung cancer in bronchoscopic specimens. Chest 2006;130:694–701.

46. Kersting M, Friedl C, Kraus A, et al. Differential frequencies of p16(INK4a) promoter hypermethylation, p53 mutation, and K-ras mutation in exfoliative material mark the development of lung cancer in symptomatic chronic smokers. J Clin Oncol 2000;18:3221–29.

47. Lynch TJ, Bell DW, Sordella R, et al. Activating mutations in the epidermal growth factor receptor underlying responsiveness of non-small-cell lung cancer to gefitinib. New Engl J Med 2004;350:2129–39.

48. Paez JG, Janne PA, Lee JC, et al. EGFR mutations in lung cancer: correlation with clinical response to gefitinib therapy. Science 2004;304:1497–500.

49. Chin TM, Anuar D, Soo R, et al. Detection of epidermal growth factor receptor variations by partially denaturing HPLC. Clin Chem 2007;53:62–70.

50. Horiike A, Kimura H, Nishio K, et al. Detection of epidermal growth factor eceptor mutation in transbronchial needle aspirates of non-small cell lung cancer. Chest 2007;131:1628–34.

51. Sauter G, Feichter G, Torhorst J, et al. Fluorescence in situ hybridization for detecting erbB-2 amplification in breast tumor fine needle aspiration biopsies. Acta Cytol 1996;40:164–73.

52. Vocaturo A, Novelli F, Benevolo M, et al. Chromogenic in situ hybridization to detect HER-2/neu gene amplification in histological and ThinPrep-processed breast cancer fine-needle aspirates: a sensitive and practical method in the trastuzumab era. Oncologist 2006;11:878–86.

53. Adduci KM, Annis CE, DeVries S, et al. Fluorescence in situ hybridization of ductal lavage samples identifies malignant phenotypes from cytologically normal cells in women with breast cancer. Cancer 2007;111:185–91.

54. Davidson B. Anatomic site-related expression of cancer-associated molecules in ovarian carcinoma. Curr Cancer Drug Targets 2007;7:109–20.

55. Davidson B, Risberg B, Reich R, et al. Effusion cytology in ovarian cancer: new molecular methods as aids to diagnosis and prognosis. Clin Lab Med 2003;23. 729–754, viii.

56. Sapio MR, Posca D, Raggioli A, et al. Detection of RET/PTC, TRK and BRAF mutations in preoperative diagnosis of thyroid nodules with indeterminate cytological findings. Clin Endocrin 2007;66:678–83.

57. Nikiforova MN, Nikiforov YE. Molecular genetics of thyroid cancer: implications for diagnosis, treatment and prognosis. Expert Rev Mol Diagn 2008;8:83–95.

58. DeLellis RA. Pathology and genetics of thyroid carcinoma. J Surg Oncol 2006;94:662–69.

59. Foukakis T, Gusnanto A, Au AY, et al. A PCR-based expression signature of malignancy in follicular thyroid tumors. Endocr Relat Cancer 2007;14:381–91.

60. Mehrotra R, Gupta A, Singh M, et al. Application of cytology and molecular biology in diagnosing premalignant or malignant oral lesions. Mol Cancer 2006;5:11.

61. Ogden GR, Cowpe JG, Wight AJ. Oral exfoliative cytology: review of methods of assessment. J Oral Pathol Med 1997;26:201–5.

62. Maraki D, Becker J, Boecking A. Cytologic and DNA-cytometric very early diagnosis of oral cancer. J Oral Pathol Med 2004;33:398–404.

63. Reis-Filho JS, de Lander Schmitt FC. Fluorescence in situ hybridization, comparative genomic hybridization, and other molecular biology techniques in the analysis of effusions. Diagn Cytopathol 2005;33:294–99.

64. Blum HE. Molecular diagnosis of microbial infections. Biologicals 1996;24:193–95.

65. Purohit MR, Mustafa T, Sviland L. Detection of Mycobacterium tuberculosis by polymerase chain reaction with DNA eluted from aspirate smears of tuberculous lymphadenitis. Diagn Mol Pathol 2008;17:174–78.

66. Nagel H, Schulten HJ, Gunawan B, et al. The potential value of comparative genomic hybridization analysis in effusion-and fine needle aspiration cytology. Mod Pathol 2002;15:818–25.

67. Ibanez de Caceres I, Battagli C, Esteller M, et al. Tumor cell-specific BRCA1 and RASSF1A hypermethylation in serum, plasma, and peritoneal fluid from ovarian cancer patients. Cancer Res 2004;64:6476–81.

68. Dulaimi E, Uzzo RG, Greenberg RE, et al. Detection of bladder cancer in urine by a tumor suppressor gene hypermethylation panel. Clin Cancer Res 2004;10:1887–93.

69. Pu RT, Laitala LE, Alli PM, et al. Methylation profiling of benign and malignant breast lesions and its application to cytopathology. Mod Pathol 2003;16:1095–101.

70. Gustafson KS, Furth EE, Heitjan DF, et al. DNA methylation profiling of cervical squamous intraepithelial lesions using liquid-based cytology specimens: an approach that utilizes receiver-operating characteristic analysis. Cancer 2004;102:259–68.

71. Apostolidou S, Hadwin R, Burnell M, et al. DNA methylation in liquid based cytology for cervical screening. Int J Cancer 2009;125:2995–3002.

72. Alizadeh AA, Eisen MB, Davis RE, et al. Distinct types of diffuse large B-cell lymphoma identified by gene expression profiling. Nature 2000;403:503–11.

73. Goy A, Stewart J, Barkoh BA, et al. The feasibility of gene expression profiling generated in fine-needle aspiration specimens from patients with follicular lymphoma and diffuse large B-cell lymphoma. Cancer 2006;108:10–20.

74. Holloway AJ, Diyagama DS, Opeskin K, et al. A molecular diagnostic test for distinguishing lung adenocarcinoma from malignant mesothelioma using cells collected from pleural effusions. Clin Cancer Res 2006;12:5129–35.

75. Symmans WF, Ayers M, Clark EA, et al. Total RNA yield and microarray gene expression profiles from fine-needle aspiration biopsy and core-needle biopsy samples of breast carcinoma. Cancer 2003;97:2960–71.

76. Ronco G, Cuzick J, Pierotti P, et al. Accuracy of liquid based versus conventional cytology: overall results of new technologies for cervical cancer screening: randomised controlled trial. BMJ (Clin Res) 2007;335:28.

77. Longatto Filho A, Pereira SM, Di Loreto C, et al. DCS liquid-based system is more effective than conventional smears to diagnosis of cervical lesions: study in high-risk population with biopsy-based confirmation. Gynecol Oncol 2005;97:497–500.

78. Brandao GD, Rose R, McKenzie S, et al. Grading follicular lymphomas in fine-needle aspiration biopsies: the role of ThinPrep slides and flow cytometry. Cancer 2006;108:319–23.

79. Cochand-Priollet B, Prat JJ, Polivka M, et al. Thyroid fine needle aspiration: the morphological features on ThinPrep slide preparations. Eighty cases with histological control. Cytopathology 2003;14:343–49.

80. Sahebali S, Depuydt CE, Boulet GA, et al. Immunocytochemistry in liquid-based cervical cytology: analysis of clinical use following a cross-sectional study. Int J Cancer 2006;118:1254–60.

81. Haack LA, Shalkham J. Validation in the cytopathology laboratory: its time has come. Diagn Cytopathol 2007;35:529–34.

82. Rojo MG, Garcia GB, Mateos CP, et al. Critical comparison of 31 commercially available digital slide systems in pathology. Int J Surg Pathol 2006;14:285–305.

83. Katz RL, Zaidi TM, Fernandez RL, et al. Automated detection of genetic abnormalities combined with cytology in sputum is a sensitive predictor of lung cancer. Mod Pathol 2008;21:950–60.

84. Salto-Tellez M. A case for integrated morphomolecular diagnostic pathologists. Clin Chem 2007;53:1188–90.

# Index

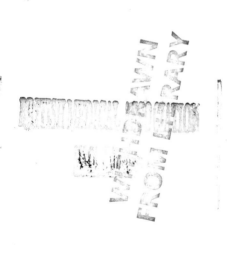